HEMATOLOGY – SCIENCE AND PRACTICE

Edited by **Charles H. Lawrie**

Hematology – Science and Practice
Edited by Charles H. Lawrie

Published by InTech
Janeza Trdine 9, 51000 Rijeka, Croatia

Publishing Process Manager Sandra Bakic

Technical Editor Teodora Smiljanic

Cover Designer InTech Design Team

Additional hard copies can be obtained from orders@intechopen.com

Hematology – Science and Practice, Edited by Charles H. Lawrie
p. cm.
ISBN 978-953-51-0174-1

For EU product safety concerns:
IN TECH d.o.o., Prolaz Marije Krucifikse Kozulić 3, 51000 Rijeka, Croatia,
info@intechopen.com or visit our website at intechopen.com.

Meet the editor

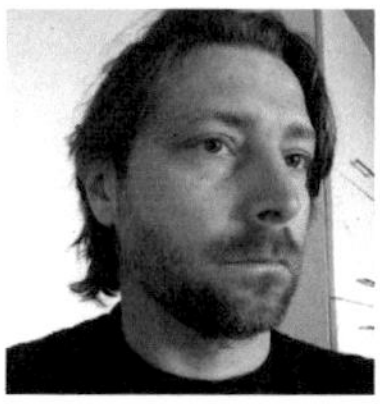

Charles H. Lawrie was awarded his BA (Hons) and MA (Oxon) in biochemistry at Trinity College, University of Oxford (1991-1995). He went on to obtain his doctorate (DPhil) in biological sciences. (Trinity College, University of Oxford (1996-2000)). From 2000 to 2003 he was a post-doctoral researcher at the Institute of Virology and Environmental Microbiology (IVEM), Oxford. He was Principal Investigator at the Lymphoid Malignancy Research Group (LMRG) and a Julian Starmer-Smith Research Fellow at the Nuffield Department of Clinical Laboratory Sciences, University of Oxford between 2004 and 2011. Charles Lawrie was awarded an Ikerbasque Research Professorship in 2011, and currently holds the position of Director of Oncology Research at the Biodonostia Research Institute in San Sebastian, Spain. He continues to be a university research lecturer at the University of Oxford and is a Julian Starmer-Smith Lymphoma Trust research fund fellow.

Contents

Preface

'Blood, blood, glorious blood,
Thicker than water and nicer than mud'

Humphrey Kay - The Hematologist's Song

Hematology encompasses the physiology and pathology of blood and of the blood-forming organs. In common with other areas of medicine, the pace of change in hematology has been breathtaking over recent years. There is now a plethora of treatment options available to the hematologist which happily coincides with a greatly improved outlook for the vast majority of patients with blood disorders, in particular those with hematological malignancies. Improvements in the clinic reflect, and in many respects are driven by, advances in our scientific understanding of hematological processes under both normal and disease conditions. This book which consists of a selection of essays aims to inform both specialist and non-specialist readers about some of the latest advances in hematology, in both laboratory and clinic.

The first section of this book (Section 1 - Blood Physiology) is concerned with the study of the molecular and cellular mechanisms behind the physiological functioning of the blood system. The first three chapters deal with the mechanisms behind early hematopoiesis, the process occurring almost exclusively in the bone marrow by which all mature blood cells are generated from multi-potent hematopoietic stem cells (HSCs). This is a finely balanced process that is tightly controlled by a complex network of inter-related signaling pathways and molecular components. In Chapter 1, Fiedler and Brunner review some of the intricate regulatory mechanisms involved in this process, in particular focusing on the role of transcription factors in early lineage control and lineage commitment. In Chapter 2, Velazquez describes the role that negative regulation plays in hematopoiesis, and in particular the function of members of the inhibitory adaptor family such as DOK, Lnk and SOCS, their role in cytokine signaling pathways and hematological pathologies. This chapter also explores the potential therapeutic use of these inhibitors and associated regulators. Expanding upon the theme of hematopoiesis, Goossens and Jody, in Chapter 3, discuss the role of modulators of the epithelial to mesenchymal transition (EMT) pathway focusing on the function of SNAI family members, snail and slug, and interestingly how they can be involved in leukemic transformation.

The ability of the HSC (and other cells along the hematopoietic pathway) to divide into two functionally distinct daughter cells, one that is differentiated whilst the other retains self-renewal properties and can continue to proliferate, is crucial to the maintenance of the hematopoietic system. So-called asymmetric division is discussed in Chapter 4 by Jimenez-Teja *et al.* The authors outline the historical perspective behind this field before going into a detailed review of the function of asymmetric division in both hematopoietic and immune systems, as well as the latest evidence to suggest that asymmetric division and in particular abnormal functioning of cell fate determinant molecules can lead to cancer.

After the initial commitment step the HSC loses its ability to self-renew and the hematopoietic pathway bifurcates with formation of either the common lymphoid progenitor (CLP) or common myeloid-erythroid progenitor (CMEP) cells. CLPs can give rise to mature NK, B and T cells, whilst the CMEPs can form erythrocyte, megakaryocyte, granulocyte and monocyte populations. In Chapter 5, Čokić *et al.* describe the role of nitric oxide/cyclic nucleotide regulation in erythropoiesis, the formation of red blood cells (erythrocytes). In this chapter the authors provide an overview of the erythropoietic pathway including the crucial role that GATA1/2 plays in hemoglobin switching. They present some novel findings whereby they used microarrays to measure changes in expression levels of globin-related genes during ontogenesis, and later on provide evidence to show that NO and cGMP can induce globin gene expression.

Platelets play an essential role in hemostasis and thrombosis, initiating clot formation in response to cellular damage. Central to the clotting process is platelet aggregation mediated by the cross-linking of intergrin αIIbβ3 to fibrinogen, von Willebrand factor and other soluble ligands. Aside from their role in physiological processes, platelets may also form pathological thrombi which can lead to myocardial infarction or stroke. Therefore inhibitors of αIIbβ3 are of great clinical interest. In Chapter 6, Chen *et al.* use a proteomic approach to identify binding partners to αIIb and the αIIbβ3 heterodimer expressed in cord-blood derived megakaryocytes. Using this technique they identified and validated DNAJC10 as a novel binding partner of the immature form of αIIbβ3, and showed that it binds early on in the biogenic pathway. Furthermore, the authors found that silencing of *DNAJC10* could modulate levels of αIIbβ3 in megakaryocytes as well as HEK293 cells transfected with aIIb and b3 cDNA constructs.

Chapter 7 by Gottimukkala, Burute and Galande concerns the role of the transcription factor SATB1 in the development and differentiation of T-cells, in particular, the key role that this molecule plays in T_H differentiation. The authors also describe how the loss of SATB1 function may be associated with the T-cell lymphoma, Sézary syndrome.

Cell polarization is necessary for the migration of cells in many processes including embryogenesis, inflammation and tumor metastasis. Chemoattractant recruitment of neutrophils to trauma sites is an essential process of the inflammatory response.

Neutrophil polarization involves directional sensing of external stimuli via cell surface receptors resulting in a reorganization of the cortical cytoskeleton. In Chapter 8, Cerecedo discusses the molecular mechanisms behind neutrophil migration focusing on the role of proteins and protein complexes that promote cell polarization. This theme is expanded in Chapter 9 where Massena and Philipson review leukocyte recruitment during inflammation, particularly the mechanisms behind the recently described phenomenon of intravascular leukocyte chemotaxis.

The formation of new blood vessels, or neovascularization, can occur either *de novo* (vasculogenesis) or arise from pre-existing vasculature (angiogenesis). Angiogenesis is a vital process in growth and development as well as in wound healing. It is also fundamental in the transition of tumors to a malignant state. Angiogenesis involves multiple cellular processes including cell proliferation, migration, adhesion and morphogenesis. This process is controlled by a multitude of signaling proteins. Their membrane trafficking and associated endothelial-cell dynamics are reviewed in Chapter 10 by Tiwari *et al*.

In the second section of this book (Section 2 - Hematological Pathologies), the focus shifts onto discussion of the diseases of the blood system. This section starts with a chapter by Khanna-Gupta and Abayasekara (Chapter 11) that reviews diseases of the myeloid system/lineage. This chapter focuses on the role that translational control plays in myeloid cells under normal and disease conditions. In particular the role C/EBPα, PU.1, and components of the mTOR pathway are described as well as the role of post-transcriptional regulation by microRNAs in these processes. Myeloproliferative neoplasms (MPNs) are a subset of clonal disorders of the myeloid system that includes diseases of the granulocytes (chronic myeloid leukemia), erythrocytes (polycythemia vera) and platelets (essential thrombocythemia). Although essentially chronic in clinical progression, patients have a finite risk of undergoing evolution to acute leukemic disease. In Chapter 12, Rinaldi *et al.* review these diseases and provide a detailed discussion about the role of constitutive activation of tyrosine kinases, in particularly members of the JAK2 pathway, and how these discoveries are translating into new therapeutic options.

The next chapters in this section concern malignancies of the lymphoid lineage. In Chapter 13 Vitale *et al.* review physiological and pathological features of NK (natural killer) cells. NK cells are a fascinating lymphoid subset which, relative to the more commonly studied B and T cells, are very poorly understood. They are a major component of the innate immune system and play an important role in tumor immunity and viral defenses. This chapter describes what is known of cellular interactions between NK cells and other immune components such as dendritic cells, as well as the molecular pathways involved in these interactions including the pivotal role of TRAIL. Although rare, NK neoplasms represent a very distinct class of disorders that can range in their clinical presentation from very indolent to very aggressive. The latest advances in understanding these diseases are presented in this chapter along with a discussion of current and future therapeutic options.

Lymphomas are classified as malignancies of NK cells, B lymphocytes or T lymphocytes. Lymphoma is the fifth most common cancer type in the Western world and, worryingly, its incidence appears to have steadily increased during recent years. Chapter 14 concerns the most common form of low-grade lymphoma, follicular lymphoma (FL). FL accounts for approximately one third of lymphomas in the US and consequently is a common encounter in the hematology clinic. Despite its high frequency surprisingly there is no consensus regarding the best treatment protocol for FL patients, and patients will eventually succumb to the disease with a heterogeneous range of survival times ranging from less than one year to more than 20 years (median OS ~10 years). Consequently, a more robust grading and/or stratification scheme would help refine and define treatment options for FL patients. Chapter 14 reviews the various techniques currently used in the clinic in respect of FL patients including clinical, cytogenetic and molecular methods as well as the various algorithms used, and discusses their relative strengths and weaknesses.

Approximately 30% of FL cases will undergo high-grade transformation to an aggressive lymphoma that is histologically indistinguishable from diffuse large B-cell lymphoma (DLBCL). Transformed FL patients have a particularly poor outcome with a median survival of less than 14 months. The molecular basis of FL transformation is only poorly understood and importantly to date there are no reliable biomarkers that can identify FL patients at risk of transformation. Chapter 15 poses the tantalizing possibility that microRNAs may prove to be suitable biomarkers for these at-risk patients. The chapter presents the author's (largely) microarray data suggesting that biopsies from FL patients that undergo transformation have a microRNA signature that differs from those that do not undergo transformation. The implication being that patients can be tested for the presence of this signature and so those that might benefit from a more aggressive therapy regimen up-front can be identified.

Despite only formally being recognized for just over 10 years, the field of microRNAs is a useful illustration of the speed of scientific discovery today. In the first two years after microRNAs were first named (I.e. 2003), there were just over 50 publications; this number has been growing exponentially since, and there are now more than 15,000 publications (source PubMed; search string= "microRNA"; date="11/01/12"). MicroRNAs are now known to play key regulatory roles in virtually every physiological and pathological aspect of human biology including that of the hematological system (discussed briefly in Chapter 15). In addition to their utility in higher organisms, microRNAs also form part of the armory of many pathogens including viruses. Chapter 16 reviews the function and characterization of microRNAs encoded by Epstein-Barr virus (EBV), a pathogen intimately involved in lymphogenesis. As with other herpesvirus family members, the genome of EBV encodes for multiple microRNAs that are differentially expressed at various stages of the infectious cycle. EBV-encoded microRNAs have been shown to direct modulate host cells, for example changing the immune response to favor infection. Indeed, it has been suggested that these microRNAs play a fundamental role in the maintenance (though not necessarily establishment) of EBV-associated cancers such as Burkitt's lymphoma and Hodgkin's disease.

Lymphoproliferative disorders (LPD) is a term used to describe a heterogeneous group of disorders characterized by the presence of monoclonal or oligoclonal lymphoid cell expansion. The LPDs includes lymphomas, lymphoid leukemias, multiple myeloma as well as more rarely encountered entities such as post-transplant lymphoproliferative disorders (PTLD) and Waldenström's macroglobulinemia. An essential tool in understanding the pathogenesis of these diseases is the availability of a suitable animal model. In Chapter 17 Tsingotjidou tackles this subject with particular focus on a murine model of Waldenström's macroglobulinemia developed in the laboratory of the author.

Systemic mastocytosis (SM) is rare disorder characterized by the presence of excess mast cells in internal organs in addition to involvement of the skin. SM is a clonal disorder and can occur in association with hematological malignancies. The most frequently observed partner malignancies are myeloid in origin. By contrast, there are very few instances in the literature of SM presenting in concert with lymphoid malignancies. In Chapter 18, Antonia *et al.* present a thorough review of what little is known about SM and its pathology as well as discussing the treatment options available to the hematologist.

In the third and final section of the book (Section 3 - Hematology in the Clinic), we turn our attention to the practice of clinical hematology. Essays in this section include proposals to advance the current treatment regimens of blood disorders as well as possible novel therapeutics for these diseases. Chapter 19 considers the use of adoptive immunotherapy in order to target minimal residual disease (MRD) in acute myeloid leukemia (AML). Although improvements in chemotherapy have greatly advanced complete remission rates in this malignancy, a significant proportion of responders retain MRD that is refractory to further treatment interventions, eventually leading to relapse and disease progression. This chapter presents some novel solutions to this problem focusing on the use of NK cells as vehicles of adoptive immunotherapy against AML tumor cells. In addition, the use of leukemia vaccines is discussed including the various pros and cons of promising antigens identified by the latest research studies.

The ubiquitin-proteasome system (UPS) is essential for many cellular processes including cell cycle regulation, gene expression, cellular stress responses and regulation of immune function. The UPS system is also associated with many different disease types including inflammatory, cardiovascular and cancer. As a consequence, inhibitors of the UPS system, and proteosome inhibitors in particular, have been targeted as useful anti-cancer therapeutics. Chapter 20 by Mao reviews the functioning of the UPS system with particular emphasis on its involvement in hematological malignancies. The author discusses the discovery, mechanism and use of the most widely available proteosome inhibitor, bortezomib. Bortezomib is licensed as second line therapy for patients with relapsed multiple myeloma and mantle cell lymphoma in the US. Although bortezomib is effective in achieving remission for 35% of relapsed and refractory myeloma patients, complete remission is only achieved in less than 5% of patients and 65% of patients do not respond at all. Therefore the need for alternative therapies is clear and in the final part of this chapter the authors review some of the latest research looking at the development of novel proteasome inhibitors.

Heparin is a very widely available anticoagulant used to prevent the formation of venous thromboembolism, particularly in patients with angina, acute myocardial infarction and patients that have undergone vascular surgery, as well as in the treatment of venous thrombosis and pulmonary embolism. However, heparin treatment in five to 10% of patients can in itself lead to potentially fatal heparin-induced thrombocytopenia (HIT). HIT is characterized by a low platelet count and predisposition to thrombosis. Chapter 21 reviews this phenomenon, including the epidemiology, pathophysiology and diagnosis of HIT in patients as well as current and future treatment options for patients.

Chapter 22 considers the flip side of the ever increasing range of treatment options and patient data available to the modern day hematologist; how to prioritize and deal with potential information overload in the context of an ever-increasing workload, efficiency audits and accountability practices. The interface between the diagnostic instrument and the physician is known as middleware. This chapter considers the optimal way to achieve clarity in presentation of data to the clinician through proper design of middleware and its output. Bernstein *et al.* review this subject thoroughly in the context of data generated by the most commonly used diagnostic test of all, the hematocrit.

Chapters 23 and 24 move away from human clinical hematology to its use in the veterinary field. Chapter 23 describes the use of a porcine model as a surrogate investigative tool for the human surgical procedures, splenectomy and the still controversial procedure, autologous spleen transplantation. The authors carried out these procedures and measured the effect on blood count and cell morphology and well as spleen tissue functionality via measurements of rates of erythrocyte having Howell-Jolly bodies from the blood stream. Chapter 24 considers the use of hematological measurements in the veterinary treatment and management of horses, with special emphasis on race horses. Satué *et al.* consider the variability in equine hematological profiles in the context of physiological differences including the influence of gender, age, season, circadian rhythm, training and race history etc., as well as technical variability induced by sample handling, method of venipuncture, accuracy of measurement and so on. The authors conclude that although widely used as an indicator of general health in routine equine veterinary practice, the interpretation of data should be treated with caution due to the many exogenous and endogenous factors that can influence these measurements.

In summary, these essays cover a wide range of subjects pertaining to hematology, both theoretical and clinical, and aptly illustrate both the complexity and challenges that face the hematologist today and in the future.

This book is dedicated to my wonderful and understanding wife María, and my two beautiful children, Julia and Carlos. Special thanks should also be given to Dr. Chris Hatton (Director of Clinical Medicine at the John Radcliffe Hospital, Oxford) for his inspiration and continual support over the years.

Charles H. Lawrie
Biodonostia Research Institute,
San Sebastián,
Spain

Part 1

Blood Physiology

1

Mechanisms Controlling Hematopoiesis

Katja Fiedler and Cornelia Brunner
University Ulm
Germany

1. Introduction

Hematopoiesis – the generation of blood cells that proceeds mainly in the bone marrow - is a well-controlled process constantly occurring throughout the live of the mammalian organism. Generally, blood cells are relatively short-lived cells with a life span ranging from few hours to several weeks causing the need for a sustained replenishment of functional erythroid, lymphoid and myeloid cells. The development of mature hematopoietic cells in a hierarchical manner from a pluripotent hematopoietic stem cell over multipotent progenitors that further develop to oligopotent and then to lineage-restricted progenitors requires several control mechanisms at different levels. Transcription factors important for the expression of lineage-specific genes play a major role in the regulation of hematopoietic stem cell maintenance as well as hematopoietic lineage decision. Moreover, the discovery of so-called master transcription factors determining the fate of a terminally differentiated cell population indicates on one side the coordinated processes of hematopoietic cell differentiation but on the other side the complex mechanisms of transcriptional activation and/or repression of specific genes. However, what in turn regulates the expression of transcription factors that finally determine the lineage and differentiation choice of a certain progenitor or immature cell? Is the development into one or another cell type a definitive event or is there some plasticity observed? Which factors are necessary and which sufficient for hematopoietic cell differentiation? These and several other important questions concerning the regulation of development and differentiation of blood cells will be discussed. This chapter summarizes the current knowledge about cell intrinsic, environmental as well as epigenetic mechanisms involved in the control of hematopoiesis under homeostatic as well as infectious conditions.

1.1 Hematopoiesis

The hematopoietic system is traditionally categorized into two separate lineages, the lymphoid lineage responsible for adaptive immunity and the myeloid lineage embracing morphologically, phenotypically and functionally distinct cell types like innate immune cells as well as erythrocytes and platelets. Mature hematopoietic cells, except some rare lymphoid cell types, are relatively short-lived with life spans ranging from few hours for granulocytes to a couple of weeks for erythrocytes demanding a continued replenishment of functional cells. This process is named hematopoiesis and takes place primarily in the bone marrow, where few hematopoietic stem cells give rise to a differentiated progeny following a series of more or less well-defined steps of multipotent progenitors and lineage-restricted precursors leading to a hierarchical structure of the process. During the course of hematopoiesis cells lose their proliferative potential as well as multi-lineage differentiation capacity and progressively acquire characteristics of terminally differentiated mature cells.

1.2 Hematopoietic stem cells

In the hematopoietic differentiation hierarchy, the most primitive cells with highest multipotent activity are long-term repopulating hematopoietic stem cells (LT-HSC). One of the first definitions of true HSC meaning LT-HSC came from bone marrow transplantation experiments in mice determining HSC by their capacity to reconstitute several times the hematopoietic system of lethally irradiated adult organisms. Such experiments have demonstrated that HSC possess multi-potentiality as well as the ability to produce exact replicas upon cell division, named self-renewal capacity. In contrast to real HSC, short-term repopulating HSC (ST-HSC) defined by their ability to contribute transiently to the production of lymphoid and myeloid cells in lethally irradiated recipients, are often described misleadingly as self-renewing cells. The contemporary model of hematopoietic stem cells proposes the affiliation of ST-HSC to the group of multipotent progenitors (MPP), which are characterized by a more limited proliferative potential, but retained ability to differentiate into various hematopoietic lineages (Kondo et al., 2003; Weissman & Shizuru, 2008). Concerning MPP hierarchy, a defined model is not available at the moment, because several studies have demonstrated different types of multipotent progenitors with myelo-lymphoid or myelo-erythroid potential, such as the lymphoid-primed multipotent progenitor (LMPP) (Iwasaki & Akashi, 2007).

Additionally, a lot of research concerning prospective isolation and characterization of HSC and multipotent progenitors has provided insight into the surface marker expression on these types of cells leading to the definition of HSC and multipotent progenitors as cells being mainly negative for lineage markers but positive for the surface markers Sca1 and Kit. This fraction of bone marrow cells is also named LSK-fraction ($Lin^-Sca1^+Kit^+$) and comprises all stem cell capacity of the hematopoietic system, whereby HSC are defined as $Lin^-Kit^+Sca1^+Flt3^-$ and MPP as $Lin^-Kit^+Sca1^+Flt3^+$. Furthermore, the Slam (signaling lymphocyte activation molecule) family receptors CD150 and CD48 are useful surface markers allowing to distinguish inside the LSK-fraction between HSC ($CD150^+CD48^-$) and multipotent progenitors ($CD150^-CD48^-$) as well as the most restricted progenitors ($CD48^+$) (Kiel et al., 2005).

Under homeostatic conditions, the number of HSC remains relatively constant and the majority of HSC stays in a quiescent state that contributes not only to their long-term maintenance, but also allows a rapid cell cycle entry upon a variety of differentiation cues. The minority of HSC is in an active and dividing state and gives rise to all hematopoietic cells meaning that these few active HSC not only have to self-renew, but also have to produce all differentiated progeny. These different cell fates can only be achieved by an asymmetric division of the HSC, which allows the generation of two non-identical daughter cells, one maintaining stem cell identity and the other becoming a differentiated cell. Two different mechanisms are proposed by which asymmetry could be achieved: first by divisional asymmetry that is introduced by unequally redistributed cell-fate determinants in the cytoplasm (Florian & Geiger, 2010). An alternative possibility would be the environmental asymmetry, which is caused by different extrinsic signals provided by distinct local microenvironments and provokes different cell fate decisions of two identical daughter cells (Wilson, A. & Trumpp, 2006).

1.3 Lineage-committed progenitors

Downstream of the HSC and MPP populations with high proliferative and self-renewal capacity starts the differentiation process in hematopoiesis leading to oligopotent and later on to lineage-committed progenitors with a diminished proliferation but increased differentiation. The contemporary model of hematopoiesis (Figure 1) assumes that the decision for differentiation into the lymphoid/myeloid or megakaryocyte/erythrocyte lineages probably occurs very early in hematopoiesis. Several studies have demonstrated that multipotent progenitors like the lymphoid-primed multipotent progenitor (LMPP, $Lin^{-}Kit^{+}Sca1^{+}CD150^{-}CD34^{+}Flt3^{hi}$) retain only minor megakaryocyte/erythrocyte lineage potential, whereas the vast majority of progenitors appears to be committed to the granulocyte/monocyte as well as the lymphoid lineage (Iwasaki & Akashi, 2007).

In the next step of ongoing differentiation oligopotent progenitors with differentiation capacity for several hematopoietic lineages develop from an ancestor, the common lymphoid progenitor (CLP) (Kondo et al., 1997) and the common myeloid progenitor (CMP) (Akashi et al., 2000). The CLP is the earliest population in the lineage-negative fraction that upregulates the receptor for interleukin 7 (IL-7), an essential cytokine for T and B cell development. Furthermore, the CLP carries differentiation potential for all types of lymphoid cells including B cells, T cells and NK cells. The surface marker profile of CLP is defined as $Lin^{-}Sca1^{lo}Kit^{lo}IL7R\alpha^{+}$ (Kondo et al., 1997). In contrast to CLP, the CMP resides in the $Lin^{-}Sca1^{-}Kit^{+}$ population in bone marrow that can be further fractioned by expression of the Fcγ receptor II/III (FcγRII/III) and CD34 leading to three distinct progenitor populations.

The CMP is defined as $Fc\gamma RII/III^{lo}CD34^{+}$ and can give rise to all types of myeloid colonies in clonogenic assays, while the $Fc\gamma RII/III^{hi}CD34^{+}$ granulocyte-monocyte progenitor (GMP) is restricted to granulocytes and macrophages. The $Fc\gamma RII/III^{lo}CD34^{-}$ megakaryocyte-erythrocyte progenitor (MEP) is delimitated to megakaryocytes and erythrocytes (Akashi et al., 2000).

Still a matter of dispute is the dendritic cell (DC) development, because DC mainly are the progeny of GMP, but can also be generated from lymphoid progenitors such as CLP and pro T cells under certain conditions (Manz et al., 2001). However, the majority of plasmacytoid DC (pDC) and conventional or myeloid DC (mDC) develop successively by several commitment steps downstream of the GMP in the bone marrow. The first step is the development of the monocyte/macrophage and DC precursor (MDP) (Fogg et al., 2006) (MDP) out of the GMP that has lost differentiation potential for granulocytes and expresses the FcγRII/III and CD34 at a comparable level to the GMP, but is also $Kit^{lo}CX_3CR1^{+}$. Further differentiation of MDP, which is accompanied by the loss of monocyte potential, leads to the common DC precursor (CDP) defined as $Lin^{-}Kit^{int}Flt3^{+}M\text{-}CSFR^{+}$ population that can only give rise to pDC and mDC (Geissmann et al., 2010; Naik et al., 2007; Onai et al., 2007).

Besides the characterization of MDP and CDP by several studies, further progenitor populations for eosinophils, basophils and mast cells have been isolated downstream of the GMP and their position in the hematopoietic hierarchy is depicted in Figure 1. Moreover,

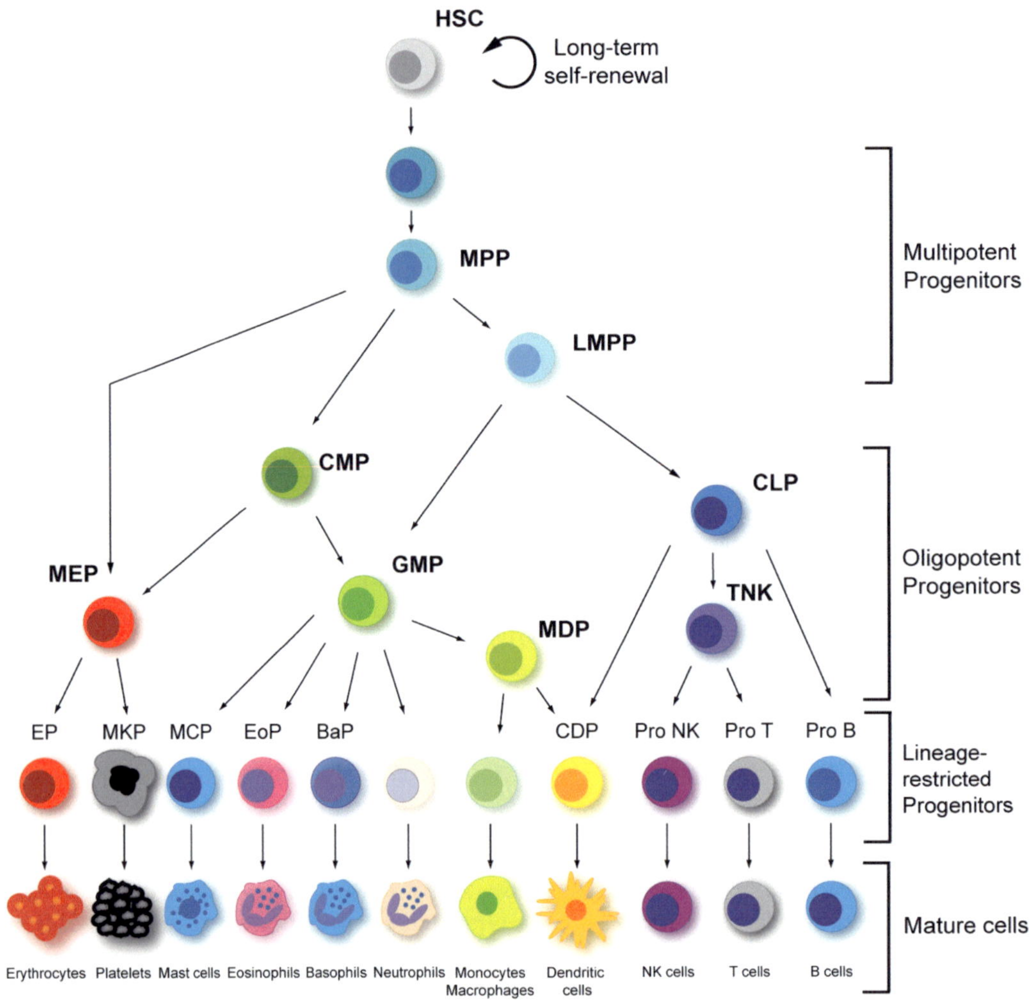

Fig. 1. Model of the hematopoietic hierarchy in the mouse.
The developmental course shown in the scheme is proposed using results generated by prospective isolation and characterization of different progenitors. HSC, hematopoietic stem cell; MPP, multipotent progenitor; LMPP, lymphoid-primed multipotent progenitor; CLP, common lymphoid progenitor; CMP, common myeloid progenitor; MEP, megakaryocyte-erythrocyte progenitor; GMP, granulocyte-macrophage progenitor; MDP, monocyte-dendritic cell progenitor; TNK, T cell NK cell progenitor; EP, erythroid progenitor; MKP, megakaryocyte progenitor; MCP, mast cell progenitor; EoP, eosinophil progenitor; BaP, basophil progenitor; CDP, common dendritic cell progenitor.

the monopotent megakaryocyte lineage-committed progenitor (MKP) (Pronk et al., 2007) and erythroid progenitor (EP) (Terszowski et al., 2005) have been described downstream of the MEP. Only for the monocyte/macrophage lineage and the neutrophil granulocytes, a putative committed precursor downstream of the GMP has not been identified to date (Iwasaki & Akashi, 2007). With regard to lymphoid development one committed precursor downstream of the CLP is the bipotent T/NK cell progenitor that resides in the bone marrow and is able to generate thymic- and bone marrow-dependent NK cells as well as T cells (Nozad Charoudeh et al., 2010).

1.4 Factors involved in the regulation of hematopoiesis

The highly regulated differentiation process of quiescent HSC towards different progeny of mature hematopoietic cells is associated with a variety of cell fate choices at every single step of hematopoiesis. These different choices comprise quiescence, self-renewal or differentiation at HSC level as well as proliferation, lineage commitment and terminal differentiation at the progenitor or precursor level. Of course, different cell fate choices require at each step in the hematopoietic hierarchy a process of decision-making that is presumed to be dependent on and regulated by a combination of intrinsic factors that embrace lineage-determining transcription factors and their epigenetic regulation as well as extrinsic regulators such as cytokines.

1.4.1 Maintenance of HSC characteristics

For the maintenance of HSC with respect to quiescence, self-renewal and suppression of differentiation, the major intrinsic factors belong to the Bmi1-p53 axis of cell cycle regulators and the PI3K signaling pathway. Bmi1 is a member of the Polycomb group gene family that controls cell proliferation via repression of the *Ink4/Arf* locus. Therefore, Bmi1 supports self-renewal by suppressing transcription of the cell cycle inhibitors $p16^{Ink4a}$ and $p19^{ARF}$, which are encoded in the *Ink4/Arf* locus, whereas the tumor suppressor p53 contributes to the regulation of HSC quiescence via inhibition of cell cycle (Warr et al., 2011). In contrast, the PI3K signaling pathway controls cell proliferation, growth and survival via integration of numerous upstream signals, including growth factors, nutrients and oxygen status.

Additionally, several extrinsic factors have been identified that are necessary for preservation of HSC stemness. The extrinsic regulators embrace soluble membrane-bound extrinsic factors including cytokines (fms-related tyrosine kinase 3-ligand, stem cell factor), chemokines (CXCL12) and growth factors (Angiopoietin-1, granulocyte-CSF, granulocyte-macrophage-CSF), as well as Wnt (wingless type), Notch, Hedgehog and the TGFβ (transforming growth factor β) family of cytokines. These extrinsic factors are provided by a specialized microenvironment in the bone marrow, the so-called stem cell niche that resides in the endosteal and vascular compartments of the bone. In these areas, the bone marrow cells of hematopoietic and non-hematopoietic origin like megakaryocytes, osteoblasts, endothelial cells and CXCL12-abundant reticular (CAR) cells create a supportive microenvironment via physical interaction with HSC and production of soluble factors (Warr et al., 2011).

1.4.2 Transcription factors involved in lineage commitment

At the cellular level the differentiation process from HSC into lineage-committed hematopoietic cells involves the selective activation of lineage-specific genes as well as the silencing of lineage-foreign genes and developmental regulators in a defined order. The orchestration of such complex lineage-determining programs is dependent on several factors, but extensive research has emphasized the essential role of gene regulatory networks in directing cell fate choice and lineage restriction. These gene regulatory networks are composed of several master transcription factors that join special features, such as mutual regulation of transcriptional activity by antagonism as well as lineage-determining functions via activation of lineage-specific genes and repression of lineage-foreign genes. The first example pointing out the importance of such transcription factors is the transition from self-renewing HSC towards more committed MPP that is dependent on the transcription factor CCAAT-enhancer binding protein α (C/EBPα). The prototype of the C/EBP family displays all characteristic features of the transcription factor family, such as the N-terminal transactivation domain as well as the C-terminal DNA-binding domain consisting of a highly conserved basic region and a leucine zipper dimerization domain. Prerequisite for binding of C/EBPα to the cognate DNA-site is the homo- or heterodimerization with another transcription factor via the leucine zipper domain that in turn allows the basic region to bind to the CCAAT motif (Johnson, 2005; Lekstrom-Himes, J. & Xanthopoulos, 1998). Evidences for the function of C/EBPα in hematopoietic differentiation revealed from studies on conditional C/EBPα-deficient mice, which demonstrated a competitive advantage of C/EBPα-deficient HSC over wild type HSC in reconstitution experiments. Further analyses of the transcriptome of C/EBPα-deficient HSC have confirmed that the expression of the self-renewal factor Bmi1 is increased in these cells, suggesting C/EBPα as a pro-differentiation factor in HSC fate decision (Zhang et al., 2004).

1.4.2.1 Erythroid-megakaryocyte lineage commitment

Probably, the next step in decision-making during differentiation is the choice for erythroid versus myeloid-lymphoid lineage restriction at the transition from MPP to LMPP or MEP that is regulated by the E-twenty six (Ets) family transcription factor PU.1 and the transcription factor GATA-binding protein 1 (GATA-1). GATA-1 is expressed in erythroid, megakaryocyte and mast cell as well as eosinophil lineages and contains zinc fingers, which mediate DNA binding to the WGATAR DNA sequence as well as protein-protein interaction (Bresnick et al., 2010; Morceau et al., 2004). In contrast to GATA-1, PU.1 is restricted to monocyte as well as B lymphoid lineages and consists of a N-terminal transactivation domain, a PEST-domain (proline, glutamic acid, serine and threonine rich sequence) and the eponymous Ets-domain at the C-terminus, which mediate DNA binding to an 11 bp sequence with a central GGAA motif (Gangenahalli et al., 2005; Sharrocks, 2001). Additionally, both transcription factors are detectable in MPP and gene disruption studies have demonstrated the indispensable functions of GATA-1 and PU.1 for megakaryocyte/erythrocyte and myeloid/lymphoid development, respectively. Analyses of systemic PU.1-deficient mice revealed a complete loss of CMP, GMP and CLP populations but normal numbers of MEP causing impaired lymphoid and myeloid cell development as well as retained megakaryocyte/erythrocyte development (Scott et al., 1994). In contrast, GATA-1-deficient mice die between embryonic day 10.5 and 11.5 due to severe anemia resulting from a maturation arrest of erythroid cells (Fujiwara et al., 1996). Further support for the lineage instructive role of GATA-1 originated from the forced expression of GATA-1 in lineage-committed progenitors like GMP and CLP that exclusively leads to megakaryocyte/erythrocyte development (Iwasaki et al., 2003). Several other studies dealing with certain aspects of the molecular interaction of PU.1 and GATA-1 as well as their gene regulatory capacity revealed the cross-antagonism between these proteins involving direct physical interaction of both factors that results in an inhibition of the transactivation potential of the counterpart (Laslo et al., 2008). Based on these findings,

GATA-1 is prospected as the erythrocyte/megakaryocyte lineage determinant, whereas PU.1 is regarded as the myeloid/lymphoid lineage determinant. Regarding the regulation of erythrocyte versus megakaryocyte development, the detailed molecular mechanisms are not fully understood, but several transcription factors involved in this process are described such as Friend of GATA-1 (FOG-1), Fli-1 or Krueppel-like factor 1 (KLF1) (Kerenyi & Orkin, 2010; Szalai et al., 2006).

1.4.2.2 Myeloid lineage commitment

Downstream of LMPP, lineage choice embraces myeloid, as well as B or T lymphoid lineage and mainly depends on the transcription factors PU.1, early B cell factor 1 (EBF1) and Notch. For myeloid lineage restriction, a high expression level of PU.1 is necessary, whereas low levels of PU.1 plus EBF1 expression establish the B lymphoid lineage restriction and Notch instructs the T lymphoid lineage choice. Regarding granulocyte and monocyte development, besides PU.1, the transcription factor C/EBPα has to be enumerated. Studies have demonstrated that conditional deletion of C/EBPα in bone marrow cells of mice using the Mx1-Cre system leads to a total lack of mature granulocytes and a partial lack of monocytes due to a differentiation block at the transition from CMP to GMP (Zhang et al., 2004). Moreover, lineage choice between monocytes and granulocytes depends on the expression level of PU.1 and C/EBPα, which has been shown by studies using different mouse as well as *in vitro* models for diminished PU.1 expression in the hematopoietic system. In all experimental setups, reduced expression of PU.1 is followed by an augmented granulopoiesis to the disadvantage of monopoiesis. Additionally, gene expression analyses of PU.1-deficient progenitors have demonstrated a decreased or even absent expression of several monocyte-specific genes, like the macrophage scavenger receptor or the M-CSF receptor. Furthermore, the need for C/EBPα during the transition from CMP to GMP is possibly due to the transcriptional upregulation of PU.1, since forced C/EBPα expression in hematopoietic progenitors favors monopoiesis and not granulopoiesis, whereas exogenous C/EBPα in myeloid cell lines directs granulopoiesis (Friedman, 2007). Nevertheless, C/EBPα is probably indispensable for granulocyte development due to the transcriptional upregulation of several granulocyte-specific factors. One of these factors is the transcriptional repressor growth factor independent 1 (Gfi1), which is necessary for the repression of proliferation and of monocyte lineage-promoting factors such as M-CSF (Borregaard, 2010). Another important target of C/EBPα is the transcription factor C/EBPε that is important for terminal granulocyte differentiation, because of the transcriptional control of granule-specific genes (lactoferrin and gelatinase) as well as genes necessary for cell cycle regulation (Borregaard, 2010).

Besides the upregulation of other transcription factors, C/EBPα forces granulocyte development additionally by transactivation of various genes, such as G-CSF receptor (Hohaus et al., 1995; Smith, L. T. et al., 1996) or myeloperoxidase (MPO) (Wang, W. et al., 2001), and downregulation of proliferation by direct interaction with the cell cycle regulator E2F (D'Alo et al., 2003; Theilgaard-Monch et al., 2005). In line with these experimental results is the association of inactivating C/EBPα mutations with hematopoietic malignancies like acute myeloid leukemia and high-risk myelodysplastic syndrome proposing that C/EBPα possesses the ability to arrest cell proliferation and to drive terminal differentiation (Koschmieder et al., 2009). Taken together, the plethora of studies implicates the following model for monocyte versus granulocyte lineage choice: First

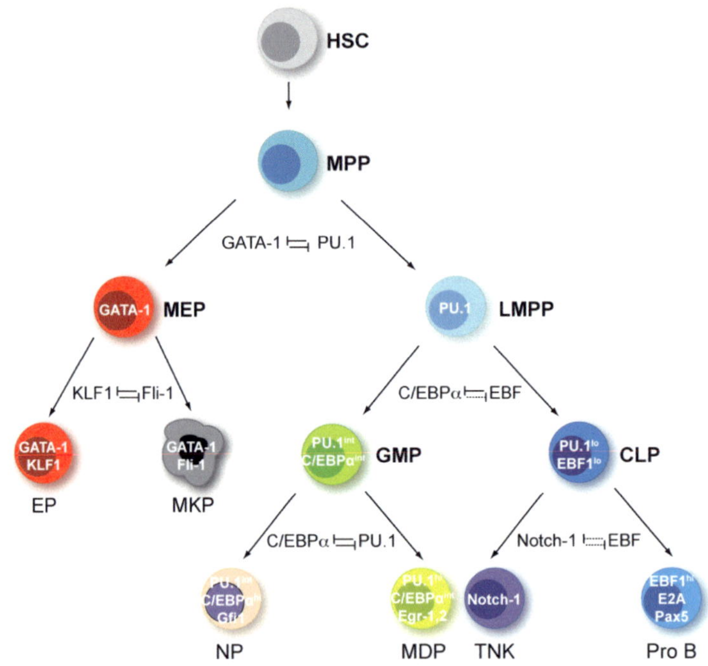

Fig. 2. Transcription factor network regulating lineage commitment.
The scheme displays a simplified overview of gene regulatory networks, which have a major influence on hematopoietic lineage choice during hematopoiesis. Supposed (dashed lines) and proved (continuous lines) cross-antagonisms between key transcription factors which function to regulate binary cell fate choices are noted in the scheme. Additionally, transcription factors that are important for the generation of particular intermediates are noted in white. HSC, hematopoietic stem cell; MPP, multipotent progenitor; LMPP, lymphoid-primed multipotent progenitor; CLP, common lymphoid progenitor; CMP, common myeloid progenitor; MEP, megakaryocyte-erythrocyte progenitor; GMP, granulocyte-macrophage progenitor; NP, neutrophil progenitor; MDP, monocyte-dendritic cell progenitor; TNK, T cell NK cell progenitor; EP, erythroid progenitor; MKP, megakaryocyte progenitor.

of all, C/EBPα is needed for the transition from CMP to GMP by induction of PU.1 expression. High protein levels of PU.1 induce monopoiesis via interaction with other transcription factors like interferon regulatory factor 8 (IRF8) or activating protein-1 family transcription factors (AP-1/Jun proteins) and the transcriptional activation of monocyte-specific genes (Friedman, 2007). However, AP-1 family transcription factors are also able to heterodimerize with C/EBPα (Cai et al., 2008) implicating an inhibition mechanism of PU.1 for granulocyte development by sequestering the binding partners of C/EBPα. In contrast to the high protein levels of PU.1 that favor monopoiesis, insufficient activation of PU.1 transcription allows C/EBPα to induce the granulopoiesis program accompanied by suppression of monopoiesis (Figure 2).

Terminal granulopoiesis starts with the myeloblast and promyelocyte state, where the switch from proliferation to differentiation takes place, displayed by the loss of ability for cell division after the promyelocyte state. Moreover, the formation of the first granules starts, which are named primary or azurophilic granules. The most important transcription factors at myeloblast/promyelocyte stage are C/EBPα and Gfi1, which are necessary for the suppression of monocyte development and proliferation as well as for the transcriptional activation of granulocyte-specific genes like *MPO*, *ELANE* or *CEBPE* (Borregaard, 2010; Koschmieder et al., 2009; Theilgaard-Monch et al., 2005). The importance of Gfi1 and ELANE has been demonstrated by studies analyzing the genetic background of severe congenital neutropenia (SCN) and other forms of neutropenia. These studies revealed that one of the major causes for loss of neutrophil differentiation beyond promyelocyte state are mutations in the *ELANE* gene (Dale et al., 2000; Horwitz et al., 1999), but in rare cases of SCN also mutations of the *GFI1* gene have been described (Person et al., 2003). Detailed analyses of Gfi1 in mice further supported the function of Gfi1 as molecular switch towards granulocyte development by suppression of monocyte-specific genes, like *Csf1* (M-CSF) and *Csf1r* (M-CSFR) (Zarebski et al., 2008).

Ongoing differentiation beyond promyelocytes leads to the development of myelocytes and metamyelocytes, which are defined by the beginning of nuclear segmentation and the appearance of secondary (also called specific) granules as well as the exit from cell cycle. The regulation of secondary granule protein expression and the exit from cell cycle mainly depends on the transcription factor C/EBPε, whose expression peaks in myelocytes and metamyelocytes (Bjerregaard et al., 2003; Theilgaard-Monch et al., 2005). Based on studies using C/EBPε-deficient mice, which displayed neutrophil-specific defects including bilobed nuclei, abnormal respiratory burst and compromised bactericidal activity as well as impaired chemotaxis (Lekstrom-Himes, J. & Xanthopoulos, 1999; Yamanaka et al., 1997), the genetic cause of a very rare congenital disorder named neutrophil specific granule deficiency (SGD) has been delineated to the *CEBPE* locus (Lekstrom-Himes, J. A. et al., 1999). Additional studies have revealed the essential functions of C/EBPε for the expression of secondary and tertiary granule proteins (Verbeek et al., 1999; Yamanaka et al., 1997) and demonstrated the direct interaction of C/EBPε with E2F1 and Rb protein, finally leading to cell cycle exit (Gery et al., 2004).

The last step of terminal granulopoiesis, the differentiation into band and segmented neutrophils leads to mature neutrophils with finally segmented nuclei and tertiary as well as secretory granules. In the course of neutrophil terminal differentiation, C/EBPα expression gradually diminishes during the myeloblast stage. C/EBPε peaks at the myelocyte/metamyelocyte stage, whereas the expression level of the transcription factors PU.1, C/EBPβ, C/EBPδ and C/EBPγ increases subsequently to the metamyelocyte stage (Bjerregaard et al., 2003). However, gene deletion studies using C/EBPβ- or C/EBPδ-deficient mice revealed no hematopoietic abnormalities with regard to terminal granulopoiesis. Still, Hirai and colleagues have demonstrated the indispensable role of C/EBPβ during emergency granulopoiesis in response to cytokine treatment or fungal infection in contrast to C/EBPα and C/EBPε, which were not upregulated under these conditions (Hirai et al., 2006). In the case of the transcription factor PU.1, a conditional gene deletion model has evidenced a PU.1-dependent transcriptional activation of *gp91*^{phox}, a component of the NADPH oxidase, as well as of *Mac-1/CD11b* (Dakic et al., 2005) (Figure 3).

Terminal differentiation during monopoiesis leads to monocytes, macrophages as well as dendritic cells and involves again the selection of specific gene expression programs to

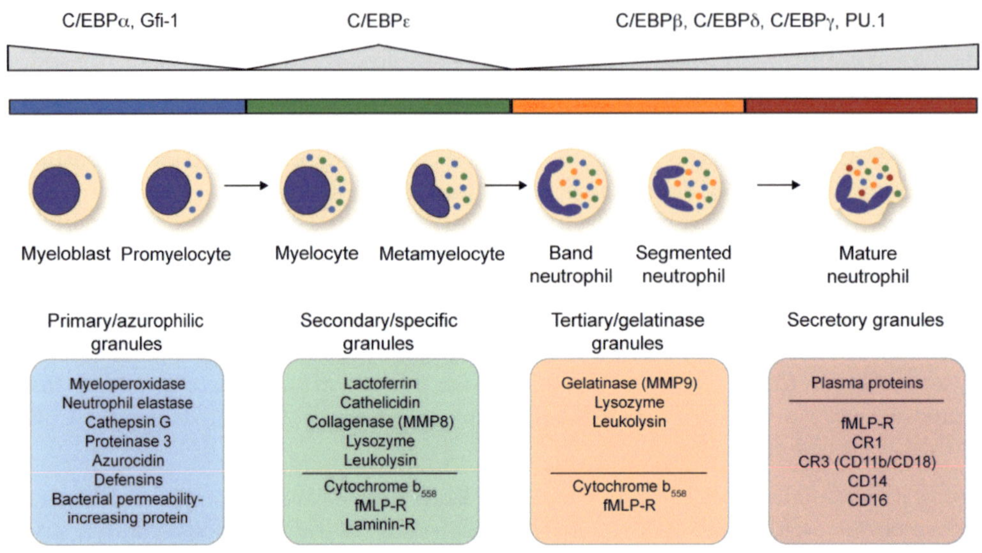

Fig. 3. Terminal granulopoiesis in the bone marrow.
The terminal granulopoiesis that is characterized by sequential formation of different granule types and segmentation of the nucleus starts at the myeloblast/promyelocyte stage and ends with mature neutrophils. Granule types not only differ in the time point at which they are formed, but also in their specific content, which is described at the bottom of the figure. Above the line in the boxes matrix content is depicted and beneath the proteins that are located to the vesicle membrane. At different stages of terminal granulopoiesis several transcription factors, which are indicated on top of the figure, are important for the regulation of maturation and timed expression of granule proteins.

determine cell fates. Additionally, several subtypes of macrophages or DC have been described in recent years bringing more complexity into monopoietic differentiation. Nevertheless, some key transcription factors with indispensable functions for monopoiesis are known already. For example, PU.1 is not only required for myeloid lineage commitment, but also for macrophage versus DC lineage choice during late myelopoiesis. Intermediate PU.1 expression at GMP stage results in the activation of the macrophage-specific transcription factors Egr-1 and Egr-2 (Laslo et al., 2006), whereas high expression of PU.1 promotes the induction of DC fate via repression of the macrophage-inducing transcription factors c-Maf and MafB (Bakri et al., 2005). In addition, gain-of-function experiments have demonstrated that ectopic expression of MafB, c-Maf, Egr-1 or IRF8 in early progenitors can drive monocyte or macrophage lineage commitment. In contrast, RelB induces DC differentiation and SpiB pDC differentiation in monocytic intermediates (Auffray et al., 2009; Geissmann et al., 2010). However, the detailed molecular mechanisms driving terminal monopoiesis remains to be elucidated.

1.4.2.3 B cell lineage commitment

B cells develop from CLP in the bone marrow, where several stages of B cell development have been defined. The earliest B lineage precursors are the pre/pro B cells, which begin to express the B lineage specific marker B220 at their surfaces. The transition of pre/pro B cells to the pre B cell stage is characterized by the upregulation of the surface marker CD19 as well as by the rearrangement of the immunoglobulin (Ig) heavy chain gene locus. Successful rearrangement of the Ig light chain locus is the prerequisite for the development to immature IgM expressing B cells. At this stage the antigen-independent phase of B cell development is almost complete. IgM^+ cells are ready to leave the bone marrow to enter peripheral secondary lymphoid organs where they first develop via the IgM^+IgD^+ stage to mature IgD^+ B cells. These cells undergo final maturation during the antigen-dependent phase of B cell development.

In addition to cytokines and cytokine receptors, several key transcription factors have been identified necessary for the B lineage commitment as well as for the maintenance of the B cell fate, like Ikaros, Gfi1, PU.1, E2A, EBF1 and Pax5. Prior to the differentiation of CLP, PU.1 is involved in the expression of components of the IL-7 signaling pathways (DeKoter et al., 2007) essential for EBF1-dependent lineage restriction in early lymphoid progenitors (Tsapogas et al., 2011). Additionally, the level of PU.1 expression predicts the decision between the myeloid and the B cell lineage. Low levels of PU.1 favors B cell development whereas high levels promote myeloid cell differentiation (DeKoter & Singh, 2000). The upregulation of the transcriptional repressor Gfi1 was suggested to be responsible for the down-modulation of PU.1 expression in early progenitors by displacing PU.1 from its upstream autoregulatory element and therefore for the promotion of B lineage decision (Spooner et al., 2009). In MPP, Gfi1 is upregulated by Ikaros to antagonize PU.1 expression, thus favoring B cell development (Spooner et al., 2009). CLP begin to express genes associated with committed B cells including E2A as well as EBF1 at the onset of B lymphopoiesis (Roessler et al., 2007; Seet et al., 2004; Smith, E. M. et al., 2002). The deficiency of these factors leads to a block of B cell development at a very early stage, even before D_H-J_H rearrangement of the IgH gene (Bain et al., 1994; Lin, H. & Grosschedl, 1995; Zhuang et al., 1994). In contrast, forced expression of E2A and EBF1 revealed that both factors cooperate in the upregulation of several B cell-specific genes, like Pax5, the surrogate light chain *λ5* gene, the *VpreB*, *Igα* and *Igβ* genes, plus the genes coding for *Rag1* and *Rag2* (Kee & Murre, 1998; O'Riordan & Grosschedl, 1999; Sigvardsson et al., 1997). In addition, the transcriptional co-activator *Pou2af1 (BOB.1/OBF.1; OCA-B)* and the transcription factor *FoxO1* were identified as direct targets of EBF1 (Zandi et al., 2008). In CLP the expression of Pax5 is still low. Consistent with the observation that Pax5 is essential for B lineage commitment, CLP still retain T cell developmental potential. The expression of Pax5 is detectable at the pro B cell where Pax5 antagonizes T cell development by blocking Notch1 (Souabni et al., 2002). Additionally, Pax5 interferes with the developmental potential to differentiate into several other hematopoietic lineages, since in the absence of Pax5 but in the presence of appropriate cytokines pro B cells are able to differentiate *in vitro* into NK cells, dendritic cells, macrophages, granulocytes and osteoclasts (Nutt, S. L. et al., 1999) indicating that the expression E2A and EBF1 is not sufficient to commit B cell progenitors to the B cell lineage in the absence of Pax5. Therefore, Pax5 plays an essential and dual role in B lineage development, it represses non-B cell-specific genes, like the genes coding for the M-CSFR or for MPO (Nutt, S. L. et al., 1999), whereas in the same time it activates the B lineage-specific gene program (Nutt, S. L. et al., 1998; Schebesta et al., 2002). Thus, Pax5 controls the pre-BCR signaling by promoting the V to DJ recombination at the *IgH* locus (Nutt, S. L. et al., 1997) and also by regulating directly the expression of the signaling molecule BLNK (Schebesta et al., 2002). Additionally, Pax5 is essential for the upregulation of *CD19* and *Igα* gene expression (Kozmik et al., 1992; Nutt, S. L. et al., 1997). Pax5-deficient

B cells are arrested at the pro B cell stage while expressing normal levels of E2A and EBF1 as well as of their target genes (Nutt, S. L. et al., 1998; Nutt, S.L. et al., 1997), indicating that E2A and EBF1 are upstream of Pax5 in the hierarchical order of lineage-determining transcription factor expression.

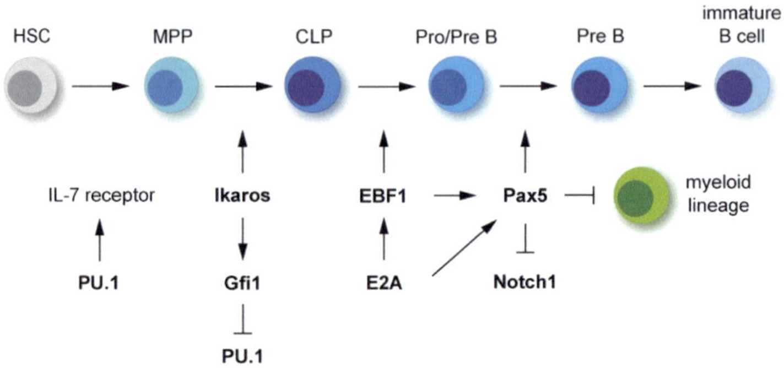

Fig. 4. Key transcription factors involved in B lymphopoiesis.
B cell development is driven by the consecutive activation of lineage-determining transcription factors like E2A, EBF1 and Pax5 and the repression of lineage-foreign genes. Transcription factors are highlighted in bold. HSC, hematopoietic stem cell; MPP, multipotent progenitor; CLP, common lymphoid progenitor.

However, sustained expression of EBF1 in Pax5-deficient hematopoietic precursor cells efficiently blocks myeloid and T lineage potential *in vivo*. Moreover, overexpression of EBF1 in Pax5-deficient pro B cells represses alternative lineage potential indicating that EBF1 promotes the commitment of the B cell lineage independently of Pax5 (Pongubala et al., 2008) (Figure 4). E2A in turn is required for the initiation but also for the maintenance of the expression of EBF1, Pax5 and the B cell-specific gene program at the pro B cell stage (Kwon et al., 2008). E2A exerts its instructive role not only in the bone marrow at the pro and pre B cell stage as well as at the immature B cell stage, but also in peripheral lymphatic organs during the formation of germinal center B cells (Kwon et al., 2008). In contrast, E2A is dispensable for Ig class switch recombination as well as for the generation of mature splenic subpopulations, like marginal zone B cells, follicular B cells and B1 cells. Also, the memory B cell subpopulation and the plasma cell generation is unaffected by the loss of E2A (Kwon et al., 2008).

Conditional inactivation of Pax5 revealed its requirement for the maintenance of B cell identity also during late B cell development in peripheral lymphatic organs (Horcher et al., 2001). Upon exposure to an antigen B lymphocytes can either maintain their B cell identity and differentiate into memory B cells or rapidly change their gene expression program and develop into germinal center (GC) and plasma cells (PC). During GC formation pre GC B cells upregulate the expression of the transcriptional repressor Bcl6 that controls the GC B cell differentiation. Bcl6-deficiency results in a complete block of GC B cell reaction, necessary for the generation of high-affinity antibodies by somatic hypermutation and class-switch recombination. In contrast, plasma cell generation occurs normally in Bcl6-deficient mice (Dent et al., 1997; Fukuda et al., 1997). The transcription factor IRF8 directly regulates, possibly in concert with other transcription factors, Bcl6 upregulation in GC B cells (Lee, C. H. et al., 2006). Bcl6 is able to repress several targets including the transcriptional repressor Blimp1 (B lymphocyte induced maturation protein 1) (Shaffer et al., 2000; Tunyaplin et al.,

2004). Therefore, during the GC reaction, Bcl6 represses the gene program for plasma cell generation in GC B cells (Shaffer et al., 2000).

Blimp1 is a key transcription factor for plasma cell (PC) differentiation, where it initiates a gene program, which leads to the inhibition of cell division, to the repression of genes defining the identity of GC B cells, and to the induction of genes necessary for Ig secretion (Kallies et al., 2007; Shaffer et al., 2002). Besides Blimp1, the transcription factors XBP-1 and IRF4 play an essential role for PC differentiation (Sciammas et al., 2006; Shaffer et al., 2004). During PC generation the GC gene program should be downregulated, which is achieved by Blimp1 that represses the expression of Bcl6 and also Pax5 (Diehl et al., 2008; Lin, K. I. et al., 2002) (Figure 5).

In general, the hierarchical expression and the cooperative action of transcription factors as well as epigenetic modulators cause the initiation of a gene program characteristic and irreversible for a certain committed lineage. However, under certain conditions, committed lineages exhibit a high degree of plasticity. For example, TLR engagement drives lymphoid progenitor cells to differentiate into dendritic cells (Nagai et al., 2006), a mechanism that possibly ensures the generation of sufficient numbers of myeloid cells during an acute infection. Today we know that the overexpression of few transcription factors Oct3/4, Sox2, c-Myc and Klf4 in adult murine or human fibroblasts can re-differentiate these cells into multipotent embryonic stem cell-like cells with pluripotent potential *in vitro* as well as *in vivo* (Takahashi et al., 2007; Takahashi & Yamanaka, 2006; Wernig et al., 2007). Therefore, it is not longer surprising that in the hematopoietic system the overexpression of lineage-determining transcription factors in committed cells leads to re-differentiation and lineage conversion. Thus, T cell progenitors could be converted into dendritic cells and mast cells by ectopic expression of PU.1 or GATA-3, respectively (Laiosa et al., 2006; Taghon et al., 2007). Also B cells could be re-differentiated into macrophages upon overexpression of C/EBPα (Xie et al., 2004). Nevertheless, these studies revealed the high instructive capacity of lineage-determining transcription factors.

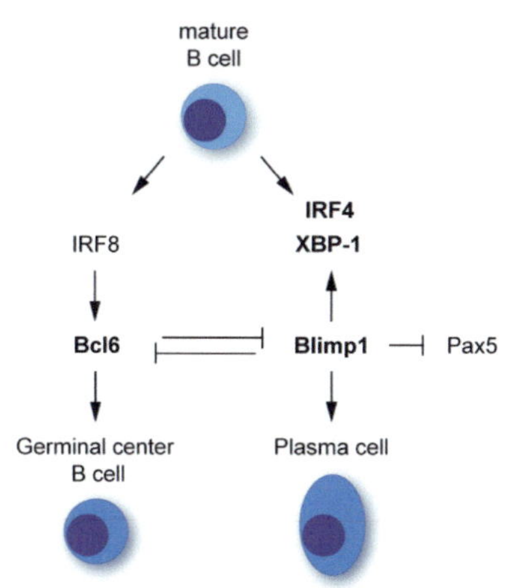

Fig. 5. Cross-regulatory control of germinal center B cell versus plasma cell fate.
Cell fate decision of mature B cells upon antigen exposure is regulated by key transcription factors (bold) that activate cell-specific genes and mutually repress transcription factors necessary for alternative cell differentiation.

In B cells, the lineage commitment and the maintenance of the B cell fate throughout B cell development is achieved by a single transcription factor - Pax5 (Cobaleda et al., 2007; Nutt, S. L. et al., 1999). As already mentioned, deletion of Pax5 leads to a block of B cell development at the pro B cell stage and $Pax5^{-/-}$ pro B cells can be re-differentiate in the presence of appropriate cytokines into osteoclasts, NK cells, dendritic cells, macrophages and granulocytes (Nutt, S. L. et al., 1999). More recently it was shown, that the conditional deletion of Pax5 in mature B cells from peripheral lymphoid organs, despite their advanced differentiation state, leads to a de-differentiation back to early uncommitted progenitors in the bone marrow, which even rescued T cell development in T cell-deficient mice (Cobaleda et al., 2007). However, the molecular mechanisms for these reprogramming processes are not finally clear. Since the complete loss of Pax5 in mature B cells also caused the development of aggressive lymphomas, Pax5 was identified as a tumor suppressor for the B cell lineage (Cobaleda et al., 2007).

1.4.2.4 T cell lineage commitment

Multiple bone marrow-derived hematopoietic precursor populations that belong mainly to the MPP or the CLP subsets are able to enter the thymus (Saran et al., 2010; Serwold et al., 2009), where they represent the population of early thymic progenitors (ETP), the initial source for the development of T cells. At this developmental stage the ETP still retain beside the T cell developmental potential also the capability to develop into B cells, macrophages, granulocytes, dendritic cells, and NK cells. Thymic environmental factors, like IL-7, Kit-ligand as well as ligands activating Notch signaling, operate in an inductive manner to force T cell development (Petrie & Zuniga-Pflucker, 2007) and at the same time to down-modulate the capacity to develop into the NK, B or myeloid lineage. Notch signaling blocks these alternative developmental processes and, in addition, is necessary to maintain T cell specification and differentiation (Feyerabend et al., 2009; Franco et al., 2006; Laiosa et al., 2006; Schmitt et al., 2004; Taghon et al., 2007). Very recently it became evident, that besides blocking alternative lineage development Notch signaling drives T cell lineage commitment by upregulating the expression of T lineage-specific transcription factors like TCF-1 necessary for the induction of several T cell-specific genes, like *GATA-3*, *Bcl11b*, and genes coding for components of the T cell receptor (Weber et al., 2011). The Krueppel-like C2H2 type zinc finger transcription factor Bcl11b in turn is required for the repression of NK cell associated genes as well as for the downregulation of stem cell or progenitor cell genes not longer required for committed T cells (Li, L. et al., 2010) (Figure 6).

After initial T lineage commitment a subsequent lineage decision is made - the choice to develop into either αβ or γδ T cell sub-lineages. At the double negative stage (DN; $CD4^-CD8$) thymocytes begin to rearrange their TCRβ, γ and δ genes. These cells that productively rearranged their TCRγ and δ genes develop to γδ T cells, which remain largely $CD4^-CD8^-$. Thymocytes that rearranged efficiently their TCRβ locus are committed to the αβ lineage and express a pre-TCR complex composed of functional TCRβ chains paired with the invariant pre-TCRα (pTα) chain. Committed αβ T cells undergo a strong proliferative burst and develop further to $CD4^+CD8^+$ double positive (DP) thymocytes that start to rearrange their TCRα locus. The precise mechanisms by which DN thymocytes develop into αβ or γδ T cells are not well understood. Currently mainly two models are discussed: the stochastic and the TCR signal strength model, where strong TCR signals favor γδ and weak signals αβ lineage choice (reviewed in (Kreslavsky et al., 2010)). Beside TCR signaling also the

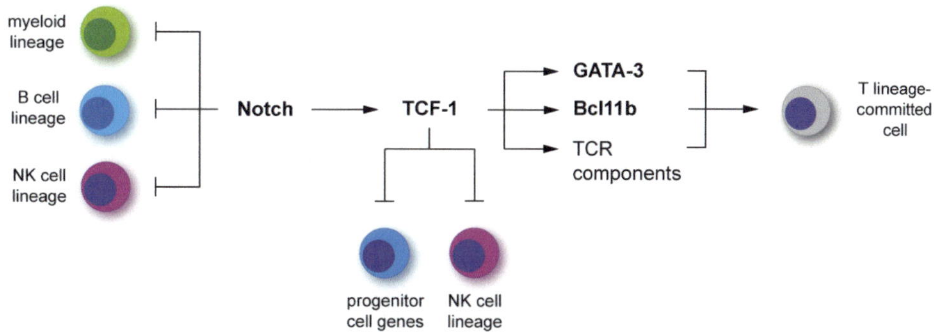

Fig. 6. T lineage-determining transcription factors.
The key transcription factor for T lineage commitment is Notch that suppresses lineage-foreign gene programs and upregulates the lineage-determining transcription factor TCF-1. Finally, lineage commitment is achieved by upregulation of the transcription factors GATA-3 and Bcl11b. Transcription factors are highlighted in bold.

Lymphotoxin-mediated as well as Notch signaling are important for the αβ versus γδ lineage commitment (Ciofani et al., 2004; Garbe et al., 2006; Garcia-Peydro et al., 2003; Hayes et al., 2005; Kang et al., 2001; Silva-Santos et al., 2005; Van de Walle et al., 2009). Additionally, several transcription factors were identified as important regulators of αβ versus γδ lineage decision. The high-mobility group transcription factor Sox13, for example, promotes γδ T cell development while opposing αβ T cell differentiation by antagonizing TCF-1 (Melichar et al., 2007), which is required, similar to RORγt (Guo, J. et al., 2002), for the survival of $CD4^+CD8^+$ αβ thymocytes (Ioannidis et al., 2001). Also, the TCR-signal strength dependent upregulation of the Zn-finger transcription factor ThPOK (T-helper inducing POZ-Krueppel factor) was shown to be an important regulator of γδ T cell development and maturation (Park, K. et al., 2010). Additionally, by integrating TCR and Notch signals as well as by interacting with and thereby suppressing E protein targets, also the helix-loop-helix transcription factor Id3 promotes γδ T cell fate (Lauritsen et al., 2009). The AP-1 family member c-Jun in turn controls directly the expression of the *IL-7Rα* gene important for thymocyte development. Deletion of c-Jun results in an enhanced γδ T cell generation indicating the importance of IL-7 receptor signaling for the regulation of αβ/γδ T cell fate decision (Riera-Sans & Behrens, 2007).

$CD4^+CD8^+$ DP cells expressing a mature αβTCR further undergo positive and negative selection processes based on their ability to recognize self-peptide:self-MHC-complexes as well as their affinity to such complexes. During these selection processes DP cells develop to functionally competent single positive $CD4^+CD8^-$ or $CD4^-CD8^+$ T cells equipped with a specific gene expression program characteristic for $CD4^+$ T helper or $CD8^+$ cytotoxic T lymphocytes. Mainly two transcription factors - ThPOK and Runx3 - are important for directing the development of DP thymocytes either into the $CD4^+$ T helper or $CD8^+$ cytotoxic T cell population (Egawa & Littman, 2008; He et al., 2008; Taniuchi et al., 2002; Wang, L. et al., 2008). Therefore, ThPOK is required for the commitment to $CD4^+$ T helper cells by repressing the characteristic genes for $CD8^+$ cells including Runx3, whereas Runx3 mediates the silencing of the *CD4* locus in $CD8^+$ cells. These dual regulative processes, leading to the exclusion of Runx3 expression in $CD4^+$ cells by ThPOK as well as the exclusion of the expression of ThPOK in $CD8^+$ cells by Runx3, result finally in CD4-CD8 lineage commitment. Transcription factors involved in ThPOK upregulation in MHCII-restricted T lymphocytes are GATA-3 (Wang, L. et al., 2008) together with the HMG protein Tox (Aliahmad & Kaye, 2008). In contrast, IL-7-mediated activation of the STAT5 transcription factor promotes the upregulation of Runx3 in $CD8^+$ cells (Park, J. H. et al., 2010) indicating a differential requirement of cytokine signaling for CD4 and CD8 lineage development. After $CD4^+$ or $CD8^+$ single positive αβ T cells are generated they are ready to leave the thymus and enter via the blood stream peripheral lymphatic organs, where their terminal differentiation occurs.

From the $CD4^+CD8^+$ DP pool of thymocytes not only conventional αβ T cells arise, but also natural killer (NK) T cells. In contrast to conventional αβ T cells that are restricted by MHCI or MHCII molecules, invariant NK T cells undergo positive and negative selection processes during their thymic maturation, which are mediated by the recognition of glycolipids presented by the MHCI-like molecule CD1d. Additionally, they also require signals from the Slam family of receptors. Different types of NK T cells are described. However, the most common and best-studied NK T cells are the invariant NK (iNK) T cells expressing an invariant TCR that is composed of a common α-chain in combination with a certain number of β-chains. After antigen recognition iNK T cells secrete high amounts of a large variety of cytokines and chemokines within minutes. Therefore, these cells exhibit rather an innate than an adaptive immune function. Several transcription factors were identified to be important for iNK T cell lineage choice. Among them, the transcription factor PLZF (promyelocytic leukemia zinc finger) is a key regulator for the development of this particular cell type (Kovalovsky et al., 2008; Savage et al., 2008), since in the thymus it is exclusively expressed by iNK T cells. In addition, several other transcription factors like NF-κB (Sivakumar et al., 2003; Stanic et al., 2004), Ets-1 (Lacorazza et al., 2002; Walunas et al., 2000), GATA-3 (Kim, P. J. et al., 2006), T-bet (Matsuda et al., 2006) and Runx proteins (Egawa et al., 2007) contribute to the development, differentiation and survival of iNK T cells. Because these transcription factors are also expressed in other thymic subpopulations they are not exclusively important for the iNK T cell lineage. However, PLZF-deficiency did not prevent iNK T cell development in general but severely interfered with iNK T cell effector differentiation and therefore with their functionality (Kovalovsky et al., 2008; Savage et al., 2008).

In the thymus, a subpopulation of MHC-II-restricted $CD4^+$ T cells further differentiates into $CD25^+$ naturally occurring regulatory T cells (nTregs) characterized by the expression of the transcription factor FoxP3 (Fontenot et al., 2003; Hori et al., 2003). They comprise about 5 to 10% of peripheral $CD4^+$ T cell and play a crucial role for maintaining peripheral tolerance. nTregs are able to suppress the proliferation, cytokine secretion as well as activation of autoreactive effector T cells thereby preventing autoimmunity. FoxP3 plays an essential function for the regulation of nTregs suppressive activity, since the deficiency of a functional FoxP3 leads to a severe autoimmune pathology in mouse (Godfrey et al., 1991; Lyon et al., 1990) and man (Bennett et al., 2001; Wildin et al., 2001). Several transcription factors are implicated in the *FoxP3* gene regulation and therefore for the development and function of nTregs. After activation of PKCθ and/or CD28 engagement, Notch3 together with NF-κB heterodimers composed of p50/p65 are able to bind and to trans-activate the FoxP3 promoter *in vivo* (Barbarulo et al., 2011; Soligo et al., 2011). Also NF-κB c-Rel was identified as a factor able to initiate FoxP3 transcription in thymic Treg precursors (Deenick et al., 2010; Isomura et al., 2009; Long et al., 2009; Ruan et al., 2009). Additionally, the FoxP3 promoter contains several functional NFAT/AP-1 binding sites, which are occupied *in vivo* (Mantel et al., 2006). Moreover, the transcription factor Bcl11b is also able to promote directly FoxP3 as well as IL-10 expression. Deletion of Bcl11b at the DP stage of thymic T cell development or solely in Tregs causes inflammatory bowel disease - a severe autoimmune disorder - due to reduced Treg suppressor activity accompanied with reduced FoxP3 and IL-10 expression (Vanvalkenburgh et al., 2011).

Conventional $\alpha\beta$ T cells leave the thymus and settle peripheral lymphatic organs as naïve T cells. After activation by exposure to their cognate antigens naïve $CD4^+$ cells differentiate into an appropriate T helper cell (TH) lineage that plays an essential role in acquired immunity. Depending on the cytokine milieu produced by antigen presenting cells naïve CD4+ cells undergo differentiation processes resulting in the expression of master transcription factors defining the ability to secrete a certain set of cytokines. Initially, two main TH subpopulations were described (Mosmann et al., 1986). The generation of TH1 cells depends on the presence of IFNγ and/or IL-12 inducing the expression of the master transcription factor T-bet essential for the TH1 phenotype characterized by the production of large amounts of IFNγ, IL-2 and TNFα. TH1 cells mediate the defense against infections by intracellular microbes and the isotype switching to IgG2a and IgG2b. In contrast, TH2 cells are generated in the presence of IL-4 and also secrete, depending on the upregulation of the transcription factor GATA-3, IL-4 together with IL-5 and IL-13. Thereby, humoral responses against parasites and extracellular pathogens are supported and also the class switching to IgG1 and IgE (Mosmann et al., 1986; Mowen & Glimcher, 2004; Szabo et al., 2003). A third TH subpopulation was described, the TH17 cells that is characterized by the secretion mainly of IL-17A and IL17F, but also IL-21 and IL-22, protecting the host against bacterial and fungal infections. Their differentiation is induced by TGFβ together with IL-6 or IL-21, which prompts the expression of the master transcription factor essential for TH17-development - RORγt (Ivanov et al., 2006). More recently, two additional TH subsets were described - TH9 and TH22 expressing predominantly the cytokines IL-9 or IL-22, respectively. The development of TH9 cells is initiated upon antigen receptor stimulation in the presence of IL-4 and TGFβ (Dardalhon et al., 2008; Veldhoen et al., 2008) and requires the upregulation of the transcription factor PU.1 (Chang et al., 2010). TH22, identified in the human skin, are characterized by the expression of the chemokine receptors CCR6, CCR4 and CCR10 as well as by the transcription factor aryl hydrocarbon receptor (AHR) that might be involved in the regulation of *IL-22* gene expression (Duhen et al., 2009; Trifari et al., 2009).

Another T helper subtype that differentiates in the periphery from naïve $CD4^+$ cells is the follicular T helper (TFH) cell subpopulation, characterized by the expression of CXCR5, ICOS and PD-1 as surface markers. They synthesize large quantities of IL-21 and require the upregulation of the transcriptional repressor Bcl6 for their development and also for their function to promote germinal center B cell maturation (Johnston et al., 2009; Nurieva et al., 2009; Yu et al., 2009). Bcl6 expression is regulated by IL-6 and IL-21 (Nurieva et al., 2009) and drives not only the TFH differentiation but also inhibits the development of other $CD4^+$ differentiation pathways by blocking Blimp1 (Johnston et al., 2009).

In the periphery, $CD4^+$ effector T cells can be converted by exposure to TGFβ and IL-2 to inducible regulatory T cells (iTregs) expressing CD25 at the surface and, like nTregs, FoxP3 as a master transcription factor necessary for Treg function (Davidson et al., 2007; Zheng et al., 2007) (Figure 7).

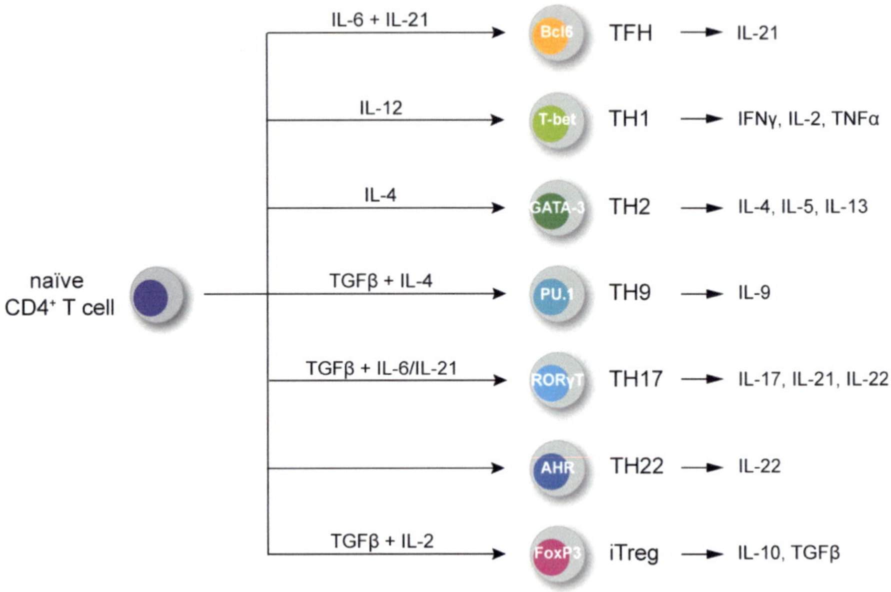

Fig. 7. Terminal Differentiation of CD4$^+$ T cells.
Differentiation of CD4$^+$ T cells into different T helper cell subpopulations after antigen exposure is driven by the specific cytokine milieu and results in the expression of specific transcription factors (noted in white). Every T helper cell subset releases distinct cytokines, which modulate the immune response of the host.

CD4$^+$ T cell master transcription factors as well as lineage-specific cytokines characteristic for the appropriate TH subpopulations are able to block the differentiation of other TH subsets. For example, T-bet in cooperation with Runx3 suppresses the generation of TH2 cells by physical interaction with GATA-3 thereby inhibiting GATA-3 activity (Djuretic et al., 2007; Hwang et al., 2005). Additionally, T-bet also actively represses TH17 differentiation by preventing Runx1-mediated upregulation of RORγt expression (Lazarevic et al., 2011). Also, as already noted, Bcl6 expressed by TFH antagonizes Blimp1 and thereby it inhibits the developmental program necessary for alternative TH cell differentiation (Johnston et al., 2009). However, several studies suggest certain plasticity in the expression of master transcription factors as well in the set of cytokines that differentiated T helper cells secrete. The conversion of peripheral effector CD4$^+$ cells to iTregs expressing FoxP3 like nTregs that developed in the thymus was a first hint indicating plasticity of CD4$^+$ TH cells (Jonuleit et al., 2001). Moreover, in the presence of TGFβ TH2 cells can acquire IL-9 producing capacity (Veldhoen et al., 2008). Additionally, several studies described the acquisition of IFNγ-producing potential by TH17 cells *in vivo* in mouse and man (Kurschus et al., 2010; Wilson, N. J. et al., 2007) and even a complete conversion of TH17 cells into IFNγ-producers (Bending et al., 2009; Lee, Y. K. et al., 2009; Shi et al., 2008). When stimulated with IL-4, TH17 cells can change into IL4-secreting TH2 cells (Yi et al., 2009). Also, Tregs stimulated with IL-6 can express IL-17 and downregulate FoxP3 expression (Xu et al., 2007). Together, these data indicate the high flexibility of peripheral CD4+ cells in their potential to secrete a certain set of cytokines and therefore to modulate and/or influence the outcome of an ongoing immune response. However, the mechanism(s) underlying the plasticity of "committed" TH cells remain largely unclear.

1.4.3 Epigenetic mechanisms controlling hematopoiesis

The highly coordinated program needed to pass through the diverse developmental stages that comprise hematopoiesis can only be achieved by tight regulation. In fact, every cellular transition and differentiation step is characterized by the activation of a new, lineage-specific, genetic program and the extinction of the previous one. This is achieved by the action of well-defined networks of transcription factors at each developmental step as already described. However, transcription factors are not the only players in the complex differentiation process of hematopoiesis, since there is an increasing body of evidence demonstrating that the regulation of hematopoietic stemness and lineage commitment is dependent on epigenetic mechanisms. Chromatin, the higher order structure of DNA and nucleosomes, can adopt different structural conformations depending on epigenetic modifications, which influence the accessibility of DNA for the gene transcription machinery. Four types of epigenetic regulation can take place: DNA methylation, histone modification, chromatin remodeling and gene silencing via microRNAs.

1.4.3.1 DNA methylation

DNA methylation of cytosines at CpG dinucleotides, except for CpG islands, is established during early embryogenesis by DNA methyltransferases (Dnmt) and is maintained in somatic cells to repress transcription. The DNA methyltransferases Dnmt3a and Dnmt3b are supposed to convey *de novo* methylation, whereas Dnmt1 conserves previously installed methylation states during replication. First hints depicting the importance of DNA methylation for hematopoietic development arose from gene deletion studies in mice revealing the indispensable functions of Dnmt1 for HSC self-renewal and lineage-commitment. The ablation or reduced expression of Dnmt1 in murine HSC led to diminished repopulating capacity of HSC and decreased production of lymphoid progenitors accompanied with retained myelo-erythroid progenitor development (Broske et al., 2009; Trowbridge et al., 2009). Additionally, the examination of genome-wide methylation profiles of the mouse hematopoietic system demonstrated methylation pattern changes during differentiation resulting in the activation of silent genes and the silencing of active genes. Moreover, the study could show that myeloid commitment involved less global DNA methylation than lymphoid commitment (Ji et al., 2010) in line with the findings from the Dnmt1 deletion studies. In contrast to Dnmt1, Dnmt3a/3b deficiency affected only the long-term reconstitution ability of HSC, but not their differentiation into committed progenitors (Tadokoro et al., 2007). Nevertheless, the molecular mechanisms mediating DNA methylation and demethylation during hematopoietic development have not been deciphered, although chromatin-remodeling factors as well as Polycomb group/Dnmt3a/3b complexes recruited by transcription factors were supposed to be involved (Gao et al., 2009; Kirillov et al., 1996; Vire et al., 2006).

1.4.3.2 Histone modification

Another crucial epigenetic mechanism is the posttranslational modification of histones, which embraces acetylation, methylation, phosphorylation and sumoylation among others. These modifications occur at the tails of histones and change the direct interactions between nucleosomes and DNA, thereby affecting gene expression (Campos & Reinberg, 2009). In terms of hematopoietic regulation the methylation of lysine 4 (K4) and 27 (K27) of histone 3 (H3) particularly have to be stressed, since they can serve as repressing, activating and poising marks dependent on the methylation pattern. The concomitant trimethylation of H3K27 (repressing mark) and H3K4 (activating mark) as well as the mono- and dimethylation of H3K4 introduce a bivalent epigenetic modification leading to poised chromatin that is primed for activation of gene transcription (Bernstein, B. E. et al., 2006; Heintzman et al., 2009; Orford et al., 2008). Several studies have demonstrated that a plethora of lineage-specific genes are poised at the beginning of hematopoiesis or achieve poising marks during hematopoietic differentiation. After commitment of the cell to a specific lineage, lineage-foreign genes lose their poising marks and repression of gene transcription occurs (Orford et al., 2008; Weishaupt et al., 2010). Moreover, genome-wide analysis of poised chromatin sites revealed a tight correlation of bivalent histone methylation sites with binding sites of lineage-determining transcription factors such as EBF1, E2A, GATA-1 or PU.1. These sites are independent of the transcription start site and are probably enhancer sites that are involved in the priming for transcriptional activation in later stages of hematopoietic development (Heintzman et al., 2009; Heinz et al., 2010; Lin, Y. C. et al., 2010; Treiber et al., 2010). Similar to DNA methylation, the molecular mechanisms underlying histone modifications have not yet been identified.

1.4.3.3 Chromatin remodeling

Additional epigenetic modifiers of DNA accessibility that were recruited through lineage-specific transcription factors are chromatin-remodeling complexes. Such chromatin remodelers are multi-protein complexes that are able to change nucleosome location or conformation in an ATP-dependent manner, but they additionally contain interchangeable histone modifying enzymes such as deacetylase or acetylase to produce functionally distinct complexes (Bowen et al., 2004). For example, Ikaros, a lymphoid-specific transcription factor crucial for the commitment of LMPP into CLP can recruit Mi2/NuRD complexes in order to repress genes (Kim, J. et al., 1999; Koipally et al., 1999; Sridharan & Smale, 2007). Whereas, EBF1 and E2A are involved in the recruitment of the SWI/SNF complex to the upstream enhancer of the *CD19* locus as well as to the *CD79a* promoter region facilitating the transcriptional activation of these B cell-specific genes (Gao et al., 2009; Walter et al., 2008).

1.4.3.4 MicroRNAs

Besides the already mentioned epigenetic mechanisms established at the level of DNA, the recent discovery of microRNAs (miRNAs) added a further layer of epigenetic regulation that guides the hematopoietic differentiation process. These mRNAs are small, single-stranded, non-coding RNAs, which are able to repress mRNA transcription by the promotion of mRNA degradation due to direct binding to the 3′ untranslated regions (UTR) of specific target mRNAs. The first evidences for the importance of miRNAs during hematopoietic development revealed from the deletion of Dicer, an RNase-III-like enzyme that is indispensable for miRNA biogenesis, in mice. These gene ablation leads to embryonal lethality at day 7.5 due to a lack of detectable multipotent stem cells, whereas the conditional deletion in murine embryonic stem cells blocks the ability to differentiate (Bernstein, E. et al., 2003; Kanellopoulou et al., 2005) and the lineage-specific ablation of Dicer in lymphoid progenitors results in severe defects in the B as well as T cell development (Cobb et al., 2005; Koralov et al., 2008; Muljo et al., 2005). Moreover, analyses of miRNA expression in several subsets of human $CD34^+$ HSC and progenitors cells as well as murine hematopoietic tissues have demonstrated the modulated transcription of different miRNA during hematopoiesis (Chen et al., 2004; Georgantas et al., 2007; Liao et al., 2008). With regard to the relative young field of miRNA research, only limited data about the detailed role of single miRNAs in the different steps of HSC maintenance or hematopoietic differentiation are available, but some regulatory mechanisms are already described. At the level of HSC, where decision-making comprises self-renewal and differentiation into committed progenitors, miRNAs of the miR-196 and miR-10 family are highly expressed, which are able to modulate HSC homeostasis and lineage commitment through the regulation of certain *HOX* genes (Mansfield et al., 2004; Yekta et al., 2004), whereas miR-125a has been shown to mediate self-renewal of LT-HSC by targeting the pro-apoptotic protein *Bak-1* (Guo, S. et al., 2010). In contrast, miR-126 conferring lineage commitment and progenitor production via down-modulation of *HOXA9* and the tumor suppressor polo-like kinase 2 that has to be downregulated during differentiation towards multipotent progenitors (Shen et al., 2008).

Downstream of HSC, the introduction of lineage commitment is the most important task of a regulatory mechanism and several miRNAs are involved in these processes in the different progenitor populations. For example, during erythroid lineage differentiation starting from the MEP a progressive downregulation of miR-24, miR-221, miR-222 and miR-223 as well as a upregulation of miR-451 and miR-16 has been reported in differentiating human erythroid progenitors (Bruchova et al., 2007). The down-modulation of miR-221 and miR-222 is necessary for the expression of Kit that in turn allows the expansion of erythroblasts (Felli et al., 2005), whereas the repression of miR-24 permit the expression of activin type I receptor, which promotes erythropoiesis in cooperation with erythropoietin (Wang, Q. et al., 2008). A further activator of erythroid differentiation is the transcription factor and miR-223-target LIM-only protein 2 that along with GATA-1 and others constitutes a multi-protein complex (Felli et al., 2009). In contrast to these down-modulated miRNAs, miR-451 upregulation is indispensable for erythroid maturation and effective erythropoiesis in response to oxidative stress. Several studies have demonstrated that miR-451 targets 14-3-3ζ, a chaperone protein modulating intracellular growth factor signals, and therefore regulating the expression of several genes associated with late erythropoiesis (Patrick et al., 2010; Rasmussen et al., 2010; Zhan et al., 2007). But also megakaryocyte differentiation occurs downstream of the MEP and several studies revealed the importance of miR-150 for lineage commitment during megakaryocyte-erythroid differentiation, since the ectopic expression of miR-150 in MEP drives the differentiation towards megakaryocytes at the expense of erythroid cells by targeting the transcription factor *c-Myb* (Lu et al., 2008). Further support for the lineage-determining function of miR-150 has arose from a study demonstrating the regulation of miR-150 and c-Myb through the megakaryocyte-specific cytokine TPO (Barroga et al., 2008). Other miRNAs downregulated during megakaryopoiesis are miR-130 targeting *MafB* that in turn together with GATA-1 is needed for the induction of the *GbIIb* gene (Garzon et al., 2006) as well as miR-155 that targets the transcription factors *Ets-1* and *Meis-1* (Romania et al., 2008).

With respect to the role of miRNAs in myelopoiesis miR-223 has to be enumerated, which also functions as lineage-determining factor that is upregulated during granulopoiesis and downregulated during monopoiesis (Fazi et al., 2005; Johnnidis et al., 2008). Targets of miR-223 are the cell cycle regulator *E2F1* and the monocyte lineage-promoting gene *Mef2c* leading to suppression of proliferation and induction of granulocyte differentiation (Johnnidis et al., 2008). Moreover, the transcription of miR-223 is activated by the master transcription factor for granulopoiesis C/EBPα that replaces the transcriptional repressor NFI-A upon activation of granulocytic differentiation (Fazi et al., 2005). A similar mechanism has been recently described for miR-34a that is also increased expressed during granulopoiesis by C/EBPα-mediated transcription and targets the cell cycle regulator *E2F3* (Pulikkan et al., 2010). Another lineage-determining mechanism displays the repression of miR-21 and miR-196b by the transcriptional repressor Gfi1 during granulopoiesis, since ectopic expression of both miRNAs in myeloid progenitors results in a complete block of G-CSF induced granulopoiesis (Velu et al., 2009). In favor of monocytic development acts the activation of miR-424 transcription via PU.1 that in turn targets the negative regulator of monopoiesis *NFI-A* (Forrest et al., 2010). Whereas the miR-17/miR-20/miR-106 cluster is repressed during monopoiesis in humans, probably to allow expression of the target AML-1 that consecutively promotes monocyte-macrophage differentiation and maturation (Fontana et al., 2007).

Concerning the function of single miRNAs during lymphopoiesis only few data are available, despite the astonishing effects of Dicer deletion on lymphoid development. However, one study partially explains the phenotype of Dicer deletion by the defective expression of the miR17-92 cluster. This miRNA cluster that is highly expressed in progenitor cells targets the pro-apoptotic factors *Bim* and *Pten*. In line with these findings,

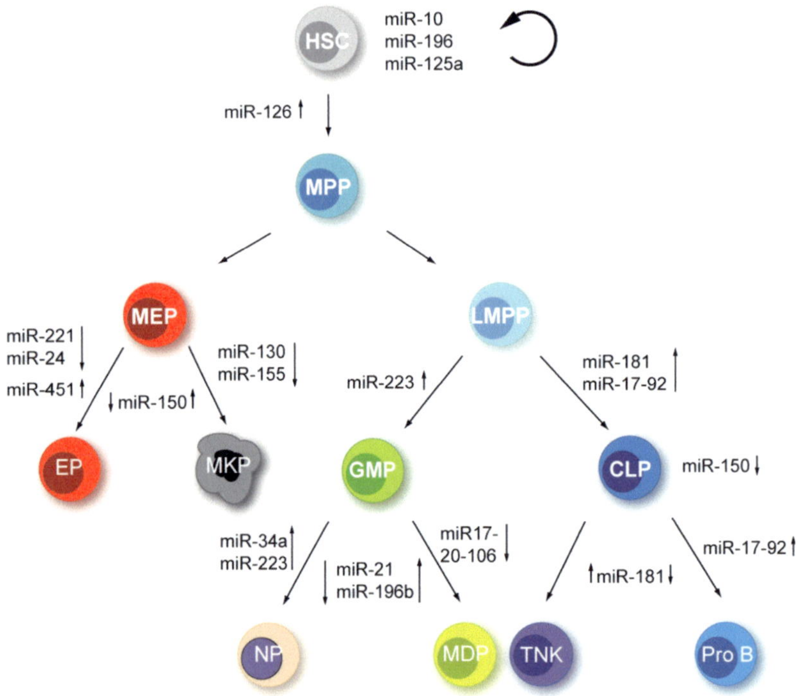

Fig. 8. The regulatory network of miRNAs during hematopoiesis.
Several miRNAs are involved in maintenance of HSC self-renewal, whereas other miRNAs are associated with lineage commitment and development towards differentiated progeny. HSC, hematopoietic stem cell; MPP, multipotent progenitor; LMPP, lymphoid-primed multipotent progenitor; CLP, common lymphoid progenitor; CMP, common myeloid progenitor; MEP, megakaryocyte-erythrocyte progenitor; GMP, granulocyte-macrophage progenitor; NP, neutrophil progenitor; MDP, monocyte-dendritic cell progenitor; TNK, T cell NK cell progenitor; EP, erythroid progenitor; MKP, megakaryocyte progenitor.

ablation of the miR17-92 cluster in mice results in a severe block of B cell development at the pro B to pre B transition due to increased apoptosis of pro B cells (Ventura et al., 2008). A similar block in B cell development at the pro B to pre B transition is caused by the ectopic expression of miR-150 in lymphoid progenitors due to the repression of the transcriptional repressor *c-Myb* (Xiao et al., 2007). The best-described miRNA involved in T lymphocyte development is miR-181, which promotes T cell differentiation through increasing signaling strength of the TCR signaling. In detail, miR-181 targets multiple phosphatases such as *PTPN22* or *DUSP5* and *DUSP6*, which are negative regulators of distinct steps of the TCR signaling pathway leading to an upregulation of ERK1/2 phosphorylation upon TCR engagement. This increased sensitivity of TCR signaling is needed during the positive selection of double-positive T cells in the thymus (Li, Q. J. et al., 2007) (Figure 8).

1.4.4 Role of cytokines in guiding hematopoiesis

Cytokines are a large family of extracellular ligands that stimulate several responses after binding to structurally and functionally conserved cytokine receptors. Biological responses provoked by cytokines cover a broad spectrum of different biological activities, for example survival, proliferation, differentiation, or maturation. In the case of the hematopoietic system, the most important cytokines are interleukins and colony-stimulating factors with supportive functions for several lineages as well as erythropoietin (EPO) and thrombopoietin (TPO) that act on single lineages (Metcalf, 2008). Besides the requirement of cytokines for regulation of basal hematopoiesis, they are also essential for controlling emergency hematopoiesis in response to infections or blood loss. This is reflected by the different origins of cytokines, secreted for example by activated immune cells or by stroma cells as well as by organs, like liver and kidney.

In steady-state conditions, serum concentrations of cytokines are low, but they can be elevated up to 1000-fold by challenging the immune system and possess high picomolar affinities for their corresponding receptors (Metcalf, 2008). On the binding of cytokine molecules follows the activation of the receptor via homodimerization (G-CSFR), oligomerization with a common signaling subunit (GM-CSFR, IL-6R) or conformational changes in preformed receptor dimers (EPOR), which finally leads to activation of Janus kinases (JAK). Upon activation of the tyrosine kinases of JAK family, the cytokine receptors as well as the kinases themselves are phosphorylated to generate docking sites for SH2 domain containing proteins. One example is the STAT protein family that promotes transcriptional activation of target genes after phosphorylation by JAK (Robb, 2007; Smithgall et al., 2000). Additionally, other signaling molecules can be recruited to the cytokine receptors, such as Src kinases, protein phosphatases or PI3K, which mediate the activation of numerous signaling pathways like MAPK-ERK, Ras or PI3K (Baker et al., 2007).

To date, basically two hypotheses exist concerning the role of cytokines in hematopoiesis. The instructive model proposes that cytokines transmit specific signals to multipotent progenitors to direct their lineage commitment. In contrast, the permissive or stochastic model suggests that cytokines only provide permissive growth and survival signals to intrinsically determined and lineage-committed progenitors. Supportive data for the permissive as well as the instructive model of cytokine function originated from different studies, where cytokine receptors were ectopically expressed in lineage-committed progenitors. Studies in favor of the permissive model have demonstrated that viral transduction of fetal liver cells with the M-CSF receptor results in the generation of erythroid colonies upon M-CSF administration (McArthur et al., 1994). Similar results have been obtained by the restoration of definitive erythropoiesis in EPOR-deficient fetal liver cells via the expression of the human GM-CSFR plus GM-CSF treatment (Hisakawa et al., 2001). Furthermore, replacement of the intracellular domain of the G-CSFR with the intracellular domain of EPOR induces no alterations in lineage commitment (Semerad et al., 1999). Oppositional results emanated from the ectopic expression of IL-2Rβ in CLP, which results in rapid generation of granulocytes and macrophages in the presence of IL-2 (Kondo et al., 2000).

Additionally, ectopic expression of the human GM-CSFR in IL-7-deficient CLP was not able to restore lymphopoiesis upon GM-CSF administration (Iwasaki-Arai et al., 2003). Experiments with single GMP cultured in the presence of M-CSF or G-CSF have further supported the hypothesis of lineage instruction by cytokines due to the almost solely development of either macrophages or granulocytes, respectively (Rieger et al., 2009). Nevertheless, gene deletion studies for several cytokine receptors have shown the indispensable function of the most cytokines for hematopoiesis. For example, the knockout of EPO and EPOR in mice leads to embryonic death at E13.5 due to severe anemia, even if erythroid progenitor cells were present (Lin, C. S. et al., 1996; Wu, H. et al., 1995). Analysis of IL-7Rα-deficient mice revealed a lethal phenotype as a result of a severe hypoplasia of all lymphoid lineages, but retained development of the earliest unipotent T and B cell precursors (Peschon et al., 1994). In contrast, mice bearing deletions of colony-stimulating factor receptors demonstrated no lethal phenotypes. Disruption of the G-CSFR in mice results in ineffective granulopoiesis, with chronic neutropenia due to a decrease of mature myeloid cells in the bone marrow and a modest reduction of progenitor cells (Liu et al., 1996), whereas deletion of the common β-chain of IL-3, IL-5 and GM-CSF receptor in mice only lead to reduced numbers of eosinophils (Nishinakamura et al., 1996; Nishinakamura et al., 1996).

Taken together, the present available data do not resolve the question if cytokines only have permissive functions in the guidance of hematopoiesis, especially with regard to differentiation from HSC to restricted progenitors or not. But the plasticity of the transition from multipotent progenitor cells to restricted progenitor cells, especially regarding adaption of hematopoiesis in emergency situations suggests that cytokines have to some extend instructive functions. Furthermore, almost nothing is known about potential functions of cytokines and cytokine signaling regarding gene expression or posttranslational regulation of lineage-determining transcription factors, which would provide a possible link between intrinsic and extrinsic regulation of hematopoiesis (Figure 9).

1.5 Perspectives

The unique property of the hematopoietic system to replenish permanently all hematopoietic cells together with the ongoing progress in the understanding of hematopoietic differentiation processes allows the development of new therapy approaches to treat hemic diseases such as hematologic malignancies, immunodeficiencies or autoimmune diseases. These new therapies are mainly based on the transplantation of hematopoietic stem cells (HSC). Two basic findings promoted the clinical use of HSC transplantation (HSCT) in the last twenty years. First, the definition of human HSC as

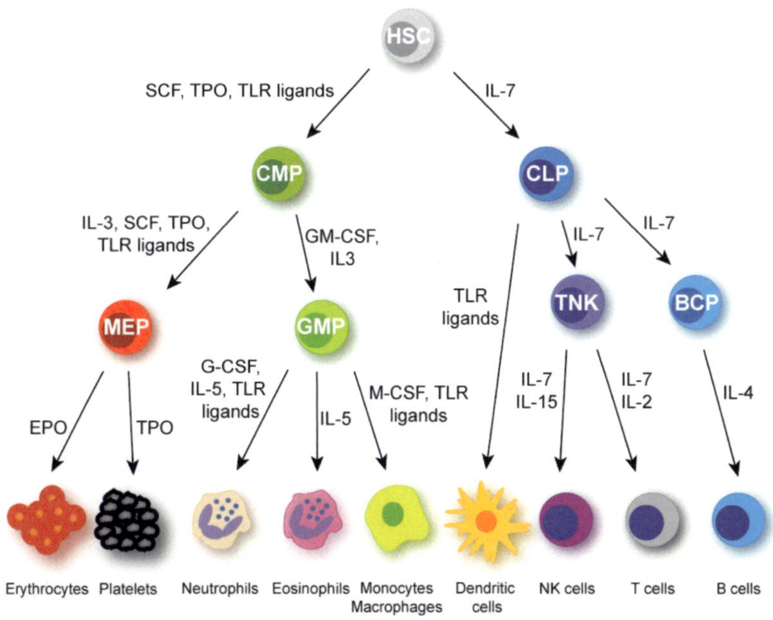

Fig. 9. The role of cytokines in hematopoiesis.
Cytokines act on both multipotent progenitors as well as committed progenitors and provide survival and proliferation signals. HSC, hematopoietic stem cell; CLP, common lymphoid progenitor; CMP, common myeloid progenitor; MEP, megakaryocyte-erythrocyte progenitor; GMP, granulocyte-macrophage progenitor; TNK, T cell NK cell progenitor; BCP, B cell progenitor.

$CD34^+/CD38^-$ cells that can be found in the bone marrow as well as in the umbilical cord blood (Weissman & Shizuru, 2008), and second, the discovery of the potent function of the cytokine G-CSF in mobilization of stem cells from the bone marrow into peripheral blood (Weaver et al., 1993). In most cases, this method provides several advantages in comparison to bone marrow transplantation, since the isolation of stem cells from peripheral blood via leukapheresis is less invasive for the donor and the recovery of the hematopoietic system occurs faster (Gertz, 2010).

Currently, only two possibilities of HSCT for the treatment of life-threatening hemic diseases or immunodeficiencies are available: the autologous transplantation or the allogeneic transplantation of HSC from a healthy donor. Autologous transplantation of HSC is often used during the cure of hematologic malignancies like myeloma or some types of lymphoma to restore the hematopoietic system after aggressive chemotherapy (Gertz et al., 2000; Linch et al., 1993; Moreau et al., 2011; Philip et al., 1995). In contrast, allogeneic HSC transplantation (HSCT) is the treatment of choice for many otherwise fatal hematologic malignancies (chronic myeloid leukemia, acute leukemia) and genetic disorders such as aplastic anemia, β-thalassemia as well as primary immunodeficiencies (severe combined immunodeficiency, Wiskott-Aldrich syndrome) and requires an almost perfect human leukocyte antigen (HLA) match of donor and recipient (Roncarolo et al., 2011). Additionally, recent trails of allogeneic HSCT provided good results in the cure of autoimmune diseases like multiple sclerosis and rheumatoid arthritis (Sullivan et al., 2010). Nevertheless, the need for an almost perfect HLA match to avoid graft-versus-host reactions, the restricted availability of donors as well as pre-transplant conditioning limits the application of allogeneic HSCT today (Roncarolo et al., 2011).

One possible approach to circumvent the potential risks of allogeneic HSCT is the gene therapy, where defective genes are restored by the introduction of functional counterparts in autologous HSC. The first trails of gene therapy for primary immunodeficiencies employed the retroviral transduction of isolated HSC for gene delivery and afterwards the re-transplantation into patients. But in some of this trails, a certain amount of patients developed hematologic malignancies due to random integration of the transgene into the genome that can lead to the trans-activation of proto-oncogenes when the virus sequence is integrated in their vicinity. Recent efforts for the improvement of viral vectors by the use of retro- and lentiviral vectors with cell-specific promoter sequences may provide gene therapy with a decreased incidence for undesired trans-activation of oncogenes. Another approach could be the development of robust methods for homologous recombination in HSC, which would not only avoid the cancer risk, but also allow the endogenous regulation of the corrected gene (Kohn, 2010). Additionally, new perspectives offered the groundbreaking findings of Takahashi and Yamanaka demonstrating the induction of pluripotent stem cells from mouse fibroblasts by the viral transduction of Oct3/4, Sox2, c-Myc and Klf4 (Takahashi & Yamanaka, 2006). Moreover, several recent improvements in induction of pluripotency in several cell types like dermal fibroblasts, keratinocytes and blood cells by the use of virus-free and/or vector-free techniques render reprogrammed somatic cells to a possible future technology for stem cell plus gene therapy (Wu, S. M. & Hochedlinger, 2011). Some of the advantages of iPS (inducible pluripotent stem) cells are the independency of the cell source, the possibility of prolonged culturing *ex vivo* allowing genetic manipulation, and the differentiation into all cell types. A first proof of principle for use of iPS cells in gene therapy supplied the successful treatment of sickle cell anemia in a mouse model. In this study, autologous skin fibroblasts from humanized sickle cell anemia mice were reprogrammed into iPS cells and the genetic defect was repaired via homologous recombination, afterwards the iPS cells were differentiated into hematopoietic progenitors in vitro and finally transplanted into irradiated recipient mice (Hanna et al., 2007). Nevertheless, these types of therapies need a lot of extensive research before they can be applied in the clinic in future, but our increasing knowledge of the regulation of hematopoietic processes provides the basis for the individual treatment of patients with life-threatening hematologic disorders with autologous cells to abolish side effects associated with allogeneic HSCT, or to cure diseases currently not treatable with peripheral stem cell transplantation.

2. Conclusion

The process of differentiation and lineage commitment during hematopoietic development depends strongly on the defined activation of lineage-determining gene programs as well as the repression of lineage-foreign gene programs. This concerted regulation of genetic programs can only be achieved by the integration of several mechanisms such as activation of lineage-specific transcription factors, modulation of epigenetic marks and extrinsic signals that provide a supportive environment. Moreover, the described mechanisms of hematopoiesis illustrate the complex network involving the synergistic effects of a certain number of key transcription factors that not only induce transcription but also guide epigenetic changes to allow or deny the access of the transcriptional machinery to the DNA or the repression of important genes via gene silencing. Additionally, some of these transcription factors are often involved in several lineage decisions were they induce quite different cell fates depending on the presence of other transcription factors co-expressed in the cell or on the level of protein expression. Therefore, the hematopoietic differentiation process clearly demonstrates the importance of regulatory networks that integrate several intrinsic and extrinsic signals for the outcome of differentiation and cell fate decisions.

3. References

Akashi, K., Traver, D., Miyamoto, T. & Weissman, I.L. (2000). A clonogenic common myeloid progenitor that gives rise to all myeloid lineages. *Nature,* 404, 6774, pp. 193-197.

Aliahmad, P. & Kaye, J. (2008). Development of all CD4 T lineages requires nuclear factor TOX. *J Exp Med,* 205, 1, pp. 245-256.

Auffray, C., Sieweke, M.H. & Geissmann, F. (2009). Blood monocytes: development, heterogeneity, and relationship with dendritic cells. *Annu Rev Immunol,* 27, pp. 669-692.

Bain, G., Maandag, E.C., Izon, D.J., Amsen, D., Kruisbeek, A.M., Weintraub, B.C., Krop, I., Schlissel, M.S., Feeney, A.J., van Roon, M. & et al. (1994). E2A proteins are required for proper B cell development and initiation of immunoglobulin gene rearrangements. *Cell,* 79, 5, pp. 885-892.

Baker, S.J., Rane, S.G. & Reddy, E.P. (2007). Hematopoietic cytokine receptor signaling. *Oncogene,* 26, 47, pp. 6724-6737.

Bakri, Y., Sarrazin, S., Mayer, U.P., Tillmanns, S., Nerlov, C., Boned, A. & Sieweke, M.H. (2005). Balance of MafB and PU.1 specifies alternative macrophage or dendritic cell fate. *Blood,* 105, 7, pp. 2707-2716.

Barbarulo, A., Grazioli, P., Campese, A.F., Bellavia, D., Di Mario, G., Pelullo, M., Ciuffetta, A., Colantoni, S., Vacca, A., Frati, L., Gulino, A., Felli, M.P. & Screpanti, I. (2011). Notch3 and canonical NF-kappaB signaling pathways cooperatively regulate Foxp3 transcription. *J Immunol,* 186, 11, pp. 6199-6206.

Barroga, C.F., Pham, H. & Kaushansky, K. (2008). Thrombopoietin regulates c-Myb expression by modulating micro RNA 150 expression. *Exp Hematol,* 36, 12, pp. 1585-1592.

Bending, D., De la Pena, H., Veldhoen, M., Phillips, J.M., Uyttenhove, C., Stockinger, B. & Cooke, A. (2009). Highly purified Th17 cells from BDC2.5NOD mice convert into Th1-like cells in NOD/SCID recipient mice. *J Clin Invest,* 119, 3, pp. 565-572.

Bennett, C.L., Christie, J., Ramsdell, F., Brunkow, M.E., Ferguson, P.J., Whitesell, L., Kelly, T.E., Saulsbury, F.T., Chance, P.F. & Ochs, H.D. (2001). The immune dysregulation, polyendocrinopathy, enteropathy, X-linked syndrome (IPEX) is caused by mutations of FOXP3. *Nat Genet,* 27, 1, pp. 20-21.

Bernstein, B.E., Mikkelsen, T.S., Xie, X., Kamal, M., Huebert, D.J., Cuff, J., Fry, B., Meissner, A., Wernig, M., Plath, K., Jaenisch, R., Wagschal, A., Feil, R., Schreiber, S.L. & Lander, E.S. (2006). A bivalent chromatin structure marks key developmental genes in embryonic stem cells. *Cell,* 125, 2, pp. 315-326.

Bernstein, E., Kim, S.Y., Carmell, M.A., Murchison, E.P., Alcorn, H., Li, M.Z., Mills, A.A., Elledge, S.J., Anderson, K.V. & Hannon, G.J. (2003). Dicer is essential for mouse development. *Nat Genet,* 35, 3, pp. 215-217.

Bjerregaard, M.D., Jurlander, J., Klausen, P., Borregaard, N. & Cowland, J.B. (2003). The in vivo profile of transcription factors during neutrophil differentiation in human bone marrow. *Blood,* 101, 11, pp. 4322-4332.

Borregaard, N. (2010). Neutrophils, from marrow to microbes. *Immunity,* 33, 5, pp. 657-670.

Bowen, N.J., Fujita, N., Kajita, M. & Wade, P.A. (2004). Mi-2/NuRD: multiple complexes for many purposes. *Biochim Biophys Acta,* 1677, 1-3, pp. 52-57.

Bresnick, E.H., Lee, H.Y., Fujiwara, T., Johnson, K.D. & Keles, S. (2010). GATA switches as developmental drivers. *J Biol Chem,* 285, 41, pp. 31087-31093.

Broske, A.M., Vockentanz, L., Kharazi, S., Huska, M.R., Mancini, E., Scheller, M., Kuhl, C., Enns, A., Prinz, M., Jaenisch, R., Nerlov, C., Leutz, A., Andrade-Navarro, M.A., Jacobsen, S.E. & Rosenbauer, F. (2009). DNA methylation protects hematopoietic stem cell multipotency from myeloerythroid restriction. *Nat Genet,* 41, 11, pp. 1207-1215.

Bruchova, H., Yoon, D., Agarwal, A.M., Mendell, J. & Prchal, J.T. (2007). Regulated expression of microRNAs in normal and polycythemia vera erythropoiesis. *Exp Hematol,* 35, 11, pp. 1657-1667.

Cai, D.H., Wang, D., Keefer, J., Yeamans, C., Hensley, K. & Friedman, A.D. (2008). C/EBP alpha:AP-1 leucine zipper heterodimers bind novel DNA elements, activate the PU.1 promoter and direct monocyte lineage commitment more potently than C/EBP alpha homodimers or AP-1. *Oncogene,* 27, 19, pp. 2772-2779.

Campos, E.I. & Reinberg, D. (2009). Histones: annotating chromatin. *Annu Rev Genet,* 43, pp. 559-599.

Chang, H.C., Sehra, S., Goswami, R., Yao, W., Yu, Q., Stritesky, G.L., Jabeen, R., McKinley, C., Ahyi, A.N., Han, L., Nguyen, E.T., Robertson, M.J., Perumal, N.B., Tepper, R.S., Nutt, S.L. & Kaplan, M.H. (2010). The transcription factor PU.1 is required for the development of IL-9-producing T cells and allergic inflammation. *Nat Immunol,* 11, 6, pp. 527-534.

Chen, C.Z., Li, L., Lodish, H.F. & Bartel, D.P. (2004). MicroRNAs modulate hematopoietic lineage differentiation. *Science,* 303, 5654, pp. 83-86.

Ciofani, M., Schmitt, T.M., Ciofani, A., Michie, A.M., Cuburu, N., Aublin, A., Maryanski, J.L. & Zuniga-Pflucker, J.C. (2004). Obligatory role for cooperative signaling by pre-TCR and Notch during thymocyte differentiation. *J Immunol,* 172, 9, pp. 5230-5239.

Cobaleda, C., Jochum, W. & Busslinger, M. (2007). Conversion of mature B cells into T cells by dedifferentiation to uncommitted progenitors. *Nature,* 449, 7161, pp. 473-477.

Cobb, B.S., Nesterova, T.B., Thompson, E., Hertweck, A., O'Connor, E., Godwin, J., Wilson, C.B., Brockdorff, N., Fisher, A.G., Smale, S.T. & Merkenschlager, M. (2005). T cell lineage choice and differentiation in the absence of the RNase III enzyme Dicer. *J Exp Med,* 201, 9, pp. 1367-1373.

D'Alo, F., Johansen, L.M., Nelson, E.A., Radomska, H.S., Evans, E.K., Zhang, P., Nerlov, C. & Tenen, D.G. (2003). The amino terminal and E2F interaction domains are critical for C/EBP alpha-mediated induction of granulopoietic development of hematopoietic cells. *Blood,* 102, 9, pp. 3163-3171.

Dakic, A., Metcalf, D., Di Rago, L., Mifsud, S., Wu, L. & Nutt, S.L. (2005). PU.1 regulates the commitment of adult hematopoietic progenitors and restricts granulopoiesis. *J Exp Med,* 201, 9, pp. 1487-1502.

Dale, D.C., Person, R.E., Bolyard, A.A., Aprikyan, A.G., Bos, C., Bonilla, M.A., Boxer, L.A., Kannourakis, G., Zeidler, C., Welte, K., Benson, K.F. & Horwitz, M. (2000). Mutations in the gene encoding neutrophil elastase in congenital and cyclic neutropenia. *Blood,* 96, 7, pp. 2317-2322.

Dardalhon, V., Awasthi, A., Kwon, H., Galileos, G., Gao, W., Sobel, R.A., Mitsdoerffer, M., Strom, T.B., Elyaman, W., Ho, I.C., Khoury, S., Oukka, M. & Kuchroo, V.K. (2008). IL-4 inhibits TGF-beta-induced Foxp3+ T cells and, together with TGF-beta, generates IL-9+ IL-10+ Foxp3(-) effector T cells. *Nat Immunol,* 9, 12, pp. 1347-1355.

Davidson, T.S., DiPaolo, R.J., Andersson, J. & Shevach, E.M. (2007). Cutting Edge: IL-2 is essential for TGF-beta-mediated induction of Foxp3+ T regulatory cells. *J Immunol,* 178, 7, pp. 4022-4026.

Deenick, E.K., Elford, A.R., Pellegrini, M., Hall, H., Mak, T.W. & Ohashi, P.S. (2010). c-Rel but not NF-kappaB1 is important for T regulatory cell development. *Eur J Immunol,* 40, 3, pp. 677-681.

DeKoter, R.P., Schweitzer, B.L., Kamath, M.B., Jones, D., Tagoh, H., Bonifer, C., Hildeman, D.A. & Huang, K.J. (2007). Regulation of the interleukin-7 receptor alpha promoter by the Ets transcription factors PU.1 and GA-binding protein in developing B cells. *J Biol Chem,* 282, 19, pp. 14194-14204.

DeKoter, R.P. & Singh, H. (2000). Regulation of B lymphocyte and macrophage development by graded expression of PU.1. *Science,* 288, 5470, pp. 1439-1441.

Dent, A.L., Shaffer, A.L., Yu, X., Allman, D. & Staudt, L.M. (1997). Control of inflammation, cytokine expression, and germinal center formation by BCL-6. *Science,* 276, 5312, pp. 589-592.

Diehl, S.A., Schmidlin, H., Nagasawa, M., van Haren, S.D., Kwakkenbos, M.J., Yasuda, E., Beaumont, T., Scheeren, F.A. & Spits, H. (2008). STAT3-mediated up-regulation of BLIMP1 Is coordinated with BCL6 down-regulation to control human plasma cell differentiation. *J Immunol,* 180, 7, pp. 4805-4815.

Djuretic, I.M., Levanon, D., Negreanu, V., Groner, Y., Rao, A. & Ansel, K.M. (2007). Transcription factors T-bet and Runx3 cooperate to activate Ifng and silence Il4 in T helper type 1 cells. *Nat Immunol,* 8, 2, pp. 145-153.

Duhen, T., Geiger, R., Jarrossay, D., Lanzavecchia, A. & Sallusto, F. (2009). Production of interleukin 22 but not interleukin 17 by a subset of human skin-homing memory T cells. *Nat Immunol,* 10, 8, pp. 857-863.

Egawa, T. & Littman, D.R. (2008). ThPOK acts late in specification of the helper T cell lineage and suppresses Runx-mediated commitment to the cytotoxic T cell lineage. *Nat Immunol,* 9, 10, pp. 1131-1139.

Egawa, T., Tillman, R.E., Naoe, Y., Taniuchi, I. & Littman, D.R. (2007). The role of the Runx transcription factors in thymocyte differentiation and in homeostasis of naive T cells. *J Exp Med,* 204, 8, pp. 1945-1957.

Fazi, F., Rosa, A., Fatica, A., Gelmetti, V., De Marchis, M.L., Nervi, C. & Bozzoni, I. (2005). A minicircuitry comprised of microRNA-223 and transcription factors NFI-A and C/EBPalpha regulates human granulopoiesis. *Cell,* 123, 5, pp. 819-831.

Felli, N., Fontana, L., Pelosi, E., Botta, R., Bonci, D., Facchiano, F., Liuzzi, F., Lulli, V., Morsilli, O., Santoro, S., Valtieri, M., Calin, G.A., Liu, C.G., Sorrentino, A., Croce, C.M. & Peschle, C. (2005). MicroRNAs 221 and 222 inhibit normal erythropoiesis and erythroleukemic cell growth via kit receptor down-modulation. *Proc Natl Acad Sci U S A,* 102, 50, pp. 18081-18086.

Felli, N., Pedini, F., Romania, P., Biffoni, M., Morsilli, O., Castelli, G., Santoro, S., Chicarella, S., Sorrentino, A., Peschle, C. & Marziali, G. (2009). MicroRNA 223-dependent expression of LMO2 regulates normal erythropoiesis. *Haematologica,* 94, 4, pp. 479-486.

Feyerabend, T.B., Terszowski, G., Tietz, A., Blum, C., Luche, H., Gossler, A., Gale, N.W., Radtke, F., Fehling, H.J. & Rodewald, H.R. (2009). Deletion of Notch1 converts pro-T cells to dendritic cells and promotes thymic B cells by cell-extrinsic and cell-intrinsic mechanisms. *Immunity,* 30, 1, pp. 67-79.

Florian, M.C. & Geiger, H. (2010). Concise review: polarity in stem cells, disease, and aging. *Stem Cells,* 28, 9, pp. 1623-1629.

Fogg, D.K., Sibon, C., Miled, C., Jung, S., Aucouturier, P., Littman, D.R., Cumano, A. & Geissmann, F. (2006). A clonogenic bone marrow progenitor specific for macrophages and dendritic cells. *Science,* 311, 5757, pp. 83-87.

Fontana, L., Pelosi, E., Greco, P., Racanicchi, S., Testa, U., Liuzzi, F., Croce, C.M., Brunetti, E., Grignani, F. & Peschle, C. (2007). MicroRNAs 17-5p-20a-106a control monocytopoiesis through AML1 targeting and M-CSF receptor upregulation. *Nat Cell Biol,* 9, 7, pp. 775-787.

Fontenot, J.D., Gavin, M.A. & Rudensky, A.Y. (2003). Foxp3 programs the development and function of CD4+CD25+ regulatory T cells. *Nat Immunol,* 4, 4, pp. 330-336.

Forrest, A.R., Kanamori-Katayama, M., Tomaru, Y., Lassmann, T., Ninomiya, N., Takahashi, Y., de Hoon, M.J., Kubosaki, A., Kaiho, A., Suzuki, M., Yasuda, J., Kawai, J., Hayashizaki, Y., Hume, D.A. & Suzuki, H. (2010). Induction of microRNAs, mir-155, mir-222, mir-424 and mir-503, promotes monocytic differentiation through combinatorial regulation. *Leukemia,* 24, 2, pp. 460-466.

Franco, C.B., Scripture-Adams, D.D., Proekt, I., Taghon, T., Weiss, A.H., Yui, M.A., Adams, S.L., Diamond, R.A. & Rothenberg, E.V. (2006). Notch/Delta signaling constrains reengineering of pro-T cells by PU.1. *Proc Natl Acad Sci U S A,* 103, 32, pp. 11993-11998.

Friedman, A.D. (2007). Transcriptional control of granulocyte and monocyte development. *Oncogene,* 26, 47, pp. 6816-6828.

Fujiwara, Y., Browne, C.P., Cunniff, K., Goff, S.C. & Orkin, S.H. (1996). Arrested development of embryonic red cell precursors in mouse embryos lacking transcription factor GATA-1. *Proc Natl Acad Sci U S A,* 93, 22, pp. 12355-12358.

Fukuda, T., Yoshida, T., Okada, S., Hatano, M., Miki, T., Ishibashi, K., Okabe, S., Koseki, H., Hirosawa, S., Taniguchi, M., Miyasaka, N. & Tokuhisa, T. (1997). Disruption of the Bcl6 gene results in an impaired germinal center formation. *J Exp Med,* 186, 3, pp. 439-448.

Gangenahalli, G.U., Gupta, P., Saluja, D., Verma, Y.K., Kishore, V., Chandra, R., Sharma, R.K. & Ravindranath, T. (2005). Stem cell fate specification: role of master regulatory switch transcription factor PU.1 in differential hematopoiesis. *Stem Cells Dev,* 14, 2, pp. 140-152.

Gao, H., Lukin, K., Ramirez, J., Fields, S., Lopez, D. & Hagman, J. (2009). Opposing effects of SWI/SNF and Mi-2/NuRD chromatin remodeling complexes on epigenetic reprogramming by EBF and Pax5. *Proc Natl Acad Sci U S A,* 106, 27, pp. 11258-11263.

Garbe, A.I., Krueger, A., Gounari, F., Zuniga-Pflucker, J.C. & von Boehmer, H. (2006). Differential synergy of Notch and T cell receptor signaling determines alphabeta versus gammadelta lineage fate. *J Exp Med,* 203, 6, pp. 1579-1590.

Garcia-Peydro, M., de Yebenes, V.G. & Toribio, M.L. (2003). Sustained Notch1 signaling instructs the earliest human intrathymic precursors to adopt a gammadelta T-cell fate in fetal thymus organ culture. *Blood,* 102, 7, pp. 2444-2451.

Garzon, R., Pichiorri, F., Palumbo, T., Iuliano, R., Cimmino, A., Aqeilan, R., Volinia, S., Bhatt, D., Alder, H., Marcucci, G., Calin, G.A., Liu, C.G., Bloomfield, C.D., Andreeff, M. & Croce, C.M. (2006). MicroRNA fingerprints during human megakaryocytopoiesis. *Proc Natl Acad Sci U S A,* 103, 13, pp. 5078-5083.

Geissmann, F., Manz, M.G., Jung, S., Sieweke, M.H., Merad, M. & Ley, K. (2010). Development of monocytes, macrophages, and dendritic cells. *Science,* 327, 5966, pp. 656-661.

Georgantas, R.W., 3rd, Hildreth, R., Morisot, S., Alder, J., Liu, C.G., Heimfeld, S., Calin, G.A., Croce, C.M. & Civin, C.I. (2007). CD34+ hematopoietic stem-progenitor cell microRNA expression and function: a circuit diagram of differentiation control. *Proc Natl Acad Sci U S A,* 104, 8, pp. 2750-2755.

Gertz, M.A. (2010). Current status of stem cell mobilization. *Br J Haematol,* 150, 6, pp. 647-662.

Gertz, M.A., Lacy, M.Q., Inwards, D.J., Gastineau, D.A., Tefferi, A., Chen, M.G., Witzig, T.E., Greipp, P.R. & Litzow, M.R. (2000). Delayed stem cell transplantation for the management of relapsed or refractory multiple myeloma. *Bone Marrow Transplant,* 26, 1, pp. 45-50.

Gery, S., Gombart, A.F., Fung, Y.K. & Koeffler, H.P. (2004). C/EBPepsilon interacts with retinoblastoma and E2F1 during granulopoiesis. *Blood,* 103, 3, pp. 828-835.

Godfrey, V.L., Wilkinson, J.E., Rinchik, E.M. & Russell, L.B. (1991). Fatal lymphoreticular disease in the scurfy (sf) mouse requires T cells that mature in a sf thymic environment: potential model for thymic education. *Proc Natl Acad Sci U S A,* 88, 13, pp. 5528-5532.

Guo, J., Hawwari, A., Li, H., Sun, Z., Mahanta, S.K., Littman, D.R., Krangel, M.S. & He, Y.W. (2002). Regulation of the TCRalpha repertoire by the survival window of CD4(+)CD8(+) thymocytes. *Nat Immunol,* 3, 5, pp. 469-476.

Guo, S., Lu, J., Schlanger, R., Zhang, H., Wang, J.Y., Fox, M.C., Purton, L.E., Fleming, H.H., Cobb, B., Merkenschlager, M., Golub, T.R. & Scadden, D.T. (2010). MicroRNA miR-125a controls hematopoietic stem cell number. *Proc Natl Acad Sci U S A,* 107, 32, pp. 14229-14234.

Hanna, J., Wernig, M., Markoulaki, S., Sun, C.W., Meissner, A., Cassady, J.P., Beard, C., Brambrink, T., Wu, L.C., Townes, T.M. & Jaenisch, R. (2007). Treatment of sickle cell anemia mouse model with iPS cells generated from autologous skin. *Science,* 318, 5858, pp. 1920-1923.

Hayes, S.M., Li, L. & Love, P.E. (2005). TCR signal strength influences alphabeta/gammadelta lineage fate. *Immunity,* 22, 5, pp. 583-593.

He, X., Park, K., Wang, H., Zhang, Y., Hua, X., Li, Y. & Kappes, D.J. (2008). CD4-CD8 lineage commitment is regulated by a silencer element at the ThPOK transcription-factor locus. *Immunity,* 28, 3, pp. 346-358.

Heintzman, N.D., Hon, G.C., Hawkins, R.D., Kheradpour, P., Stark, A., Harp, L.F., Ye, Z., Lee, L.K., Stuart, R.K., Ching, C.W., Ching, K.A., Antosiewicz-Bourget, J.E., Liu, H., Zhang, X., Green, R.D., Lobanenkov, V.V., Stewart, R., Thomson, J.A., Crawford, G.E., Kellis, M. & Ren, B. (2009). Histone modifications at human enhancers reflect global cell-type-specific gene expression. *Nature,* 459, 7243, pp. 108-112.

Heinz, S., Benner, C., Spann, N., Bertolino, E., Lin, Y.C., Laslo, P., Cheng, J.X., Murre, C., Singh, H. & Glass, C.K. (2010). Simple combinations of lineage-determining transcription factors prime cis-regulatory elements required for macrophage and B cell identities. *Mol Cell,* 38, 4, pp. 576-589.

Hirai, H., Zhang, P., Dayaram, T., Hetherington, C.J., Mizuno, S., Imanishi, J., Akashi, K. & Tenen, D.G. (2006). C/EBPbeta is required for 'emergency' granulopoiesis. *Nat Immunol,* 7, 7, pp. 732-739.

Hisakawa, H., Sugiyama, D., Nishijima, I., Xu, M.J., Wu, H., Nakao, K., Watanabe, S., Katsuki, M., Asano, S., Arai, K., Nakahata, T. & Tsuji, K. (2001). Human granulocyte-macrophage colony-stimulating factor (hGM-CSF) stimulates primitive and definitive erythropoiesis in mouse embryos expressing hGM-CSF receptors but not erythropoietin receptors. *Blood,* 98, 13, pp. 3618-3625.

Hohaus, S., Petrovick, M.S., Voso, M.T., Sun, Z., Zhang, D.E. & Tenen, D.G. (1995). PU.1 (Spi-1) and C/EBP alpha regulate expression of the granulocyte-macrophage colony-stimulating factor receptor alpha gene. *Mol Cell Biol,* 15, 10, pp. 5830-5845.

Horcher, M., Souabni, A. & Busslinger, M. (2001). Pax5/BSAP maintains the identity of B cells in late B lymphopoiesis. *Immunity,* 14, 6, pp. 779-790.

Hori, S., Nomura, T. & Sakaguchi, S. (2003). Control of regulatory T cell development by the transcription factor Foxp3. *Science,* 299, 5609, pp. 1057-1061.

Horwitz, M., Benson, K.F., Person, R.E., Aprikyan, A.G. & Dale, D.C. (1999). Mutations in ELA2, encoding neutrophil elastase, define a 21-day biological clock in cyclic haematopoiesis. *Nat Genet,* 23, 4, pp. 433-436.

Hwang, E.S., Szabo, S.J., Schwartzberg, P.L. & Glimcher, L.H. (2005). T helper cell fate specified by kinase-mediated interaction of T-bet with GATA-3. *Science,* 307, 5708, pp. 430-433.

Ioannidis, V., Beermann, F., Clevers, H. & Held, W. (2001). The beta-catenin--TCF-1 pathway ensures CD4(+)CD8(+) thymocyte survival. *Nat Immunol,* 2, 8, pp. 691-697.

Isomura, I., Palmer, S., Grumont, R.J., Bunting, K., Hoyne, G., Wilkinson, N., Banerjee, A., Proietto, A., Gugasyan, R., Wu, L., McNally, A., Steptoe, R.J., Thomas, R., Shannon, M.F. & Gerondakis, S. (2009). c-Rel is required for the development of thymic Foxp3+ CD4 regulatory T cells. *J Exp Med,* 206, 13, pp. 3001-3014.

Ivanov, II, McKenzie, B.S., Zhou, L., Tadokoro, C.E., Lepelley, A., Lafaille, J.J., Cua, D.J. & Littman, D.R. (2006). The orphan nuclear receptor RORgammat directs the differentiation program of proinflammatory IL-17+ T helper cells. *Cell,* 126, 6, pp. 1121-1133.

Iwasaki, H. & Akashi, K. (2007). Hematopoietic developmental pathways: on cellular basis. *Oncogene,* 26, 47, pp. 6687-6696.

Iwasaki, H. & Akashi, K. (2007). Myeloid lineage commitment from the hematopoietic stem cell. *Immunity,* 26, 6, pp. 726-740.

Iwasaki, H., Mizuno, S., Wells, R.A., Cantor, A.B., Watanabe, S. & Akashi, K. (2003). GATA-1 converts lymphoid and myelomonocytic progenitors into the megakaryocyte/erythrocyte lineages. *Immunity,* 19, 3, pp. 451-462.

Iwasaki-Arai, J., Iwasaki, H., Miyamoto, T., Watanabe, S. & Akashi, K. (2003). Enforced granulocyte/macrophage colony-stimulating factor signals do not support lymphopoiesis, but instruct lymphoid to myelomonocytic lineage conversion. *J Exp Med,* 197, 10, pp. 1311-1322.

Ji, H., Ehrlich, L.I., Seita, J., Murakami, P., Doi, A., Lindau, P., Lee, H., Aryee, M.J., Irizarry, R.A., Kim, K., Rossi, D.J., Inlay, M.A., Serwold, T., Karsunky, H., Ho, L., Daley, G.Q., Weissman, I.L. & Feinberg, A.P. (2010). Comprehensive methylome map of lineage commitment from haematopoietic progenitors. *Nature,* 467, 7313, pp. 338-342.

Johnnidis, J.B., Harris, M.H., Wheeler, R.T., Stehling-Sun, S., Lam, M.H., Kirak, O., Brummelkamp, T.R., Fleming, M.D. & Camargo, F.D. (2008). Regulation of progenitor cell proliferation and granulocyte function by microRNA-223. *Nature,* 451, 7182, pp. 1125-1129.

Johnson, P.F. (2005). Molecular stop signs: regulation of cell-cycle arrest by C/EBP transcription factors. *J Cell Sci,* 118, Pt 12, pp. 2545-2555.

Johnston, R.J., Poholek, A.C., DiToro, D., Yusuf, I., Eto, D., Barnett, B., Dent, A.L., Craft, J. & Crotty, S. (2009). Bcl6 and Blimp-1 are reciprocal and antagonistic regulators of T follicular helper cell differentiation. *Science,* 325, 5943, pp. 1006-1010.

Jonuleit, H., Schmitt, E., Steinbrink, K. & Enk, A.H. (2001). Dendritic cells as a tool to induce anergic and regulatory T cells. *Trends Immunol,* 22, 7, pp. 394-400.

Kallies, A., Hasbold, J., Fairfax, K., Pridans, C., Emslie, D., McKenzie, B.S., Lew, A.M., Corcoran, L.M., Hodgkin, P.D., Tarlinton, D.M. & Nutt, S.L. (2007). Initiation of plasma-cell differentiation is independent of the transcription factor Blimp-1. *Immunity,* 26, 5, pp. 555-566.

Kanellopoulou, C., Muljo, S.A., Kung, A.L., Ganesan, S., Drapkin, R., Jenuwein, T., Livingston, D.M. & Rajewsky, K. (2005). Dicer-deficient mouse embryonic stem cells are defective in differentiation and centromeric silencing. *Genes Dev,* 19, 4, pp. 489-501.

Kang, J., Volkmann, A. & Raulet, D.H. (2001). Evidence that gammadelta versus alphabeta T cell fate determination is initiated independently of T cell receptor signaling. *J Exp Med,* 193, 6, pp. 689-698.

Kee, B.L. & Murre, C. (1998). Induction of early B cell factor (EBF) and multiple B lineage genes by the basic helix-loop-helix transcription factor E12. *J Exp Med,* 188, 4, pp. 699-713.

Kerenyi, M.A. & Orkin, S.H. (2010). Networking erythropoiesis. *J Exp Med,* 207, 12, pp. 2537-2541.

Kiel, M.J., Yilmaz, O.H., Iwashita, T., Terhorst, C. & Morrison, S.J. (2005). SLAM family receptors distinguish hematopoietic stem and progenitor cells and reveal endothelial niches for stem cells. *Cell,* 121, 7, pp. 1109-1121.

Kim, J., Sif, S., Jones, B., Jackson, A., Koipally, J., Heller, E., Winandy, S., Viel, A., Sawyer, A., Ikeda, T., Kingston, R. & Georgopoulos, K. (1999). Ikaros DNA-binding proteins direct formation of chromatin remodeling complexes in lymphocytes. *Immunity,* 10, 3, pp. 345-355.

Kim, P.J., Pai, S.Y., Brigl, M., Besra, G.S., Gumperz, J. & Ho, I.C. (2006). GATA-3 regulates the development and function of invariant NKT cells. *J Immunol,* 177, 10, pp. 6650-6659.

Kirillov, A., Kistler, B., Mostoslavsky, R., Cedar, H., Wirth, T. & Bergman, Y. (1996). A role for nuclear NF-kappaB in B-cell-specific demethylation of the Igkappa locus. *Nat Genet,* 13, 4, pp. 435-441.

Kohn, D.B. (2010). Update on gene therapy for immunodeficiencies. *Clin Immunol,* 135, 2, pp. 247-254.

Koipally, J., Renold, A., Kim, J. & Georgopoulos, K. (1999). Repression by Ikaros and Aiolos is mediated through histone deacetylase complexes. *EMBO J,* 18, 11, pp. 3090-3100.

Kondo, M., Scherer, D.C., Miyamoto, T., King, A.G., Akashi, K., Sugamura, K. & Weissman, I.L. (2000). Cell-fate conversion of lymphoid-committed progenitors by instructive actions of cytokines. *Nature,* 407, 6802, pp. 383-386.

Kondo, M., Wagers, A.J., Manz, M.G., Prohaska, S.S., Scherer, D.C., Beilhack, G.F., Shizuru, J.A. & Weissman, I.L. (2003). Biology of hematopoietic stem cells and progenitors: implications for clinical application. *Annu Rev Immunol,* 21, pp. 759-806.

Kondo, M., Weissman, I.L. & Akashi, K. (1997). Identification of clonogenic common lymphoid progenitors in mouse bone marrow. *Cell,* 91, 5, pp. 661-672.

Koralov, S.B., Muljo, S.A., Galler, G.R., Krek, A., Chakraborty, T., Kanellopoulou, C., Jensen, K., Cobb, B.S., Merkenschlager, M., Rajewsky, N. & Rajewsky, K. (2008). Dicer ablation affects antibody diversity and cell survival in the B lymphocyte lineage. *Cell,* 132, 5, pp. 860-874.

Koschmieder, S., Halmos, B., Levantini, E. & Tenen, D.G. (2009). Dysregulation of the C/EBPalpha differentiation pathway in human cancer. *J Clin Oncol,* 27, 4, pp. 619-628.

Kovalovsky, D., Uche, O.U., Eladad, S., Hobbs, R.M., Yi, W., Alonzo, E., Chua, K., Eidson, M., Kim, H.J., Im, J.S., Pandolfi, P.P. & Sant'Angelo, D.B. (2008). The BTB-zinc finger transcriptional regulator PLZF controls the development of invariant natural killer T cell effector functions. *Nat Immunol,* 9, 9, pp. 1055-1064.

Kozmik, Z., Wang, S., Dorfler, P., Adams, B. & Busslinger, M. (1992). The promoter of the CD19 gene is a target for the B-cell-specific transcription factor BSAP. *Mol Cell Biol,* 12, 6, pp. 2662-2672.

Kreslavsky, T., Gleimer, M., Garbe, A.I. & von Boehmer, H. (2010). alphabeta versus gammadelta fate choice: counting the T-cell lineages at the branch point. *Immunol Rev,* 238, 1, pp. 169-181.

Kurschus, F.C., Croxford, A.L., Heinen, A.P., Wortge, S., Ielo, D. & Waisman, A. (2010). Genetic proof for the transient nature of the Th17 phenotype. *Eur J Immunol,* 40, 12, pp. 3336-3346.

Kwon, K., Hutter, C., Sun, Q., Bilic, I., Cobaleda, C., Malin, S. & Busslinger, M. (2008). Instructive role of the transcription factor E2A in early B lymphopoiesis and germinal center B cell development. *Immunity,* 28, 6, pp. 751-762.

Lacorazza, H.D., Miyazaki, Y., Di Cristofano, A., Deblasio, A., Hedvat, C., Zhang, J., Cordon-Cardo, C., Mao, S., Pandolfi, P.P. & Nimer, S.D. (2002). The ETS protein

MEF plays a critical role in perforin gene expression and the development of natural killer and NK-T cells. *Immunity,* 17, 4, pp. 437-449.

Laiosa, C.V., Stadtfeld, M., Xie, H., de Andres-Aguayo, L. & Graf, T. (2006). Reprogramming of committed T cell progenitors to macrophages and dendritic cells by C/EBP alpha and PU.1 transcription factors. *Immunity,* 25, 5, pp. 731-744.

Laslo, P., Pongubala, J.M., Lancki, D.W. & Singh, H. (2008). Gene regulatory networks directing myeloid and lymphoid cell fates within the immune system. *Semin Immunol,* 20, 4, pp. 228-235.

Laslo, P., Spooner, C.J., Warmflash, A., Lancki, D.W., Lee, H.J., Sciammas, R., Gantner, B.N., Dinner, A.R. & Singh, H. (2006). Multilineage transcriptional priming and determination of alternate hematopoietic cell fates. *Cell,* 126, 4, pp. 755-766.

Lauritsen, J.P., Wong, G.W., Lee, S.Y., Lefebvre, J.M., Ciofani, M., Rhodes, M., Kappes, D.J., Zuniga-Pflucker, J.C. & Wiest, D.L. (2009). Marked induction of the helix-loop-helix protein Id3 promotes the gammadelta T cell fate and renders their functional maturation Notch independent. *Immunity,* 31, 4, pp. 565-575.

Lazarevic, V., Chen, X., Shim, J.H., Hwang, E.S., Jang, E., Bolm, A.N., Oukka, M., Kuchroo, V.K. & Glimcher, L.H. (2011). T-bet represses T(H)17 differentiation by preventing Runx1-mediated activation of the gene encoding RORgammat. *Nat Immunol,* 12, 1, pp. 96-104.

Lee, C.H., Melchers, M., Wang, H., Torrey, T.A., Slota, R., Qi, C.F., Kim, J.Y., Lugar, P., Kong, H.J., Farrington, L., van der Zouwen, B., Zhou, J.X., Lougaris, V., Lipsky, P.E., Grammer, A.C. & Morse, H.C., 3rd. (2006). Regulation of the germinal center gene program by interferon (IFN) regulatory factor 8/IFN consensus sequence-binding protein. *J Exp Med,* 203, 1, pp. 63-72.

Lee, Y.K., Turner, H., Maynard, C.L., Oliver, J.R., Chen, D., Elson, C.O. & Weaver, C.T. (2009). Late developmental plasticity in the T helper 17 lineage. *Immunity,* 30, 1, pp. 92-107.

Lekstrom-Himes, J. & Xanthopoulos, K.G. (1998). Biological role of the CCAAT/enhancer-binding protein family of transcription factors. *J Biol Chem,* 273, 44, pp. 28545-28548.

Lekstrom-Himes, J. & Xanthopoulos, K.G. (1999). CCAAT/enhancer binding protein epsilon is critical for effective neutrophil-mediated response to inflammatory challenge. *Blood,* 93, 9, pp. 3096-3105.

Lekstrom-Himes, J.A., Dorman, S.E., Kopar, P., Holland, S.M. & Gallin, J.I. (1999). Neutrophil-specific granule deficiency results from a novel mutation with loss of function of the transcription factor CCAAT/enhancer binding protein epsilon. *J Exp Med,* 189, 11, pp. 1847-1852.

Li, L., Leid, M. & Rothenberg, E.V. (2010). An early T cell lineage commitment checkpoint dependent on the transcription factor Bcl11b. *Science,* 329, 5987, pp. 89-93.

Li, Q.J., Chau, J., Ebert, P.J., Sylvester, G., Min, H., Liu, G., Braich, R., Manoharan, M., Soutschek, J., Skare, P., Klein, L.O., Davis, M.M. & Chen, C.Z. (2007). miR-181a is an intrinsic modulator of T cell sensitivity and selection. *Cell,* 129, 1, pp. 147-161.

Liao, R., Sun, J., Zhang, L., Lou, G., Chen, M., Zhou, D., Chen, Z. & Zhang, S. (2008). MicroRNAs play a role in the development of human hematopoietic stem cells. *J Cell Biochem,* 104, 3, pp. 805-817.

Lin, C.S., Lim, S.K., D'Agati, V. & Costantini, F. (1996). Differential effects of an erythropoietin receptor gene disruption on primitive and definitive erythropoiesis. *Genes Dev,* 10, 2, pp. 154-164.

Lin, H. & Grosschedl, R. (1995). Failure of B-cell differentiation in mice lacking the transcription factor EBF. *Nature,* 376, 6537, pp. 263-267.

Lin, K.I., Angelin-Duclos, C., Kuo, T.C. & Calame, K. (2002). Blimp-1-dependent repression of Pax-5 is required for differentiation of B cells to immunoglobulin M-secreting plasma cells. *Mol Cell Biol,* 22, 13, pp. 4771-4780.

Lin, Y.C., Jhunjhunwala, S., Benner, C., Heinz, S., Welinder, E., Mansson, R., Sigvardsson, M., Hagman, J., Espinoza, C.A., Dutkowski, J., Ideker, T., Glass, C.K. & Murre, C. (2010). A global network of transcription factors, involving E2A, EBF1 and Foxo1, that orchestrates B cell fate. *Nat Immunol,* 11, 7, pp. 635-643.

Linch, D.C., Winfield, D., Goldstone, A.H., Moir, D., Hancock, B., McMillan, A., Chopra, R., Milligan, D. & Hudson, G.V. (1993). Dose intensification with autologous bone-marrow transplantation in relapsed and resistant Hodgkin's disease: results of a BNLI randomised trial. *Lancet,* 341, 8852, pp. 1051-1054.

Liu, F., Wu, H.Y., Wesselschmidt, R., Kornaga, T. & Link, D.C. (1996). Impaired production and increased apoptosis of neutrophils in granulocyte colony-stimulating factor receptor-deficient mice. *Immunity,* 5, 5, pp. 491-501.

Long, M., Park, S.G., Strickland, I., Hayden, M.S. & Ghosh, S. (2009). Nuclear factor-kappaB modulates regulatory T cell development by directly regulating expression of Foxp3 transcription factor. *Immunity,* 31, 6, pp. 921-931.

Lu, J., Guo, S., Ebert, B.L., Zhang, H., Peng, X., Bosco, J., Pretz, J., Schlanger, R., Wang, J.Y., Mak, R.H., Dombkowski, D.M., Preffer, F.I., Scadden, D.T. & Golub, T.R. (2008). MicroRNA-mediated control of cell fate in megakaryocyte-erythrocyte progenitors. *Dev Cell,* 14, 6, pp. 843-853.

Lyon, M.F., Peters, J., Glenister, P.H., Ball, S. & Wright, E. (1990). The scurfy mouse mutant has previously unrecognized hematological abnormalities and resembles Wiskott-Aldrich syndrome. *Proc Natl Acad Sci U S A,* 87, 7, pp. 2433-2437.

Mansfield, J.H., Harfe, B.D., Nissen, R., Obenauer, J., Srineel, J., Chaudhuri, A., Farzan-Kashani, R., Zuker, M., Pasquinelli, A.E., Ruvkun, G., Sharp, P.A., Tabin, C.J. & McManus, M.T. (2004). MicroRNA-responsive 'sensor' transgenes uncover Hox-like and other developmentally regulated patterns of vertebrate microRNA expression. *Nat Genet,* 36, 10, pp. 1079-1083.

Mantel, P.Y., Ouaked, N., Ruckert, B., Karagiannidis, C., Welz, R., Blaser, K. & Schmidt-Weber, C.B. (2006). Molecular mechanisms underlying FOXP3 induction in human T cells. *J Immunol,* 176, 6, pp. 3593-3602.

Manz, M.G., Traver, D., Miyamoto, T., Weissman, I.L. & Akashi, K. (2001). Dendritic cell potentials of early lymphoid and myeloid progenitors. *Blood,* 97, 11, pp. 3333-3341.

Matsuda, J.L., Zhang, Q., Ndonye, R., Richardson, S.K., Howell, A.R. & Gapin, L. (2006). T-bet concomitantly controls migration, survival, and effector functions during the development of Valpha14i NKT cells. *Blood,* 107, 7, pp. 2797-2805.

McArthur, G.A., Rohrschneider, L.R. & Johnson, G.R. (1994). Induced expression of c-fms in normal hematopoietic cells shows evidence for both conservation and lineage restriction of signal transduction in response to macrophage colony-stimulating factor. *Blood,* 83, 4, pp. 972-981.

Melichar, H.J., Narayan, K., Der, S.D., Hiraoka, Y., Gardiol, N., Jeannet, G., Held, W., Chambers, C.A. & Kang, J. (2007). Regulation of gammadelta versus alphabeta T lymphocyte differentiation by the transcription factor SOX13. *Science,* 315, 5809, pp. 230-233.

Metcalf, D. (2008). Hematopoietic cytokines. *Blood,* 111, 2, pp. 485-491.

Morceau, F., Schnekenburger, M., Dicato, M. & Diederich, M. (2004). GATA-1: friends, brothers, and coworkers. *Ann N Y Acad Sci,* 1030, pp. 537-554.

Moreau, P., Avet-Loiseau, H., Harousseau, J.L. & Attal, M. (2011). Current trends in autologous stem-cell transplantation for myeloma in the era of novel therapies. *J Clin Oncol,* 29, 14, pp. 1898-1906.

Mosmann, T.R., Cherwinski, H., Bond, M.W., Giedlin, M.A. & Coffman, R.L. (1986). Two types of murine helper T cell clone. I. Definition according to profiles of lymphokine activities and secreted proteins. *J Immunol,* 136, 7, pp. 2348-2357.

Mowen, K.A. & Glimcher, L.H. (2004). Signaling pathways in Th2 development. *Immunol Rev,* 202, pp. 203-222.

Muljo, S.A., Ansel, K.M., Kanellopoulou, C., Livingston, D.M., Rao, A. & Rajewsky, K. (2005). Aberrant T cell differentiation in the absence of Dicer. *J Exp Med,* 202, 2, pp. 261-269.

Nagai, Y., Garrett, K.P., Ohta, S., Bahrun, U., Kouro, T., Akira, S., Takatsu, K. & Kincade, P.W. (2006). Toll-like receptors on hematopoietic progenitor cells stimulate innate immune system replenishment. *Immunity,* 24, 6, pp. 801-812.

Naik, S.H., Sathe, P., Park, H.Y., Metcalf, D., Proietto, A.I., Dakic, A., Carotta, S., O'Keeffe, M., Bahlo, M., Papenfuss, A., Kwak, J.Y., Wu, L. & Shortman, K. (2007). Development of plasmacytoid and conventional dendritic cell subtypes from single precursor cells derived in vitro and in vivo. *Nat Immunol,* 8, 11, pp. 1217-1226.

Nishinakamura, R., Miyajima, A., Mee, P.J., Tybulewicz, V.L. & Murray, R. (1996). Hematopoiesis in mice lacking the entire granulocyte-macrophage colony-stimulating factor/interleukin-3/interleukin-5 functions. *Blood,* 88, 7, pp. 2458-2464.

Nishinakamura, R., Wiler, R., Dirksen, U., Morikawa, Y., Arai, K., Miyajima, A., Burdach, S. & Murray, R. (1996). The pulmonary alveolar proteinosis in granulocyte macrophage colony-stimulating factor/interleukins 3/5 beta c receptor-deficient mice is reversed by bone marrow transplantation. *J Exp Med,* 183, 6, pp. 2657-2662.

Nozad Charoudeh, H., Tang, Y., Cheng, M., Cilio, C.M., Jacobsen, S.E. & Sitnicka, E. (2010). Identification of an NK/T cell-restricted progenitor in adult bone marrow contributing to bone marrow- and thymic-dependent NK cells. *Blood,* 116, 2, pp. 183-192.

Nurieva, R.I., Chung, Y., Martinez, G.J., Yang, X.O., Tanaka, S., Matskevitch, T.D., Wang, Y.H. & Dong, C. (2009). Bcl6 mediates the development of T follicular helper cells. *Science,* 325, 5943, pp. 1001-1005.

Nutt, S.L., Heavey, B., Rolink, A.G. & Busslinger, M. (1999). Commitment to the B-lymphoid lineage depends on the transcription factor Pax5. *Nature,* 401, 6753, pp. 556-562.

Nutt, S.L., Morrison, A.M., Dorfler, P., Rolink, A. & Busslinger, M. (1998). Identification of BSAP (Pax-5) target genes in early B-cell development by loss- and gain-of-function experiments. *Embo J,* 17, 8, pp. 2319-2333.

Nutt, S.L., Urbanek, P., Rolink, A. & Busslinger, M. (1997). Essential functions of Pax5 (BSAP) in pro-B cell development: difference between fetal and adult B lymphopoiesis and reduced V- to DJ recombination at the IgH locus. *Genes Dev.,* 11, pp. 476-491.

Nutt, S.L., Urbanek, P., Rolink, A. & Busslinger, M. (1997). Essential functions of Pax5 (BSAP) in pro-B cell development: difference between fetal and adult B lymphopoiesis and reduced V-to-DJ recombination at the IgH locus. *Genes Dev,* 11, 4, pp. 476-491.

O'Riordan, M. & Grosschedl, R. (1999). Coordinate regulation of B cell differentiation by the transcription factors EBF and E2A. *Immunity,* 11, 1, pp. 21-31.

Onai, N., Obata-Onai, A., Schmid, M.A., Ohteki, T., Jarrossay, D. & Manz, M.G. (2007). Identification of clonogenic common Flt3+M-CSFR+ plasmacytoid and conventional dendritic cell progenitors in mouse bone marrow. *Nat Immunol,* 8, 11, pp. 1207-1216.

Orford, K., Kharchenko, P., Lai, W., Dao, M.C., Worhunsky, D.J., Ferro, A., Janzen, V., Park, P.J. & Scadden, D.T. (2008). Differential H3K4 methylation identifies developmentally poised hematopoietic genes. *Dev Cell,* 14, 5, pp. 798-809.

Park, J.H., Adoro, S., Guinter, T., Erman, B., Alag, A.S., Catalfamo, M., Kimura, M.Y., Cui, Y., Lucas, P.J., Gress, R.E., Kubo, M., Hennighausen, L., Feigenbaum, L. & Singer, A. (2010). Signaling by intrathymic cytokines, not T cell antigen receptors, specifies CD8 lineage choice and promotes the differentiation of cytotoxic-lineage T cells. *Nat Immunol,* 11, 3, pp. 257-264.

Park, K., He, X., Lee, H.O., Hua, X., Li, Y., Wiest, D. & Kappes, D.J. (2010). TCR-mediated ThPOK induction promotes development of mature (CD24-) gammadelta thymocytes. *EMBO J,* 29, 14, pp. 2329-2341.

Patrick, D.M., Zhang, C.C., Tao, Y., Yao, H., Qi, X., Schwartz, R.J., Jun-Shen Huang, L. & Olson, E.N. (2010). Defective erythroid differentiation in miR-451 mutant mice mediated by 14-3-3zeta. *Genes Dev,* 24, 15, pp. 1614-1619.

Person, R.E., Li, F.Q., Duan, Z., Benson, K.F., Wechsler, J., Papadaki, H.A., Eliopoulos, G., Kaufman, C., Bertolone, S.J., Nakamoto, B., Papayannopoulou, T., Grimes, H.L. & Horwitz, M. (2003). Mutations in proto-oncogene GFI1 cause human neutropenia and target ELA2. *Nat Genet,* 34, 3, pp. 308-312.

Peschon, J.J., Morrissey, P.J., Grabstein, K.H., Ramsdell, F.J., Maraskovsky, E., Gliniak, B.C., Park, L.S., Ziegler, S.F., Williams, D.E., Ware, C.B., Meyer, J.D. & Davison, B.L. (1994). Early lymphocyte expansion is severely impaired in interleukin 7 receptor-deficient mice. *J Exp Med,* 180, 5, pp. 1955-1960.

Petrie, H.T. & Zuniga-Pflucker, J.C. (2007). Zoned out: functional mapping of stromal signaling microenvironments in the thymus. *Annu Rev Immunol,* 25, pp. 649-679.

Philip, T., Guglielmi, C., Hagenbeek, A., Somers, R., Van der Lelie, H., Bron, D., Sonneveld, P., Gisselbrecht, C., Cahn, J.Y., Harousseau, J.L. & et al. (1995). Autologous bone marrow transplantation as compared with salvage chemotherapy in relapses of chemotherapy-sensitive non-Hodgkin's lymphoma. *N Engl J Med,* 333, 23, pp. 1540-1545.

Pongubala, J.M., Northrup, D.L., Lancki, D.W., Medina, K.L., Treiber, T., Bertolino, E., Thomas, M., Grosschedl, R., Allman, D. & Singh, H. (2008). Transcription factor EBF restricts alternative lineage options and promotes B cell fate commitment independently of Pax5. *Nat Immunol,* 9, 2, pp. 203-215.

Pronk, C.J., Rossi, D.J., Mansson, R., Attema, J.L., Norddahl, G.L., Chan, C.K., Sigvardsson, M., Weissman, I.L. & Bryder, D. (2007). Elucidation of the phenotypic, functional, and molecular topography of a myeloerythroid progenitor cell hierarchy. *Cell Stem Cell,* 1, 4, pp. 428-442.

Pulikkan, J.A., Peramangalam, P.S., Dengler, V., Ho, P.A., Preudhomme, C., Meshinchi, S., Christopeit, M., Nibourel, O., Muller-Tidow, C., Bohlander, S.K., Tenen, D.G. & Behre, G. (2010). C/EBPalpha regulated microRNA-34a targets E2F3 during granulopoiesis and is down-regulated in AML with CEBPA mutations. *Blood,* 116, 25, pp. 5638-5649.

Rasmussen, K.D., Simmini, S., Abreu-Goodger, C., Bartonicek, N., Di Giacomo, M., Bilbao-Cortes, D., Horos, R., Von Lindern, M., Enright, A.J. & O'Carroll, D. (2010). The miR-144/451 locus is required for erythroid homeostasis. *J Exp Med,* 207, 7, pp. 1351-1358.

Rieger, M.A., Hoppe, P.S., Smejkal, B.M., Eitelhuber, A.C. & Schroeder, T. (2009). Hematopoietic cytokines can instruct lineage choice. *Science,* 325, 5937, pp. 217-218.

Riera-Sans, L. & Behrens, A. (2007). Regulation of alphabeta/gammadelta T cell development by the activator protein 1 transcription factor c-Jun. *J Immunol,* 178, 9, pp. 5690-5700.

Robb, L. (2007). Cytokine receptors and hematopoietic differentiation. *Oncogene,* 26, 47, pp. 6715-6723.

Roessler, S., Gyory, I., Imhof, S., Spivakov, M., Williams, R.R., Busslinger, M., Fisher, A.G. & Grosschedl, R. (2007). Distinct promoters mediate the regulation of Ebf1 gene expression by interleukin-7 and Pax5. *Mol Cell Biol,* 27, 2, pp. 579-594.

Romania, P., Lulli, V., Pelosi, E., Biffoni, M., Peschle, C. & Marziali, G. (2008). MicroRNA 155 modulates megakaryopoiesis at progenitor and precursor level by targeting Ets-1 and Meis1 transcription factors. *Br J Haematol,* 143, 4, pp. 570-580.

Roncarolo, M.G., Gregori, S., Lucarelli, B., Ciceri, F. & Bacchetta, R. (2011). Clinical tolerance in allogeneic hematopoietic stem cell transplantation. *Immunol Rev,* 241, 1, pp. 145-163.

Ruan, Q., Kameswaran, V., Tone, Y., Li, L., Liou, H.C., Greene, M.I., Tone, M. & Chen, Y.H. (2009). Development of Foxp3(+) regulatory t cells is driven by the c-Rel enhanceosome. *Immunity,* 31, 6, pp. 932-940.

Saran, N., Lyszkiewicz, M., Pommerencke, J., Witzlau, K., Vakilzadeh, R., Ballmaier, M., von Boehmer, H. & Krueger, A. (2010). Multiple extrathymic precursors contribute to T-cell development with different kinetics. *Blood,* 115, 6, pp. 1137-1144.

Savage, A.K., Constantinides, M.G., Han, J., Picard, D., Martin, E., Li, B., Lantz, O. & Bendelac, A. (2008). The transcription factor PLZF directs the effector program of the NKT cell lineage. *Immunity,* 29, 3, pp. 391-403.

Schebesta, M., Pfeffer, P.L. & Busslinger, M. (2002). Control of pre-BCR signaling by Pax5-dependent activation of the BLNK gene. *Immunity,* 17, 4, pp. 473-485.

Schmitt, T.M., Ciofani, M., Petrie, H.T. & Zuniga-Pflucker, J.C. (2004). Maintenance of T cell specification and differentiation requires recurrent notch receptor-ligand interactions. *J Exp Med,* 200, 4, pp. 469-479.

Sciammas, R., Shaffer, A.L., Schatz, J.H., Zhao, H., Staudt, L.M. & Singh, H. (2006). Graded expression of interferon regulatory factor-4 coordinates isotype switching with plasma cell differentiation. *Immunity,* 25, 2, pp. 225-236.

Scott, E.W., Simon, M.C., Anastasi, J. & Singh, H. (1994). Requirement of transcription factor PU.1 in the development of multiple hematopoietic lineages. *Science*, 265, 5178, pp. 1573-1577.

Seet, C.S., Brumbaugh, R.L. & Kee, B.L. (2004). Early B cell factor promotes B lymphopoiesis with reduced interleukin 7 responsiveness in the absence of E2A. *J Exp Med*, 199, 12, pp. 1689-1700.

Semerad, C.L., Poursine-Laurent, J., Liu, F. & Link, D.C. (1999). A role for G-CSF receptor signaling in the regulation of hematopoietic cell function but not lineage commitment or differentiation. *Immunity*, 11, 2, pp. 153-161.

Serwold, T., Ehrlich, L.I. & Weissman, I.L. (2009). Reductive isolation from bone marrow and blood implicates common lymphoid progenitors as the major source of thymopoiesis. *Blood*, 113, 4, pp. 807-815.

Shaffer, A.L., Lin, K.I., Kuo, T.C., Yu, X., Hurt, E.M., Rosenwald, A., Giltnane, J.M., Yang, L., Zhao, H., Calame, K. & Staudt, L.M. (2002). Blimp-1 orchestrates plasma cell differentiation by extinguishing the mature B cell gene expression program. *Immunity*, 17, 1, pp. 51-62.

Shaffer, A.L., Shapiro-Shelef, M., Iwakoshi, N.N., Lee, A.H., Qian, S.B., Zhao, H., Yu, X., Yang, L., Tan, B.K., Rosenwald, A., Hurt, E.M., Petroulakis, E., Sonenberg, N., Yewdell, J.W., Calame, K., Glimcher, L.H. & Staudt, L.M. (2004). XBP1, downstream of Blimp-1, expands the secretory apparatus and other organelles, and increases protein synthesis in plasma cell differentiation. *Immunity*, 21, 1, pp. 81-93.

Shaffer, A.L., Yu, X., He, Y., Boldrick, J., Chan, E.P. & Staudt, L.M. (2000). BCL-6 represses genes that function in lymphocyte differentiation, inflammation, and cell cycle control. *Immunity*, 13, 2, pp. 199-212.

Sharrocks, A.D. (2001). The ETS-domain transcription factor family. *Nat Rev Mol Cell Biol*, 2, 11, pp. 827-837.

Shen, W.F., Hu, Y.L., Uttarwar, L., Passegue, E. & Largman, C. (2008). MicroRNA-126 regulates HOXA9 by binding to the homeobox. *Mol Cell Biol*, 28, 14, pp. 4609-4619.

Shi, G., Cox, C.A., Vistica, B.P., Tan, C., Wawrousek, E.F. & Gery, I. (2008). Phenotype switching by inflammation-inducing polarized Th17 cells, but not by Th1 cells. *J Immunol*, 181, 10, pp. 7205-7213.

Sigvardsson, M., O'Riordan, M. & Grosschedl, R. (1997). EBF and E47 collaborate to induce expression of the endogenous immunoglobulin surrogate light chain genes. *Immunity*, 7, 1, pp. 25-36.

Silva-Santos, B., Pennington, D.J. & Hayday, A.C. (2005). Lymphotoxin-mediated regulation of gammadelta cell differentiation by alphabeta T cell progenitors. *Science*, 307, 5711, pp. 925-928.

Sivakumar, V., Hammond, K.J., Howells, N., Pfeffer, K. & Weih, F. (2003). Differential requirement for Rel/nuclear factor kappa B family members in natural killer T cell development. *J Exp Med*, 197, 12, pp. 1613-1621.

Smith, E.M., Gisler, R. & Sigvardsson, M. (2002). Cloning and characterization of a promoter flanking the early B cell factor (EBF) gene indicates roles for E-proteins and autoregulation in the control of EBF expression. *J Immunol*, 169, 1, pp. 261-270.

Smith, L.T., Hohaus, S., Gonzalez, D.A., Dziennis, S.E. & Tenen, D.G. (1996). PU.1 (Spi-1) and C/EBP alpha regulate the granulocyte colony-stimulating factor receptor promoter in myeloid cells. *Blood*, 88, 4, pp. 1234-1247.

Smithgall, T.E., Briggs, S.D., Schreiner, S., Lerner, E.C., Cheng, H. & Wilson, M.B. (2000). Control of myeloid differentiation and survival by Stats. *Oncogene,* 19, 21, pp. 2612-2618.

Soligo, M., Camperio, C., Caristi, S., Scotta, C., Del Porto, P., Costanzo, A., Mantel, P.Y., Schmidt-Weber, C.B. & Piccolella, E. (2011). CD28 costimulation regulates FOXP3 in a RelA/NF-kappaB-dependent mechanism. *Eur J Immunol,* 41, 2, pp. 503-513.

Souabni, A., Cobaleda, C., Schebesta, M. & Busslinger, M. (2002). Pax5 promotes B lymphopoiesis and blocks T cell development by repressing Notch1. *Immunity,* 17, 6, pp. 781-793.

Spooner, C.J., Cheng, J.X., Pujadas, E., Laslo, P. & Singh, H. (2009). A recurrent network involving the transcription factors PU.1 and Gfi1 orchestrates innate and adaptive immune cell fates. *Immunity,* 31, 4, pp. 576-586.

Sridharan, R. & Smale, S.T. (2007). Predominant interaction of both Ikaros and Helios with the NuRD complex in immature thymocytes. *J Biol Chem,* 282, 41, pp. 30227-30238.

Stanic, A.K., Bezbradica, J.S., Park, J.J., Matsuki, N., Mora, A.L., Van Kaer, L., Boothby, M.R. & Joyce, S. (2004). NF-kappa B controls cell fate specification, survival, and molecular differentiation of immunoregulatory natural T lymphocytes. *J Immunol,* 172, 4, pp. 2265-2273.

Sullivan, K.M., Muraro, P. & Tyndall, A. (2010). Hematopoietic cell transplantation for autoimmune disease: updates from Europe and the United States. *Biol Blood Marrow Transplant,* 16, 1 Suppl, pp. S48-56.

Szabo, S.J., Sullivan, B.M., Peng, S.L. & Glimcher, L.H. (2003). Molecular mechanisms regulating Th1 immune responses. *Annu Rev Immunol,* 21, pp. 713-758.

Szalai, G., LaRue, A.C. & Watson, D.K. (2006). Molecular mechanisms of megakaryopoiesis. *Cell Mol Life Sci,* 63, 21, pp. 2460-2476.

Tadokoro, Y., Ema, H., Okano, M., Li, E. & Nakauchi, H. (2007). De novo DNA methyltransferase is essential for self-renewal, but not for differentiation, in hematopoietic stem cells. *J Exp Med,* 204, 4, pp. 715-722.

Taghon, T., Yui, M.A. & Rothenberg, E.V. (2007). Mast cell lineage diversion of T lineage precursors by the essential T cell transcription factor GATA-3. *Nat Immunol,* 8, 8, pp. 845-855.

Takahashi, K., Tanabe, K., Ohnuki, M., Narita, M., Ichisaka, T., Tomoda, K. & Yamanaka, S. (2007). Induction of pluripotent stem cells from adult human fibroblasts by defined factors. *Cell,* 131, 5, pp. 861-872.

Takahashi, K. & Yamanaka, S. (2006). Induction of pluripotent stem cells from mouse embryonic and adult fibroblast cultures by defined factors. *Cell,* 126, 4, pp. 663-676.

Taniuchi, I., Osato, M., Egawa, T., Sunshine, M.J., Bae, S.C., Komori, T., Ito, Y. & Littman, D.R. (2002). Differential requirements for Runx proteins in CD4 repression and epigenetic silencing during T lymphocyte development. *Cell,* 111, 5, pp. 621-633.

Terszowski, G., Waskow, C., Conradt, P., Lenze, D., Koenigsmann, J., Carstanjen, D., Horak, I. & Rodewald, H.R. (2005). Prospective isolation and global gene expression analysis of the erythrocyte colony-forming unit (CFU-E). *Blood,* 105, 5, pp. 1937-1945.

Theilgaard-Monch, K., Jacobsen, L.C., Borup, R., Rasmussen, T., Bjerregaard, M.D., Nielsen, F.C., Cowland, J.B. & Borregaard, N. (2005). The transcriptional program of terminal granulocytic differentiation. *Blood,* 105, 4, pp. 1785-1796.

Treiber, T., Mandel, E.M., Pott, S., Gyory, I., Firner, S., Liu, E.T. & Grosschedl, R. (2010). Early B cell factor 1 regulates B cell gene networks by activation, repression, and transcription- independent poising of chromatin. *Immunity,* 32, 5, pp. 714-725.

Trifari, S., Kaplan, C.D., Tran, E.H., Crellin, N.K. & Spits, H. (2009). Identification of a human helper T cell population that has abundant production of interleukin 22 and is distinct from T(H)-17, T(H)1 and T(H)2 cells. *Nat Immunol,* 10, 8, pp. 864-871.

Trowbridge, J.J., Snow, J.W., Kim, J. & Orkin, S.H. (2009). DNA methyltransferase 1 is essential for and uniquely regulates hematopoietic stem and progenitor cells. *Cell Stem Cell,* 5, 4, pp. 442-449.

Tsapogas, P., Zandi, S., Ahsberg, J., Zetterblad, J., Welinder, E., Jonsson, J.I., Mansson, R., Qian, H. & Sigvardsson, M. (2011). IL-7 mediates Ebf-1-dependent lineage restriction in early lymphoid progenitors. *Blood,* 118, 5, pp. 1283-1290.

Tunyaplin, C., Shaffer, A.L., Angelin-Duclos, C.D., Yu, X., Staudt, L.M. & Calame, K.L. (2004). Direct repression of prdm1 by Bcl-6 inhibits plasmacytic differentiation. *J Immunol,* 173, 2, pp. 1158-1165.

Van de Walle, I., De Smet, G., De Smedt, M., Vandekerckhove, B., Leclercq, G., Plum, J. & Taghon, T. (2009). An early decrease in Notch activation is required for human TCR-alphabeta lineage differentiation at the expense of TCR-gammadelta T cells. *Blood,* 113, 13, pp. 2988-2998.

Vanvalkenburgh, J., Albu, D.I., Bapanpally, C., Casanova, S., Califano, D., Jones, D.M., Ignatowicz, L., Kawamoto, S., Fagarasan, S., Jenkins, N.A., Copeland, N.G., Liu, P. & Avram, D. (2011). Critical role of Bcl11b in suppressor function of T regulatory cells and prevention of inflammatory bowel disease. *J Exp Med,* pp.

Veldhoen, M., Uyttenhove, C., van Snick, J., Helmby, H., Westendorf, A., Buer, J., Martin, B., Wilhelm, C. & Stockinger, B. (2008). Transforming growth factor-beta 'reprograms' the differentiation of T helper 2 cells and promotes an interleukin 9-producing subset. *Nat Immunol,* 9, 12, pp. 1341-1346.

Velu, C.S., Baktula, A.M. & Grimes, H.L. (2009). Gfi1 regulates miR-21 and miR-196b to control myelopoiesis. *Blood,* 113, 19, pp. 4720-4728.

Ventura, A., Young, A.G., Winslow, M.M., Lintault, L., Meissner, A., Erkeland, S.J., Newman, J., Bronson, R.T., Crowley, D., Stone, J.R., Jaenisch, R., Sharp, P.A. & Jacks, T. (2008). Targeted deletion reveals essential and overlapping functions of the miR-17 through 92 family of miRNA clusters. *Cell,* 132, 5, pp. 875-886.

Verbeek, W., Lekstrom-Himes, J., Park, D.J., Dang, P.M., Vuong, P.T., Kawano, S., Babior, B.M., Xanthopoulos, K. & Koeffler, H.P. (1999). Myeloid transcription factor C/EBPepsilon is involved in the positive regulation of lactoferrin gene expression in neutrophils. *Blood,* 94, 9, pp. 3141-3150.

Vire, E., Brenner, C., Deplus, R., Blanchon, L., Fraga, M., Didelot, C., Morey, L., Van Eynde, A., Bernard, D., Vanderwinden, J.M., Bollen, M., Esteller, M., Di Croce, L., de Launoit, Y. & Fuks, F. (2006). The Polycomb group protein EZH2 directly controls DNA methylation. *Nature,* 439, 7078, pp. 871-874.

Walter, K., Bonifer, C. & Tagoh, H. (2008). Stem cell-specific epigenetic priming and B cell-specific transcriptional activation at the mouse Cd19 locus. *Blood,* 112, 5, pp. 1673-1682.

Walunas, T.L., Wang, B., Wang, C.R. & Leiden, J.M. (2000). Cutting edge: the Ets1 transcription factor is required for the development of NK T cells in mice. *J Immunol,* 164, 6, pp. 2857-2860.

Wang, L., Wildt, K.F., Zhu, J., Zhang, X., Feigenbaum, L., Tessarollo, L., Paul, W.E., Fowlkes, B.J. & Bosselut, R. (2008). Distinct functions for the transcription factors GATA-3 and ThPOK during intrathymic differentiation of CD4(+) T cells. *Nat Immunol,* 9, 10, pp. 1122-1130.

Wang, Q., Huang, Z., Xue, H., Jin, C., Ju, X.L., Han, J.D. & Chen, Y.G. (2008). MicroRNA miR-24 inhibits erythropoiesis by targeting activin type I receptor ALK4. *Blood,* 111, 2, pp. 588-595.

Wang, W., Wang, X., Ward, A.C., Touw, I.P. & Friedman, A.D. (2001). C/EBPalpha and G-CSF receptor signals cooperate to induce the myeloperoxidase and neutrophil elastase genes. *Leukemia,* 15, 5, pp. 779-786.

Warr, M.R., Pietras, E.M. & Passegue, E. (2011). Mechanisms controlling hematopoietic stem cell functions during normal hematopoiesis and hematological malignancies. *Wiley Interdiscip Rev Syst Biol Med,* pp.

Weaver, C.H., Buckner, C.D., Longin, K., Appelbaum, F.R., Rowley, S., Lilleby, K., Miser, J., Storb, R., Hansen, J.A. & Bensinger, W. (1993). Syngeneic transplantation with peripheral blood mononuclear cells collected after the administration of recombinant human granulocyte colony-stimulating factor. *Blood,* 82, 7, pp. 1981-1984.

Weber, B.N., Chi, A.W., Chavez, A., Yashiro-Ohtani, Y., Yang, Q., Shestova, O. & Bhandoola, A. (2011). A critical role for TCF-1 in T-lineage specification and differentiation. *Nature,* 476, 7358, pp. 63-68.

Weishaupt, H., Sigvardsson, M. & Attema, J.L. (2010). Epigenetic chromatin states uniquely define the developmental plasticity of murine hematopoietic stem cells. *Blood,* 115, 2, pp. 247-256.

Weissman, I.L. & Shizuru, J.A. (2008). The origins of the identification and isolation of hematopoietic stem cells, and their capability to induce donor-specific transplantation tolerance and treat autoimmune diseases. *Blood,* 112, 9, pp. 3543-3553.

Wernig, M., Meissner, A., Foreman, R., Brambrink, T., Ku, M., Hochedlinger, K., Bernstein, B.E. & Jaenisch, R. (2007). In vitro reprogramming of fibroblasts into a pluripotent ES-cell-like state. *Nature,* 448, 7151, pp. 318-324.

Wildin, R.S., Ramsdell, F., Peake, J., Faravelli, F., Casanova, J.L., Buist, N., Levy-Lahad, E., Mazzella, M., Goulet, O., Perroni, L., Bricarelli, F.D., Byrne, G., McEuen, M., Proll, S., Appleby, M. & Brunkow, M.E. (2001). X-linked neonatal diabetes mellitus, enteropathy and endocrinopathy syndrome is the human equivalent of mouse scurfy. *Nat Genet,* 27, 1, pp. 18-20.

Wilson, A. & Trumpp, A. (2006). Bone-marrow haematopoietic-stem-cell niches. *Nat Rev Immunol,* 6, 2, pp. 93-106.

Wilson, N.J., Boniface, K., Chan, J.R., McKenzie, B.S., Blumenschein, W.M., Mattson, J.D., Basham, B., Smith, K., Chen, T., Morel, F., Lecron, J.C., Kastelein, R.A., Cua, D.J., McClanahan, T.K., Bowman, E.P. & de Waal Malefyt, R. (2007). Development, cytokine profile and function of human interleukin 17-producing helper T cells. *Nat Immunol,* 8, 9, pp. 950-957.

Wu, H., Liu, X., Jaenisch, R. & Lodish, H.F. (1995). Generation of committed erythroid BFU-E and CFU-E progenitors does not require erythropoietin or the erythropoietin receptor. *Cell,* 83, 1, pp. 59-67.

Wu, S.M. & Hochedlinger, K. (2011). Harnessing the potential of induced pluripotent stem cells for regenerative medicine. *Nat Cell Biol,* 13, 5, pp. 497-505.

Xiao, C., Calado, D.P., Galler, G., Thai, T.H., Patterson, H.C., Wang, J., Rajewsky, N., Bender, T.P. & Rajewsky, K. (2007). MiR-150 controls B cell differentiation by targeting the transcription factor c-Myb. *Cell,* 131, 1, pp. 146-159.

Xie, H., Ye, M., Feng, R. & Graf, T. (2004). Stepwise reprogramming of B cells into macrophages. *Cell,* 117, 5, pp. 663-676.

Xu, L., Kitani, A., Fuss, I. & Strober, W. (2007). Cutting edge: regulatory T cells induce CD4+CD25-Foxp3- T cells or are self-induced to become Th17 cells in the absence of exogenous TGF-beta. *J Immunol,* 178, 11, pp. 6725-6729.

Yamanaka, R., Barlow, C., Lekstrom-Himes, J., Castilla, L.H., Liu, P.P., Eckhaus, M., Decker, T., Wynshaw-Boris, A. & Xanthopoulos, K.G. (1997). Impaired granulopoiesis, myelodysplasia, and early lethality in CCAAT/enhancer binding protein epsilon-deficient mice. *Proc Natl Acad Sci U S A,* 94, 24, pp. 13187-13192.

Yekta, S., Shih, I.H. & Bartel, D.P. (2004). MicroRNA-directed cleavage of HOXB8 mRNA. *Science,* 304, 5670, pp. 594-596.

Yi, T., Chen, Y., Wang, L., Du, G., Huang, D., Zhao, D., Johnston, H., Young, J., Todorov, I., Umetsu, D.T., Chen, L., Iwakura, Y., Kandeel, F., Forman, S. & Zeng, D. (2009). Reciprocal differentiation and tissue-specific pathogenesis of Th1, Th2, and Th17 cells in graft-versus-host disease. *Blood,* 114, 14, pp. 3101-3112.

Yu, D., Rao, S., Tsai, L.M., Lee, S.K., He, Y., Sutcliffe, E.L., Srivastava, M., Linterman, M., Zheng, L., Simpson, N., Ellyard, J.I., Parish, I.A., Ma, C.S., Li, Q.J., Parish, C.R., Mackay, C.R. & Vinuesa, C.G. (2009). The transcriptional repressor Bcl-6 directs T follicular helper cell lineage commitment. *Immunity,* 31, 3, pp. 457-468.

Zandi, S., Mansson, R., Tsapogas, P., Zetterblad, J., Bryder, D. & Sigvardsson, M. (2008). EBF1 is essential for B-lineage priming and establishment of a transcription factor network in common lymphoid progenitors. *J Immunol,* 181, 5, pp. 3364-3372.

Zarebski, A., Velu, C.S., Baktula, A.M., Bourdeau, T., Horman, S.R., Basu, S., Bertolone, S.J., Horwitz, M., Hildeman, D.A., Trent, J.O. & Grimes, H.L. (2008). Mutations in growth factor independent-1 associated with human neutropenia block murine granulopoiesis through colony stimulating factor-1. *Immunity,* 28, 3, pp. 370-380.

Zhan, M., Miller, C.P., Papayannopoulou, T., Stamatoyannopoulos, G. & Song, C.Z. (2007). MicroRNA expression dynamics during murine and human erythroid differentiation. *Exp Hematol,* 35, 7, pp. 1015-1025.

Zhang, P., Iwasaki-Arai, J., Iwasaki, H., Fenyus, M.L., Dayaram, T., Owens, B.M., Shigematsu, H., Levantini, E., Huettner, C.S., Lekstrom-Himes, J.A., Akashi, K. & Tenen, D.G. (2004). Enhancement of hematopoietic stem cell repopulating capacity and self-renewal in the absence of the transcription factor C/EBP alpha. *Immunity,* 21, 6, pp. 853-863.

Zheng, S.G., Wang, J., Wang, P., Gray, J.D. & Horwitz, D.A. (2007). IL-2 is essential for TGF-beta to convert naive CD4+CD25- cells to CD25+Foxp3+ regulatory T cells and for expansion of these cells. *J Immunol,* 178, 4, pp. 2018-2027.

Zhuang, Y., Soriano, P. & Weintraub, H. (1994). The helix-loop-helix gene E2A is required for B cell formation. *Cell,* 79, 5, pp. 875-884.

2

Negative Regulation of Haematopoiesis: Role of Inhibitory Adaptors

Laura Velazquez
UMR U978 Inserm/Université Paris 13, UFR SMBH, Bobigny
France

1. Introduction

Cytokine signalling is initiated through ligand interaction with specific members of the cytokine receptor superfamily. The subsequent receptor oligomerization and conformational change result in activation of either an intrinsic kinase domain or receptor associated kinases, notably the Janus (JAK) family of cytoplasmic tyrosine kinases. The activated JAKs phosphorylate tyrosine residues in the receptor and subsequently downstream substrates, such as the signal transducers and activators of transcription (STAT) proteins. Once recruited to the receptor complex, STAT proteins are themselves phosphorylated on tyrosine, dimerize and translocate into the nucleus, where they activate the transcription of genes mediating cytokine-induced responses (Ortmann et al., 2000). Cytokines also activate other signaling cascades, such as the Ras/Mitogen-Activated Protein Kinase (MAPK) and the Phosphoinositide 3-kinase (PI3K)/Akt pathways. These cascades have been implicated in the proliferation, survival, and differentiation of several cell types in the haematopoietic system (Geest and Coffer, 2009; Leevers et al., 1999. However, all these signalling pathways require precise cellular control and their deregulation has been implicated in haematopoietic disorders, autoimmune and chronic inflammatory diseases and cancer, making it important to understand the mechanisms by which these cytokine-mediated signalling pathways are controlled (Schade et al., 2006; Khwaja, 2006).

It is therefore not surprising that multiple levels of control have evolved to finely modulate the threshold, magnitude and specific responses elicited by cytokine stimulation. This regulation is achieved through both positive and negative mechanisms. The aim of the present chapter is to review the current advances in the regulation of haematopoiesis, with special interest on inhibitory pathways. Understanding how haematopoiesis is modulated is essential to provide useful information on its physiological functioning, the pathological origin of many related haematological disorders and to yield potential therapeutic targets.

2. Regulation of cytokine signalling pathways: Role of adaptor proteins

Cytokine binding to their receptors results in tyrosine autophosphorylation of the associated tyrosine kinase and of the receptor cytoplasmic domain at sites where specific signalling molecules can bind. In this way, the cytoplasmic domain of these cytokine receptors serves to initially localize the signalling response to the plasma membrane. It is the combination of the signalling proteins that are recruited to the receptor that then determines the quality of the response that is generated. Indeed, the location of the proteins inside the cell and the kinetics of their activation are important features of signal-transduction pathways. How the signalling molecules are localized in the cell and how the strength and quality of the signal is regulated is an area of intense research, and increasing attention has focused on the so-called adaptor proteins as key molecules controlling these more complex aspects of signal transduction.

Adaptor proteins lack enzymatic activity or other direct effector function. Adaptors can be transmembrane proteins, reside in the cytoplasm under resting conditions and be recruited to the membrane upon activation, or be localized by specific interactions in intracellular compartments. Regardless of their cellular localization, they possess an array of binding sites and modules that allow them to mediate specific protein-protein and protein-lipid interactions. Examples of binding domains in adaptors include Src-homology 2 (SH2) and Phosphotyrosine-binding (PTB) domains that bind to phosphotyrosine motifs, SH3 domains that bind to proline-rich sequences and Pleckstrin homology (PH) domain that recognizes phospholipids (Pawson and Scott, 1996). With an assemblage of modules and binding sequences, a single adaptor can serve as a scaffold protein for the binding of multiple proteins into complexes, bringing in this way effectors into close proximity to their targets. However, the general ability of adaptor proteins to amplify or inhibit signalling, highly depends on their cell-specific expression and level, as well as on that of their binding partners, their location in the cell, the stability of the interactions between the adaptor and its targets and in certain conditions, on the basal kinase/phosphatase activity in the cell.

Lastly, it should be noted that the domains and motifs found in adaptors are also frequently present in enzymatically active molecules, such as tyrosine phosphatases of the SH2-containing phosphatase (SHP) family and the ubiquitin ligases Casitas B-cell lineage lymphoma (c-Cbl) proteins, where they can mediate true adaptor-like functions and also orchestrate signalling complex formation.

3. Inhibitory adaptors in cytokine signalling regulation

New insights into the biology of adaptor protein function have been possible with the use of a variety of biochemical, cellular and imaging techniques, as well as *in vivo* genetic approaches. All these techniques have helped establish that adaptor proteins can affect the thresholds and the dynamics of signalling reactions by coordinating positive and negative feedback signals. Over the years, the majority of investigations on cytokine signalling pathways have mainly focused on the mechanisms of cytokine-receptor activation, whereas our knowledge of negative regulation has been less explored. However, the most recent research has placed increasing emphasis on the mechanisms by which cytokine signals are attenuated or terminated. Indeed, stringent mechanisms of signal attenuation are essential for ensuring an appropriate, controlled cellular response following cytokine stimulation. One could imagine how the aberrant assembly of macromolecular active signalling complexes could lead to disease: excess positive signalling or insufficient negative signalling may lead to autoimmunity, chronic inflammation or malignant transformation, while excess negative signalling or insufficient positive signalling may lead to immunodeficiency or certain haematological disorders.

A number of mechanisms have been proposed to regulate the initiation, duration, magnitude and specificity of cytokine signalling at multiple levels: 1) receptor internalization and inhibition mediated by soluble receptor antagonists and/or specific inhibitors (such as the Lnk and Dok adaptor proteins); 2) tyrosine dephosphorylation of the receptor and signalling intermediates mediated by tyrosine phosphatases; 3) proteosomal degradation of signalling molecules mediated by the suppressors of cytokine signalling (SOCS) proteins and the Cbl E3 ubiquitin ligases proteins; and lastly 4) transcriptional suppression mediated by specific inhibitors such as the protein inhibitors of activated STATs (PIAS) proteins. In this section, we review what is currently known about the function and regulation of four families of inhibitory adaptor proteins that are key players in some of the regulatory mechanisms mentioned above. These families are the DOK, the Lnk/SH2B3, the Cbl and the SOCS proteins. We first discuss the adaptors without catalytic activity (DOK and Lnk), followed by those possessing an enzymatic function (Cbl and SOCS). The latter ones are also known as scaffold proteins; however we will refer to them as adaptors in hopes that this distinction provides a clear picture on the different properties of each.

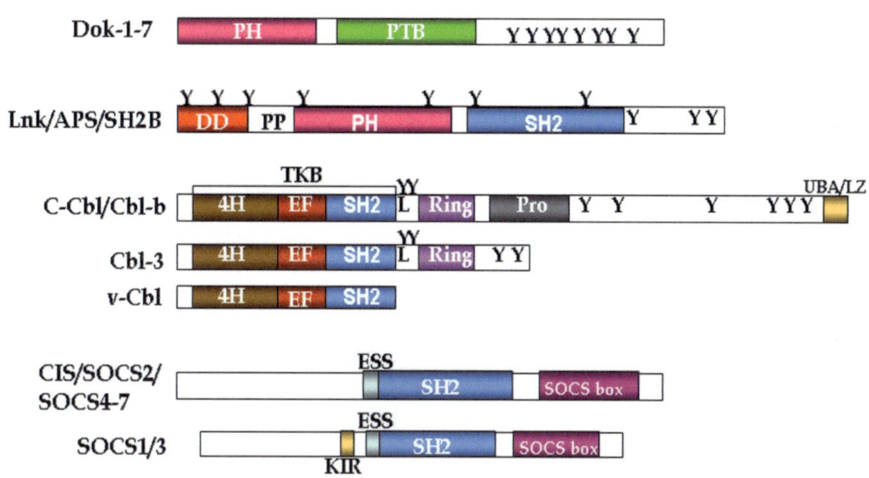

Fig. 1. Schematic representation of the domain structure of inhibitory adaptors

3.1 The DOK family

3.1.1 Structure and cell expression

The Dok (Downstream Of Tyrosine Kinases) family of adaptor proteins consists of seven members, Dok 1 to Dok-7, that differ in the length of their C-terminal region. They are all characterized by an N-terminal PH domain, a central PTB domain and multiple SH2 and SH3 binding motifs in the C-terminal region (Figure 1). Dok-1 ($p62^{dok}$), Dok-2 ($p56^{dok-2}$, also called Dok-R, or FRIP) and Dok-3 (also called DokL) are preferentially expressed in the haematopoietic compartment, as well as co-expressed in haematopoietic progenitors (Carpino et al., 1997; Yamanashi et al., 1997; Di Cristofano et al., 1998; Lemay et al., 2000). All three Dok proteins are expressed in myeloid cells, but differ in their lymphoid lineage expression. While Dok-1 and Dok-2 are highly expressed in T cells, Dok-3 is little or not detected at all. In contrast, Dok-1 and Dok-3 are expressed in B cells, while Dok-2 is not normally detected in these cells. Moreover, several studies have demonstrated that Dok-1 and Dok-2 expression was up or down-regulated, respectively, by different signalling pathways in immune cells. Dok-1 expression was upregulated in response to the glucocorticoid dexamethasone in RBL-2H3 mast cells (Hiragun et al., 2005). By contrast, its expression was downregulated in bone marrow-derived macrophages in response to lipopolysaccharide (LPS) [Shinohara et al., 2005]. As for Dok-2, its expression increased in response to cytokines such as M-CSF, granulocyte–macrophage colony stimulating factor (GM-CSF), and interleukin-3 (IL-3) in NFS-60 myeloid leukemia cells, suggesting its implication in a negative feedback loop for the regulation of these cytokine pathways (Suzu et al., 2000). The other Dok proteins, Dok-4 (IRS5), Dok-5 (IRS6), Dok-6 and Dok-7 are mainly expressed in non-haematopoietic cells, notably in neural cells. However, Dok-4 was reported to function as negative regulator in human T cells (Favre et al., 2003).

Dok protein	Binding domain	Binding partner	Signalling Receptor
Dok-1	PTB	Abl	BCR
		SHIP-1	FcγRIIB
		Dok-1, Dok-2	CD2
		TCRε	idem
	pY	CD3ε	idem
		p120RasGap	BCR, CD2+CD28, FcεRI
		Abl, Lyn	BCR
		Nck	FcεRI
		SHIP-1	FcγRIIB, FcεRI
Dok-2	PTB	SHIP-1	FcγRIIB
		Dok-1, Dok-2	CD2
		TCRε, CD3ε	idem
	pY	p120RasGAP,Abl	BCR
		Nck	TCR
Dok-3	PTB	SHIP-1, Abl	FcγRIIB
		Dok-3	BCR
	pY	Grb2	BCR
		SHIP-1	FcγRIIB

Table 1. Signalling partners bound to the different domains and motifs of Dok proteins

3.1.2 Signalling partners

The biological functions of the Dok proteins have been defined with the identification and functional analysis of their binding partners, as well as of their subcellular localization. Dok-1 was the first member of this family identified as a tyrosine-phosphorylated 62 kDa substrate of both v-ABL and BCR-ABL and associated with p120RasGap, a negative regulator of Ras. Several studies have later shown that Dok-1/2/3 can be tyrosine phosphorylated by a variety of growth factors, cytokines and immuno receptors, providing multiple docking sites for SH2 and PTB-containing proteins such as Nck, SHP-1, SHIP-1 and p120RasGap (Table 1). The interaction between p120RasGap and Dok-1/2 has been the most extensively studied and the one likely responsible for the negative regulation of the Ras/Erk pathway mediated by the Dok adaptors. It involves the SH2 domain of p120RasGap and its binding motifs present in the C-terminal moiety of Dok-1/2 (Songyang et al., 2001). In contrast, Dok-3 protein has no YxxP motifs and therefore is unable to associate with p120 RasGap. However, it can negatively regulate Erk activation through its binding with Grb2 (Honma et al., 2006). Fewer signalling molecules have been reported to associate with the PTB domain of Dok-1/2/3 (Table 1). Interestingly, these Dok proteins show homotypic and heterotypic (for Dok-1/2) oligomerization that is dependent on their tyrosine phosphorylation and PTB domains. Moreover, this oligomerization appears crucial to their function, at least for Dok-1/2 (Boulay et al., 2005). Instead, the functional relevance of Dok-3 oligomerization is not yet clear (Stork et al., 2007). The presence of a PH domain in the structure of Dok proteins suggests an important role for this domain in the localization or translocation of the Dok adaptors to cellular membranes. Indeed, it seems that Dok-1 and PI3K activity are required for the recruitment of the adaptor to the membrane and its negative effect on PDGF-mediated ERK activation. Furthermore, Dok-1/2 PH domain can bind tightly to PI(5)P and modulate the negative function and tyrosine phosphorylation of the adaptors in T-cells (Guittard et al., 2009). Conversely, the PH domain of Dok-3 is important for its localization to the membrane in B cells (Stork et al., 2007).

3.1.3 Signalling pathways in immune cells

Studies with Dok-1/2/3 deficient mice and/or cells have helped demonstrate the physiological importance of these inhibitory adaptors to the function and development of immune cells. Using *Dok-1*-deficient splenic B cells, Yamanashi et al. demonstrated a negative role of Dok-1 in antigen receptor-mediated signalling through suppression of MAPK activity and cell proliferation (Yamanashi et al., 2000). Moreover, co-cross-linking of the B-cell receptor (BCR) and FcγRIIB receptor induces the tyrosine phosphorylation of Dok-1 and its subsequent association with RasGap (Vuica et al., 1997). In FcγRIIB signalling, Dok-1 is recruited to the receptor complex at the membrane via SHIP, and in this way, contributes to the negative regulation of the Erk pathway [Figure 2.] (Tamir et al., 2000). On the other hand, Dok-3 is also expressed in B cells and therefore, one can expect a functional redundancy between Dok-1/3 in these cells. Indeed, it was reported that Dok-3 can function as a negative regulator of BCR-mediated responses (Ng et al., 2007). Furthermore, both Dok-1 and Dok-3 were shown to be phosphorylated by Lyn kinase after stimulation of the BCR, suggesting that Lyn can activate these Dok proteins to then function as negative regulators in B cells (Yamanashi et al., 2000; Stork et al., 2007). However, B cells from *Dok-3*-deficient mice exhibited augmented proliferation and $Ca2^{+}$ influx upon BCR stimulation (Ng et al., 2007), while these responses are not observed in the absence of Dok-1 (Yamanashi et al., 2000). These phenotypic differences could be attributed to Dok-1, but not Dok-3, recruiting p120RasGAP, which can inhibit Ras/Erk signalling; by contrast, Dok-3, but not Dok-1, can recruit Grb2, which can then inhibit $Ca2^{+}$ signalling in B cells.

Dok-1 and Dok-2 adaptor proteins have been also shown to play a role in the maintenance of T-cell homeostasis. In some cell line systems, Dok-1 is phosphorylated by Lck kinase and associates with RasGap upon CD2 and CD28 stimulation, but not CD3-TCR engagement, indicating a possible role of Dok-1 in T cell signalling (Nemorin & Duplay, 2000). Furthermore, overexpression of Dok-2 results in a dramatic reduction in both thymocytes and splenic T-cell numbers, suggesting a negative role of Dok-2 in T-cell development

(Gugasyan et al., 2002). Although the molecular mechanisms underlying the Dok-mediated inhibition are unclear, Dok proteins can bind to the ITAM motifs of TCRζ and CD3ε through their PTB domain. As these ITAMs are essential for the binding and activation of ZAP-70, interference between the Dok proteins and ZAP-70 might occur through their binding to the ITAMs (Figure 2). Recently, Nunès and colleagues reported that the PH domain of Dok-1 and Dok-2 is necessary for the tyrosine phosphorylation of these Dok proteins and their negative functions in T cells (Guittard et al., 2009). These results demonstrate the functional relevance of the membrane localization of the Dok adaptors.

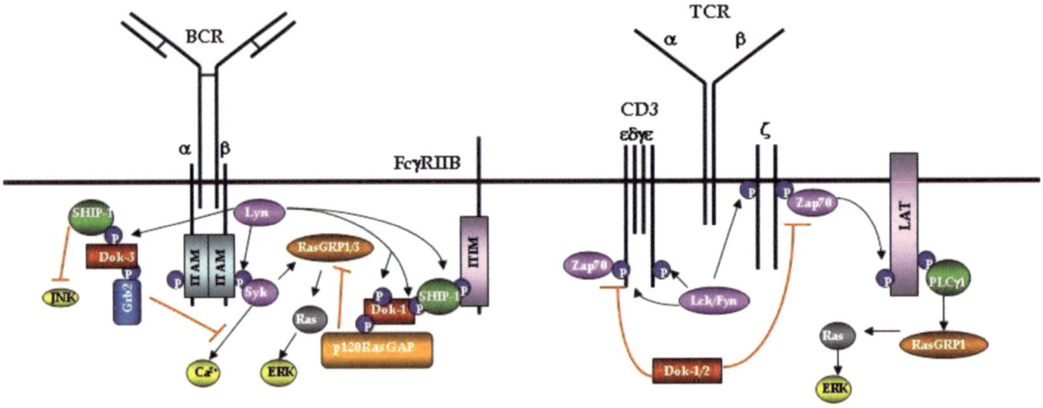

Fig. 2. Dok-mediated signalling pathways in immune cells

Unlike lymphoid cells, myeloid cells express all the immune cell Dok proteins. However, the loss of Dok-1 and Dok-2 causes mainly neoplastic abnormalities in myeloid cells, suggesting an important role in immune and cytokine receptor signalling in these cells. Analysis of *Dok-1* and *Dok-2* deficient myeloid cells showed enhanced proliferation and survival in response to Stem Cell Factor (SCF), IL-3, macrophage-colony stimulating factor (M-CSF), and granulocyte-monocyte-colony stimulating factor (GM-CSF), which are cytokines crucial for myelopoiesis. These findings indicate that Dok-1 and Dok-2 act as key negative regulators of signalling downstream of these cytokine receptors. Indeed, the activation of Erk and Akt in macrophages deficient for *Dok-1* and *Dok-2* was strongly augmented compared with that in wild type controls upon M-CSF receptor stimulation, confirming the role of Dok adaptors as negative regulators for these pathways. On the other hand, the role of Dok-1 and Dok-2 was examined in innate immune signalling in macrophages. Stimulation of macrophages by LPS induces rapid tyrosine phosphorylation of Dok-1 and Dok-2, suggesting the involvement of these adaptors in TLR4 signalling (Shinohara et al., 2005). In addition, the stimulation of *Dok-1* or *Dok-2*-deficient macrophages promoted the activation of Erk and hyperproduction of TNF-α and nitric oxide, two major signalling mediators of innate immunity, indicating that the Dok proteins are key negative regulators of TLR4 signalling in macrophages. The Dok adaptors are also expressed in mast cells where they have been shown to interact exclusively with negative regulators of FcεRI signalling. FcεRI stimulation leads to the tyrosine phosphorylation of only Dok-1 and Dok-2. Nevertheless, Dok-3 associates with tyrosine-phosphorylated proteins upon FcεRI stimulation, implicating a yet undefined function for this adaptor protein downstream of the receptor (Abramson et al., 2003). A complex of Dok-1, RasGAP, and SHIP-1, similar to the one described in B cells after co-aggregation of the BCR with FcγRIIB, was also described in mast cells after FcεRI and FcγRIIB co-aggregation (Ott et al., 2002). Moreover, Dok-1 has also been involved downstream of activating receptors, like FcεRI, by associating with and negatively regulating signals without the involvement of inhibitory receptors (Ott et al., 2002; Abramson et al., 2003). However, *Dok-1*-deficiency did not affect mast cell activation, suggesting a possible functional redundancy among the different isoforms expressed in these cells.

Recently, two groups have reported the expression and function of the Dok proteins in human platelets. Using a proteomic approach in these cells, it was shown that Dok proteins are tyrosine phosphorylated downstream of main platelet activation receptors (Garcia et al., 2004; Hughan et al., 2007; Senis et al., 2009). Tyrosine phosphorylation of Dok-1 and Dok-3 was primarily Src kinase-independent downstream of the integrin pathway, whereas it was Src-dependent downstream of glycoprotein VI (GPVI) pathway. Both proteins interact in an inducible-fashion with Grb-2 and SHIP-1 in fibrinogen-spread platelets, suggesting that the formation of a multi-molecular negative signalling complex may be a mechanism of down-regulating αIIbβ3 outside-in signalling.

3.2 The Lnk/SH2B family

3.2.1 Structure, origin and cell expression

The Lnk (or SH2B) family of adaptor proteins is composed of 3 members, SH2-B [also known as PSM (proline-rich, PH and SH2 domain-containing signalling mediator) or SH2B1], APS (for Adaptor protein with PH and SH2 domain, also known as SH2B2) and Lnk (SH2B3). They all possess a dimerization (DD) domain and proline-rich motifs at the N-terminus, followed by a PH and SH2 domains, and several potential tyrosine phosphorylation sites, notably a conserved tyrosine residue at the C-terminus [Figure 1](Rudd, 2001). The *SH2B1* gene encodes four isoforms (α, β, γ, δ) resulting from alternative mRNA splicing at their 3′ terminus giving rise to proteins differing at their C-terminus (Nelms et al., 1999). SH2-Bα and β isoforms were originally cloned from yeast tribrid and two-hybrid systems screening, respectively, using different proteins as baits (Osborne et al., 1995; Riedel et al, 1997; Rui et al., 1997). Despite its initial identification in immune cells, SH2-B isoforms are mainly expressed and functional, as shown by gene inactivation in mice, in non-haematopoietic tissues. The *APS/SH2B2* gene encodes for two isoforms, SH2B2α and recently identified SH2B2β (Li et al., 2007). The APS protein was also identified in a two-hybrid system screening of human B cells or adipocytes (Yokouchi et al., 1997; Moodie et al., 1999). Like SH2-B, APS adaptor protein is also highly expressed in non-haematopoietic tissues. However, it is also expressed in haematopoietic cells, notably in mature B and mast cells. As for Lnk, it has only one form in mammalians and one invertebrate orthologue in *Drosophila melanogaster* (D-Lnk) to date (Werz et al., 2009). The Lnk adaptor protein was the first member of this family identified (Huang et al., 1995; Takaki et al., 1997). However, it was later found that the Lnk protein was much larger than initially reported (Li et al., 2000; Takaki et al., 2000; Velazquez et al., 2002). In contrast to SH2-B and APS, Lnk is mainly expressed in haematopoietic cells, notably in haematopoietic stem cells (HSC), and haematopoietic (lymphoid and myeloid) progenitors. Moreover, Lnk expression is up-regulated by certain cytokines important for the development and function of these haematopoietic cells, such as SCF, thrombopoietin [TPO], and erythropoietin [EPO] (Kent et al., 2008; Buza-Vidas et al., 2006; Gerry et al., 2009a, 2009b; Baran-Marszak et al., 2010). Interestingly, Lnk is also highly expressed in endothelial cells and its expression is also induced by Tumor Necrosis Factor (TNF)-α (Fitau et al., 2006; Kwon et al., 2009). These findings suggest the implication of Lnk adaptor in a negative feedback loop for the regulation of these cytokine pathways.

3.2.2 Signalling partners

Over the last years, much effort has gone into understanding the role of the Lnk family as signalling regulators through the identification of the molecules binding to their different functional domains and motifs, as well as their signalling pathways (Table. 2). The SH2 domain of the Lnk adaptor proteins is implicated in most of the key molecular interactions between the adaptors and their partners/effectors and their biological functions. The fist identified binding partner of the Lnk protein was the SCF receptor, Kit. The primary Kit-binding site for Lnk SH2 domain has been identified as phosphotyrosine 567 (pTyr567), which resides in the juxtamembrane region of the receptor (Simon et al., 2008; Gueller et al., 2008). Similarly, the SH2 domain of APS was reported to bind to Y568 and Y936 in the human c-Kit receptor (Wollberg et al., 2003). Interestingly, this region of Kit contains critical tyrosine (Y) residues (Y567/69) for the recruitment of different regulatory signalling molecules (Chan et al., 2003). In this system, a proposed mode of action of Lnk is that once bound to the juxtamembrane region of Kit, it will then block the association of activators with the receptor, resulting in down-regulation of SCF-mediated pathways. Indeed, expression of an SH2-inactive Lnk protein abolishes Lnk-mediated negative regulation of SCF-induced cell proliferation and migration (Simon et al., 2008). Lnk has been also reported to bind through its SH2 domain to other tyrosine kinase receptors, such as the PDGFR and the M-CSF receptor (c-Fms); however the physiological implication of these associations is not yet clear (Gueller et al., 2010, 2011).

The JAK2 tyrosine kinase was the first characterized binding partner of SH2-B and APS, and subsequently of Lnk. This association results in activation of the kinase in the case of SH2-B and APS or in its inhibition when bound to Lnk. Different biochemical studies have shown that the interaction of the SH2 domains of SH2-B and APS occurs preferentially with kinase-active, tyrosyl phosphorylated JAK2 (Rui et al., 1997). The primary JAK2-binding site for the SH2 domain of the Lnk family has been identified as pTyr813, which resides within the regulatory JH2 pseudokinase domain of JAK2 (Kurzer et al., 2004, 2006). Crystallographic studies have demonstrated that the SH2 domain of APS dimerizes when binding to the insulin receptor, whereas the SH2 domain of SH2-B, binds JAK2 as a monomer (Hu et al., 2003; Hu & Hubbard, 2006). Less is known on how the Lnk SH2 domain binds JAK2. However, it has been shown that Lnk is capable of binding JAK2 wild-type form, as well as the constitutive active JAK2-V617F form present in myeloproliferative neoplasms (Bersenev et al., 2008; Gery et al., 2009; Baran-Marszak et al., 2010). In addition to the SH2-dependent interaction of the Lnk adaptor family with pTyr813 in JAK2, there appears to be one low-affinity interaction involving amino acids outside the SH2 domain in the adaptors and inactive JAK2 that might prevent abnormal activation of the kinase. (Rui et al., 2000; Kurzer et al., 2006; Baran-Marzak et al., 2010).

The N-terminal region of the Lnk adaptor family contains a dimerization domain whose crystal structure has revealed a "phenylalanine zipper" motif. This domain mediates SH2-B

Lnk proteins	Binding domain	Binding partner	Cells System
Lnk	N-term	Lnk	COS
	Inter PH-SH2	ABP-280	COS, T cells (TCR)
	SH2	Kit	Mast (SCF)
		JAK2	Myeloid (EPO, TPO)
		c-Fms	Myeloid (M-CSF)
		PDGFR	COS (PDGF)
APS	N-term	APS, SH2B	HEK293, CHO (In)
	PH	Vav3	NIH3T3
	SH2	Kit	Mast (SCF)
		JAK2	Myeloid (GH)
		IR	Adipocyte (In)
	pY618	Cbl	Adipocyte (In)
SH2B	N-term	SH2B, APS	CHO (In), COS
		Rac	CHO, COS (GH)
	SH2	JAK2	Myeloid (GH)
		GHR, IR	Adipocyte (GH, In)

GHR, growth hormone receptor; IR, insulin receptor; In, insulin

Table 2. Signalling partners bound to the different domains and motifs of Lnk proteins.

and APS homo and heterodimerization that appears crucial to their function (Dhe-Paganon et al., 2004). Instead, Lnk homodimerization has only been shown in an over-expressed system (Takizawa et al., 2006) and therefore, its functional relevance is not yet clear.

The presence of a PH domain in the structure of Lnk proteins suggests an important role for this domain in the localization or translocation of these adaptor proteins to cellular membranes. Indeed, previous reports showed that Lnk PH mutants (W191A or W270A) proteins moderately affected Lnk modulation of TPO-, EPO- or SCF-dependent biological responses (Tong & Lodish, 2004; Tong et al., 2005; Simon et al., 2008). Moreover, the Lnk PH domain seemed to display moderate affinity and little specificity to phosphoinositides *in vitro*. It is therefore possible that the Lnk PH domain may down-regulate membrane targeting of Lnk in the absence of docking site for the SH2 domain and increase binding stability to membrane receptors when the SH2 domain is engaged.

Association of Lnk, APS and SH2-B with growth factor, cytokine receptors or the JAK2 kinase allows phosphorylation of these adaptors and their proper localization at the signalling complex. The conserved C-terminal tyrosine residue present in all members of this family has been shown to be a main site for phosphorylation upon growth factor or cytokine stimulation. In Lnk, this residue, Y536, was suggested to be phosphorylated upon SCF stimulation in a mast cell line (Takaki et al., 2002). However, an Lnk form mutated at this tyrosine still gets phosphorylated upon Kit activation in primary mast cells (Simon et al., 2008). This result suggested that Lnk could be phosphorylated at sites other than Y536. Indeed, a similar result was reported with human Lnk mutated at this residue (Li et al., 2000). On the other hand, the biological relevance of Lnk Y536 seems to depend on the signalling pathway analyzed. Lnk Y536 is dispensable for lymphoid development, TPO- or SCF-dependent signalling pathways, but it might play a regulatory role in IL3- and EPO-mediated proliferation (Takaki et al., 2003; Tong & Lodish, 2004; Simon et al., 2008).

However, no Lnk binding partners for this site has so far been identified. In contrast, APS C-terminal tyrosine, Y618, has been shown to get phosphorylated by activated growth factor (IR), cytokine (EPO) and immune (BCR) receptors and then serve as binding site for the Cbl protein (Moodie et al., 1999; Yokouchi et al., 1997; Wakioka et al., 1999). The APS/Cbl association plays an important role in down-regulation of IR signalling (Kishi et al., 2007). Other binding proteins have been identified that associate with other regions of Lnk, APS and SH2-B that are involved in actin regulation. In particular, an amino acid sequence in the N-terminal region of SH2-B has been shown to bind to Rac, a mayor actin regulating protein, while a similar sequence in APS can associate with Vav3, a guanine nucleotide exchange factor for Rac (Diakonova et al., 2002; Yabana and Shibuya, 2002). Lnk was demonstrated to associate with the actin binding protein ABP-280 via a sequence between the PH and SH2 domains of human Lnk in Jurkat T cells (He et al., 2000). These findings suggest a role for the Lnk family members in the regulation of actin cytoskeleton and cell motility.

3.2.3 Signalling pathways in haematopoietic cells

The initial *in vitro* biochemical analysis was done on SH2-B and APS and showed that these adaptors were phosphorylated and became positive mediators of receptor and protein tyrosine kinases cascades. However, APS can also function as negative regulator in the BCR and JAK2 signalling pathways (Yokouchi et al., 1997; Wakioka et al., 1999). Conversely, Lnk is considered as a negative regulator of growth factor and cytokine receptor-induced proliferation and migration (Takaki et al., 2000, 2002; Velazquez et al., 2002; Tong & Lodish, 2004; Tong et al., 2005; Fitau et al., 2006; Simon et al., 2008; Gueller et al., 2010, 2011). Nonetheless, Lnk seems to play a positive role in mouse platelets for the stabilization of thrombus through the integrin αIIbβ3 outside-in signalling and in human vascular endothelial cells via the PI3K/Akt pathway activated by TNF-α (Takizawa et al., 2010; Fitau et al., 2006). Together with data on *in vivo* ablation of these adaptors, these findings demonstrate that these adaptor proteins can function as positive and/or negative regulators depending on their cell expression and on the growth factor or cytokine receptor–mediated pathway.

The generation of mice and cell lines deficient for members of this family has confirmed Lnk and APS, but not SH2-B, specific function in the haematopoietic system, while establishing SH2-B implication in other tissues. As stated before, Lnk is highly expressed in HSC, so as expected, *Lnk*$^{-/-}$-derived HSC show an increased capacity to proliferate and to self-renew together with an increase in the quiescent fraction. These effects on HSC homeostasis are due to abnormal TPO signalling in these cells, that results from an enhanced TPO hypersensibility, increased TPO-dependent activation of Akt, STAT5 and down-regulation of p38MAPK (Ema et al., 2005; Buza-Vidas et al., 2006; Seita et al., 2007; Bersenev et al., 2008). These findings therefore confirm that Lnk controls TPO-induced self-renewal, quiescence and proliferation of HSC. Moreover, *Lnk* deficiency enhances the ability of HSC and haematopoietic progenitors to reconstitute the haematopoietic system in irradiated hosts. Indeed, transient inhibition of endogenous Lnk significantly increased the repopulating capacity of the transduced cells and thereby, engraftment (Takizawa et al., 2006). Moreover, analysis of *Lnk*$^{-/-}$-derived haematopoietic progenitors show an hypersensibility to several cytokines resulting in sustained MAPK, JAK/STAT activation and cell proliferation (Takaki et al., 2000; Velazquez et al., 2002; Tong, 2005; Takizawa et al., 2008).

Lnk-deficient mice have also revealed an essential role for Lnk in B cell lymphopoiesis with the selective expansion of pro-/pre-B and immature B cells in bone marrow and spleen. This abnormal proliferation is partly due to hypersensitivity to SCF and IL-7 (Takaki et al., 2000; Velazquez et al., 2002). Alternatively, Lnk over-expression in transgenic mice show impaired B production in an Lnk dose-dependent manner confirming the negative control mediated by this adaptor in B-lineage cell production (Takaki et al., 2003). However, no evident effect on mature B cells was observed in the absence of Lnk, suggesting either a lack of role for Lnk in this population or a functional compensation by APS in these cells. APS has also been shown to play a role in B cell development and function. Ablation of *APS* in mice caused an increase in B-1 cell number and an enhanced humoral immune response against a thymus-independent type 2 antigen, suggesting a role for APS in mature B cell proliferation (Iseki et al., 2004). Accordingly, APS transgenic mice showed reduced numbers of peritoneal B-1 and splenic B cells and impaired BCR-induced proliferation of mature B cells (Iseki et al., 2005). In these cells, APS co-localized with pre-activated capped BCR complexes and filamentous actin, indicating a negative regulatory role for APS in BCR signalling and actin reorganization.

Lnk has been also shown to control erythropoiesis and megakaryopoiesis. Studies on primary *Lnk*$^{-/-}$ erythrocytes and megakaryocytes indicate an abnormal proliferation due to the absence of negative regulation of EPO and TPO signalling pathways (Figure 3). Indeed, Lnk, through its SH2 domain, negatively modulates MPL, and EPO receptor (EPOR) signalling by attenuating three major signalling pathways: JAK2/STAT, MAPK and Akt (Tong et al., 2005; Tong & Lodish, 2004). Moreover, Lnk is capable of binding and regulating MPL-W515L and JAK2-V617F, the mutated forms expressed in Myeloproliferative Neoplasms [MPN] (Gery et al., 2007, 2009; Bersenev et al., 2008; Baran-Marszak et al., 2010). In addition, Lnk also regulates thrombopoiesis through control of crosstalk between integrin- and TPO-mediated pathways implicated in the megakaryocyte maturation and platelet release process (Takizawa et al., 2008). Furthermore, Lnk plays an important role in stabilizing thrombus formation through positive regulation of integrin signalling pathways. In this way, it contributes to platelet cytoskeleton rearrangement and spreading (Takizawa et al., 2010).

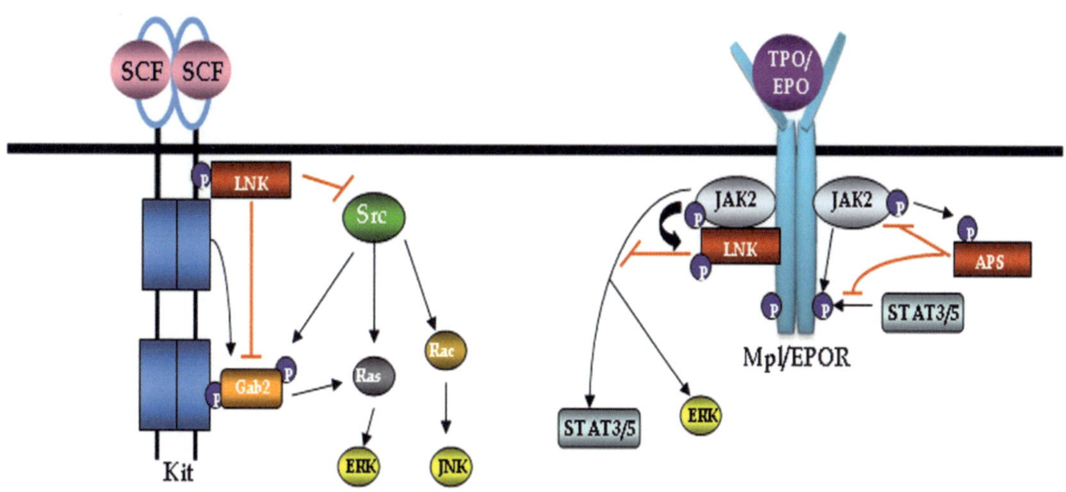

Fig. 3. Lnk family signalling pathways in haematopoietic cells

Studies on *Lnk-/-* and *APS-/-* mast cells demonstrated their physiological implication in mast-cell functions. Lnk regulates SCF-mediated signalling pathways controlling proliferation (MAPK and JNK) and migration (Rac and p38MAPK) in these cells (Takizawa et al., 2006; Simon et al., 2008). These functions are mainly mediated by binding of its SH2 domain to specific effectors involved in actin rearrangement. On the other hand, APS controls actin cytoskeleton and magnitude of degranulation induced by FcεRI receptor cross-linking (Kubo-Akashi et al., 2004). Besides its specific expression in the haematopoietic system, Lnk is also highly expressed in endothelial-like cells in the aorta-gonad-mesonephros (AGM) region and in endothelial progenitor (EPC) and mature cells [EC](Nobuhisa et al., 2003; Fitau et al., 2006; Kwon et al., 2009). Fitau *et al.* have shown that the pro-inflammatory cytokine TNF-α rapidly evokes Lnk phosphorylation together with down-regulation of vascular cell adhesion molecule 1 (VCAM-1) expression in activated vascular ECs. These results implicate Lnk as an important negative regulator of TNF-α signalling pathway (Fitau et al., 2006).

3.3 The Cbl family

3.3.1 Origin, cell expression and structure

The Cbl (for Casitas B-lineage Lymphoma) family comprises multidomain regulators with dual function, as E3 ubiquitin ligases and adaptor proteins. It consists of three mammalian homologues, c-Cbl, Cbl-b and Cbl-c/Cbl-3 (Blake et al., 1991; Keane et al., 1995, 1999), as well as invertebrate orthologues (Thien & Langdon, 2001). The first isoform of this family identified was the oncogenic protein v-Cbl, a Gag-fusion transforming protein of Cas NS-1 retrovirus, which induces pre- and pro-B lymphomas and the transformation of rodent fibroblasts (Langdon et al., 1989). The cellular form, c-Cbl was subsequently cloned and revealed that v-Cbl was a result of a large truncation of its C-terminal portion and that overexpression of c-Cbl did not promote tumorigenesis. The 120 kDa c-Cbl protein is ubiquitously expressed, primarily cytoplasmic, with highest expression levels in haematopoietic organs (thymus) and testis. In contrast, Cbl-3 is expressed mainly in epithelial cells of the gastrointestinal system.

All Cbl proteins share highly conserved N-terminal regions, but their C-terminal sequence differs and is less well-conserved (Figure 1). The N-terminal half encompasses two important domains: a tyrosine kinase-binding (TKB) and a C3HC4 zinc-binding RING finger domains, both separated by a small linker sequence. The TKB domain contains three distinct subdomains comprising a four-helix bundle (4H), a calcium-binding EF hand and a modified SH2 domain, all necessary for its function as phosphotyrosine-binding (PTB) module. The second conserved domain in the N-terminal region is a zinc-binding RING finger domain responsible for the E3 ubiquitin ligase activity of c-Cbl (Joazeiro et al., 1999). The C-terminal sequences are less homologous among Cbl proteins; however, they all have proline-rich regions that are involved in numerous SH3-domain interactions (Keane et al., 1995) and the major sites of tyrosine phosphorylation, which enable interactions of Cbl with SH2 domain containing proteins. The C-terminus of c-Cbl, Cbl-b contains a sequence homologous to both the leucine zipper (LZ) and the ubiquitin associated (UBA) domain. The LZ domain has been shown to mediate Cbl dimerization (Bartkiewicz et al., 1999; Liu et al., 2003), while only Cbl-b and not c-Cbl can bind to ubiquitin through its UBA domain (Davies et al., 2004).

3.3.2 Signalling binding partners

The TKB domain is unique to Cbl proteins and its feature role is to determine Cbl substrate specificity by engaging specific phosphorylated tyrosine residues on proteins that are to be ubiquitylated by Cbl. Some of Cbl TKB domain targets include: receptor tyrosine kinases (RTKs), non-receptor protein tyrosine kinases (PTKs) of the Syk family, several adaptors and regulatory proteins (Table 3). In contrast to SH2 binding motif, the TKB phosphotyrosine recognition consensus sequence displays an specificity conferred by amino acid residues C-terminal to the tyrosine (Lupher et al., 1997). These findings argue that interaction of the TKB domain with RTKs may then primarily be to ensure the appropriate orientation of the receptor such that Cbl's E3 ligase activity can promote the transfer of ubiquitin. TKB domain interactions may therefore determine the number of ubiquitin molecules transferred to the substrate and thus regulate the extent to which activated RTKs are ubiquitylated. Thus the TKB domain appears to have at least two important roles in regulating E3 ligase activity, and, as such, it is functionally more complex than classical SH2 or PTB domains.

Binding domain	Binding partner	Signalling receptor
TKB	Syk, Zap-70	AgR
	c-Src	AgR, GFR, CyR
	APS	HR
	EGFR, PDGFR	GFR
RING	E2s(Ub-conjugated enzyme)	GFR, AgR, CyR
Pro-rich	Grb2	GFR
	Nck	GFR, AgR
	Src kinases	GFR, AgR, CyR
pY	Vav, CrkL, Src kinases	AgR
	p85 (only with c-Cbl)	AgR, GFR
UBA	Ub (only with Cbl-b)	GFR
LZ	c-Cbl, Cbl-b	GFR, HR

AgR, antigen receptor; GFR, growth factor receptor; CyR, cytokine receptor; HR, hormone receptor.

Table 3. Signalling proteins bound to the different domains and motifs of c-Cbl/Cbl-b proteins.

Separating the TKB and the RING domains, a short linker sequence extends which has been shown crucial for Cbl ubiquitin ligase activity (Thien et al., 2001). The TKB domain makes intramolecular contacts with the linker α-helix and these contacts are centred on conserved residues Y368 and Y371 in human c-Cbl (Zheng et al., 2000). Interestingly, deletion of these tyrosines causes c-Cbl to become oncogenic (Thien et al., 2001). Molecular modelling data predicted that this structural alteration, in addition to loss of E3 activity, is required to activate fully the oncogenic potential of Cbl proteins. The second highly conserved domain among all Cbl proteins is the RING finger. *In vitro* ubiquitylation assays proved that the highly conserved Cbl RING finger has intrinsic E3 ligase activity and can independently recruit E2s or ubiquitin-conjugating (Ubc) enzymes for the transfer of ubiquitin to substrates (Joazeiro et al., 1999). The structural integrity of the RING finger domain is an absolute requirement for Cbl proteins to function as E3 ligases. Moreover, the RING finger domain acts in concert with the TKB domain to facilitate ubiquitylation and degradation of activated

PTKs, with the TKB domain conferring substrate specificity and the RING finger bringing in an E2 ubiquitin-conjugating enzyme. The carboxy-terminal half of c-Cbl is rich in proline residues, which contributes at least 15 and 17 potential SH3-domain-binding sites in c-Cbl and Cbl-b respectively, while Cbl-3 encodes five potential SH3-binding sites. Moreover, the proline-rich region in c-Cbl is also required for the ubiquitylation and proteasomal degradation of activated forms of Src (Yokouchi et al., 2001). In this case, the Cbl substrate is targeted by proline sequence interactions, rather than the TKB domain.

c-Cbl and Cbl-b are prominent substrates of RTKs and PTKs following stimulation of diverse cell surface receptors, as they possess major sites of tyrosine phosphorylation at their C-terminal part that enable them to interact with different SH2 domain containing proteins. Indeed, several studies have demonstrated the important role of tyrosine phosphorylation of Cbl proteins for their adaptor function, as well as for their E3 activity. The best-characterized phosphorylation sites are Y700, Y731 and Y774 in human c-Cbl and Y709 and Y665 in Cbl-b (Tsygankov et al., 1996; Keane et al., 1995). These residues are efficiently phosphorylated by Syk and the Src-family kinases Fyn, Yes and Lyn, but not by Lck or ZAP-70. An important difference between c-Cbl and Cbl-b is the unique presence of Y731 in c-Cbl which binds the SH2 domain of the p85 regulatory subunit of PI3K. Surprisingly, this association enables c-Cbl to function as a positive regulator by recruiting PI3K to the cell membrane (Hunter et al., 1999).

3.3.3 E3 ligase activity and adaptor function

The multi-domain nature of Cbl allows it to interact, directly or indirectly, with a wide range of signalling molecules. In this way, activated Cbl proteins act essentially as attenuators of cellular signals by exerting their function as E3 ubiquitin ligases or as adaptors/inhibitors proteins towards PTK pathways.

Cbl E3 ligase activity. Extensive biochemical studies have demonstrated Cbl-mediated ubiquitylation of its substrates (Figure 4). It is clear that ubiquitylation of a targeted receptor occurs in parallel to the onset of receptor internalization and continues to occur throughout the endosomal pathway. One of the best-studied examples of how Cbl-mediated ubiquitylation affects receptor trafficking, and helps terminate the signal from the activated receptor complex, is the EGF receptor (EGFR). This multistep process was initially described in *C. elegans*, where SLI-1 (the Cbl orthologue) was shown to negatively regulate signalling downstream of the LET-23 receptor [the EGFR orthologue] (reviewed in Thien and Langdon, 2001). This mechanism has become a model for the regulation of other RTKs by Cbl.

Cbl as an adaptor/inhibitor protein. An alternative way for Cbl to ubiquitylate EGFR is indirect and utilises its adaptor/inhibitor function by binding to the adaptor protein growth factor- receptor bound-2 (Grb2). One of the first proteins to be recruited into the complex is Grb2, which can recruit Cbl proteins from the cytoplasm to the plasma membrane through interactions between the proline-rich region of Cbl proteins and the N-terminal SH3 domain of Grb2. In this way, Cbl competes with the guanine-nucleotide-exchange factor son-of-sevenless (SOS) to bind Grb2, thereby blocking signalling through the Ras–mitogen-activated protein kinase (MAPK) pathway and inhibiting proliferation.

3.3.4 Signalling pathways in the haematopoietic and immune systems

Cbl gene deletions primarily affected the haematopoietic, immune and metabolic systems. A recent study on *c-Cbl*$^{-/-}$ HSC showed that the number and ability to reconstitute the haematopoietic system was increased in these cells compared to wild-type HSC. These results suggested that Cbl ubiquitin-mediated protein degradation is important for HSC homeostasis (Rathinam et al., 2008). Furthermore, it was shown that c-Cbl is capable of controlling HSC development and function through negative regulation of TPO-dependent STAT5 activation, an important pathway for HSC maintenance. Indeed, *c-Cbl*-deficient HSC displayed TPO hypersensibility, as well as increased levels of STAT5 and its activated form, phospho-STAT5. Thus, these findings underline the role of c-Cbl as important modulator of the TPO/Mpl/JAK/STAT5 signalling pathway in HSCs.

The importance of c-Cbl and Cbl-b in immunity and immune receptor signalling pathways has been demonstrated clearly by the phenotypes of their respective gene knockout mice. Both *c-Cbl*$^{-/-}$ and *Cbl-b*$^{-/-}$ mice display hyperactive signalling downstream of the TCR. Loss of either Cbl protein results in lower activation threshold for signalling through the TCR, hypersensitivity to low affinity/avidity engagement of the receptor, and activation of downstream signalling pathways without the normal requirement for co-receptor stimulation (Figure 4) (Murphy et al., 1998; Naramura et al., 1998; Bachmaier et al., 2000; Chiang et al., 2007). Interestingly, these c-Cbl and Cbl-b phenotypes are restricted to thymocytes and T-cells, respectively, reflecting a difference in tissue distribution with c-Cbl more prominent in the thymus and Cbl-b highly expressed in peripheral T-cells. Loss of Cbl-b dramatically increases T-cell activation threshold and uncouples T-cell activation from the requirement for CD28 co-stimulation, thus leading to spontaneous autoimmunity (Gronski et al., 2004).

Cbl proteins have been also shown to differentially modulate BCR-dependent signalling. Loss of c-Cbl in primary B cells showed a significant inhibition of BCR-mediated signalling mainly caused, not by down-regulation of Syk, but instead by up-regulation of Lyn kinase (Shao et al., 2004). In contrast, Cbl-b negatively regulates BCR-mediated signalling, this time, by down-regulating Syk in primary B cells (Sohn et al., 2003). Furthermore, the activity of Cbl proteins as adaptors was also implicated in the effect of Cbl proteins on B-cell activation. In this case, it has been shown that c-Cbl negatively regulates the phospholipase C-γ2 (PLC-γ2) pathway in B cells, while Cbl-b was shown to positively regulate this same pathway (Yasuda et al., 2002).

Studies carried out with cell lines have demonstrated that both c-Cbl and Cbl-b negatively regulated FcεRI-mediated mast cell activation (Figure 4). However, experiments on primary mast cells derived from *c-Cbl* and *Cbl-b*-deficient mice revealed a more profound effect with the lack of Cbl-b than of c-Cbl (Zhang et al., 2004). Cbl-dependent FcεRI down-regulation occurs mainly via Cbl E3 ubiquitin ligase activity that promotes receptor β and γ multiubiquitination, providing signals for receptor internalization and sorting into lysosomal compartments for degradation. Interestingly, Syk activity is required for c-Cbl-dependent ubiquitylation of FcεRI receptor (Paolini et al., 2002). On the other hand, Cbl proteins can also down-modulate engaged FcεRI through its adaptor function by interacting with molecules involved in clathrin-mediated endocytosis (Molfetta et al., 2005). Remarkably, Cbl proteins also negatively regulate mast cell activation by selectively ubiquitinating and degrading the activated kinase form of Lyn and Syk proteins (Paolini et al., 2002; Kyo et al., 2003; Qu et al., 2004).

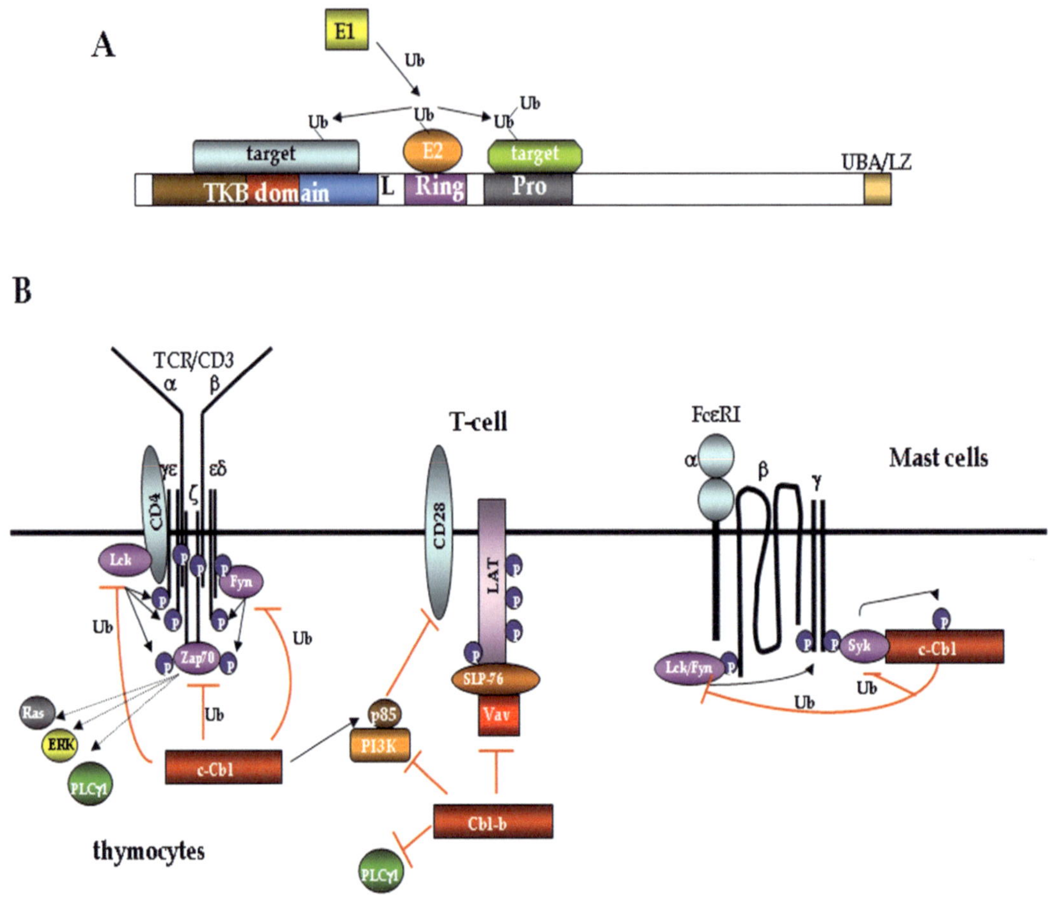

Fig. 4. A) Model of Cbl ligase activity. B) Schematic model of Cbl signalling pathways in T and mast cells

c-Cbl also participates in the modulation of monocyte/macrophage signalling mediated by Fcγ and Colony Stimulating Factor (CSF)-1 receptors through its adaptor functions. c-Cbl is capable of attenuating CSF-1-mediated signalling by binding to a phosphotyrosine residue of this receptor and then ubiquitylating and targeting it for degradation. Lastly, c-Cbl also appears to play a negative regulatory role in platelets as well. This is not so surprising considering that Syk kinase has a biological function in these cells, a known substrate of c-Cbl. The contribution of c-Cbl-dependent ubiquitylation of Syk to the negative effect of c-Cbl on platelet functions is not yet understood, however, it is possible that the biological role of c-Cbl in platelets consists in preventing unwanted platelet activation *in vivo* by increasing the threshold of platelet activation.

3.3.5 Regulation of Cbl function

Cbl proteins are potent regulators of cell function and development through their adaptor function and ligase activity. It is therefore necessary that the Cbl proteins are at their turn, subject to complex and sophisticated regulatory mechanisms that fine-tune the effects that these proteins have on signalling (Ryan et al., 2006). These include: *cis*-acting structural elements that prevent inappropriate E3 activity until the Cbl proteins interact with their substrate, degradation of the Cbl proteins, inhibition of Cbl protein function mediated by protein interactions, deubiquitination of the Cbl substrates, and negative regulation of trafficking of the ubiquitinated Cbl substrates. Therefore, abnormal Cbl regulation can lead to pathological conditions such as immunological and malignant diseases, thus underscoring the essential role of Cbl in normal homeostasis.

3.4 The SOCS family

3.4.1 Origin, structure and cellular expression

The SOCS (for Suppressors Of Cytokine Signalling) proteins are a family of intracellular molecules that negatively regulate the strength and duration of cytokine receptor signalling cascades, notably the JAK/STAT pathway. This family consists of eight members, CIS and SOCS1-7 that share structural and functional homology. The first family member identified was CIS (for Cytokine-Inducible SH2-containing protein) cloned as an early gene differentially induced following IL-3 and EPO exposure (Yoshimura et al., 1995). The second member identified, SOCS1 (also known as JAB for JAK-Binding protein or SSI for STAT-induced STAT Inhibitor) was identified simultaneously by three separate groups (Starr et al., 1997; Endo et al., 1997; Naka et al., 1997). SOCS-2 and SOCS-3 were cloned using distantly related expressed sequence tags [ESTs] and the rest of the members (SOCS4-7) were identified on the basis of a conserved C-terminal amino acid sequence using various DNA databases (Starr et al. 1997; Minamoto et al., 1997; Hilton et al., 1998). All members of the SOCS family have a similar tripartite domain organization composed of a variable N-terminal region, followed by a central SH2 domain and a conserved C-terminal SOCS box domain (Fig. 1). SOCS1 and SOCS3 differ from other family members in that they possess an extended SH2 domain at the N-terminus (for SOCS1 and SOCS3) or the C-terminus (for SOCS3) of this domain. Additionally, they also present at their N-terminal region and adjacent to their SH2 domain, a Kinase-Inhibitory Region (KIR) required for inhibition of JAK kinase activity (Yasukawa et al., 1999; Sasaki et al., 1999). Another exception is SOCS7 which is unique in its possession of a proline-rich N-terminus and a nuclear localisation signal.

SOCS molecules expression is controlled at the transcriptional, translational and post-translational levels. Many *SOCS* genes contain STAT-binding sequences in their promoter region and their STAT-dependent transcription can be differentially regulated in a factor- and tissue specific manner. SOCS proteins are often low or undetectable at the basal level in unstimulated cells and their expression is rapidly induced to a variable extent in different cell types and tissues by immunoregulatory cytokines, colony stimulating factors, growth factors and hormones that signal via JAK-STAT pathway or via RTK [Table 4] (Starr et al., 1997). Certain cytokines that do not signal via JAK kinases or RTKs, and a number of non-cytokine ligands can also induce *SOCS* gene expression, such as TNF signalling and bacterial products such as LPS and CpG DNA which signal via Toll-like receptors (TLR). Because *SOCS* genes are induced by cytokines and the corresponding proteins inhibit further cytokine-induced signalling, SOCS proteins are believed to form part of a classical negative feedback loop mechanism. Northern blot analysis of murine tissues has shown that *CIS* and *SOCS2* mRNA was ubiquitously expressed, with expression being particularly strong (CIS) or weak (SOCS2) in kidney, lung, liver, heart, testis and male spleen (Yoshimura et al., 1995; Starr et al., 1997). *SOCS1* and *SOCS3* mRNA was detected at different levels in adult haematopoietic organs such as the thymus and spleen and to some extent in other organs like lung, spleen and testis (Starr et al., 1997). However, *SOCS3* show high expression in fetal liver (Marine et al., 1999). Although some of the SOCS members appear to be co-expressed in only a few organs, the *in vivo* expression of *SOCS* genes may be more pronounced than is detectable by Northern hybridisation, since most cell types seem to depend on cytokine stimuli for SOCS induction.

3.4.2 Signalling targets

The different domains in the SOCS proteins allow them to bind to the cytokine receptors, associated JAKs or other signalling molecules and to attenuate signal transduction directly or indirectly by targeting the receptor complex for ubiquitin-mediated degradation in proteosomes. The N-terminal region of the SOCS proteins is variable in length and sequence. In SOCS1 and SOCS3, there is a 12 amino acid sequence adjacent to the SH2 domain that is essential for the inhibition of JAK2 kinase called KIR. This sequence is supposed to function via a conserved tyrosine residue as a pseudo-substrate, lodging in the catalytic cleft to block further JAK kinase activity. Removal of this tyrosine does not affect binding of the SOCS proteins to the kinase, but does abrogate its inhibition (Sasaki et al., 1999). Inded, a SOCS1-KIR mimetic peptide is sufficient to inhibit IFNγ-mediated JAK2 activity in primary cells (Waiboci et al., 2007). The role of the remaining N-terminal region among the SOCS family members has yet to be elucidated.

The central SH2 domain determines the target protein for degradation of each SOCS protein. It binds to distinct phosphorylated tyrosine motifs on SOCS target proteins (Table 4). Once the SH2 domain binds to its specific target, it brings other domains in proximity to the target protein, directing degradation of the appropriate protein. Mutagenesis studies allowed the identification of small regions at the N-termini of SOCS1 and SOCS3, and at the C-terminus of SOCS3 SH2 domains, critical for phosphotyrosine binding. These regions have been defined as an N- and C-extended SH2 domain (N-ESS and C-ESS, respectively). The solved structure of SOCS3 SH2 domain had shown that the N-ESS sequence directly contacts the phosphotyrosine-binding loop of the kinase and determines its orientation (Babon et al., 2006). The C-ESS of SOCS3 forms part of the SH2 domain that is spatially displaced by a 35 amino acid PEST [for Proline, Glutamic acid (E), Serine and Threonine rich sequence] insertion. This sequence is thought to signal for rapid proteolytic degradation. It is therefore not surprising that removal of this sequence lowers SOCS3 turnover without affecting the SH2 domain folding and function (Babon et al., 2006). Since other SOCS members contain putative PEST sequences, this may prove to be a common mechanism for regulation of SOCS protein levels.

The SOCS proteins are substrate recognition factors for an E3 ligase that targets their specific cargo for ubiquitin-mediated degradation. They serve this function by binding to the E3 complex via the highly conserved SOCS box domain at their C-terminus. The SOCS box is a 40 amino acid motif found not only in the SOCS family members, but also in a vast number of proteins. The SOCS box consists of a three-α-helical structure bound to an E3 ubiquitin ligase complex that in turn covalently binds ubiqutin to lysines in the target protein. The N-terminus of the SOCS box mediates interaction with Elongin C/B, while the C-terminus of

SOCS proteins	SH2 partner	Inducer system	Signalling system inhibited
CIS	EPOR, PRLR, Leptin R	EPO, IL-2/3/6, IFNα, PRL, GH, Leptin	EPO, PRL, IL-2/3, GH
SOCS1	JAK2, IFNGRI	EPO, TPO, GM-CSF, G-CSF,M-CSF,IL-2/4/6/7/9/10/13/15, PRL, LPS, TNFα, GH, In, CpG DNA	IL-2/4/6/7/12/15, IFNα/β/γ, LIF, TNFα, EPO, TPO, GH, PRL, In, Leptin
SOCS2	GHR, Leptin R	GH, IL-6, IFNα/γ, LIF	IL-6, GH, IGF-1
SOCS3	EPOR, gp130, G-CSFR, IL-12Rβ2, Leptin R	IL-1, TGF-β, IL-2/6/9/10/13, GH, LPS, EGF, IFNα/γ, LIF, EPO, GM-CSF, PRL, In, Leptin	IL-2/4/6/9/11, IFNα/β/γ, LIF, EPO, GH, PRL, In, Leptin
SOCS4, SOCS5	EGFR	EGF, IL-6	EGF, IL-4/6
SOCS6, SOCS7	IRS2/4, IR	In, IGF	In, IGF

In, insulin; PRL, prolacftin.

Table 4. Signalling partners, transduction pathways and factors regulating SOCS protein expression and function.

the SOCS box directs the SOCS/Elongin C/B association with Cullin 5 (Cul5) scaffold protein (Zhang et al., 1999). The latter one recruits the stabilizing RING finger protein Rbx and allows Cul5 to bind to an E2 ubiquitin-conjugating enzyme. The resulting complex SOCS/Elongin B/C/Cul5/Rbx/E2 forms a functional E3 ubiquitin ligase (Figure 5a). The SOCS1-SOCS box has been shown to be capable of driving the ubiquitination of specific proteins such as TEL-JAK2 fusion and Vav1, and only in very few cases the receptor complex for subsequent degradation through the proteosome (Frantsve et al., 2001; De Sepulveda et al., 2000; Irandoust et al., 2007; Verdier et al., 1998). The importance of the SOCS box has been further shown by *in vivo* targeted deletion of SOCS1 and SOCS3 in mice that resulted in partial loss of SOCS function with enhanced IFNγ and G-CSF signalling, respectively (Zhang et al., 2001).

3.4.3 Regulation of cytokine receptor signalling pathways

The structural analysis of the SOCS molecules revealed they can control cytokine receptor signalling by several mechanisms (Figure 5):

(1) Direct inhibition of intrinsic kinase activity by binding to JAKs. Immunoprecipitation assays revealed that both SOCS1 and SOCS3 were able to co-precipitate with JAK kinases upon cytokine stimulation, and that this association blocked JAK kinase activity, although with a different affinity and kinetics (Endo et al., 1997; Sasaki et al., 1999). Structure-function studies using truncated versions of SOCS1 identified the regions essential for SOCS-JAK association and for inhibition of JAK activity. SOCS1 inhibits tyrosine kinase activity upon interaction with phosphorylated tyrosine Y1007 located in the activation loop of JAK.

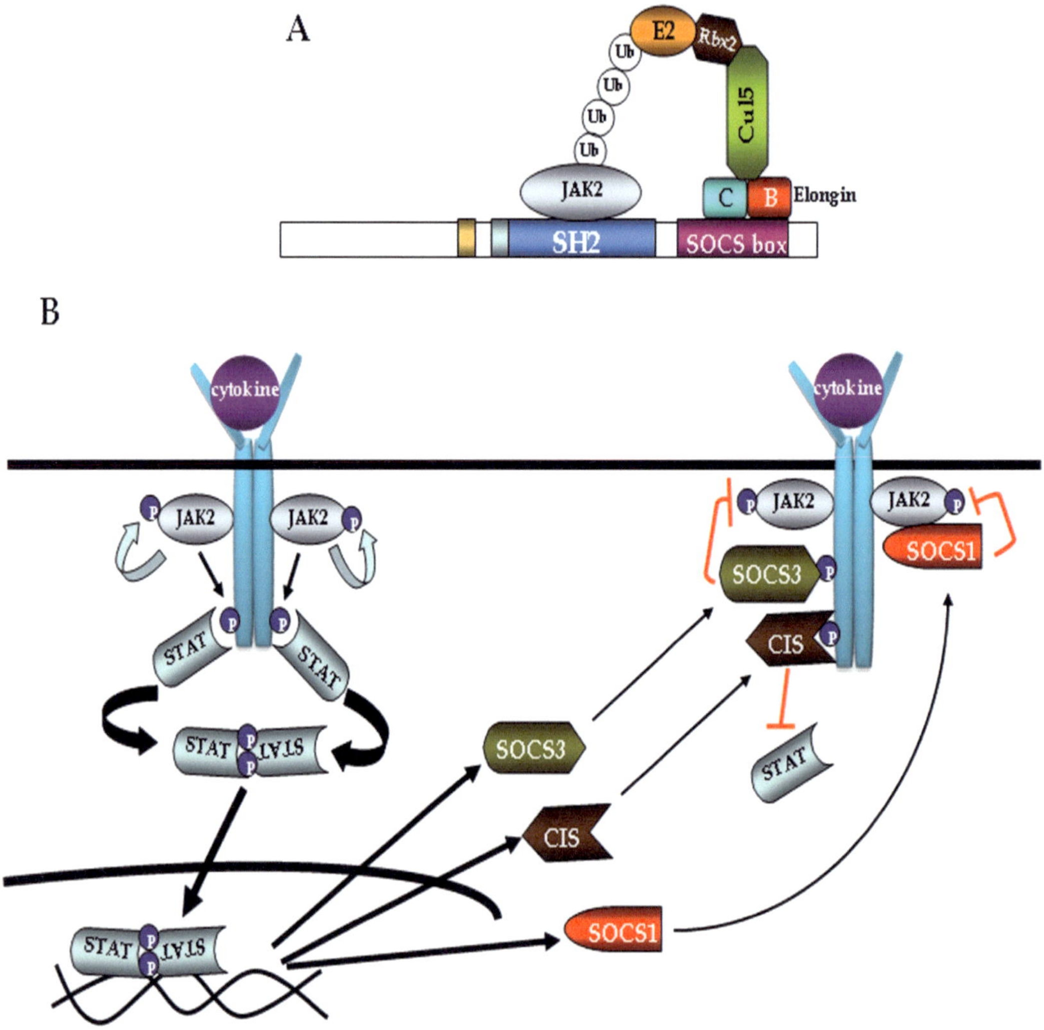

Fig. 5. A) Schematic representation of the SOCS box function, B) Mechanisms of suppression by the SOCS proteins.

However, complete inhibition of the kinase activity requires not only the SH2 domain but also the KIR region (Narazaki et al., 1998; Nicholson et al., 1999). The critical amino acids for the KIR region's function are conserved between SOCS1 and SOCS3, suggesting a common inhibitory mechanism for these two family members.

(2) Indirect inhibition of JAKs by binding to the receptor. As with SOCS1, the SOCS3 SH2 domain was initially shown to interact with Y1007 in JAK2, albeit with lower affinity than SOCS1. However, subsequent studies demonstrated that SOCS3 SH2 domain exhibited a higher affinity for phosphotyrosine residues located within the receptor subunits than for JAK2 (Sasaki et al., 1999). Accordingly, it was found that SOCS3 associated with higher affinity with phosphorylated residues in the IL-6 receptor subunit, gp130, notably Y759, than with the activation loop of JAKs (Nicholson et al., 2000). SOCS3, therefore, in contrast to SOCS1, has to be recruited to the receptor complex in order to inhibit IL-6 signal transduction (Schmitz et al., 2000). Subsequently, SOCS3 might inhibit the kinase activity of JAKs through the pseudo-substrate, KIR, in the same way as SOCS1, but only after recruitment and binding to critical phosphotyrosine residues in the cytokine receptor. Given that SOCS1 and SOCS3 can interact with both receptor and JAK, a two-step interaction model has been proposed, whereby the SOCS1/3 SH2 domains are first recruited to the receptor and subsequent bi-modal binding to nearby JAK through the SH2 domain and KIR region results in a high affinity interaction, inhibition of JAK kinase activity and potential proteosomal degradation.

(3) Blocking binding of downstream signalling molecules to the receptor. This mechanism has been shown for CIS and SOCS2 for EPO and GH signalling inhibition, respectively. Upon stimulation of the receptors, the SOCS proteins bind to tyrosine residues at the membrane distal region of receptor chains that are docking sites for downstream signalling molecules, such as STAT5 or SHP-2. By masking these phosphorylated residues, CIS/SOCS2 competes with STAT thereby down-modulating the signalling (Yoshimura et al., 1995; Ram & Waxman, 1999). On the other hand, SOCS3-mediated inhibition of signalling via EpoR, gp130 and LeptinR could partially result from competitive inhibition of SHP-2 binding to gp130, LeptinR, and EpoR, resulting in the blockade of SHP-2-mediated ERK activation (Schmitz et al., 2000; Bjorbaek et al., 2001; Sasaki et al., 2000).

(4) Ubiquitination and subsequent proteasomal degradation of JAKs and receptor. Studies on EPO receptor using proteasome inhibitors showed that these compounds protected the EpoR and STAT5 from the normal reduction in phosphorylation upon CIS expression, indicating proteasome involvement of both EPO-receptor and STAT5 inactivation (Verdier et al., 1998). These results allow proposing a model where the phosphorylated target molecules may become a substrate of the proteolytic machinery by binding to SOCS. In this situation, the SOCS box acts as an adaptor molecule, bringing into this complex the Elongin B/C/E3 ligase for ubiquitination of the target protein. Subsequently, the substrate and the associated SOCS proteins may be destroyed, and the cell is ready to respond again to stimulation. Therefore, targeting the signalling proteins for degradation by the SOCS box seems to be another mechanism by which cytokine signalling might be inhibited under physiological levels of SOCS proteins.

3.4.4 Regulation of SOCS proteins

Besides elaborate transcriptional regulation, another control point of the expression of SOCS molecules is their protein stability. SOCS proteins exhibit a rapid turnover rate, and the half lives of SOCS1, SOCS2 and SOCS3 have been estimated to be less than 2 h (Siewert et al., 1999). Several mechanisms have been proposed to regulate SOCS expression. The presence of a PEST sequence in SOCS3 appears to mediate non-proteosomal degradation, while SOCS box-dependent ubiquitination of SOCS3 on lysine 6, at least *in vitro,* contributes to proteosomal degradation of the SOCS3 protein (Sasaki et al., 2003). Furthermore, SOCS3 is uniquely phosphorylated within the SOCS box on Y204 and Y221 and this appears to have two consequences, interaction with the Elongin B/C complex is lost, destabilizing the SOCS3 protein, and signalling through the Ras/MAPK pathway can be potentiated (Haan et al., 2003; Cacalano et al., 2001). Nevertheless, the full implication of SOCS3 phosphorylation on its regulation remains to be explored.

4. Animal models of inhibitory adaptors: Definition of their physiological significance

Central to understanding the physiological role of families of inhibitory adaptors in the haematopoietic and immune systems, has been the generation of mice deficient for these proteins when possible. This has also helped dissect regulatory and/or compensatory mechanisms through the functional, complete or partial, reconstitution in these mice, in particular for members of multi-gene families. These approaches have allowed 1) analyse changes in the expression level of the adaptor that can also affect its signalling pathway; 2) establish how deficiency of an adaptor can have dramatically different effects in different cell lineages; 3) understand the functional synergy between members of the same family of adaptors; 4) identify null mutations leading to the complete absence of some cell types, while leaving others with no discernable defect and 5) define how some deficiencies are selective within a cell type, disrupting only particular pathways while leaving others intact. Mice deficient for the different families of inhibitory adaptors discussed in this chapter have certainly provided important new insights into the biology and function of these adaptors. However, in some cases, these animal models have also raised important questions regarding the mechanisms of action of these regulators and their potential therapeutic application.

4.1 *Dok* deficient mice

Although Dok-1, Dok-2, and Dok-3 have been shown to act as negative regulators downstream of a wide range of immunoreceptors, cytokine, and LPS receptors mediated signalling, insights into their physiological importance in immune cells have and will continue to come from studies with mice or cells lacking individually or in combination Dok-1, Dok-2, and Dok-3. *Dok-1* or *Dok-2*-deficient mice displayed normal steady-state haematopoiesis. By contrast, mice lacking both *Dok-1* and *Dok-2* succumbed to a myeloproliferative disease resembling human chronic myelogenous leukaemia (CML) and chronic myelomonocytic leukaemia (CMMoL) at around one year of age (Yasuda et al., 2004; Niki et al., 2004) [Table 5]. These animals displayed medullary and extramedullary hyperplasia of granulocyte/macrophage progenitors with leukemic potential, and their myeloid cells showed hyperproliferation and hypo-apoptosis upon treatment and deprivation of cytokines, respectively. Consistently, the mutant myeloid cells showed aberrant Ras/MAP kinase and Akt activation upon cytokine stimulation. Strikingly, ablation of *Dok-1* and *Dok-2* markedly accelerated leukaemia and blastic crisis onset in *bcr-abl* transgenic mice known to develop a CML-like disease. These results demonstrate the critical role of Dok-1 and Dok-2 in myeloid homeostasis and suppression of leukaemia. Interestingly, half of the double-deficient mice also developed histiocytic sarcoma (HS) of macrophage origin. These results suggest an involvement of additional genetic changes.

Similar to *Dok-1* and *Dok-2* deficiency, *Dok-3* inactivation did not result in development of aggressive tumors in haematopoietic cells (Ng et al., 2007). However, ablation of all three Dok proteins (Dok-1/2/3) in mice has recently shown drastic phenotypic consequences. These mice showed earlier mortality due to development of aggressive HS with multiple organ invasions, but no incidence of other types of tumors (Mashima et al., 2010). This disease is a haematological malignancy characterized by cells displaying a tissue macrophage-like (histiocytic) morphology (Grogan et al., 2008). Indeed, loss of *Dok-1/2/3* causes aberrant proliferation of macrophages in the lung, already detectable before the onset of morphologically recognizable HS. These cells displayed an exaggerated proliferative response to M-CSF or GM-CSF compared to wild type littermates. These results suggest that Dok proteins can mutually compensate and inhibit macrophage proliferation and therefore suppress the aggressive transformation of HS.

4.2 *Lnk/APS/SH2-B* deficient mice

Mice deficient for members of this family have demonstrated the positive (SH2-B) and negative (Lnk and APS) physiological role of these adaptors in growth factor, cytokine, and immune receptors signalling (Table 5). Deletion of the *SH2B1* gene resulted in severe obesity, hyperphagia and both leptin and insulin resistance as well as infertility, which might be a consequence of resistance to IGF-1 (Ohtsuka et al., 2002; Ren et al., 2005). Thus, *SH2-B*-deficient mice support a role for this adaptor as a positive regulator of JAK2 signalling pathways initiated by leptin, insulin and potentially, by IGF-1.

Interestingly, *APS*-deficient mice also displayed an insulin-related phenotype. They showed a hypersensibility to insulin and enhanced glucose tolerance, a finding that is consistent with APS playing a negative role in insulin signalling (Minami et al., 2003). Moreover, these mice present also a haematopoietic phenotype with defects in degranulation of mast cells and cytoskeleton rearrangement in both mast and B-1 cells (Kubo-Akashi et al, 2004; Iseki et

Gene	Approach	System	Mouse phenotype/Human disease
Dok-1 Dok-2	KO	mu	Impaired immunoreceptor signaling in lymphocytes, allergic responses in mast cells, enhanced ERK signaling, hyperresponsiveness to LPS
Dok-1/2	KO	mu	MPN, Lupus Renal disease/CML, CMMoL
Dok-1/2/3	KO	mu	HS
Lnk	KO	mu	MPN-like (ET/PMF), CML (aged mice)
	Tg	mu	Impaired lymphopoiesis
	Mu (SNP)	hu	MPN, autoimmune, cardiovascular and inflammatory diseases
APS	KO	mu	Insulin hypersensitivity, enhanced glucose tolerance, enhanced B1 cells proliferation
	Tg	mu	Reduced B1 and B2 cell number, impaired B-cell development and BCR-dependent proliferation, reduced mast cell degranulation and actin assembly
SH2B	KO	mu	Severe obesity, hyperphagia, increased leptin and insulin resistance, infertility
c-Cbl	KO	mu	Enlarged thymus, splenomegaly, extramedullar haematopoiesis, enhanced thymocyte function/ myeloid malignancies
	Mu	mu	Oncogenesis, mastocytosis, myeloid leukemia, tumourigenesis

Gene	Approach	System	Mouse phenotype/Human disease
c-Cbl	Mu	hu	AML, MPD/MPN, aCML, JMML
Cbl-b	KO	mu	Impaired immunological tolerance, autoimmune diseases with inflammatory organ and tissue damage, enhanced peripheral T-cell function, rejection of certain tumours
c-Cbl/ Cbl-b	KO	mu	Embryonic lethal
	T-cell KO	mu	Autoimmune-like vasculitis, SLE-like autoimmune disease
CIS	KO	mu	No specific phenotype
	Tg	mu	Fewer T-cells, NK, and NK-T cells, lactation deficiency, similar phenotype to STAT5 KO
SOCS1	KO	mu	perinatal lethality, enhanced IFNγ production and responsiveness, lymphopenia and inflammation with multi-organ infiltration
	Tg(Tcell)	mu	Inhibited T-cell response to IFNγ, IL-6 and IL-7, increased CD4+T-cells, reduced peripheral T-cell activation
		hu	Increased expression in Th-driven inflammatory diseases (RA, UC, Crohn, dermatitis), decreased expression and/or hyper-methylation in certain cancers
SOCS2	KO	mu	Gigantism, deregulated GH signalling
	Tg	mu	Gigantism
SOCS3	KO	mu	Embryonic lethality due to placental deficiency, erythrocytosis, deregulated LIF response
	Tg	mu	Embryonic lethality due to anemia
	Tg(Tcell)	mu	High TGFβ1 and IL-10 production
	Mu (SNP)	hu	Allergic diseases
		hu	Increased expression in Th2-driven asthma patients and inflammatory diseases, hyper-phosphorylation in MPN
SOCS5	KO	mu	No specific phenotype
	Tg	mu	Reduced IL-4-mediated STAT6 activation, reduced Th2 development and cytokine production
SOCS6	KO	mu	Mild growth retardation
SOCS7	KO	mu	Growth retardation (strain-dependent), hypoglucemia, hydrocephalus, altered glucose homeostasis, enlarged pancreatic islets

KO, knock out; Tg, transgenic; Mu, mutations; hu, human; mu, murine, RA, theumatoid arthritis; UC, ulcer colitis.

Table 5. Mouse phenotype and human diseases related to deficiencies in inhibitory adaptors.

al., 2004). These results suggest a negative role for APS in controlling actin dynamics in these cells. Furthermore, *APS*-deficient mice display an increase in B-1 cells in the peritoneal cavity and humoral responses to type-2 antigen, indicating a negative regulatory role for APS in BCR-mediated cell proliferation and cytoskeletal regulation.

By contrast, mice deficient for *Lnk* display a profound perturbation in haematopoiesis that confirmed its role as a key negative regulator of cytokine signalling in the haematopoietic system. Indeed, these mice exhibit splenomegaly together with fibrosis, expansion of HSC, B lymphoid and myeloid progenitors that confer an enhanced repopulating ability. *Lnk*-deficient mice have also revealed an important role for Lnk in B-cell lymphopoiesis, megakaryopoiesis and erythropoiesis, as a result of the absence of negative regulation of SCF, TPO and EPO signalling pathways. One important feature of the *Lnk*-/- mice phenotype is its resemblance to human myeloproliferative neoplasms (MPN): hypersensitivity to cytokines, increased number of haematopoietic progenitors, high platelet counts, splenomegaly together with fibrosis and extramedullary hematopoiesis (Velazquez et al., 2002; Campbell & Green, 2008). This has suggested an important role for Lnk in the development of these diseases. Indeed, loss of Lnk cooperates with oncogenes, such as JAK2 and BCR-ABL, to induce MPN in mice. These animals exhibit a disproportionate expansion of myeloid progenitors and immature precursors *in vitro* and *in vivo* (Bersenev et al., 2010). Moreover, aged *Lnk*-/- mice seem to spontaneously develop a Chronic Myeloid Leukemia (CML)-like MPN, suggesting a role for Lnk in myeloid expansion *in vivo*. However, this myeloid cell hyperproliferation fails to trigger blast crises, reflecting the need of *Lnk*-deficiency for additional oncogenic events to promote blast transformation. *Lnk*-deficient mice also exhibited an increase in endothelial progenitor cells (EPC) numbers that display an enhance capacity for colony formation. Different molecular, physiological and morphological approaches have shown that *Lnk* deficiency promotes vasculogenesis/angiogenesis and osteogenesis through the mobilization and recruitment of HSCs/EPCs via activation of the SCF/Kit signalling pathway in the ischemic and perifracture zone, respectively, thereby establishing an optimal environment for neovascularisation, bone healing and remodelling (Kwon et al., 2009, Matsumoto, et al., 2010). Taken together, these findings strongly suggest that Lnk regulates bone marrow EPC kinetics during vascular and bone regeneration.

4.3 *Cbl*-deficient mice

Mice deficient for *c-Cbl* and *Cbl-b* have been invaluable in demonstrating the important roles played by these proteins in fine-tuning signalling thresholds in immune cells. Despite close structural similarities, loss of c-Cbl and Cbl-b proteins evokes prominent phenotypic differences (Table 5). *c-Cbl*-null mice have an enlarged thymus, expanded hematopoietic progenitor pools with increased repopulating capacity, splenomegaly with extramedullary hematopoiesis, as well as changes in energy metabolism, and reduced fertility of male mice (Murphy et al., 1998; Naramura et al., 1998; Molero et al., 2004; El Chami et al., 2005, Rathinam et al., 2008). However, the most marked alteration in *c-Cbl* and *Cbl-b*-deficient animals is being associated with thymocyte and peripheral T-cell activation, respectively. *c-Cbl*-/- mice exhibit strong effects on thymocytes, with increase cell numbers in the thymus of the young adult and enhanced signal strength following TCR engagement. Moreover, perturbed thymocyte signalling does not depend on the TKB domain of c-Cbl, as a TKB knock-in did not rescue the phenotype (Thien et al., 2003). In contrast, *Cbl-b* ablation results in an impaired immunological tolerance induction and animals succumb to spontaneous and/or induced autoimmune diseases with widespread inflammatory organ (pancreas, lung) and tissue (adipose) damage (Bachmaier et al., 2000, 2007; Hirasaka et al., 2007). Importantly, *Cbl-b*-null mice are able to reject multiple types of tumours spontaneously (Chiang et al., 2007; Loeser et al., 2007).

The redundant and overlapping functions of Cbl family proteins are more evident from the striking phenotypes of *Cbl, Cbl-b* double-deficient mice. Deletion of both proteins in the germline leads to early embryonic lethality (Naramura et al., 2002). In contrast, T-cell specific double knock-out mice are viable, however, their T-cells develop independent of MHC-restricted thymic selection and these mice eventually succumb to autoimmune-like vasculitis early in adult life (Huang et al., 2006; Naramura et al., 2002). Similarly, B-cell specific *Cbl, Cbl-b* double deficiency leads to a failure to acquire tolerance to self antigens and the animals developed Systemic Lupus Erythematosus (SLE)-like autoimmune diseases (Kitaura et al., 2007). At the molecular level, cells from these double knock-out mice display delayed down-modulation of cell surface antigen receptors and prolonged activation of downstream signalling pathways.

Loss of *c-Cbl*, but not of *Cbl-b*, led to a significant expansion of HSC and haematopoietic progenitors. Strikingly, ablation of both proteins enhanced this phenotype and eventually all mice succumbed to aggressive myeloproliferative disease-like leukemia with peripheral organ involvement within two to three months after birth (Naramura et al., 2010). Moreover, blastic transformation of chronic myelogeneous leukemia in a *bcr/abl*-transgenic model is accelerated in the *c-Cbl* null background (Sanada et al., 2009). Combined, these observations support that c-Cbl can act as a tumor suppressor and that complete loss of Cbl functions is required to promote myeloid malignancy. In contrast to the tumor suppressor function of the wild-type c-Cbl, c-Cbl mutants isolated from human and murine neoplasms, as well as v-Cbl, show clear transforming capacity in terms of anchorage-independent growth in soft agar *in vitro* and tumour generation in nude mice *in vivo* (Sanada et al., 2009; Thien et al., 2001). Bone marrow cells transduced with c-Cbl mutants in the linker (70Z) or in the RING finger domain (R420Q) generate generalized mastocytosis, a myeloproliferative disease, and myeloid leukemia in lethally irradiated mice with long latency but high penetrance (Bandi et al., 2009). The transforming activity of these mutant forms of c-Cbl seems to be mediated by alteration of the E3 ubiquitin ligase activity. Most c-Cbl mutations in myeloid neoplasms are missense changes at highly conserved amino acid positions within the linker and RING finger domains, or involve splice-site sequences, leading to amino acid deletions within them. Supporting these findings, the generation of knock-in mutants carrying single point mutations in the TKB, linker or RING domains of c-Cbl protein has further validated the importance of these domains in Cbl-mediated tumorigenesis. Interestingly, mice with an equivalent RING finger domain mutation in *Cbl-b* do not show comparable changes in the haematopoietic compartment, indicating that Cbl-b is not capable of inhibiting c-Cbl functions (Rathinam et al., 2010). Taken together, mouse models with Cbl family ablation or point mutations have convincingly established the role of these proteins as important E3 ubiquitin ligases for the homeostasis of the haematopoietic and immune systems and as tumour suppressors.

4.4 *SOCS*-deficient mice

Since the discovery of SOCS proteins, much attention has been drawn to their physiological roles and their involvement in human diseases. Many of their common inhibitory activities on cytokine signalling demonstrated *in vitro*, do not seem to be essential *in vivo* as genetic ablation of CIS, SOCS1, SOCS2 and SOCS3 genes has demonstrated remarkable cytokine specificity for different SOCS molecules (Table 5).

SOCS1-deficient mice are growth retarded and died within 3 weeks of birth with a syndrome characterized by severe lymphopenia, activation of peripheral T cells, fatty degeneration and necrosis of the liver and multi-organ failure with rampant inflammation due to macrophage infiltration of major organs (Alexander et al., 1999; Marine et al., 1999a, Starr et al., 1998). The neonatal phenotypes appear primarily as the result of deregulated IFNγ signalling, because *SOCS1*$^{-/-}$ mice that are also deficient for IFNγ, do not die neonatally. Moreover, constitutive STAT1 activation and IFNγ-inducible genes were observed in *SOCS1* deficient mice, indicating that IFNγ signalling is regulated by SOCS1 and that its deregulation contributes to the lethal phenotype. However, the *SOCS1, IFNγ* double deficient mice ultimately died 6 months after birth with inflammation and polycystic kidneys, which suggests that SOCS1 regulation is not exclusive to IFNγ (Metcalf et al., 2002). The lethality in *SOCS1*$^{-/-}$ mice is also significantly delayed in the *RAG2*$^{-/-}$, *STAT1*$^{-/-}$, *STAT6*$^{-/-}$ and *STAT4*$^{-/-}$ backgrounds, thus implicating SOCS1 as a critical regulator of IFNγ, IL-4 and IL-12 signalling pathways (Alexander and Hilton, 2004).

In recent years, it has become clear that some of the SOCS members play critical roles in regulating T-cell differentiation, maturation and function by controlling different signalling events, as shown by the phenotypes displayed by *SOCS1* and *SOCS3* deficient mice. In this sense, T-cell specific conditional deletion of *SOCS1* showed that it is not sufficient to induce the lethal multi-organ disease; however it does cause T-cell specific abnormalities that include increased numbers of CD8^{+} T cells and increased sensitivity to cytokines with common γ-chain receptors. SOCS1 also plays an important role in the regulation of Tregs. Higher number of Tregs is observed in the thymus and spleen of T-cell-specific *SOCS1*-deficient mice (Horino et al., 2008). This is probably due to higher IL-2 responses, because IL-2 enhances Tregs proliferation. Moreover, Lu and colleagues have recently showed that SOCS1-specific ablation in Tregs induced the development of spontaneous dermatitis, splenomegaly and lymphoadenopathy in these mice (Lu et al., 2009). These results point out SOCS1 as an important controller of Tregs.

Analysis of mice bearing the deletion of the SOCS box of *SOCS1* demonstrated the *in vivo* importance of the SOCS box for inhibition of IFNγ signalling by SOCS1. SOCS box deleted-deficient mice also die prematurely and suffer from reduced body weight. Inflammatory lesions are observed in skeletal and heart muscle, cornea, pancreas and dermis.

SOCS2 is thought to play a major role in the regulation of GH signalling. Indeed, mice deficient for *SOCS2* develop gigantism with enlargement of visceral organs and 3 months after birth weight 30-40% more than control mice, elevated mRNA levels of insulin-like growth factor (IGF-1) and enhanced responses to exogenous GH (Metcalf et al., 2000; Greenhalgh et al., 2005). Interestingly, over-expression of SOCS2 increases GH signalling and *SOCS2* transgenic mice develop mild gigantism (Favre et al., 1999). These results suggest a more complex role of SOCS2 in regulating GH signalling. To date, there are no evidences on the role of SOCS2 in the regulation of immune responses.

Deletion of *SOCS3* leads to embryonic lethality with embryos dying between 12 and 16 days of gestation (Marine et al., 1999b). Lethality was initially thought to result from excessive erythropoiesis due to enhanced EPO signalling. However, further studies showed that lethality was in fact due to placental insufficiency with poor development of embryonic vessels, spongiotrophoblasts, as well as increase in trophoblast giant cell differentiation (Roberts et al., 2001). Tetraploid aggregation assays resulting in *SOCS3*-deficient foetal components with SOCS3 sufficient placental tissues, generated live birth *SOCS3*$^{-/-}$ mice. These mice were smaller than littermates, exhibited cardiac hyperthrophy and finally succumbed by 25 days. Importantly, SOCS3 lethality could be rescued if mice were also deficient for Leukemia-Inhibitory factor (LIF) or its receptor (LIFR), indicating that SOCS3 is required for modulating LIF signalling in giant trophoblast cell differentiation (Takahashi et al., 2003, Robb et al., 2005).

SOCS3 has also been shown to play an important role in Th1 and Th2 cell differentiation. Indeed, blocking SOCS3 either by a dominant-negative mutant or in heterozygous *SOCS3* mice diminishes the differentiation of Th2 cells, resulting in the skewing of T-cells towards the Th1 phenotype and reduced allergic responses (Seki et al., 2003; Kubo et al., 2006). Furthermore, over-expression of SOCS3 in T-cells provokes exacerbating Th2 cell-mediated eye-allergy, with inhibition of SOCS3 ameliorating the severity of the disease.

The receptors to which SOCS3 binds mostly activate STAT3, therefore, SOCS3 has been considered as a negative regulator of inflammation and an inhibitor relatively specific to STAT3. Indeed, mice with a conditional deletion of SOCS3 in haematopoietic and endothelial cells die as young adults due to severe inflammatory lesions in the peritoneal and pleural cavities (Croker et al., 2004, Robb et al., 2005). If G-CSF is administered to these mice, mimicking emergency granulopoiesis during infection, they exhibit massive neutrophil infiltration and destruction of liver, lung, muscle and spinal tissue, resulting from increased intensity and duration of G-CSF-induced STAT3 activation. These results thus indicate SOCS3 as a negative regulator of G-CSF and STAT3 in myeloid cells. Mice with *SOCS3*-deficient haematopoiesis display also high susceptibility to inflammatory joint disease in an IL-1-induced inflammatory model (Wong et al., 2006). Adenoviral gene transfer of SOCS3 or dominant negative STAT3 indeed reduced the proliferation of RA synovial fibroblasts and the severity of the disease in a mouse model that is also dependent on Th17 cells (Shouda et al., 2001). The generation of these same cells is enhanced in T-cell specific *SOCS3*-deficient mice and abrogation of SOCS3 binding site in gp130 knock-in mutant mice results in Th17-like arthritis (Taleb et al., 2009; Ogura et al., 2008). Together, these results show that the absence of SOCS3 has dramatic pro-inflammatory effects by promoting Th17 development and Th17-mediated disease.

Mice lacking *CIS* did not display any specific phenotype (Marine et al., 1999a). However, CIS-over-expressing transgenic mice recreate a phenotype quite similar to *STAT5*-deficient mice with defects in growth and lactation, GH and prolactin signalling, as well as in natural killer, natural killer T-cell and T-cell development (Matsumoto et al., 1999). These results support its role in JAK/STAT5 pathway.

The role of SOCS4 *in vivo* or in immune responses is to date unknown. However, *in vivo* studies on SOCS5 reveal its possible role in adaptive immunity, notably in Th1 and Th2 cell differentiation. *SOCS5* transgenic mice show attenuation of IL-4-mediated STAT6 signalling, as well as reduced Th2 cell development and production of Th2-type-cytokines (Seki et al., 2002). Interestingly, SOCS5 over-expression augmented eosinophilic airway inflammation and septic peritonitis in mice (Ohshima et al., 2007; Watanabe et al., 2006). In contrast, *SOCS5*-deficent mice appear to have normal T-cell development and differentiation to both Th1 and Th2 cells (Brender et al., 2004). These contradictory phenotypes might be explained with the high homology between SOCS4 and SOCS5 denoting a redundant role of these proteins *in vivo*.

SOCS6-deficient mice do not display overt abnormalities, but just mild growth retardation, suggesting its role in cell growth (Krebs et al., 2002). However, SOCS6 over-expression results in inhibited insulin signalling and improvement in glucose tolerance, similarly to *p85*-deficient mice (Li et al., 2004). *SOCS7* ablation *in vivo* has mainly delineated its essential role in insulin signalling. *SOCS7*-deficient mice shows multiple defects at an early age with half of the homozygous progeny displaying severe hydrocephalus and growth retardation concomitant with hypoglycaemia and enhanced glucose metabolism that resulted in perinatal lethality (Banks et al., 2005; Krebs et al., 2004). On the other hand, SOCS7 seems to have a role in the regulation of allergic inflammatory disease. *SOCS7*-deficient mice have a propensity toward spontaneous development of cutaneous disease with infiltration of degranulated mast cells (Knisz et al., 2009). Thus, these studies suggest a role for SOCS7 in modulating the development of allergic diseases.

5. Inhibitory adaptors in human haematological diseases

As described in the previous section, animal models for the Dok, Lnk, Cbl and SOCS families have been invaluable in demonstrating the important roles played by these adaptor proteins in fine-tuning signalling thresholds in haematopoietic and immune cells. Some of these *in vivo* models recapitulate exactly or almost, essential features of different haematological and immune diseases, allowing us to identify new molecular players and mechanisms implicated in the initiation and progression of these malignancies.

Dok proteins

Studies on *Dok-1* and *Dok-2*-deficient mice demonstrated that these adaptors are essential to suppress the blastic transformation of the Bcr-Abl–induced CML-like disease. However, it is of note that in case of patients with CML, blast crisis mostly results in myeloid or B cell leukemia/lymphoma, usually not in the T cell variety. That Bcr-Abl mice carrying a p53 mutation also developed T cell lymphoma suggests involvement of genetic background (Honda et al., 2000). Moreover, as double *Dok-1/2* knockout mice developed myeloproliferative disease in the absence of Bcr-Abl, Dok-1 and Dok-2 may oppose a wide range of myeloid leukemogenesis in humans. Consistently, undetectable or marginal levels of their expression was observed in about half of the leukemic cell lines established from patients with myeloid leukaemia, regardless of whether it is CML or not (Yasuda et al., 2004). Further investigation of the tumour suppressive function of Dok-1 and Dok-2 in human malignancies, especially myeloid leukaemia including CML and CMMoL, might lead to an understanding of the molecular mechanisms of such diseases and contribute to designing effective therapies against them (Table 5).

Histiocytic sarcoma (HS) is a malignant proliferation of cells showing morphological and immunophenotypic features of mature histiocytes, which represent tissue-resident macrophages. Until recently, HS, which was also known as malignant histiocytosis, was often confused with anaplastic large B-cell lymphoma or with other malignant lymphomas

(Weiss et al., 2009). As the molecular etiology of this disease is unknown, there remains a need for realistic animal models. Mouse models that have been reported for HS frequently show multiple lesions including lymphomas and severe renal failure. The syndrome elicited in mice lacking all the three proteins, Dok-1, Dok-2, and Dok-3, more specifically resembles the disease found in humans and hence may serve as a useful model for the study of HS. Although elucidation of the mechanisms by which the ablation of Dok proteins specifically causes HS and how the tumour gains its aggressive phenotype awaits further studies, such studies will help unveil the hidden etiology of this rare aggressive human malignancy.

Lnk proteins

Lnk-deficient mice display a phenotype reminiscent of BCR-ABL negative (Ph^-) MPNs, notably Essential Thrombocythemia (ET) and Primary Myelofibrosis (PMF) that has suggested a role for Lnk in the development of these diseases (Table 5). All MPNs are clonal disorders of HSC characterized by excessive proliferation of haematopoietic cells due to hypersensibility to normal cytokine regulation and absence of negative feed back regulation. The recent discovery of the Val617Phe acquired mutation of the *JAK2* gene (*JAK2*-V617F) represents the first reliable molecular marker of Ph^- MPN (Campbell & Green, 2008). The pathogenic role of JAK2-V617F constitutive active kinase and more recently of mutated Mpl (*MPL*W-515L) most likely will go through abnormal activation of signalling molecules, among which Lnk likely plays an important negative regulatory role through its binding to JAK2-V617F and MPL-W515L forms. Indeed, recent work has demonstrated a modulation of Lnk level in megakaryocyte/platelets and $CD34^+$ cells from MPNs patients (Baran-Marszak et al., 2010). Recently, the first *LNK* mutations in JAK2-V617F-negative MPN patients (ET and PMF) were identified (Oh et al., 2010). Both mutations are on exon 2, one (E208Q) is a missense mutation in the PH domain (ET patient), while the second mutation lead to a premature stop codon resulting in the absence of the protein (PMF patient). The prevalence of such mutations is rare (5% or less). However, other *LNK* mutations have been identified in leukemic transformation of MNP at a higher frequency [13%] (Pardani et al., 2010). Moreover, *LNK* exon 2 mutations were also found in pure erythrocytosis (Lasho et al., 2010). In this case, one mutation (A215V) was previously described in PMF blast crisis and another (E208X) results in absence of the protein. This finding suggests that the *LNK* mutations induce an MPN phenotype that may depend on different parameters, such as the presence of other mutations (Lasho et al., 2011).

Genome-wide association studies (GWAS) have recently revealed that different diseases share susceptibility variants. The *LNK/SH2B3* gene maps on chromosome 12q24 and a non-synonymous single nucleotide polymorphisms (SNP) in this gene has been reported in exon 2 resulting in a missense mutation at position 262 leading to a R262W amino acid substitution in the PH domain. Surprisingly, this nsSNP has recently been associated with inflammatory disorders, such as celiac disease (Hunt et al., 2008; Zhernakova et al., 2010), type 1 diabetes (Lavrikova et al., 2010), asthma (Gudbjartsson et al., 2009) multiple sclerosis (Alcina et al., 2010), and also to eight clinically relevant haematological parameters (Soranzo et al., 2009; Ganesh et al., 2009) in different populations. Furthermore, the *LNK* R262W variant has also been associated to cardiovascular diseases such as myocardial infarction, coronary heart disease and hypertension (Gudbjartsson et al., 2009; Ikram et al., 2010). All these data suggests that Lnk nsSNP could be a risk variant for these diseases contributing to their pathogenesis, and in consequence, providing a useful diagnostic marker.

Cbl proteins

Animal models have demonstrated the enhanced biological responses in the haematopoietic and immune system of Cbl family members when they are either genetically ablated or point mutated. It is in this context that the recent identification of mutations in CBL in patients with myeloid malignancies provides an important milestone (Table 5). Two groups simultaneously identified CBL mutations in Acute Myeloid Leukaemia (AML) patient samples (Sargin et al., 2007; Caligiuri et al., 2007). CBL mutations are most frequently observed in a distinct group of myeloid disorders named myelodysplastic syndromes/myeloproliferative neoplasms (MDS/MPN) that include: the Chronic Myelomonocytic Leukaemia (CMML), atypical Chronic Myeloid Leukaemia (aCML) and Juvenile Myelomonocytic Leukaemia (JMML). They originate from immature haematopoietic progenitors and are characterized by the production of dysplastic blood cells and myeloproliferative features. In most adult cases, mutations seem to be somatic, but germline mutations were reported in some JMML cases in children (Loh et al., 2009; Niemeyer et al., 2010; Martinelli et al., 2010). Genetic alterations in these haematological malignancies are strongly associated with hyperactivation of the Ras/MAPK signalling pathway due to activating mutations in signalling molecules involved in this pathway accounting for approximately 75%cases of JMML (Schubbert, et al., 2007). Strikingly, *CBL* mutations are found in 5% of aCML and up to 15% of JMML and CMML (Grand et al., 2009; Loh et al., 2009; Muramatsu et al., 2010; Shiba et al., 2010; Dunbar et al., 2008; Sanada et al., 2009). Most *CBL* mutations associated with myeloid malignancies are clustered around the linker and the RING finger domains and *in vitro* studies with these mutants have shown their lack of E3 ubiquitin ligase activity (Sargin et al., 2007; Grand et al., 2009; Sanada et al., 2009). Complete loss of *CBL*, deletions or mutations outside the linker/RING finger domains are rare, as well as mutations in *CBLB*. These findings suggest that expression of mutant Cbl proteins act as dominant negative inhibitor of wild-type Cbl or even of lost Cbl expression. A remarkable genetic feature of *c-CBL* mutations in these myeloid neoplasms is that mutations are homozygous in most cases, as a result of duplication of the mutated parental copy of 11q (where the *CBL* gene resides) and loss of the remaining wild-type allele, a genetic process called "acquired uniparental disomy" (aUPD) (Grand et al., 2009). This feature underlies the gain-of-function nature, rather than a loss-of-function, of the CBL mutations and may represent a defining oncogenic event. Indeed, mutations involving *RUNX1, JAK2, FLT3* and *TP53* have been shown to coexist with CBL mutations in myeloid neoplasms (Sanada et al., 2009; Perez et al., 2010; Tefferi, 2010; Makishima et al., 2011) suggesting that additional oncogenic events may contribute to the mutant Cbl-driven leukemogenic process.

SOCS proteins

There is now emerging evidence that SOCS expression is differentially regulated during Th cell differentiation and in Th-driven inflammatory diseases (Table 5). In Th1 inflammatory diseases (rheumatoid arthritis, ulcerative colitis, Crohn disease, contact and atopic dermatitis), SOCS1 expression is observed in lymphocytes and macrophages, as well as keratinocytes and stromal cells that are capable of antigen presentation, but granulocytes are negative (Egan et al., 2003; Federici et al., 2002). Importantly, SOCS3 expression levels seem to correlate with the severity of this type of inflammatory diseases (Seki et al., 2003; Shouda et al., 2001; Suzuki et al., 2001). The same is true for Th2-driven asthma that promotes lymphocyte, basophile and mast cell infiltration, where SOCS3 expression in Th2 lymphocytes is elevated. Furthermore, the association of the function of SOCS molecules in the allergic response has been supported by human studies analyzing the association of polymorphisms in *SOCS* genes with allergic disease in people. Interestingly, an association of a promoter polymorphism leads to a promoter with modified activity *in vitro*, suggesting that changes in *SOCS1* expression can have considerable effects on disease manifestations in patients (Harada et al., 2007). SOCS1 expression has been found decreased in some human cancers including hepatocellular carcinoma and myeloproliferative neoplasms and this is frequently associated with hyper-methylation of one or more *SOCS* genes (Yoshikawa et al., 2001; Watanabe et al., 2004; Quentmeier et al., 2008; Chaligné et al., 2009). In some cases, this methylation has been correlated to the degree of malignancy (Okochi et al., 2003; Yoshida et al., 2004). These observations strongly suggest that SOCS proteins may be tumour suppressors. Loss of SOCS expression may then contribute or favour tumour progression in synergy with other oncogenes. SOCS expression has also been implicated in the resistance to interferon in haematopoietic malignancies, such as leukaemia, lymphomas and multiple myeloma (Sakamoto et al., 2000, Sakai et al., 2002). Persistent expression of SOCS1 and/or SOCS3 has been detected in cutaneous T-cell lymphoma (CTCL), chronic myeloid leukaemia (CML), and some acute leukaemia (Brender et al., 2001b; Cho-Vega et al., 2004; Roman-Gomez et al., 2004). In these circumstances, elevated expression of SOCS coincides with constitutive activation of JAK/STAT pathways. Moreover, in certain myeloproliferative neoplasm, SOCS3 has been found hyper-phosphorylated, which enhances the half-life of the protein but interferes with its regulatory function (Hookham et al., 2007; Elliott et al., 2009; Suessmuth et al., 2009). These data suggests that perturbed SOCS expression may contribute to the malignant phenotype and favour disease progression, rather than being an early event in the oncogenic process.

6. Therapeutic application of inhibitory adaptors

Given the central role played by inhibitory adaptors in the regulation of different aspects of haematopoietic and immune cell function, they are predicted to serve as excellent new targets in the development of anti-oncogenic, anti-inflammatory and immunosuppressor reagents. The advantage of these adaptors as targets is their restricted expression in cells of the haematopoietic and immune system, at least of some of the members in the different families discussed here. The disadvantage for some of them (Dok, Lnk) is their lack of enzymatic activity for drug targeting. However, this can be surpassed by utilizing strategies based in the direct inhibition or blockade of their specific protein-protein interactions for targeting a particular signalling pathway. This approach relies on the current information available on the molecular structure of the adaptor functional domains and the identification of specific sequences or residues involved in the adaptor/partner interaction. In some pathological contexts, the association of the inhibitory adaptor with mutated or oncogenic forms of its targets is modified from that engaged with its normal counterpart (Baran-Marszak et al., 2010). These findings open the possibility to use the binding sequence in the adaptor to exclusively inhibit the oncogenic protein and signalling pathway, while sparing the normal cell signalling cascades. Indeed, successful development of small molecule inhibitors of protein-protein interaction has begun to emerge, validating it as a practical approach (Azmi & Mohammad, 2009). The use of dominant negative forms of these inhibitory proteins has also proved to be advantageous, notably for adaptors that have shown dual functions, as positive and negative regulators, as they allow modulate specifically their function depending on the cell type and biological response to be addressed. In the case of Lnk, its loss or inhibition causes the abnormal expansion and enhanced ability for engraftment of HSC (Takizawa et al., 2006); this feature can be used for bone marrow transplantation where the scarce number of these cells is always the limiting factor for the use of this therapy.

On the other hand, adaptors with catalytic activity, like the Cbl and SOCS proteins, have the double advantage of being used as adaptors and as E3 ligase. In the case of Cbl, it is clear that its ligase activity is central to the regulation of many oncogenic proteins, so drugs that could enhance this activity may provide new therapeutic strategies for limiting their constitutive signalling. A potential strategy is the screening for molecules that could mimic the activation of its E3 activity while retaining its targets binding. This can be use in basophile and mast cells of allergic patients as a therapy to treat allergy diseases. In the case of SOCS, a strategy based in the delivery of the SOCS3 protein using a recombinant cell penetrating moiety has proved to increase the concentration and activity of SOCS3 in the cells and suppressed the effects of acute inflammation (Jo et al., 2005). Moreover, therapeutic trials using SOCS antisense oligonucleotide, small hairpin RNA and peptide mimetics are currently investigated in animal models (Yoshimura et al., 2007). Importantly, a better understanding of the spectrum of signalling alterations provoked by mutant forms of the inhibitory adaptors identified in human pathologies is likely to reveal therapeutic strategies for patients with these mutations. In this context, the association of single nucleotide polymorphisms (SNP) in the genes of some of these adaptors (*LNK, SOCS*) with different inflammatory, myeloproliferative and vascular diseases suggests the implication of these molecules as risk factor and their potential use as biomarkers in these diseases. Lastly, future challenges in the study of inhibitory adaptors lie also in the development of performing techniques that will allow accurate monitoring of their signalling complexes at the molecular level. Indeed, precise regulation of protein interactions is of medical relevance, as modifications in the composition or localization of crucial components of these signalling networks can lead to the development of human diseases.

7. Conclusions

Over the past decade, it has become clear the pivotal role that cytokines play in the development and pathology of human diseases, including those of the haematopoietic and immune system. They perform their actions by regulating essential biological functions, such as cell proliferation, differentiation, cell morphology and migration. It is therefore not surprising that cytokine signal transduction pathways are tightly regulated. To achieve this, they have set up a variety of mechanisms and the rate at which the signal is turned off will be due to the net effect of all of these regulatory pathways. Although initially identified and best understood as mediators of positive signalling, adaptors have also shown an equally critical role in the negative control of signalling events. Inhibitory adaptors have been demonstrated important for maintaining homeostasis by preventing inappropriate cellular activation (Lnk, Cbl), by localizing enzymatically active regulatory molecules to specific subcellular compartments (Dok), and/or by terminating signalling cascades once they are initiated through targeting activated mediators to degradative pathways (Cbl, SOCS). In doing so, these molecules act upon three key signalling intermediates (the receptor,

JAK/other kinases, and STATs/downstream effectors) to completely switch off the signal. In contrast to SOCS and Lnk, which are induced in response to cytokines, Cbl and Dok (with the exception of Dok-2 in some cases) are constitutively present in the cell and may therefore function as more acute, early response regulators. The timing and specificity of each of these mechanisms, as well as how the inhibitors interact and cooperate with each other, is still an area for future investigation. Furthermore, the fact that the expression of these adaptors is itself regulated, points out further the complexity of the regulatory system. While gene-targeting studies have highlighted critical roles for the inhibitory adaptors in immune function, haematological malignancy and inflammation, the complexity of the mouse models, particularly with regard to multi-gene families, suggests that these studies should be carefully interpreted, and certainly more work is required before we can predict the consequences of using these molecules or their agonists/antagonists in a clinical setting. Thus, one of the challenges for the future is sorting out the roles of negative regulators of cytokine signalling in all the existing pathways activated in response to cytokines. This knowledge is likely to yield both new and confirmatory findings, with the anticipation of a better understanding of how these adaptors orchestrate the functional activity and fate of many partners to produce the desired intensity of a signalling response. Although a great deal of research remains to be done to clarify the roles of these inhibitors and their mutant forms in human diseases such as cancer and inflammation, it can be foreseen that it will lead to the development of strategies based on the up- or down-regulation of their properties for therapeutic purposes.

8. Acknowledgments

I thank the members of my laboratory and of the U978 Inserm for sharing their data and support. This work was supported by grants from the Institut National de la Santé et la Recherche Médicale (Inserm) and the Association pour la Recherche contre le Cancer (ARC, contrat no. SFI20101201732).

9. References

Abramson, J., Rozenblum, G., & Pecht, I. (2003). Dok protein family members are involved in signaling mediated by the type 1 Fcepsilon receptor. *Eur J Immunol.*, Vol.33, pp. 85–91

Alcina, A., Vandenbroeck, K., Otaegui, D., Saiz, A., Gonzalez, J.R., Fernandez, O., Cavanillas, M.L., Cénit, M.C., Arroyo, R., Alloza, I., García-Barcina, M., Antigüedad, A., Leyva, L., Izquierdo, G., Lucas, M., Fedetz, M., Pinto-Medel, M.J., Olascoaga, .J, Blanco, Y., Comabella, M., Montalban, X., Urcelay, E., & Matesanz, F. (2010). The autoinmune disease-associated KIF5A, CD226 and SH2B3 gene variants confer susceptibility for multiple sclerosis. *Genes and Immun.*, Vol.11, pp. 439-445

Alexander, W.S., Starr, R., Fenner, J.E., Scott, C.L., Handman, E., Sprigg, N.S., Corbin, J.E., Cornisa, A.L., Darwiche, R., Owczarek, C.M., Kay, T.W., Incola, N.A., Hertzog, P.J., Metcalf, D., & Milton, D.J. (1999). SOCS1 is a critical inhibitor of interferon □ signalling and prevents the potentially fatal neonatal actions of this cytokine. *Cell*, Vol.9, pp. 597–608

Alexander WS, & Hilton DJ. (2004). The role of suppressors of cytokine signaling (SOCS) proteins in regulation of the immune response. *Annu Rev Immunol*, Vol.22, pp. 503–29

Azmi, A.S., & Mohammad, R.M. (2009). Non-peptidic small molecule inhibitors against Bcl-2 for cancer therapy. *J. Cell. Physiol.*, Vol.218, pp. 13-21

Babon, J.J., McManus, E., Yao, S., DeSouza, D.P., Mielke, L.A., Sprigg, N.S., Wilson, T.A., Hilton, D.J., Nicola, N.A., Baca, M., Nicholson, S.E., & Norton, R.S. (2006). The structure of SOCS3 reveals the basis of the extended SH2 domain function and identifies an unstructured insertion that regulates stability. *Mol. Cell.*, Vol.22, No.2, pp. 205-216

Bachmaier, K., Krawczyk, C., Kozieradzki, I., Kong, Y.-Y., Sasaki, T., Oliveira-dos-Santos, A., Mariathasan, S., Bouchard, D., Wakeham, A., Itie, A., Le, J., Ohashi, P.S., Sarosi, I., Nishina, H., Lipkowitz, S., & Penninger, J.M. (2000). Negative regulation of lymphocyte activation and autoimmunity by the molecular adaptor Cbl-b. *Nature*, Vol.403, pp. 211–216

Bachmaier, K., Toya, S., Gao, X., Triantafillou, T., Garrean, S., Park, G.Y., Frey, R.S., Vogel, S., Minshall, R., Christman, J.W., Tiruppathi, C., & Malik, A.B. (2007). E3 ubiquitin ligase Cbl-b regulates the acute inflammatory response underlying lung injury. *Nat. Med.*, Vol.13, pp. 920-926

Bandi, S.R., Brandts, C., Rensinghoff, M., Grundler, R., Tickenbrock, L., Kohler, G., Duyster, J., Berdel, W.E., Muller-Tidow, C., Serve, H., & Sargin, B. (2009). E3 ligase-defective Cbl mutants lead to a generalized mastocytosis and myeloproliferative disease. *Blood*, Vol.114, pp. 4197–208

Banks, A.S., Li, J., McKeag, L., Hribal, M.L., Kashiwada, M., Accili, D., & Rothman, P.B. (2005). Deletion of SOCS7 leads to enhanced insulin action and enlarged islets of Langerhans. *J Clin Invest.*, Vol.115, No.9, pp. 2462-2471

Baran-Marszak, F., Magdoud, H., Desterke, C., Alvarado, A., Roger, C., Harel, S., Mazoyer, E., Cassinat, B., Chevret, S., Tonetti, C., Giraudier, S., Fenaux, P., Cymbalista, F., Varin-Blank, N., LeBousse-Kerdilès, M.C., Kiladjian, J.J., & Velazquez, L. (2010). Expression level and differential JAK2-V617F-binding of the adaptor protein Lnk regulates JAK2-mediated signals in myeloproliferative neoplasms. *Blood*, Vol.116, No.26, pp. 5961-5971

Bartkiewicz, M., Houghton, A., & Baron, R. (1999). Leucine zipper-mediated homodimerization of the adaptor protein c-Cbl. A role in c-Cbl's tyrosine phosphorylation and its association with epidermal growth factor receptor. *J. Biol. Chem.*, Vol.274, No.43, pp. 30887–30895

Bersenev, A., Wu, C., Balcerek, J., & Tong, W. (2008). Lnk controls mouse hematopoietic stem cell self-renewal and quiescence through direct interactions with JAK2. *J. Clin. Invest.*, Vol.118, No.8, pp. 2832-2844

Bersenev, A., Wu, C., Balcerek, J., Jing, J., Kundu, M., Blobel, G.A., Chikwave, K.R., & Tong, W. (2010). Lnk constraints myeloproliferative diseases in mice. *J. Clin. Invest.*, Vol.120, No. 6, pp. 2058-2069

Bjorbaek, C., Buchholz, R.M., Davis, S.M., Bates, S.H., Pierroz, D.D., Gu, H., Neel, B.G., Myers, M.G. Jr, & Flier, J.S. (2001). Divergent roles of SHP-2 in ERK activation by leptin receptors. *J Biol Chem.*, Vol.276, pp. 4747–4755

Blake, T.J., Shapiro, M., Morse, H.C. III., & Langdon, W.Y. (1991). The sequences of the human and mouse *c-cbl* proto-oncogenes show *v-cbl* was generated by a large truncation encompassing a proline-rich domain and a leucine zipper-like motif. *Oncogene*, Vol.6, pp. 653-657

Boulay, I., Némorin, J.G., & Duplay, P. (2005). Phosphotyrosine binding-mediated oligomerization of downstream of tyrosine kinase (Dok)-1 and Dok-2 is involved in CD2-induced Dok phosphorylation. *J Immunol*, Vol.175, pp. 4483–4489

Boyle, K., Egan, P., Rakar, S., Wilson, T.A., Wicks, I.P., Metcalf, D., Hilton, D.J., Nicola, N.A., Alexander, W.S., Roberts, A.W., & Robb, L. (2007). The SOCS box of suppressor of cytokine signaling-3 contributes to the control of G-CSF responsiveness in vivo. *Blood*, Vol.110, pp. 1466-1474

Brender, C., Nielsen, M., Kaltoft, K., Mikkelsen, G., Zhang, Q., Wasik, M., Billestrup, N., & Odum, N. (2001b). STAT3-mediated constitutive expression of SOCS-3 in cutaneous T-cell lymphoma. *Blood.*, Vol.97, No.4, pp. 1056-1062.

Brender, C., Columbus, R., Metcal, D., Handman, E., Starr, R., Huntington, N., Tarlinton, D., Ødum, N., Nicholson, S.E., Nicola, N.A., Hilton, D.J., & Alexander, W.S. (2004). SOCS5 is expressed in primary B and T lymphoid cells but is dispensable for lymphocyte production and function. *Mol Cell Biol.*, Vol.24, No.13, pp. 6094-6103

Buza-Vidas, N., Antonchuk, J., Qian, H., Mansson, R., Luc, S., Zandi, S., Anderson, K., Takaki, S., Nygren, J.M., Jensen, C.T., & Jacobsen, S.E.W. (2006). Cytokines regulate postnatal hematopoietic stem cell expansion: opposing roles of thrombopoietin and LNK. *Genes & Dev.*, Vol.20, pp. 2018-2023

Cacalano, N.A., Sanden, D., & Johnston, J.A. (2001). Tyrosine-phosphorylated SOCS-3 inhibits STAT activation but binds to p120 RasGap and activates Ras. *Nat. Cell Biol.*, Vol.3, pp. 460-465

Caligiuri, M.A., Briesewitz, R., Yu, J., Wang, L., Wei, M., Arnoczky, K.J., Marburger, T.B., Wen, J., Perroti, D., Bloomfield, C.D., & Whitman, S.P. (2007). Novel c-CBL and CBL-b ubiquitin ligase mutations in human acute myeloid leukemia. *Blood*, Vol.110, pp. 1022–1024

Campbell, P.J., & Green, A.R. (2008). The myeloproliferative disorders. N Engl J Med., Vol. 355, pp. 2452-2466.

Carpino, N., Wisniewski, D., Strife, A., Marshak, D., Kobayashi, R., Stillman, B., & Clarkson, B. (1997). p62^{dok}: a constitutively tyrosine-phosphorylated, GAP-associated protein in chronic myelogenous leukemia progenitor cells. *Cell*, Vol.88, pp. 197–204

Chaligné, R., Tonetti, C., Besancenot, R., Marty, C., Kiladjian, J.J., Socié, G., Bordessoule, D., Vainchenker, W., & Giraudier, S. (2009). SOCS3 inhibits TPO-stimulated, but not spontaneous, megakaryocytic growth in primary myelofibrosis. *Leukemia.*, Vol.23, No.6, pp. 1186-1190

Chan, M.P., Ilangumaran, S., La Rose, J., Chakrabartty, A., & Rottapel, R. (2003). Autoinhibition of the Kit receptor tyrosine kinase by the cytosolic juxtamembrane region. *Mol. Cell. Biol.*, Vol.23, pp. 3067-3078

Chiang, Y.J., Jang, I.K., Hodes, R., & Gu, H. (2007). Ablation of Cbl-b provides protection against transplanted and spontaneous tumors. *J. Clin. Invest.*, Vol.117, pp.1029-1036

Cho-Vega, J.H., Rassidakis, G.Z., Amin, H.M., Tsioli, P., Spurgers, K., Remache, Y.K., Vega, F., Goy, A.H., Gilles, F., & Medeiros, L.J. (2004). Suppressor of cytokine signaling 3 expression in anaplastic large cell lymphoma. *Leukemia.*, Vol.18, No.11, pp. 1872-1878

Croker, B.A., Metcalf, D., Robb, L., Wei, W., Mifsud, S., DiRago, L., Cluse, L.A., Sutherland, K.D., Hartley, L., Williams, E., Zhang, J.G., Hilton, D.J., Nicola, N.A., Alexander,

W.S., & Roberts, A.W. (2004). SOCS3 is a critical physiological negative regulator of G-CSF signaling and emergency granulopoiesis. *Immunity*, Vol.20, pp. 153-165

Crowder R.J., Enomoto, H., Yang, M., Johnson, E.M. Jr, & Milbrandt, J. (2004). Dok-6, a Novel p62 Dok family member, promotes Ret-mediated neurite outgrowth. *J Biol Chem*, Vol. 279, pp. 42072–42081

Davies, G.C., Ettenberg, S.A., Coats, A.O., Mussante, M., Ravichandran, S., Collins, J., Nau, M.M., & Lipkowitz, S. (2004). Cbl-b interacts with ubiquitinated proteins; differential functions of the UBA domains of c-Cbl and Cbl-b. *Oncogene*, Vol.23, No.42, pp. 7104–7115

De Sepulveda, P., Ilangumaran, S., & Rottapel, R. (2000). Suppressor of cytokine signaling-1 inhibits VAV function through protein degradation. *J Biol Chem*, Vol.275, pp. 14005–14008

Dhe-Paganon, S., Werner, E.D., Nishi, M., Hansen, L., Chi, Y.I., & Shoelson, S.E. (2004). A phenylalanine zipper mediates APS dimerization. *Nat. Struct. Mol. Biol.*, Vol. 11, No.10, pp. 968-974

Diakonova, M., Gunter, D.R., Herrington, J., & Carter-Su, C. (2002). SH2-B□ is a Rac-binding protein that regulates cell motility. *J. Biol. Chem.*, Vol.277, No.12, pp. 10669-10677

Di Cristofano, A., Carpino, N., Dunant, N., Friedland, G., Kobayashi, R., Strife, A., Wisniewski, D., Clarkson, B., Pandolfi, P.P., & Resh, M.D. (1998). Molecular cloning and characterization of p56^{dok-2} defines a new family of RasGAP-binding proteins. *J. Biol. Chem.*, Vol.273, pp. 4827–4830

Dunbar, A.J., Gondek, L.P., O'Keefe, C.L., Makishima, H., Rataul, M.S., Szpurka, H., Sekeres, M.A., Wang, X.F., McDevitt, M.A., & Maciejewski, J.P. (2008). 250K single nucleotide polymorphism array karyotyping identifies acquired uniparental disomy and homozygous mutations, including novel missense substitutions of c-Cbl, in myeloid malignancies. *Cancer Res*, Vol.68, pp. 10349–10357

Egan, P.J., Lawlor, K.E., Alexander, W.S., & Wicks, I.P. (2003). Suppressor of cytokine signaling-1 regulates acute inflammatory arthritis and T cell activation. *J Clin Invest.*, Vol.111, No.6, pp. 915-924

El Chami N, Ikhlef F, Kaszas K, Yakoub S, Tabone E, Siddeek B, Cunha S, Beaudoin C, Morel L, Benahmed M, Régnier DC. (2005). Androgen-dependent apoptosis in male germ cells is regulated through the proto-oncoprotein Cbl. *J Cell Biol.*, Vol.171, No.4, pp.651-61

Elliott, J., Suessmuth, Y., Scott, L.M., Nahlik, K., McMullin, M.F., Constantinescu, S.N., Green, A.R., & Johnston, J.A. (2009). SOCS3 tyrosine phosphorylation as a potential bio-marker for myeloproliferative neoplasms associated with mutant JAK2 kinases. *Haematologica.*, Vol.94, No.4, pp. 576-80

Ema, H., Sudo, K., Seita, J., Matsubara, A., Morita, Y., Osawa, M., Takatsu, K., Takaki, S., & Nakauchi, H. (2005). Quantification of self-renewal capacity in single hematopoietic stem cells from normal and Lnk-deficient mice. *Develop. Cell*, Vol.8, pp. 907-914

Endo, T.A., Masuhara, M., Yokochi, M., Suzuki, R., Sakamoto, H., Mitsui, K., Matsumoto, A., Tanimura, S., Ohtsubo, M., Misawa, H., Miyazaki, T., Leonor, N., Taniguchi, T., Fujita, T., Kanakura, Y., Komiya, S., & Yoshimura, A. (1997). A new protein containing an SH2 domain that inhibits JAK kinases. *Nature*, Vol.387, pp. 921–924

Favre, H., Benhamou, A., Finidori, J., Kelly, P.A., & Edery, M. (1999). Dual effects of suppressor of cytokine signaling (SOCS-2) on growth hormone signal transduction. *FEBS Lett*, Vol.453, 63–66.

Favre, C., Gerard, A., Clauzier, E., Pontarotti, P., Olive, D., & Nunes, J.A. (2003). DOK4 and DOK5: new Dok-related genes expressed in human T cells. *Genes Immun.*, Vol.4, pp. 40–45

Federici M, Giustizieri ML, Scarponi C, Girolomoni G, & Albanesi C. (2002). Impaired IFN-gamma-dependent inflammatory responses in human keratinocytes overexpressing the suppressor of cytokine signaling 1. *J Immunol*, Vol.169, No.1, pp. 434-442

Fitau, J., Boulday, G., Coulon, F., Quillard, T. & Charreau, B. (2006). The adaptor molecule Lnk negatively regulates TNFalpha-dependent VCAM-1 expression in endothelial cells through inhibition of the ERK1 and 2 pathways. *J. Biol. Chem.*, Vol.281, No.29, pp. 20148-59

Frantsve, J., Schwaller, J., Sternberg, D.W., Kutok, J., & Gilliland, D.G. (2001). Socs-1 inhibits TEL-JAK2-mediated transformation of hematopoietic cells through inhibition of JAK2 kinase activity and induction of proteasome- mediated degradation. *Mol Cell Biol*, Vol.21, pp. 3547–3557

Garcia, A., Prabhakar, S., Hughan, S., Anderson, T.W., Brock, C.J., Pearce, A.C., Dwek, R.A., Watson, S.P., Heberstreit, H.F., & Zitzmann, N.A. (2004). Differential proteome analysis of TRAP-activated platelets: involvement of DOK-2 and phosphorylation of RGS proteins. *Blood*, Vol.103, pp. 2088-2095

Ganesh, S.K., Zakai, N.A., Van Rooij, F.J.A., Soranzo, N., Smith, A.V., Nalls, M.A., Chen, M.H., Kottgen, A., Glazer, N.L., Dehghan, A., Kuhnel, B., Aspelund, T., Yang, Q., Tanaka, T., Jaffe, A., Bis, J.C., Verwoert, G.C., Teumer, A., Fox, C.S., Guralnik, J.M., Ehret, G.B., Rice, K., Felix, J.F., Rendon, A., Eiriksdottir, G., Levy, D., Patel, K.V., Boerwinkle, E., Rotter, J.I., Hofman, A., Sambrook, J.G., Hernandez, D.G., Zheng, G., Bandinelli, S., Singleton, A.B., Coresh, J., Lumley, T., Uitterlinden, A.G., Vangils, J.M., Launer, L.J., Cupples, L.A., Oostra, B.A., Zwaginga, J.J., Ouwehand, W.H., Thein, S.L., Meisinger, C., Deloukas, P., Nauck, M., Spector, T.D., Gieger, C., Gudnason, V., van Duijn, C.M., Psaty, B.M., Ferrucci, L., Chakravarti, A., Greinacher, A., O'Donnell, C.J., Witteman, J.C., Furth, S., Cushman, M., Harris, T.B., & Lin, J.P. (2009). Multiple loci influence erythrocyte phenotypes in the CHARGE Consortium. *Nat. Genet.*, Vol.41, No.11, pp. 1191-1198

Geest, C.R. & Coffer, P. J. (2009). MAPK signaling pathways in the regulation of hematopoiesis. *J. Leuk. Biol.*, Vol.86, pp. 237-250

Gery, S., Gueller, S., Chumakova, K., Kawamata, N., Liu, L., & Koeffler, H.P. (2007). Adaptor protein Lnk negatively regulates the mutant MPL, MPLW515L associated with myeloproliferative disorders. *Blood*, Vol.110, No.9, pp. 3360-3364

Gery, S., Qi, C., Gueller, S., Hongtao, X., Tefferi, A., & Koeffler, H.P. (2009a). Lnk inhibits myeloproliferative disorder-associated JAK2 mutant, JAK2V617F. *J Leuk Biol.*, Vol.85, pp. 957-965

Gery, S., Gueller, S., Nowak, V., Sohn, J., Hofman, W.K., & Koeffler, H.P. (2009b). Expression of the adaptor protein Lnk in leukemia cells. *Exp Hematol.*, Vol.37, pp. 585-592

Grand, F.H., Hidalgo-Curtis, C.E., Ernst, T., Zoi, K., Zoi, C., McGuire, C., Kreil, S., Jones, A., Score, J., Metzgeroth, G., Oscier, D., Hall, A., Brandts, C., Serve, H., Reiter, A., Chase, A.J., & Cross, N.C.P. (2009). Frequent CBL mutations associated with 11q acquired uniparental disomy in myeloproliferative neoplasms. *Blood*, Vol.113, pp. 6182–6192

Greenhalgh, C.J., Metcalf, D., Thaus, A.L., Corbin, J.E., Uren, R., Morgan, P.O., Fabri, L.J., Zhang, J.G., Martin, H.M., Willson, T.A., Billestrup, N., Nicola, N.A., Baca, M.,

Alexander, W.S., & Hilton, D.J. (2002). Biological evidence that SOCS-2 can act either as an enhancer or suppressor of growth hormone signaling. *J Biol Chem*, Vol.277, pp. 40181–4

Grogan, T.M., Pileri, S.A., Chan, J.K.C., Helgadottir, A., Sulem, P., Jonsdottir, G.M., Thorleifsson, G., Helgadottir, H, Steinthorsdottir, V., Stefansson, H., Williams, C., Hui, J., Beilby, J., Warrington, N.M., James, A., Palmer, L.J., Koppelman, G.H., Heinzmann, A., Krueger, M., Boezen, H.M., Wheatley, A., Altmuller, J., Shin, H.D., Uh, S.T., Cheong, H.S., Jonsdottir, B., Gislason, D., Park, C.S., Rasmussen, L.M., Porsbjerg, C., Hansen, J.W., Backer, V., Werge, T., Janson, C., Jönsson, U.B., Ng, M.C., Chan, J., So, W.Y., Ma, R., Shah, S.H., Granger, C.B., Quyyumi, A.A., Levey, A.I., Vaccarino, V., Reilly, M.P., Rader, D.J., Williams, M.J., van Rij, A.M., Jones, G.T., Trabetti, E., Malerba, G., Pignatti, P.F., Boner, A., Pescollderungg, L., Girelli, D., Olivieri, O., Martinelli, N., Ludviksson, B.R., Ludviksdottir, D., Eyjolfsson, G.I., Arnar, D., Thorgeirsson, G., Deichmann, K., Thompson, P.J., Wjst, M., Hall, I.P., Postma, D.S., Gislason, T., Gulcher, J., Kong, A., Jonsdottir, I., Thorsteinsdottir, U., & Stefansson, K. Histiocytic sarcoma. In: Swerdlow SH, Campo E, Harris NL, et al. (eds). WHO Classification of Tumours of Haematopoietic and Lymphoid Tissues. 4th edn. International Agency for Research on Cancer: Lyon, 2008, pp 356–357

Gronski, M.A., Boulter, J.M., Moskophidis, D., Nguyen, L.T., Holmberg, K., Elford, A.R., Deenick, E.K., Kim, H.O., Penninger, J.M., Odermatt, B., Gallimore, A., Gascoigne, N.R., & Ohashi, P.S. (2004). TCR affinity and negative regulation limit autoimmunity. *Nat Med*, Vol.10, No.11, pp.1234–1239

Gudbjartsson, D. F., Bjornsdottir, U. S., Halapi, E., et al. (2009). Sequence variants affecting eosinophil numbers associate with asthma and myocardial infarction. *Nat. Genet.*, Vol.41, No.3, pp. 342-347

Gueller, S., Goodrigde, H.S., Niebuhr, B., Xing, H., Koren-Michowitz, M., Serve, H., Underhill, H.D., Brandts, C.H., & Koeffler, H.P. (2010). Adaptor protein Lnk inhibits c-fms-mediated macrophage function. *J. Leuk. Biol.*, Vol.88, pp. 699-706

Gueller, S., Hehn, S., Nowak, V., Gery, S., Serve, H., Brandts, C.H., & Koeffler, H.P. (2011). Adaptor protein Lnk binds to PDGF receptor and inhibits PDGF-dependent signaling. *Exp. Hematol.*, Vol.39, No.5, pp.591-600

Gueller, S., Gery, S., Nowak, V., Liu, L., Serve, H., & Koeffler, H.P. (2008). Adaptor protein Lnk associates with Y568 in c-Kit. *Biochem. J.*, Vol.415, pp. 241-245

Gueller, S., Hehn, S., Nowak, V., Gery, S., Serve, H., Brandts, C.H., & Koeffler, H.P. (2011). Adaptor protein Lnk binds to PDGF receptor and inhibits PDGF-dependent signaling. *Exp. Hematol.*, doi: 10.1016/j.exphem.2011.02.001

Gueller, S., Goodridge, H.S., Niebuhr, B., Xing, H., Koren-Michowitz, M., Serve, H., Underhill, D.M., Brandts, C.H., & Koeffler, H.P. (2010). Adaptor protein Lnk inhibits c-Fms-mediated macrophage function. *J. Leukoc. Biol.*, Vol.88, pp. 699-706

Guittard, G., Gérard, A., Dupuis-Coronas, S., Tronchère, H., Mortier, E., Favre, C., Olive, D., Zimmermann, P., Payrastre, B., & Nunès, J. (2009). Dok-1 and Dok-2 adaptor molecules are regulated by phosphatidylinositol 5-phosphate production in T cells. *J Immunol*, Vol.182, pp. 3974–3978

Gugasyan, R., Quilici, C., Grail, S.T.T.I., Verhagen, A.M., Roberts, A., Kitamura, T., Dunn, A.R., & Lock, P. (2002). Dok-related protein negatively regulates T cell development via its RasGTPase-activating protein and Nck docking sites. *J. Cell. Biol.*, Vol.158, pp. 115-125

Haan, S., Ferguson, P., Sommer, U., Hiremath, M., McVicar, D.W., Heinrich, P.C., Johnston, J.A., & Cacalano, N.A. (2003). Tyrosine phosphorylation disrupts elongin interaction and accelerates SOCS3 degradation. *J Biol Chem.*, Vol.278, No.34, pp.31972-31979

Harada M, Nakashima K, Hirota T, Shimizu M, Doi S, Fujita K, Shirakawa T, Enomoto T, Yoshikawa M, Moriyama H, Matsumoto K, Saito H, Suzuki Y, Nakamura Y, & Tamari M. (2007). Functional polymorphism in the suppressor of cytokine signaling 1 gene associated with adult asthma. *Am J Respir Cell Mol Biol.*, Vol.36, No.4, 491-496

He, X., Li, Y., Schembri-King, J., Jakes, S., & Hayashi, J. (2000). Identification of actin binding protein, ABP-280, as a binding partner of human Lnk adaptor protein. *Mol. Immunol.*, Vol.37, pp. 603-612

Hiragun, T., Peng, Z., & Beaven, M.A. (2005). Dexamethasone up-regulates the inhibitory adaptor protein Dok-1 and suppresses downstream activation of the mitogen-activated protein kinase pathway in antigen-stimulated RBL-2H3 mast cells. *Mol Pharmacol,* Vol.67, pp. 598–603

Hirasaka, K., Kohno, S., Goto, J., Furochi, H., Mawatari, K., Harada, N., Hosaka, T., Nakaya, Y., Ishidoh, K., Obata, T., Ebina, Y., Gu, H., Takeda, S., Kishi, K., & Nikawa, T. (2007). Deficiency of Cbl-b gene enhances infiltration and activation of macrophages in adipose tissue and causes peripheral insulin resistance in mice. *Diabetes,* Vol.56, pp. 2511-2522

Hilton, D.J., Richardson, R.T., Alexander, W.S., Viney, E.M., Willson, T.A., & Sprigg, N.S. (1998). Twenty proteins containing a C-terminal SOCS box form five structural classes. *Proc Natl Acad Sci* USA, Vol.95, pp.114–9

Honda, H., Ushijima, T., Wakazono, K., Oda, H., Tanaka, Y., Aizawa, S., Ishikawa, T., Yazaki, Y., & Hirai, H. (2000). Acquired loss of p53 induces blastic transformation in p210(bcr/abl)-expressing hematopoietic cells: a transgenic study for blast crisis of human CML. *Blood,* Vol.95, No.4, pp. 1144-1150

Honma M, Higuchi, O., Shirakata, M., Yasuda, T., Shibuya, H., Iemura, S., Natsume, T., & Yamanashi, Y. (2006). Dok-3 sequesters Grb2 and inhibits the Ras–Erk pathway downstream of protein-tyrosine kinases. *Genes Cells,* Vol.11, pp. 143–151

Hookham, M.B., Elliott, J., Suessmuth, Y., Staerk, J., Ward, A.C., Vainchenker, W., Percy, M.J., McMullin, M.F., Constantinescu, S.N., & Johnston, J.A. (2007). The myeloproliferative disorder-associated JAK2 V617F mutant escapes negative regulation by suppressor of cytokine signaling 3. *Blood,* Vol.109, No.11, pp. 4924-4929

Horino, J., Fujimoto, M., Terabe, F., serada, S., Takahashi, T., Soma, Y., Tanaka, K., Chinen, T., Yoshimura, A., Nomura, S., Kawase, I., Hayashi, N., Kishimoto, T., & Naka, T. (2008). Suppressor of cytokine signaling-1 ameliorates dextran sulfate sodium-induced colitis in mice. *Int. Immunol.*, Vol.20, pp. 753-762

Hu, J., & Hubbard, S.R. (2006). Structural basis for phosphotyrosine recognition by the Src Homology-2 domains of the adapter proteins SH2-B and APS. *J. Mol. Biol.*, Vol.361, pp. 69-79

Hu, J., Liu, J., Ghirlando, R., Saltiel, A.R., & Hubbard, S.R. (2003). Structural basis for recruitment of the adaptor protein APS to the activated Insulin receptor. *Mol. Cell.*, Vol.12, pp. 1379-1389

Huang, X., Li, Y., Tanaka, K., Moore, G., & Hayashi, J. (1995). Cloning and characterization of Lnk, a signal transduction protein that links T-cell receptor activation signal to phospholipase C1, Grb2, and phosphatidylinositol 3-kinase. *Proc. Natl. Acad. Sci.* USA. Vol.92, pp. 11618–11622

Huang, F., Kitaura, Y., Jang, I., Naramura, M., Kole, H.H., Liu, L., Qin, H., Schlissel, M.S., & Gu, H. (2006). Establishment of the major compatibility complex-dependent development of CD4+ and CD8+ T cells by the Cbl family proteins. *Immunity*, Vol.25, pp. 571-581

Hughan, S.C., & Watson, S.P. (2007). Differential regulation of adapter proteins Dok2 and Dok1 in platelets, leading to an association of Dok2 with integrin □IIb□3. *J. Thromb Haemost*, Vol.5, pp. 387-394

Hunt, K., Zhernakova, A., Turner, G., Heap, G.A., Franke, L., Bruinenberg, M., Romanos, J., Dinesen, L.C., Ryan, A.W., Panesar, D., Gwilliam, R., Takeuchi, F., McLaren, W.M., Holmes, G.K., Howdle, P.D., Walters, J.R., Sanders, D.S., Playford, R.J., Trynka, G., Mulder, C.J., Mearin, M.L., Verbeek, W.H., Trimble, V., Stevens, F.M., O'Morain, C., Kennedy, N.P., Kelleher, D., Pennington, D.J., Strachan, D.P., McArdle, W.L., Mein, C.A., Wapenaar, M.C., Deloukas, P., McGinnis, R., McManus, R., Wijmenga, C., & van Heel, D.A. (2008). Newly identified genetic risk variants for celiac disease related to the immune response. *Nat. Genet.*, Vol.40, No.4, pp. 395-402

Hunter, S., Burton, E. A., Wu, S. C. & Anderson, S. M. (1999). Fyn associates with Cbl and phosphorylates tyrosine 731 in Cbl, a binding site for phosphatidylinositol 3-kinase. *J. Biol. Chem.*, Vol.274, pp. 2097–2106

Ikram, M.K., Xueking, S., Jensen, R.A., Cotch, M.F., Hewitt, A.W., Ikram, M.A., Wang, J.J., Klein, R., Klein, B.E., Breteler, M.M., Cheung, N., Liew, G., Mitchell, P., Uitterlinden, A.G., Rivadeneira, F., Hofman, A., de Jong, P.T., van Duijn, C.M., Kao, L., Cheng, C.Y., Smith, A.V., Glazer, N.L., Lumley, T., McKnight, B., Psaty, B.M., Jonasson, F., Eiriksdottir, G., Aspelund, T.; Global BPgen Consortium, Harris, T.B., Launer, L.J., Taylor K.D., Li, X., Iyengar, S.K., Xi, Q, Sivakumaran, T.A., Mackey, D.A., Macgregor, S, Martin, ,N..G., Young, T.L., Bis, J.C., Wiggins, K.L., Heckbert, S.R., Hammond, C.J., Andrew, T, Fahy S, Attia, J., Holliday E.G, Scott, R.J., Islam, F.M., Rotter, J.I., McAuley, A.K., Boerwinkle, E, Tai, E.S., Gudnason, V., Siscovick, D. S, Vingerling, J.R., & Wong.TY (2010). Four novel loci (19q13, 6q24, 12q24, and 5q14) influence the microcirculation in vivo. *PLoS Genet.*, Vol.6, No.10, e1001184

Irandoust, M.I., Aarts, L.H., Roovers, O., Gits, J., Erkeland, S.J., & Touw, I.P. (2007). Suppressor of signaling 3 controls lysosomal routing of G-CSF receptor. *EMBO J.*, Vol.26, pp. 1782-1793

Iseki, M., Kubo, C., Kwon, S.M., Yamaguchi, A., Kataoka, Y., Yoshida, N., Takatsu, S., & Takaki, S. (2004). Increased numbers of B-1 cells and enhanced responses against TI-2 antigen in mice lacking APS and adaptor molecule containing PH and SH2 domains. *Mol. Cell. Biol.*, Vol.24, pp. 2243-2250

Iseki, M., Kubo-Akashi, C., Kwon, S.M., Yamaguchi, A., Takatsu, K., & Takaki, S. (2005). APS, an adaptor molecule containing PH and SH2 domains, has a negative regulatory role in B cell proliferation. *Biochem. Biophys. Research. Commun.*, Vol.330, pp. 1005-1013

Jo, D., Liu, D., Yao, S., Collins, R.D., & Hawiger, J. (2005). Intracellular protein therapy with SOCS3 inhibits inflammation and apoptosis. *Nat Med.*, Vol.11, No.8, pp. 892-898

Joazeiro, C. A. P., Wing, S. S., Huang, H.-K., Leverson, J. D., Hunter, T. & Liu, Y.-C. (1999) The tyrosine kinase negative regulator c-Cbl as a RING-type, E2-dependent ubiquitin-protein ligase. *Science*, Vol.286, pp. 309–312

Kamura, T., Sato, S., Haque, D., Liu, L., Kaelin, W.G. Jr., Conaway, R.C., & Conaway, J.W. (1998). The elongin BC complex interacts with the conserved SOCS-box motif present in members of the SOCS, ras, WD- 40 repeat, and ankyrin repeat families. *Genes Dev.*, Vol.12, pp. 3872–3881

Keane, M.M., Rivero-Lezcano, O., Mitchell, J.A., Robbins, K.C., & Lipkowitz, S. (1995). Cloning and characterization of cbl-b: a SH3 binding protein with homology to the c-cbl proto-oncogene. *Oncogene*, Vol.10, pp. 2367-2377

Keane, M.M., Ettenberg, S.A., Nau, M.M., Banerjee, P., Cuello, M., Penninger, J., & Lipkowitz, S. (1999). Cbl-3: a new mammalian cbl family protein. *Oncogene*, Vol.18, pp. 3365-3375

Kent, D.G., Dykstra, B.J., Cheyne, J., Ma, E., & Eaves, C.J. (2008). Steel factor coordinately regulates the molecular signature and biologic function of hematopoietic stem cells. *Blood.*, Vol.112, pp. 560-567

Khwaja, A. (2006). The role of Janus kinases in haemopoiesis and haematological malignancy. *British Journal of Haematology*, Vol.134, pp. 366–384

Kitaura, Y., Jang, I.K., Wang, Y., Han, Y.C., Inazu, T., Cadera, E.J., Schlissel, M., Hardy, R.R., & Gu, H. (2007). Control of the B cell-intrinsic tolerance programs by ubiquitin ligases Cbl and Cbl-b. *Immunity*, Vol.26, pp. 567-578

Kimura, A., Kinjyo, I., Matsumara, Y., Mori, H., Mashima, R., Harada, M., Chien, K.R., Yasukawa, H., & Yoshimura, A. (2004). SOCS3 is a physiological negative regulator for granulopoiesis and granulocyte colony-stimulating factor receptor signaling. *J. Biol. Chem.*, Vol.279, pp. 6905-6910

Kinjyo, I., Hanada, T., Inagaki-Ohara, Mori, K., H., Aki, D., Ohishi, M., Yoshida, H., Kubo, M., & Yoshimura, A. (2002). SOCS1/JAB is a negative regulator of LPS-induced macrophage activation. *Immunity*, Vol.17, pp. 583–591

Kishi, K., Mawatari, K., Sakai-Wakamatsu, K., Yuasa, T., Wang, M., Ogura-Sawa, M., Nakaya, Y., Hatakeyama, S., & Ebina, Y. (2007). APS-mediated ubiquitination of the insulin receptor enhances its internalization, but does not induce its degradation. *Endocrinology*, Vol.54, No.1, pp. 77-88

Knisz, J., Banks, A., McKeag, L., Metcalfe, D.D., Rothman, P.B., & Brown, J.M. (2009). Loss of SOCS7 in mice results in severe cutaneous disease and increased mast cell activation. *Clin Immunol.*, Vol.132, No.2, pp. 277-284

Krawczyk, C., Bachmaier, K., Sasaki, T., Jones, R.G., Snapper, S.B., Bouchard, D., Kozieradzki, I., Ohashi, P.S., Alt, F.W., & Penninger, J.M. (2000). Cbl-b is a negative regulator of receptor clustering and raft aggregation in T cells. *Immunity*, Vol.13, pp. 463–473

Krebs, D.L., Uren, R.T., Metcalf, D., Rakar, S., Zhang, J.G., Starr, R., De Souza, D.P., Hanzinikolas, K., Eyles, J., Connolly, L.M., Simpson, R.J., Nicola, N.A., Nicholson, S.E., Baca, M., Hilton, D.J., & Alexander, W.S. (2002). SOCS-6 binds to insulin receptor substrate 4, and mice lacking the SOCS-6 gene exhibit mild growth retardation. *Mol Cell Biol.*, Vol.22, No.13, pp. 4567-4578.

Krebs, D.L., Metcalf, D., Merson, T.D., Voss, A.K., Thomas, T., Zhang, J.G., Rakar, S., O'bryan, M.K., Willson, T.A., Viney, E.M., Mielke, L.A., Nicola, N.A., Hilton, D.J., &

Alexander, W.S. (2004). Development of hydrocephalus in mice lacking SOCS7. *Proc Natl Acad Sci* U S A., Vol.101, No.43, pp. 15446-15451

Kwon, S.M., Suzuki, T., Kawamoto, A., Ii, M., Eguchi, M., Akimaru, H., Wada, M., Matsumoto, T., Masuda, H., Nakagawa, Y., Nishimura, H., Kawai, K., Takaki, S. & Asahara, T. (2009). Pivotal role of Lnk adaptor protein in endothelial progenitor cell biology for vascular regeneration. *Circ Res.* Vol.104, pp. 969-977

Kubo, M., Ozaki, A., Tanaka, S., Okamoto, M., & Fukushima, A. (2006). Role of suppressor of cytokine signaling in ocular allergy. *Curr. Opin. Allergy Clin. Immunol.*, Vol.6, pp. 361-366

Kubo-Akashi, C., Seki, M., Kwon, S.M., Takizawa, H., Takatsu, K., & Takaki, S. (2004). Roles of a conserved family of adaptor proteins, Lnk, SH2-B, and APS, for mast cell development, growth, and functions: APS-deficiency causes augmented degranulation and reduced actin assembly. *Biochem. Biophys. Research. Commun.*, Vol.315, pp. 356-362

Kurzer., J.H., Argetsinger, L.S., Zhou, Y.J., Kouadio, J.L.K., O'Shea, J.J., & Carter-Su, C. (2004). Tyrosine 813 is a site of JAK2 autophosphorylation critical for activation of JAK2 by SH2-B□. *Mol. Cell. Biol.*, Vol.24, No.10, pp. 4557-4570

Kurzer, J.H., Saharinen, P., Silvennoinen, O., & Carter-Su, C. (2006). Binding of SH2-B family members within a potencial negative regulatory region maintains JAK2 in an active state. *Mol. Cell. Biol.*, Vol.26, No.17, pp. 6381-6394

Kyo, S., Sada, K., Qu, X., Maeno, K., Miah, S.M., Kawauchi-Kamata, K., & Yamamura, H. (2003). Negative regulation of Lyn protein-tyrosine kinase by c-Cbl ubiquitin protein ligase in Fc epsilon RI-mediated mast cell activation. *Genes Cells*, Vol.8, No.10, pp. 825–836

Langdon, W.Y., Hartley, J.W., Klinken, S.P., Ruscetti, S.K., & Morse, H.C. (1989). V-cbl, an oncogene from a dual-recombinant murine retrovirus that induces early B-lineage lymphomas. *Proc. Natl. Acad. Sci.* USA, Vol.86, pp. 1168-1172

Lasho, T.L., Pardanani, A., & Tefferi, A. (2010). *LNK* mutations in *JAK2* mutation-negative erythrocytosis. *N. Engl. J. Med.*, Vol.363, No.12, pp. 1189-1190

Lasho, T.L., Tefferi, A., Finke, C., & Pardanani, A. (2011). Clonal hierarchy and allelic mutation segregation in a myelofibrosis patient with two distinct LNK mutations. *Leukemia*, Vol. 25; No.6, pp. 1056-1058

Lavrikova, E. Y., Nikitin, A. G., Kuraeva, T.L. Peterkova, V.A., Tsitlidze, N.M., Chistiakov, D.A., & Nosikov, V.V. (2011). The carriage of the type I diabetes-associated R262W variant of human LNK correlates with increased proliferation of peripheral blood monocytes in diabetic patients. *Pediatric Diabetes*, Vol.12, No.2, pp. 127-32

Leevers, S.J., Vanhaesebroeck, B., & Waterfield, M.D. (1999). Signalling through phosphoinositide 3-kinases: the lipids take centre stage. *Curr. Opin. Cell Biol.*, Vol.11, pp. 219–225

Lemay, S., Davidson, D., Latour, S., & Veillette, A. (2000). Dok-3, a novel adaptor molecule involved in the negative regulation of immunoreceptor signaling. *Mol. Cell. Biol.*, Vol.20, pp. 2743–2754

Li, Y., He, X., Schembri-King, J., Jakes, S., & Hayashi, J. (2000). Cloning and characterization of human Lnk, an adaptor protein with pleckstrin homology and Src homology 2 domains that can inhibit T cell activation. *J. Immunol.*, Vol.164, pp. 5199–5206

Li, L., Grønning, L.M., Anderson, P.O., Li, S., Edvardsen, K., Johnston, J., Kioussis, D., Shepherd, P.R., & Wang, P. (2004). Insulin induces SOCS-6 expression and its binding to the p85 monomer of phosphoinositide 3-kinase, resulting in improvement in glucose metabolism. *J Biol Chem.*, Vol.279, No.33, pp. 34107-34114

Li, M., Li, Z., Morris, D.L., & Rui, L. (2007). Identification of SH2B2□ as an inhibitor for SH2B1- and SH2B2□-promoted Janus kinase-2 activation and insulin signaling. *Endocrinology*, Vol.148, pp. 1615-1621

Liu, J., DeYoung, S.M., Hwang, J.B., O'Leary, E.E., & Saltiel, A.R. (2003). The roles of Cbl-b and c-Cbl in insulin-stimulated glucose transport. *J. Biol. Chem.*, Vol.278, No.38, pp. 36754–36762

Loeser, S., Loser, K., Bijker, S.M., Rangachari, M., van der Burg, S.H., Wada, T., Beissert, S., Melief, C.J., & Penninger, J.M. (2007). Spontaneous tumor rejection by cbl-b-deficient CD8+ T cells. *J. Exp. Med.*, Vol.204, pp. 879-891

Loh, M.L., Sakai, D.S., Flotho, C., Kang, M., Fliegauf, M., Archambeault, S., Mullighan, C.G., Chen, L., Bergstraesser, E., Bueso-Ramos, C.E., Emanuel, P.D., Hasle, H., Issa, J.P., van den Heuvel-Eibrink, M.M., Locatelli, F., Starý, J., Trebo, M., Wlodarski, M., Zecca, M., Shannon, K.M., & Niemeyer, C.M. (2009). Mutations in CBL occur frequently in juvenile myelomonocytic leukemia. *Blood*, Vol.114, pp. 1859-1863

Lu, L.F., Thai, T.H., Calado, D.P., Chaudhry, A., Kubo, M., Tanaka, K., Loeb, G.B., Lee, H., Yoshimura, A., Rajewsky, K., & Rudensky, A.Y. (2009). Foxp3-dependent microRNA155 confers competitive fitness to regulatory T cells by targeting SOCS1 protein. *Immunity.*, Vol.30, No.1, pp. 80-91

Lupher, M.L., Jr. Songyang, Z., Shoelson, S.E., Cantley, L.C., & Band, H. (1997). The Cbl phosphotyrosine-binding domain selects a D(N/D)XpY motif and binds to the Tyr292 negative regulatory phosphorylation site of ZAP-70. *J Biol Chem*, Vol.272, No.52, pp. 33140–33144

Makishima, H., Jankowska, A.M., McDevitt, M.A., O'Keefe, C., Dujardin, S., Cazzolli, H., Przychodzen, B., Prince, C., Nicoll, J., Siddaiah, H., Shaik, M., Szpurka, H., His, E., Advani, A., Paquette, R., & Maciejewski, J.P. (2011). CBL, CBLB, TET2, ASXLi, and IDH1/2 mutations and additional chromosomal aberrations constitute molecular events in chronic myelogenous leukemia. *Blood*, Vol. 117, No.21, pp. e198-e206

Marine, J.C., Topham, D.J., McKay, C., Wang, D., Parganas, E., Stravopodis, D., Yoshimura, A., & Ihle, J.N. (1999a). SOCS1 deficiency causes a lymphocyte-dependent perinatal lethality. *Cell*, Vol.98, pp. 609–16

Marine, J.C., McKay, C., Wang, D., Topham, D.J., Parganas, E., Nakajima, H., Penderville, H., Yasukawa, H., Sasaki, A., Yoshimura, A., & Ihle, J.N. (1999b). SOCS3 is essential in the regulation of fetal liver erythropoiesis. *Cell*, Vol.98, pp. 617–627

Martinelli, S., de Luca, A., Stellacci, E., Rossi, C., Checquolo, S., Lepri, F., Caputo, C., Silvano, M., Buscherini, F., Consoli, F., ferrara, G., Digilio, M.C., Cavaliere, M.L., van Hagen, J.M., Zampino, G., van der Burgt, I., Ferrero, G.B., Mazzanti, L., Screpanti, I., Yntema, H.G., Nillesen, W.M., Savarirayan, R., Zenker, M., Dallapiccola, B., Gelb, B.D., & Tartaglia, M. (2010). Heterozygous germline mutations in the CBL tumor-suppressor gene cause a Noonan syndrome-like phenotype. *Am. J. Hum. Genet.*, Vol.87, pp. 250-257

Mashima, R., Honda, K., Yang, Y., Morita, Y., Inoue, A., Arimura, S., Nishina, H., Ema, H., Nakauchi, H., Seed, B., Oda, H., & Yamanashi, Y. (2010). Mice lacking Dok-1, Dok-2, and Dok-3 succumb to aggressive histiocytic sarcoma. *Lab Invest.* Vol.90, No.9, pp. 1357-1364

Matsumoto, A., Seki, Y., Kubo, M., Ohtsuka, S., Suzuki, A., Hayashi, I., Tsuji, K., Nakahata, T., Okabe, M., Yamada, S., & Yoshimura, A. (1999). Suppression of STAT5 functions in liver, mammary glands, and T cells cytokine-inducible SH2-containing protein 1 transgenic mice. *Mol. Cell. Biol.*, Vol.9, No.9, pp. 6396-6407

Matsumoto, T., Ii, M., Nishimura, H., Shoji, T., Mifune, Y., Kawamoto, A., Kuroda, R., Fukui, T., Kawakami, Y., Kuroda, T., Kwon, S.M., Iwasaki, H., Horii, M., Yokoyama, A., Oyamada, A., Lee, S.Y., Hayashi, S., Kurosaka, M., Takaki, S., & Asahara, T. (2010). Lnk-dependent axis of SCF-cKit signal for osteogenesis in bone fracture healing. *J. Exp. Med.*, Vol.207, pp. 2207-2223

Metcalf, D., Greenhalgh, C.J., Viney, E., Willson, T.A., Starr, R., Nicola, N.A., Hilton, D.J., & Alexander, W.S. (2000). Gigantism in mice lacking suppressor of cytokine signalling-2. *Nature*, Vol.405, pp. 1069–1073

Metcalf, D.S., Mifsud, L., Di Rago, N., Nicola, N. A., Hilton, D.J., & Alexander, W.S. (2002). Polycistic kidneys and chronic inflammatory lesions are the delayed consequences of loss of the suppressor of cytokine signaling-1 (SOCS-1). *Proc. Natl. Acad. Sci.* U.S.A., Vol.99, pp. 943-948

Minami, A., Iseki, M., Kishi, K., Wang, M., Ogura, M., Furukawa, N., Hayashi, S., Yamada, M., Obata, T., Takeshita, Y., Nakaya, Y., Bando, Y., Izumi, K., Moodie, S.A., Kajiura, f., Matsumoto, M., Takatsu, K., Takaki, S., & Ebina, Y. (2003). Increased insulin sensitivity and hypoinsulinemia in APS knockout mice. *Diabetes*, Vol.52, pp. 2657-2665

Minamoto, S., Ikegame, K., Ueno, K., Narazaki, M., Naka, T., Yamamoto, H., Matsumoto, T., Saito, H., Hosoe, S., & Kishimoto, T. (1997). Cloning and functional análisis of new members of STAT induced STAT inhibitor (SSI) family: SSI-2 and SSI-3. *Biochem. Biophys. Res. Commun.*, Vol.237, No.1, pp. 79-83

Molero JC, Jensen TE, Withers PC, Couzens M, Herzog H, Thien CB, Langdon WY, Walder K, Murphy MA, Bowtell DD, James DE, Cooney GJ. (2004). c-Cbl-deficient mice have reduced adiposity, higher energy expenditure, and improved peripheral insulin action. *J Clin Invest.*, Vol.114, No.9, pp.1326-33

Molfetta, R., Belleudi, F., Peruzzi, G., Morrone, S., Leone, L., Dikic, I., Piccoli, M., Frati, L., Torrisi, M.R., Santoni, A., & Paolini, R. (2005). CIN85 regulates the ligand-dependent endocytosis of the IgE receptor: a new molecular mechanism to dampen mast cell function. *J Immunol*, Vol.175, pp. 4208-4216

Moodie, S.A., Alleman-Sposeto, J., & Gustafson, T.A. (1999). Identification of the APS protein as a novel insulin receptor substrate. *J. Biol. Chem.*, Vol.274, pp. 11186-11193

Muramatsu H, Makishima H, Jankowska AM, Yoshida, N., Xu, Y., Nishio, N., Hama, A., Yagasaki, H., Takahashi, Y., Kato, K., Manabe, A., Kojima, S., & Maciejewski, J.P. (2010). Mutations of E3 ubiquitin ligase Cbl family members but not TET2 mutations are pathogenic in juvenile myelomonocytic leukemia. *Blood*, Vol.15, pp. 1969–1975

Murphy, M. A., Schnall, R. G., Venter, D. J., Barnett, L., Bertoncello, I., Thien, C. B. F., Langdon, W. Y., & Bowtell, D. D. L. (1998). Tissue hyperplasia and enhanced T cell signalling via ZAP-70 in c-Cbl deficient mice. *Mol. Cell. Biol.*, Vol.18, pp. 4872–4882

Naka, T., Narazaki, M., Hirate, M., Matsumoto, T., Minamoto, S., Aono, A., Nishimoto, N., Kajita, T., Taga, T., Yoshizaki, K., Akira, S., & Kishimoto, T. (1997). Structure and function of a new STAT-induced STAT inhibitor. *Nature*, Vol.387, pp. 924–929

Nakagawa, R., Naka, T., Tsutsui, H., Fujimoto, M., Kimura, A., Abe, T., Seki, E., Sato, S., Takeuchi, O., Takeda, K., Akira, S., Yamanishi, K., Kawase, I., Nakanishi, K., & Kishimoto, T. (2002). SOCS-1 participates in negative regulation of LPS responses, *Immunity*, Vol.17, pp. 677–687

Naramura, M., Kole, H. K., Hu, R.-J., & Gu, H. (1998). Altered thymic positive selection and intracellular signals in Cbl-deficient mice. *Proc. Natl. Acad. Sci.* U.S.A., Vol.95, pp. 15547–15552

Naramura, M., Jang, I.K., Kole, H., Huang, F., Haines, D., & Gu, H. (2002). c-Cbl and Cbl-b regulate T cell responsiveness by promoting ligand-induced TCR downmodulation. *Nat. Immunol.*, Vol.3, pp. 1192–1199

Naramura, M., Nandwani, N., Gu, H., Band, V., & Band, H. (2010). Rapidly fatal myeloproliferative disorders in mice with deletion of Casitas B-cell lymphoma (Cbl) and Cbl-b in hematopoietic stem cells. *Proc. Natl. Acad. Sci.* U.S.A., Vol.107, N0. 37, pp. 16274-16279

Narazaki, M., Fujimoto, M., Matsumoto, T., Morita, Y., Saito, H., Kajita, T., Yoshizaki, K., Naka, T., & Kishimoto, T. (1998). Three distinct domains of SSI-1/SOCS-1/JAB protein are required for its suppression of interleukin 6 signaling. *Proc Natl Acad Sci* USA, Vol.95, pp. 13130–13134

Nelms, K., O'Neill, T.J., Li, S., Hubbard, S.R., Gustafson, T.A., & Paul, W.E. (1999). Alternative splicing, gene localization, and binding of SH2-B to the insulin receptor kinase domain. *Mamm Genome*, Vol.10, pp. 1160-1167

Némorin , J.G., & Duplay, P. (2000). Evidence that Lck-mediated phosphorylation of p56dok-2 and p62dok may play a role in CD2 signalling. *J. Biol. Chem.*, Vol.275, pp. 14590-14597

Nicholson, S.E., Willson, T.A., Farley, A., Starr, R., Zhang, J.G., Baca, M., Alexander, W.S., Metcalf, D., Hilton, D.J., & Nicola, N.A. (1999). Mutational analyses of the SOCS proteins suggest a dual domain requirement but distinct mechanisms for inhibition of LIF and IL-6 signal transduction. *EMBO J.*, Vol.18, pp. 375–385.

Nicholson, S.E., De Suoza, D., Fabri, L.J,, Corbin, J., Willson, T.A., Zhang, J.G., Silva, A., Asimakis, M., Farley, A., Nash, A.D., Metcalf, D., Hilton, D.J., Nicola, N.A., & Baca, M. (2000). Suppressor of cytokine signalling-3 preferentially binds to the SHP-2-binding site on the shared cytokine receptor subunit gp 130. *Proc Natl Acid Sci* USA, Vol.97, pp. 6493–6498

Niemeyer, C., Kang, M.W., Shin, D.H., Furlan, I., Erlacher, M., Bunin, N.J., Bunda, S., Finklestein, J.Z., Sakamoto, K.M., Gorr, T.A., Mehta, P., Schmid, I., Kropshofer, G., Corbacioglu, S., Lang, P.J., Klein, C., Schlegel, P.G., Heinzmann, A., Schneider, M., Starý, J., van den Heuvel-Eibrink, M.M., Hasle, H., Locatelli, F., Sakai, D., Archambeault, S., Chen, L., Russell, R.C., Sybingco, S.S., Ohh, M., Braun, B.S., Flotho, C., & Loh, M.L. (2010). Germline CBL mutations cause developmental abnormalities and predispose to juvenile myelomonocytic leukemia. *Nat. Genet.*, Vol.42, No.9, pp. 794-800

Niki, M., Di Cristofano, A., Zhao, M., Honda, H., Hirai, H., Van Aelst, L., Cordon-Cardo, C., & Pandolfi, P.P. (2004). Role of Dok-1 and Dok-2 in leukemia suppression. *J. Exp. Med.*, Vol.200, No.12, pp. 1689-1695

Ng, C.H., Xu, S., & Lam, K.P. (2007). Dok-3 plays a non redundant role in negative regulation of B-cell activation. *Blood*, Vol.110, pp. 259–266

Nobuhisa, I., Takizawa, M., Takaki, S., Inoue, H., Okita, K., Ueno, M., Takatsu, K., & Taga, T. (2003). Regulation of hematopoietic development in the Aorta-Gonad-Mesonephros region mediated by Lnk adaptor protein. *Mol. Cell. Biol.*, Vol.23, No.23, pp. 8486-8494

Ogura, H., Murakami, M., Okuyama, Y., Tsuruoka, M., Kitabayashi, C., Kanamoto, M., Nishihara, M., Iwakura, Y., & Hirano, T. (2008). Interleukin-17 promotes autoimmunity by triggering a positive-feedback loop via interleukin-6 induction. *Immunity*, Vol.29, pp. 628-636

Oh, S.T., Simonds, E.F., Jones, C., Hale, M.B., Goltsev, Y., Gibbs Jr, K.D., Merker, J.D., Zehnder, J.L., Nolan, G.P., & Gotlib, J. (2010). Novel mutations in the inhibitory adaptor protein LNK drive JAK-STAT signaling in patients with myeloproliferative neoplasms. *Blood*, 116, No.6, pp. 988-992

Ohshima, M., Yokoyama, A., Ohnishi, H., Hamada, H., Kohno, N., Higaki, J., & Naka, T. (2007). Overexpression of suppressor of cytokine signalling-5 augments eosinophilic airway inflammation in mice. *Clin Exp Allergy.*, Vol.37, No.5, pp. 735-742

Ohtsuka, S., Takaki, S., Iseki, M., Miyoshi, K., Nakagata, N., Kataoka, Y., Yoshida, N., Takatsu, K., & Yoshimura, A. (2002). SH2-B is required for both male and female reproduction. *Mol. Cell. Biol.*, Vol.22, pp. 3066-3077

Okochi O, Hibi K, Sakai M, Inoue S, Takeda S, Kaneko T, & Nakao A. (2003). Methylation-mediated silencing of SOCS-1 gene in hepatocellular carcinoma derived from cirrhosis. *Clin Cancer Res.*, Vol.9, No.14, pp. 5295-5298

Ortmann, R. A., Cheng, T., Visconti, R., Frucht, D. M. & O'Shea, J.J. (2000). Janus kinases and signal transducers and activators of transcription: their roles in cytokine signaling, development and immunoregulation. *Arthritis Res*, Vol.2, pp. 16-32

Osborne, M.A., Dalton, S., & Kochan, J.P. (1995). The yeast tribrid system: genetic detection of trans-phosphorylated ITAM-SH2-interactions. *Biotechnology*, Vol.13, pp. 1474-1478

Ott, V.L., Tamir, I., Niki, M., Pandolfi, P.P., & Cambier, J.C. (2002). Downstream of kinase, p62(dok), is a mediator of Fc gamma IIB inhibition of Fc epsilon RI signaling. *J Immunol.*, Vol.168, pp. 4430–4439

Paolini, R., Molfetta, R., Beitz, L.O., Zhang, J., Scharenberg, A.M., Piccoli, M., Frati, L., Siraganian, R., & Santoni, A. (2002). Activation of Syk tyrosine kinase is required for c-Cbl-mediated ubiquitination of Fcepsilon RI and Syk in RBL cells. *J Biol Chem*, Vol.277, No.40, pp. 36940–36947

Pardani, A., Lasho, T., Finke, C., Oh, S.T., Gotlib, J., & Tefferi, A. (2010). LNK mutation studies in blast-phase myeloproliferative neoplasms, and in chronic-phase disease with TET2, IDH, JAK2 or MPL mutations. *Leukemia*, Vol.24, No.10, pp. 1713-1718

Pawson, T. & Scott, J. D. (1996). Signaling Through Scaffold, Anchoring, and Adaptor Proteins. *Science*, Vol.278, pp. 2075-2080

Perez, B., Kosmider, O., Cassinat, B., Renneville, A., Lachenaud, J., Kaltenbach, S., Bertrand, Y., Chomienne, C., Fontenay, M., Preudhomme, C., & Cavé, H. (2010). Genetic typing of CBL, ASXL1, RUNX1, TET2, and JAK2 in juvenile myelomonocytic leukaemia reveals a genetic profile distinct from chronic myelomonocytic leukaemia. *Br. J. Haematol.*, Vol.151, pp. 460-468

Qu, X., Sada, K., Kyo, S., Maeno, K., Miah, S.M., & Yamamura, H. (2004). Negative regulation of FcepsilonRI-mediated mast cell activation by a ubiquitin-protein ligase Cbl-b. *Blood*, Vol.103, No.5, pp. 1779–1786

Quentmeier, H., Geffers, R., Jost, E., Macleod, R.A., Nagel, S., Röhrs, S., Romani, J., Scherr, M., & Zaborski, M., & Drexler, H.G. (2008). SOCS2: inhibitor of JAK2V617F-mediated signal transduction. *Leukemia.*, Vol.22, No.12, pp. 2169-2175

Ram, P.A., & Waxman, D.J. (1999). SOCS/CIS protein inhibition of growth hormone-stimulated STAT5 signaling by multiple mechanisms. *J Biol Chem.*, Vol.274, pp. 35553–35561

Rathinam, C., Thien, C.B.F., Langdon, W.Y., Gu, H., & Flavell, R.A. (2008). The E3 ubiquitin ligase c-Cbl restricts development and functions of hematopoietic stem cells. *Genes Dev.*, Vol.22, pp. 992-997

Rathinam, C., Thien, C.B.F., Flavell, R.A., & Langdon, W.Y. (2010). Myeloid leukemia development in c-Cbl RING finger mutant mice is dependent on FLT3 signaling. *Cancer Cell*, Vol.18, pp. 341-352

Reichsteiner, M., & Rogers, S.W. (1996). PEST sequences and regulation by proteolysis. *Trends Biochem. Sci.*, Vol.21, pp. 267-271

Ren, D., Li, M., Duan, C., & Rui, L. (2005). Identification of SH2-B as a key regulator of leptin sensitivity, energy balance, and body weight in mice. *Cell. Metab.*, Vol.2, pp. 95-104

Riedel, H., Wang, J., Hansen, H., & Yousaf, N. (1997). PSM, an insulin-dependent, pro-rich, PH, SH2 domain containing partner of the insulin receptor. *J. Biochem.*, Vol.122, pp. 1105-1113

Robb, L., Boyle, K., Rakar, S., Hartley, R., Lochland, J., & Roberts, A.W. (2005). Genetic reduction of embryonic leukemia-inhibitory factor production rescues placentation in SOCS3-null embryos but does not prevent inflammatory disease. *Proc Natl Acad Sci* USA, Vol.102, pp.16333-16338

Roberts, A.W., Robb, L., Rakar, S., Hartley, L., Cluse, L., Nicola, N.A., Metcalf, D., Hilton, D.H., & Alexander, W.S. (2001). Placental defects and embryonic lethality in mice lacking suppressor of cytokine signaling 3. *Proc Natl Acad Sci* USA, Vol.98, pp. 9324–9329

Roman-Gomez, J., Jimenez-Velasco, A., Castillejo, J.A., Cervantes, F., Barrios, M., Colomer, D., Heiniger, A., & Torres, A. (2004). The suppressor of cytokine signaling-1 is constitutively expressed in chronic myeloid leukemia and correlates with poor cytogenetic response to interferon-alpha. *Haematologica.*, Vol.89, No.1, pp. 42-48

Rudd, E.C. (2001). Lnk adaptor: novel negative regulator of B cell lymphopoiesis. *Science's STKE*: PE1.

Rui, L., Mathews, L.S., Hotta, K., Gustafson, T.A., & Carter-Su, C. (1997). Identification of SH2-B□ as a substrate of the tyrosine kinase JAK2 involved in Growth hormone signaling. *Mol. Cell. Biol.*, Vol.17, No.11, pp- 6633-6644

Rui, L., Gunter, D.R., Herrington, J., & Carter-Su, C. (2000). Differential binding to and regulation of JAK2 by the SH2 domain and N-terminal region of SH2-B□. *Mol. Cell. Biol.*, Vol.20, No.9, pp. 3168-3177

Rui, L., Yuan, M., Frantz, D., Shoelson, S., & White, M.F. (2002). SOCS-1 and SOCS-3 block insulin signaling by ubiquitin-mediated degradation of IRS1 and IRS2. *J Biol Chem*, Vol.277, pp. 42394–42398

Ryan, P., Davies, G.C., Nau, M.M., & Lipkowitz, S. (2006). Regulating the regulator: negative regulation of Cbl ubiquitin ligases. *Trends Biochem. Sci.*, Vol.31, No.2, pp. 79-88

Sakai, I., Takeuchi, K., Yamauchi, H., Narumi, H., & Fujita, S. (2002). Constitutive expression of SOCS3 confers resistance to IFN-alpha in chronic myelogenous leukemia cells. *Blood.*, Vol.100, No.8, pp.2926-31

Sakamoto, H., Kinjyo, I., & Yoshimura, A. (2000). The Janus kinase inhibitor, Jab/SOCS-1, is an interferon-gamma inducible gene and determines the sensitivity to interferons. *Leuk Lymphoma.*, Vol.38, No.1-2, pp.49-58

Sargin, B., Choudhary, C., Crosetto, N., Schmidt, M.H.H., Grundler, R., Rensinghoff, M., Thiessen, C., Tickenbrock, L., Schwäble, J., Brandts, C., August, B., Koschmieder, S., Bandi, S.R., Duyster, J., Berdel, W.E., Müller-Tidow, C., Dikic, I., & Serveet, H. (2007). Flt3-dependent transformation by inactivating c-Cbl mutations in AML. *Blood*, Vol.110, pp. 1004–12

Sanada, M., Suzuki, T., Shih, L.Y., Otsu, M., Kato, M., Yamazaki, S., Tamura, A., Honda, H., Sakata-Yamagimoto, M., Kumano, K., Oda, H., Yamagata, T., Takita, J., Gotoh, N., Nakazaki, K., Kawamanta, N., Onodera, M., Nobuyoshi, M., Hayashi, Y., Harada, H., Kurokawa, M., Chiba S., Mori, H., Ozawa, K., Omine, M., Hirai, H., Nakauchi, H., Koeffler, H. P. & Ogawa, S. (2009). Gain-of-function of mutated c-CBL tumour suppressor in myeloid neoplasms. *Nature*, Vol.460, pp. 904–908

Sasaki, A., Yasukawa, H., Susuki, A., Kamizono, S., Syoda, T., Kinyo, I, Sasaki, M., Johnston, J.A., & Yoshimura, A. (1999). Cytokine-inducible SH2 protein-3 (CIS3/SOCS3) inhibits Janus tyrosine kinase by binding through the N-terminal kinase inhibitory region as well as SH2 domain. *Genes Cells*, Vol.4, pp. 339-351

Sasaki, A., Yasukawa, H., Shouda, T., Kitamura, T., Dikic, I., & Yoshimura, A. (2000). CIS3/SOCS-3 suppresses erythropoietin (EPO) signaling by binding the EPO receptor and JAK2. *J Biol Chem.*, Vol.275, pp. 29338–29347

Sasaki, A., Inagaki-Ohara, K., Yoshida, T., Yamanaka, A., Sasaki, M., Yasukawa, H., Koromilas, A.E., & Yoshimura, A. (2003). The N-terminal truncated isoform of SOCS3 translated from an alternative initiation AUG codon under stress conditions is stable due to the lack of a major ubiquitination site, Lys-6. *J Biol Chem*, Vol.278, pp. 2432–2436

Schade, A.E., Wlodarski, M.W. & Maciejewski, J.P. (2006). Pathophysiology Defined by Altered Signal Transduction Pathways. The Role of JAK-STAT and PI3K Signaling in Leukemic Large Granular Lymphocytes. *Cell Cycle*, Vol.5, No.22, pp. 2571-2574

Schmitz, J.,Weissenbach, M., Haan, S., Heinrich, P.C., & Schaper, F. (2000). SOCS3 exerts its inhibitory functions on interleukin-6 signal transduction through the SHP2 recruitment site of gp130. *J Biol Chem.*, Vol.275, pp. 12848–12856

Schubbert, S., Shannon, K., & Bollag, G. (2007). Hyperactive Ras in developmental disorders and cancer. *Nat. Rev. Cancer.*, Vol.7, pp. 295-308

Seita, J., Ema, H., Ooehara, J., Ymazaki, S., Tadokoro, Y., Yamasaki, A., Eto, K., Takaki, S., Takatsu, S., & Nakauchi, H. (2007). Lnk negatively regulates self-renewal of hematopoietic stem cells by modifying thrombopoietin-mediated signal transduction. *Proc. Natl. Acad. Sci.* USA., Vol.104, No.7, pp. 2349-2354

Seki, Y., Hayashi, K., Matsumoto, A., Seki, N., Tsukada, J., Ransom, J., Naka, T., Kishimoto, T., Yoshimura, A., & Kubo, M. (2002). Expression of the suppressor of cytokine signaling-5 (SOCS5) negatively regulates IL-4-dependent STAT6 activation and Th2 differentiation. *Proc Natl Acad Sci* USA., Vol.99, No.20, pp. 13003-13008

Seki, Y., Inoue, H., Nagata, N., Hayashi, K., Fukuyama, S. Matsumoto, K., Komine, O. , Hamano, S., Himeno, K., Inagaki-Ohara, K., Cacalano, N., O'Garra, A., Oshida, T.,

Saito, H., Johnston, J.A., Yoshimura, A., & Kubo, M. (2003). SOCS-3 regulates onset and maintenance of T(H)2-mediated allergic responses, *Nat Med*, Vol.9, pp. 1047–1054

Senis, Y.A., Antrobus, R., Severin, S., Parguiña, A.F., Rosa, I., Zitzmann, N., Watson, S.P., & Garcia, A. (2009). Proteomic analysis of integrin □IIb□3 outside-in signaling reveals Src-kinase-independent phosphorylation of Dok-1 and Dok-3 leading to SHIP-1 interactions. *J. Thromb Haemost*, Vol.7, pp. 1718-1726

Shao, Y., Yang, C., Elly, C., & Liu, Y.C. (2004). Differential regulation of the B cell receptor-mediated signaling by the E3 ubiquitin ligase Cbl. *J Biol Chem*, Vol.279, No.42, pp. 43646–43653

Shiba N, Kato M, Park, M.J., Sanada, M., Ito, E., Fukushima, K., Sako, M., Arakawa, H., Ogawa, S., & Hayashi, Y. (2010). CBL mutations in juvenile myelomonocytic leukemia, but not in pediatric myelodysplastic syndrome. *Leukemia*, Vol.24, No.4, pp. 1090-1092

Shinohara, H., Inoue, A., Toyama-Sorimachi, N., Nagai, Y., Yasuda, T., Suzuki, H., Horai, R., Iwakura, Y., Yamamoto, T., Karasuyama, H., Miyake, K., & Yamanashi, Y. (2005). Dok-1 and Dok-2 are negative regulators of lipopolysaccharide induced signaling. *J Exp Med*, Vol.201, pp. 333–339

Shouda, T., Yoshida, T., Hanada, T., Wakioka, T., Oishi, M., Miyoshi, K., Komiya, S., Kosai, K., Hanakawa, Y., Hashimoto, K., Nagata, K., & Yoshimura, A. (2001). Induction of the cytokine signal regulator SOCS3/CIS3 as a therapeutic strategy for treating inflammatory arthritis. *J. Cin. Invest.* 108, pp. 1781-1788

Simon, C., Dondi, E., Chaix, A., De Sepulveda, P., Kubiseski, T.J., Varin-Blank, N., & Velazquez L. (2008). Lnk adaptor protein down-regulates specific Kit-induced signaling pathways in primary mast cells. *Blood.*, Vol.112, pp. 4039-4047

Siewert, E., Muller-Esterl, W., Starr, R., Heinrich, P.C., & Schape, F. (1999). Different protein turnover of interleukin-6-type cytokine signaling components. *Eur J Biochem*, Vol.265, pp. 251–257

Sohn, H.W., Gu, H., & Pierce, S.K. (2003). Cbl-b negatively regulates B cell antigen receptor signaling in mature B cells through ubiquitination of the tyrosine kinase Syk. *J Exp Med*, Vol.197, No.11, pp. 1511–1524.

Songyang, Z., Yamanashi, Y., Liu, D., & Baltimore, D. (2001). Domain-dependent function of the ras-GAP-binding protein p62Dok in cell signaling. *J Biol Chem*, Vol.276, pp. 2459–2465

Soranzo, N., Spector, T. D., Mangino, M., Kühnel, B., Rendon, A., Teumer, A., Willenborg, C., Wright, B., Chen, L., Li, M., Salo, P., Voight, B.F., Burns, P., Laskowski, R.A,, Xue, Y., Menzel, S., Altshuler, D., Bradley, J.R., Bumpstead, S., Burnett, M.S., Devaney, J., Döring, A., Elosua, R., Epstein, S.E., Erber, W., Falchi, M., Garner, S.F., Ghori, M.J., Goodall, A.H., Gwilliam, R., Hakonarson, H.H., Hall, A.S., Hammond, N., Hengstenberg, C., Illig, T., König, I.R., Knouff, C.W., McPherson, R., Melander, O., Mooser, V., Nauck, M., Nieminen, M.S., O'Donnell, C.J., Peltonen, L., Potter, S.C., Prokisch, H., Rader, D.J., Rice, C.M., Roberts, R., Salomaa, V., Sambrook, J., Schreiber, S., Schunkert, H., Schwartz, S.M., Serbanovic-Canic, J., Sinisalo, J., Siscovick, D.S., Stark, K., Surakka, I., Stephens, J., Thompson, J.R., Völker, U., Völzke, H., Watkins, N.A., Wells, G.A., Wichmann, H.E., Van Heel, D.A., Tyler-Smith, C., Thein, S.L., Kathiresan, S., Perola, M., Reilly, M.P., Stewart, A.F., Erdmann, J., Samani, N.J., Meisinger, C., Greinacher, A., Deloukas, P., Ouwehand, W.H., Gieger, C. (2009). A genome-wide meta-analysis identifies 22 loci associated with eight haematological parameters in the HaemGen consortium. *Nat. Genet.*, Vol.41, No.11, pp. 1182-1190

Starr, R., Willson, T.A., Viney, E.M., Murra, L.J.L., Rayner, J.R., Jenkins, B.J., Gonda, T.J., Alexander, W.S., Metcalf, D., Nicola, N.A., & Hilton, D.J. (1997). A family of cytokine-inducible inhibitors of signalling. *Nature*, Vol.387, pp. 917–921

Starr, R., Metcalf, D., Elefanty, A.G., Brysha, M., Willson, T.A., Nicola, N.A., Hilton, D.J., & Alexander, W.S. (1998). Liver degeneration and lymphoid deficiencies in mice lacking suppressor of cytokine signaling-1. *Proc. Natl. Acad. Sci.* USA, Vol.95, No.24, pp. 14395-14399

Stork, B., Neumann, K., Goldbeck, I., Alers, S., Kähne, T., Naumann, M., Engelke, M., & Wienands, J. (2007). Subcellular localization of Grb2 by the adaptor protein Dok-3 restricts the intensity of Ca2+ signaling in B cells. *EMBO J*, Vol.26, pp. 1140–1149

Suessmuth, Y., Elliott, J., Percy, M.J., Inami, M., Attal, H., Harrison, C.N., Inokuchi, K., McMullin, M.F., & Johnston, J.A. (2009). A new polycythaemia vera-associated SOCS3 SH2 mutant (SOCS3F136L) cannot regulate erythropoietin responses. *Br J Haematol.*, Vol.147, No.4, pp. 450-458

Suzu S, Tanaka-Douzono, M., Nomaguchi, K., Yamada, M., Hayasawa, H., Kimura, F., & Motoyoshi, K. (2000). p56^{dok-2} as a cytokine-inducible inhibitor of cell proliferation and signal transduction. *EMBO J*, Vol.19, pp. 5114–5122

Suzuki A, Hanada T, Mitsuyama K, Yoshida T, Kamizono S, Hoshino T, Kubo M, Yamashita A, Okabe M, Takeda K, Akira S, Matsumoto S, Toyonaga A, Sata M, & Yoshimura A. (2001). CIS3/SOCS3/SSI3 plays a negative regulatory role in STAT3 activation and intestinal inflammation. *J Exp Med.*, Vol.193, No.4, pp. 471-481

Takaki, S., Watts, J.D., Forbush, K.A., Nguyen, N.T., Hayashi, J., Alberola-Ila, J., Aebersold, R., & Perlmutter, R.M. (1997). Characterization of Lnk. An adaptor protein expressed in lymphocytes. *J. Biol. Chem.*, Vol.272, pp. 14562–14570

Takaki, S., Sauer, K., Iritani, B.M., Chien, S., Ebihara, Y., Tsuji, K.I., Takatsu, K., & Perlmutter, R.M. (2000). Control of B cell production by the adaptor protein Lnk: definition of a conserved family of signal-modulating proteins. *Immunity*. Vol.13, pp. 599–609

Takaki, S., Morita, H., Tezuka, Y., & Takatsu, K. (2002). Enhanced hematopoiesis by hematopoietic progenitor cells lacking intracellular adaptor protein, Lnk. *J Exp Med.*, Vol.195, pp. 151-160

Takaki, S., Tezuka, Y., Sauer, K., Kubo, C., & Kwon, S.M., Armstead, E., Nakao, K., Katsuki, M., Perlmutter, R.M., & Takatsu, K. (2003). Impaired lymphopoiesis and altered B cell subpopulations in mice overexpressing Lnk adaptor protein. *J Immunol*, Vol.170, pp. 703-710

Takahashi, Y., Carpino, N., Cross, J.C., Torres, M., Parganas, E. & Ihle, J.N. (2003). SOCS3: an essential regulator of LIF receptor signaling in trophoblast giant cell differentiation, *EMBO J*, Vol.22, pp. 372–384

Takizawa, H., Kubo-Akashi, C., Nobuhisa, I., Kwon, S.M., Iseki, M., Taga, T., Takatsu, K., & Takaki, S. (2006). Enhanced engraftment of hematopoietic stem/progenitor cells by the transient inhibition of an adaptor protein, Lnk. *Blood*, Vol.107, No.7, pp. 2968-2975

Takizawa, H., Eto, K., Yoshikawa, A., Nakauchi, H., Takatsu, K., & Takaki, S. (2008). Growth and maturation of megakaryocytes is regulated by Lnk/SH2B3 adaptor protein through crosstalk between cytokine- and integrin-mediated signals. *Exp. Hematol.*, Vol.36, No.7, pp. 897-906

Takizawa, H., Nishimura, S., Takayama, N., Oda, A., Nishikii, H., Morita, Y., Kakimura, S., Yamazaki, S., Okamura, S., Tamura, N., Goto, S., Sawaguchi, A., Manabe, I., Takatsu, K., Nakauchi, H., Takaki, S., & Eto, K. (2010). Lnk regulates integrin aIIb□3 outside-in signaling in mouse platelets, leading to stabilization of thrombus development in vivo. *J. Clin. Invest.*, Vol.120, No.1, pp. 179-190

Taleb, S., Romain, M., Ramkhelawon, B., Uyttenhove, C., Pasterkamp, G., Herbin, O., Esposito, B., Perez, N., Yasukawa, H., Van Snick, J., Yoshimura, A., Tedgui, A., & Mallat, Z. (2009). Loss of SOCS3 expression in T cells reveals a regulatory role for interleukin-17 in atherosclerosis. *J Exp Med*, Vol.206, pp. 2067-2077

Tamir, I., Stolpa, J.C., Helgason, C.D., Nakamura, K., Bruhns, P., Daeron, M., & Cambier, J. (2000). The RasGap-binding protein p62dok is a mediator of inhibitory Fc□RIIB signals in B cells. *Immunity*, Vol.12, pp. 347-358

Tefferi, A. (2010). Novel mutations and their functional and clinical relevance in myeloproliferative neoplasms: JAK2, MPL, TET2, ASXL1, CBL, IDH and IKZF1. *Leukemia*, Vol.24, pp. 1128-1138

Thien, C.B., Bowtell, D.D., & Langdon, W.Y. (1999). Perturbed regulation of ZAP-70 and sustained tyrosine phosphorylation of LAT and SLP-76 in c-Cbl-deficient thymocytes. *J Immunol*, Vol.162, No.12, pp. 7133–7139.

Thien, C. B. F., Walker, F. & Langdon, W. Y. (2001) Ring finger mutations that abolish c-Cbl-directed polyubiquitination and downregulation of the EGF receptor are insufficient for cell transformation. *Mol. Cell*, Vol.7, pp. 355–365

Thien, C.B.F., & Langdon, W.Y. (2001). Cbl: many adaptations to regulate protein tyrosine kinases. *Nat. Rev. Mol. Cell. Biol.*, Vol. 2, pp. 294-305.

Thien, C.B.F., Scaife, R.M., Papadimitriou, J.M., Murphy, M.A., Bowtell, D.D.L. & Langdon, W.Y. (2003). A mouse with a loss-of-function mutation in the c-Cbl TKB domain shows perturbed thymocyte signaling without enhancing the activity of the ZAP-70 tyrosine kinase. *J. Exp. Med.*, Vol.197, pp. 503–513

Tong, W., & Lodish, F.H. (2004). Lnk inhibits Tpo-mpl signaling and Tpo-mediated megakaryocytopoiesis. *J Exp Med.*, Vol.200, pp. 569-580

Tong, W., Zhang, J., & Lodish, F.H. (2005). Lnk inhibits erythropoiesis and Epo-dependent JAK2 activation and downstream signaling pathways. *Blood.*, Vol.105, pp. 4604-4612

Tsygankov, A. Y., Mahajan, S., Fincke, J. E. & Bolen, J. B. (1996). Specific association of tyrosine-phosphorylated c-Cbl with Fyn tyrosine kinase in T cells, *J. Biol. Chem.*, Vol.271, pp. 27130–27137

Velazquez, L., Cheng, A.M., Fleming, H.E., Furlonger, C., Vesely, S., Bernstein, A., Paige, C.J., & Pawson, T. (2002). Cytokine Signaling and Hematopoietic Homeostasis Are Disrupted in Lnk-deficient Mice. *J. Exp. Med.*, Vol.195, No. 12, pp. 1599-1611

Verdier, F., Chretien, S., Muller, O., Varlet, P., Yoshimura, A., Gisselbrecht, S., Lacombe, C., & Mayeux, P. (1998). Proteasomes regulate erythropoietin receptor and signal transducer and activator of transcription 5 (STAT5) activation. Possible involvement of the ubiquitinated Cis protein. *J Biol Chem*, Vol.273, pp. 28185–28190

Vuica, M., Desiderio, S., & Schneck, J.P. (1997). Differential effects of B cell receptor and B cell receptor-Fc□RIIB1 engagement on Docking of Csk to GTPase-activating protein (GAP)-associated p62. *J. Exp. Med.*, Vol.186, pp. 259-267

Wakioka, T., Sasaki, A., Mitsui, K., Yokouchi, M., Inoue, A., Komiya, S., & Yoshimura, A. (1999). APS, an adaptor protein containing Pleckstrin homology (PH) and Src homology-2 (SH2) domains inhibits the JAK-STAT pathway in collaboration with c-Cbl. *Leukemia.*, Vol.13, pp. 760–767

Waiboci, L.W., Ahmed, C.M., Mujtaba, M.G., Flowers, L.O., Martin, J.P., Haider, M.I., & Johnson, H.M. (2007). Both the suppressor of cytokine 1 (SOCS-1) kinase-inhibitory region and SOCS-1 mimetic bind to JAK2 autophosphorylation site: implications for the development of a SOCS-1 antagonist. *J. Immunol.*, Vol.178, pp. 5058-5068

Wan, M., Li, Y., Xue, H., Li, Q., & Li, J. (2006). TNF-□ induces Lnk expression through PI3K-dependent signaling pathway in human umbilical vein endothelial cells. *J. Surg. Research.*, Vol.136, pp. 53-57

Watanabe, H., Kubo, M., Numata, K., Takagi, K., Mizuta, H., Okada, S., Ito, T., & Matsukawa, A. (2006). Overexpression of suppressor of cytokine signaling-5 in T cells augments innate immunity during septic peritonitis. *J Immunol.*, Vol.177, No.12, pp. 8650-8657

Weiss, L.M., & Chang, K.L. Pathology of Langerhans cell histiocytosis and other histiocytic proliferations. In: Greer JP, Foerster J, Rodgers GM, et al. (eds). Wintrobe's Clinical Hematology. 12th edn. Lippincott Williams & Wilkins: Philadelphia, 2009, pp 1582–1588

Werz, C., Köhler, K., Hafen, E., & Stocker, H. (2009). The Drosophila SH2B family adaptor Lnk acts in parallel to Chico in the Insulin signaling pathway. *PLos Genet.*, Vol.5, No.8, e1000596, doi: 10.1371/journal.pgen.1000596

White, G.E., Cotterill, A., Addley, M.R., Soilleux, E.J., & Greaves, D.R. (2001). Suppressor of cytokine signaling protein SOCS3 expression is increased at sites of acute and chronic inflammation. *J. Mol. Hist.*, Vol.42, pp. 137-151

Wollberg, P., Kennartsson, J., Gottridsson, E., Yoshimura, A., & Rönnstrand, L. (2003). The adapter protein APS associates with the multifunctional docking sites Tyr-568 and Tyr-936 in c-Kit. *Biochem. J.*, Vol.370, pp. 1033-1038

Wong, P.K., Egan, P.J., Croker, B.A., O'Donnell, K., Sims, N.A., Drake, S., Kiu, H., McManus, E.J., Alexander, W.S., Roberts, A.W., & Wicks, I.P. (2006). SOCS-3 negatively regulates innate and adaptive immune mechanisms in acute IL-1 dependent inflammatory arthritis. *J. Clin. Invest.*, Vol.116, pp. 1571-1581

Yabana, N., & Shibuya, M. (2002). Adaptor protein APS binds the NH2-terminal autoinhibitory domain of guanine exchange factor Vav3 and augments its activity. *Oncogene*, Vol.21, pp. 7720-7729

Yamanashi, Y., & Baltimore, D. (1997). Identification of the Abl- and rasGAP-associated 62 kDa protein as a docking protein, Dok. *Cell*, Vol.88, pp. 205–211

Yamanashi, Y., Tamura, T., Kanamori, T., Yamane, H., Nariuchi, H., Yamamoto, T., & Baltimore, D. (2000). Role of the rasGAP-associated docking protein p62dok in negative regulation of B cell receptor-mediated signaling. *Genes Dev*, Vol.14, pp. 11–16

Yasuda, T., Maeda, A., Kurosaki, M., Tezuka, T., Hironaka, K., Yamamoto, T., & Kurosaki, T. (2000). Cbl suppresses B cell receptor-mediated phospholipase C (PLC)-gamma2 activation by regulating B cell linker protein-PLC-gamma2 binding. *J Exp Med*, Vol.191, pp. 641–650

Yasuda, T., Tezuka, T., Maeda, A., Inazu, T., Yamanashi, Y., Gu, H., Kurosaki, T., & Yamamoto, T. (2002). Cbl-b positively regulates Btk-mediated activation of phospholipase C-gamma2 in B cells. *J Exp Med*, Vol.196, pp. 51–63

Yasuda, T., Shirakata, M., Iwama, A., Ishii, A., Ebihara, Y., Osawa, M., Honda, K., Shinohara, H., Sudo, K, Tsuji, K., Nakauchi, H., Iwakura, Y., Hirai, H., Oda, H., Yamamoto, T., &

Yamanashi, Y. (2004). Role of Dok-1 and Dok-2 in myeloid homeostasis and suppression of leukemia. *J. Exp. Med.*, Vol.200, No.12, pp. 1681-1687

Yasukawa, H., Misawa, H., Sakamoto, H., Masuhara, M., Sasaki, A., & Wakioka, T. (1999). The JAK-binding protein JAB inhibits Janus tyrosine kinase activity through binding in the activation loop. *EMBO J*, Vol.18, pp. 1309–20

Yokouchi, M., Suzuki, R., Masuhara, M., Komiya, S., Inoue, A., & Yoshimura, A. (1997). Cloning and characterization of APS, an adaptor molecule containing PH and SH2 domains that is tyrosine phosphorylated upon B-cell receptor stimulation. *Oncogene*, Vol.15, pp. 7-15

Yokouchi, M., Kondo, T., Sanjay, A., Houghton, A., Yoshimura, A., Komiya, S., Zhang, H. & Baron, R. (2001). Src-catalyzed phosphorylation of c-Cbl leads to the interdependent ubiquitination of both proteins. *J. Biol. Chem.*, Vol.276, pp. 35185–35193

Yoshida, T., Ogata, H., Kamio, M., Joo, A., Shiraishi, H., Tokunaga, Y., Sata, M., Nagai, H., & Yoshimura, A. (2004). SOCS1 is a suppressor of liver fibrosis and hepatitis-induced carcinogenesis. *J Exp Med.*, Vol.199, No.12, pp. 1701-1707

Yoshikawa, H., Matsubara, K., Qian, G.S., Jackson, P., Groopman, J.D., Manning, J.E., Harris, C.C., & Herman, J.G. (2001). SOCS-1, a negative regulator of the JAK/STAT pathway, is silenced by methylation in human hepatocellular carcinoma and shows growth-suppression activity. *Nat Genet.*, Vol.28, No.1, pp. 29-35

Yoshimura, A., Ohkubo, T., Kiguchi, T., Jenkins, N.A., Gilbert, D.J., Copeland, N.G.,Hara, T., & Miyajima, A. (1995). A novel cytokine-induced gene CIS encodes an SH2-containing protein that binds to tyrosine-phosphorylated interleukin 3 and erythropoietin receptors. *EMBO J.*, Vol.14, pp. 2816–26

Yoshimura, A., Naka, T., & Kubo, M. (2007). SOCS proteins, cytokine signalling and immune regulation. *Nat Rev Immunol.*, Vol.7, No.6, pp. 454-65

Zhang, J.G., Farley, A., Nicholson, S.E., Wilson, T.A., Zugaro, L.M., simpson, R.J., Moritz, R.L., Cary, D., Richardson, R., Hausmann, G., Kile, B.J., Kent, S.B., Alexander, W.S., Metcalf, D., Hilton, D.J., Nicola, N.A., & Baca, M. (1999). The conserved SOCS box motif in suppressors of cytokine signaling binds to elongins B and C and may couple bound proteins to proteasomal degradation. *Proc. Natl. Acad. Sci.* USA, Vol.96, No.5, pp. 2071-2076

Zhang, J.G., Metcalf, D., Rakar, S., Asimakis, M., Greenhalgh, C.J., Willson, T.A., Starr, R., Nicholson, S.E., Carter, W., Alexander, W.S., Hilton, D.J., Nicola, N.A. (2001). The SOCS box of suppressor of cytokine signaling-1 is important for inhibition of cytokine action in vivo. *Proc Natl Acad Sci* USA, Vol.98, pp.13261–13265

Zhang, J., Chiang, Y.J., Hodes, R.J., & Siraganian, R.P. (2004). Inactivation of c-Cbl or Cbl-b differentially affects signaling from the high affinity IgE receptor. *J Immunol*, Vol.173, No.3, pp. 1811–1818

Zheng, N., Wang, P., Jeffrey, P. D. & Pavletich, N. P. (2000) Structure of a c-Cbl–UbcH7 complex: RING domain function in ubiquitin-protein ligases. *Cell*, Vol.102, pp. 533–539

Zhernakova, A., Elbers, C.C., Ferwerda, B., Romanos, J., Trynka, G., Dubois, P.C., de Kovel, C.G., Franke, L., Oosting, M., Barisani, D., Bardella, M.T.; Finnish Celiac Disease Study Group, Joosten, L.A., Saavalainen, P., van Heel, D.A., Catassi, C., Netea, M.G., & Wijmenga, C. (2010). Evolutionary and functional analysis of Celiac risk loci reveals SH2B3 as a protective factor against bacterial infection. *Am. J. Hum. Genet.*, Vol.86, pp. 970-977

3

The Role of EMT Modulators in Hematopoiesis and Leukemic Transformation

Goossens Steven and Haigh J. Jody
VIB and Ghent University
Belgium

1. Introduction

Mature blood cells arise from hematopoietic stem cells (HSCs) capable of generating every hematopoietic cell type; including the various lymphoid and myeloid lineages. To maintain the steady state levels of hematopoietic cells in the circulation, each HSC has the capacity to generate large numbers of mature cells daily via various multi- and oligopotent lineage-committed progenitors (Kondo et al., 2003; Orkin, 2000). Finely tuned self-renewal and differentiation programs, controlled by essential transcriptional regulatory networks (Miranda-Saavedra & Gottgens, 2008), determine the HSC and progenitor pool sizes in adults. These regulatory networks include both positive and negative transcriptional regulators that control lineage specific gene expression and ensure normal hematopoietic cell differentiation. Deregulation of these transcriptional networks caused by aberrant upstream signalling, point mutations as well as chromosomal translocations of key transcriptional regulators particularly within the HSC compartment (Bonnet & Dick, 1997) can lead to various blood related disorders including anemia and hematological malignancies or leukemia.

The origins of HSCs during the development of a mammalian embryo are only beginning to be understood. Tracing of the true stem cells via marker analysis is difficult and the 'gold standard' for identifying these cells is based on their ability to reconstitute lethally irradiated hosts over a long term. Various transplantation studies in the mouse (Dzierzak & Medvinsky, 2008) have revealed that HSCs arise in a complex developmental process during which multipotent progenitors sequentially migrate to several anatomical sites (Dzierzak & Speck, 2008; Orkin & Zon, 2008), including the yolk sac, the aorta-gonadomesonephros (AGM) region, placenta, fetal liver and finally the bone marrow in the adult (Palis et al., 2001). Lately, it is thought that the first definitive adult-type of HSCs are generated in the AGM region at embryonic day (E) 10.5 in the mouse (de Bruijn et al., 2002). It was demonstrated through fate mapping that the first HSCs arise as part of the hematopoietic progenitor clusters that emerge from the hemogenic endothelium and subendothelial layers at the ventral part of the dorsal aorta and in the vitelline artery (Rybtsov et al., 2011; Yokomizo et al., 2011). These small cell clusters of hematopoietic progenitors are closely associated with the endothelium and originate from vascular remodelling and extravascular budding (Boisset et al., 2010; Robin et al., 2011; Zovein et al., 2010). This involves changes in endothelial cell shape and loss of cellular adhesion that have been likened to the changes in cell adhesion that epithelial cells undergo during epithelial to mesenchymal transition (**EMT**). EMT encompasses a series of events in which well-polarized epithelial cells round up in shape, lose their cell contacts and acquire the motile, migratory properties of mesenchymal cells (Greenburg & Hay, 1982). EMT is essential for many developmental processes including mesoderm formation during gastrulation and neural crest delamination and migration (Kalluri & Weinberg, 2009; Thiery et al., 2009). Similar EMT-like changes in cellular morphology can be observed during tumor progression and allow tumor cells to acquire the capacity to invade into the surrounding tissue and ultimately metastasize to a distant site (Berx et al., 2007). Subsequent tissue colonization occurs via a reverse transitional mechanism, called mesenchymal to epithelial transition (MET) (Kalluri, 2009). Significant cross talk and interactions between members of the Snai family and Zeb family of transcription factors have been documented to be involved in the regulation of these EMT/MET processes (Thiery & Sleeman, 2006). More recently, it has been suggested that the expression of the EMT regulators are also involved in the formation/acquisition of (cancer) stem cell properties (Gupta et al., 2009). In addition to their roles in epithelial/mesenchymal biology there is accumulating evidence that these EMT inducers may be involved in several aspects of hematopoietic differentiation and hematological malignancies that is the main focus of this chapter and are reviewed below.

2. EMT regulators of the Snai family

Members of Snai family encode for transcription factors with a common structural organization consisting of a highly conserved C-terminal region with four to six C_2H_2 zinc-fingers (Knight & Shimeld, 2001) and a more divergent N-terminal region (Fig. 1). This zinc-finger domain serves as a sequence-specific DNA binding domain that recognizes consensus E2-box type elements C/A(CAGGTG) (Batlle et al., 2000; Cano et al., 2000; Mauhin et al., 1993). All vertebrate Snai family members share as well an evolutionary conserved 7-9 AA N-terminus, the SNAG (Snail/Gfi) domain (Grimes et al., 1996). This domain was originally identified as a repressor domain in the zinc-finger protein Gfi1 that acts as a molecular hook to recruit co-regulators and/or demethylases and is essential for their Snai transcriptional repressive function (Lin et al., 2010).

Snail (also known as Snai1, Sna, Snah, Slugh2, Snail1.) represents the founding member of the superfamily (Manzanares et al., 2001; Nieto, 2002) and was first described in *Drosophila melanogaster* (Grau et al., 1984). In mammals, besides Snail two other Snail family members were identified **Slug** (aka Snai2, Slugh1, Slugh, Snail2) and **Smuc** (aka Snai3, Zfp293, Znf293). Snail and Slug are the best characterized and have been implicated in the formation of the mesoderm (Boulay et al., 1987; Sefton et al., 1998) and neural crest cell migration (del Barrio & Nieto, 2002; LaBonne & Bronner-Fraser, 2000) as well as with the loss of epithelial features associated with the acquisition of a fibroblast-like motile and invasive phenotype of tumor cells. Induced expression of Snail or Slug in various epithelial cancer cell lines either by FGF, Wnt, Notch or TGFβ administration (De Craene et al., 2005) or directly via ectopic expression of the repressors is sufficient to adopt a more mesenchymal morphology (Cano et al., 2000). This phenotypic switch is characterized by the downregulation of a number of epithelial marker genes (E-cadherin, desmoplakin, Muc-1, cytokeratin-18) (Batlle et al., 2000; Cano et al., 2000) and the induction of various mesenchymal marker genes (vimentin, fibronectin) (Cano et al., 2000), which can vary dependent on the cellular context. Several lines of evidence indicated that Snail family members not only regulate cellular adhesion and motility or invasion but as well can bind and regulate genes that participate in other processes (Wu Y. & Zhou, 2010) like proliferation (CyclinD1) (Liu J. et al. 2010), cell survival/apoptosis (BID, caspase-6) (Kajita et al., 2004), inflammation (Lyons et al., 2008; Yang & Wolf, 2009) and angiogenesis (Gill et al. 2011).

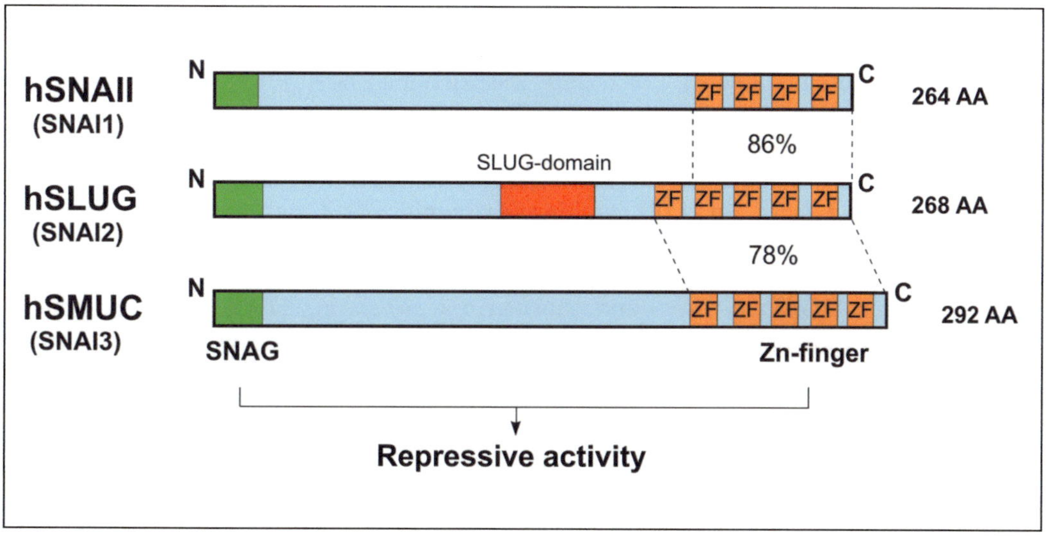

Fig. 1. Schematic diagram of conserved functional domains of the three members of the Snai family of transcription factors. All members contain an N-terminal SNAG domain and a C-terminal zinc-finger (ZF) domain. The central SLUG-domain is unique for Slug (Figure based on Cobaleda et al., 2007)

Besides this, Snai gain-of-function is correlated with the acquisition of (cancer) stem cell properties (Gupta et al., 2009). Studies of various neoplastic tissues have demonstrated the existence of cancer stem cells (CSC) or tumor-initiating-cells with self-renewal capacity that exhibit an ability to induce new tumors when transplated into nude and/or syngeneic mouse strains (Schatton et al., 2009). The existence of CSCs was initially discovered in leukemia samples (Bonnet & Dick, 1997), but subsequently they have been identified in various solid tumor types as well (Al-Hajj et al., 2003; Ricci-Vitiani et al., 2007; Singh et al., 2004). The origin of these stem cells is until now unclear but compelling results from Mani and colleagues (Mani et al., 2008) now link EMT processes with the formation of CSCs. Ectopic expression of Snail in an immortalized human mammary epithelial cell line resulted in the acquisition of mesenchymal traits, expression of stem cell markers and enhanced capacity to form mammospheres, a property previously and exclusively associated with mammary epithelial stem cells. For now it is unclear whether this is restricted to cancer stem cells of an epithelial origin or can be generalized to all (cancer) stem cells. Somewhat contradictory to this, is the recent findings that suppression of EMT inducers and the expression of E-cadherin is one of the first essential steps during the reprogramming of fibroblasts for the generating induced pluripotent stem cells (Li et al., 2010; Redmer et al., 2011; Wang et al., 2010). This may reflect the fact that stemness properties and totipotency are not equivalent and may be controlled by divergent molecular mechanisms.

Recently, the *in vivo* functions of Snail and Slug could be further analyzed by the generation of novel gain/loss-of-function mouse models. Here we shall focus more on the hematopoietic phenotypes observed in these mouse models.

2.1 Slug is an important downstream mediator of SCF/cKit signaling and plays pivotal roles in stress-induced hematopoietic stem/progenitor cell survival and self-renewal

The first evidence of an important role for Slug in hematopoiesis and leukemia came from study by Inukai et al. (1999) in which Slug was identified as a downstream target of the E2A-HLF oncogene in leukemic B-cells. The E2A-HLF fusion gene transforms human pro-B lymphocytes by interfering with the apoptotic signaling pathway at an early step. Moreover, Slug expression in IL3-dependent Baf-3 cells prolonged the survival of these cells significantly after deprivation of the cytokine. These initial data suggested a pivotal role for Slug in the cell survival pathway of lymphocyte progenitor cells and possibly as well in other hematopoietic progenitors, based on its expression profile. Endogenous Slug is normally expressed in both long- and short-term repopulating HSCs and in committed progenitors of the myeloid lineage but not in differentiated myeloid cells or pro-B or pro-T cells. Its role in other lineages was further investigated *in vivo* by the generation of Slug deficient mice. Mice lacking Slug survive and are fertile, but display postnatal growth retardation phenotypes (Inoue et al., 2002). Upon loss of Slug, normal circulating blood cell counts were observed but the number of hematopoietic colony-forming progenitors in the bone marrow and spleen were significantly (2-4-fold) increased. This suggested that in the absence of Slug, hematopoietic progenitor pools must expand to maintain normal levels of differentiated blood cells in the circulation. In addition, Slug deficient mice are more radio-sensitive; these mice not only died earlier upon γ-irradiation, but as well showed accentuated decreases in peripheral blood cell counts and marked increases in apoptotic (TUNEL+) bone marrow progenitors cells compared to their control littermates. These data implicated an important role for Slug in protecting hematopoietic progenitor cells from apoptosis after DNA damage (Inoue et al., 2002). By crossing the Slug knockout mice with various other mouse models it was demonstrated that Slug directly represses the proapoptotic factor Puma and in this way is able to antagonize the p53-mediated upregulation of Puma in γ-irradiated myeloid progenitor cells, allowing them to survive (Wu W.S. et al., 2005). All together these data suggest that Slug governs a pivotal checkpoint that controls cell survival/apoptosis decisions upon exposure to genotoxic stress.

The role of Slug in the regulation of the bone marrow stem cell compartment was further investigated under both normal steady-state and stress conditions via competitive repopulating assays and serial bone marrow transplants (Sun et al., 2010). Under normal conditions, Slug deficiency seems to have no effect on proliferation or differentiation of HSC or progenitors. However, if transplanted, Slug null HSCs demonstated increased repopulating potential that was not a result of altered differentiation nor homing ability, suggesting Slug deficiency alters HSC self-renewal. Indeed this was confirmed under the stress conditions of serial bone marrow transplantation. Consistently, 5-FU treatment of Slug knockout mice showed an expansion of the Lin-Sca1+ cell population, not by changing their cell survival capacity but by increasing their proliferation rates (Sun et al., 2010).

More detailed analysis of Slug deficient mice revealed macrocytic anemia as well as pigmentation deficiency and gonadal defects (Perez-Losada et al., 2002). These phenotypes are very similar to the defects reported in the white-spotting (W) and Steel (Sl) mutant mice with mutations in the c-Kit receptor (Chabot et al., 1988; Geissler et al., 1988) and its Stem Cell Factor (SCF) ligand (Copeland et al., 1990; Huang et al., 1990; Zsebo et al., 1990). The SCF/c-Kit signaling pathway has pleiotrophic functions in hematopoiesis and beyond. The primary function of SCF/c-Kit in early hematopoiesis seems to induce the growth of quiescent progenitor/stem cells through synergistic interactions with other early-acting cytokines (Migliaccio et al., 1991; Williams N. et al., 1992). Ample evidence indicates that in the absence of other cytokines, SCF selectively promotes viability rather than proliferation of primitive murine progenitor cells (Fleming et al., 1993) and confirms previous findings of Slug playing a role in both cell cycle/proliferation and cell survival/apoptosis. Next to its role in hematopoiesis, SCF/c-Kit signaling has been implicated in the development/migration of melanocytes (Nishikawa et al., 1991). In human piebaldism patients, c-Kit signaling has been demonstrated to be involved in congenital depigmented patches and poliosis, (Giebel & Spritz, 1991). Interestingly in some piebaldism patients, also heterozygous SLUG deletions could be detected, providing further genetic evidence that Slug may play crucial roles in the SCF/c-Kit signaling pathway (Sanchez-Martin et al., 2003). The importance of Slug as a putative downstream mediator of c-Kit signaling was further tested by means of a complementation study in which transduction with TAT-Slug protein was sufficient to rescue the radio-sensitivity of c-Kit deficient mice. Taken together these data clearly demonstrate that Slug is an important mediator downstream of c-Kit receptor activation (Perez-Losada et al., 2003).

The observed macrocytic anemia observed in the Slug mutant mice resemble in some ways human congenital anemias such as Diamond-Blackfan anemia (Perez-Losada et al., 2002), however more research is necessary to explore the involvement of Slug in this disease.

2.2 Snail and Smuc in normal hematopoiesis

Mice deficient for Snail are embryonic lethal at E7.5-8.5 due to defects in mesoderm formation (Carver et al., 2001) as well as vascular defects (Lomeli et al., 2009). Consequently, due to the early embryonic lethality, the effects of Snail loss on hematopoiesis could not be further investigated in these mice. Although some evidence exists that Snail is expressed in the hematopoietic system, more detailed research is necessary and final proof of its potential role in hematpoiesis will come from breeding the conditional floxed Snail mice (Murray S.A. et al., 2006) to mice with hematopoietic-specific transgenic Cre lines.

Based upon the fact that *in vitro* Snail binds similar E-box binding domains and in general shows more drastic phenotypes both *in vitro* as *in vivo* compared to Slug, Snail may also play crucial roles in hematopoiesis. Interestingly, Snail and Slug in most cases can complement each other and differences in phenotypes can be explained by differences in expression patterns as exemplified by the aggravated phenotypes of the Snail/Slug double knockouts (Murray S.A. et al., 2007). In addition, loss of one Snai family member often induces or increases the expression of the other(s). In this way hematopoietic-specific double knockouts may reveal even more functions for Snail and Slug in normal hematopoiesis.

More recently a third family member of the Snail family was identified in vertebrates, Smuc. Until now, little is known about its functions but it is abundantly expressed in thymocytes (Zhuge et al., 2005), specifically in the early CD4-CD8- double negative (DN) and

CD4+CD8+ double positive (DP) stages of thymocyte maturation and then solely expressed in the CD8+ T lymphocyte lineage both in the thymus and peripheral immune system. In macrophages, Smuc is able to interact with PU.1, a master regulator of myeloid differentiation, and binds the negative regulatory element within the Pactolus promoter. These data suggests that Smuc is modulating the PU.1 transcriptional activity and lack of Smuc leads to aberrant PU.1 transactivation (Hale et al., 2006).

2.3 Overexpression of Snail or Slug induces leukemia

Based on the prominent roles of Snail and Slug in stress-induced hematopoiesis, and their roles in the progression of solid tumours, as well as acquisition of cancer stem cell characteristics, it is therefore surprising that only a limited number of studies have addressed the roles of Snai family members in hematopoietic malignancies.

Nevertheless, strong evidence that Snail and Slug are involved in leukemia formation and/or progression comes from the gain-of-function mouse models that were previously developed. CombiTA-Snail mice, carrying a hypermorphic tetracycline-repressible Snail transgene, showed increased Snail expression up to 20% above normal levels (Perez-Mancera et al., 2005b). These mice survive and are fertile and although no morphological alterations were observed, their thymus were smaller and showed reduced differentiation towards CD4+CD8+ DP thymocytes. From 5-7 months onwards, CombiTA-Snail mice started to develop various types of epithelial and non-epithelial cancers especially lymphomas and acute leukemias (> 75% in two separate transgenic lines). Suppression of the Snail transgene expression by tetracycline administration did not ameliorate the malignant phenotype, suggesting that the effect of Snail overexpression is irreversible. As well, CombiTA-Snail transgene expression resulted in increased *in vivo* radioprotection, suggesting similar roles for Snail in hematopoietic cell survival upon genotoxic stress as was previously shown for Slug.

Similar experiments were performed for *in vivo* overexpression of Slug. In a similar setup as described above for Snail, CombiTA-Slug mice were generated. To prove transgene functionality, these mice were crossed with Slug deficient mice, which rescued the null phenotype. Again these mice were born without overt morphological abnormalities (Perez-Mancera et al., 2006). Only after 6-8 months 20% of the transgenic mice died as a consequence of congestive heart failure. The surviving mice started to develop various tumors from 9 months of age with highest incidence of (90%) acute leukemias (Perez-Mancera et al., 2005a). Similar as to the CombiTA-Snail mice this malignant phenotype was irreversible after tetracycline administration. As well, c-Kit signaling has been implicated both in solid tumors as well as leukemias, e.g. constitutive activating mutations of the receptor have been described in AML (Jung et al., 2011) Furthermore, the BCR–ABL oncogene did not induce leukaemia in Slug-deficient mice, implicating Slug in BCR–ABL leukemogenesis *in vivo* (Perez-Mancera et al., 2005a). As well, in an independent study it was shown that the increased Slug expression upon Bcr-Abl mutations is involved in the prolonged survival of chronic myeloid leukemia cells (Mancini et al., 2010).

From the Slug knockout mice it appears that it is governing a pivotal role in cell survival upon DNA damage by repressing the pro-apoptotic factor Puma. These results may be highly relevant for cancer therapy. Analyzing or controlling Slug levels before or during treatment may be useful as a prognostic marker for sensitivity to genotoxic agents and can be helpful for limiting therapeutic doses or increasing the efficiency of radiation or chemotherapy.

3. EMT regulators of the Zeb family

The **Z**inc finger **E-B**ox binding (**ZEB**) family of DNA-binding transcriptional regulators consists of two structurally related proteins (Fortini et al., 1991)(Fig. 2): **Zeb1** (also known as δEF-1, TCF8, BZP, ZEB, AREB6, NIL-2-A, Zfhep, and Zfhx1a) and **Zeb2** (also known as Sip1, KIAA0569 and Zfhx1b). Both genes have a very similar genomic structures (Fortini et al., 1991; Vandewalle et al., 2009) and encode for large multi-domain proteins that possess N-terminal and C-terminal zinc finger DNA binding domains along with more centrally located homeo (HD), Smad protein binding (SBD) and CtBP interaction (CID) domains; and in the case of Zeb2, an N-terminal NuRD interaction domain (Verstappen et al., 2008). ¶

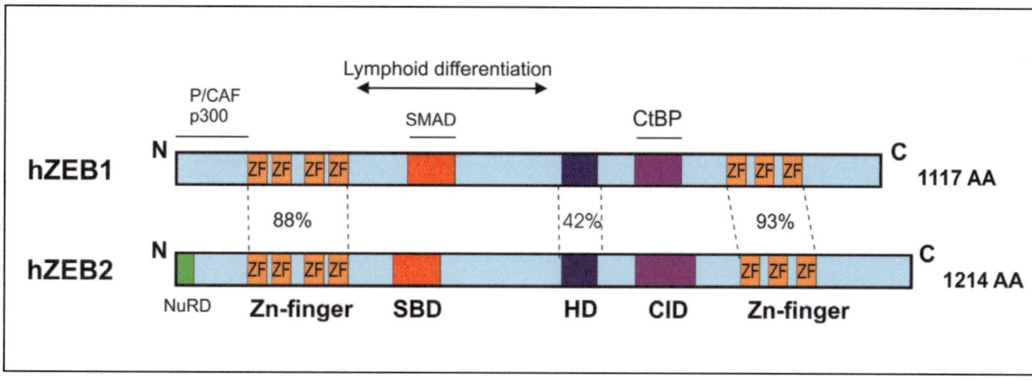

Fig. 2. Schematic diagram of conserved functional domains of the two members of the Zeb family of transcription factors. Both possess 2 zinc-finger domains, a homeodomain (HD), Smad (SBD) and CtBP (CID) binding domain (Figure based on Vandewalle et al., 2009)

Especially within the Zn-finger domains there exists a high degree of sequence similarity/identity between the two Zeb proteins, suggesting they bind similar target sequences (Verschueren et al., 1999). Each Zn-finger cluster independently can bind a 5′-CACCT(G)-3′ sequence located in the target promotor region (Remacle et al., 1999). The domains outside the Zn-finger clusters seem less conserved and may be essential for the recruitment of various co-repressors, like CtBP (Grooteclaes & Frisch, 2000;Postigo & Dean, 1999b; van Grunsven et al., 2007) or co-activators like p300 or P/CAF (van Grunsven et al., 2006). Still a lot of controversy exists over whether Zeb proteins can only act as transcriptional repressors or as well as activators. The molecular mechanism underlying the choice between repression or activation are currently unknown and may include cell-type specific differences and/or posttranslational modifications (Costantino et al., 2002). Similarly, the roles of Zeb proteins in TGFβ/BMP signaling are not well understood; both Zebs have been shown to be able to bind receptor activated R-Smads (Postigo, 2003; Verschueren et al., 1999). Postigo et al. (Postigo, 2003) postulated Zeb proteins as putative important downstream mediators of this signaling pathway however with opposing effects. While Zeb1 would synergize with Smad proteins to activate transcription of TGFβ responsive reporter constructs, the structurally very similar Zeb2 would inhibit transcriptional activation donwstream of TGFβ (Postigo, 2003). These antagonistic effects were hypothesized to result from differential recruitment of co-activators and co-repressors to the Smads by Zeb1 or Zeb2 respectively (Postigo et al., 2003).

The Zeb family of zinc finger/homeodomain proteins genes was first idenfied in *Drosphila melanogaster* (Fortini et al., 1991) and shown to be essential for myogenesis (Postigo et al., 1999) and the organization of the central nervous system (Clark & Chiu, 2003). As well in vertebrates a vast number of muscle master regulatory genes have been shown to be repressed directly by Zeb1/2 (α7 integrin, δ crystalin enhancer, Mef2c) (Postigo & Dean, 1997, 1999a) as well as genes essential for cartilage and bone formation (Col2α1) (Murray D. et al., 2000). The first functional studies in Xenopus proved Zeb1 to be essential for the expression of XBra (Xenopus Brachyury) (Papin et al., 2002), a member of T-box family of transcription factor essential for mesoderm formation and notochord differentiation and previously been implicated in EMT processes. Subsequently various *in vitro* studies using multiple epithelial cancer cell lines, it was demonstrated that both Zeb1/2 are able to bind and downregulate E-cadherin (Comijn et al., 2001; Eger et al., 2005) and other epithelial-specific marker genes via binding bipartite E-boxes in their promotor regions. Exogeneous Zeb1/2 overexpression results in EMT-like phenotypes similarly as described above for the Snai family members of EMT inducers (Comijn et al., 2001; Vandewalle et al., 2005). Increased *in vivo* Zeb1/2 expression has been correlated in various tumor types with increased invasion, metastasis, dedifferentiation, cancer stem cell characteristics, recurrence and bad prognosis (Spaderna et al., 2006; Spoelstra et al., 2006; Wellner et al., 2009; Yoshihara et al., 2009).

Besides their roles in suppression of epithelial marker genes more and more studies revealed their participation in other cellular processes like cell division (Mejlvang et al., 2007), apoptosis and senescence (Liu Y. et al., 2008; Ozturk et al., 2006; Sayan et al., 2009) and inflammation (Chua et al., 2007).

From expression analysis it was clear that both Zeb proteins are also expressed in the hematopoietic system. Actually, Zeb1 has been demonstrated to be more expressed during T-lymphocyte development, while Zeb2 expression has been seen more in splenic B cells (Postigo & Dean, 2000). Using various novel mouse models recent data clearly indicated that this family of EMT inducers also plays pivotal roles in various steps of hematopoietic differentiation and progression of hematopoietic malignancies, which are discussed in detail below.

3.1 Role of Zeb2 in hematopoietic stem/progenitor differentiation and mobilization

Moderate to high Zeb2 expression is reported in all hematopoietic cells with highest levels in stem (HSC) and progenitor (HPC) populations (Goossens et al., 2011) and lowest expression in mature T cells (Postigo & Dean, 2000). Through the use of a conditional Zeb2 knockout mouse (Higashi et al., 2002) model we could show that it is not essential for the initial formation of HSCs in the embryo but it is crucial for HSC differentiation and mobilization/homing (Goossens et al., 2011). Hematopoietic-specific Zeb2 loss-of-function resulted in embryonic lethality resulting from bleedings occurring in the developing brain. The observed phenotype is very reminiscent of the phenotypes associated with ubiquitous loss of the hematopoietic transcriptional regulators AML/Runx1 (Okuda et al., 1996). Runx1 knockout embryos are deficient in AGM HSCs and lack intra-arterial hematopoietic clusters, suggesting that Zeb2 deletion may also affect hematopoietic cluster formation. However, no changes in the number of hematopoietic progenitor clusters was detected for the Zeb2 null AGM regions (Goossens et al., 2011) indicating that the formed stem cells are not functional at later stages of development. Zeb2 seems to be more involved in stem/progenitor differentiation properties as isolated progenitors from various developing hematopoietic organs were unable to differentiate *in vitro*. As well, significant decreases in fully differentiated hematopoietic cells were observed. Next to this differentiation block, an increased adhesion/clustering of hematopoietic cells in the fetal liver and less mobile progenitors in the peripheral blood were observed. It was hypothesized that the increased levels of Cxcr4 within the Zeb2 null progenitors lead to their retention in the fetal liver that resulted in less progenitors in the embryonic circulation. This decreased mobilization of hematopoietic progenitors likely contributed to the decreased levels of angiogenic factors (like Ang1) within the circulation, thereby resulting in less maturation and pericyte recruitment towards the newly formed vessels in the developing brain. Most probably this defect contributed to the observed cephalic bleeding phenotype. From this initial data it has become clear that Zeb2 is not only a crucial transcriptional regulator of hematopoietic differentiation but as well plays pivotal roles in the mobilization and homing of HSCs within the embryo (Goossens et al., 2011). More experiments need to be performed to analyze whether this also holds true in adult haematopoiesis.

3.2 Role of Zeb1 in T cell development

Neonatal Zeb1 total knockout mice die shortly after birth. Drastic skeletal abnormalities (Takagi et al., 1998) and serious thymic atrophy were observed. Through the use of a second Zeb1 loss-of-function mouse model, expressing a C-terminal zinc finger truncation allowed survival to adulthood, it was feasible to further investigate the *in vivo* role of Zeb1 in adult hematopoiesis (Higashi et al., 1997). In these ΔC-fin mice no skeletal phenotypes were observed. On the other hand T lymphocyte differentiation was drastically impaired. This observation points towards the hypothesis that different domains of Zeb1 are responsible for alternative/synergistic functions, which as well was hypothesized previously by Postigo and colleagues via their *in vitro* approaches described above (Postigo & Dean, 1999a). More detailed FACS analysis of Zeb1 ΔC-fin mutant thymocytes revealed a block at a very early stage in the cKit+ $CD4^-CD8^-$DN population, before rearrangements of the T cell receptor (TCR) locus (Higashi et al., 1997). Only a very small proportion of the intrathymic T cell precursors (<1%compared of the normal T cell development) was able to differentiate further and expressed differentiated T cell markers. These differentiated cells were skewed mainly towards $CD4^+CD8^-$SP cells, indicated that also at later stages of T cell development Zeb1 expression may play essential roles. More recently it was shown that Zeb1 binds the 5′ E-boxes in the proximal enhancer of the CD4 promoter and competes with the transcriptional activators E12 and HEB for DNA binding. Therefore it was concluded that overexpression of Zeb1 in T cells converts the CD4 proximal enhancer into a silencer element leading to a reduction of CD4 expression. This data shows that the CD4 gene is a direct target of the transcriptional repressor Zeb1 and can explain the increased proportion of $CD4^+CD8^-$SP mature T cells in Zeb1 mutant mice (Brabletz et al., 1999).

Another known downstream target of Zeb1 during myogenesis is α4-integrin. Also in hematopoietic differentiation of various lineages α4-integrin is known to play crucial roles through its interaction with fibronectin and V-CAM in the stromal matrix and stromal cells of the bone marrow and fetal liver. α4-integrin is highly expressed in stem and progenitor cells and upon further differentiation its expression is restricted to lymphocytes and myeloid subpopulations. Zeb1 binds and directly represses α4-integrin expression (Postigo & Dean, 1999a). Previously it was shown that α4 integrin expression depends on C-Myb and Ets family of transcription factors. Based on *in vitro* α4-intregrin promotor analysis, Postigo (Postigo & Dean, 1997) concluded that Zeb1 blocks activity of c-Myb and Ets individually but together these synergize to overcome Zeb1 repression. Next to CD4 and α4 integrin, Zeb1 has been suggested to repress a number of other genes implicated in proper T cell differentiation like Gata3 (Gregoire & Romeo, 1999), immunoglobin heavy chain enhancer (Genetta et al.,1994) and interleukin-2 (Williams T.M. et al., 1991; Yasui et al., 1998).

Within B-lymphocytes a functional cooperation between FoxO transcription factors and Zeb1 has been revealed. Zeb1 binds and activates two promotors of known FoxO target genes cyclin G2 and retinoblastoma-like 2. Both have been implicated in cell cycle arrest and Foxo-dependent quiescence in fibroblasts (Chen et al., 2006). However a role of Zeb1 in B-cell development has not been reported

3.3 Role of Zeb1/2 in T and B cell acute lymphoblastic leukemia

Using the same ΔC-fin Zeb1 mutant mice described above it was demonstrated that expression of the truncated Zeb1 protein resulted in the development of spontaneous $CD4^+$ T-cell lymphomas with a median onset at 30 weeks of age. This is consistent with the fact that ZEB1 expression is frequently lost in human adult T-cell leukemia/lymphoma (T-ALL) patients (Hidaka et al., 2008; Vermeer et al., 2008). In T-ALL cell lines it was demonstrated that the tumour cell's resistance to TGF-β mediated growth suppression is via up-regulation of the inhibitory Smad7 (Nakahata et al., 2010). Here the role of Zeb proteins in the regulation of Smad7 remains needs to be better understood. Similarly the actual role of the other above described Zeb1 targets remains to be determined in T cell lymphomas.

The role of Zeb1 in B-Cell leukemia has not been reported. However, in terms of hematological malignancy, some independent genome-wide retroviral insertional mutagenesis screens have identified Zeb2 and not Zeb1 as a possible gene involved in mouse B-cell lymphoma progression (Lund et al., 2002; Mikkers et al., 2002; Shin et al., 2004). From these initial studies it was not clear if Zeb2 expression is lost due to retroviral integration and translocation events or enhanced during the transformation process. More recently in CALM-AF10 transgenic mice, enhanced Zeb2 expression was found to correlate with increased leukemia progression (Caudell et al., 2010). Additionally, knockdown of Zeb2 in a B-ALL cell line resulted in decreased proliferation rates. However *in vivo* Zeb2 overexpression studies are missing to be conclusive concerning the role of Zeb2 in leukemogenesis. Nevertheless, ZEB2 genomic locus rearrangements are commonly associated with aggressive B cell lymphomas in humans as well (Matteucci et al., 2008).

4. Conclusions

From the above literature survey it is clear that EMT inducers of the Snai and Zeb families play crucial and yet specific roles during various stages of hematopoiesis and leukemic transformation. These specific roles are in some way surprising given that they all bind similar E box-containing DNA sequences and a significant overlap in target genes has been reported. This can in some ways be explained by differences in their expression patterns and/or the recruitment of other cell-specific co-repressors and/or activators.

As well, the above reviewed data clearly indicate crucial roles for the EMT inducers of the Zeb and Snai family in different aspects of hematopoiesis: differentiation, proliferation, apoptosis/survival, mobilization, stemness, as well as quiescence. All of this suggests that these two family of proteins might be excellent targets for developing novel and improved cancer therapies not only as was suggested before for solid tumours but as well for blood-borne cancers and other haematological defects associated with improper lineage differentiation.

5. Acknowledgment

This work was partially supported by the European Hematology Association (EHA Young Investigator Fellowship 2009/26 to SG). SG is a postdoctoral fellow of the Basic Science Research Foundation-Flanders (FWO).

6. References

Al-Hajj, M., Wicha, M.S., Benito-Hernandez, A., Morrison, S.J. & Clarke, M.F. (2003) Prospective identification of tumorigenic breast cancer cells. *Proceedings of the National Academy of Sciences of the United States of America,* Vol.100, No.7, pp. 3983-3988

Batlle, E., Sancho, E., Franci, C., Dominguez, D., Monfar, M., Baulida, J. & Garcia De Herreros, A. (2000) The transcription factor snail is a repressor of e-cadherin gene expression in epithelial tumour cells. *Nature cell biology,* Vol.2, No.2, pp. 84-89

Berx, G., Raspe, E., Christofori, G., Thiery, J.P. & Sleeman, J.P. (2007) Pre-emting metastasis? Recapitulation of morphogenetic processes in cancer. *Clinical & experimental metastasis,* Vol.24, No.8, pp. 587-597

Boisset, J.C., van Cappellen, W., Andrieu-Soler, C., Galjart, N., Dzierzak, E. & Robin, C. In vivo imaging of haematopoietic cells emerging from the mouse aortic endothelium. *Nature,* Vol.464, No.7285, pp. 116-120

Bonnet, D. & Dick, J.E. (1997) Human acute myeloid leukemia is organized as a hierarchy that originates from a primitive hematopoietic cell. *Nature medicine,* Vol.3, No.7, pp. 730-737

Boulay, J.L., Dennefeld, C. & Alberga, A. (1987) The drosophila developmental gene snail encodes a protein with nucleic acid binding fingers. *Nature,* Vol.330, No.6146, pp. 395-398

Brabletz, T., Jung, A., Hlubek, F., Lohberg, C., Meiler, J., Suchy, U. & Kirchner, T. (1999) Negative regulation of cd4 expression in t cells by the transcriptional repressor zeb. *International immunology,* Vol.11, No.10, pp. 1701-1708

Cano, A., Perez-Moreno, M.A., Rodrigo, I., Locascio, A., Blanco, M.J., del Barrio, M.G., Portillo, F. & Nieto, M.A. (2000) The transcription factor snail controls epithelial-mesenchymal transitions by repressing e-cadherin expression. *Nature cell biology,* Vol.2, No.2, pp. 76-83

Carver, E.A., Jiang, R., Lan, Y., Oram, K.F. & Gridley, T. (2001) The mouse snail gene encodes a key regulator of the epithelial-mesenchymal transition. *Molecular and cellular biology,* Vol.21, No.23, pp. 8184-8188

Caudell, D., Harper, D.P., Novak, R.L., Pierce, R.M., Slape, C., Wolff, L. & Aplan, P.D. (2010) Retroviral insertional mutagenesis identifies zeb2 activation as a novel leukemogenic collaborating event in calm-af10 transgenic mice. *Blood,* Vol.115, No.6, pp. 1194-1203

Chabot, B., Stephenson, D.A., Chapman, V.M., Besmer, P. & Bernstein, A. (1988) The proto-oncogene c-kit encoding a transmembrane tyrosine kinase receptor maps to the mouse w locus. *Nature,* Vol.335, No.6185, pp. 88-89

Chen, J., Yusuf, I., Andersen, H.M. & Fruman, D.A. (2006) Foxo transcription factors cooperate with delta ef1 to activate growth suppressive genes in b lymphocytes. *Journal of immunology,* Vol.176, No.5, pp. 2711-2721

Chua, H.L., Bhat-Nakshatri, P., Clare, S.E., Morimiya, A., Badve, S. & Nakshatri, H. (2007) Nf-kappab represses e-cadherin expression and enhances epithelial to mesenchymal transition of mammary epithelial cells: Potential involvement of zeb-1 and zeb-2. *Oncogene,* Vol.26, No.5, pp. 711-724

Clark, S.G. & Chiu, C. (2003) C. Elegans zag-1, a zn-finger-homeodomain protein, regulates axonal development and neuronal differentiation. *Development,* Vol.130, No.16, pp. 3781-3794

Cobaleda, C., Perez-Caro, M., Vicente-Duenas, C. & Sanchez-Garcia, I. (2007) Function of the zinc-finger transcription factor snai2 in cancer and development. *Annual review of genetics,* Vol.41, pp. 41-61

Comijn, J., Berx, G., Vermassen, P., Verschueren, K., van Grunsven, L., Bruyneel, E., Mareel, M., Huylebroeck, D. & van Roy, F. (2001) The two-handed e box binding zinc finger protein sip1 downregulates e-cadherin and induces invasion. *Molecular Cell,* Vol.7, No.6, pp. 1267-1278

Copeland, N.G., Gilbert, D.J., Cho, B.C., Donovan, P.J., Jenkins, N.A., Cosman, D., Anderson, D., Lyman, S.D. & Williams, D.E. (1990) Mast cell growth factor maps near the steel locus on mouse chromosome 10 and is deleted in a number of steel alleles. *Cell,* Vol.63, No.1, pp. 175-183

Costantino, M.E., Stearman, R.P., Smith, G.E. & Darling, D.S. (2002) Cell-specific phosphorylation of zfhep transcription factor. *Biochemical and biophysical research communications,* Vol.296, No.2, pp. 368-373

de Bruijn, M.F., Ma, X., Robin, C., Ottersbach, K., Sanchez, M.J. & Dzierzak, E. (2002) Hematopoietic stem cells localize to the endothelial cell layer in the midgestation mouse aorta. *Immunity,* Vol.16, No.5, pp. 673-683

De Craene, B., van Roy, F. & Berx, G. (2005) Unraveling signalling cascades for the snail family of transcription factors. *Cellular signalling,* Vol.17, No.5, pp. 535-547

del Barrio, M.G. & Nieto, M.A. (2002) Overexpression of snail family members highlights their ability to promote chick neural crest formation. *Development,* Vol.129, No.7, pp. 1583-1593

Dzierzak, E. & Medvinsky, A. (2008) The discovery of a source of adult hematopoietic cells in the embryo. *Development,* Vol.135, No.14, pp. 2343-2346

Dzierzak, E. & Speck, N.A. (2008) Of lineage and legacy: The development of mammalian hematopoietic stem cells. *Nature immunology,* Vol.9, No.2, pp. 129-136

Eger, A., Aigner, K., Sonderegger, S., Dampier, B., Oehler, S., Schreiber, M., Berx, G., Cano, A., Beug, H. & Foisner, R. (2005) Deltaef1 is a transcriptional repressor of e-cadherin and regulates epithelial plasticity in breast cancer cells. *Oncogene,* Vol.24, No.14, pp. 2375-2385

Fleming, W.H., Alpern, E.J., Uchida, N., Ikuta, K. & Weissman, I.L. (1993) Steel factor influences the distribution and activity of murine hematopoietic stem cells in vivo. *Proceedings of the National Academy of Sciences of the United States of America,* Vol.90, No.8, pp. 3760-3764

Fortini, M.E., Lai, Z.C. & Rubin, G.M. (1991) The drosophila zfh-1 and zfh-2 genes encode novel proteins containing both zinc-finger and homeodomain motifs. *Mechanisms of development,* Vol.34, No.2-3, pp. 113-122

Geissler, E.N., Ryan, M.A. & Housman, D.E. (1988) The dominant-white spotting (w) locus of the mouse encodes the c-kit proto-oncogene. *Cell,* Vol.55, No.1, pp. 185-192

Genetta, T., Ruezinsky, D. & Kadesch, T. (1994) Displacement of an e-box-binding repressor by basic helix-loop-helix proteins: Implications for b-cell specificity of the immunoglobulin heavy-chain enhancer. *Molecular and cellular biology,* Vol.14, No.9, pp. 6153-6163

Giebel, L.B. & Spritz, R.A. (1991) Mutation of the kit (mast/stem cell growth factor receptor) protooncogene in human piebaldism. *Proceedings of the National Academy of Sciences of the United States of America,* Vol.88, No.19, pp. 8696-8699

Gill, J.G., Langer, E.M., Lindsley, R.C., Cai, M., Murphy, T.L. & Murphy, K.M. (2011) Snail promotes the cell-autonomous generation of flk1+ endothelial cells through the repression of the mir-200 family. *Stem cells and development,* in press.

Goossens, S., Janzen, V., Bartunkova, S., Yokomizo, T., Drogat, B., Crisan, M., Haigh, K., Seuntjens, E., Umans, L., Riedt, T., Bogaert, P., Haenebalcke, L., Berx, G., Dzierzak, E., Huylebroeck, D. & Haigh, J.J. (2011) The emt regulator zeb2/sip1 is essential for murine embryonic hematopoietic stem/progenitor cell differentiation and mobilization. *Blood,* Vol.117, No.21, pp. 5620-5630

Grau, Y., Carteret, C. & Simpson, P. (1984) Mutations and chromosomal rearrangements affecting the expression of snail, a gene involved in embryonic patterning in drosophila melanogaster. *Genetics,* Vol.108, No.2, pp. 347-360

Greenburg, G. & Hay, E.D. (1982) Epithelia suspended in collagen gels can lose polarity and express characteristics of migrating mesenchymal cells. *The Journal of cell biology,* Vol.95, No.1, pp. 333-339

Gregoire, J.M. & Romeo, P.H. (1999) T-cell expression of the human gata-3 gene is regulated by a non-lineage-specific silencer. *The Journal of biological chemistry,* Vol.274, No.10, pp. 6567-6578

Grimes, H.L., Chan, T.O., Zweidler-McKay, P.A., Tong, B. & Tsichlis, P.N. (1996) The gfi-1 proto-oncoprotein contains a novel transcriptional repressor domain, snag, and inhibits g1 arrest induced by interleukin-2 withdrawal. *Molecular and cellular biology,* Vol.16, No.11, pp. 6263-6272

Grooteclaes, M.L. & Frisch, S.M. (2000) Evidence for a function of ctbp in epithelial gene regulation and anoikis. *Oncogene,* Vol.19, No.33, pp. 3823-3828

Gupta, P.B., Chaffer, C.L. & Weinberg, R.A. (2009) Cancer stem cells: Mirage or reality? *Nature medicine,* Vol.15, No.9, pp. 1010-1012

Hale, J.S., Dahlem, T.J., Margraf, R.L., Debnath, I., Weis, J.J. & Weis, J.H. (2006) Transcriptional control of pactolus: Evidence of a negative control region and comparison with its evolutionary paralogue, cd18 (beta2 integrin). *Journal of leukocyte biology,* Vol.80, No.2, pp. 383-398

Hidaka, T., Nakahata, S., Hatakeyama, K., Hamasaki, M., Yamashita, K., Kohno, T., Arai, Y., Taki, T., Nishida, K., Okayama, A., Asada, Y., Yamaguchi, R., Tsubouchi, H., Yokota, J., Taniwaki, M., Higashi, Y. & Morishita, K. (2008) Down-regulation of tcf8 is involved in the leukemogenesis of adult t-cell leukemia/lymphoma. *Blood,* Vol.112, No.2, pp. 383-393

Higashi, Y., Moribe, H., Takagi, T., Sekido, R., Kawakami, K., Kikutani, H. & Kondoh, H. (1997) Impairment of t cell development in deltaef1 mutant mice. *The Journal of experimental medicine,* Vol.185, No.8, pp. 1467-1479

Higashi, Y., Maruhashi, M., Nelles, L., Van de Putte, T., Verschueren, K., Miyoshi, T., Yoshimoto, A., Kondoh, H. & Huylebroeck, D. (2002) Generation of the floxed allele of the sip1 (smad-interacting protein 1) gene for cre-mediated conditional knockout in the mouse. *Genesis,* Vol.32, No.2, pp. 82-84

Huang, E., Nocka, K., Beier, D.R., Chu, T.Y., Buck, J., Lahm, H.W., Wellner, D., Leder, P. & Besmer, P. (1990) The hematopoietic growth factor kl is encoded by the sl locus and is the ligand of the c-kit receptor, the gene product of the w locus. *Cell,* Vol.63, No.1, pp. 225-233

Inoue, A., Seidel, M.G., Wu, W., Kamizono, S., Ferrando, A.A., Bronson, R.T., Iwasaki, H., Akashi, K., Morimoto, A., Hitzler, J.K., Pestina, T.I., Jackson, C.W., Tanaka, R., Chong, M.J., McKinnon, P.J., Inukai, T., Grosveld, G.C. & Look, A.T. (2002) Slug, a highly conserved zinc finger transcriptional repressor, protects hematopoietic progenitor cells from radiation-induced apoptosis in vivo. *Cancer cell,* Vol.2, No.4, pp. 279-288

Inukai, T., Inoue, A., Kurosawa, H., Goi, K., Shinjyo, T., Ozawa, K., Mao, M., Inaba, T. & Look, A.T. (1999) Slug, a ces-1-related zinc finger transcription factor gene with antiapoptotic activity, is a downstream target of the e2a-hlf oncoprotein. *Molecular Cell,* Vol.4, No.3, pp. 343-352

Jung, C.L., Kim, H.J., Kim, D.H., Huh, H., Song, M.J. & Kim, S.H. (2011) Ckit mutation in therapy-related acute myeloid leukemia with mllt3/mll chimeric transcript from t(9;11)(p22;q23). *Annals of clinical and laboratory science,* Vol.41, No.2, pp. 193-196

Kajita, M., McClinic, K.N. & Wade, P.A. (2004) Aberrant expression of the transcription factors snail and slug alters the response to genotoxic stress. *Molecular and cellular biology,* Vol.24, No.17, pp. 7559-7566

Kalluri, R. (2009) Emt: When epithelial cells decide to become mesenchymal-like cells. *The Journal of clinical investigation,* Vol.119, No.6, pp. 1417-1419

Kalluri, R. & Weinberg, R.A. (2009) The basics of epithelial-mesenchymal transition. *The Journal of clinical investigation,* Vol.119, No.6, pp. 1420-1428

Knight, R.D. & Shimeld, S.M. (2001) Identification of conserved c2h2 zinc-finger gene families in the bilateria. *Genome biology,* Vol.2, No.5, pp. RESEARCH0016

Kondo, M., Wagers, A.J., Manz, M.G., Prohaska, S.S., Scherer, D.C., Beilhack, G.F., Shizuru, J.A. & Weissman, I.L. (2003) Biology of hematopoietic stem cells and progenitors: Implications for clinical application. *Annual review of immunology,* Vol.21, pp. 759-806

LaBonne, C. & Bronner-Fraser, M. (2000) Snail-related transcriptional repressors are required in xenopus for both the induction of the neural crest and its subsequent migration. *Developmental biology,* Vol.221, No.1, pp. 195-205

Li, R., Liang, J., Ni, S., Zhou, T., Qing, X., Li, H., He, W., Chen, J., Li, F., Zhuang, Q., Qin, B., Xu, J., Li, W., Yang, J., Gan, Y., Qin, D., Feng, S., Song, H., Yang, D., Zhang, B., Zeng, L., Lai, L., Esteban, M.A. & Pei, D. (2010) A mesenchymal-to-epithelial transition initiates and is required for the nuclear reprogramming of mouse fibroblasts. *Cell stem cell,* Vol.7, No.1, pp. 51-63

Lin, Y., Wu, Y., Li, J., Dong, C., Ye, X., Chi, Y.I., Evers, B.M. & Zhou, B.P. (2010) The snag domain of snail1 functions as a molecular hook for recruiting lysine-specific demethylase 1. *The EMBO journal,* Vol.29, No.11, pp. 1803-1816

Liu, J., Uygur, B., Zhang, Z., Shao, L., Romero, D., Vary, C., Ding, Q. & Wu, W.S. (2010) Slug inhibits proliferation of human prostate cancer cells via downregulation of cyclin d1 expression. *The Prostate,* Vol.70, No.16, pp. 1768-1777

Liu, Y., El-Naggar, S., Darling, D.S., Higashi, Y. & Dean, D.C. (2008) Zeb1 links epithelial-mesenchymal transition and cellular senescence. *Development,* Vol.135, No.3, pp. 579-588

Lomeli, H., Starling, C. & Gridley, T. (2009) Epiblast-specific snail deletion results in embryonic lethality due to multiple vascular defects. *BMC research notes,* Vol.2, pp. 22

Lund, A.H., Turner, G., Trubetskoy, A., Verhoeven, E., Wientjens, E., Hulsman, D., Russell, R., DePinho, R.A., Lenz, J. & van Lohuizen, M. (2002) Genome-wide retroviral insertional tagging of genes involved in cancer in cdkn2a-deficient mice. *Nature genetics,* Vol.32, No.1, pp. 160-165

Lyons, J.G., Patel, V., Roue, N.C., Fok, S.Y., Soon, L.L., Halliday, G.M. & Gutkind, J.S. (2008) Snail up-regulates proinflammatory mediators and inhibits differentiation in oral keratinocytes. *Cancer research,* Vol.68, No.12, pp. 4525-4530

Mancini, M., Petta, S., Iacobucci, I., Salvestrini, V., Barbieri, E. & Santucci, M.A. (2010) Zinc-finger transcription factor slug contributes to the survival advantage of chronic myeloid leukemia cells. *Cellular signalling,* Vol.22, No.8, pp. 1247-1253

Mani, S.A., Guo, W., Liao, M.J., Eaton, E.N., Ayyanan, A., Zhou, A.Y., Brooks, M., Reinhard, F., Zhang, C.C., Shipitsin, M., Campbell, L.L., Polyak, K., Brisken, C., Yang, J. & Weinberg, R.A. (2008) The epithelial-mesenchymal transition generates cells with properties of stem cells. *Cell,* Vol.133, No.4, pp. 704-715

Manzanares, M., Locascio, A. & Nieto, M.A. (2001) The increasing complexity of the snail gene superfamily in metazoan evolution. *Trends in genetics,* Vol.17, No.4, pp. 178-181

Matteucci, C., Bracci, M., Barba, G., Carbonari, M., Casato, M., Visentini, M., Pulsoni, A., Varasano, E., Roti, G., La Starza, R., Crescenzi, B., Martelli, M.F., Fiorilli, M. & Mecucci, C. (2008) Different genomic imbalances in low- and high-grade hcv-related lymphomas. *Leukemia,* Vol.22, No.1, pp. 219-222

Mauhin, V., Lutz, Y., Dennefeld, C. & Alberga, A. (1993) Definition of the DNA-binding site repertoire for the drosophila transcription factor snail. *Nucleic acids research,* Vol.21, No.17, pp. 3951-3957

Mejlvang, J., Kriajevska, M., Vandewalle, C., Chernova, T., Sayan, A.E., Berx, G., Mellon, J.K. & Tulchinsky, E. (2007) Direct repression of cyclin d1 by sip1 attenuates cell cycle progression in cells undergoing an epithelial mesenchymal transition. *Molecular biology of the cell,* Vol.18, No.11, pp. 4615-4624

Migliaccio, G., Migliaccio, A.R., Valinsky, J., Langley, K., Zsebo, K., Visser, J.W. & Adamson, J.W. (1991) Stem cell factor induces proliferation and differentiation of highly enriched murine hematopoietic cells. *Proceedings of the National Academy of Sciences of the United States of America,* Vol.88, No.16, pp. 7420-7424

Mikkers, H., Allen, J., Knipscheer, P., Romeijn, L., Hart, A., Vink, E. & Berns, A. (2002) High-throughput retroviral tagging to identify components of specific signaling pathways in cancer. *Nature genetics,* Vol.32, No.1, pp. 153-159

Miranda-Saavedra, D. & Gottgens, B. (2008) Transcriptional regulatory networks in haematopoiesis. *Current opinion in genetics & development,* Vol.18, No.6, pp. 530-535

Murray, D., Precht, P., Balakir, R. & Horton, W.E., Jr. (2000) The transcription factor deltaef1 is inversely expressed with type ii collagen mrna and can repress col2a1 promoter activity in transfected chondrocytes. *The Journal of biological chemistry,* Vol.275, No.5, pp. 3610-3618

Murray, S.A., Carver, E.A. & Gridley, T. (2006) Generation of a snail1 (snai1) conditional null allele. *Genesis,* Vol.44, No.1, pp. 7-11

Murray, S.A., Oram, K.F. & Gridley, T. (2007) Multiple functions of snail family genes during palate development in mice. *Development,* Vol.134, No.9, pp. 1789-1797

Nakahata, S., Yamazaki, S., Nakauchi, H. & Morishita, K. (2010) Downregulation of zeb1 and overexpression of smad7 contribute to resistance to tgf-beta1-mediated growth suppression in adult t-cell leukemia/lymphoma. *Oncogene,* Vol.29, No.29, pp. 4157-4169

Nieto, M.A. (2002) The snail superfamily of zinc-finger transcription factors. *Nature reviews,* Vol.3, No.3, pp. 155-166

Nishikawa, S., Kusakabe, M., Yoshinaga, K., Ogawa, M., Hayashi, S., Kunisada, T., Era, T., Sakakura, T. & Nishikawa, S. (1991) In utero manipulation of coat color formation by a monoclonal anti-c-kit antibody: Two distinct waves of c-kit-dependency during melanocyte development. *The EMBO journal,* Vol.10, No.8, pp. 2111-2118

Okuda, T., van Deursen, J., Hiebert, S.W., Grosveld, G. & Downing, J.R. (1996) Aml1, the target of multiple chromosomal translocations in human leukemia, is essential for normal fetal liver hematopoiesis. *Cell,* Vol.84, No.2, pp. 321-330

Orkin, S.H. (2000) Diversification of haematopoietic stem cells to specific lineages. *Nature reviews,* Vol.1, No.1, pp. 57-64

Orkin, S.H. & Zon, L.I. (2008) Hematopoiesis: An evolving paradigm for stem cell biology. *Cell,* Vol.132, No.4, pp. 631-644

Ozturk, N., Erdal, E., Mumcuoglu, M., Akcali, K.C., Yalcin, O., Senturk, S., Arslan-Ergul, A., Gur, B., Yulug, I., Cetin-Atalay, R., Yakicier, C., Yagci, T., Tez, M. & Ozturk, M. (2006) Reprogramming of replicative senescence in hepatocellular carcinoma-derived cells. *Proceedings of the National Academy of Sciences of the United States of America,* Vol.103, No.7, pp. 2178-2183

Palis, J., Chan, R.J., Koniski, A., Patel, R., Starr, M. & Yoder, M.C. (2001) Spatial and temporal emergence of high proliferative potential hematopoietic precursors during murine embryogenesis. *Proceedings of the National Academy of Sciences of the United States of America,* Vol.98, No.8, pp. 4528-4533

Papin, C., van Grunsven, L.A., Verschueren, K., Huylebroeck, D. & Smith, J.C. (2002) Dynamic regulation of brachyury expression in the amphibian embryo by xsip1. *Mechanisms of development,* Vol.111, No.1-2, pp. 37-46

Perez-Losada, J., Sanchez-Martin, M., Rodriguez-Garcia, A., Sanchez, M.L., Orfao, A., Flores, T. & Sanchez-Garcia, I. (2002) Zinc-finger transcription factor slug contributes to the function of the stem cell factor c-kit signaling pathway. *Blood,* Vol.100, No.4, pp. 1274-1286

Perez-Losada, J., Sanchez-Martin, M., Perez-Caro, M., Perez-Mancera, P.A. & Sanchez-Garcia, I. (2003) The radioresistance biological function of the scf/kit signaling pathway is mediated by the zinc-finger transcription factor slug. *Oncogene,* Vol.22, No.27, pp. 4205-4211

Perez-Mancera, P.A., Gonzalez-Herrero, I., Perez-Caro, M., Gutierrez-Cianca, N., Flores, T., Gutierrez-Adan, A., Pintado, B., Sanchez-Martin, M. & Sanchez-Garcia, I. (2005a) Slug in cancer development. *Oncogene,* Vol.24, No.19, pp. 3073-3082

Perez-Mancera, P.A., Perez-Caro, M., Gonzalez-Herrero, I., Flores, T., Orfao, A., de Herreros, A.G., Gutierrez-Adan, A., Pintado, B., Sagrera, A., Sanchez-Martin, M. & Sanchez-Garcia, I. (2005b) Cancer development induced by graded expression of snail in mice. *Human Molecular Genetics,* Vol.14, No.22, pp. 3449-3461

Perez-Mancera, P.A., Gonzalez-Herrero, I., Maclean, K., Turner, A.M., Yip, M.Y., Sanchez-Martin, M., Garcia, J.L., Robledo, C., Flores, T., Gutierrez-Adan, A., Pintado, B. & Sanchez-Garcia, I. (2006) Slug (snai2) overexpression in embryonic development. *Cytogenetic and Genome Research,* Vol.114, No.1, pp. 24-29

Postigo, A.A. & Dean, D.C. (1997) Zeb, a vertebrate homolog of drosophila zfh-1, is a negative regulator of muscle differentiation. *The EMBO journal,* Vol.16, No.13, pp. 3935-3943

Postigo, A.A. & Dean, D.C. (1999a) Independent repressor domains in zeb regulate muscle and t-cell differentiation. *Molecular and cellular biology,* Vol.19, No.12, pp. 7961-7971

Postigo, A.A. & Dean, D.C. (1999b) Zeb represses transcription through interaction with the corepressor ctbp. *Proceedings of the National Academy of Sciences of the United States of America,* Vol.96, No.12, pp. 6683-6688

Postigo, A.A., Ward, E., Skeath, J.B. & Dean, D.C. (1999) Zfh-1, the drosophila homologue of zeb, is a transcriptional repressor that regulates somatic myogenesis. *Molecular and cellular biology,* Vol.19, No.10, pp. 7255-7263

Postigo, A.A. & Dean, D.C. (2000) Differential expression and function of members of the zfh-1 family of zinc finger/homeodomain repressors. *Proceedings of the National Academy of Sciences of the United States of America,* Vol.97, No.12, pp. 6391-6396

Postigo, A.A. (2003) Opposing functions of zeb proteins in the regulation of the tgfbeta/bmp signaling pathway. *The EMBO journal,* Vol.22, No.10, pp. 2443-2452

Postigo, A.A., Depp, J.L., Taylor, J.J. & Kroll, K.L. (2003) Regulation of smad signaling through a differential recruitment of coactivators and corepressors by zeb proteins. *The EMBO journal,* Vol.22, No.10, pp. 2453-2462

Redmer, T., Diecke, S., Grigoryan, T., Quiroga-Negreira, A., Birchmeier, W. & Besser, D. (2011) E-cadherin is crucial for embryonic stem cell pluripotency and can replace oct4 during somatic cell reprogramming. *EMBO reports,* Vol.12, No.7, pp. 720-726

Remacle, J.E., Kraft, H., Lerchner, W., Wuytens, G., Collart, C., Verschueren, K., Smith, J.C. & Huylebroeck, D. (1999) New mode of DNA binding of multi-zinc finger transcription factors: Deltaef1 family members bind with two hands to two target sites. *The EMBO journal,* Vol.18, No.18, pp. 5073-5084

Ricci-Vitiani, L., Lombardi, D.G., Pilozzi, E., Biffoni, M., Todaro, M., Peschle, C. & De Maria, R. (2007) Identification and expansion of human colon-cancer-initiating cells. *Nature,* Vol.445, No.7123, pp. 111-115

Robin, C., Ottersbach, K., Boisset, J.C., Oziemlak, A. & Dzierzak, E. (2011) Cd41 is developmentally regulated and differentially expressed on mouse hematopoietic stem cells. *Blood,* Vol.117, No.19, pp. 5088-5091

Rybtsov, S., Sobiesiak, M., Taoudi, S., Souilhol, C., Senserrich, J., Liakhovitskaia, A., Ivanovs, A., Frampton, J., Zhao, S. & Medvinsky, A. (2011) Hierarchical organization and early hematopoietic specification of the developing hsc lineage in the agm region. *The Journal of experimental medicine,* Vol.208, No.6, pp. 1305-1315

Sanchez-Martin, M., Perez-Losada, J., Rodriguez-Garcia, A., Gonzalez-Sanchez, B., Korf, B.R., Kuster, W., Moss, C., Spritz, R.A. & Sanchez-Garcia, I. (2003) Deletion of the slug (snai2) gene results in human piebaldism. *American journal of medical genetics,* Vol.122A, No.2, pp. 125-132

Sayan, A.E., Griffiths, T.R., Pal, R., Browne, G.J., Ruddick, A., Yagci, T., Edwards, R., Mayer, N.J., Qazi, H., Goyal, S., Fernandez, S., Straatman, K., Jones, G.D., Bowman, K.J., Colquhoun, A., Mellon, J.K., Kriajevska, M. & Tulchinsky, E. (2009) Sip1 protein protects cells from DNA damage-induced apoptosis and has independent prognostic value in bladder cancer. *Proceedings of the National Academy of Sciences of the United States of America,* Vol.106, No.35, pp. 14884-14889

Schatton, T., Frank, N.Y. & Frank, M.H. (2009) Identification and targeting of cancer stem cells. *BioEssays,* Vol.31, No.10, pp. 1038-1049

Sefton, M., Sanchez, S. & Nieto, M.A. (1998) Conserved and divergent roles for members of the snail family of transcription factors in the chick and mouse embryo. *Development,* Vol.125, No.16, pp. 3111-3121

Shin, M.S., Fredrickson, T.N., Hartley, J.W., Suzuki, T., Akagi, K. & Morse, H.C., 3rd (2004) High-throughput retroviral tagging for identification of genes involved in initiation and progression of mouse splenic marginal zone lymphomas. *Cancer research,* Vol.64, No.13, pp. 4419-4427

Singh, S.K., Clarke, I.D., Hide, T. & Dirks, P.B. (2004) Cancer stem cells in nervous system tumors. *Oncogene,* Vol.23, No.43, pp. 7267-7273

Spaderna, S., Schmalhofer, O., Hlubek, F., Berx, G., Eger, A., Merkel, S., Jung, A., Kirchner, T. & Brabletz, T. (2006) A transient, emt-linked loss of basement membranes indicates metastasis and poor survival in colorectal cancer. *Gastroenterology,* Vol.131, No.3, pp. 830-840

Spoelstra, N.S., Manning, N.G., Higashi, Y., Darling, D., Singh, M., Shroyer, K.R., Broaddus, R.R., Horwitz, K.B. & Richer, J.K. (2006) The transcription factor zeb1 is aberrantly expressed in aggressive uterine cancers. *Cancer research,* Vol.66, No.7, pp. 3893-3902

Sun, Y., Shao, L., Bai, H., Wang, Z.Z. & Wu, W.S. (2010) Slug deficiency enhances self-renewal of hematopoietic stem cells during hematopoietic regeneration. *Blood,* Vol.115, No.9, pp. 1709-1717

Takagi, T., Moribe, H., Kondoh, H. & Higashi, Y. (1998) Deltaef1, a zinc finger and homeodomain transcription factor, is required for skeleton patterning in multiple lineages. *Development,* Vol.125, No.1, pp. 21-31

Thiery, J.P. & Sleeman, J.P. (2006) Complex networks orchestrate epithelial-mesenchymal transitions. *Nature reviews,* Vol.7, No.2, pp. 131-142

Thiery, J.P., Acloque, H., Huang, R.Y. & Nieto, M.A. (2009) Epithelial-mesenchymal transitions in development and disease. *Cell,* Vol.139, No.5, pp. 871-890

van Grunsven, L.A., Taelman, V., Michiels, C., Opdecamp, K., Huylebroeck, D. & Bellefroid, E.J. (2006) Deltaef1 and sip1 are differentially expressed and have overlapping activities during xenopus embryogenesis. *Developmental dynamics,* Vol.235, No.6, pp. 1491-1500

van Grunsven, L.A., Taelman, V., Michiels, C., Verstappen, G., Souopgui, J., Nichane, M., Moens, E., Opdecamp, K., Vanhomwegen, J., Kricha, S., Huylebroeck, D. & Bellefroid, E.J. (2007) Xsip1 neuralizing activity involves the co-repressor ctbp and occurs through bmp dependent and independent mechanisms. *Developmental biology,* Vol.306, No.1, pp. 34-49

Vandewalle, C., Comijn, J., De Craene, B., Vermassen, P., Bruyneel, E., Andersen, H., Tulchinsky, E., Van Roy, F. & Berx, G. (2005) Sip1/zeb2 induces emt by repressing genes of different epithelial cell-cell junctions. *Nucleic acids research,* Vol.33, No.20, pp. 6566-6578

Vandewalle, C., Van Roy, F. & Berx, G. (2009) The role of the zeb family of transcription factors in development and disease. *Cellular and molecular life sciences,* Vol.66, No.5, pp. 773-787

Vermeer, M.H., van Doorn, R., Dijkman, R., Mao, X., Whittaker, S., van Voorst Vader, P.C., Gerritsen, M.J., Geerts, M.L., Gellrich, S., Soderberg, O., Leuchowius, K.J., Landegren, U., Out-Luiting, J.J., Knijnenburg, J., Ijszenga, M., Szuhai, K., Willemze, R. & Tensen, C.P. (2008) Novel and highly recurrent chromosomal alterations in sezary syndrome. *Cancer research,* Vol.68, No.8, pp. 2689-2698

Verschueren, K., Remacle, J.E., Collart, C., Kraft, H., Baker, B.S., Tylzanowski, P., Nelles, L., Wuytens, G., Su, M.T., Bodmer, R., Smith, J.C. & Huylebroeck, D. (1999) Sip1, a novel zinc finger/homeodomain repressor, interacts with smad proteins and binds to 5'-cacct sequences in candidate target genes. *The Journal of biological chemistry,* Vol.274, No.29, pp. 20489-20498

Verstappen, G., van Grunsven, L.A., Michiels, C., Van de Putte, T., Souopgui, J., Van Damme, J., Bellefroid, E., Vandekerckhove, J. & Huylebroeck, D. (2008) Atypical mowat-wilson patient confirms the importance of the novel association between zfhx1b/sip1 and nurd corepressor complex. *Human Molecular Genetics,* Vol.17, No.8, pp. 1175-1183

Wang, Y., Mah, N., Prigione, A., Wolfrum, K., Andrade-Navarro, M.A. & Adjaye, J. (2010) A transcriptional roadmap to the induction of pluripotency in somatic cells. *Stem cell reviews,* Vol.6, No.2, pp. 282-296

Wellner, U., Schubert, J., Burk, U.C., Schmalhofer, O., Zhu, F., Sonntag, A., Waldvogel, B., Vannier, C., Darling, D., zur Hausen, A., Brunton, V.G., Morton, J., Sansom, O., Schuler, J., Stemmler, M.P., Herzberger, C., Hopt, U., Keck, T., Brabletz, S. & Brabletz, T. (2009) The emt-activator zeb1 promotes tumorigenicity by repressing stemness-inhibiting micrornas. *Nature cell biology,* Vol.11, No.12, pp. 1487-1495

Williams, N., Bertoncello, I., Kavnoudias, H., Zsebo, K. & McNiece, I. (1992) Recombinant rat stem cell factor stimulates the amplification and differentiation of fractionated mouse stem cell populations. *Blood,* Vol.79, No.1, pp. 58-64

Williams, T.M., Moolten, D., Burlein, J., Romano, J., Bhaerman, R., Godillot, A., Mellon, M., Rauscher, F.J., 3rd & Kant, J.A. (1991) Identification of a zinc finger protein that inhibits il-2 gene expression. *Science,* Vol.254, No.5039, pp. 1791-1794

Wu, W.S., Heinrichs, S., Xu, D., Garrison, S.P., Zambetti, G.P., Adams, J.M. & Look, A.T. (2005) Slug antagonizes p53-mediated apoptosis of hematopoietic progenitors by repressing puma. *Cell,* Vol.123, No.4, pp. 641-653

Wu, Y. & Zhou, B.P. (2010) Snail: More than emt. *Cell adhesion & migration,* Vol.4, No.2, pp. 199-203

Yang, C.C. & Wolf, D.A. (2009) Inflamed snail speeds metastasis. *Cancer cell,* Vol.15, No.5, pp. 355-357

Yasui, D.H., Genetta, T., Kadesch, T., Williams, T.M., Swain, S.L., Tsui, L.V. & Huber, B.T. (1998) Transcriptional repression of the il-2 gene in th cells by zeb. *Journal of immunology,* Vol.160, No.9, pp. 4433-4440

Yokomizo, T., Ng, C.E., Osato, M. & Dzierzak, E. (2011) Three-dimensional imaging of whole midgestation murine embryos shows an intravascular localization for all hematopoietic clusters. *Blood,* Vol.117, No.23, pp. 6132-6134

Yoshihara, K., Tajima, A., Komata, D., Yamamoto, T., Kodama, S., Fujiwara, H., Suzuki, M., Onishi, Y., Hatae, M., Sueyoshi, K., Fujiwara, H., Kudo, Y., Inoue, I. & Tanaka, K. (2009) Gene expression profiling of advanced-stage serous ovarian cancers distinguishes novel subclasses and implicates zeb2 in tumor progression and prognosis. *Cancer science,* Vol.100, No.8, pp. 1421-1428

Zhuge, X., Kataoka, H., Tanaka, M., Murayama, T., Kawamoto, T., Sano, H., Togi, K., Yamauchi, R., Ueda, Y., Xu, Y., Nishikawa, S., Kita, T. & Yokode, M. (2005) Expression of the novel snai-related zinc-finger transcription factor gene smuc during mouse development. *International journal of molecular medicine,* Vol.15, No.6, pp. 945-948

Zovein, A.C., Turlo, K.A., Ponec, R.M., Lynch, M.R., Chen, K.C., Hofmann, J.J., Cox, T.C., Gasson, J.C. & Iruela-Arispe, M.L. (2010) Vascular remodeling of the vitelline artery initiates extravascular emergence of hematopoietic clusters. *Blood,* Vol.116, No.18, pp. 3435-3444

Zsebo, K.M., Williams, D.A., Geissler, E.N., Broudy, V.C., Martin, F.H., Atkins, H.L., Hsu, R.Y., Birkett, N.C., Okino, K.H., Murdock, D.C. & et al. (1990) Stem cell factor is encoded at the sl locus of the mouse and is the ligand for the c-kit tyrosine kinase receptor. *Cell,* Vol.63, No.1, pp. 213-224

4

Asymmetric Division in the Immuno-Hematopoietic System

Daniel Jimenez-Teja, Nadia Martin-Blanco and Matilde Canelles
Instituto de Parasitología y Biomedicina, CSIC, P. T. Ciencias de la Salud, Granada
Spain

1. Introduction

Asymmetric division is a process by which stem cells asymmetrically segregate certain proteins, called "cell fate determinants", in order to generate two functionally different cells. Normally, one of the daughter cells terminally differentiates while the other retains stem cell properties and continues proliferating. Asymmetric division has been found in virtually all developing systems where stem cells need to simultaneously proliferate and generate differentiated cells: brain, skin, gut, mammary gland, hematopoiesis, also in plants and algae. As a consequence of these studies, it has been established that, by virtue of asymmetric division, both developing and adult organs maintain the delicate equilibrium between proliferation and differentiation. The recent discovery of links to cancer has added momentum to an already very dynamic research area. This review article will discuss the latest developments in the asymmetric division field, with a focus on the immuno-hematopoietic system.

2. Historical perspective

The hypothesis about the existence of asymmetric division was postulated in 1878 based on studies of leech development, where certain cytoplasmic domains of the egg are differentially segregated to the descendants (Whitman, 1878). In the 1980s asymmetric division was described and analyzed in many other organisms, like yeasts, nematode, algae and *Drosophila* (see Horvitz and Herskowitz 1992 for a comprehensive review). At this stage, it was thought that each organism had a different means to undergo asymmetric division. Daughter cells acquired the differences that made them differentiate into various lineages either intrinsically (by differential inheritance of cytoplasmic or chromosomal factors) or extrinsically, by differential segregation of soluble factors. Intrinsic differences were described in expression of transcription factors, chromatin components, nucleases, receptors, cytoskeletal proteins and others; however, at this point it was not clear which of them were involved in generating asymmetry or were subject to asymmetric segregation themselves to influence differentiation. Extrinsic asymmetric cell division seemed to be the result of either direct cell-cell contact, or secretion of soluble factors. We will focus on intrinsic asymmetric division, which has been most widely studied.

In the 1990s, *Drosophila* asymmetric division was analyzed in detail and visualized by confocal microscopy (Rhyu, Jan, and Jan 1994). Two proteins with antagonistic function,

Numb and Notch, were pointed out as the main characters in this complicated process. This was followed by the description of asymmetric division in mammalian brain, with a similar mechanism and also involving asymmetric segregation of Numb (Zhong et al. 1996). At this point, Numb function was unknown, however it was discovered that it could bind (and antagonize) the transmembrane receptor Notch. During the following years, efforts in the two main invertebrate model systems, *C. elegans* and *Drosophila*, were focused on the mechanisms to set up cell polarity previous to division, spindle positioning and asymmetric localization of cell fate determinants (Betschinger and Knoblich 2004). Studies on vertebrates showed that many of the proteins involved were conserved, and that there may be a general mechanism for asymmetric division, conserved from the most ancient organisms up to our own brain and muscles. These discoveries resulted on a shift of research in the direction of vertebrates and, concretely, mammalians, and soon asymmetric division was first described in the hematopoietic system (Wu et al. 2007; Schroeder 2007). Studies in *Drosophila* were still ahead, thus the first link between cancer and asymmetric division was discovered in *Drosophila* earlier than in mammalians (Caussinus and Gonzalez 2005). In the following years, an important role for phosphorylation of cell fate determinants during mitosis was described (Wirtz-Peitz, Nishimura, and Knoblich 2008). Additionally, the mechanisms for asymmetric inheritance of centrioles (mediated by microtubules), DNA and vesicles were discovered [reviewed in (Neumuller and Knoblich 2009)]. It was realized that, although the proteins involved in asymmetric division are conserved, their roles are different in vertebrates. However, *Drosophila* studies were vey helpful in the case of the link to cancer, and a molecular mechanism involving Numb and p53 was discovered (Colaluca et al. 2008). The challenge for the next decade will be to integrate all this knowledge at the systems level to understand how asymmetric division works in health and disease, with enormous implications for stem cell research.

3. Molecular mechanisms of asymmetric division

Although the mechanism of asymmetric cell division has been intensively studied, there is no general model of how it occurs, because the data have been obtained studying different organisms that normally have their own specificity. Besides, different techniques, depending on the field, have been used to obtain the data, making it difficult to discern real differences from those arising as a result of using different techniques. Another problem, even when dealing with a single model system, is that there are data on asymmetric segregation of different proteins and organelles of the cell, but these data are not connected either temporally or mechanistically. A considerable effort to unify this knowledge into a common model has been made by J. Knoblich, who has continually summarized the data from diverse model systems in a series of excellent reviews [specifically (Knoblich 2010) (Neumuller and Knoblich 2009) are of great help in understanding the underlying mechanisms of asymmetric division]. We will first summarize the current knowledge on how different components of the cell are asymmetrically segregated.

Membrane adaptors- The first stage of asymmetric division in *Drosophila* neuroblasts is polarization of the cell fate determinants Numb (an endocytic adaptor) and Miranda (an adaptor that recruits other proteins to the membrane), as a result of asymmetric phosphorylation by aPKC (Wirtz-Peitz, Nishimura, and Knoblich 2008). If Numb and Miranda are phosphorylated by aPKC, they cannot localize to the membrane and exert their function (Wirtz-Peitz, Nishimura, and Knoblich 2008). During interphase, aPKC is bound to

PAR6 and Numb to L(2)GL, which allows Numb to be at the membrane. When the cell enters mitosis, Aurora A phosphorylates PAR6, resulting in L(2)GL phosphorylation and decoupling from Numb, allowing the adaptor PAR3 to bind simultaneously to both Numb and aPKC. Numb is then phosphorylated by aPKC and excluded from the membrane as a consequence (Smith et al. 2007; Wirtz-Peitz, Nishimura, and Knoblich 2008). Since aPKC is asymmetrically positioned in a constitutive fashion, this automatically results in asymmetric membrane distribution of Numb. This mechanism seems to be conserved in mammalians.

Vesicular compartments- Both endocytic adaptors (like Numb) and vesicles have been described to segregate asymmetrically both in *Drosophila* and mammalians (Zhong et al. 1996; Le Borgne and Schweisguth 2003). Most transmembrane receptors are subject to constant internalization, degradation and recycling, and the balance between these defines signaling levels at each moment. It is also known that receptors inside the endosomes do not only undergo degradation, but are also able to signal, sometimes even at a stronger level than on the membrane (Miaczynska and Bar-Sagi, 2010). This indicates that asymmetric segregation of vesicular compartments is a means to enhance signaling by certain receptors in one of the daughter cells at the expense of the other. Interestingly, such asymmetric segregation of vesicles or proteins involved in endocytosis has been shown to exist in the hematopoietic system (Aguado et al. 2010; Giebel and Beckmann 2007).

Microtubules- During telophase, microtubules play a role in spindle orientation and maintenance of Numb and Miranda asymmetric segregation, although the mechanism is not completely understood (Knoblich 2010).

Centrioles- It has been shown that centrioles are asymmetrically segregated in neuroblasts (the old centriole normally remains with the cell retaining progenitor potential) and this may play a role in cell fate determination (Yamashita et al. 2007).

DNA- There is evidence in some model systems of asymmetric DNA segregation, where the "template" DNA strand is retained by the less differentiated cell. This seems to be true for intestinal epithelium (Potten et al. 1978), muscle (Shinin et al. 2006), and neural stem cells (Karpowicz et al. 2005) but not for hair follicle (Sotiropoulou, Candi, and Blanpain 2008) or hematopoietic (Kiel et al. 2007) stem cells. However, it is not clear whether these disparities arise from looking at cells with different specifics in terms of lag between divisions.

Ribosomal components- In *Drosophila*, the cell that retains stem cell properties has been shown to present both increased size and enhanced protein synthesis. This seems to be related to asymmetric segregation of ribosomes (Neumuller et al. 2008) and other factors involved in protein synthesis (Fichelson et al. 2009). This has not yet been demonstrated in mammalians, but nevertheless is very intriguing and may be the mechanism by which the capacity to keep proliferating is asymmetrically inherited by just one of the precursors during development.

At this point, the data indicate that the main mechanism of asymmetric division consists on asymmetric inheritance of diverse proteins and subcellular structures, which in its turn helps to enhance the difference between the two daughter cells, so that one can retain stem cell capabilities while the other terminally differentiates. In this way, asymmetric segregation of endocytic adaptors, vesicles and microtubules may contribute to differential signaling in the two daughter cells, while differential inheritance of centrioles, DNA and ribosomes may help preserve stem cell capabilities in just one of the cells.

Two other important aspects that influence asymmetric division are polarization and spindle orientation during cell division. Polarization has been most extensively studied in *C. elegans*, where a complex formed by the proteins Par-3, Par-6 and aPKC are already polarized during interphase (Suzuki and Ohno 2006). This mechanism is conserved in *Drosophila* and is involved in all processes that depend on cell polarity. The mentioned complex is located in the apical part of the cell and, in mammalian cells, is combined with Cadherin and mediates adhesion. Thus, when the spindle forms during cell division, its orientation is crucial to determine symmetry or asymmetry. If the spindle is positioned perpendicular to the Par complex, the cell divides asymmetrically, and the daughter cell that inherits the complex remains a stem cell (probably through adhesion to the stem cell niche), while the other daughter cell abandons the cell niche and differentiates. On the contrary, if the spindle axis parts the Par complex, both daughter cells inherit it and the division is symmetric (Knoblich 2010; Fig. 1).

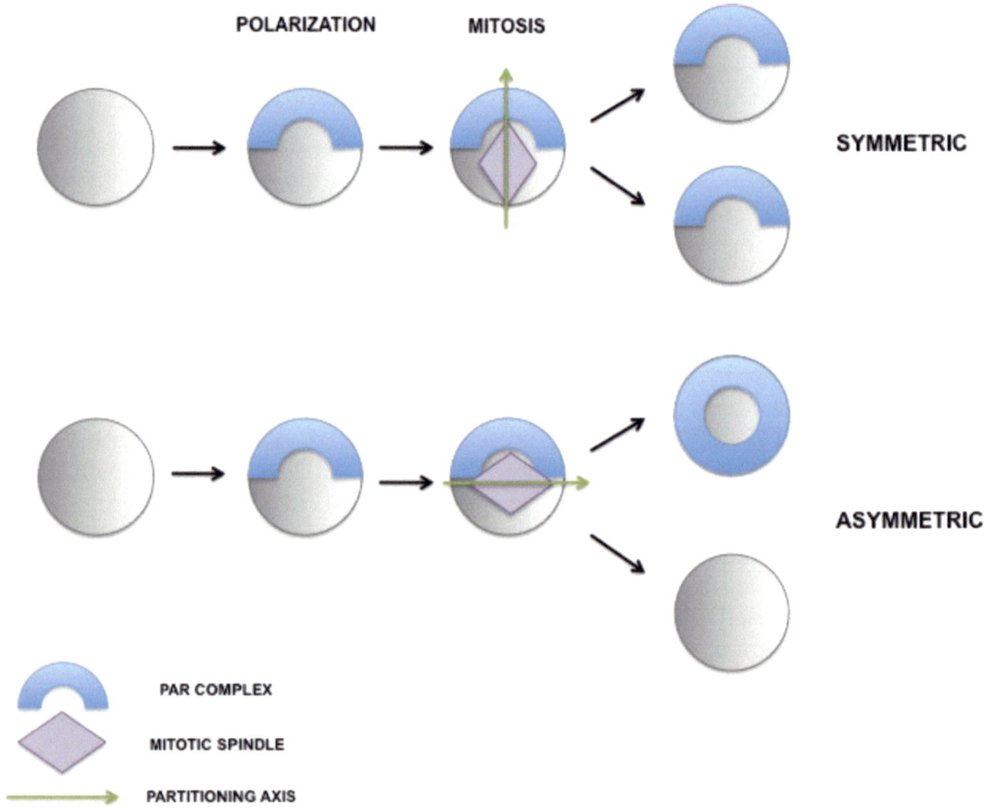

Fig. 1. Polarization and spindle orientation during symmetric or asymmetric division in *C. elelgans*.

Undoubtedly, in the future all these facts will be unified in a single model explaining how and when things happen during asymmetric division, independently of individual differences among the various model systems used to obtain the data.

4. Asymmetric division during normal hematopoiesis

Hematopoiesis is the process by which about $7x10^9$ blood cells are replaced everyday and per kg to maintain the Hematopoietic Stem Cell (HSC) pool in an organism. On the other hand, a HSC can be defined as a clonogenic cell that has the capacity to self-renew and differentiate into the progenitors of mature blood cells through a symmetric or an asymmetric division, respectively.

The hematopoietic system in mammalians shows a hierarchical structure. There is a wide range of distinct mature cells, such as erythrocytes, megacaryocytes, myeloid cells, mast cells, NK cells, monocytes, B and T cells, and others (Figure 2). All these different cells share a common progenitor cell, the Hematopoietic Stem Cell (HSC). HSCs can divide trough a symmetric process to self-renew or through an asymmetric division process to generate daughter cells with different fates: one daughter cell with the same fate as the progenitor cell, and the second one with Multipotent Progenitor cell fate (MPP). Later, MPPs go downstream through the hierarchy and can divide into three different Oligopotent Progeitors (OPPs). These three different OPPs are Common Lymphoid Progenitors (CLPs), megakaryocyte/erythrocyte progenitors (MEPs) and Common Myeloid Progenitors (CMPs). The last type of OPPs can generate other OPPs such as granulocyte/macrophage progenitors (GMPs) or MEPs. Then, these OPPs derive in a wide range of Lineage Restricted Progenitors, such as pro-B lymphoid cells, pro-T lymphoid cells, pro-NK cells, etc., to finally generate Mature Effector Cells (platelets, dendritic cells, macrophages, erytorocytes, NK, B & T cells, etc). It must be emphasized that multipotency is lost during this process, therefore, the potency to generate two daughter cells with different fates is reduced from HSCs to mature effector cells (Seita and Weissman 2010).

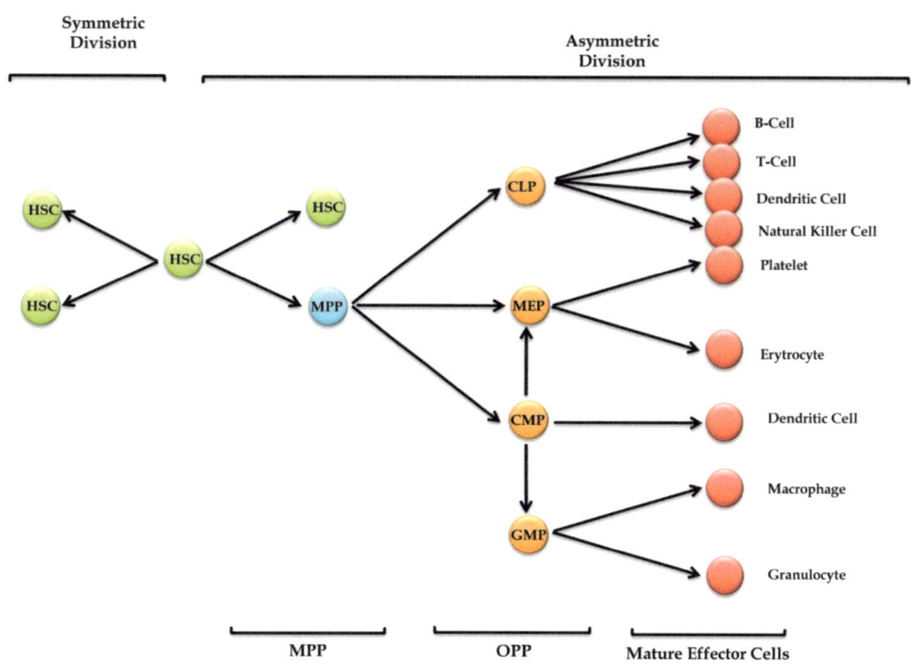

Fig. 2. Schematic representation of precursor decisions during hematopoiesis.

In symmetric divisions, identical copies of the progenitor cell are generated, maintaining the pool of HSCs. On the other hand, asymmetric divisions contribute to generate diversity. Although it is accepted that the capacity to generate cells with different fates is an intrinsic property of HSCs, and studies with fluorescent proteins have shown that several determinant factors can be asymmetrically distributed during mitosis (Congdon and Reya 2008), the environment has an important role in asymmetric division, as well. Thus, several studies have indicated that the stroma plays an important role in differentiation of HSCs into all blood cell types (Purton and Scadden 2008). In this study, different cell lineages with various fates were obtained culturing the HSCs in the presence of different stromas. Other studies indicate that osteoblasts and endothelial cells act as stem cell niches and may play an important role in progenitor diversity generation. Some experiments show that when HSCs are cultured in the presence of osteoblasts asymmetric division is induced, and symmetric division is more frequent when HSCs are cultured on stromal cells. In addition, experiments where HSCs were cultured in presence or not of Lnk, trombopoeitin (TPO) and several interleukins such as IL-3, IL-6 and IL-11 showed effects in self-renewal and differentiation processes. For instance, Lnk is considered a negative regulator of self-renewal while TPO is a negative regulator of differentiation. In addition, there are other cell types with a potential role as regulators of the HSC niche. One of them is the sympathetic nervous system (Katayama et al. 2006). Therefore, it seems that asymmetric division is an important process for hematopoiesis, although the molecular details remain to be elucidated.

5. Role of cell fate determinants in hematopoietic malignant proliferation

The plasma membrane receptor Notch in directly implicated in the proliferative/ differentiative balance of stem cells. Thus, deregulation in Notch signaling is related with several diseases, such as cancer. An increase in Notch signaling results in the development of adenocarcinomas in lung and mammary gland (Allen et al. 2010; Farnie and Clarke 2007). Notch1 can be found in many hematopoietic tissues, such as peripheral T and B cells, neutrophils and bone marrow precursors (Stier et al. 2002), and activation of Notch1 increases self-renewal of HSCs while inhibiting the generation of mature cells. This supports previous *in vitro* studies where Notch activation produced immortalized clones of multipotent cells (Stier et al. 2002; Varnum-Finney et al. 2000), however Notch1 did not completely block the generation of mature cells.

The first proof of the relationship between Notch signaling and cancer was found in acute T lymphoblastic leukemia (T-ALL), and afterwards Notch signaling was shown to be involved in generation of solid tumors, including melanoma, colorectal cancer, breast cancer, non-small cell lung carcinoma and others (Ranganathan, P., et al. 2011). Currently, Notch signaling is receiving increased attention in the development of new therapies against cancer. Some studies have shown that its ligands (specifically Dll4, involved in angiogenesis and T cell fate specification) are overexpressed in different kinds of cancer (Stylianou S, et al. 2006). As a result, several ways of inhibiting Notch signaling are being tested at different levels:

Synthetic inhibitors. The Notch pathway is inhibited by small compounds, which arrest the proteolysis of Notch receptors by the γ-secretases-presenilin complex or interfere with the activity of the Notch intracellular domain. The most common γ-secretases (GSIs) are DAPT and DBZ (dibenzazepine). In addition, specific inhibitors for Dll4-Notch signaling have been developed as well. Although different versions of these inhibitors can be found, all of them present the same disadvantage. Initially, these drugs were developed to arrest proteolysis of the amyloid precursor protein (APP) in Alzehimer's disease and therefore, they are not specific and normally interfere with a wide range of different pathways. On the other hand, dnMAML1, a dominant negative of Mastermind-like 1 (MAML1) represents a more selective option. dnMAML1 blocks the transduction of the four known Notch receptors (Notch 1-4). Although dnMAML1 is a potent inhibitor, it shows low levels of cell permeability; for this reason, similar compounds with a better cell permeability have been developed. All these inhibitors down-regulate Notch signaling and have shown good results in treating T-ALL.

Endogenous inhibitors. Endogenous inhibitors, such as Fwb (an E3 ligase), Cbl, Numb and Numblike can be used to regulate Notch signaling by targeting Notch receptors, however, an important disadvantage is their poor specifity. On the other hand, soluble inhibitors such as the extracellular domains of Jagged1, DLk1 and EGFL7 can offer a more specific alternative. However, it must be considered that the mechanism of these inhibitors is not well known and their role in Notch signaling must be studied in detail.

Antibodies. Antibodies against Notch receptors can be used to regulate Notch signaling. Some antibodies have been already developed against Notch1 and Notch3 receptors (Asano N., et al. 2008, Elyaman W., et al 2007, Jurynczyk M., et al 2008, Maekawa Y., et al 2003, Schaller MA., et al. 2007 and Li K., et al. 2008). Antibodies can block specific Notch receptors with a high selectivity, leaving other Notch receptors activated. For example, an anti-Dll4 antibody has been developed against Dll4-Notch signaling and it is showing promising perspectives in anti-angiogenic cancer therapy because of its low toxicity (Ridgway J, et al. 2006). A similar strategy uses molecules called decoys. Decoys are soluble extracellular domains of Notch receptors or ligands. They compete with Notch receptors, inhibiting Notch signaling by binding to endogenous molecules. These associations do not trigger Notch signaling because of lacking the transmembrane region. Notch signaling in endothelial cells has been inhibited using a decoy of Notch1, successfully reducing tumor growth. Other decoys of Dll1, Dll4 and Jagged1 have been successfully developed (Funahashi Y., et al. 2008, Varnum-Finney B., et al. 2000 and Small D., et al. 2001). However, decoys show an important disadvantage. It has been observed that they can be switched from inhibitors into activators easily. The association of decoys with extracellular matrix can produce an activator and trigger Notch proteolysis and activation. The process by which a decoy can be transformed into an activator is not yet fully understood, and this feature makes decoys unpredictable and not valid as therapeutics (Hicks C., et al. 2002).

Notch is regulated by Numb, and loss of this regulation has been described in more than 50% of human mammary carcinomas. When Numb is lost, Notch signaling is increased, and the balance between self-renewal and differentiation is affected, which results in uncontrolled proliferation. Loss of Numb may be due to ubiquitylation and subsequent proteosomal degradation.

Recent studies carried out by Colaluca et al. (Colaluca et al. 2008) showed that Numb plays an important role in the regulation of the protein p53, also called TP53, an important tumor suppressor involved in 50% of breast cancers and in 70% of colon cancers. Numb binds to p53 and the E3 ubiquitin ligase HDM2 (or MDMD2 ligase) to form a triple complex, inhibiting p53 ubiquitylation and, therefore, its degradation. As a consequence, p53 levels are higher and the apparition of breast cancer is diminished. When there is loss of Numb, p53 degradation is higher, allowing higher expression of Notch, which results in chemoresistance to the drugs used to combat the disease and in uncontrolled cellular proliferation. Besides, p53 regulates the expression of genes implicated in cell-cycle arrest and apoptosis upon cellular stress. Additionally, it acts as transcriptional factor. Therefore, it seems clear that there is a relationship between Numb deregulation and uncontrolled cellular proliferation via the tumor suppressor p53. However, the mechanism by which Numb regulates p53 remains still unclear (Carter and Vousden 2008).

In some cases, such as in breast cancers, deficiency in Numb expression is due to an increase in ubiquitylation resulting in higher proteasomal degradation. This may be related to increased levels or activity of E3-ligases such as LNK, Siah-1 and MDM2. Another explanation for Numb loss may be ubiquitylation after over-phosphorylation. Restoration of Numb normal levels could be achieved pharmacologically using substances with antiproteasomal activity such as PS-341 or enzymatic inhibitors of Numb degradation (Pece et al. 2004). These investigations have a clear practical application: hopefully, in the future some of the resulting knowledge will be applied to the clinic.

6. Asymmetric division in the immune system

During immune system development and function, progenitor cells undergo a series of proliferation and differentiation processes in order to generate the different mature cell populations that protect the body from foreign pathogens. T cells develop in the thymus from bone marrow precursors through a series of intermediate stages. Double negative cells (DN) undergo some division rounds before differentiating into double positive cells (DP), afterwards T cell progenitors do not divide again in the thymus: only after exiting the thymus and populating the periphery will mature T cells be able to proliferate again. During the immune response, naive T lymphocytes (T lymphocytes recently created that have not encountered antigen) are activated by antigen-presenting cells. Naive T cell activation, through the T cell receptor (TCR), leads to proliferation and differentiation, triggering a massive expansion of differentiated effector cells, as well as a small number of memory cells (these will remain undifferentiated until subsequent antigen encounters). Thus, after T cell activation, a single naïve T cell is able to generate many different T cell types in order to orchestrate an effective immune response (Stemberger et al. 2007). How can a single cell generate all the T lymphocyte types that are required for immunity? This question has fascinated immunologists over the past years. Several models have been suggested to explain the generation of subset diversity during the immune response. Some studies suggest a progressive differentiation model (Sallusto, Geginat, and Lanzavecchia 2004), while others suggest an early bifurcation between effector and memory phenotypes, more consistent with asymmetric division, but the question remains controversial. Despite asymmetric division being the most widespread process that regulates the generation of a variety of cell types, this process has only started to be studied in the immune system in the last few years, and it still remains controversial.

Nothing suggests, *a priori*, that the widespread principle of asymmetric division should not be applied to the thymus, where DN cell proliferation does regulate the total number of cells in the whole organ, and during this process, precursor cells resulting from such divisions must decide between differentiation and proliferation. In this respect, three different aspects should have been studied before making statements about the role of asymmetrically segregated cell fate determinants in thymocytes. First, demonstration of the existence of asymmetric division itself (including an assessment of the effect of manipulating asymmetric division); second, identification of cell fate determinants that are asymmetrically segregated and their signaling pathways; finally, elucidation of the mechanisms that lead to asymmetric localization of these determinants, including external cues that regulate cell polarization, as well as intracellular processes that mediate asymmetric segregation of proteins and organelles (as has been described before for studies of both *Drosophila* and mammalian neural system).

However, the first studies related to asymmetric division in the thymus used either transgenic or knockout mice to over-express or delete Numb (French et al. 2002; Anderson et al. 2005; Wilson et al. 2007). In these studies, investigators used classical assessments of thymocyte differentiation in order to determine whether or not Numb played a role in thymocyte differentiation (they never examined asymmetric division). The conclusion drawn by the three studies was that Numb plays no role in thymus differentiation. However, there are three important considerations that were not taken into account. First, both Numb and its homologue Numblike are expressed in mammalians (the thymus included), and if their levels are reduced so that just 1% of endogenous levels of either Numb or Numblike remain in the cells, this is still enough to maintain normal asymmetric division (Petersen et al. 2002; Petersen et al. 2006). Second, four different isoforms of Numb are expressed in mammalians (Dho et al. 1999). Third, knockout studies in the immune system must be taken with caution, since there is accumulating evidence that the absence of phenotype does not necessarily mean that the protein does not have a function (Saveliev and Tybulewicz 2009). If Numb acts as a cell fate determinant during asymmetric division in the thymus, one would expect an effect in precursor proliferation rate and the total number of thymocytes, however none of these were examined in these first studies. Nevertheless, the existence of three studies claiming no role for Numb in the thymus predisposed the whole field against the notion of asymmetric division.

Fortunately, over the past few years, the first studies on asymmetric division in the thymus and peripheral T lymphocytes performed following a more logical order (i.e., examining in the first place asymmetric segregation of determinants) have provided exciting data about asymmetric division in the immune system (Aguado et al. 2010; Chang et al. 2007). In the first study, our group showed by confocal microscopy that Numb is segregated asymmetrically during thymocyte division. By inhibiting Numb (using a dominant negative), or overexpressing it, we showed that functional Numb levels determine DN thymocyte proliferation rate and, ultimately, thymus size. Furthermore, we showed that Numb can regulate pre-TCR localization and signaling, acting as an endocytic protein. As a result, a model was proposed where thymocytes divide by asymmetric division to generate one daughter cell that inherits Numb and keeps precursor properties and a second that does not inherit Numb and receives pre-TCR signaling as a consequence, which results in differentiation (Fig. 3). The second study showed that peripheral $CD8^+$ T cells do indeed undergo asymmetric division, and this process regulates the choice between effector and memory differentiation (Chang et al. 2007). The authors showed that after the first naïve $CD8^+$ T cell division, the proximal and distal daughter cells have different phenotypes. Thus, proximal daughter cells expressed low CD62L levels and higher CD69, CD43 and CD25 levels. Furthermore, when these cells were transferred into naïve secondary recipients, they provided protection against acute infection, but poor long-term protection, a profile consistent with the effector lineage. However, distal daughters expressed high levels of CD62L and lower levels of CD69, CD43, CD25 and CD44 and these cells provided a good long-term protection *in vivo*, a profile more consistent with the central memory cells. This is clear evidence that asymmetric division occurs, at least during the first division.

As we have explained before, for asymmetric division to occur, the progenitor cell needs to receive an external cue to dictate the axis of polarity, recruit cell fate determinants and align the mitotic spindle with a correct position that ensures asymmetric segregation of the determinants. During mature T cell division, the axis of polarity and mitotic spindle alignment are established by the formation of the immunological synapse. The immunological synapse has been extensively studied as a site of clustered signaling molecules, and can be considered as a marker of the polarized T cell and a mechanism for asymmetric division regulation. Recent studies showed that asymmetric cell division is not observed either during non antigen-dependent activation or the second and subsequent cell divisions following antigen stimulation, and that the polarity cue for asymmetric cell division requires the contact with antigen-presenting cells (Chang et al. 2007; Oliaro et al. 2010; Fig. 3). One problem with this model is that if it is just the first division that is

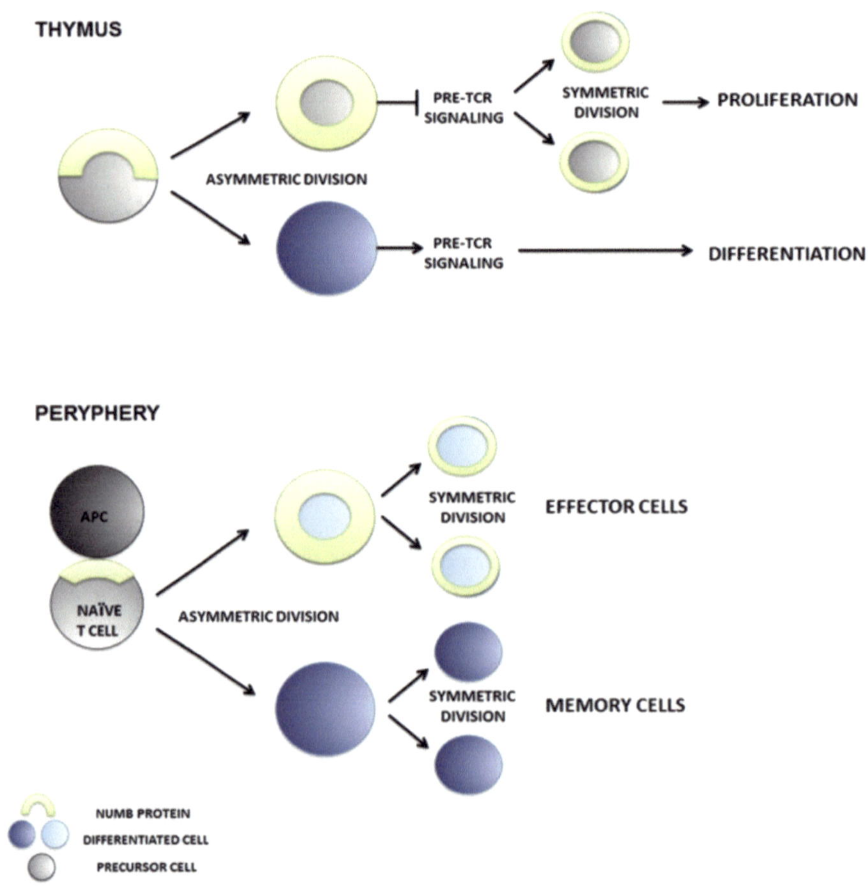

Fig. 3. Schematic representation of the current models for asymmetric division in thymus and periphery.

asymmetric during the immune response, and all the subsequent divisions are symmetric, it is not clear how the final numbers of memory and effector cells are achieved. In any case, these data on thymus and peripheral T cells demonstrate that the immunological system is not a remarkable exception to the principle of asymmetric division as the universal mechanism to ensure a correct balance between expansion and differentiation during development. The mechanistic details on how asymmetric division is orchestrated in the immune system in order to achieve correct numbers of mature cells will surely be elucidated soon.

7. Future directions of the field

Asymmetric division has transitioned from being an intriguing but unexplained anomaly of neural development into a fertile field where scientists working on different developmental biology areas converge to exchange methods and ideas. The recently discovered link to cancer stresses out the importance of these studies in the immuno-hematopoietic system.

An important current challenge for the field of asymmetric division is unification of knowledge. A general model for the functioning of asymmetric division that applies to all organisms and tissues needs to be postulated, even if it is very schematic at the beginning. Next, unification of methods should be achieved: the same phenomenon in different organisms should not be studied using different techniques simply because researchers of different areas feel more comfortable with a certain approach. To avoid this, more joint scientific meetings on asymmetric division must be organized, so that researchers can exchange views and knowledge, besides funding should be available for those willing to assume the risk of applying new techniques to old model systems. If the field does not evolve in this way, it risks loosing its current novelty and drive. Hopefully, new exciting discoveries will keep the area alive, and the many open questions about how organisms and tissues orchestrate growth and differentiation will be answered soon.

8. References

Aguado, R., N. Martin-Blanco, M. Caraballo, and M. Canelles. 2010. The endocytic adaptor Numb regulates thymus size by modulating pre-TCR signaling during asymmetric division. *Blood* 116 (10):1705-14.

Allen, T. D., E. M. Rodriguez, K. D. Jones, and J. M. Bishop. 2010. Activated notch1 induces lung adenomas in mice and cooperates with myc in the generation of lung adenocarcinoma. *Cancer Res* 71 (18):6010-8.

Anderson, A. C., E. A. Kitchens, S. W. Chan, C. St Hill, Y. N. Jan, W. Zhong, and E. A. Robey. 2005. The Notch regulator Numb links the Notch and TCR signaling pathways. *J Immunol* 174 (2):890-7.

Asano N., Watanabe T., Kitani A., et al. 2008. Notch1 signaling and regulatory T cell function. J Immunol 180: 2796–804.

Betschinger, J., and J. A. Knoblich. 2004. Dare to be different: asymmetric cell division in *Drosophila, C. elegans* and vertebrates. *Curr Biol* 14 (16):R674-85.

Carter, S., and K. H. Vousden. 2008. A role for Numb in p53 stabilization. *Genome Biol* 9 (5):221.

Caussinus, E., and C. Gonzalez. 2005. Induction of tumor growth by altered stem-cell asymmetric division in *Drosophila melanogaster*. *Nat Genet* 37 (10):1125-9.

Chang, J. T., V. R. Palanivel, I. Kinjyo, F. Schambach, A. M. Intlekofer, A. Banerjee, S. A. Longworth, K. E. Vinup, P. Mrass, J. Oliaro, N. Killeen, J. S. Orange, S. M. Russell, W. Weninger, and S. L. Reiner. 2007. Asymmetric T lymphocyte division in the initiation of adaptive immune responses. *Science* 315 (5819):1687-91.

Colaluca, I. N., D. Tosoni, P. Nuciforo, F. Senic-Matuglia, V. Galimberti, G. Viale, S. Pece, and P. P. Di Fiore. 2008. NUMB controls p53 tumour suppressor activity. *Nature* 451 (7174):76-80.

Congdon, K. L., and T. Reya. 2008. Divide and conquer: how asymmetric division shapes cell fate in the hematopoietic system. *Curr Opin Immunol* 20 (3):302-7.

Dho, S. E., M. B. French, S. A. Woods, and C. J. McGlade. 1999. Characterization of four mammalian numb protein isoforms. Identification of cytoplasmic and membrane-associated variants of the phosphotyrosine binding domain. *J Biol Chem* 274 (46):33097-104.

Elyaman W., Bradshaw E. M., Wang Y., et al. 2007. JAGGED1 and delta1 differentially regulate the outcome of experimental autoimmune encephalomyelitis. J Immunol 179: 5990–98.

Farnie, G., and R. B. Clarke. 2007. Mammary stem cells and breast cancer--role of Notch signalling. *Stem Cell Rev* 3 (2):169-75.

Fichelson, P., C. Moch, K. Ivanovitch, C. Martin, C. M. Sidor, J. A. Lepesant, Y. Bellaiche, and J. R. Huynh. 2009. Live-imaging of single stem cells within their niche reveals that a U3snoRNP component segregates asymmetrically and is required for self-renewal in *Drosophila*. *Nat Cell Biol* 11 (6):685-93.

French, M. B., U. Koch, R. E. Shaye, M. A. McGill, S. E. Dho, C. J. Guidos, and C. J. McGlade. 2002. Transgenic expression of numb inhibits notch signaling in immature thymocytes but does not alter T cell fate specification. *J Immunol* 168 (7):3173-80.

Funahashi Y., Hernandez S. L., Das I., et al. 2008. A notch1 ectodomain construct inhibits endothelial notch signaling, tumor growth, and angiogenesis. Cancer Res 68: 4727–35.

Giebel, B., and J. Beckmann. 2007. Asymmetric cell divisions of human hematopoietic stem and progenitor cells meet endosomes. *Cell Cycle* 6 (18):2201-4.

Hicks C., Ladi E., Lindsell C., et al. 2002. A secreted Delta1-Fc fusion protein functions both as an activator and inhibitor of Notch1 signaling. J Neurosci Res 68: 655–67.

Horvitz, H. R., and I. Herskowitz. 1992. Mechanisms of asymmetric cell division: two Bs or not two Bs, that is the question. *Cell* 68 (2):237-55.

Jurynczyk M., Jurewicz A., Raine C. S., et al. 2008. Notch3 inhibition in myelin-reactive T cells down-regulates protein kinase C theta and attenuates experimental autoimmune encephalomyelitis. J Immunol 180: 2634– 40.

Karpowicz, P., C. Morshead, A. Kam, E. Jervis, J. Ramunas, V. Cheng, and D. van der Kooy. 2005. Support for the immortal strand hypothesis: neural stem cells partition DNA asymmetrically in vitro. *J Cell Biol* 170 (5):721-32.

Katayama, Y., M. Battista, W. M. Kao, A. Hidalgo, A. J. Peired, S. A. Thomas, and P. S. Frenette. 2006. Signals from the sympathetic nervous system regulate hematopoietic stem cell egress from bone marrow. *Cell* 124 (2):407-21.

Kiel, M. J., S. He, R. Ashkenazi, S. N. Gentry, M. Teta, J. A. Kushner, T. L. Jackson, and S. J. Morrison. 2007. Haematopoietic stem cells do not asymmetrically segregate chromosomes or retain BrdU. *Nature* 449 (7159):238-42.

Knoblich, J. A. 2010. Asymmetric cell division: recent developments and their implications for tumour biology. *Nat Rev Mol Cell Biol* 11 (12):849-60.

Le Borgne, R., and F. Schweisguth. 2003. Unequal segregation of Neuralized biases Notch activation during asymmetric cell division. *Dev Cell* 5 (1):139-48.

Li K., Li Y., Wu W., et al. 2008. Modulation of Notch signaling by antibodies specific for the extracellular negative regulatory region of NOTCH3. J Biol Chem 283: 8046–54.

Maekawa Y., Tsukumo S., Chiba S., et al. 2003. Delta1-Notch3 inter- actions bias the functional differentiation of activated CD4þ T cells. Immunity 19: 549–59.

Miaczynska, M., and D. Bar-Sagi. 2010. Signaling endosomes: seeing is believing. *Curr Opin Cell Biol* 22 (4):535-40.

Neumuller, R. A., and J. A. Knoblich. 2009. Dividing cellular asymmetry: asymmetric cell division and its implications for stem cells and cancer. *Genes Dev* 23 (23):2675-99.

Neumuller, R. A., J. Betschinger, A. Fischer, N. Bushati, I. Poernbacher, K. Mechtler, S. M. Cohen, and J. A. Knoblich. 2008. Mei-P26 regulates microRNAs and cell growth in the *Drosophila* ovarian stem cell lineage. *Nature* 454 (7201):241-5.

Oliaro, J., V. Van Ham, F. Sacirbegovic, A. Pasam, Z. Bomzon, K. Pham, M. J. Ludford-Menting, N. J. Waterhouse, M. Bots, E. D. Hawkins, S. V. Watt, L. A. Cluse, C. J. Clarke, D. J. Izon, J. T. Chang, N. Thompson, M. Gu, R. W. Johnstone, M. J. Smyth, P. O. Humbert, S. L. Reiner, and S. M. Russell. 2010. Asymmetric cell division of T cells upon antigen presentation uses multiple conserved mechanisms. *J Immunol* 185 (1):367-75.

Pece, S., M. Serresi, E. Santolini, M. Capra, E. Hulleman, V. Galimberti, S. Zurrida, P. Maisonneuve, G. Viale, and P. P. Di Fiore. 2004. Loss of negative regulation by Numb over Notch is relevant to human breast carcinogenesis. *J Cell Biol* 167 (2):215-21.

Petersen, P. H., H. Tang, K. Zou, and W. Zhong. 2006. The enigma of the numb-Notch relationship during mammalian embryogenesis. *Dev Neurosci* 28 (1-2):156-68.

Petersen, P. H., K. Zou, J. K. Hwang, Y. N. Jan, and W. Zhong. 2002. Progenitor cell maintenance requires numb and numblike during mouse neurogenesis. *Nature* 419 (6910):929-34.

Potten, C. S., W. J. Hume, P. Reid, and J. Cairns. 1978. The segregation of DNA in epithelial stem cells. *Cell* 15 (3):899-906.

Purton, L. E., and D. T. Scadden. 2008. The hematopoietic stem cell niche.

Rhyu, M. S., L. Y. Jan, and Y. N. Jan. 1994. Asymmetric distribution of numb protein during division of the sensory organ precursor cell confers distinct fates to daughter cells. *Cell* 76 (3):477-91.

Sallusto, F., J. Geginat, and A. Lanzavecchia. 2004. Central memory and effector memory T cell subsets: function, generation, and maintenance. *Annu Rev Immunol* 22:745-63.

Saveliev, A., and V. L. Tybulewicz. 2009. Lymphocyte signaling: beyond knockouts. *Nat Immunol* 10 (4):361-4.

Schaller M. A., Neupane R., Rudd B. D., et al. 2007. Notch ligand Delta-like 4 regulates disease pathogenesis during respiratory viral infections by modulating Th2 cytokines. J Exp Med 204: 2925–34.

Schroeder, T. 2007. Asymmetric Cell Division in Normal and Malignant Hematopoietic Precursor Cells. *Cell Stem Cell* 1 (5):479-481.

Seita, J., and I. L. Weissman. 2010. Hematopoietic stem cell: self-renewal versus differentiation. *Wiley Interdiscip Rev Syst Biol Med* 2 (6):640-53.

Shinin, V., B. Gayraud-Morel, D. Gomes, and S. Tajbakhsh. 2006. Asymmetric division and cosegregation of template DNA strands in adult muscle satellite cells. *Nat Cell Biol* 8 (7):677-87.

Small D., Kovalenko D., Kacer D., et al. 2001. Soluble Jagged 1 represses the function of its transmembrane form to induce the formation of the Src- dependent chord-like phenotype. J Biol Chem 276: 32022–30.

Smith, C. A., K. M. Lau, Z. Rahmani, S. E. Dho, G. Brothers, Y. M. She, D. M. Berry, E. Bonneil, P. Thibault, F. Schweisguth, R. Le Borgne, and C. J. McGlade. 2007. aPKC-mediated phosphorylation regulates asymmetric membrane localization of the cell fate determinant Numb. *EMBO J* 26 (2):468-80.

Sotiropoulou, P. A., A. Candi, and C. Blanpain. 2008. The majority of multipotent epidermal stem cells do not protect their genome by asymmetrical chromosome segregation. *Stem Cells* 26 (11):2964-73.

Stemberger, C., K. M. Huster, M. Koffler, F. Anderl, M. Schiemann, H. Wagner, and D. H. Busch. 2007. A single naive CD8+ T cell precursor can develop into diverse effector and memory subsets. *Immunity* 27 (6):985-97.

Stier, S., T. Cheng, D. Dombkowski, N. Carlesso, and D. T. Scadden. 2002. Notch1 activation increases hematopoietic stem cell self-renewal in vivo and favors lymphoid over myeloid lineage outcome. *Blood* 99 (7):2369-78.

Suzuki A. and Ohno S. 2006. The PAR-aPKC systme: lessons in polarity. *J.Cell Sci.* 119: 979-987.

Varnum-Finney, B., L. Xu, C. Brashem-Stein, C. Nourigat, D. Flowers, S. Bakkour, W. S. Pear, and I. D. Bernstein. 2000. Pluripotent, cytokine-dependent, hematopoietic stem cells are immortalized by constitutive Notch1 signaling. *Nat Med* 6 (11):1278-81.

Whitman, C.. 1878. The embryology of *Clepsine*. *Q.J. Microsc. Sci.* 18: 215.

Wilson, A., D. L. Ardiet, C. Saner, N. Vilain, F. Beermann, M. Aguet, H. R. Macdonald, and O. Zilian. 2007. Normal hemopoiesis and lymphopoiesis in the combined absence of numb and numblike. *J Immunol* 178 (11):6746-51.

Wirtz-Peitz, F., T. Nishimura, and J. A. Knoblich. 2008. Linking cell cycle to asymmetric division: Aurora-A phosphorylates the Par complex to regulate Numb localization. *Cell* 135 (1):161-73.

Wu, M., H. Y. Kwon, F. Rattis, J. Blum, C. Zhao, R. Ashkenazi, T. L. Jackson, N. Gaiano, T. Oliver, and T. Reya. 2007. Imaging hematopoietic precursor division in real time. *Cell Stem Cell* 1 (5):541-54.

Yamashita, Y. M., A. P. Mahowald, J. R. Perlin, and M. T. Fuller. 2007. Asymmetric inheritance of mother versus daughter centrosome in stem cell division. *Science* 315 (5811):518-21.

Zhong, W., J. N. Feder, M. M. Jiang, L. Y. Jan, and Y. N. Jan. 1996. Asymmetric localization of a mammalian numb homolog during mouse cortical neurogenesis. *Neuron* 17 (1):43-53.

5

Nitric Oxide / Cyclic Nucleotide Regulation of Globin Genes in Erythropoiesis

Vladan P. Čokić[1], Bojana B. Beleslin-Čokić[2], Gordana Jovčić[1], Raj K. Puri[3] and Alan N. Schechter[4]

[1]Laboratory of Experimental Hematology, Institute for Medical Research, Belgrade,
[2]Clinic of Endocrinology, Diabetes and Diseases of Metabolism, School of Medicine, University Clinical Center, Belgrade,
[3]Division of Cellular and Gene Therapies, Center for Biologics Evaluation and Research, Food and Drug Administration, Bethesda,
[4]Molecular Medicine Branch, National Institute of Diabetes and Digestive and Kidney Diseases, National Institutes of Health, Bethesda,
[1,2]Serbia
[3,4]USA

1. Introduction

1.1. Hemoglobin synthesis

The human hematopoiesis initiates in the second to third embryonic weeks with formation of mesoderm-derived blood islands in the extraembryonic mesoderm of the developing secondary yolk sac (Migliaccio et al., 1986). Erythropoiesis involves proliferation and differentiation of committed erythroid progenitors to mature red blood cells (erythrocytes). Although globins represents <0.1% of proteins at the proerythroblast level, it reaches 95% of all proteins at the level of reticulocytes (Nienhuis & Benz, 1977). Physiologically, the expression of the globin genes is generally regulated in such a way that at any point in development the output of the beta (β)-globin-like chains equals the alpha (α)-globin chains (Lodish & Jacobsen, 1972). The α-globin gene cluster contains three genes and several pseudogenes arranged from the telomere toward the centromere in the following order: 5'-ξ2-ψξ1-ψα2-ψα1-α2-α1-θ1-3' (Higgs et al., 1998). The human β-globin locus consists of five functional β-like globin genes, that are arranged in the order of their expression during development (5′-ε-^{G}γ-^{G}γ-δ-β-3′), and an upstream regulatory element, the locus control region (LCR), that is physically composed of five DNase I-hypersensitive sites (HSs) (Grosveld et al., 1987). The most widely studied changes during red cell ontogeny are the shifts or "switches" in globin types. Embryonic erythroblasts are characterized by the synthesis of the unique hemoglobins Gower I ($\zeta_2\varepsilon_2$), Gower II ($\alpha_2\varepsilon_2$), and Hb Portland ($\zeta_2\gamma_2$). The zeta (ζ)- and epsilon (ε)-globin chains are embryonic α-like and β-like chains, respectively. Thus, a switch from ζ- to α- and ε- to gamma (γ)-globin gene production begins during the embryonic phase of erythropoiesis but is not complete until fetal erythropoiesis is well established. During the transition from yolk sac to fetal liver erythropoiesis (5–8 weeks), erythroid precursors within the fetal liver co-express embryonic (ζ- or ε-) and fetal (α- or γ-) globins both in vivo and in vitro (Peschle et al., 1984). The predominant type of hemoglobin synthesized during fetal liver erythropoiesis is fetal hemoglobin (HbF, $\alpha_2\gamma_2$). HbF is formed by γ-globin chain A or G according to the amino acid at the 136 position in the γ chain, i.e., alanine or glycine. The proportion of $^G\gamma$ to $^A\gamma$ is constant throughout fetal development: about 75% of $^G\gamma$ and 25% of $^A\gamma$. However, in adult red cells, the small amount of HbF is composed mainly of $^A\gamma$ (60% *vs.* 40% of $^G\gamma$) (Jensen et al., 1982). α- and β-globin chains combine as a tetramer of two α- and two β-globin polypeptides along with a heme moiety to form the adult hemoglobin molecule (HbA, $\alpha_2\beta_2$). HbA, detectable at the earliest stages of fetal liver erythropoiesis, is also synthesized as a minor component throughout this period, but HbA_2 ($\alpha_2\delta_2$), minor hemoglobin in the adult, is undetectable in these early stages. From about the 30th gestational week onward, β-globin synthesis steadily increases, so that by term 50%–55% of hemoglobin synthesized is HbA. By 4-5 weeks of postnatal age, 75% of the hemoglobin is HbA, this percentage increasing to 95% by 4 months as the fetal-to-adult hemoglobin switch is completed. HbF levels in circulating red cells are in a plateau for the first 2–3 weeks (as a result of the decline in total erythropoiesis that follows birth), but HbF gradually declines and normal levels (<1%) are achieved by 200 days after birth.

1.2 The GATA-1/2 and Krüppel-like factors role in hemoglobin switching

The regulation of globin gene switching is a very complex process requiring the coordination of different signaling pathways and molecular reactions. Many transcription factors controlling globin gene expression have been identified and characterized. These factors form a complex network of protein-protein and protein-DNA interactions with each other, globin gene promoters, LCR HSs, and other *cis*-acting intergenic regions (Stamatoyannopoulos, 2005). The GATA family of proteins (GATA1–6) comprises zinc finger transcription factors that both activate and repress target genes containing a consensus GATA binding motif (Orkin, 1992). Binding sites with this motif are present in many positions in the α- and β-globin loci, as well as many other erythroid-expressed genes. The founding member of this family, GATA1, was discovered as a β-globin locus-binding protein (Pruzina et al., 1991). GATA1 is essential for erythroid cell maturation in vivo (Pevny et al., 1989). In addition, GATA1 homodimerizes and interacts with other transcription factors, such as SP-1 and erythroid Krüppel-like factor (EKLF/KLF1), further contributing to the complex network of GATA factor interactions (Gregori et al., 1996). GATA2 is primarily expressed in primitive erythropoiesis, but later in development GATA1 expression predominates (Leonard et al., 1993). Downregulation of GATA2 is important for progression of erythroid cell differentiation (Persons et al., 1999). The protein Friend of GATA1 (FOG) is co-expressed with GATA1 during embryonic development in erythroid cells (Tsang et al., 1997). GATA1 binds a region upstream of both the HBG1- and HBG2-promoter, necessary for HbF silencing, in a FOG1 dependent manner leading to recruitment of the suppressive NuRD-complex (Harju-Baker et al., 2008). GATA-1, together with FOG-1, functions as an anchor in the formation of chromatin looping, and is required for physical interactions between the β LCR and β globin promoter (Vakoc et al., 2005).

The Krüppel-like factors are a family of C2H2 zinc finger DNA binding proteins that are important in controlling developmental programs. KLF1 gene is an erythroid cell-specific zinc finger transcription factor, containing a DNA-binding domain located at its C-terminus, composed of three 'Krüppel-like' C2H2 zinc finger motifs, and a proline-rich transactivation domain at its N-terminus (Miller & Bieker, 1993). KLF1 preferentially activates the β-globin gene promoter by binding with high affinity to the CACCC element (Bieker & Southwood, 1995). KLF1 is essential for adult β-globin gene transcription and binds to the βLCR and β-globin promoters, required for direct interactions between the βLCR and the β-globin gene in humans (Donze et al., 1995, Scheme 1). Patients with hereditary persistence of HbF, with elevated levels of HbF, have mutations in the gene encoding erythroid transcription factor KLF1 (Borg et al., 2010). Recent findings demonstrate that KLF1, and the co-activator BRG1, are designated by short-chain fatty acid derivatives to activate the fetal globin genes. The SWI/SNF complex chromatin-modifying core ATPase BRG1 is required for γ-globin induction by short-chain fatty acid derivatives, and is actively recruited to the γ-globin promoter in the KLF1-dependent manner (Perrine et al., 2009). KLF1-GATA1 fusion proteins activated δ-, γ-, and β-globin promoters, and significantly up-regulated delta (δ)- and γ-globin RNA transcript and protein expression in human erythroleukemic cells (Zhu et al., 2011). DRED (direct repeat erythroid-definitive) was identified as a repressor of the ε-globin gene, it appears to prevent binding of KLF1 to the ε-globin gene promoter and silences ε-globin expression during definitive erythropoiesis (Tanimoto et al., 2000). KLF2 also regulates the expression of the human embryonic ε-globin gene but not the adult β-globin gene (Basu et al., 2005). Another erythroid-specific transcription factor, called fetal Krüppel-like factor (KLF11), activates γ- and ε-globin genes in human erythroleukemic cells (Asano et al., 1999, Scheme 1). KLF11 also activates γ-globin transcription via the CACCC element in the promoter (Asano et al., 2000). The protein encoded by this gene is a zinc finger transcription factor that binds to SP1-like sequences in ε- and γ-globin gene promoters.

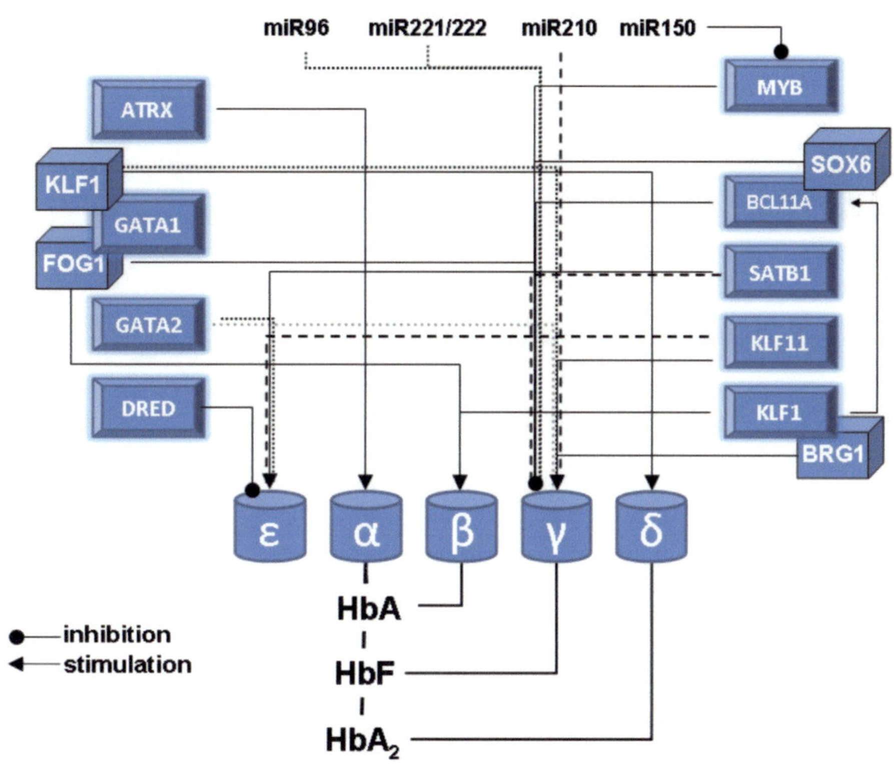

Sheme 1. Overview of globin genes control by examined transcription factors.

1.3 Other factors that participate in hemoglobin switching

A nuclear protein, special AT-rich binding protein 1 (SATB1), regulates genes through targeting chromatin remodeling and its overexpression increases ε-globin and decreases γ-globin gene expression (Wen et al., 2005, Scheme 1). Global changes to chromatin, including acetylation, phosphorylation, and methylation play roles in LCR activation. Histone acetylation occurs during chromatin remodeling and hyperacetylation is associated with transcriptional activation of a locus (Pazin & Kadonaga, 1997). Similar to acetylation, phosphorylation of histone H3 disrupts DNA-nucleosome interaction and increases transcription factor accessibility to DNA. SATB1 overexpression increased ε-globin and decreased γ-globin gene expression accompanied by histone hyperacetylation and hypomethylation in chromatin from the ε-globin promoter and HS2, and histone hypoacetylation and hypermethylation associated with the γ-globin promoter (Wen et al., 2005). Mitogen activated protein kinase (MAPK) pathways, as well as the stress activated p38 pathway, activate histone H3 phosphorylation (Cheung et al., 2000). Studies on p38 knockout mice established a role for the p38 stress pathway in the switch from primitive to definitive erythropoiesis (Tamura et al., 2000). Mutations in the transcription factor alpha thalassemia/mental retardation syndrome X-linked (ATRX), nearly always downregulate α-globin expression, provide potentially important insight into the trans-regulation of globin gene expression (Gibbons et al., 1995). Alpha hemoglobin stabilizing protein (AHSP) is an erythroid-specific protein that forms a stable complex with free alpha-hemoglobin (Kihm et al., 2002). It has been found that AHSP expression was highly dependent on the larger subunit of nuclear factor erythroid-derived 2 (NFE2) (Guo-wei et al., 2010). The transcription factor NFE2 activation of globin production was stimulated by cAMP-dependent protein kinase (PKA) in erythroid cells (Casteel et al., 1998).

BCL11A gene (encoding the transcription factor B-cell lymphoma/leukemia 11A) maintains silencing of γ-globin expression in adult erythroid cells and functions as a direct transcriptional regulator of the fetal to adult hemoglobin switch in humans. BCL11A protein levels vary in erythroid progenitors over the course of human ontogeny. BCL11A is expressed as short variant proteins in primitive erythroid progenitors that largely express γ-globin and as full-length forms at the adult stage with silenced γ-globin genes (Sankaran et al., 2008). In erythroid progenitors, BCL11A physically interacts with the NuRD chromatin remodelling complex, and the erythroid transcription factors, GATA1 and FOG1. In addition, KLF1, as a key activator of BCL11A, controls globin gene switching by directly activating β-globin and indirectly repressing γ-globin gene expression (Zhou et al., 2010). BCL11A binds the upstream LCR, ε-globin, and the intergenic regions between γ-globin and δ-globin genes. BCL11A and SOX6 co-occupy the human β-globin cluster along with GATA1, and cooperate in silencing γ-globin transcription in adult human erythroid progenitors (Xu et al., 2010, Scheme 1). SOX6 has also been suggested to enhance definitive erythropoiesis in mouse by stimulating erythroid cell survival, proliferation and terminal maturation (Dumitriu et al., 2006). A broad genome expression profile studies led to the identification of common genetic polymorphisms in the locus of the β-globin gene, a region between the HBS1-like gene HBS1L and the oncogene MYB, as well as within the gene BCL11A (Galarneau et al., 2010). HBS1L-MYB intergenic polymorphism on chromosome 6q23 is associated with elevated HbF levels. MYB and HBS1L expression was significantly reduced in erythroid cultures of individuals with high HbF levels, whereas overexpression of MYB in human erythroleukemic cells inhibited γ-globin expression supporting role of MYB in HbF regulation (Jiang et al., 2006). The human erythroid precursor cells from individuals with higher HbF and higher F cell levels have lower MYB expression associated with lower erythrocyte count but higher erythrocyte volume (Jiang et al., 2006).

MicroRNAs (miRNAs or miRs) are small, 19 to 25 nucleotide long, non-coding RNAs, which target mRNAs in a sequence-specific manner, inducing translational repression or decay. Increased miRNA-210 levels elevated γ-globin levels in hereditary persistence of HbF (Bianchi et al., 2009), while the let-7 family has been associated with hemoglobin switching (Noh et al., 2009). Recently, two miRNAs, miR-221 and miR-222, have been identified to regulate HbF expression in erythropoietic cells via the kit receptor (Gabbianelli et al., 2010). miRNA-150 repression of MYB in hematopoietic progenitor cells, of human bone marrow origin, supported MYB's importance in erythroid and megakaryocytic differentiation (Lu et al., 2008). It has been reported that miRNA-96, miRNA-146a, let-7a, miR-888 and miR-330a-3p are significantly more abundant in reticulocytes obtained from adults than from umbilical cord blood and therefore are potential inhibitors of γ-globin expression. The miR-96 has been identified as a direct inhibitor of γ-globin expression (Azzouzi et al., 2011, Scheme 1). These findings demonstrate that miRNAs contribute to HbF regulation by the post-transcriptional inhibition of γ-globin expression during adult erythropoiesis.

2. Microarray analysis of globin related genes during ontogenesis

2.1 Introduction

Several groups have examined the gene expression profile of human CD34$^+$ hematopoietic progenitor cells from bone marrow (BM), peripheral blood (PB) and cord blood (CB) using microarray technology (He et al., 2005; Ng et al., 2004; Steidl et al., 2002). The modulation of gene expression during ontogeny, in fetal liver (FL)- and CB-derived CD34$^+$CD38$^-$ hematopoietic progenitor cells, appears to overlap broadly with early response genes of growth factor stimulated adult (BM) hematopoietic progenitor cells (Oh et al., 2000). Recent studies have begun to define a general gene expression profiling for human erythroid cells from different origins - adult BM and PB (Goh et al., 2007; Gubin et al., 1999; Fujishima et al., 2004). In general, it has been hypothesized that globin gene switching may be mediated by proteins expressed during different stages of ontogeny.

Following the same intention, we have performed serial gene expression profiling in human differentiating erythroid cells by oligonucleotide microarrays. The several expressed genes (GATA1, ALAS2, EPOR, globins, etc.) linked to known erythroid differentiation confirms the validity of our approach in establishing the appropriate in vitro cell culture conditions. To study the mechanism of globin gene switching, we have performed gene expression profiling of erythroid progenitor cells derived from hematopoietic tissues during ontogeny, using a large Gene Array to gain insight into the associated molecular pathways. Gene expression patterns of CD71$^+$ erythroid progenitor cells, differentiated from human FL, CB, BM, PB and granulocyte colony-stimulating factor (G-CSF) mobilized PB (mPB), were compared to establish the expression patterns of representative genes.

2.2 Material and methods

2.2.1 Liquid erythroid cell cultures

$CD34^+$ hematopoietic progenitor cells were purified by positive immunomagnetic selection using the MACS cell isolation system (Miltenyi Biotec, Auburn, CA). Fresh BM, PB and G-CSF stimulated mPB $CD34^+$ cells were collected (AllCells LLC, Berkeley, CA) and proceeded with selection. CB $CD34^+$ cells (AllCells LLC) and FL $CD34^+$ cells (Cambrex Bio Science, Inc., Walkersville, MD) were collected and frozen. For analysis, $CD34^+$ cells were resuspended in medium with erythropoietin (EPO), as already described (Cokic et al., 2003). After 6 days of EPO treatment, $5x10^5$ cells were washed and incubated for 20 minutes in the presence of the monoclonal antibody anti-CD71 Tricolor for cell staining (Beckman-Coulter, Miami, FL). Cells were then washed, fixed and acquired on an LSRII flow cytometer (BD Biosciences, San Jose, CA). Data were analyzed with Flowjo software (Tree Star, San Carlos, CA). After 6 days of erythropoietin treatment and incubation at 37°C (5% CO_2, 95% humidity), we used the RNeasy protocol for isolation of total RNA from erythroid progenitor cells (Qiagen, Valencia, CA) according to the manufacturer's instructions. Concentration and integrity of total RNA was assessed using an 8453 UV/Visible Spectrophotometer (Hewlett-Packard GmbH, Waldbronn, Germany) and Agilent 2100 Bioanalyzer Software (Agilent Technologies, Waldbronn, Germany).

2.2.2 Microarray studies

In microarray studies, the numbers of total genes overexpressed in erythroid cells of CB, BM and PB origin were determined from three independent samples as biological repeats. FL and mPB-derived samples were analyzed in independent duplicate samples at day 6 of erythroid liquid culture. High quality oligonucleotide glass arrays were produced containing a total of 16,659 seventy-mer oligonucleotides (Operon Inc. Valencia, CA). The array includes probes for 2121 hypothetical proteins and 18-expressed sequence tags (ESTs) and spans approximately 50% of the human genome (Operon Inc.). The arrays were produced in house by spotting oligonucleotides on poly-L-lysine coated glass slides by Gene Machines robotics (Omnigrid, San Carlos, CA).

Total human universal RNA (HuURNA) isolated from a collection of adult human tissues to represent a broad range of expressed genes from both male and female donors (BD Biosciences, Palo Alto, CA) served as a universal reference control in the competitive hybridization. Labeled cDNA probes were produced as described (Risinger et al., 2003). cDNA was purified by the MinElute column (Qiagen). Binding buffer PB was added to the coupled cDNA, and the mixture applied to the MinElute column and centrifuged. After discharging the flow-through, washing buffer PE was added to the column, and centrifuged. Then the columns were placed into a fresh eppendorf tube and elution buffer added to the membrane, incubated and centrifuged and probe collected. The probe was dried in speed-vac. Finally, 5 μl of 2X coupling buffer and 5 μl Cy3 and Cy5 dye (GE Healthcare Bio-Sciences Corp., Piscataway, NJ) were mixed into the control (HuURNA) and experimental cDNAs (huES cell-derived) respectively and incubated at room temperature in dark for 90 minutes. After incubation, the volume was raised to 60 μl by DEPC water and then cDNA was purified by the MinElute column and eluted with 13 μl elution buffer by centrifugation. For hybridization, 36 μl hybridization mixture was pre-heated at 100°C for 2 minutes and cooled for 1 minute. Total volume of probe was added on the array and covered with cover slip. Slides are placed in hybridization chamber and 20μl water was added to the slide, and incubated overnight at 65°C. Slides were then washed for 2 minutes each in 2X SSC, 1X SSC and 0.1X SSC and spin-dried. Microarray slides were scanned in both Cy3 (532nm) and Cy5 (635nm) channels using Axon GenePix 4000B scanner (Axon Instruments, Inc., Foster City, CA) with a 10-micron resolution. Scanned microarray images were exported as TIFF files to GenePix Pro 3.0 software for image analysis. The average of the total Cy3 and Cy5 signal gave a ratio that was used to normalize the signals. Each microarray experiment was globally normalized to make the median value of the log2-ratio equal to zero. The Loess normalization process corrects for dye bias, photo multiplier tube voltage imbalance, and variations between channels in the amounts of the labeled cDNA probes hybridized. The data files representing the differentially expressed genes were then created. For advanced data analysis, gpr and jpeg files were imported into microarray database, and normalized by software tools provided by NIH Center for Information Technology (http://nciarray.nci.nih.gov/). Spots with confidence interval of 99 (≥ 2 fold) with at least 150-fluorescence intensity for both channel and 30 μm spot size were considered as good quality spots for analysis. Paired t test was used in microarray analysis.

2.3 Results

2.3.1 Predominantly elevated genes expression in ontogenic tissues

In the presence of EPO and other cytokines, $CD34^+$ cells were differentiated in vitro into erythroid progenitor cells. Besides flow cytometry for analysis of *in vitro* erythroid differentiation, we already reported measurement of hemoglobin content by benzidine staining and high-performance liquid chromatography in erythroid progenitor cells during their *in vitro* differentiation in same culture conditions (Cokic et al., 2003, 2008). The transferrin receptor (CD71) is present on early erythroid cells but is lost as reticulocytes differentiate into mature erythrocytes (Cokic et al., 2003). At day 6 of erythroid cell culture, the erythroid progenitor cells were sorted as 100% $CD71^+$, a well-known early marker of erythroid differentiation. In microarray studies, the quantities of tissue specific overexpressed genes were determined from two to four independent samples (biological repeats). During microarray analysis genes are upregulated or downregulated versus HuURNA, what we used as a control alongside each sample. We observed largely upregulated genes in all tissues (Table 1).

Besides common highly expressed genes in erythroid progenitor cells: CD71, Rh-associated glycoprotein (RHAG), SERPINE1 mRNA binding protein 1 (SERBP1); the highly expressed genes in erythroid cells of FL origin are ribonuclease, RNase A family 2 and 3 (RNASE2/3) and serpin peptidase inhibitor, clade B (SERPINB1, Table 1).

The highly expressed genes in erythroid cells of CB origin are hemoglobin gamma A (HBG1), NFE2 and eosinophil peroxidase (EPX). The greatly expressed genes in erythroid cells of BM origin are latexin (LXN), coproporphyrinogen oxidase (CPOX) and carbonic anhydrase II (CA2). The highly expressed genes in erythroid cells of mPB origin are KLF1, aminolevulinate, delta-, synthase 2 (ALAS2) and THO complex 2 (THOC2). The genes with reduced expressed in erythroid cells of PB origin are proteoglycan 2 (PRG2), Charcot-Leyden crystal protein (CLC), EPX and v-myb myeloblastosis viral oncogene homolog

Gene Name	Description	Fold induction vs. HuURNA (±SD)				
		FL	CB	BM	mPB	PB
HBG1	hemoglobin, gamma A	4.2±0.7	4.5±0.9	4.1±1	4.3±0.2	4.7±0.6
CLC	Charcot-Leyden crystal protein	4.3±0.4	4.3±0.7	4.6±0.6	4.8±0.4	2.9±0.6
PRG2	proteoglycan 2, bone marrow	5±0.3	4.2±0.9	4.7±0.5	4.1±0.7	2.9±0.4
RNASE2	ribonuclease, RNase A family, 2	**4.3±0.7**	3.7±0.9	3.1±0.6	3.5±0.7	1.4±0.8
HBD	hemoglobin, delta	2±1.3	3.5±0.3	4.3±0.4	4.2±0.4	3.2±0.5
EPX	eosinophil peroxidase	**4±0.2**	**3.4±0.8**	2.9±0.7	2.6±1.1	0.9±0.5
SRGN	serglycin	4.3±1	2.8±1	4.4±1.3	4.6±0.4	2.1±0.5
TFRC	transferrin receptor (p90, CD71)	3.1±1	3.3±1.2	4.4±0.3	4.3±0.03	3±0.9
HBE1	hemoglobin, epsilon 1	3±1.2	2.6±1.5	**4.4±1.7**	**4.6±0.01**	3.4±1.3
RHAG	Rh-associated glycoprotein	2.7±1.3	3.2±1.2	2.1±0.9	3.1±0.7	2.1±0.5
MPO	myeloperoxidase	3.8±0.2	3.2±0.6	3.4±0.1		
MYB	v-myb myeloblastosis viral oncogene homolog	3±0.3	3.1±0.7	2.6±0.4	3.5±0.4	1.7±1
RNASE3	ribonuclease, RNase A family, 3	**3.6±1.2**	2.7±1.5	2±1	3.1±0.7	0.6±0.2
LXN	latexin	1.5±0.4	1.9±0.7	**4.7±1**	**4.1±0.5**	2.7±0.2
CD36	CD36 molecule (thrombospondin rec)	1.6±1.1	2.6±0.5	**4±1**	3.2±0.5	2.1±0.8
CPOX	coproporphyrinogen oxidase	2±0.8	2.7±0.6	**3.5±0.7**	2.9±0.4	1.8±0.6
CA2	carbonic anhydrase II	0.15	1±0.3	**3.3±0.6**	1.8±0.2	1.7±0.5
CYTL1	cytokine-like 1	1.4±0.8	1.7±0.4	2.8±0.4	**3.7±0.3**	2.4±0.3
KLF1	Kruppel-like factor 1 (erythroid)	1±0.4	1.7±0.5	2.5±0.9	**3.6±0.3**	2.3±0.2
ALAS2	aminolevulinate, delta-, synthase 2	1.5±0.4	1.4±0.3	2.5±0.9	**3.5±0.7**	2.7±0.3
CPA3	carboxypeptidase A3 (mast cell)	1	0.9±0.3	1.9±0.7	**3.2±0.4**	1.2±0.5
THOC2	THO complex 2	0.6±0.4	0.9±0.5	1.4±0.7	**3.1±0.2**	1.6±0.5
GATA1	globin transcription factor 1	0.9	2.1±0.4	2.7±0.6	2.5±0.3	2.3±0.3
NFE2	nuclear factor (erythroid-derived 2)	1.4±0.4	1.9±0.5	2.6		1.6±0.5
SERPINB1	serpin peptidase inhibitor, clade B	**2.5±0.2**	1.8±0.3	1.7±0.4	0.9±0.3	0.7±0.3
SERBP1	SERPINE1 mRNA binding protein 1	2.1±0.4	2.4±0.5	1.9±0.7	1.9±0.5	1.6±0.6

Table 1. Largely up-regulated genes vs. HuURNA among different tissues: FL, CB, BM, mPB, PB. Bolded black values represent increased genes expression, whereas bolded gray values represent decreased genes expression in comparison to other tissues.

(MYB). Presence of certain gene in the least two samples (66% filtering), in one group of tissues, reduced largely the total gene expression in all tissues. Using the range of microarray analysis and filtering reduction, the erythroid cells of FL tissue origin expressed 1772 genes, CB-derived erythroid cells expressed 3846 genes, BM derived erythroid cells expressed 1827 genes, mPB derived erythroid cells expressed 4008 genes, and PB derived erythroid cells expressed 1320 genes. The observed gene expression is more than doubled in CB and mPB tissues in comparison to other tissues.

2.3.2 A comparison in genes expression of erythroid cells during subsequent stages of development

Using Venn diagrams we compared total gene expression, determined by microarray analysis, among all examined ontogenic tissues. By 66% filtering, we analyzed only genes

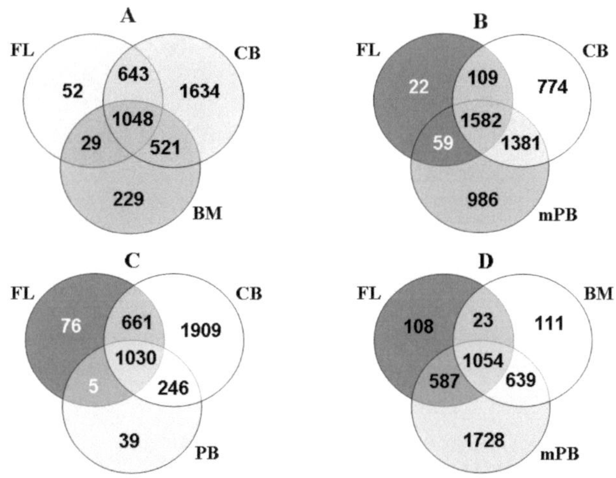

Fig. 1. **Venn diagram of genes expression in erythroid progenitor cells between FL and other developmental tissues.** A: Comparison among FL, CB and BM tissues; B: Comparison among FL, CB and mPB tissues; C: Comparison among FL, CB and PB tissues; D: Comparison among FL, BM and mPB tissues.

present in at least two donor samples per tissue. We compared gene expression of FL-derived erythroid cell with other ontogenic derived tissues in Figure 1. Shared genes expression was more prominent between CB and FL/mPB derived erythroid cells, than between FL and BM/PB tissues (Figure 1A-C). Moreover, the FL- and CB-derived erythroid cells have the more common genes with mPB-derived erythroid cells than with BM and PB tissues (Figures 1D, 2C). The genes related to FL tissue shared the similar expression with BM- and PB-derived cells (Figure 2A). In addition, the genes expression in mPB-derived erythroid cells contains the majority of genes expressed in FL, BM and PB tissues (Figure 2B,

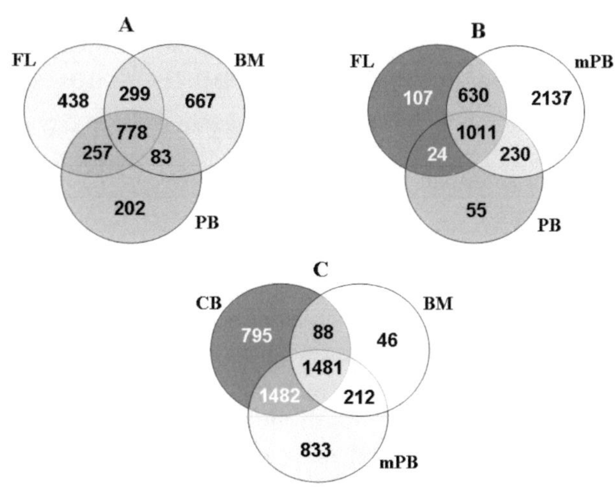

Fig. 2. **Venn diagram of genes expression in erythroid progenitor cells among ontogenic tissues.** A: Comparison among FL, BM and PB tissues; B: Comparison among FL, mPB and PB tissues; C: Comparison among CB, BM and mPB tissues.

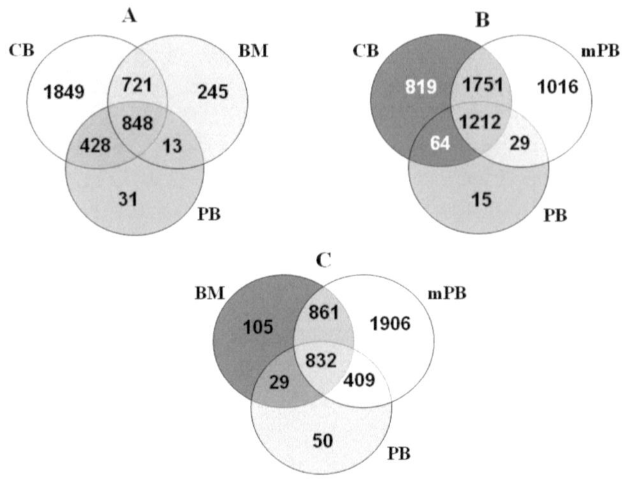

Fig. 3. **Venn diagram of genes expression in erythroid progenitor cells between PB and other ontogenic tissues.** A: Comparison among CB, BM and PB tissues; B: Comparison among CB, mPB and PB tissues; C: Comparison among BM, mPB and PB tissues.

3C), but not in CB tissue (Figures 2C, 3B). Also, mPB-derived erythroid cells shared more genes with BM tissue than with PB tissue (Figure 3C). The genes expression in CB-derived erythroid cells overwhelmed the gene expression in BM tissues and almost completely in PB tissue (Figure 3A).

Comparison in genes expression between FL- and CB-derived erythroid cells revealed couple statistically significant genes ($p<0.01$, Table 2): POLE3 and BRP44. Negative values in Tables represent downregulated genes expression in ontogenic tissues in contrast to HuURNA, whereas positive values represent upregulated genes.

Gene	Description	p value	FL Mean±SD	CB Mean±SD	Tissue presence
POLE3	polymerase epsilon 3	0.0022	0.4±0.22	0.8±0.4	FL, CB, mPB, PB
SNRPD3	small nuclear ribonucleoprotein D3	0.0036	0.8±0.02	1.6±0.4	FL, CB, mPB
ZFP36	zinc finger protein 36	0.0072	-1.6±0.07	-2.3±0.6	FL, CB, mPB
BRP44	brain protein 44	0.0063	-0.14±0.09	0.5±0.1	All tissues

Table 2. Comparison of statistically significant ($p<0.01$) genes between FL and CB tissues.

Brain protein 44 (BRP44) gene expressions was highly significantly increased in CB-derived erythroid cells vs. FL-derived cells (Table 2), but was reduced in comparison to PB-derived cells (Table 8). BRP44 gene was stable expression in all examined ontogenic tissues, whereas POLE 3 gene expression was absent in BM tissue (Table 2). Comparison in genes expression between FL- and BM-derived erythroid cells exposed more statistically significant genes (Table 3): SBNO2, WDR1 and CTAG2 present in all tissues.

WD repeat domain 1 (WDR1) gene expressions was significantly increased in BM- vs. PB-derived erythroid cells (Table 10), but was reduced in comparison to FL-derived cells (Table

3). Evaluation in genes expression between FL- and mPB-derived erythroid cells exposed also statistically significant genes (Table 4): ME2 present just in FL and mPB tissues, highly upregulated EEF1B2 expressed in all tissues. IFI30 was downregulated in mPB-derived erythroid cells, but was upregulated in FL-derived cells (Table 4).

Gene	Description	p value	FL Mean±SD	BM Mean±SD	Tissue presence
SPRR2B	small proline-rich protein 2B	0.0001	-0.8±0.03	-0.9±0.5	FL, CB, BM,mPB
SRI	sorcin	0.0014	0.9±0.04	1.1±0.2	All tissues
KPNA2	karyopherin alpha 2	0.002	0.5±0.005	1 ±0.2	All tissues
SDHC	succinate dehydrogenase complex, subunit C	0.0021	0.1±0.05	0.2±0.2	All tissues
NCOA4	nuclear receptor coactivator 4	0.0048	2±0.3	1.8±0.4	All tissues
SBNO2	strawberry notch homolog 2	0.005	-1.5±0.02	-1.1±0.6	All tissues
TTC3	tetratricopeptide repeat domain 3	0.0057	0.3±0.08	0.6±0.1	FL, CB, BM,mPB
PTTG1	pituitary tumor-transforming1	0.0078	0.7±0.05	1±0.2	All tissues
WDR1	WD repeat domain 1	0.0079	0.5±0.002	0.3±0.1	All tissues
MINK1	Misshapen-like kinase 1	0.0089	-1.2±0.1	-0.9±0.5	All tissues
CTAG2	cancer/testis antigen 2	0.0094	-0.1±0.25	-0.2±0.54	All tissues

Table 3. Comparison of statistically significant (p<0.01) genes between FL and BM tissues.

Gene	Description	p value	FL Mean±SD	mPB Mean±SD	Tissue presence
ME2	malic enzyme 2, NAD(+)-dependent, mitochondrial	0.0068	1.19±0.15	0.9±0.14	FL, mPB
INSIG1	insulin induced gene 1	0.0073	-0.08±0.4	-0.01±0.4	FL, mPB
EEF1B2	eukaryotic translation elongation factor 1 beta 2	0.0009	1.77±0.12	2.3±0.12	All tissues
ZNF224	zinc finger protein 224	0.0015	-0.2±0.06	0.9±0.06	FL, CB, BM, mPB
CSDE1	cold shock domain containing E1, RNA-binding	0.004	0.56±0.08	0.6± 0.02	All tissues
IFI30	Interferon, gamma-inducible protein 30	0.0059	0.06±0.05	-2±0.07	FL, CB, BM, mPB
PSMD11	proteasome 26S, non-ATPase,11	0.0091	0.67±0.17	0.18±0.16	All tissues
PGAM1	phosphoglycerate mutase 1	0.0093	0.87±0.15	0.06±0.16	FL, CB, mPB, PB
PTPRC	protein tyrosine phosphatase, receptor type, C	0.0093	1.42±0.75	1.5±0.75	FL, CB, BM, mPB

Table 4. Comparison of statistically significant (p<0.01) genes between FL and mPB tissues.

Comparison between FL- and PB-derived erythroid cells revealed just two significant genes: TOP1 and CAT (Table 5). TOP1 and CAT genes have higher levels in FL tissue than in PB.

Gene	Description	p value	FL Mean±SD	PB Mean±SD	Tissue presence
TOP1	topoisomerase I	0.0017	1.3±0.34	0.9±0.7	All tissues
CAT	catalase	0.0042	1.8±0.18	1.3±0.26	FL, CB, mPB, PB

Table 5. Comparison of statistically significant ($p<0.01$) genes between FL and PB tissues.

Evaluation in genes expression between CB- and BM-derived erythroid cells exposed several genes: WAPAL, GRB2, GOLIM4, etc. (Table 6). CTDSP1 has the elevated expression in CB tissue, while TPST2 has the higher expression in BM tissue (Table 6).

Gene	Description	p value	CB Mean±SD	BM Mean±SD	Tissue presence
SCAMP2	secretory carrier membrane protein 2	0.0022	0.4±0.22	0.8±0.4	CB, BM, PB
ABCF2	ATP-binding cassette, sub-family F	0.0075	-0.2±0.17	0.22±0.08	CB, BM, PB
ZNF16	zinc finger protein 16	0.0093	0.2±0.2	0.6±0.18	CB, BM, PB
GRIPAP1	GRIP1 associated protein 1	0.0014	-0.6±0.45	-0.06±0.45	All tissues
WAPAL	wings apart-like homolog	0.0023	1.3±0.1	1.7±0.1	All tissues
TPST2	tyrosylprotein sulfotransferase 2	0.0029	0.8±0.26	1.6±0.21	All tissues
TPSB2	tryptase beta 2	0.0035	-0.7±0.43	1±0.33	All tissues
CCNB2	cyclin B2	0.0037	1.3±0.21	1.7±0.19	All tissues
RPS13	ribosomal protein S13	0.0041	1.9±0.23	1.5±0.21	All tissues
GRB2	growth factor receptor-bound protein 2	0.0067	-0.06±0.4	0.4±0.38	All tissues
GSK3A	glycogen synthase kinase 3α	0.0071	-1±0.04	-0.8±0.06	All tissues
CTDSP1	carboxy-terminal domain, A polypeptide small phosphatas 1	0.0077	0.4±0.23	-0.05±0.01	All tissues
ZNF43	zinc finger protein 43	0.0086	0.9±0.11	1.2±0.09	All tissues
GOLIM4	golgi integral membrane protein 4	0.0094	0.4±0.04	0.85±0.07	All tissues

Table 6. Comparison of statistically significant ($p<0.01$) genes between CB and BM tissues.

Zinc finger protein 43 (ZNF43) has also significantly increased gene expressions in BM-derived erythroid cells compared to CB- and PB-derived erythroid cells (Tables 6, 10). Golgi integral membrane protein 4 (GOLIM4) gene has also significantly increased expressions in BM-derived erythroid cells compared to CB- and mPB-derived erythroid cells (Tables 6, 9). Assessment in genes expression between CB- and mPB-derived erythroid cells uncovered several genes: ARF4, PHIP, ACIN1, etc. (Table 7). ARF4 has highly upregulated gene expression in CB-derived cells compared to mPB tissue.

Measurement in genes expression profile between CB and PB tissues revealed the downregulated genes PPFIA4 and WIPI2, as well as upregulated genes FBL and BRP44 (Table 8). WIPI2 was less downregulated in PB tissue than in CB tissue.

Determination of statistical significance between BM and mPB tissues showed the prevalent quantity of genes: MYCL2, ADIPOR2 and POP7 present in CB, BM and mPB tissues; NFATC3, YY1, GCA present in all tissues except PB; YWHAZ, TACC3, UBE2D3 present in BM, mPB and PB tissues (Table 9).

Gene	Description	P value	CB Mean±SD	mPB Mean±SD	Tissue presence
GRN	granulin	0.0007	-1.1±0.35	-1.5±0.16	All tissues
PHIP	pleckstrin homology domain interacting protein	0.0009	0.5±0.38	1.4±0.29	All tissues
ARF4	ADP-ribosylation factor 4	0.0037	0.4±0.3	0.04±0.15	FL, CB, BM, mPB
UBE2V1	ubiquitin-conjugating enzyme E2 variant 1	0.0044	0.7±0.06	0.4±0.04	All tissues
ACIN1	apoptotic chromatin condensation inducer 1	0.0058	0.6±0.11	0.3±0.05	All tissues
XRCC6	X-ray repair complementing defective repair in Chinese hamster cells 6	0.0067	1.2±0.13	0.8±0.11	All tissues
F2R	coagulation factor II (thrombin) receptor	0.0072	-0.2±0.22	-0.9±0.21	FL, CB, BM, mPB
SNRPA	small nuclear ribonucleoprotein polypeptide A	0.008	1.6±0.37	1.1±0.02	FL, CB, mPB
LGALS1	lectin, galactoside-binding, soluble, 1	0.0093	-1.3±0.48	-0.5±0.57	FL, CB, mPB

Table 7. Comparison of statistically significant (p<0.01) genes between CB and mPB tissues.

Gene	Description	p value	CB Mean±SD	PB Mean±SD	Tissue presence
PPFIA4	protein tyrosine phosphatase, f polypeptide, interacting protein α 4	0.0016	-1.3±0.37	-0.06±0.44	All tissues
WIPI2	WD repeat domain, phosphoinositide interacting 2	0.0043	-0.3±0.08	-0.02±0.14	All tissues
FBL	fibrillarin	0.0056	1.5±0.29	0.9±0.36	All tissues
BRP44	brain protein 44	0.0059	0.5±0.13	1±0.14	All tissues

Table 8. Comparison of statistically significant (p<0.01) genes between CB and PB tissues.

Gene	Description	p value	BM Mean±SD	mPB Mean±SD	Tissue presence
MYCL2	v-myc avian myelocytomatosis viral oncogene homolog 2	0.0006	-0.7±0.26	-1.4±0.26	CB, BM, mPB
SKAP2	src kinase associated phosphoprotein 2	0.0012	-1.1±0.3	-1.6±0.31	CB, BM, mPB
MPHOSPH9	Mphase phosphoprotein mpp9	0.0012	-0.7±0.18	-1.3±0.19	CB, BM, mPB
SLC25A39	solute carrier family 25, member 39	0.0013	1.5±0.13	0.9±0.07	CB, BM, mPB

Gene	Description	p value	BM Mean±SD	mPB Mean±SD	Tissue presence
UBE2NL	ubiquitin-conjugating enzyme E2N-like	0.0015	0.9±0.17	0.6±0.17	CB, BM, mPB
POP7	Processing of precursor 7, ribonuclease P/MRP subunit	0.0027	-0.4±0.21	0.28±0.12	CB, BM, mPB
ANKH	ankylosis, progressive homolog	0.0031	-0.5±0.22	-1.2±0.21	CB, BM, mPB
ADIPOR2	adiponectin receptor 2	0.0045	0.6±0.32	0.6±0.01	CB, BM, mPB
ZBTB43	zinc finger and BTB domain containing 43	0.0041	-0.9±0.22	-1.4±0.21	CB, BM, mPB
RBM8A	RNA binding motif protein 8A	0.0048	-0.9±0.45	-0.3±0.13	CB, BM, mPB
ZYG11B	zyg-11 homolog B	0.0062	-0.2±0.28	-0.9±0.23	CB, BM, mPB
APBB2	amyloid beta precursor protein-binding, family B, member 2	0.0074	-0.8±0.16	-1.1±0.17	CB, BM, mPB
CEP97	centrosomal protein 97kDa	0.0082	-0.6±0.09	-1.4±0.1	CB, BM, mPB
KLRD1	killer cell lectin-like receptor subfamily D	0.0011	-0.4±0.16	-1.3±0.16	FL, CB, BM, mPB
TOMM34	translocase of outer mitochondrial membrane 34	0.0035	-0.5±0.21	-0.6±0.15	FL, CB, BM, mPB
NFATC3	nuclear factor of activated T-cells, cytoplasmic, calcineurin-dependent 3	0.0045	1.3±0.19	0.9±0.23	FL, CB, BM, mPB
YY1	YY1 transcription factor	0.0047	1.4±0.18	0.8±0.22	FL, CB, BM, mPB
SSB	Sjogren syndrome antigen B	0.0050	2.7±0.72	2.3±0.003	FL, CB, BM, mPB
UBC	ubiquitin C	0.0069	-1±0.53	-1.3±0.08	FL, CB, BM, mPB
UBA1	ubiquitin-like modifier activating enzyme 1	0.0083	-0.4±0.6	-0.6±0.17	FL, CB, BM, mPB
LRRC59	leucine rich repeat containing59	0.0086	1.9±0.25	1.5±0.03	FL, CB, BM, mPB
GCA	grancalcin, EF-hand calcium binding protein	0.0098	1.2±0.21	0.4±0.17	FL, CB, BM, mPB
TACC3	transforming, acidic coiled-coil containing protein 3	0.0011	0.02±0.01	-0.3±0.03	BM, mPB, PB
LMNB1	lamin B1	0.0014	1±0.1	-0.1±0.04	BM, mPB, PB
SREBF2	sterol regulatory element binding	0.0019	-0.6±0.05	-2.1±0.18	BM, mPB, PB
UBE2D3	ubiquitin-conjugating enzyme E2D 3	0.0032	1.02±0.06	0.5±0.001	BM, mPB, PB
YWHAZ	tyrosine 3-mono oxygenase/tryptophan 5-monooxygenase activation protein, zeta polypeptide	0.0042	1.4±0.08	0.7±0.04	BM, mPB, PB

Gene	Description	p value	BM Mean±SD	mPB Mean±SD	Tissue presence
GOLIM4	golgi integral membrane protein 4	0.0044	0.8±0.02	0.29±0.05	BM, mPB, PB
GLE1	GLE1 RNA export mediator homolog	0.0049	-0.4±0.02	0.29±0.12	BM, mPB, PB
CORO1C	coronin actin binding protein 1C	0.0049	1.4±0.1	0.6±0.08	BM, mPB, PB
ARHGDIB	Rho GDPdissociation inhibitorβ	0.0075	1.4±0.02	1.2±0.03	BM, mPB, PB
TMEM187	transmembrane protein 187	0.0082	-0.4±0.08	-0.9±0.03	BM, mPB, PB
TIMM23	translocase of inner mitochon-drial membrane 23 homolog	0.0088	0.9±0.1	0.3±0.05	BM, mPB, PB
PSMB5	proteasome subunit, β type, 5	0.0092	0.3±0.02	0.02±0.02	BM, mPB, PB

Table 9. Comparison of statistically significant ($p<0.01$) genes between BM and mPB tissues.

YY1 transcription factor has significantly increased gene expressions in BM-derived erythroid cells compared to PB- and mPB-derived erythroid cells (Tables 9, 10). Measurement of statistical significance between BM and PB tissues revealed the following significant genes: NUCKS1 and KDM3B prevalent in BM tissue, ATF5 and ATP5L prevalent in BM tissue (Table 10).

Gene	Description	p value	BM Mean±SD	PB Mean±SD	Tissue presence
NUCKS1	nuclear casein kinase and cyclin-dependent kinase substrate 1	0.0092	1.1±0.62	0.7±0.12	CB, BM,PB
KDM3B	lysine (K)-specific demethylase 3B	0.0002	0.8±0.01	0.15±0.03	BM, mPB, PB
WDR1	WD repeat domain 1	0.0018	0.3±0.1	-0.2±0.03	BM, mPB, PB
YY1	YY1 transcription factor	0.0018	1.4±0.2	0.25±0.14	BM, mPB, PB
FEN1	flap structure-specific endonuclease 1	0.004	2.7±0.1	1.13±0.2	BM, mPB, PB
ATF5	activating transcription factor 5	0.0057	-0.8±0.1	-0.2±0.14	BM, mPB, PB
ZNF43	zinc finger protein 43	0.0058	1.2±0.08	0.5±0.15	BM, mPB, PB
ATP5L	ATP synthase, H+ transporting, mitochondrial F0 complex, subunit G	0.0071	0.3±0.08	0.78±0.09	BM, mPB, PB
HLA-C	MHC class I human leukocyte antigen	0.0046	-2.7±0.7	-2.1±0.88	CB,BM,PB

Table 10. Comparison in statistically significant ($p<0.01$) gene between BM and PB tissues.

Flap structure-specific endonuclease 1 (FEN1) gene has significantly decreased expressions in PB-derived erythroid cells compared to BM- and mPB-derived erythroid cells (Tables 10, 11). Similarity in genes expression between mPB and PB tissues was limited on four significant genes: TXNIP, EIF3E, FEN1 and FECH (Table 11). TXNIP was present and downregulated just in mPB and PB tissues, whereas EIF3E and FEN1 was highly upregulated in all tissues and predominantly in mPB-derived erythroid cells. FECH has more prominent expression in PB- than in mPB-derived cells.

Gene	Description	p value	mPB Mean±SD	PB Mean±SD	Tissue presence
TXNIP	Brain-expressed HHCPA78 homolog VDUP1	0.0063	-1.3±0.05	-0.14±0.18	mPB, PB
EIF3E	eukaryotic translation initiation factor 3, subunit E	0.0003	2.5±0.14	1.2±0.24	All tissues
FEN1	flap structure-specific endonuclease 1	0.0028	2±0.21	1.13±0.21	All tissues
FECH	ferrochelatase	0.0074	1.6±0.7	2.5±0.59	FL, CB, mPB, PB

Table 11. Comparison in statistically significant ($p<0.01$) gene between mPB and PB tissues.

2.3.3 Signaling pathways related to globin genes expression

It has been already reported that γ globin genes expression is regulated by nitric oxide (NO) and p38 MAPK signaling pathways (Cokic et al., 2003; Ramakrishnan & Pace, 2011). We examined the genes related to those pathways in erythroid progenitor cells during ontogeny in succeeding tissues (Figure 4). Protein kinase, cAMP-dependent, regulatory, type II, beta (PRKAR2B) has the highest expression in NO signaling pathways linked genes throughout the ontogeny reaching the top in PB-derived erythroid cells. Calmodulin 2 (CALM2) gene demonstrates decline in expression during ontogeny, as well as protein phosphatase 3 beta isoform (PPP3CB, Figure 4A). Downregulation in gene expression during ontogeny was shown for protein kinase, cAMP-dependent, regulatory, type I, alpha (PRKAR1A) and calmodulin 3 (CALM3). Regarding p38 MAPK signaling pathway, transforming growth factor, beta 1 (TGFB1) gene expression was predominant in FL- and BM-derived erythroid cells, while heat shock 27kDa protein 1 (HSPB1) was decreased in BM-derived erythroid cells (Figure 4B). Linked to p38 MAPK, v-myc myelocytomatosis viral oncogene homolog (MYC) has the most upregulated gene expression throughout the ontogeny (Figure 4B).

2.3.4 Discussion

To recognize sets of genes that reveal the essential mechanisms in hematopoiesis, as potential novel therapeutic targets, several groups have performed individual gene expression profiling in erythroid cells from certain tissues during ontogenesis. We extended those studies, of gene expression pattern of ontogenic tissues, to compare gene expression from fetal to adult hematopoiesis as a more reflective and comprehensive overview of erythropoiesis. Gene expression in normal human erythroid progenitor cells has been described and generally static expression analysis was performed on cultured human erythroid progenitor $CD71^+$ cells derived from $CD34^+$ cells in the presence of EPO and cocktail of cytokines. We presented the number of total genes overexpressed in evaluated tissues, the most dominant in CB and mPB tissues. Also, the highly expressed genes are SERPINE1, PRG2, CLC, HBG1, NFE2 and EPX. General genes expression was more present between CB and FL/mPB derived erythroid cells, than between FL and adult tissues.

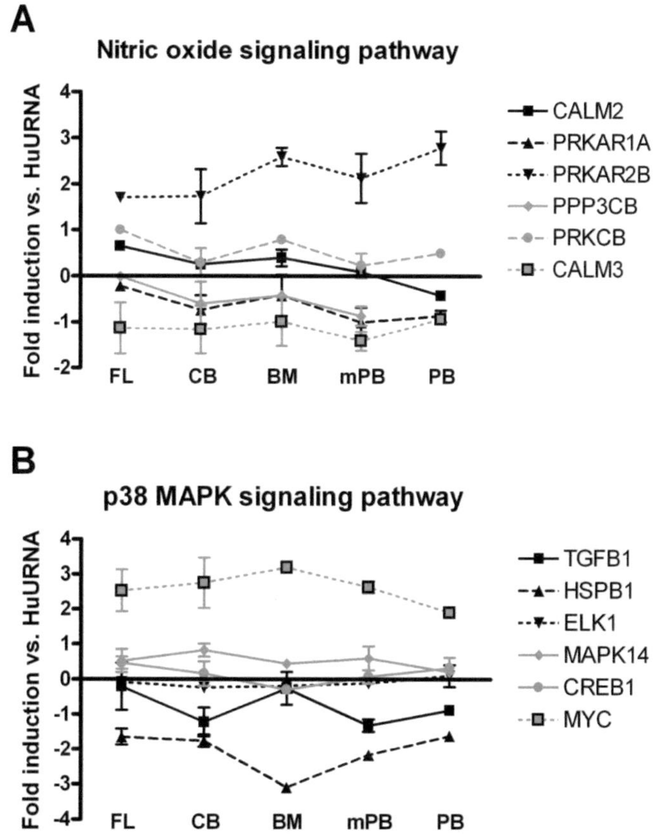

Fig. 4. **Gene expression in signaling pathways related to globins stimulation determined by microarray analysis.** A: Induction of Nitric oxide signaling pathway related genes in erythroid progenitor cells during human ontogeny. B: Induction of p38 MAPK signaling pathway related genes in erythroid progenitor cells during human ontogeny.

Comparison between certain tissues revealed the statistically significant genes: TOP1, CAT, IFI30 in FL tissue, ARF4, CTDSP1 in CB tissue, WDR1, ATF5, YWHAZ in BM tissue, EIF3E and FEN1 in mPB tissue, FECH in PB tissue. PRKAR2B has the highest expression in NO signaling pathways, while MYC has the most upregulated gene expression in p38 MAPK signaling pathway in erythroid progenitor cells throughout ontogeny.

3. Nitric oxide interaction with signaling pathways related to erythropoiesis

It has been found that proliferation of erythropoietic cells is more related to activation of JAK-STAT and MAPK p42/44 signaling pathways, whereas the survival of erythropoietic cells correlated better with activation of PI-3K-AKT, JAK-STAT and MAPK p42/44 pathways (Ratajczak et al., 2001). During erythroid maturation, the p38 MAPK regulates γ-globin transcription through its downstream effector cAMP response element binding protein 1 (CREB1) which binds the Gγ-globin 3′,5′-cyclic adenosine monophosphate (cAMP) response element (Ramakrishnan & Pace, 2011). NO is a diffusible free radical that plays a role as a chemical messenger involved in vasodilator, neurotransmitter, and anti-platelet aggregation. NO is produced and released from three different isoforms of NO synthase (NOS) that convert the l-arginine and molecular oxygen to citrulline and NO in cells: endothelial (eNOS), inducible (iNOS), and neuronal (nNOS) (Cokic & Schechter, 2008). NO readily diffuses across cell membranes into neighboring cells, or may produce effects distant from its site of production transported by vehicles such as low-molecular weight S-nitrosotiols, S-nitrosylated proteins including hemoglobin and albumin, and nitrosyl-metal complexes which liberate NO spontaneously or after cleavage by ectoenzymes (Bogdan, 2001). A significance of NO in erythroid differentiation has been founded on demonstration that NO donors inhibit growth of erythroid primary cells and colony cultures (Maciejewski et al., 1995). Besides observation that NO inhibited erythroid differentiation induced by butyric acid, antitumour drugs aclarubicin and doxorubicin, but not by hemin (Chénais et al., 1999), additional study demonstrated inhibitory effect of NO in the hemin-induced erythroid differentiation (Kucukkaya et al., 2006). NO decreased colony-forming unit-erythrocytes (CFU-E) and CFU-granulocyte macrophage (CFU-GM) formation derived from human bone marrow mononuclear cells. Moreover, NO increased CFU-GM and decreased CFU-E formation derived from $CD34^+$ hematopoietic progenitor cells (Shami & Weinberg, 1996). Although NO increased intracellular levels of guanosine 3′,5′-cyclic monophosphate (cGMP) in bone marrow cells, addition of a membrane permeable cGMP analogue did not reproduce previously mentioned effects of NO in bone marrow derived colonies (Shami & Weinberg, 1996). We have previously shown that HbF stimulation is dependent on NO/cGMP signaling pathway in erythroid progenitor cells (Cokic et al., 2003). NO-releasing agents and cGMP analogues inhibit murine erythroleukemia cell differentiation and suppress erythroid-specific gene expression such as beta-globin and delta-aminolevulinate synthetase (Suhasini et al., 1995). Serum nitrate and nitrite (NOx) concentrations correlated inversely with hemoglobin levels (Choi et al., 2002).

EPO increased the level of phosphorylated eNOS and stimulated NO production and cGMP activity during hypoxia (Beleslin-Cokic et al., 2004; Su et al., 2006). Phospho-eNOS and eNOS were significantly induced by hypoxia (Beleslin-Čokić et al., 2011). NO participates in stability control of hypoxia inducible factor (HIF)-1α and induces HIF-1α accumulation and HIF-1-DNA binding (Kovacević-Filipović et al., 2007). Hypoxia and EPO increased erythropoietin receptor (EPOR) gene expression and protein level (Beleslin-Čokić et al., 2011). The physiologically low oxygenation of bone marrow is a regulator of hematopoiesis maintenance, and physiological levels of O_2 should be considered as an important environmental factor that significantly influences cytokine activity (Brüne & Zhou, 2007; Krstic et al., 2009a). The proportion of γ-globin mRNA (the $\gamma/(\gamma+\beta)$ mRNA ratio) increased with reduced oxygen, reaching a maximum value at 5% O_2 of 1.5 to 4-fold higher than at 20% O_2, and then decreased as the O_2 dropped to 2%. In parallel, the proportion of HbF (the HbF/(HbF+HbA) ratio) also peaked at 5% O_2. Reported increase in the HbF was generally lower than that of the γ-globin mRNA, suggesting that although globin mRNA accumulation is primarily under transcriptional regulation, additional post-transcriptional processing such as globin chain stability contribute to the amount of produced hemoglobins (Rogers et al., 2008).

4. Nitric oxide influence on hematopoietic microenvironment in bone marrow

Various growth factors, cytokines, and chemokines are secreted by human hematopoietic progenitor cells, myeloblasts, erythroblasts, and megakaryoblasts to regulate normal hematopoiesis in an autocrine/paracrine manner. Furthermore, each stromal cell in the bone marrow may provide the preferable microenvironment for a rapid expansion of the lineage-restricted progenitor cells (Kameoka et al., 1995; Majka et al., 2001). We showed that the human endothelial cells and macrophages contain NOS activity, representing the potential pool for NO production. The erythroid progenitor cell co-cultures with either macrophages or endothelial cells, stimulated by NO-inducers, demonstrated more elevated levels of γ-globin gene expression than in the erythroid cells only (Čokić et al., 2009). This observation suggests that NO could come out of the bone marrow stromal cells and diffuse into the erythroid progenitor cells largely participating in γ-globin gene induction, linked to stromal cells augmented capability for NO production. This supplemented NO production, in the hematopoietic microenvironment, has the potential to enhance HbF synthesis in erythroid progenitor cells, which still have low hemoglobin levels and presumably low scavenging activity. Accumulating evidence emphasized the involvement and important role of NO in the regulation of hematopoiesis (Krstić et al., 2009, 2010). Spleen is also an active hematopoietic organ where response of hematopoietic cells to cytokines depends on the tissue microenvironment (Jovčić et al., 2007). Improper signaling inside bone marrow stromal cells can lead to their failure and inconsistent microenvironmental niche for hematopoietic stem cells. It has been recently shown that basal NO/cGMP/cGMP-dependent protein kinase (PKG) activity is necessary for preserving bone marrow stromal cell survival and promoting cell proliferation and migration (Wong & Fiscus, 2011). Co-culture studies of human macrophages, as well as human bone marrow endothelial cell line, with erythroid progenitor cells resulted in induction of γ-globin mRNA expression in the presence of cytostatic hydroxyurea. NOS-dependent stimulation of NO by lipopolysaccharide and interferon-γ has been observed in human macrophages. In addition, lipopolysaccharide and interferon-γ together increased γ-globin gene expression in human macrophage/erythroid cell co-cultures (Čokić et al., 2009). These observations are in accord to the intimate contact between erythroid and stromal cells, effects and associations in physiological hematopoietic microenvironment. The endothelial cells as well as macrophages, normal components of bone marrow stroma, play an active role in the modulation of human hematopoietic stem cell growth (Ascensao et al., 1984; Davis et al., 1005; Hanspal & Hanspal, 2004). The murine endothelial cell lines also stimulate the proliferation and differentiation of erythroid precursors, where close cell contact is necessary for erythropoiesis (Ohneda & Bautch, 1997). Mice deficient in eNOS, expressed by bone marrow stromal cells, demonstrated a defect in progenitor cell mobilization (Aicher et al., 2003). Hemoglobin synthesis of erythroleukemia cells line was increased after co-culture with endothelial cells and monolayers of bone-marrow-derived macrophages, as well as with cell-free culture media conditioned by blood-monocyte-derived macrophages (Zuhrie et al., 1988). NO has also an important role in bone marrow angiogenesis, together with vascular endothelial growth factor (VEGF), with implications in patients with leukemic malignancies (Antic et al., 2010, 2011). NO-cGMP pathway stimulates the proliferation and osteoblastic differentiation of primary mouse bone marrow-derived mesenchymal stem cells and osteoblasts (Hikiji et al., 1997). NO donors, as well as proteasome inhibitors, inhibited cytokine induced intercellular adhesion molecule 1 (ICAM-1) and vascular cell adhesion molecule 1 (VCAM-1) expression (Cobb et al., 1996; De Caterina et al., 1995). The proteasome inhibition also significantly enhanced endothelial-dependent vasorelaxation of rat aortic rings (Stangl et al., 2004), as well as NO production in endothelial cells (Cokic et al., 2007).

5. Cyclic nucleotides induction of globin genes expression

5.1 NO/cGMP stimulation of γ-globin gene expression

We demonstrated that NO increases γ-globin gene expression in erythroid cells during differentiation. Inhibition of soluble guanylate cyclase (sGC) prevents NO-induced increase in γ-globin gene expression (Cokic et al., 2003). In addition, we have shown that the well known γ-globin gene inducer hydroxyurea stimulated HbF by the NO-dependent activation of sGC in human erythroid progenitor cells (Cokic et al., 2003). It has been shown that both sGC activators and cGMP induce γ-globin gene expression in human erythroleukemic cell line and primary erythroblasts (Ikuta et al., 2001). Therefore, intracellular pathway including sGC and PKG induced expression of the γ-globin gene (Ikuta et al., 2001). Moreover, it has been reported that hydroxyurea increased NOx levels and NOS-dependent γ-globin transcription in erythroleukemic and primary erythroid cells. This γ-globin gene activation demonstrated cGMP-dependence (Lou et al., 2009). We found that during human erythroid differentiation in vitro, eNOS mRNA and protein levels were initially high but then declined steadily, as did the production of NO derivatives, in contrast with steady elevation of hemoglobin levels, a potent scavenger of NO (Cokic et al., 2008). According to our previous results, hydroxyurea dose- and time-dependently induced rapid but transient activation of eNOS in endothelial cells (Cokic et al., 2006). Hydroxyurea stimulated NO production in endothelial cells, both as short and long term effects (Cokic et al., 2006, 2007). Chronic hydroxyurea therapy significantly increased NO, cGMP, and HbF levels in patients with sickle cell anemia (Nahavandi et al., 2002). cGMP levels were found to be significantly higher in red blood cells (RBCs) of sickle cell patients than in RBCs of normal individuals, and were further increased in RBCs of sickle cell patients on hydroxyurea therapy (Conran et al., 2004). NOS activity was also higher in RBCs of sickle cell disease patients on hydroxyurea therapy than in untreated patients (Iyamu et al., 2005). It is in accordance with results that l-arginine alone does not increase serum NOx production in steady-state patients, however it does when given together with hydroxyurea (Morris et al., 2003). Neither l-arginine alone nor l-arginine in combination with NOS inhibitor effected hydroxyurea-mediated induction of HbF synthesis in erythroid progenitors (Haynes et al., 2004). L-arginine did not change the suppression of burst forming unit-erythroid (BFU-E) colony growth and stimulation of HbF synthesis by hydroxyurea in erythroid progenitors (Baliga et al., 2010). Inhibition of NOS attenuated the hydroxyurea and l-arginine effects on BFU-E colony growth and HbF synthesis (Baliga et al., 2010), but did not decrease NOx production in RBCs during incubation with hydroxyurea (Nahavandi et al., 2006).

5.2 Nitric oxide synthase levels in red blood cells

It has been demonstrated that human RBCs contain iNOS and eNOS as well as calmodulin, suggesting that RBCs may synthesize its own NO (Jubelin & Gierman, 1996). This notion was supported by the observation that RBCs have an active eNOS protein (Chen & Mehta, 1998). Addition of l-arginine to RBCs stimulated NO production (measured as plasma nitrite) in a dose-dependent manner (Nahavandi et al., 2006), whereas it did not significantly change NOx levels (Chen & Mehta, 1998). However, it was later reported that RBCs possess iNOS and eNOS, but the proteins are without catalytic activity (Kang et al., 2000). Recent studies, revealed eNOS protein activity in the cytosol and in the internal side of membrane RBCs, serving essential regulatory functions for RBCs deformability and platelet aggregation (Kleinbongard et al., 2006). In vitro NOx production by RBCs (normal and sickle) is increased by treatment with hydroxyurea, but it's not decreased by NOS inhibition (Nahavandi et al., 2006). In difference to this result, we showed that hydroxyurea increased NO production via induction of eNOS activity in endothelial cells (Cokic et al., 2006). Thus, hydroxyurea may increase the plasma concentration of NO by combining endothelial cell NOS activity and interaction with oxy/deoxy hemoglobin in RBCs. We found previously that hydroxyurea increased cAMP and cGMP levels in human endothelial cells (Cokic et al., 2006), as well as NO levels via activation of eNOS and proteasome inhibition (Cokic et al., 2007). Previous reports indicated that cAMP elevation activated the L-arginine/NO system and induced vasorelaxation in rabbit femoral artery in vivo and human umbilical vein in vitro (Xu et al., 2000). It is known that agents that increase cAMP stimulate eNOS activity in human umbilical vein endothelial cells (Ferro et al., 1999). A recent report revealed that a rapid increase in endothelial NO production by bradykinin is mediated exclusively by PKA signaling pathway (Bae et al., 2003). PKA signaling acts by increasing phosphorylation of Ser1177 and dephosphorylation of Thr495 to activate eNOS (Michell et al., 2001). Shear stress stimulates phosphorylation of bovine eNOS at the corresponding serine in a PKA-dependent, but PKB/Akt-independent, manner, whereas NO production is regulated by the mechanisms dependent on both PKA and PKB/Akt (Boo et al., 2002).

5.3 A role of cAMP-dependent pathway in γ-globin gene induction

During erythroid differentiation adenylate cyclase and cAMP phosphodiesterase activity, as well as cellular cAMP concentrations, decline in a synchronized manner (Setchenska et al., 1981). The cAMP-dependent pathway plays a negative role in a γ-globin gene expression in K562 erythroleukemic cell line, in contrast to a cGMP positive role (Inoue et al., 2004). It has been also found that, upon activation of the cAMP pathway, expression of the γ-globin gene is induced in adult erythroblasts (Kuroyanagi et al., 2006). The subsequent study found that the cAMP-dependent pathway efficiently induced γ-globin expression in adult erythroblasts of beta-thalassaemia (Bailey et al., 2007). In patients with beta-thalassaemia intermedia, cAMP levels were elevated in both RBCs and nucleated erythroblasts but no consistent elevation was found with cGMP levels. The transcription factor cAMP response element binding protein (CREB) was phosphorylated in nucleated erythroblasts and its phosphorylation levels correlated with γ-globin gene expression of the patients (Bailey et al., 2007). According to previous study, guanylate cyclase inhibition minimally reduced HbF induction, whereas adenylate cyclase inhibition markedly decreased HbF induction by hydroxyurea in $CD34^{+}$-derived erythroid cells. Activation of the adenylate cyclase modestly induced HbF production, while hydroxyurea failed to significantly stimulate adenylate cyclase activity on days 7 to 10 of erythroid cells liquid culture (Keefer et al., 2006). However, in our cultures we found that in early erythroid progenitor cell cultures (day 4), hydroxyurea stimulated cAMP production (Cokic et al., 2008). It has been also postulated that cJun activates the $^{G}\gamma$-globin promoter via an upstream cAMP response element in a way equivalent to CREB1 (Kodeboyina et al., 2010).

5.4 Cyclic nucleotides interaction with phosphodiesterases

It has been shown that nitrite increased blood flow in the human circulation as well as vasodilatation of rat aortic rings. Formation of both NO gas and NO-modified hemoglobin resulted from the nitrite reductase activity of deoxyhemoglobin and deoxygenated erythrocytes levels (Cosby et al., 2003). Studies of nitrite activation of sGC demonstrated that nitrite alone activated sGC in solution (Jeffers et al., 2005). In our performed in vitro studies nitrite failed to induce cGMP, in purified form of sGC in solution, what confirmed a major role of NO molecule in hydroxyurea interaction with sGC (Cokic et al., 2008). It has been also demonstrated that eNOS is rapidly activated and phosphorylated on both Ser1177 and Thr495 in the presence of cGMP-dependent protein kinase II and the catalytic subunit of PKA in endothelial cells. These processes are more prominent in the presence of Ca^{2+}/calmodulin (Butt et al., 2000). The transient rises of cGMP levels induced by bradykinin and endothelin-1, which caused release of Ca^{2+} from internal stores, were similarly enhanced by activation of adenylate cyclase and increased cAMP levels. The cAMP seems to enhance NO formation, which depends on Ca^{2+} release from internal stores (Reiser, 1992). An elevated cGMP level attenuated the store-operated Ca^{2+} entry in vascular endothelial cells (Kwan et al., 2000). The cGMP-mediated $[Ca^{2+}]$i-reducing mechanisms may operate as a negative reaction to protect endothelial cells from the damaging effect of excessive $[Ca^{2+}]$i. The main targets of cGMP are phosphodiesterases (PDEs), resulting in interference with the cAMP-signaling pathway (Vaandrager & de Jonge, 1996). cAMP hydrolyzing PDE isozymes in endothelial cells are represented by PDE2 and PDE4 as cGMP-stimulated and cGMP-insensitive PDE, respectively. In endothelial cells, PDE4 inhibition may up-regulate basal production of NO, being supported by PDE2 inhibition (Lugnier et al., 1999). cGMP-inhibited PDE3 was expressed in K562 erythroleukemic cells at a high level (Inoue et al., 2004), while PDE3/4 inhibitor treatment reduced asymmetrical dimethylarginine, an endogenous NOS inhibitor, and elevated NO/cGMP levels (Pullamsetti et al., 2011). In addition, PDE9A gene expression is increased in $CD34^+$-derived erythroid cells and K562 erythroleukemic cells. Inhibition of PDE9A enzyme significantly increased production of the γ-globin gene in K562 cells (Almeida et al., 2008).

6. Nitric oxide-related therapy in hemoglobinopathies

NO inhibits HbS polymer formation and has anti-sickling properties. NO may disrupt HbS polymers by abolishing the excess positive charge of HbS, resulting in increased oxygen affinity in patients with sickle cell disease (Ikuta et al., 2011). In sickle cell disease, HbS polymerization and intravascular sickling lead to reperfusion injury, hemolysis, decreased NO bioavailability and oxidative stress. Increased expression of HbF decreased intravascular sickling, accompanied by decreased hemolysis, oxidative stress and increased NO metabolites (NOx) levels (Dasgupta et al., 2010). Nitrite can react similarly with adult oxy- and deoxy-hemoglobin (HbA), resulting in oxidative denitrosylation of nitrosyl-hemoglobin and rapid dissociation of NO. RBCs containing oxy-HbF (F-cells) had accelerated oxidative denitrosylation. So, induction of HbF present in sickle cell disease may enhance vasodilatation in addition to direct inhibition of polymerization of deoxy sickle hemoglobin (Salhany, 2008). The role of NO in erythrocyte function, sickle cell anemia, malaria, and damage to banked blood has been already reviewed, as well as the use of NO targeted therapies for erythrocyte disease (Maley et al., 2010). Pain from vaso-occlusive crisis is the major cause of hospitalization in patients with sickle cell disease, where beneficial therapeutic effects of inhaled NO have been demonstrated (Head et al., 2010). Decreased exhaled nitric oxide levels (FE_{NO}) have been described in patients with sickle cell disease, together with deficiency in plasma arginine. Additional study shows that sickle cell disease patients, with and without a history of acute chest syndrome, have similar FE_{NO} at baseline when compared with healthy controls (Sullivan et al., 2010).

The protecting effects of exogenous NO on murine cerebral malaria are associated with decreased brain vascular expression of inflammatory markers, ICAM-1 and P-selectin, resulting in attenuated endothelial damage and facilitating blood flow (Zanini et al., 2011). Previous reports demonstrated reduced NO levels in severe malaria related to impaired production of NO, reduced mononuclear cell iNOS expression and NOS substrate arginine (Anstey et al., 1996; Lopansri et al., 2003). Responsible factors for low NO levels in malaria include scavenging of NO by free hemoglobin and superoxide anion, and reduced levels of nitrate, a NO precursor molecule (Lopansri et al., 2003). Endothelial activation plays a central role in the pathogenesis of severe malaria with angiopoietin-2 as a key regulator. NO is a major inhibitor of angiopoietin-2 release from endothelium and has been shown to decrease endothelial inflammation and reduce the adhesion of parasitized RBCs. Low-flow inhaled NO is an attractive new candidate for the adjunctive treatment of severe malaria (Hawkes et al., 2011). Exhaled NO was also lower in severe malaria in comparison to moderately severe falciparum malaria and controls. Intravenous administration of l-arginine increased exhaled NO in moderately severe malaria (Yeo et al., 2007).

7. Conclusion: Nitric oxide and soluble guanylate cyclase

Besides direct stimulation of sGC in erythroid cells, NO is produced by stromal cells of bone marrow hematopoietic microenvironment. NOS enzymes in stromal cells are activated via PKA, supported by intracellular Ca^{2+} elevation. NO has been released into the intercellular space and then passed through the plasma membrane of erythroid cells, where it binds directly to ferrous-deoxy heme of sGC, activating the enzyme. Activation of NO-sGC increases conversion of GTP to cGMP, resulting in elevation of cGMP and subsequent activation of cGMP-dependent protein kinases (PKG) and cGMP-hydrolyzing PDEs. Activation of sGC and PKG increases expression of the γ-globin gene in erythroid cells. NO reduces cAMP levels in erythroid cells, whereas cAMP appears to enhance NO formation. The NO-mediated cAMP-reducing mechanisms may operate as a negative feedback in control of cAMP levels. In addition, cGMP enhances cAMP level and cAMP-signalling pathway by competing for the PDEs active site that has modest cyclic nucleotides selectivity (e.g., PDE3 isozymes). By this way, cGMP inhibits the activity of cAMP-specific PDE3, which results in the increase in intracellular cAMP levels and thereby leads to the activation of PKA. Activation of the cAMP-dependent pathway also induces expression of the γ-globin gene in erythroblasts. The phosphorylation levels of CREB correlated with elevated γ-globin gene expression. Moreover, inhibition of PDE9A enzyme significantly increases production of the γ-globin gene. Therefore, it appears that activation of the linked cGMP- and cAMP-signalling pathways regulates γ-globin expression.

Presented results contribute to the understanding of the significance of NO participation in γ-globin induction. These results should support future studies, with the emphasis focused on the hematopoietic microenvironment, in search of therapy of sickle cell disease. In addition to the possibility of NOS presence and activity in mature RBCs, our data show strong eNOS protein levels and function in more primitive human erythroid progenitor and precursor cells, where control of gene expression occurs. While mechanisms involved in globin gene expression have been recognized at different levels within the regulatory hierarchy, relations between molecular pathways are only emerging. Our presented microarray results demonstrated the broad gene expression profile and related pathways linked to stimulation of globin genes during ontogeny. The presented genes and signaling pathways, involved in the mechanism of globin genes activation, might be targets for therapeutic agents that upregulate γ-globin gene expression and HbF levels in hemoglobinopathies. This ontogenic overview linked to specific genes and transcriptional programs in normal erythropoiesis may contribute to further understanding of erythroid progenitor cell development.

8. Acknowledgments

This research was supported by the Intramural Research Program of the NIH and NIDDK and by grant from the Serbian Ministry of Education and Science (175053).

9. References

Aicher, A., Heeschen, C., Mildner-Rihm, C., Urbich, C., Ihling, C., Technau-Ihling, K., Zeiher, A.M., & Dimmeler, S. (2003). Essential role of endothelial nitric oxide synthase for mobilization of stem and progenitor cells. *Nature medicine*, Vol. 9, No. 11, (Nov 2003), pp.1370-1376, ISSN 1078-8956

Almeida, C.B., Traina, F., Lanaro, C., Canalli, A.A., Saad, S.T., Costa, F.F., & Conran, N. (2008). High expression of the cGMP-specific phosphodiesterase, PDE9A, in sickle cell disease (SCD) and the effects of its inhibition in erythroid cells and SCD neutrophils. *British journal of haematology*, Vol. 142, No. 5, (Sep 2008), pp. 836-844, ISSN 1365-2141

Anstey, N.M., Weinberg, J.B., Hassanali, M.Y., Mwaikambo, E.D., Manyenga, D., Misukonis, M.A., Arnelle, D.R., Hollis, D., McDonald, M.I., & Granger, D.L. (1996). Nitric oxide in Tanzanian children with malaria: inverse relationship between malaria severity and nitric oxide production/nitric oxide synthase type 2 expression. *The Journal of experimental medicine*, Vol. 184, No. 2, (Aug 1996), pp. 557-567, ISSN 0022-1007

Antic, D., Perunicic Jovanovic, M., Dencic Fekete, M., & Cokic, V.P. Assessment of bone marrow microvessel density in chronic lymphocytic leukemia. (2010). *Applied immunohistochemistry & molecular morphology*, Vol. 18, No. 4, (Jul 2010), pp. 353-356, ISSN 1533-4058

Antic, D., Mihaljevic, B., Cokic, V., Fekete, M.D., Djurasevic, T.K., Pavlovic, S., Milic, N., & Elezovic, I. (2011). Patients with early stage chronic lymphocytic leukemia: new risk stratification based on molecular profiling. *Leukemia & Lymphoma*, Vol. 524, No. 7, (Jul 2011), pp. 1394-1397, ISSN 1029-2403

Asano, H., Li, X.S., & Stamatoyannopoulos, G. (1999). FKLF, a novel Krüppel-like factor that activates human embryonic and fetal beta-like globin genes. *Molecular and cellular biology*, Vol. 19, No. 5, (May 1999), pp. 3571-3579, ISSN 0270-7306

Asano, H., Li, X.S., & Stamatoyannopoulos, G. (2000). FKLF-2: a novel Krüppel-like transcriptional factor that activates globin and other erythroid lineage genes. *Blood*, Vol. 95, No.6, (Jun 2000), pp.3578-3584, ISSN 0006-4971

Ascensao, J.L., Vercellotti, G.M., Jacob, H.S., & Zanjani, E.D. (1984). Role of endothelial cells in human hematopoiesis: modulation of mixed colony growth in vitro. *Blood*, Vol. 63, No. 3, (Mar 1984), pp. 553-558, ISSN 0006-4971

Azzouzi, I., Moest, H., Winkler, J., Fauchère, J.C., Gerber, A.P., Wollscheid, B., Stoffel, M., Schmugge, M., & Speer, O. (2011). MicroRNA-96 Directly Inhibits γ-Globin Expression in Human Erythropoiesis. *PLoS One*, Vol. 6, No.7, (2011), e22838, ISSN 1932-6203

Bae, S.W., Kim, H.S., Cha, Y.N., Park, Y.S., Jo, S.A., & Jo, I. (2003). Rapid increase in endothelial nitric oxide production by bradykinin is mediated by protein kinase A signaling pathway. *Biochemical and Biophysical Research Communications*, Vol. 306, No. 4, (Jul 2003), pp. 981-987, ISSN 0006-291X

Bailey, L., Kuroyanagi, Y., Franco-Penteado, C.F., Conran, N., Costa, F.F., Ausenda, S., Cappellini, M.D., & Ikuta, T. (2007). Expression of the gamma-globin gene is sustained by the cAMP-dependent pathway in beta-thalassaemia. *British Journal of Haematology*, Vol. 138, No. 3, (Aug 2007), pp. 382-395, ISSN 0007-1048

Baliga, B.S., Haynes, J. Jr, Obiako, B., & Mishra, N. (2010). Combined effects of arginine and hydroxyurea on BFU-E derived colony growth and HbF synthesis in erythroid progenitors isolated from sickle cell blood. *Cellular and Molecular Biology (Noisy-le-grand)*, Vol. 56, Suppl, (Jun 2010), pp. OL1290-1298, ISSN 1165-158X

Basu, P., Morris, P.E., Haar, J.L., Wani, M.A., Lingrel, J.B., Gaensler, K.M., & Lloyd, J.A. (2005). KLF2 is essential for primitive erythropoiesis and regulates the human and murine embryonic {beta}-like globin genes in vivo. *Blood*, Vol. 106, No. 7, (Oct 2005), pp. 2566-2571, ISSN 0006-4971

Beleslin-Cokic, B.B., Cokic, V.P., Yu, X., Weksler, B.B., Schechter, A.N., & Noguchi, C.T. (2004). Erythropoietin and hypoxia stimulate erythropoietin receptor and nitric oxide production by endothelial cells. *Blood*, Vol. 104, No. 7, (Oct 2004), pp. 2073-2080, ISSN 0006-4971

Beleslin-Cokic, B.B., Cokic, V.P., Wang, L., Piknova, B., Teng, R., Schechter, A.N., & Noguchi, C.T. (2011). Erythropoietin and hypoxia increase erythropoietin receptor and nitric oxide levels in lung microvascular endothelial cells. *Cytokine*, Vol. 54, No. 2, (May 2011), pp. 129-135, ISSN 1096-0023

Bianchi, N., Zuccato, C., Lampronti, I., Borgatti, M., & Gambari, R. (2009). Expression of miR-210 during erythroid differentiation and induction of gamma-globin gene expression. *BMB Reports*, Vol. 42, No. 8, (Aug 2009), pp. 493-499, ISSN 1976-6696

Bieker, J.J., & Southwood, C.M. (1995). The erythroid Kruppel-like factor transactivation domain is a critical component for cell-specific inducibility of a beta-globin promoter. *Molecular and Cellular Biology*, Vol. 15, No. 2, (Feb 1995), pp. 852-860, ISSN 0270-7306

Bogdan, C. (2001). Nitric oxide and the immune response. *Nature Immunology*, Vol. 2, No. 10, (Oct 2001), pp. 907-916, ISSN 1529-2908

Boo, Y.C., Sorescu, G., Boyd, N., Shiojima, I., Walsh, K., Du, J., & Jo, H. (2002). Shear stress stimulates phosphorylation of endothelial nitricoxide synthase at Ser1179 by Akt-independent mechanisms: role of protein kinase A. *The Journal of Biological Chemistry*, Vol. 277, No. 5, (Feb 2002), pp. 3388-3396, ISSN 0021-9258

Borg, J., Papadopoulos, P., Georgitsi, M., Gutiérrez, L., Grech, G., Fanis, P., Phylactides, M., Verkerk, A.J., van der Spek, P.J., Scerri, C.A., Cassar, W., Galdies, R., van Ijcken, W., Ozgür, Z., Gillemans, N., Hou, J., Bugeja, M., Grosveld, F.G., von Lindern, M., Felice, A.E., Patrinos, G.P., & Philipsen, S. (2010). Haploinsufficiency for the erythroid transcription factor KLF1 causes hereditary persistence of fetal hemoglobin. *Nature Genetics*, Vol. 42, No. 9, (Sep 2010), pp. 801-805, ISSN 1546-1718

Brüne, B., & Zhou, J. (2007). Hypoxia-inducible factor-1alpha under the control of nitric oxide. *Methods in Enzymology*, Vol. 435, (2007), pp. 463-478, ISSN 0076-6879

Butt, E., Bernhardt, M., Smolenski, A., Kotsonis, P., Fröhlich, L.G., Sickmann, A., Meyer, H.E., Lohmann, S.M., & Schmidt, H.H. (2000). Endothelial nitric-oxide synthase (type III) is activated and becomes calcium independent upon phosphorylation by cyclic nucleotide-dependent protein kinases. *The Journal of Biological Chemistry*, Vol. 275, No. 7, (Feb 2000), pp. 5179-5187, ISSN 0021-9258

Casteel, D., Suhasini, M., Gudi, T., Naima, R., & Pilz, R.B. (1998). Regulation of the erythroid transcription factor NF-E2 by cyclic adenosine monophosphate- dependent protein kinase. *Blood*, Vol. 91, No. 9, (May 1998), pp. 3193-3201, ISSN 0006-4971

Chen, L.Y., & Mehta, J.L. (1998). Evidence for the presence of L-arginine-nitric oxide pathway in human red blood cells: relevance in the effects of red blood cells on platelet function. *Journal of Cardiovascular Pharmacology*, Vol. 32, No. 1, (Jul 1998), pp. 57-61, ISSN 0160-2446

Chénais, B., Molle, I., & Jeannesson, P. (1999). Inhibitory effect of nitric oxide on chemically induced differentiation of human leukemic K562 cells. *Biochemical Pharmacology*, Vol. 58, No. 5, (Sep 1999), pp. 773-778, ISSN 0006-2952

Cheung, P., Allis, C.D., & Sassone-Corsi, P. Signaling to chromatin through histone modifications. *Cell*, Vol. 103, No. 2, (Oct 2000), pp. 263-271, ISSN 0092-8674

Choi, J.W., Pai, S.H., Kim, S.K., Ito, M., Park, C.S., & Cha, Y.N. Iron deficiency anemia increases nitric oxide production in healthy adolescents. *Annals of Hematology*, Vol. 81, No. 1, (Jan 2002), pp. 1-6, ISSN 0939-5555

Cobb, R.R., Felts, K.A., Parry, G.C., & Mackman, N. (1996). Proteasome inhibitors block VCAM-1 and ICAM-1 gene expression in endothelial cells without affecting nuclear translocation of nuclear factor-kappa B. *European Journal of Immunology*, Vol. 26, No. 4, (Apr 1996), pp. 839-845, ISSN 0014-2980

Cokic, V.P., Smith, R.D., Beleslin-Cokic, B.B., Njoroge, J.M., Miller, J.L., Gladwin, M.T., & Schechter, A.N. (2003). Hydroxyurea induces fetal hemoglobin by the nitric oxide-dependent activation of soluble guanylyl cyclase. *Journal of Clinical Investigation*, Vol. 111, No. 2, (Jan 2003), pp. 231-239, ISSN 0021-9738

Cokic, V.P., Beleslin-Cokic, B.B., Tomic, M., Stojilkovic, S.S., Noguchi, C.T., & Schechter, A.N. (2006). Hydroxyurea induces the eNOS-cGMP pathway in endothelial cells. *Blood*, Vol. 108, No. 1, (Jul 2006), pp. 184-191, ISSN 0006-4971

Cokic, V.P., Beleslin-Cokic, B.B., Noguchi, C.T., & Schechter, A.N. (2007). Hydroxyurea increases eNOS protein levels through inhibition of proteasome activity. *Nitric Oxide: Biology and Chemistry*, Vol. 16, No. 3, (May 2007), pp. 371-378, ISSN 1089-8603

Cokic, V.P., Andric, S.A., Stojilkovic, S.S., Noguchi, C.T., & Schechter, A.N. (2008). Hydroxyurea nitrosylates and activates soluble guanylyl cyclase in human erythroid cells. *Blood*, Vol. 111, No. 3, (Feb 2008), pp. 1117-1123, ISSN 0006-4971

Cokic, V.P., & Schechter, A.N. (2008). Effects of nitric oxide on red blood cell development and phenotype. *Current Topics in Developmental Biology*, Vol. 82, (2008), pp. 169-215, ISSN 0070-2153

Cokic, V.P., Beleslin-Cokic, B.B., Smith, R.D., Economou, A.P., Wahl, L.M., Noguchi, C.T., & Schechter, A.N. (2009). Stimulated stromal cells induce gamma-globin gene expression in erythroid cells via nitric oxide production. *Experimental Hematology*, Vol. 37, No. 10, (Oct 2009), pp. 1230-1237, ISSN 1873-2399

Conran, N., Oresco-Santos, C., Acosta, H.C., Fattori, A., Saad, S.T., & Costa, F.F. (2004). Increased soluble guanylate cyclase activity in the red blood cells of sickle cell patients. *British Journal of Haematology*, Vol. 124, No. 4, (Feb 2004), pp. 547-554, ISSN 0007-1048

Cosby, K., Partovi, K.S., Crawford, J.H., Patel, R.P., Reiter, C.D., Martyr, S., Yang, B.K., Waclawiw, M.A., Zalos, G., Xu, X., Huang, K.T., Shields, H., Kim-Shapiro, D.B., Schechter, A.N., Cannon, R.O. 3rd, & Gladwin, M.T. (2003). Nitrite reduction to nitric oxide by deoxyhemoglobin vasodilates the human circulation. *Nature Medicine*, Vol. 9, No. 12, (Dec 2003), pp. 1498-1505, ISSN 1078-8956

Dasgupta, T., Fabry, M.E., & Kaul, D.K. (2010). Antisickling property of fetal hemoglobin enhances nitric oxide bioavailability and ameliorates organ oxidative stress in transgenic-knockout sickle mice. *American Journal of Physiology*, Vol. 298, No. 2, (Feb 2010), R394-402, ISSN 1522-1490

Davis, T.A., Robinson, D.H., Lee, K.P., & Kessler, S.W. (1995). Porcine brain microvascular endothelial cells support the in vitro expansion of human primitive hematopoietic bone marrow progenitor cells with a high replating potential: requirement for cell-to-cell interactions and colony-stimulating factors. *Blood*, Vol. 85, No. 7, (Apr 1995), pp. 1751-1761, ISSN 0006-4971

De Caterina, R., Libby, P., Peng, H.B., Thannickal, V.J., Rajavashisth, T.B., Jr., Gimbrone, M.A., Shin, W.S., & Liao, J.K. (1995). Nitric oxide decreases cytokine induced endothelial activation. Nitric oxide selectively reduces endothelial expression of adhesion molecules and proinflammatory cytokines. *The Journal of Clinical Investigation*, Vol. 96, No. 1, (Jul 1995), pp. 60-68, ISSN 0021-9738

Donze, D., Townes, T.M., & Bieker, J.J. (1995). Role of erythroid Kruppel-like factor in human gamma- to beta-globin gene switching. *The Journal of Biological Chemistry*, Vol. 270, No. 4, (Jan 1995), pp. 1955-1959, ISSN 0021-9258

Dumitriu, B., Dy, P., Smits, P., & Lefebvre, V. (2006). Generation of mice harboring a Sox6 conditional null allele. *Genesis*, Vol. 44, No. 5, (May 2006), pp. 219-224, ISSN 1526-954X

Ferro, A., Queen, L.R., Priest, R.M., Xu, B., Ritter, J.M., Poston, L., Ward, J.P. (1999). Activation of nitric oxide synthase by beta 2-adrenoceptors in human umbilical vein endothelium in vitro. *British Journal of Pharmacology*, Vol. 126, No. 8, (Apr 1999), pp. 1872-1880, ISSN 0007-1188

Fujishima, N., Hirokawa, M., Aiba, N., Ichikawa, Y., Fujishima, M., Komatsuda, A., Suzuki, Y., Kawabata, Y., Miura, I., & Sawada, K. (2004). Gene expression profiling of human erythroid progenitors by micro-serial analysis of gene expression. *International Journal of Hematology*, Vol. 80, No. 3, (Oct 2004), pp. 239-245, ISSN 0925-5710

Gabbianelli, M., Testa, U., Morsilli, O., Pelosi, E., Saulle, E., Petrucci, E., Castelli, G., Giovinazzi, S., Mariani, G., Fiori, M.E., Bonanno, G., Massa, A., Croce, C.M., Fontana, L., & Peschle, C. (2010). Mechanism of human Hb switching: a possible role of the kit receptor/miR 221-222 complex. *Haematologica*, Vol. 95, No. 8, (Aug 2010), pp. 1253-1260, ISSN 1592-8721

Galarneau, G., Palmer, C.D., Sankaran, V.G., Orkin, S.H., Hirschhorn, J.N., & Lettre, G. (2010). Fine-mapping at three loci known to affect fetal hemoglobin levels explains additional genetic variation. *Nature Genetics*, Vol. 42, No. 12, (Dec 2010), pp. 1049-1051, ISSN 1546-1718

Gibbons, R.J., Picketts, D.J., Villard, L., & Higgs, D.R. (1995). Mutations in a putative global transcriptional regulator cause X-linked mental retardation with alpha-thalassemia (ATR-X syndrome). *Cell*, Vol. 80, No. 6, (Mar 1995), pp. 837-845, ISSN 0092-8674

Goh, S.H., Josleyn, M., Lee, Y.T., Danner, R.L., Gherman, R.B., Cam, M.C., & Miller, J.L. (2007). The Human Reticulocyte Transcriptome. *Physiological Genomics*, Vol. 30, No. 2, (Jul 2007), pp. 172-178, ISSN 1531-2267

Gregory, R.C., Taxman, D.J., Seshasayee, D., Kensinger, M.H., Bieker, J.J., & Wojchowski, D.M. (1996). Functional interaction of GATA1 with erythroid Krüppel-like factor and Sp1 at defined erythroid promoters. *Blood*, Vol. 87, No. 5, (Mar 1996), pp. 1793-1801, ISSN 0006-4971

Grosveld, F., van Assendelft, G.B., Greaves, D.R., & Kollias, G. (1987). Position-independent, high-level expression of the human beta-globin gene in transgenic mice. *Cell*, Vol. 51, No. 6, (Dec 1987), pp. 975-985, ISSN 0092-8674

Gubin, A.N., Njoroge, J.M., Bouffard, G.G., & Miller, J.L. (1999). Gene Expression in Proliferating Human Erythroid Cells. *Genomics*, Vol. 59, No. 2, (Jul 1999), pp. 168-177, ISSN 0888-7543

Guo-wei, Z., Rui-feng, Y., Xiang, L., Mitchell, W.J., De-pei, L., & Chih-chuan, L. (2010). NF-E2: a novel regulator of alpha-hemoglobin stabilizing protein gene expression. *Chinese Medical Sciences Journal*, Vol. 25, No. 4, (Dec 2010), pp. 193-198, ISSN 1001-9294

Hanspal, M., & Hanspal, J.S. (1994). The association of erythroblasts with macrophages promotes erythroid proliferation and maturation: a 30-kD heparin-binding protein is involved in this contact. *Blood*, Vol. 84, No. 10, (Nov 1994), pp. 3494-3504, ISSN 0006-4971

Harju-Baker, S., Costa, F.C., Fedosyuk, H., Neades, R., & Peterson, K.R. (2008). Silencing of Agamma-globin gene expression during adult definitive erythropoiesis mediated by GATA-1-FOG-1-Mi2 complex binding at the -566 GATA site. *Molecular and Cellular Biology*, Vol. 28, No. 10, (May 2008), pp. 3101-3113, ISSN 1098-5549

Hawkes, M., Opoka, R.O., Namasopo, S., Miller, C., Thorpe, K.E., Lavery, J.V., Conroy, A.L., Liles, W.C., John, C.C., & Kain, K.C. (2011). Inhaled nitric oxide for the adjunctive therapy of severe malaria: protocol for a randomized controlled trial. *Trials*, Vol. 12, (Jul 2011), pp. 176, ISSN 1745-6215

Haynes, J. Jr., Baliga, B.S., Obiako, B., Ofori-Acquah, S., & Pace, B. (2004). Zileuton induces hemoglobin F synthesis in erythroid progenitors: role of the L-arginine-nitric oxide signaling pathway. *Blood*, Vol. 103, No. 10, (May 2004), pp. 3945-3950, ISSN 0006-4971

He, X., Gonzalez, V., Tsang, A., Thompson, J., Tsang, T.C., & Harris, D.T. (2005). Differential Gene Expression Profiling of CD34+ CD133+ Umbilical Cord Blood Hematopoietic Stem Progenitor Cells. *Stem Cells and Development*, Vol. 14, No. 2, (Apr 2005), pp. 188-198, ISSN 1547-3287

Head, C.A., Swerdlow, P., McDade, W.A., Joshi, R.M., Ikuta, T., Cooper, M.L., & Eckman, J.R. (2010). Beneficial effects of nitric oxide breathing in adult patients with sickle cell crisis. *American Journal of Hematology*, Vol. 85, No. 10, (Oct 2010), pp. 800-802, ISSN 1096-8652

Higgs, D.R., Sharpe, J.A., & Wood, W.G. (1998). Understanding alpha globin gene expression: a step towards effective gene therapy. *Seminars in Hematology*, Vol. 35, No. 2, (Apr 1998), pp. 93-104, ISSN 0037-1963

Hikiji, H., Shin, W. S., Oida, S., Takato, T., Koizumi, T., & Toyo-oka, T. (1997). Direct action of nitric oxide on osteoblastic differentiation. *FEBS Letters*, Vol. 410, No. 2-3, (Jun 1997), pp. 238-242, ISSN 0014-5793

Ikuta, T., Ausenda, S., & Cappellini, M.D. (2001). Mechanism for fetal globin gene expression: role of the soluble guanylate cyclase-cGMP-dependent protein kinase pathway. *Proceedings of the National Academy of Sciences of the USA*, Vol. 98, No. 4, (Feb 2001), pp. 1847-1852, ISSN 0027-8424

Ikuta, T., Thatte, H.S., Tang, J.X., Mukerji, I., Knee, K., Bridges, K.R., Wang, S., Montero-Huerta, P., Joshi, R.M., & Head, C.A. (2011). Nitric oxide reduces sickle hemoglobin polymerization: potential role of nitric oxide-induced charge alteration in depolymerization. *Archives of Biochemistry and Biophysics*, Vol. 510, No. 1, (Jun 2011), pp. 53-61, ISSN 1096-0384

Inoue, A., Kuroyanagi, Y., Terui, K., Moi, P., & Ikuta, T. (2004). Negative regulation of gamma-globin gene expression by cyclic AMP-dependent pathway in erythroid cells. *Experimental Hematology*, Vol. 32, No. 3, (Mar 2004), pp. 244-253, ISSN 0301-472X

Iyamu, E.W., Cecil, R., Parkin, L., Woods, G., Ohene-Frempong, K., & Asakura, T. Modulation of erythrocyte arginase activity in sickle cell disease patients during hydroxyurea therapy. (2005). *British Journal of Haematology*, Vol. 131, No. 3, (Nov 2005), pp. 389-394, ISSN 0007-1048

Jeffers, A., Xu, X., Huang, K.T., Cho, M., Hogg, N., Patel, R.P., & Kim-Shapiro, D.B. (2005). Hemoglobin mediated nitrite activation of soluble guanylyl cyclase. *Comparative Biochemistry and Physiology. Part A, Molecular and Integrative Physiology*, Vol. 142, No. 2, (Oct 2005), pp. 130-135, ISSN 1095-6433

Jensen, M., Attemberg, H., Schneider, C.H., & Walter, J.U. (1982). The developmental change in the G gamma and A gamma globin proportions in hemoglobin F. *European Journal of Pediatrics*, Vol. 138, No. 4, (Jul 1982), pp. 311-314, ISSN 0340-6199

Jiang, J., Best, S., Menzel, S., Silver, N., Lai, M.I., Surdulescu, G.L., Spector, T.D.,& Thein, S.L. (2006). cMYB is involved in the regulation of fetal hemoglobin production in adults. *Blood*, Vol. 108, No. 3, (Aug 2006), pp. 1077-1083, ISSN 0006-4971

Jovcic, G., Bugarski, D., Krstic, A., Vlaski, M., Petakov, M., Mojsilovic, S., Stojanovic, N., & Milenkovic, P. (2007). The effect of interieukin-17 on hematopoietic cells and cytokine release in mouse spleen. *Physiological Research*, Vol. 56, No. 3, (2007), pp. 331-339, ISSN 0862-8408

Jubelin, B.C., & Gierman, J.L. (1996). Erythrocytes may synthesize their own nitric oxide. *American Journal of Hypertension*, Vol. 9, No. 12, (Dec 1996), pp. 1214-1219, ISSN 0895-7061

Kameoka, J., Yanai, N., & Obinata, M. (1995). Bone marrow stromal cells selectively stimulate the rapid expansion of lineage-restricted myeloid progenitors. *Journal of Cellular Physiology*, Vol. 164, No. 1, (Jul 1995), pp. 55-64, ISSN 0021-9541

Kang, E.S., Ford, K., Grokulsky, G., Wang, Y.B., Chiang, T.M., & Acchiardo, S.R. (2000). Normal circulating adult human red blood cells contain inactive NOS proteins. *Journal of Laboratory and Clinical Medicine*, Vol. 135, No. 6, (Jun 2000), pp. 444-451, ISSN 0022-2143

Keefer, J.R., Schneidereith, T.A., Mays, A., Purvis, S.H., Dover, G.J., & Smith, K.D. (2006). Role of cyclic nucleotides in fetal hemoglobin induction in cultured CD34+ cells. *Experimental Hematology*, Vol. 34, No. 9, (Sep 2006), pp. 1151-1161, ISSN 0301-472X

Kihm, A.J., Kong, Y., Hong, W., Russell, J.E., Rouda, S., Adachi, K., Simon, M.C., Blobel, G.A., & Weiss, M.J. (2002). An abundant erythroid protein that stabilizes free alpha-haemoglobin. *Nature*, Vol. 417, No. 6890, (Jun 2002), pp. 758-763, ISSN 0028-0836

Kleinbongard, P., Schulz, R., Rassaf, T., Lauer, T., Dejam, A., Jax, T., Kumara, I., Gharini, P., Kabanova, S., Ozuyaman, B., Schnurch, H.G., Godecke, A., Weber, A.A., Robenek, M., Robenek, H., Bloch, W., Rosen, P., & Kelm, M. (2006). Red blood cells express a functional endothelial nitric oxide synthase. *Blood*, Vol. 107, No. 7, (Apr 2006), pp. 2943-2951, ISSN 0006-4971

Kodeboyina, S., Balamurugan, P., Liu, L., & Pace, B.S. (2010). cJun modulates Ggamma-globin gene expression via an upstream cAMP response element. *Blood cells, molecules & diseases*, Vol. 44, No. 1, (Jan 2010), pp. 7-15, ISSN 1096-0961

Kovacevic-Filipovic, M., Petakov, M., Hermitte, F., Debeissat, C., Krstic, A., Jovcic, G., Bugarski, D., Lafarge, X., Milenkovic, P., Praloran, V., & Ivanovic, Z. (2007). Interleukin-6 (IL-6) and low O2 concentration (1%) synergize to improve the maintenance of hematopoietic stem cells (pre-CFC). *Journal of Cellular Physiology*, Vol. 212, No. 1, (Jul 2007), pp. 68-75, ISSN 0021-9541

Krstic, A., Ilic, V., Mojsilovic, S., Jovcic, G., Milenkovic, P., & Bugarski, D. (2009). p38 MAPK signaling mediates IL-17-induced nitric oxide synthase expression in bone marrow cells. *Growth Factors*, Vol. 27, No. 2, (Apr 2009), pp. 79-90, ISSN 1029-2292

Krstic, A., Vlaški, M., Hammoud, M., Chevaleyre, J., Duchez, P., Jovcic, G., Bugarski, D., Milenkovic, P., Bourin, P., Boiron, J.M., Praloran, V., & Ivanovic, Z. (2009). Low O2 concentrations enhance the positive effect of IL-17 on the maintenance of erythroid progenitors during co-culture of CD34+ and mesenchymal stem cells. *European Cytokine Network*, Vol. 20, No. 1, (Mar 2009), pp. 10-16, ISSN 1148-5493

Krstic, A., Santibanez, J.F., Okic, I., Mojsilovic, S., Kocic, J., Jovcic, G., Milenkovic, P., & Bugarski, D. (2010). Combined effect of IL-17 and blockade of nitric oxide biosynthesis on haematopoiesis in mice. *Acta Physiologica (Oxford, England)*, Vol. 199, No. 1, (May 2010), pp. 31-41, ISSN 1748-1716

Kucukkaya, B., Ozturk, G., & Yalcintepe, L. (2006). Nitric oxide levels during erythroid differentiation in K562 cell line. *Indian Journal of Biochemistry and Biophysics*, Vol. 43, No. 4, (Aug 2006), pp. 251-253, ISSN 0301-1208

Kuroyanagi, Y., Kaneko, Y., Muta, K., Park, B.S., Moi, P., Ausenda, S., Cappellini, M.D., & Ikuta, T. (2006). cAMP differentially regulates gamma-globin gene expression in erythroleukemic cells and primary erythroblasts through c-Myb expression. *Biochemical and Biophysical Research Communications*, Vol. 344, No. 3, (Jun 2006), pp. 1038-1047, ISSN 0006-291X

Kwan, H.Y., Huang, Y., & Yao, X. (2000). Store-operated calcium entry in vascular endothelial cells is inhibited by cGMP via a protein kinase G-dependent mechanism.*The Journal of Biological Chemistry*, Vol. 275, No. 10, (Mar 2000), pp. 6758-6763, ISSN 0021-9258

Leonard, M., Brice, M., Engel, J.D., & Papayannopoulou T. (1993). Dynamics of GATA transcription factor expression during erythroid differentiation. *Blood*, Vol. 82, No. 4, (Aug 1993), pp. 1071-1079, ISSN 0006-4971

Lodish, H.F., & Jacobsen, M. (1972). Regulation of hemoglobin synthesis. Equal rates of translation and termination of-and-globin chains. *The Journal of Biological Chemistry*, Vol. 247, No. 11, (Jun 1972), pp. 3622-3629, ISSN 0021-9258

Lopansri, B.K., Anstey, N.M., Weinberg, J.B., Stoddard, G.J., Hobbs, M.R., Levesque, M.C., Mwaikambo, E.D., & Granger, D.L. (2003). Low plasma arginine concentrations in children with cerebral malaria and decreased nitric oxide production. *Lancet*, Vol. 361, No. 9358, (Feb 2003), pp. 676-678, ISSN 0140-6736

Lou, T.F., Singh, M., Mackie, A., Li, W., & Pace, B.S. (2009). Hydroxyurea generates nitric oxide in human erythroid cells: mechanisms for gamma-globin gene activation. *Experimental Biology and Medicine (Maywood)*, Vol. 234, No. 11, (Nov 2009), pp. 1374-1382, ISSN 1535-3699

Lu, J., Guo, S., Ebert, B.L., Zhang, H., Peng, X., Bosco, J., Pretz, J., Schlanger, R., Wang, J.Y., Mak, R.H., Dombkowski, D.M., Preffer, F.I., Scadden, D.T., & Golub, T.R. (2008). MicroRNA-mediated control of cell fate in megakaryocyte-erythrocyte progenitors. *Developmental Cell*, Vol. 14, No. 6, (Jun 2008), pp. 843-853, ISSN 1878-1551

Lugnier, C., Keravis, T., & Eckly-Michel, A. (1999). Cross talk between NO and cyclic nucleotide phosphodiesterases in the modulation of signal transduction in blood vessel. *Journal of Physiology and Pharmacology*, Vol. 50, No. 4, (Dec 1999), pp. 639-652, ISSN 0867-5910

Maciejewski, J. P., Selleri, C., Sato, T., Cho, H. J., Keefer, L. K., Nathan, C. F., & Young, N. S. (1995). Nitric oxide suppression of human hematopoiesis in vitro. Contribution to inhibitory action of interferon-gamma and tumor necrosis factor-alpha. *The Journal of Clinical Investigation*, Vol. 96, No. 2, (Aug 2005), pp.1085-1092, ISSN 0021-9738

Majka, M., Janowska-Wieczorek, A., Ratajczak, J., Ehrenman, K., Pietrzkowski, Z., Kowalska, M.A., Gewirtz, A.M., Emerson, S.G., & Ratajczak, M.Z. (2001). Numerous growth factors, cytokines, and chemokines are secreted by human CD34(+) cells, myeloblasts, erythroblasts, and megakaryoblasts and regulate normal hematopoiesis in an autocrine/paracrine manner. *Blood*, Vol. 97, No. 10, (May 2001), pp. 3075-3085, ISSN 0006-4971

Maley, J.H., Lasker, G.F., & Kadowitz, P.J. (2010). Nitric oxide and disorders of the erythrocyte: emerging roles and therapeutic targets. *Cardiovascular & hematological disorders drug targets*, Vol. 10, No. 4, (Dec 2010), pp. 284-291, ISSN 1871-529X

Michell, B.J., Chen, Z., Tiganis, T., Stapleton, D., Katsis, F., Power, D.A., Sim, A.T., & Kemp, B.E. (2001). Coordinated control of endothelial nitric-oxide synthase phosphorylation by protein kinase C and the cAMP dependent protein kinase. The *Journal of biological chemistry,* Vol. 276, No. 21, (May 2001), pp. 17625-17628, ISSN 0021-9258

Migliaccio, G., Migliaccio, A.R., Petti, S., Mavilio, F., Russo, G., Lazzaro, D., Testa, U., Marinucci, M., & Peschle, C. (1986). Human embryonic hemopoiesis. Kinetics of progenitors and precursors underlying the yolk sac-liver transition. *The Journal of Clinical Investigation,* Vol. 78, No. 1, (Jul 1986), pp. 51-60, ISSN 0021-9738

Miller, I.J., & Bieker, J.J. (1993). A novel, erythroid cell-specific murine transcription factor that binds to the CACCC element and is related to the Krüppel family of nuclear proteins. *Molecular and cellular biology,* Vol.13, No. 5, (May 1993), pp. 2776-2786, ISSN 0270-7306

Morris, C.R., Vichinsky, E.P., van Warmerdam, J., Machado, L., Kepka-Lenhart, D., Morris, S.M. Jr, & Kuypers, F.A. (2003). Hydroxyurea and arginine therapy: impact on nitric oxide production in sickle cell disease. *Journal of pediatric hematology/oncology,* Vol. 25, No. 8, (Aug 2003), pp. 629-634, ISSN 1077-4114

Nahavandi, M., Tavakkoli, F., Wyche, M.Q., Perlin, E., Winter, W.P., & Castro, O. (2002). Nitric oxide and cyclic GMP levels in sickle cell patients receiving hydroxyurea. *British journal of haematology,* Vol. 119, No. 3, (Dec 2002), pp. 855-857, ISSN 0007-1048

Nahavandi, M., Tavakkoli, F., Millis, R.M., Wyche, M.Q., Habib, M.J., & Tavakoli, N. (2006) Effects of hydroxyurea and L-arginine on the production of nitric oxide metabolites in cultures of normal and sickle erythrocytes. *Hematology,* Vol. 11, No. 4, (Aug 2006), pp. 291-294, ISSN 1607-8454

Ng, Y.Y., van Kessel, B., Lokhorst, H.M., Baert, M.R., van den Burg, C.M., Bloem, A.C., & Staal, F.J. (2004). Gene-expression profiling of CD34+ cells from various hematopoietic stem-cell sources reveals functional differences in stem cell activity. *Journal of leukocyte biology,* Vol. 75, No. 2, (Feb 2004), pp. 314-323, ISSN 0741-5400

Nienhuis, A.W., & Benz, E.J. (1977). Regulation of hemoglobin synthesis during the development of the red cell. *The New England journal of medicine,* Vol. 297, No. 24, (Dec 1977), pp. 1318-1328, ISSN 0028-4793

Noh, S.J., Miller, S.H., Lee, Y.T., Goh, S.H., Marincola, F.M., Stroncek, D.F., Reed, C., Wang, E., & Miller, J.L. (2009). Let-7 microRNAs are developmentally regulated in circulating human erythroid cells. *Journal of translational medicine,* Vol. 7:98, (Nov 2009), ISSN 1479-5876

Oh, I.H., Lau, A., & Eaves, C.J. (2000). During ontogeny primitive (CD34+CD38-) hematopoietic cells show altered expression of a subset of genes associated with early cytokine and differentiation responses of their adult counterparts. *Blood,* Vol. 96, No. 13, (Dec 2000), pp. 4160-4168, ISSN 0006-4971

Ohneda, O., & Bautch, V.L. (1997). Murine endothelial cells support fetal liver erythropoiesis and myelopoiesis via distinct interactions. *British journal of haematology,* Vol. 98, No. 4, (Sep 1997), pp. 798-808, ISSN 0007-1048

Orkin, S.H. (1992). GATA-binding transcription factors in hematopoietic cells. *Blood,* Vol. 80, No. 3, (Aug 1992), pp. 575-581, ISSN 0006-4971

Pazin, M.J., & Kadonaga, J.T. (1997). What's up and down with histone deacetylation and transcription? *Cell*, Vol. 89, No. 3, (May 1997), pp. 325-328, ISSN 0092-8674

Perrine, S.P., Mankidy, R., Boosalis, M.S., Bieker, J.J., & Faller, D.V. (2009). Erythroid Kruppel-like factor (EKLF) is recruited to the gamma-globin gene promoter as a co-activator and is required for gamma-globin gene induction by short-chain fatty acid derivatives. *European journal of haematology*, Vol. 82, No. 6, (Jun 2009), pp. 466-476, ISSN 1600-0609

Persons, D.A., Allay, J.A., Allay, E.R., Ashmun, R.A., Orlic, D., Jane, S.M., Cunningham, J.M., & Nienhuis, A.W. (1999). Enforced expression of the GATA-2 transcription factor blocks normal hematopoiesis. *Blood*, Vol. 93, No. 2, (Jan 1999), pp. 488-499, ISSN 0006-4971

Peschle, C., Migliaccio, A.R., Migliaccio, G., Petrini, M., Calandrini, M., Russo, G., Mastroberardino, G., Presta, M., Gianni, A.M., & Comi, P. (1984). Embryonic fetal Hb switch in humans: studies on erythroid bursts generated by embryonic progenitors from yolk sac and liver. *Proceedings of the National Academy of Sciences of the USA*, Vol. 81, No. 8, (Apr 1984), pp. 2416-2420, ISSN 0027-8424

Pevny, L., Lin, C.S., D'Agati, V., Simon, M.C., Orkin, S.H., & Costantini, F. (1995). Development of hematopoietic cells lacking transcription factor GATA-1. *Development*, Vol. 121, No. 1, (Jan 1995), pp. 163-172, ISSN 0950-1991

Pruzina, S., Hanscombe, O., Whyatt, D., Grosveld, F., & Philipsen, S. (1991). Hypersensitive site 4 of the human beta globin locus control region. *Nucleic acids research*, Vol. 19, No. 7, (Apr 1991), pp. 1413-1419, ISSN 0305-1048

Pullamsetti, S.S., Savai, R., Schaefer, M.B., Wilhelm, J., Ghofrani, H.A., Weissmann, N., Schudt, C., Fleming, I., Mayer, K., Leiper, J., Seeger, W., Grimminger, F., & Schermuly, R.T. (2011). cAMP phosphodiesterase inhibitors increases nitric oxide production by modulating dimethylarginine dimethylaminohydrolases. *Circulation*, Vol. 123, No. 11, (Mar 2011), pp. 1194-1204, ISSN 1524-4539

Ramakrishnan, V., & Pace, B.S. (2011). Regulation of γ-globin gene expression involves signaling through the p38 MAPK/CREB1 pathway. *Blood cells, molecules & diseases*, Vol. 47, No. 1, (Jun 2011), pp. 12-22, ISSN 1096-0961

Ratajczak, J., Majka, M., Kijowski, J., Baj, M., Pan, Z.K., Marquez, L.A., Janowska-Wieczorek, A., & Ratajczak, M.Z. (2001). Biological significance of MAPK, AKT and JAK-STAT protein activation by various erythropoietic factors in normal human early erythroid cells. *British journal of haematology*, Vol. 115, No.1, (Oct 2001), pp. 195-204, ISSN 0007-1048

Reiser, G. (1992). Nitric oxide formation caused by Ca^{2+} release from internal stores in neuronal cell line isenhanced by cyclic AMP. *European journal of pharmacology*, Vol. 227, No. 1, (Sep 1992), pp. 89-93, ISSN 0014-2999

Risinger, J.I., Maxwell, G.L., Chandramouli, G.V., Aprelikova, O., Litzi, T., Umar, A., Berchuck, A., & Barrett, J.C. (2003). Microarray analysis reveals distinct gene expression profiles among different histologic types of endometrial cancer. *Cancer research*, Vol. 63, No. 1, (Jan 2003), pp. 6-11, ISSN 0008-5472

Rogers, H.M., Yu, X., Wen, J., Smith, R., Fibach, E., & Noguchi, C.T. (2008). Hypoxia alters progression of the erythroid program. *Experimental hematology*, Vol. 36, No. 1, (Jan 2008), pp. 17-27, ISSN 0301-472X

Salhany, J.M. (2010). Reaction of nitrite with human fetal oxyhemoglobin: a model simulation study with implications for blood flow regulation in sickle cell disease (SCD). *Blood cells, molecules & diseases*, Vol. 44, No. 2, (Apr 2010), pp111-114, ISSN 1096-0961

Sankaran, V.G., Menne, T.F., Xu, J., Akie, T.E., Lettre, G., Van Handel, B., Mikkola, H.K., Hirschhorn, J.N., Cantor, A.B., & Orkin, S.H. (2008). Human fetal hemoglobin expression is regulated by the developmental stage-specific repressor BCL11A. *Science*, Vol. 322, No. 5909, (Dec 2008), pp. 1839-1842, ISSN 1095-9203

Setchenska, M.S., Arnstein, H.R., & Vassileva-Popova, J.G. (1981). Cyclic AMP phosphodiesterase activity during differentiation of rabbit erythroid bone marrow cells. *The Biochemical journal*, Vol. 196, No. 3, (Jun 1981), pp. 887-892, ISSN 0264-6021

Shami, P.J., & Weinberg, J.B. (1996). Differential effects of nitric oxide on erythroid and myeloid colony growth from CD34+ human bone marrow cells. *Blood*, Vol. 87, No. 3, (Feb 1996), pp. 977-982, ISSN 0006-4971

Stamatoyannopoulos, G. (2005). Control of globin gene expression during development and erythroid differentiation. *Experimental hematology*, Vol. 33, No. 3, (Mar 2005), pp. 259-271, ISSN 0301-472X

Stangl, V., Lorenz, M., Meiners, M., Ludwig, A., Bartsch, C., Moobed, M., Vietzke, A., Kinkel, H.T., Baumann, G., & Stangl, K. (2004). Long-term up-regulation of eNOS and improvement of endothelial function by inhibition of the ubiquitin-proteasome pathway. *The FASEB journal*, Vol. 18, No. 2, (Feb 2004), pp. 272-279, ISSN 1530-6860

Steidl, U., Kronenwett, R., Rohr, U.P., Fenk, R., Kliszewski, S., Maercker, C., Neubert, P., Aivado, M., Koch, J., Modlich, O., Bojar, H., Gattermann, N., & Haas, R. (2002). Gene expression profiling identifies significant differences between the molecular phenotypes of bone marrow-derived and circulating human CD34+ hematopoietic stem cells. *Blood*, Vol. 99, No. 6, (Mar 2002), pp. 2037-2044, ISSN 0006-4971

Su, K.H., Shyue, S.K., Kou, Y.R., Ching, L.C., Chiang, A.N., Yu, Y.B., Chen, C.Y., Pan, C.C., & Lee, T.S. (2011). β common receptor integrates the erythropoietin signaling in activation of endothelial nitric oxide synthase. *Journal of cellular physiology*, (Feb 2011), doi: 10.1002/jcp.22678, ISSN 1097-4652

Suhasini, M., Boss, G.R., Pascual, F.E., & Pilz, R.B. (1995). Nitric oxide-releasing agents and cGMP analogues inhibit murine erythroleukemia cell differentiation and suppress erythroid-specific gene expression: correlation with decreased DNA binding of NF-E2 and altered c-myb mRNA expression. *Cell growth & differentiation*, Vol. 6, No. 12, (Dec 1995), pp. 1559-1566, ISSN 1044-9523

Sullivan, K.J., Kissoon, N., Sandler, E., Gauger, C., Froyen, M., Duckworth, L., Brown, M., & Murphy, S. (2010). Effect of oral arginine supplementation on exhaled nitric oxide concentration in sickle cell anemia and acute chest syndrome. *Journal of pediatric hematology/oncology*, Vol. 32, No. 7, (Oct 2010), pp. 249-258, ISSN 1536-3678

Tamura, K., Sudo, T., Senftleben, U., Dadak, A.M., Johnson, R., & Karin, M. (2000). Requirement for p38α in erythropoietin expression: a role for stress kinases in erythropoiesis. *Cell*, Vol. 102, No. 2, (Jul 2000), pp. 221-231, ISSN 0092-8674

Tanimoto, K., Liu, Q., Grosveld, F., Bungert, J., & Engel, J.D. (2000). Context dependent EKLF responsiveness defines the developmental specificity of the human epsilon-globin gene in erythroid cells of YAC transgenic mice. *Genes & development*, Vol. 14, No. 21, (Nov 2000), pp. 2778-2794, ISSN 0890-9369

Tsang, A.P., Visvader, J.E., Turner, C.A., Fujiwara, Y., Yu, C., Weiss, M.J., Crossley, M., & Orkin, S.H. (1997). FOG, a multitype zinc finger protein, acts as a cofactor for transcription factor GATA-1 in erythroid and megakaryocytic differentiation. *Cell*, Vol. 90, No. 1, (Jul 1997), pp. 109-119, ISSN 0092-8674

Vaandrager, A.B., & de Jonge, H.R. (1996). Signalling by cGMP-dependent protein kinases. *Molecular and cellular biochemistry*, Vol. 157, No. 1-2, (Apr 1996), pp. 23-30, ISSN 0300-8177

Vakoc, C.R., Letting, D.L., Gheldof, N., Sawado, T., Bender, M.A., Groudine, M., Weiss, M.J., Dekker, J., & Blobel. G.A. (2005). Proximity among distant regulatory elements at the beta-globin locus requires GATA-1 and FOG-1. *Molecular cell*, Vol. 17, No. 3, (Feb 2005), pp. 453-462, ISSN 1097-2765

Wen, J., Huang, S., Rogers, H., Dickinson, L.A., Kohwi-Shigematsu, T., & Noguchi, C.T. (2005). SATB1 family protein expressed during early erythroid differentiation modifies globin gene expression. *Blood*, Vol. 105, No. 8, (Apr 2005), pp. 3330-3339, ISSN 0006-4971

Wong, J.C., & Fiscus, R.R. (2011). Essential roles of the nitric oxide (no)/cGMP/protein kinase G type-Iα (PKG-Iα) signaling pathway and the atrial natriuretic peptide (ANP)/cGMP/PKG-Iα autocrine loop in promoting proliferation and cell survival of OP9 bone marrow stromal cells. *Journal of cellular biochemistry*, Vol. 112, No. 3, (Mar 2011), pp. 829-39, ISSN 1097-4644

Xu, B., Li, J., Gao, L., & Ferro, A. (2000). Nitric oxide-dependent vasodilatation of rabbit femoral artery by beta(2)-adrenergic stimulation or cyclic AMP elevation in vivo. *British journal of pharmacology*. Vol. 129, No. 5, (Mar 2000), pp. 969-974, ISSN 0007-1188

Xu, J., Sankaran, V.G., Ni, M., Menne, T.F., Puram, R.V., Kim, W., & Orkin, S.H. (2010). Transcriptional silencing of {gamma}-globin by BCL11A involves long-range interactions and cooperation with SOX6. *Genes & development*. Vol. 24, No. 8, (Apr 2010), pp. 783-798, ISSN 1549-5477

Yeo, T.W., Lampah, D.A., Gitawati, R., Tjitra, E., Kenangalem, E., McNeil, Y.R., Darcy, C.J., Granger, D.L., Weinberg, J.B., Lopansri, B.K., Price, R.N., Duffull, S.B., Celermajer, D.S., & Anstey, N.M. (2007). Impaired nitric oxide bioavailability and L-arginine reversible endothelial dysfunction in adults with falciparum malaria. *The Journal of experimental medicine*, Vol. 204, No. 11, (Oct 2007), pp. 2693-2704, ISSN 1540-9538

Zanini, G.M., Cabrales, P., Barkho, W., Frangos, J.A., & Carvalho, L.J. (2011). Exogenous nitric oxide decreases brain vascular inflammation, leakage and venular resistance during Plasmodium berghei ANKA infection in mice. *Journal of neuroinflammation*. (Jun 2011) Vol. 8, pp 66, ISSN 1742-2094

Zhou, D., Liu, K., Sun, C.W., Pawlik, K.M., & Townes, T.M. (2010). KLF1 regulates BCL11A expression and gamma- to beta-globin gene switching. *Nature genetics*, Vol 42, No 9, (Sep 2010), 742-744, ISSN 1546-1718.

Zhu, J., Chin, K., Aerbajinai, W., Trainor, C., Gao, P., & Rodgers, G.P. (2011). Recombinant erythroid Kruppel-like factor fused to GATA1 up-regulates delta- and gamma-globin expression in erythroid cells. *Blood*, Vol. 117, No 11, (Mar 2011), pp. 3045-3052 ISSN 1528-0020

Zuhrie, S.R., Pearson, J.D., & Wickramasinghe, S.N. (1988). Haemoglobin synthesis in K562 erythroleukaemia cells is affected by intimate contact with monolayers of various human cell types. *Leukemia research*, Vol. 12, No. 7, (Nov 1988), pp.567-574, ISSN 0145-2126

6

Mechanisms of αIIbβ3 Biogenesis in the Megakaryocyte: A Proteomics Approach

Amanda Chen[1], Haiqiang Yu[2], Haiteng Deng[2] and W. Beau Mitchell[1]
[1]Laboratory of Platelet Biology, New York Blood Center
[2]Proteomics Resources Center, The Rockefeller University
USA

1. Introduction

Platelets play a central role in hemostasis and thrombosis, initiating clot formation in response to vessel wall damage. Platelet aggregates are formed at sites of injury by the binding and crosslinking of the integrin αIIbβ3 to fibrinogen, von Willebrand factor and other soluble ligands. Platelets also form pathological thrombi, and the resulting arterial occlusion can lead to myocardial infarction or stroke. Inhibition of αIIbβ3 binding can decrease the formation of pathologic thrombi, and αIIbβ3 has become an important pharmacological target. Anti-αIIbβ3 therapies have been highly successful in preventing death following myocardial infarction and percutaneous arterial stent placement.(Topol, Lincoff et al. 2002; De Luca, Ucci et al. 2009) However, attempts to design novel, orally available anti-αIIbβ3 agents have been hampered by what appears to be paradoxical activation of αIIbβ3 by the drug, in some cases leading to an increased risk of mortality in patients who received the drug.(Quinn, Plow et al. 2002)

A novel approach to manipulating αIIbβ3 would be to perturb its post-translational processing and trafficking within the megakaryocyte, prior to platelet formation. Like most membrane proteins, αIIbβ3 is formed by concerted processes of protein sorting and trafficking. Some of the mechanisms underlying αIIbβ3 biogenesis and expression in megakaryocytes have been described, such as the calnexin cycle of protein quality control.(King and Reed 2002; Tiwari, Italiano et al. 2003; El.Golli, Issertial et al. 2005; Lo, Li et al. 2005) Clues to the stringent protein quality control of αIIbβ3 biogenesis come from the study of patients with defective or absent αIIbβ3, who manifest the mucocutaneous bleeding disorder Glanzmann thrombasthenia. A subset of patients with mutations in the αIIb gene produce full-length αIIb that retains the ability to form a complex with β3 but is retained within the cell and degraded, resulting in disease. These patients demonstrate the existence of stringent quality control mechanisms acting post-translationally to control αIIbβ3 biogenesis and expression. A clearer understanding of these mechanisms may lead to new possibilities of anti-integrin therapy.

Toward the goal of identifying proteins involved in αIIbβ3 biogenesis we performed a proteomic analysis of proteins interacting with αIIb in megakaryocytes cultured from human umbilical cord blood (UCB) and in HEK293 cells expressing αIIb and β3.

Megakaryocyte proteins were captured by poly-histidine tagged αIIb, or by photoreactive crosslinking followed by immunoprecipitation with anti-αIIb mAbs, and analyzed by mass spectrometry.

The αIIb and b3 subunits are synthesized as a single-chain precursors in the chaperone-rich folding environment of the endoplasmic reticulum (ER) (Fig 1). The precursor αIIb, pro-αIIb, is glycosylated under control of the calnexin cycle of protein folding. The β3 precursor is also glycosylated but does not appear to interact with the calnexin cycle. The two precursors heterodimerize to briefly form pro-αIIbβ3, and then pro-αIIb is cleaved by one or more members of the furin family of proteases in the Golgi. Cleavage of pro-αIIb to mature αIIb marks the exit of αIIb from the ER, and this cleavage occurs only when pro-αIIb is in complex with β3.(Bray, Rosa et al. 1986; Rosa and McEver 1989) Both αIIb and β3 are synthesized in excess of what will finally be processed to mature αIIbβ3. The calnexin cycle exerts stringent quality control over αIIb production and up to one half of all pro-αIIb is targeted to the proteasome for degradation in megakaryocytes. Excess β3 is degraded by a non-proteasomal mechanism. Inhibition of the proteasome in megakaryocytes resulted in a build-up of pro-αIIb that was not being degraded, but had no apparent effect on the level of mature αIIb in the αIIbβ3 complex. Thus, the expression level of mature αIIbβ3 is not simply a result of the stoichiometry of production vs. degradation. Rather there appears to be a concerted mechanism that controls how much pro-αIIbβ3 will be converted into mature αIIbβ3, and this mechanism is not grossly responsive to excessive levels of pro-αIIb or β3.

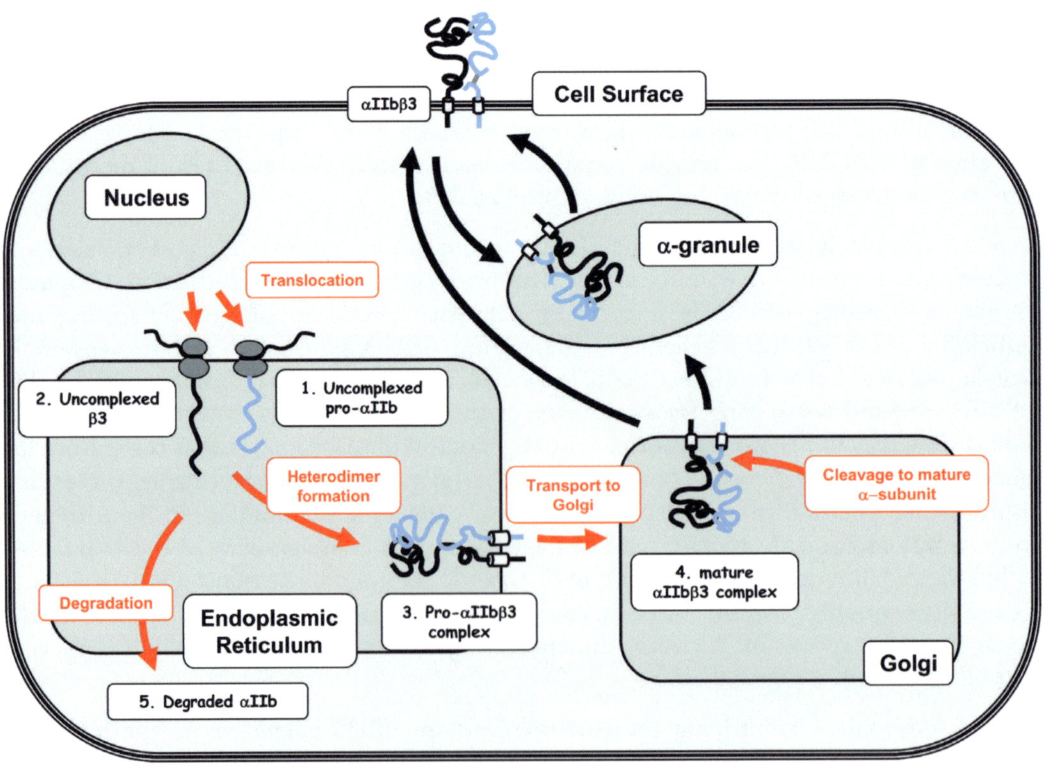

Fig. 1. Biogenesis of αIIbβ3

We hypothesized that whatever proteins underlie this mechanism must be interacting with pro-αIIb and/or pro-αIIbβ3 complex, but not with the mature αIIbβ3 complex. We chose a proteomics approach to identify these interacting proteins. In order to enrich our assay for proteins that preferentially bound pro-αIIb or pro-αIIbβ3, we used an αIIb subunit harboring R858G and R859G mutations that eliminates furin cleavage and traps αIIb in its pro-αIIb form.(Kolodziej, Vilaire et al. 1991) This αIIbR858G/R859G construct can form a complex with β3, but only in small amounts compared to normal αIIbβ3. In addition, while some of the mutant αIIbβ3 complexes reach the cell surface and can mediate adherence to immobilized fibrinogen, the proportion of αIIbR858G/R859G reaching the surface is very small compared to normal αIIb.(Kolodziej, Vilaire et al. 1991) Thus, αIIbR858G/R859G is a "nearly normal" mutant αIIb subunit that is primarily retained within the cell, making it a useful bait to capture the proteins involved in that process.

The hsp40 type chaperone protein, DNAJC10, was captured by both the normal αIIb and αIIbR858G/R859G subunits, and was evaluated as a putative αIIb interacting protein.. We report that DNAJC10 interacted with pro-αIIb and β3 in megakaryocytes, and appears to promote the degradation of pro-αIIb. Notably, while αIIbβ3-DNAJC10 interaction was evident in megakaryocytes, specific interaction was not detectable in HEK293 cells transfected with αIIb cDNA, suggesting megakaryocyte specificity. Knockdown of DNAJC10 by siRNA increased αIIbβ3 surface expression in UCB derived megakaryocytes, indicating that DNAJC10 negatively regulates αIIbβ3 surface expression. Thus, DNAJC10-αIIb interaction represents a novel post-translational mechanism regulating αIIbβ3 surface expression.

2. Materials and methods

2.1 Antibodies

The antibodies used in this study were: 10E5 (anti-αIIbβ3 complex); B1B5 (anti-αIIb);7H2 and B36 (anti-β3) (all 4 generous gifts from Dr Barry Coller); CA3 (anti-αIIb), anti-V5 epitope, and anti-Myc epitope (all three Millipore, Temecula,CA); anti-DNAJC10 (Genetex, Irvine, CA); M148 (anti-αIIb) (Santa Cruz Biotechnology, Santa Cruz, CA); mouse IgG, and rabbit IgG (both Jackson ImmunoResearch Inc, West Grove, PA).

2.2 Human Umbilical Cord Blood culture

This study used human UCB from the US National Cord Blood Bank that was deemed not suitable for clinical use due to low white blood cell number. Mothers who donate their UCB to the National Cord Blood Bank sign a consent giving permission to donate the UCB to research if it is inadequate for clinical use and will be discarded. Because the donated units are completely de-identified and are not collected prospectively specifically for research, the New York Blood Center Institutional Review Board (IRB), which oversees research ethics at the National Cord Blood Bank, considers their use exempt from IRB review. Human UCB was prepared as previously described.(Mitchell, Li et al. 2006) Briefly, leukocytes were separated from 1-3 units of human UCB judged to be inadequate for clinical purposes (generously provided by the New York Blood Center) by Dextran 70 sedimentation (Amersham Biosciences, Piscataway, NJ) for 1h, and then enriched for CD34+ progenitor cells by negative selection using a combination of antibodies against maturation/lineage-specific markers (RosetteSep, StemCell Technologies, Vancouver, BC) concomitant with density sedimentation using Ficoll-Paque Plus (Amersham Biosciences, Piscataway, NJ). These cells were cultured in serum-free medium (StemCell Technologies, Vancouver, BC) with 50 ng/ml thrombopoietin (TPO) plus 1 ng/ml SCF (both Millipore, Temecula,CA) for 3 days in 10 cm dishes in a 37°C incubator. At this point a portion of the cells will have died. The remaining living population of larger cells was gently washed and replated in fresh media with the same cytokines in 10 cm dishes and left until use (Day 8 or 9). Fresh media was added on day 6. We have previously reported that under these conditions the UCB differentiate into a population of large cells with > 90% expressing αIIbβ3, > 80% expressing GPIb, about 50% expressing α2β1.(Mitchell, Li et al. 2007) For experimental use the cells were gently harvested, pelleted at 300 rpm for 5 min, or let settle by gravity, and gently resuspended in the appropriate buffer.

2.3 HEK293 cell culture

HEK293 cell lines (American Type Culture Collection (ATCC), Manassas, VA) that stably expressed human αIIbβ3 receptors were established as previously described.(Mitchell, Li et al. 2006) Transfections were performed using Lipofectamine 2000 (Gibco-BRL, Carlsbad, CA) according to the manufacturer's instructions, followed by selection in media containing 500 μg/ml G418 for 2-4 weeks. To obtain a population of cells uniformly expressing high levels of αIIbβ3, cells were labeled with the mAb 10E5 (anti-αIIbβ3) and sorted using a MoFlo cell sorter (Beckman Coulter, Fullerton, CA).

2.4 Immunoprecipitation and biosynthetic labeling

Samples were prepared as previously described and all steps were performed on ice unless otherwise stated.(Mitchell, Li et al. 2006) Briefly, cells (either day 8 megakaryocytes derived from UCB cells or HEK293 cells) were lysed in 1% Brij 98 lysis buffer containing protease inhibitors and 20uM N-methylmaleimide (NEM). Lysates were precleared with protein-G Sepharose beads (Amersham Biosciences, Piscataway, NJ), and then equivalent amounts of protein, usually 400 μg, were incubated one h at 4°C with one or more of the antibodies listed above (4 μg/reaction). Samples were incubated with protein-G Sepharose beads for one h at 4°C, washed twice, and incubated with SDS sample buffer for 10 min at 100°C. Reduced samples contained 10% beta mercaptoethanol (Sigma, Thermo Scientific, Rockford, IL). Samples were subjected to SDS-PAGE on 7% gels, and the gels were either stained for mass spectrometry identification (described below) or transferred to PVDF membranes for immunoblotting. Non-specific binding was determined by performing parallel immunoprecipitation with mouse or rabbit IgG in each experiment. In preliminary experiments, the production of αIIbR858G/R859G and β3 was confirmed in the transfected HEK293 cell line by immunoprecipitation with both anti-αIIb and anti-β3 mAbs followed by immunoblot. For biosynthetic labeling, cells were incubated for 30 min at 37°C in methionine/cysteine-free medium, followed by pulse-labeling for 15 min at 37°C in medium containing ^{35}S-methionine/cysteine (300 μCi/10 cm plate). The pulse was terminated by incubation in medium containing unlabeled methionine/cysteine (1 mg/ml each) and the cells were incubated at 37 °C until lysis in 1% Triton-X 100 lysis buffer. Following cell lysis, supernatants were prepared as above. Gels were dried and exposed to film. For inhibition of the proteasome cells were incubated in the proteasome inhibitor MG132 (10 μM)(Sigma_Aldrich, St Louis, MO) in normal growth medium at 37C and then immediately lysed.

2.5 Histidine-tag/Nickel bead pulldown assay

HEK293 cells expressing poly-histidine tagged αIIb cDNA (in vector pEF1/V5-His) and β3 cDNA (in vector pcDNA3.1)(Mitchell, Li et al. 2007) were lysed in 1% Triton, 150 mM NaCl, 10 mM imidazole buffer (lysis buffer) on ice for 30 m, centrifuged for 30m at 4C, and then the supernatant was reacted with 50 μl of a 6:4 slurry of Ni beads:imidazole buffer (Qiagen, Inc. Valencia, CA) to bind the histidine-tagged subunits to the nickel beads. After incubating for 30 m the beads were washed four times with 10 mM imidazole lysis buffer by using a magnetic chamber to isolate the beads. Next, fresh whole cell lysates (1 mL) of UCB-derived megakaryocytes in 1% Triton, 150 mM NaCl, 10 mM imidazole buffer were incubated with the washed, Ni-bound αIIb for 1 h, and then the beads were washed twice with 1 mL lysis buffer containing 20 mM imidazole. Ni-bound proteins were eluted with 250 mM imidazole and the entire eluate was subjected to SDS-PAGE on a 7% gel followed by staining with Imperial Stain (Pierce, Thermo Scientific, Rockford, IL). Control experiments were run in parallel in which no megakaryocyte lysate was added to the beads, but all other steps remained the same. These controls aimed to identify the remaining HEK293 cell proteins still bound to either the beads or to αIIb after the washing steps, before incubation with megakaryocyte lysate. Experimental and control gels were run simultaneously, and the lanes were excised and analyzed by mass spectrometry.

2.6 Photocrosslinking amino acids

UCB cells were cultured as described above for eight days, then were washed and incubated for 24 hours in leucine- and methionine- free medium containing photoreactive methionine and leucine, dialyzed FBS (both Pierce, Thermo Scientific, Rockford, IL), and 50 ng/ml TPO (Millipore, Temecula,CA). The cells were exposed to 345 nm UV light for 15 minutes to crosslink the photoreactive amino acids, and harvested immediately, according to manufacturer's instructions. Whole cell lysates were immunoprecipitated with antibodies specific for αIIb or β3, and the proteins were separated by SDS-PAGE using the same protocol as for the histidine-tag affinity capture. Controls were simultaneously immunoprecipitated with non-immune IgG. Experimental and control lanes were excised and analyzed by mass spectrometry.

2.7 RNAi

HEK293 cells stably expressing high levels of αIIb and β3 were transfected with 100 nM siRNA duplexes (Dharmacon, Thermo Scientific, Rockford, IL and Qiagen, Valencia, CA) using Dharmafect-1 reagent (Dharmacon, Thermo Scientific, Rockford, IL), then analyzed by flow cytometry using a FacsCanto (Becton Dickenson,) at 48-96 h after transfection. Cultured UCB cells were transfected twice, on culture days 3 and 5, with 100 nM of siRNA duplexes or controls also using Dharmafect-1 reagent, and then analyzed 48 - 72 h later by flow cytometry. In order to identify individual transfected cells by FACS, cells were co-transfected with 10 nM of fluorescent-labeled non-coding siRNA (Qiagen, Valencia, CA). In some experiments, Cy3-labeled siRNA duplexes were used (Dharmacon, Thermo Scientific, Rockford, IL). Controls were: no treatment, transfection reagent but no siRNA duplex, Cy3-labeled negative control siRNA duplex only (Qiagen), siControl non targeting siRNA duplex, and siRNA duplex against cyclophillin B (positive control) (both Dharmacon).

2.8 Quantitative RT-PCR

For analysis of RNA content, cells were collected in RNAlater (Applied Biosystems, Foster City, CA) and RNA was purified using the RNEasy mini kit (Qiagen, Valencia, CA). For some analyses, siRNA transfected cells were sorted for expression of the fluorescent marker using a MoFlo sorter, and the sorted cells were subjected to QRT-PCR. Analysis was performed on an ABI 7900 or an ABI 7700 thermocycler/ fluorescence analyzer (Applied Biosystems, Foster City, CA) using the SYBR green probe (Qiagen or Invitrogen) and Quantitect primer assays (Qiagen). Relative mRNA levels were calculated using the ΔΔCt method that corrects for GAPDH expression in all samples. Fold-reduction was corrected for percent transfection in each experiment.

2.9 Immunofluorescence analysis

Mks were cytospun onto poly L-lysine-coated glass coverslips and fixed in methanol for 5 minutes at RT. Cells were then washed with saponin buffer (PBS containing 0.02% BSA, 0.005% saponin), then blocked with saponin buffer for 1 hour at RT. Cells were then incubated with the primary antibody diluted in saponin buffer for 1 hour at RT. After washing with PBS, cells were incubated with the appropriate conjugated secondary antibody in PBS for 1 hour at RT. Specimens were mounted with Prolong gold (Invitrogen). Images were acquired using a Zeiss LSM 510 META (Axiovert 200M Inverted Microscope Stand) confocal laser scanning microsope through a 100x objective. Each set of staining conditions was repeated 3 times. Background fluorescence was measured by incubating fixed cells with the secondary antibody only and then acquiring images with the exact settings used to obtain the experimental images.

2.10 Mass spectrometry data analysis

The protein gel bands were excised from the SDS-PAGE. The gel bands were reduced with 10 mM of DTT and alkylated with 55 mM iodoacetamide, and then digested with Sequence Grade Modified Trypsin (Promega, Madison, Wisconsin) in ammonium bicarbonate buffer at 37° overnight.(Kumarathasan, Mohottalage et al. 2005) The digestion products were extracted twice with 0.1% trifluoroacetic acid and 50% Acetonitrile and 1.0% trifluoroacetic acid respectively. The extracted mixture was dried by Speed-Vac and redisolved in 10 μL 0.1% trifluoroacetic acid. Half of the extracts were injected by LC-MS/MS analysis. For LC-MS/MS analysis, each digestion product was separated by a 60 min gradient elution with the Dionex U3000 capillary/nano-HPLC system (Dionex, Sunnyvale, California) at a flow rate of 0.250 μL/min that is directly interfaced with the Thermo-Fisher LTQ-Obritrap mass spectrometer (Thermo Fisher, San Jose, California) operated in data-dependent scan mode. The analytical column was a home-made fused silica capillary column (75 μm ID, 100 mm length; Upchurch, Oak Harbor, Washington) packed with C-18 resin (300 A, 5 μm, Varian, Palo Alto, California). Mobile phase A consisted of 0.1% formic acid, and mobile phase B consisted of 100% acetonitrile and 0.1% formic acid. The 60 min gradients with 250 nL/min flow rate for B solvent went from 0 to 55% in 34 minutes and then in 4 min to 80%. The B solvent stayed at 80% for another 8 min and then decreased to 5% in 8 min. Another 6 min was used for equilibration, loading and washing. The mass acquisition method was one FT-MS scan followed by 6 subsequent MS/MS scan in the ion trap. The FT-MS scan was acquired at resolution 30,000 in the Orbi-trap. The six most intense peaks from the FT full scan were selected in the ion trap for MS/MS. The selected ions were excluded for further selection for 180 seconds. The following search parameters were used in all MASCOT searches: maximum of 1 missed trypsin cleavages, cysteine carbamidomethylation, methionine oxidation. The maximum error tolerance for MS scans was 10 ppm for MS and 1.0 Da for MS/MS respectively. Proteins were designated as "hits" if they matched at least 2 distinctive peptides with a MASCOT score of at least 40. For proteins matching the same sets of peptides, only the protein with the greater percentage of coverage was selected. In the one case where 2 isoforms could not be distinguished (HSP70A/B), both proteins are reported. Proteins identified in the control gels were considered "negative," and these proteins were removed from further analysis. The interaction data were further analyzed using the Cytoscape(Cline, Smoot et al. 2007) software and publically available protein interaction databases (e.g. INTACT, NCBI, UniProt) to generate a network of first-degree interactions with αIIb. The network was further expanded to include proteins that were previously reported to interact with αIIb and known interactions between any of the proteins identified in our primary assays.

2.11 Statistical analysis

Flow cytometry data was summarized as the geographic mean fluorescence intensity (MFI) of antibody binding, and normalized to the MFI of control siRNA treated cells, so that the experimental MFI is expressed as a percentage of the control MFI. The overall percent change of the replicates was expressed as the average percent change +/- the confidence interval. The two-sided, paired t-test was used to determine whether there were differences in antibody binding between the different experimental groups. In the siRNA experiments, relative mRNA levels were calculated using the ΔΔCt method that corrects for GAPDH expression.

3. Results

3.1 The αIIb interactome

Proteins putatively interacting with αIIb were isolated from UCB derived megakaryocytes and from HEK293 cells expressing αIIbβ3, and these proteins were analyzed by mass spectrometry. Samples were processed by the two methods depicted in **Figure 2**. In the first method, recombinant αIIb or αIIbR858G/R859G subunits bearing a polyhistidine tag were expressed in HEK293 cells along with normal β3. The cells were lysed with 1% Triton buffer, and the lysates were reacted with Ni beads that bind polyhistidine. The Ni beads were washed using a magnetic separator to reduce non-specific binding to the Ni-bound αIIb, and then incubated with fresh whole cell lysate of umbilical cord blood derived megakaryocyte. Since we are interested in the early process of αIIbβ3 formation and intracellular trafficking we used megakaryocytes at day 8 or 9 of culture; at that point in our system αIIbβ3 is highly expressed but there is not yet any proplatelet formation. The Ni-bound histidine-tagged αIIb and αIIb-bound proteins were washed twice and then were eluted from the Ni beads with 250 mM imidazole in a 1% Triton buffer. Simultaneous control experiments were performed without megakaryocyte lysate in order to identify proteins non-specifically binding to either the Ni beads or the polyhistidine tag. The proteins thus collected were separated by one dimensional SDS-PAGE on a 7% gel. After staining, the experimental and control lanes were cut out and analyzed by mass spectrometry. This entire process was repeated in three separate experiments with normal αIIb, and in four separate experiments with αIIbR858G/R859G.

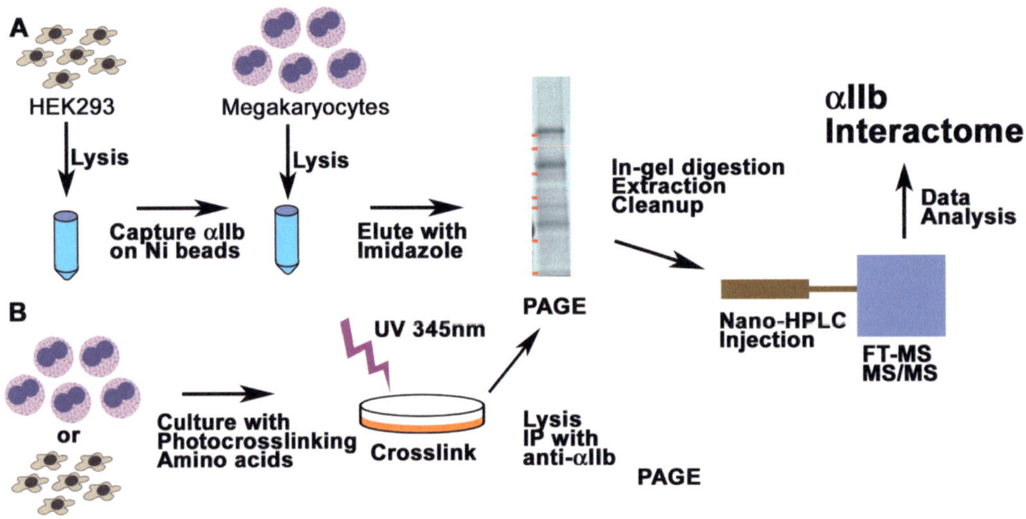

Fig. 2. Methods used to isolate and identify αIIb-interacting proteins. A): Polyhistidine-tagged αIIb subunits were captured on Ni beads and then incubated with whole cell lysate of day 8 UCB-derived megakaryocytes. Protein complexes thus captured were processed as described in the text, and then the proteins were identified by FT-MS and MS/MS. B) Crosslinking experiments were performed on day 8 UCB-derived megakaryocytes and transfected HEK293 cells. Cells were fed photoactivatable methionine and leucine, exposed to UV light and lysed immediately. Samples were processed for mass spectrometry as described.

The second strategy used photo-activated amino acids to crosslink αIIb to its binding partners (**Figure 2B**). UCB-derived megakaryocytes were starved for methionine and leucine, then fed photo-activatable methionine and leucine overnight, and then exposed to UV light to crosslink the amino acids of neighboring proteins. The megakaryocytes were immediately lysed and the αIIb-bound proteins were immunoprecipitated by anti-αIIb mAb. These proteins were separated by one dimensional SDS-PAGE and then the appropriate bands were cut out and analyzed by mass spectrometry. Because we were looking only for proteins crosslinked to αIIb, only the portions of the bands with $M_r > 120$ (M_r of the mature αIIb subunit) were analyzed. Five separate crosslinking experiments were performed with UCB-derived megakaryocytes and two on HEK293 cells expressing αIIbR858G/R859G and normal β3.

Minimum criteria for protein inclusion in data analysis were at least 2 distinctive peptides with a MASCOT score of at least 40, and absence of the protein in the control lanes. Importantly, since we were interested in proteins that are more abundant in the megakaryocyte than in HEK293 cells, even proteins known to interact with αIIbβ3, such as talin, were removed from the final results because they were present in the control lanes. Proteins identified in the Ni bead extraction experiments that are known to harbor natural polyhistidine sequences (such as the DEAH boxes) that could independently bind to the Ni beads were also excluded. Combining the results of both methods, 98 proteins were identified as potentially interacting with the normal αIIb subunit, and 79 proteins were identified as putatively interacting with the αIIbR858G/R859G subunit (Table 1). These 163 proteins putatively constitute a portion of the αIIb interactome, a network of protein-protein interactions relevant to the trafficking and function of αIIb in megakaryocytes (**Figure 3**).

Proteins Captured with αIIbR858G/R859G

Gene Symbol	Entrez Gene ID	SwissProt Acc No.	Protein Acc No.	Description	# Pep	% Cov	#. Expt
MYH9	4627	P35579 Q60FE2	gi|12667788	MYOSIN, HEAVY POLYPEPTIDE 9, NON-MUSCLE	70	45	4
LMNA	4000	P02545	gi|5031875	LAMIN A/C	37	61	3
HNRNPL*	3191	P14866 A6NIT8 Q6NTA2	gi|11527777	HETEROGENEOUS NUCLEAR RIBONUCLEOPROTEIN L	33	53	4
STIM1	6786	Q13586	gi|21070997	STROMAL INTERACTION MOLECULE 1	28	46	2
CKAP4	10970	Q07065	gi|19920317	CYTOSKELETON-ASSOCIATED PROTEIN 4	27	55	2
HSP90AB1	3326	P08238	gi|154146191	HEAT SHOCK PROTEIN 90kDa ALPHA, CLASS A MEMBER 1	21	36	1
SF3A1	10291	Q15459	gi|53831995	SPLICING FACTOR 3A, SUBUNIT 1, 120kDa	16	32	1
HSPA1A*	3303	B3KTT5 P08107 A8K5I0	gi|5123454	HEAT SHOCK 70kDa PROTEIN 1A	15	34	3
ATXN2L*	11273	Q8WWM7 A8K1R6	gi|119572372	ATAXIN 2-LIKE	14	20	2
MYH10	4628	Q6PK16 P35580 Q9BWG0	gi|41406064	MYOSIN, HEAVY POLYPEPTIDE 10, NON-MUSCLE	13	9	1
DNAJC10*	54431	Q8IXB1	gi|24308127	DNAJ (HSP40) HOMOLOG, SUBFAMILY C, MEMBER 10	13	21	3
PSPC1	55269	Q8WXF1	gi|109240550	PARASPECKLE COMPONENT 1	13	35	3
SFPQ	6421	P23246 Q86VG2	gi|119627829	SPLICING FACTOR PROLINE/GLUTAMINE-RICH (POLYPYRIMIDINE TRACT BINDING PROTEIN ASSOCIATED)	12	35	1
SF1*	7536	Q14820	gi|42544123	SPLICING FACTOR 1	12	20	2

		Q15637					
HSPA5*	3309	P11021	gi|119608027	HEAT SHOCK 70kDa PROTEIN 5 (GLUCOSE-REGULATED PROTEIN, 78kDa)	11	37	4
HLF2	4057	P02788	gi|16198357	LACTOTRANSFERRIN	11	30	1
MYH11	4629	P35749 Q3MNF1 Q3MIV8 Q3MNF0	gi|119574312	MYOSIN, HEAVY POLYPEPTIDE 11	11	9	1
LTBP1	4052	Q14766 B7ZLY3	gi|46249414	LATENT TRANSFORMING GROWTH FACTOR BETA BINDING PROTEIN 1	10	8	2
PKM2*	5315	P14618	gi|127795697	PYRUVATE KINASE, MUSCLE	10	28	1
RAVER1*	125950	Q8IY67	gi|123173757	RAVER1	10	29	2
XIRP2	129446	A4UGR9	gi|61696134	CARDIOMYOPATHY ASSOCIATED 3	10	16	1
ABCF1	23	Q8NE71 Q2L6I2 A2BF75	gi|21759807	ATP-BINDING CASSETTE, SUB-FAMILY F (GCN20), MEMBER 1	9	14	1
POTEF	728378	A5A3E0	gi|153791352	POTE ANKYRIN DOMAIN FAMILY, F	9	8	1
HSP90AA1	3320	P07900 Q86SX1	gi|153792590	HEAT SHOCK PROTEIN 90kDa ALPHA, CLASS A MEMBER 1	8	13	3
ITGA2B*	3674	P08514	gi|119571981	INTEGRIN, ALPHA 2B (PLATELET GLYCOPROTEIN IIB OF IIB/IIIA COMPLEX, ANTIGEN CD41)	8	17	2
TF*	7018	Q06AH7 P02787	gi|110590597	TRANSFERRIN	8	18	2
SAP 62	8175	A0PJA6	gi|21361376	SPLICING FACTOR 3A, SUBUNIT 2, 66kDa	8	19	1
LYZ	4069	Q05DF2 Q15428	gi|4930023	LYSOZYME (RENAL AMYLOIDOSIS)	7	70	1
SMAD4	4089	P61626 B2R4C5 Q13485	gi|4885457	SMAD, MOTHERS AGAINST DPP HOMOLOG 4 (DROSOPHILA)	7	12	2
HSP90B1	7184	P14625	gi|4507677	HEAT SHOCK PROTEIN 90kDa BETA (GRP94), MEMBER 1	7	12	2
CANX	821	P27824	gi|10716563	CALNEXIN	6	13	1
LRP2	4036	Q7Z5C1 P98164 Q7Z5C0	gi|32816595	LOW DENSITY LIPOPROTEIN-RELATED PROTEIN 2	6	1	1
CCT3	7203	A6NE14 P49368 B3KX11	gi|14124984	CHAPERONIN CONTAINING TCP1, SUBUNIT 3 (GAMMA)	6	21	2
HSPA1L	3305	P34931	gi|21759781	HEAT SHOCK 70kDa PROTEIN 1-LIKE	5	15	2
NCL	4691	P19338	gi|189306	NUCLEOLIN	5	6	1

		B3KM80					
PIP	5304	P12273	gi|4505821	PROLACTIN-INDUCED PROTEIN	5	31	1
SLPI	6590	P03973	gi|4507065	SECRETORY LEUKOCYTE PEPTIDASE INHIBITOR	5	28	1
TPM1	7168	P09493 Q9Y427 O15513	gi|854189	TROPOMYOSIN 1 (ALPHA)	5	10	1
HECTD1	25831	Q9ULT8	gi|118498337	HECT DOMAIN CONTAINING 1	5	5	3
LACRT	90070	Q9GZZ8	gi|15187164	LACRITIN	5	30	1
ACTG3	71	P63261	gi|178045		4	12	1
DMBT1	1755	Q9UGM3	gi|169218264	DELETED IN MALIGNANT BRAIN TUMORS 1	4	11	1
FLG	2312	P20930	gi|62122917	FILAGGRIN	4	2	1
HNRNPK	3190	P61978 Q6IBN1	gi|55958544	HETEROGENEOUS NUCLEAR RIBONUCLEOPROTEIN K	4	11	2
HSPA8*	3312	B3KTV0 P11142	gi|5729877	HEAT SHOCK 70kDa PROTEIN 8	4	8	1
KPNB1	3837	Q14974	gi|119615215	KARYOPHERIN (IMPORTIN) BETA 1	4	8	1
LCN1	3933	P31025	gi|4504963	LIPOCALIN 1	4	30	1
LMAN1*	3998	P49257	gi|5031873	LECTIN, MANNOSE-BINDING, 1	4	15	1
PRSS2	5645	P07478 Q5NV56	gi|74353564	PROTEASE, SERINE, 2 (TRYPSIN 2)	4	15	1
ALDH18A1	5832	P54886	gi|76779856	ALDEHYDE DEHYDROGENASE 18 FAMILY, MEMBER A1	4	5	1
NPM3	10360	O75607	gi|5801867	NUCLEOPHOSMIN/NUCLEOPLASMIN, 3	4	12	1
WAC	51322	Q9BTA9	gi|55664165	WW DOMAIN CONTAINING ADAPTOR WITH COILED-COIL	4	5	1
ANKRD24	170961	Q8TF*21	gi|16418357	ANKYRIN REPEAT DOMAIN 24	4	5	1
CALM1	801	Q96HY3 P62158 B4DJ51	gi|61680528	CALMODULIN	3	18	1
COL7A1	1294	Q02388 Q59F16	gi|119585300	COLLAGEN, TYPE VII, ALPHA 1 (EPIDERMOLYSIS BULLOSA, DYSTROPHIC, DOMINANT AND RECESSIVE)	3	1	1
HSPD1	3329	P10809	gi|14326412	HEAT SHOCK 60kDa PROTEIN 1	3	15	2
ME2	4200	P23368 Q9BWL6	gi|5822326	MALIC ENZYME 2, NAD(+)-DEPENDENT	3	5	2
PEX1	5189	O43933	gi|4505725	PEROXISOMAL BIOGENESIS FACTOR 1	3	2	1
PRKAA1	5562	Q13131	gi|29124503	PROTEIN KINASE, AMP-ACTIVATED, ALPHA 1	3	5	1

				CATALYTIC SUBUNIT			
H6PD	9563	O95479	gi|51859374	HEXOSE-6-PHOSPHATE DEHYDROGENASE (GLUCOSE 1-DEHYDROGENASE)	3	3	2
PDIA4	9601	Q549T6 P13667	gi|37182276	PROTEIN DISULFIDE ISOMERASE FAMILY A, MEMBER 4	3	2	1
COLEC10	10584	Q9Y6Z7	gi|5453619	COLLECTIN SUB-FAMILY MEMBER 10 (C-TYPE LECTIN)	3	12	1
FOXJ3	22887		gi|114555879	FORKHEAD BOX J3	3	4	1
ARS2	51593	Q9BXP5	gi|33150698	ARS2 PROTEIN	3	5	1
FOXJ2	55810	Q9P0K8	gi|8923842	FORKHEAD BOX J2	3	4	1
UBAP2	55833	Q5T6F2 Q9P0H6	gi|22325364	UBIQUITIN ASSOCIATED PROTEIN 2	3	3	1
KIAA1529*	57653	Q9P1Z9	gi|7959325	KIAA1529	3	2	3
LRRC8E	80131	B3KR78	gi|801893	LEUCINE RICH REPEAT CONTAINING 8 FAMILY, MEMBER E	3	3	1
QRICH2	84074	Q9H0J4	gi|14149793	GLUTAMINE RICH 2	3	3	1
DPP9*	91039	Q86TI2 Q1ZZB8	gi|119589606	DIPEPTIDYL-PEPTIDASE 9	3	4	2
LPLUNC1	92747	Q8TDL5	gi|40807482	NASOPHARGYNEAL RELATED	3	6	1
DOK7	285489	Q18PE1	gi|119602869	HYPOTHETICAL PROTEIN FLJ33718	3	4	1
SLFN14	342618	P0C7P3	gi|193788704	ORTHOLOG OF MOUSE SCHLAFEN 10	3	5	1
ENO1	2023	P06733	gi|4503571	ENOLASE 1	2	6	1
XRCC5	7520	P13010	gi|119590969	X-RAY REPAIR COMPLEMENTING DEFECTIVE REPAIR IN CHINESE HAMSTER CELLS 5 (DOUBLE-STRAND-BREAK REJOINING; KU AUTOANTIGEN, 80kDa)	2	4	1
WDR1	9948	O75083	gi|12652891	WD REPEAT DOMAIN 1	2	6	1
NLRP1	22861	Q9C000 Q9H5Z7	gi|37927559	NLR FAMILY, PYRIN DOMAIN CONTAINING 1	2	1	1
PPA2	27068	Q9H2U2 A6NKL9	gi|119612395	PYROPHOSPHATASE (INORGANIC) 2	2	1	1
VPS35	55737	Q96QK1	gi|7022978	VACUOLAR PROTEIN SORTING 35	2	2	1

Proteins Captured with normal αIIb

Gene Symbol	Entrez Gene ID	SwissProt Acc No.	Protein Acc No.	Description	# Pep	% Cov	# Exp
ITGB3*	3690	P05106	gi|183531	INTEGRIN, BETA 3 (PLATELET GLYCOPROTEIN IIIA, ANTIGEN CD61)	25	42	7

TUBB2C	7284	P49411	gi|20809886	TUBULIN, BETA 2C	17	35	1
DHTKD1	55526	Q96HY7	gi|119606733	DEHYDROGENASE E1 AND TRANSKETOLASE DOMAIN CONTAINING 1	15	36	1
GLUD1	2746	P00367	gi|183056	GLUTAMATE DEHYDROGENASE 1	15	67	3
DARS	1615	P14868 P78371	gi|45439306	ASPARTYL-TRNA SYNTHETASE	14	60	3
LMAN1*	3998	P49257	gi|5031873	LECTIN, MANNOSE-BINDING, 1	12	36	1
PRKAB1	5564	Q9Y478	gi|4506061	PROTEIN KINASE, AMP-ACTIVATED, BETA 1 NON-CATALYTIC SUBUNIT	12	38	1
HSPA5*	3309	P11021 P08246	gi|16507237	HEAT SHOCK 70kDa PROTEIN 5 (GLUCOSE-REGULATED PROTEIN, 78kDa)	11	30	1
SCN10A	6336	P43626 P43628 P43632	gi|110835709	SODIUM CHANNEL, VOLTAGE-GATED, TYPE X, ALPHA	11	5	1
TUBB	10383	P68371	gi|7106439	TUBULIN, BETA 5	11	44	4
TUBB4	23071	Q9BS26	gi|21361322	TUBULIN, BETA 4	10	26	1
ALDH18A1	5832	P54886	gi|76779856	ALDEHYDE DEHYDROGENASE 18 FAMILY, MEMBER A1	9	18	2
DNAJC10*	54431	Q8IXB1	gi|24308127	DNAJ (HSP40) HOMOLOG, SUBFAMILY C, MEMBER 10	9	21	4
EXOSC10	5394	Q01780 P05156	gi|50301239	EXOSOME COMPONTENT 10	9	8	1
UGP1	10352	Q9UGM6	gi|48255966	UDP-GLUCOSE PYROPHOSPHORYLASE 1	9	33	1
ADPGK	83440	Q9BRR6	gi|31542509	ADP-DEPENDENT GLUCOKINASE	8	22	1
ALAD	210	P13716	gi|248839	AMINOLEVULINATE, DELTA-, DEHYDRATASE	8	22	1
CCT2	10576	P78371	gi|5453603	CHAPERONIN CONTAINING TCP1, SUBUNIT 2 (BETA)	8	39	1
CCT4	10575	P50991	gi|38455427	CHAPERONIN CONTAINING TCP1, SUBUNIT 4 (DELTA)	8	28	1
FARS2	10667	O95363	gi|62898407	PHENYLALANINE-TRNA SYNTHETASE 2	8	24	1
HSPA1A*	3303	B3KTT5	gi|5123454	HEAT SHOCK 70kDa PROTEIN 1A	8	19	1
HSPA1B	3304	P08107	gi|167466173	HEAT SHOCK 70kDa PROTEIN 1B	8	21	1
HSPA9	3313	P38646	gi|12653415	HEAT SHOCK 70kDa PROTEIN 9B (MORTALIN-2)	8	17	2
NUDT19	390916	A8MXV4	gi|157739940	NUDIX (NUCLEOSIDE DIPHOSPHATE LINKED MOIETY X)-TYPE MOTIF 19	8	36	1

AKR7A2	8574	O43488	gi|41327764	ALDO-KETO REDUCTASE FAMILY 7, MEMBER A2 (AFLATOXIN ALDEHYDE REDUCTASE)	7	37	1
CHD9	80205	Q3L8U1	gi|95147342	CHROMODOMAIN HELICASE DNA BINDING PROTEIN 9	7	2	1
FAM175B	23172		gi|148529023	UNKNOWN PROTEIN LOC23172	7	14	1
KIF14	9928	Q15058	gi|7661878	KINESIN FAMILY MEMBER 14	7	4	1
NT5DC2	22978	A8K6K2	gi|12597653	5'-NUCLEOTIDASE DOMAIN CONTAINING 2	7	36	2
P15RS	55197	Q96P16	gi|142385371	REGULATION OF NUCLEAR pre-mRNA DOMAIN CONTAINING 1A	7	20	1
PDLIM1	9260	Q9Y3C6 Q9NR12	gi|13994151	PDZ AND LIM DOMAIN 1 (ENIGMA)	7	37	1
PM20D2	135293	Q8IYS1	gi|58082085	AMINOACYLASE 1-LIKE 2	7	15	1
POLDIP2	26073	Q9Y2S7 Q9BVV8	gi|7661672	POLYMERASE (DNA-DIRECTED), DELTA INTERACTING PROTEIN 2	7	26	1
TF*	7018	P02787	gi|553788	TRANSFERRIN	7	12	1
ACTN4	604638		gi|2804273	ACTININ, ALPHA 4	6	9	1
ATXN2L*	11273	Q8WWM7	gi|119572372	ATAXIN 2-LIKE	6	9	1
CCT7	10574	Q99832	gi|62896515	CHAPERONIN CONTAINING TCP1, SUBUNIT 7 (ETA)	6	23	1
CNDP2	55748	Q96KP4	gi|8922698	CNDP DIPEPTIDASE 2 (METALLOPEPTIDASE M20 FAMILY)	6	11	1
FLJ12529	79869	Q8N684	gi|24432016	PRE-MRNA CLEAVAGE FACTOR I, 59 kDa SUBUNIT	6	12	1
PBEF1	10135	P43490	gi|55960735	PRE-B-CELL COLONY ENHANCING FACTOR 1	6	4	1
PPP1R9A	55607	Q9ULJ8	gi|261244899	PROTEIN PHOSPHATASE 1, REGULATORY (INHIBITOR) SUBUNIT 9A, 5 isoforms	6	5	1
RB1CC1	9821	Q8TDY2	gi|134304845	RB1-INDUCIBLE COILED-COIL 1	6	3	1
SERBP1	26135	Q8NC51 Q9H707	gi|66346679	SERPINE1 MRNA BINDING PROTEIN 1	6	16	1
TXNDC4	23352	Q8WXW3 Q5T4S7 Q9NP58	gi|119579327	THIOREDOXIN DOMAIN CONTAINING 4 (ENDOPLASMIC RETICULUM)	6	35	3
ACLY	47	P53396	gi|38569423	ATP CITRATE LYASE	5	3	1
ACTB	60	Q1KLZ0	gi|14250401	ACTIN, BETA	5	22	3
CTTN	2017		gi|2498954	CORTACTIN	5	4	1
CUL-5	8065	Q93034	gi|67514034	CULLIN 5	5	5	1
FHL1	2273	Q13642	gi|3851650	FOUR AND A HALF LIM	5	3	1

				DOMAINS 1			
GPHN	10243	Q9NQX3	gi | 10880983	GEPHYRIN ISOFORM 1	5	8	1
HNRPH1	3187	P31943	gi | 5031753	HETEROGENEOUS NUCLEAR RIBONUCLEOPROTEIN H1	5	16	1
HSPA8*	3312	P11142	gi | 10880983	HEAT SHOCK 70kDa PROTEIN 8	5	8	3
IDH3A	3419	P50213	gi | 5031777	ISOCITRATE DEHYDROGENASE 3 (NAD+) ALPHA	5	13	1
PRKAG1	5571	P54619	gi | 2230863	PROTEIN KINASE, AMP-ACTIVATED, GAMMA 1 NON-CATALYTIC SUBUNIT	5	27	1
RILPL1	353116	Q5EBL4	gi | 30315660	RAB INTERACTING LYSOSOMAL PROTEIN-LIKE 1	5	12	1
SAP130	79595	Q9H0E3	gi:25579126	SIN3A-ASSOCIATED PROTEIN, 130kDa	5	3	1
WARS2	80139	Q9H7S9	gi | 7710154	TRYPTOPHANYL TRNA SYNTHETASE 2	5	19	1
ADCY6	112	O43306	gi | 168480141	ADENYLATE CYCLASE 6	4	3	1
C5orf25	375484	Q8NDZ2	gi | 196259795	FLJ44216 PROTEIN	4	8	1
CARS2	79587	Q9HA77	gi | 119618821	HYPOTHETICAL PROTEIN FLJ39378	4	10	1
CIT	11113	O14578	gi | 32698687	CITRON (RHO-INTERACTING, SERINE/THREONINE KINASE 21)	4	2	1
EEF2K	29904	O00418	gi | 9558749	EUKARYOTIC ELONGATION FACTOR-2 KINASE	4	4	1
FLJ22184	80164	Q9H6K5	gi | 239757129	HYPOTHETICAL PROTEIN FLJ22184	4	5	1
FLNA	2316	P21333	gi | 57284166	FILAMIN A, ALPHA (ACTIN BINDING PROTEIN 280)	4	2	2
FRMPD1	22844	Q5SYB0	gi | 239582740	FERM AND PDZ DOMAIN CONTAINING 1	4	3	1
GOPC	57120	Q9HD26	gi | 9966877	GOLGI ASSOCIATED PDZ AND COILED-COIL MOTIF CONTAINING	4	12	1
HMGCS1	3157	Q01581	gi | 53734504	3-HYDROXY-3-METHYLGLUTARYL-COENZYME A SYNTHASE 1 (SOLUBLE)	4	14	1
HNRNPL*	3191	P14866	gi | 133274	HETEROGENEOUS NUCLEAR RIBONUCLEOPROTEIN L	4	11	2
HTRA2	27429	O43464	gi | 21614538	HTRA SERINE PEPTIDASE 2	4	16	1
NAGK	55577	Q9UJ70	gi | 6491737	N-ACETYLGLUCOSAMINE KINASE	4	10	1
PKM2*	5315	P14618	gi | 31416989	PYRUVATE KINASE,	4	16	1

				MUSCLE			
PRDX3	10935	Q05940 P30048	gi|14250063	PEROXIREDOXIN 3	4	20	1
SF1*	7536	Q15637	gi|46362557	SPLICING FACTOR 1	4	5	1
TIMM50	92609	Q3ZCQ8	gi|48526509	TRANSLOCASE OF INNER MITOCHONDRIAL MEMBRANE 50 HOMOLOG	4	6	1
AER61	285203		gi|39930530	GLUCOSYLTRANSFERASE AER61 C3orf64	3	6	1
CSNK2A2	1459	Q14012	gi|4503097	CASEIN KINASE 2, ALPHA PRIME POLYPEPTIDE	3	6	1
DPP9*	91039	Q86TI2	gi|114657671	DIPEPTIDYL-PEPTIDASE 9	3	2	1
DVL2	1856	O14641	gi|55665917	DISHEVELLED, DSH HOMOLOG 2 (DROSOPHILA)	3	2	1
ELMO1	9844	O60895	gi|86788139	ENGULFMENT AND CELL MOTILITY 1	3	5	1
GAPDH	2597	P04406 Q16678	gi|31645	GLYCERALDEHYDE-3-PHOSPHATE DEHYDROGENASE	3	18	1
KIAA0895	23366	Q8NCT3	gi|154426319	KIAA0895 PROTEIN	3	6	1
LUC7L2	51631	Q9Y383	gi|4929587	CGI-59 PROTEIN	3	5	1
MPO	4353	P05164	gi|88180	MYELOPEROXIDASE	3	5	2
PEG10	23089	Q86TG7	gi|94421473	PATERNALLY EXPRESSED 10	3	11	1
RPLP0	6175	P05388 Q9NQX7	gi|12654583	RIBOSOMAL PROTEIN, LARGE, P0	3	12	1
SEC13	6396	A8MV37	gi|119584482	SEC13-LIKE 1 (S. CEREVISIAE)	3	11	1
SEC23A	10484	Q15436 Q92736	gi|22477159	SEC23 HOMOLOG A (S. CEREVISIAE)	3	3	1
SHROOM3	57619	Q8TF72	gi|57284166	SHROOM3 F-ACTIN BINDING PROTEIN	3	2	4
UBR4	23352		gi|9367763	ZINC FINGER, UBR1 TYPE 1	3	3	1
A2M	2	P01023	gi|177872	ALPHA-2-MACROGLOBULIN	2	1	1
ABCA13	154664	Q86UQ4	gi|8928549	ATP-BINDING CASSETTE, SUB-FAMILY A (ABC1), MEMBER 13	2	5	2
CORO1A	11151	P31146	gi|5902134	CORONIN, ACTIN BINDING PROTEIN, 1A	2	4	1
KIAA1529*	57653	Q9P1Z9	gi|7959325	KIAA1529	2	2	4
MAP3K7IP2	23118	Q9NYJ8	gi|14149669	MITOGEN-ACTIVATED PROTEIN KINASE KINASE KINASE 7 INTERACTING PROTEIN 2	2	2	1
RANBP10	57610	Q6VN20	gi|40538736	RAN BINDING PROTEIN 10	2	4	1
RAVER1*	125950	Q8IY67	gi|123173757	RAVER1	2	4	1
TUBA1A	203068	P07437	gi|340021	TUBULIN, ALPHA	2	2	3
ZNF703	80139		gi|13376610	ZINC FINGER PROTEIN 703	2	3	1

Table 1. Proteins captured with αIIb in megakaryocytes and HEK293 cells. Results are separated according to the αIIb subunit they were captured with. Column labels: Gene

Symbol, EntrezGene ID, Protein Accession Number and Description are from the NCBI database. SwissProt Accession Number is from the UniProt database. Number of Unique Peptides is cumulative from all experiments. Coverage percent is cumulative for all experiments. Tally is shown of the total number of experiments in which a protein was identified (No Expts), and whether captured by histidine tag/Ni affinity (Ni-His) or by crosslinking (X-link). Presence or absence in a recently published expression study (HaemAtlas) is indicated. * Proteins captured by both normal and mutant αIIb subunits.

3.2 Gene Ontology analysis

Gene Ontology (GO) analysis using the DAVID Bioinformatics Resources(Dennis, Sherman et al. 2003; Huang, Sherman et al. 2008) revealed enrichment for protein functions related to processing and trafficking, and ER, Golgi or vesicle components (Figure 3). Comparison of the proteins isolated with the normal αIIb subunits *vs* with the αIIbR858G/R859G subunits showed similar distributions of their localization and molecular functions (**Table 2**). Notably, the αIIbR858G/R859G subunits captured a greater percentage of these types of proteins, suggesting that a greater percentage of the αIIbR858G/R859G subunits were associated with the ER, Golgi and vesicles. Comparison of our data set to a recently published analysis of gene expression in megakaryocytes(Watkins, Gusnanto et al. 2009) showed that approximately 70% of the proteins identified herein as potentially interacting with αIIb were identified as expressed in the megakaryocyte transcriptome.

GO function/location	% of total proteins	
	αIIb	αIIbR858G/R859G
Protien transport	31	49
Stress Caperone	21	34
Vesicle part	6	14
ER or Golgi part	19	21
Organelle part	27	41
Cytoskeleton	21	29
ATP/GTP binding	31	45

Table 2. Distribution of captured proteins into Gene Ontology categories. Some proteins appear in more than one category.

Despite the similarity in distributions into GO categories pertaining to protein processing and localization, there were only 14 proteins in common between the normal αIIb and αIIbR858G/R859G captured proteins (**Table 1**). This may indicate a difference in the relative amount of time spent by the normal and mutant subunits in the protein processing environment. One protein, DNAJC10, was captured in all experiments by both αIIb and αIIbR858G/R859G. Like other DNAJ proteins, DNAJC10 contains a binding domain for the chaperone BiP, but is unique in that its second domain has four protein-disulfide-isomerase (PDI) consensus sequences. (Cunnea, Miranda-Vizuete et al. 2003; Dong, Bridges et al. 2008) Because disulfide bond rearrangement is important for both biogenesis and function of αIIbβ3, we investigated the putative interaction between αIIb and DNAJC10. To our knowledge, DNAJC10 has not previously been reported to interact with αIIb or β3.

3.3 DNAJC10 interacts with αIIbβ3 during biogenesis

DNAJC10 coimmunoprecipitated with αIIb and β3 from UCB derived megakaryocytes using anti-αIIb mAbs 10E5, B1B5, M148 and CA3, and the anti β3 mAb 7H2. DNAJC10 either interacted with αIIb and β3 directly or was part of a complex with them (**Figure 3**). Because DNAJC10 was captured by the αIIbR858G/R859G subunit, we explored the possibility that DNAJC10 interacted with αIIb prior to αIIbβ3 complex formation and αIIb cleavage to its mature form. We have previously shown that pro-αIIb is degraded by the proteasome and that proteasome inhibition leads to an increase of pro-αIIb within the cells. (Mitchell, Li et al. 2006) The undegraded pro-αIIb is trapped in a "pre-degradation" state in which normally transient protein interactions, which usually lead to degradation, may become more long-lived and may be captured by co-immunoprecipitation. Incubation of megakaryocytes with MG132 resulted in increased DNAJC10 co-immunoprecipitation with αIIb by all mAbs, but particularly M148 and CA3. Thus, DNAJC10 may associate with αIIb early in biogenesis, before excess pro-αIIb is targeted to the proteasome.

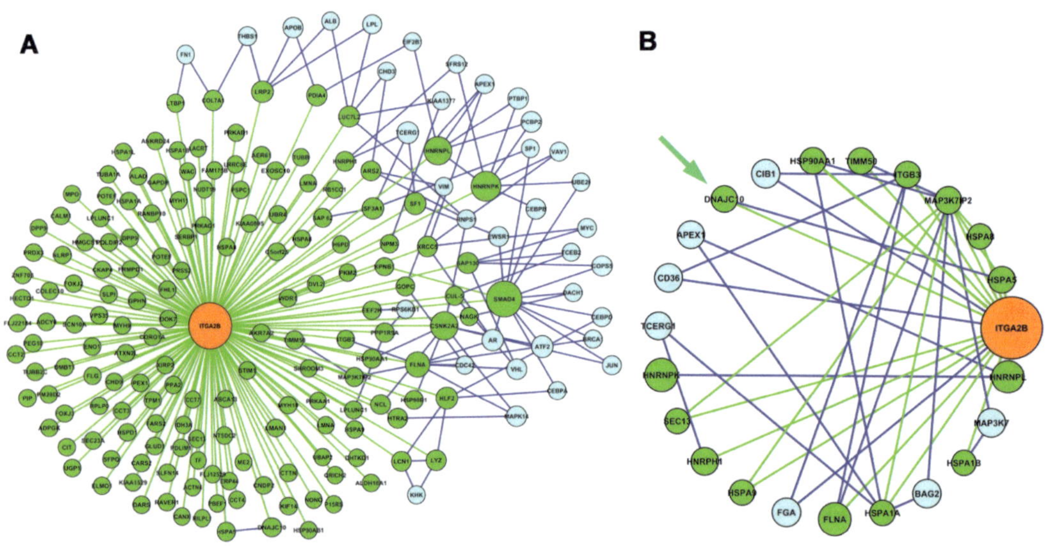

Fig. 3. Network derived from Table 1 data. Proteins are represented as nodes (circles) labeled with their gene symbol, and putative protein interactions with αIIb are indicated by thin green connecting lines. Thick blue lines and blues circles represent interactions or proteins, respectively, retrieved from online databases (Intact and NCBI) using the Cytoscape software. Arrow indicates DNAJC10. Figure prepared using Cytoscape.

To test this possibility we used a panel of conformation-specific mAbs that we have previously used to track the conformational changes of αIIb as it proceeds through biogenesis (**Figure 3**).(Mitchell, Li et al. 2007) Specifically: mAb10E5 binds to the αIIb head region and recognizes both the pro-αIIbβ3 and mature αIIbβ3 complex; mAb 7E3 binds to the β3 head region and also recognizes both the pro- and mature complex; mAb B1B5 binds to the αIIb tail and preferentially recognizes pro-αIIb and pro-αIIbβ3 complex, and mAb M148 preferentially recognizes mature αIIbβ3 but its epitope is not known.(Mitchell, Li et al.

2007) To determine whether DNAJC10 interacts with αIIb during a specific stage of biogenesis, αIIb was immunoprecipitated from megakaryocytes in the presence of MG132 using this panel of conformation-specific mAbs. DNAJC10 was most strongly coimmunoprecipitated by mAb B1B5, suggesting that DNAJC10 preferentially interacts with pro-αIIb or the pro-αIIbβ3 complex. In contrast, DNAJC10 coimmunoprecipitated less well with mAb M148, suggesting less interaction with mature αIIb. DNAJC10 also interacted with the precursor and/or mature αIIbβ3 complex, since it coimmunoprecipitated with the complex-specific mAb10E5. Since the ratio of pro-αIIbβ3 to mature αIIbβ3 is small in megakaryocytes,(Mitchell, Li et al. 2007) this binding pattern is consistent with DNAJC10 having bound preferentially to the small amount of pro-αIIbβ3 present in the cells. Together these findings suggest that DNAJC10 preferentially interacted with pro-αIIb and the pro-αIIbβ3 complex, rather than the mature complex.

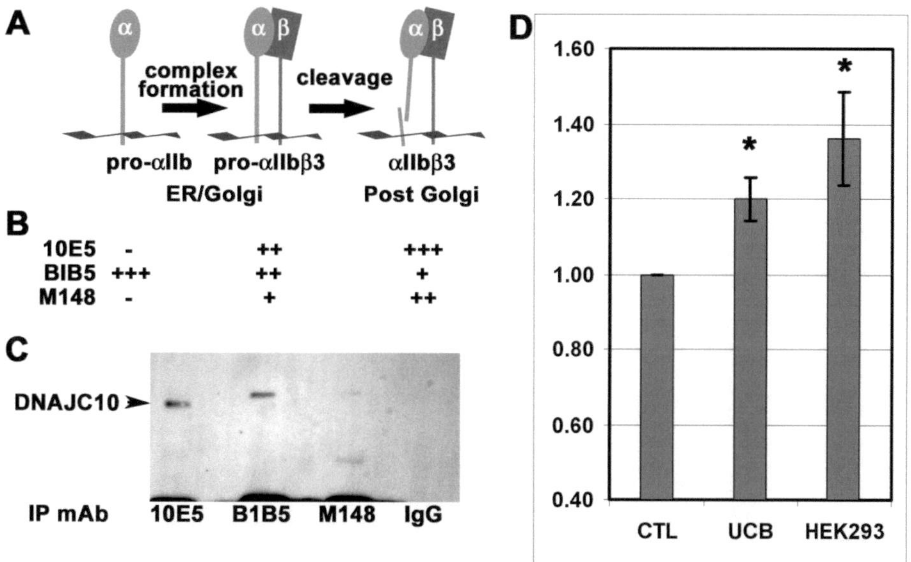

Fig. 4. Interaction of DNAJC10 with αIIbβ3 during biogenesis. A) Schematic of changing conformations of αIIbβ3 as it progresses through biogenesis. B) Changing specificity of 3 mAbs against αIIb as it progresses through distinct conformations during biogenesis. B1B5 preferentially recognizes pro-αIIb, while M148 shows preference for mature αIIb, and 10E5 recognizes the heterodimer complex.C) Immunoprecipitation and Western blot of proteins isolated from megakaryocytes, as described in text. DNAJC10 coimmunoprecipitated preferentially with αIIb that was pulled down by 10E5 and B1B5, but not M148, suggesting that DNAJC10 preferentially interacts with pro-αIIb and pro-αIIbβ3. The last lane is an IgG control. **D)** siRNA mediated knockdown of DNAJC10 increased surface expression of αIIbβ3 as measured by flow cytometry using an Alexa647-labeled anti-αIIbβ3 mAb (10E5). Expression was increased by 25 +\- 11% ($p=0.02$, $n=4$) in UCB-derived megakaryocytes (UCB) and by 35 +\- 12% ($p=0.01$, $n=3$) in HEK293 cells (HEK293) compared to control siRNA transfection (CTL).

3.4 DNAJC10 depletion increases surface expression of αIIbβ3

To determine whether the αIIb-DNAJC10 interaction had physiological relevance, we assessed its impact on the surface expression of αIIbβ3 in megakaryocytes. siRNA mediated knockdown of DNAJC10 was performed on both human megakaryocytes derived from UCB and on HEK293 cells expressing normal αIIb and β3. At least an 80% decrease in RNA level was achieved (data not shown). Knockdown of DNAJC10 increased αIIbβ3 surface expression on megakaryocytes by 25% +/- 11% (n = 4, p = 0.02), and on HEK293 cells expressing αIIbβ3 by 35% +/- 12% (n=4, p = 0.01) (**Figure 3D**).

3.5 Intracellular localization of DNAJC10 in megakaryocytes

DNAJC10 was localized within megakaryocytes by immunofluorescence microscopy (Figure 5). The distribution of DNAJC10 was compared to that of αIIb, β3, and the ER and Golgi compartments. Both αIIb and β3 were distributed throughout the ER as well as on the cell surface. DNAJC10 had a diffuse punctate distribution in the periphery of the cell, away from the nucleus, and colocalized with only a portion of aIIb and β3, consistent with their presumably transient interaction. There was partial overlap between the ER marker calnexin and DNAJC10, suggesting that part of the DNAJC10 distribution is outside the ER or at least

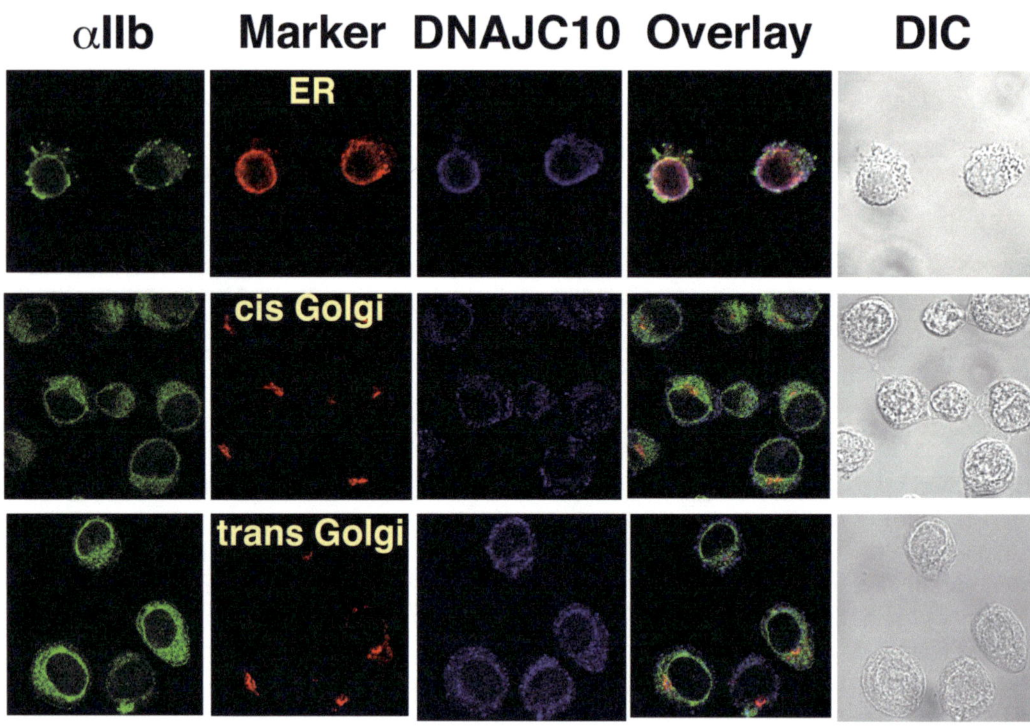

Fig. 4. Intracellular localization of DNAJC10. Cultured megakaryocytes were fixed and immunostained as described in the text. DNAJC10 (Blue) exhibited a punctate staining in the periphery of the cells, away from the nucleus. There was partial overlap of DNAJC10 with calnexin (Red) staining. αIIb (Green) was distributed throughout the ER and cell surface. While αIIb partially colocalized with the cis- and trans-Golgi, DNAJC10 did not.

separate from the distribution of calnexin in the ER. This finding was surprising since DNAJC10 has the ER-retention signal KDEL. DNAJC10 did not localize with markers for the cis- or trans-Golgi compartments.

4. Discussion

We have used a proteomics approach to identify novel proteins interacting with αIIb in megakaryocytes. Two different constructs of αIIb, representing normal αIIb and pro-αIIb subunits, were used to capture proteins interacting with both nascent and mature subunits. Megakaryocytes were derived from human UCB and used on day 8, which in our system yields high expression αIIbβ3 on the surface but no proplatelet formation.(Mitchell, Li et al. 2006) In all, 163 proteins were identified as potentially interacting with αIIb subunits; 98 were captured with normal αIIb and 79 with aIIbR858/G859G, with 14 overlapping (Table 1). Day 8 megakaryocytes express very high amounts of αIIb, most of which is mature αIIbβ3, resulting in a relatively small proportion of nascent αIIb. However, a large proportion of the mutant aIIbR858/G859G subunits are retained within the cell and degraded. Thus the difference between the two protein lists could partly be due to their differences in localization within the cell. This may be reflected in the larger proportion of ER and Golgi related proteins that were captured with the mutant subunit (**Table 2**). Only a few intracellular proteins have been reported to interact with αIIb and αIIbβ3, most notably talin, calnexin, and calreticulin (Intact and NCBI). Our two-step protein capture method was designed to isolate proteins with low affinity binding to αIIb, such as calnexin, while screening out higher affinity binding proteins, such as talin and β3. In accord with this expectation, both talin and β3 were identified in both the control and experimental lanes, and so were excluded from the final interaction list, while calnexin and calreticulin were identified only in the experimental lanes. Surprisingly, while DNAJC10 readily coimmunoprecipitates with αIIbβ3 from megakaryocytes, we have been unable to replicate this finding in HEK293 cells transfected with αIIb and β3, despite an abundance of DNAJC10 in HEK293 cells (data not shown). While this is in no way conclusive, it is suggestive of cell-specific interaction of αIIbβ3 and DNAJC10 in megakaryocytes. Comparison of our experimental results with previously reported platelet proteomic data and αIIbβ3 interaction data showed good correlation. About 70% of the proteins identified in our screens were reported as "present" in platelets in the Haem Atlas, a proteomic analysis of platelet protein content(Watkins, Gusnanto et al. 2009).

Two protein capturing strategies were used, each with strengths and weaknesses. The two-cell pull-down assay using Ni beads to capture poly-histidine-tagged αIIb, allowed the use of mutant cDNA constructs, such as αIIbR858G/R859G, as bait. However, by introducing a protein synthesized in HEK293 cells as bait, there was the potential for false positive identification of proteins that associated with αIIb in the HEK293 cells but not in megakaryocytes. Since the interactions of chaperone proteins are typically of low affinity, these proteins were most likely cleared by the washing steps and did not appear in the control lanes. Another source of false positives was non-specific binding to the Ni beads. Proteins with poly-His sequences (such as DEAH boxes) or naturally occurring Ni binding activity (such as keratin) could have bound to the beads, constituting false positives. However, virtually all of these potential false positives appeared in the control lanes as well and were excluded from analysis. The photoreactive crosslinking assay was intended to capture proteins in situ with αIIb in megakaryocytes. While crosslinking experiments typically produce high numbers of false positives, in our experiments we identified low numbers of proteins from both the experimental and control lanes. The low yield may be due in part to the short crosslinking time used. We found that more than 15 minutes of UV exposure caused excessive protein degradation, while shorter exposure resulted in low crosslinking activity.

Of the proteins captured using both αIIb and αIIbR858G/R859G the Hsp40-type chaperone protein, DNAJC10 (ERdj5), was notable due to its disulfide isomerase activity, since both αIIb and β3 require disulfide bond rearrangement for both biogenesis and function. (Shen, Meunier et al. 2002; Cunnea, Miranda-Vizuete et al. 2003; Dong, Bridges et al. 2008) Among its several functions, the ER chaperone protein BiP protects nearly-folded proteins against aggregation by binding to exposed hydrophobic patches.(Hendershot 2004) The Hsp40 chaperones bind to BiP and increase its efficiency of ATP hydrolysis, which allows BiP to release its substrate. DNAJC10 has been shown to be induced during ER stress, and may assist in delivering misfolded ER proteins to the proteasome for degradation.(Shen, Meunier et al. 2002; Cunnea, Miranda-Vizuete et al. 2003; Dong, Bridges et al. 2008)

DNAJC10 coimmunoprecipitated with both αIIb and β3 subunits in megakaryocytes, suggesting that it may bind the αIIbβ3 complex. The immunoprecipitation pattern obtained using a panel of conformation-specific mAbs(Mitchell, Li et al. 2007) indicated that DNAJC10 preferentially interacted with pro-αIIb or pro-αIIbβ3 rather than mature αIIbβ3. Together these findings suggest that DNAJC10 interacted with pro-αIIb up to the point of complex formation, but not after pro-αIIb cleavage (Figure 2). Thus DNAJC10 appears to be present and interacting with αIIb at a critical decision point during αIIbβ3 biogenesis, i.e. when pro-αIIb will either form the mature αIIbβ3 complex or be targeted to degradation.

Surprisingly, the distribution of DNAJC10, which has a KDEL ER-localization signal, was not confined to the ER, as judged by the distribution of calnexin. To determine if DNAJC10 was cycling to the Golgi and back, as many ER packaging proteins do, we looked for colocalization of DNAJC10 with cis and trans Golgi markers, and found none. The identity of the organelle(s) where DNAJC10 resides remains to be determined.

Depletion of DNAJC10 by siRNA resulted in an increase in surface expression of αIIbβ3 on both human megakaryocytes and transfected HEK293 cells (**Figure 2D**) Since DNAJC10 depletion led to an increase in αIIbβ3 surface expression, it appears to be a negative regulator of αIIbβ3 surface expression. These findings make DNAJC10 an interesting and potentially targetable protein for perturbing αIIbβ3 biogenesis.

5. Conclusion

While the details of DNAJC10-αIIb interaction remain to be investigated, the current findings provide proof of principle that manipulation of early events in αIIb biogenesis can result in altered expression levels of the mature αIIbβ3 receptor, thereby setting a precedent for a novel approach to integrin-related therapy. These studies also support the validity of the data set, although other putative interactions must be explored for greater validation. We hope that the data set created will be a useful tool for studying integrin and megakaryocyte biology.

By deciphering the αIIbβ3 biogenesis pathway we hope to gain an inroad into controlling the level of αIIbβ3 expression on platelets with the long-term goal of developing novel anti-thrombotic therapies. These types of therapy would not just inactivate the circulating platelets, but would modulate the megakaryocytes to make less adhesive platelets. One can imagine a scenario where patients at high risk of heart attack or stroke could be maintained on a drug that decreases their platelet αIIbβ3 expression. Below a certain level of expression, platelet activation and aggregation would be diminished but not completely eliminated, resulting in an overall decrease in platelet thrombus formation but not complete loss of platelet function. This type of therapy could potentially have a greater safety profile than current therapies that summarily inactivate circulating platelets.

This study also assembles some of the wide range of research methods available to hematology research. No single technique could have discovered, validated and explored the function of DNAJC10 in megakaryocytes: rather, a broad range of methods was required. This wide variety is part of what makes research exciting and underscores the benefits of collaboration.

6. Acknowledgement

We are grateful to Willem Ouwehand for helpful discussions and suggestions for data analysis, and to the National Cord Blood Bank at the New York Blood Center for providing the UCB. This work was supported in part by research funding from NIH grant KO8HL68622 (WBM).

7. References

Bray, P. F., J. P. Rosa, et al. (1986). "Biogenesis of the platelet receptor for fibrinogen: Evidence for separate precursors for glycoproteins IIb and IIIa." Proc Natl Acad Sci USA 83: 1480-1484.

Cline, M. S., M. Smoot, et al. (2007). "Integration of biological networks and gene expression data using Cytoscape." Nat. Protocols 2(10): 2366-2382.

Cunnea, P. M., A. Miranda-Vizuete, et al. (2003). "ERdj5, an Endoplasmic Reticulum (ER)-resident Protein Containing DnaJ and Thioredoxin Domains, Is Expressed in Secretory Cells or following ER Stress." Journal of Biological Chemistry 278(2): 1059-1066.

De Luca, G., G. Ucci, et al. (2009). "Benefits from small molecule administration as compared with abciximab among patients with ST-segment elevation myocardial infarction treated with primary angioplasty: a meta-analysis." J Am Coll Cardiol 53(18): 1668-73.

Dennis, G., B. Sherman, et al. (2003). DAVID: Database for Annotation, Visualization, and Integrated Discovery. Genome Biol 4(5):P3.

Dong, M., J. P. Bridges, et al. (2008). "ERdj4 and ERdj5 Are Required for Endoplasmic Reticulum-associated Protein Degradation of Misfolded Surfactant Protein C." Molecular Biology of the Cell 19(6): 2620-2630.

El.Golli, N., O. Issertial, et al. (2005). "Evidence for a Granule Targeting Sequence within Platelet Factor 4." Journal of Biological Chemistry 280(34): 30329-30335.

Hendershot, L. M. (2004). "The ER function BiP is a master regulator of ER function." Mt Sinai J Med 71(5): 289-97.

Huang, D. W., B. T. Sherman, et al. (2008). "Systematic and integrative analysis of large gene lists using DAVID bioinformatics resources." Nat. Protocols 4(1): 44-57.

King, S. M. and G. L. Reed (2002). "Development of platelet secretory granules." Seminars in Cell & Developmental Biology 13(4): 293-302.

Kolodziej, M. A., G. Vilaire, et al. (1991). "Study of the endoproteolytic cleavage of platelet glycoprotein IIb using oligonucleotide-mediated mutagenesis." J Biol Chem 266: 23499-23504.

Kumarathasan, P., S. Mohottalage, et al. (2005). "An optimized protein in-gel digest method for reliable proteome characterization by MALDI-TOF-MS analysis." Anal Biochem 346(1): 85-9.

Lo, B., L. Li, et al. (2005). "Requirement of VPS33B, a member of the Sec1/Munc18 protein family, in megakaryocyte and platelet {alpha}-granule biogenesis." Blood 106(13): 4159-4166.

Mitchell, W. B., J. Li, et al. (2006). "alphaIIbbeta3 biogenesis is controlled by engagement of alphaIIb in the calnexin cycle via the N15-linked glycan." Blood 107(7): 2713-2719.

Mitchell, W. B., J. Li, et al. (2007). "Mapping early conformational changes in alphaIIb and beta3 during biogenesis reveals a potential mechanism for alphaIIbbeta3 adopting its bent conformation." Blood 109(9): 3725-32.

Quinn, M. J., E. F. Plow, et al. (2002). "Platelet glycoprotein IIb/IIIa inhibitors: recognition of a two-edged sword?" Circulation 106(3): 379-85.

Rosa, J.-P. and R. P. McEver (1989). "Processing and assembly of the integrin, glycoprotein IIb-IIIa, in HEL cells." J Biol Chem 264: 12596-12603.

Shen, Y., L. Meunier, et al. (2002). "Identification and characterization of a novel endoplasmic reticulum (ER) DnaJ homologue, which stimulates ATPase activity of BiP in vitro and is induced by ER stress." J Biol Chem 277(18): 15947-56.

Tiwari, S., J. E. Italiano, Jr., et al. (2003). "A role for Rab27b in NF-E2-dependent pathways of platelet formation." Blood 102(12): 3970-9.

Topol, E. J., A. M. Lincoff, et al. (2002). "Multi-year follow-up of abciximab therapy in three randomized, placebo-controlled trials of percutaneous coronary revascularization." Am J Med 113(1): 1-6.

Watkins, N. A., A. Gusnanto, et al. (2009). "A HaemAtlas: characterizing gene expression in differentiated human blood cells." Blood 113(19): e1-9.

7

SATB1: Key Regulator of T Cell Development and Differentiation

Kamalvishnu P. Gottimukkala, Mithila Burute and Sanjeev Galande
Indian Institute of Science Education and Research
Sai Trinity, Garware Circle, Pashan, Pune
India

1. Introduction

Vertebrates have evolved a lymphocyte based adaptive immune system which specifically recognises antigens (Pancer and Cooper, 2006). The lymphoid progenitor cells migrate to the thymus a primary lymphoid organ for the development of T cells (Yang et al., 2010; Zlotoff and Bhandoola, 2011). Progenitor cells undergo a stringent selection process which leads to the development of T cells which have a T cell receptor that specifically reacts with the foreign antigens and not with the self antigens. The pre-T cells further differentiate into many subpopulations in the thymus or the peripheral organs, which perform different functions and are responsible for the adaptive immune responses. The maturation and development of T cells is typically defined by the expression of specific cell surface receptors. The early immature thymocytes that do not express either CD4 or CD8 are called double negative (DN) thymocytes. At these stage the cells undergo the rearrangement of T cell receptor (TCR) β chain. Subsequently, these cells express both $CD4^+$ $CD8^+$ and are referred to as the double positive (DP) cells. During this stage, the rearrangement of the α chain of TCR happens and the cells express the complete T cell receptor (Kreslavsky et al., 2010). The DP thymocytes undergo proliferation and depending on the strength of TCR signaling further develop into either $CD4^+$ or $CD8^+$ single positive (SP) T cells via repression of the gene encoding the other receptor.

The mature T cells migrate to the periphery wherein they encounter the antigens and develop into effector cells. The differentiation of naïve cells into the effector cells depends on the signaling pathways, the pathogen or the cytokines secreted by the antigen presenting cells (APCs). Naïve CD4 T cells mature into various subpopulations which secrete characterisic effector cytokines that define the functions of T cells. Based on the cytokines produced the CD4 T cells are distinguished into multiple subtypes such as T_H1, T_H2, T_H17, induced regulatory T cells (iTregs), Tfh and T_H9 (Zhu et al., 2010). Table 1 provides general overview of various lineages of $CD4^+$ T cells with their key factors and cytokines secreted. The first functionally distinct subpopulations of $CD4^+$ T cells were identified and described as the T_H1/T_H2 paradigm by Mosmann and Coffman, (Mosmann et al., 1986; Mosmann & Coffman, 1987) followed by delineation of the roles of T_H1 and T_H2 cells in cell-mediated and humoral immunity respectively. IL-12 signaling via STAT-4 results in the development of T_H1 cells. IL-4 signaling in conjunction with STAT-6 skews the cells towards T_H2

phenotype. Another major subtype of $CD4^+$ T cells that has gained considerable importance in recent years is T_H17 which produce IL-6 and IL-17. The transcription factors STAT-3 and RORγt act as master regulators for T_H17 differentiation (Park et al., 2005; Dong et al., 2008). Major function of T_H cells is to help B cells to develop antigen-specific antibody response. A subset of T_H cells enter into germinal center and interact with developing B cells and assist them for class-switching. This subset of cells is known as Follicular Helper T cells (Tfh). The Tfh cells secrete IL-4 or IFNγ depending upon their priming (King et al., 2008). Naïve peripheral $CD4^+$ T cells can be induced to give rise to iTreg cells which require FOXP3 transcription factor. These cells are shown to be involved in suppressor function of immune system and for maintainance of tolerance to self-antigens (DiPaolo et al., 2007). T_H9 is another recently discovered type of $CD4^+$ T cells which produce IL-9 and whose function is not clearly understood. However it is proposed that these cells might be involved in confering immunity against helminth infection (Staudt et al., 2010).

Subset of $CD4^+$ T cells	**Important Transcription factors**	**Hallmark cytokines secreted by cells**	**Function (Described in)**
T_H1	STAT-4, T-bet	IFN-γ	Cell mediated Immunity (Mosmann & Coffman, 1987)
T_H2	STAT-6, SATB1, GATA-3	IL-5, IL-4, IL-13	Humoral Immunity (Mosmann & Coffman, 1987)
Treg	FOXP3		Maintainance of tolerance (Sakaguchi et al., 2008)
T_H17	STAT-3, ROR γt	IL-17A, IL-17F	Inflammation, autoimmunity (Hirota et al., 2011)
Tfh	Bcl-6	IL-21	Mediate help and class switching in B cells in germinal centers (Kitano et al., 2011)
T_H9	IRF-4	IL-9	Immunity against helminth infection, most important cell type responsible for the pathogenesis of Asthma (Staudt et al., 2010)

Table 1. **Functional subtypes of $CD4^+$ T lineage.** Various characterized subtypes of $CD4^+$ T cells are listed with their reported essential factors required for lineage determination, key cytokine secreted and function of these cells. For details see text.

2. SATB1 and its role in transcriptional regulation of multiple genes

The cell signaling pathways which initiate the differentiation process ultimately lead to expression of a specific transcription factor. The key transcription factors are important for the expression of specific cytokine gene and maintenance of the phenotype. SATB1 is a T cell enriched transcription factor that regulates large number of genes involved in T cell development and is also required for the maintainance of higher-order chromatin architecture (Alvarez et al., 2000; Kumar et al., 2006; Cai et al., 2003; Cai et al., 2006, Kumar et al., 2007). Ablation of SATB1 causes dysregulation of genes required for the development of T cells and the development is stalled at the DP stage (Alvarez et al., 2000). Thymocytes from SATB1 knockout mice revealed ectopic expression of genes such as *IL-2R* and *IL-7R*. SATB1 is known to regulate genes by selectively tethering their regulatory regions and via formation of a characteristic cage-like structure around the heterochromatic regions in Thymocytes (Cai et al., 2004), presumably demarcating the active and inactive domains (Galande et al., 2007). SATB1 also acts as a docking site for chromatin remodeling/modifying factors such as ISWI, ASF1 and NURD complex containing HDAC1, leading to the repression of genes (Yasui et al., 2000). Post-translational modifications of SATB1 such as acetylation and phosphorylation act as molecular switches regulating its ability to govern gene expression. The PDZ-like domain of SATB1 undergoes phosphorylation by PKC and acetylation by PCAF acetyltransferase in signal-dependent manner (Kumar et al., 2006). Acetylation of SATB1 negatively influences the DNA binding activity of SATB1 whereas phosphorylated form of SATB1 is shown to bind tightly to the *Il-2* promoter and repress *Il-2*. Interaction of SATB1 with the CtBP1 corepressor via its N-terminal PDZ-like domain represses transcription. Upon inhibition of Wnt signaling by LiCl treatment SATB1 is acetylated, loses its interaction with CtBP1 and thus leads to activation of *Il-2* (Purbey et al., 2009). Further, SATB1 is also known to regulate chromatin loop domain organization ('loopscape') in a cell type-specific manner. In Jurkat T cells, SATB1 organizes the MHC class I locus into a 'loopscape' comprising six loops. However, CHO cells which express comparatively less SATB1 exhibit a different 'loopscape' of the MHC locus. Intersstingly, overexpression of SATB1 in CHO cells rendered the 'loopscape' similar to that in Jurkat cells underscoring the importantance of SATB1 in cell-type specific higher-order chromatin organization (Kumar et al., 2007; Galande et al., 2007). In T_H2 cells, SATB1 organizes the loop domain architecture of the T_H2 cytokine locus and governs the coordinated expression of *IL-4, IL-5* and *IL-13* and thus regulate T_H2 differentiation (Cai et al., 2006). Thus, SATB1 has emerged as an important factor orchestrating gene expression by modulating the higher-order chromatin architecture in a cell-type specific and signal-dependent manner.

Number of studies in the past few years have demonstrated the role of SATB1 in cancer. It has been shown that siRNA-mediated knockdown of SATB1 in higly aggressive breast cancer cells reversed the tumorogenic capability of cells and also inhibited the tumor growth (Han et al., 2008). Downregulation of SATB1 in cancerous cells resulted in alteration in the expression of about thousand genes. Furthermore, overexpression of SATB1 in a non-aggressive tumor cell line resulted in augmenting the tumorigenic and metastatic capacity of these cells indicating its direct role in coordinated regulation of multiple genes. SATB1 presumably reprogrammes gene expression by inducing specific epigenetic modifications at target gene loci, leading to upregulation of metastasis-associated genes and simultaneously causing downregulation of tumor suppressor genes (Han et al., 2008). These studies point to a coordinated mechanism of tumor progression.

3. SATB1 in T cell development and differentiation

3.1 Overview of T cell development

T cells arise from the hematopoietic stem cell precursors that migrate to the thymus. Early stage T cell precursors (ETPs) that migrate to the thymus lose the capability to give rise to B cells, however they have the propensity to develop into lineages other than T cells such as macrophages, dendritic cells and NKT cells (Yui et al., 2010). The ETPs also called DN1 phenotypically are $CD4^-$, $CD8^-$, $CD3^-$, $CD25^-$, $CD44^+$ cells. These cells undergo extensive proliferation and are not yet completely committed to T lineage (Rothenberg et al., 2010). The next stage of development is characterized by upregulation of CD25 and is called DN2 stage at which cells are $CD4^-$, $CD8^-$, $CD3^-$, $CD25^+$, $CD44^+$. Further, CD44 is downregulated and such cells are referred to as DN3 stage ($CD4^-$, $CD8^-$, $CD3^-$, $CD25^+$, $CD44^-$) and at this stage they are committed to the T cell lineage. The DN3 cells stop dividing and undergo rearrangement of TCRβ chain. Successful assembly of the β chain facilitates the movement of cells and this process is known as β-selection (Michie & Zuniga-Pflucker, 2002). Subsequently, these cells downregulate both CD25 (IL-2Rα) and CD44, the stage is called DN4 and these are fully committed towards T lineage and start proliferation. Following the successful rearrangement of αβ TCR, thymocytes start expressing CD4 and CD8 coreceptors on the cell surface. The DP thymocytes undergo a stringent selection process, where the TCRs that cannot bind to self antigens undergo death by neglect, whereas those which bind to self MHC with intermediate affinity undergo positive selection (Marrack & Kappler, 1997). Further, these thymocytes either develop into $CD4^+$ or $CD8^+$ SP thymocytes dependent on the TCR signals and the expression of specific transcription factor(s) (Singer et al., 2008). In the periphery, the mature T cells differentiate into effector T cells depending on the antigen encountered and cytokine signals.

3.2 Role of SATB1 in thymocyte development

SATB1 knockout mice exhibit a severe defect in T cell development. SATB1-null mice have disproportionately small thymi and spleens as compared to the wild-type mice. At the cellular level, these mice exhibit multiple defects in T-cell development. The population of immature $CD3^-$,$CD4^-$,$CD8^-$ triple negative (TN) thymocytes is greatly reduced. Most strikingly, the thymocyte development is blocked at the double positive stage and the $CD4^+$ or $CD8^+$ SP thymocytes fail to develop (Alvarez et al., 2000). Ablation of SATB1 also results in dysregulation of multiple genes such as *Il-2R* and *Il-7R* involved in T cell development and differentiation (Alvarez et al., 2000). Within the thymus majority of the DP thymocytes are eliminated via apoptosis during positive and negative selection process (Surh & Sprent, 1994). Dexamethasone-induced apoptosis of thymocytes resulted in rapid dissociation of SATB1 from chromatin. Furthermore, SATB1 is specifically cleaved by caspase-6 after the aspartate residue at position 254 which led to the identification of the PDZ-like domain in the N-terminal region of SATB1. In vitro analysis revealed that caspase-6 cleavage also abolished the DNA-binding ability of SATB1 (Galande et al., 2001). The cleavage of SATB1 during T cell apoptosis might be required for the initiation of DNA fragmentation. In SATB1- null mice peripheral $CD4^+$ T cells fail to respond to activation stimulus and undergo apoptosis demonstrating indispensible role of SATB1 during proper T cell development (Alvarez et al., 2000). Comparison of the wild-type mice with the $SATB1^{-/-}$ mice indicated that repression of *Il-2R* gene was caused specifically by recruitment of histone deacetylases by SATB1 (Yasui et al., 2002). Immunostaining of SATB1 in mouse thymocytes revealed that it forms a unique cage-like structure differentiating euchromatin from heterochromatin (Cai et al., 2003; Notani et al., 2010). In thymocytes, SATB1 is also known to cooperate with other regulatory factors such as β-catenin and CtBP-1 in signal-dependent manner and regulate gene expression (Purbey et al., 2009; Notani et al., 2010). SATB1-binding site-driven reporter assays revealed that SATB1:β-catenin interaction regulates the expression of Wnt target genes in TCF-independent manner (Notani et al., 2010). The recruitment of β-catenin to SATB1 target genes is preceded by deacetylation of SATB1 upon Wnt/β-catenin signaling in thymocytes and $CD4^+$ T cells. SATB1 directly binds to cis regulatory elements at the CD8 enhancer and required for the CD8 SP thymocyte development from the DP thymocytes (Yao et al., 2010). Thus, SATB1 which is highly expressed in thymocytes acts as a global regulator in their development.

3.3 Role of SATB1 in T_H2 differentiation

$CD4^+$ SP thymocytes from the thymus migrate to peripheral lymphoid organs, where they encounter antigen presented by the antigens presenting cells (APCs) and further differentiate into T helper (T_H) effector phenotypes. T_H1 population is involved in cellular immunity wherein they assist macrophages and cytotoxic T cells (Tc) for clearance of infected cells while T_H2 cells help B cells in generating humoral response by increasing production of neutralising antibodies against the pathogen (Zhu and Paul, 2008). T_H2 population is characterized by the effector cytokines it secretes viz., IL-5, IL-13 and IL-4. Strikingly, SATB1 which is known to have a important role during thymocyte development is upregulated during T_H2 differentiation (Lund et al., 2005; Notani et al., 2010). SATB1 was shown to regulate the expression of T_H2 cytokines by remodeling the chromatin in an actively transcribed loop form (Cai et al., 2006). T cell activation along with IL-4 cytokine stimulus showed that SATB1 forms higher-order chromatin structure of the 200 Kb T_H2 cytokine locus and regulates *Il-5, Il-13* and *Il-4.* SATB1 induces expression of these cytokines by recruiting chromatin modifying enzyme Brg1 and RNA Pol II converting the locus into transcriptionally active region (Cai et al., 2006). Furthermore, induction of SATB1 expression in $CD4^+$ cells during T_H2 differentiation is STAT-6 dependent (Lund et al., 2005 and Ahlfors et al., 2010). Transcriptome profiling of differentiating $CD4^+$ cells into T_H1/ T_H2 subtypes revealed that SATB1 is involved in regulation of over 300 genes indicating its crucial role during T_H cell differentiation (Ahlfors et al., 2010).

An important insight into the role of SATB1 in T_H differentiation was obtained when the gene expression profiles of various subsets of T_H cells were compared with the TCR-activated $CD4^+$ T cells, a condition referred to as T_H0. To ascertain whether SATB1 regulated genes are involved in T_H cell differentiation, Ahlfors et al., (2010) silenced expression of SATB1 using siRNAs in T_H cells. Their studies revealed that expression of multiple genes was altered upon SATB1 knockdown in T_H1, T_H2 and T_H0 population. The RNA expression profile revealed that in differentiating $CD4^+$ T cells, expression of 319 genes was altered. Out of these, 70 genes were selectively affected in T_H2 population while 43 genes had altered expression in T_H1 population. Thus total of 40% (43+14+43=127) genes showed altered expression upon cytokine treatment suggesting SATB1 targets were partly specific to T_H subsets. Notably, 48% of SATB1 target genes were regulated by IL-4. Furthermore, TCR stimulation alone regulated one third of SATB1 targets and only 18% of SATB1 target genes were not regulated by TCR or combination of T_H1/T_H2 polarizing cytokines. The gene expression profiling clearly indicated that SATB1 is likely to play an essential role in the development or function of various T_H subtypes (Ahlfors et al., 2010). Another important contribution of this study was the finding that IL-5 which is predominantly secreted by T_H2 cells is repressed by SATB1 during early stages of polarization. The repression of *Il-5* promoter by SATB1 was during brought about by recruiting HDAC1 corepressor to the *Il-5* locus (Figure 1). Later the course of differentiation, the competition between binding of SATB1 and GATA-3 results in binding of GATA-3 to the *Il-5* promoter which derepresses *Il-5* locus and IL-5 is produced (Ahlfors et al., 2010). IL-5 plays important role in differentiation and activation of eosinophils and dysregulation of *Il-5* results into eosinophila (Mosmann & Coffman 1987; Campbell et al., 1988; Sanderson, 1988). Hence regulation of IL-5 is not only important in proper T_H differentiation but also in understanding its role in diseases such as eosinophila.

T_H2 differentiation is also regulated by the downstream transcription factors like GATA-3 and STAT-6. GATA-3 is a transcription factor predominantly expressed in T cells and brain (Oosterwegel et al., 1992). GATA-3 has been shown to play an important role in thymocyte development and also during T_H2 differentiation (Ho et al., 2010). The essential role of GATA-3 was demonstrated by creating mice lacking GATA-3 expression. GATA-3-deficient $CD4^+$ T cells cannot differentiate into T_H2 phenotype and they produce IFNγ under T_H2 polarizing conditions (Zhu J et. al., 2004). IL-4-STAT6 signaling pathway is known to cause the upregulation of GATA-3 in T_H2 differentiating cells. However, a recent report provided an alternative view by demonstrating that $CD4^+$ T cells can differentiate to T_H2 phenotype in absence of STAT6 via notch signaling although with a reduced efficiency (Amsen et al., 2004). In this review we have focused on the newly dicovered mechanism for regulation of GATA-3 expression by SATB1 in Wnt-dependent manner.

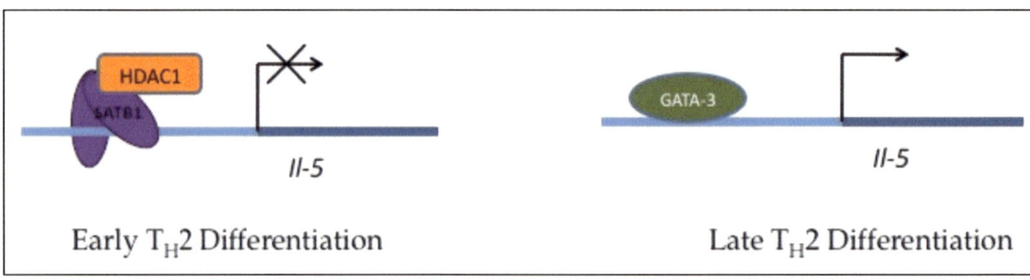

Fig. 1. **SATB1 mediated regulation of *Il-5* during T_H2 differentiation.** IL-5 is a late T_H2 cytokine. SATB1 directly binds to *Il-5* promoter and inhibits its expression by recruiting HDAC repressor complex. During allergic conditions GATA-3 displaces SATB1 bound to the *Il-5* promoter and upregulates IL-5 cytokine expression (Ahlfors et al., 2010).

3.4 SATB1 as a mediator of Wnt signaling

Recently, a new role for SATB1 has been discovered as a mediator of Wnt-signaling pathway during T_H differentiation (Notani et al., 2010). Wnt signaling is one of the well studied and highly conserved pathways responsible for various developmental processes and cell fate decisions (Logan and Nusse, 2004). β-catenin is the key transducer of canonical Wnt signaling cascade which upon Wnt signaling is stabilized in the cytoplasm, then translocates to the nucleus and interacts with T cell factor (TCF) family transcriptional factors. Asociation of β-catenin with the TCF family proteins alters the expression of Wnt-responsive genes (Logan and Nusse, 2004). SATB1 brings about T_H2 cell differentiation via Wnt signaling by recruiting β-catenin to its genomic targets (Notani et al., 2010). This study demonstrated that SATB1 represses target genes in undifferentiated cells. Upon Wnt signalling in the polarized cells, SATB1 interacts with β-catenin, recruits it to *Gata-3* promoter and derepresses it leading to T_H2 commitment (Figure 2). Several SATB1 regulated genes are activated by SATB1:β-catenin complex in Wnt-dependent manner. Post-translational modifications of SATB1 act as molecular switches regulating its DNA-binding activity and ability to interact with multiple partner proteins (Kumar et al., 2006). Upon Wnt signaling SATB1 is deacetylated and directly interacts with β-catenin through its PDZ-like domain. The physical interaction between SATB1 and β-catenin is required for T_H2 differentiation. The two prominent factors TCF and SATB1 compete for β-catenin interaction. SATB1 competitively recruits β-catenin and hence also affects the transcription of TCF regulated genes. However, TCF and SATB1 do not interact with each other suggesting that they have non-overlapping effects (Notani et al., 2010). Thus, these two mediators of Wnt signaling presumably bind to their genomic targets independent of each other. LEF/TCF family proteins were the only known β-catenin partners for number of years. Another β-catenin partner known to be involved in pituitary gland development and lineage determination is the homeodomain protein Prop-1 (Olson et al., 2006). The report by Notani et al. (2010), demonstrated that homeodomain-containing transciption regulator SATB1 is also a β-catenin-binding factor and is involved in T_H2 differentiation.

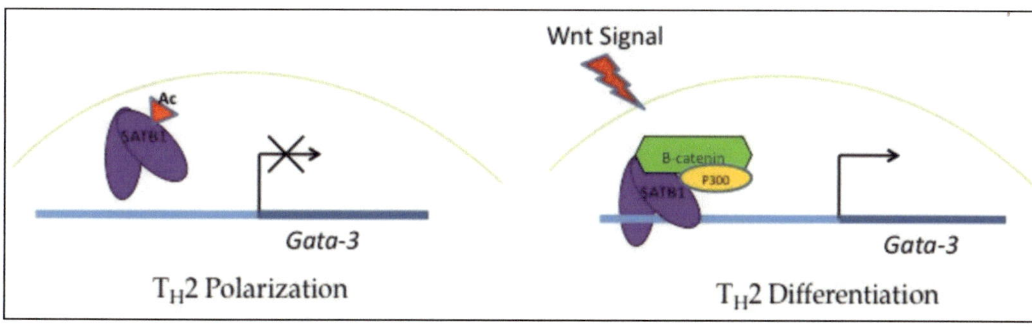

Fig. 2. **SATB1: β-catenin complex regulates *Gata-3* expression during T_H2 differentiation.** Upon Wnt signaling β-catenin translocates into the nucleus. SATB1 interacts with β-catenin and regulates multiple genes. GATA-3 is known to be a master regulator of T_H2 differentiation. In differentiating T_H2 cells, SATB1: β-catenin complex binds to the *Gata-3* promoter and upregulates Gata-3 expression by recruiting the p300 activator complex. SATB1: β-catenin complex regulates *Gata-3* expression in Wnt-dependent manner and thus regulates T_H2 differentiation (Notani et al., 2010).

Role of transcription factor GATA-3 in T_H2 polarization by upregulating IL-4 secretion and inhibiting IFN-γ expression is very well established (Avni et al., 2002; Spilianakis et al., 2004). SATB1 positively regulates GATA-3 expression in T_H2 cells by recruiting p300 acetyltransferase and β-catenin to *Gata-3* promoter upon Wnt signal (Figure 2). The role of Wnt signaling in T_H2 cell differentiation was further demonstrated by using DKK1, an inhibitor of Wnt signaling. Upon DKK1 treatment in T_H cells, GATA-3 expression was suppressed and also T_H2 cytokines were downregulated. Quantitative transcript profiling revealed that expression of GATA-3 was suppressed upon Dkk1 treatment in T_H2 subset, suggesting that Wnt signaling is necessary for the upregulation of GATA-3 during differentiation of T_H2 cells. Overexpression and siRNA mediated silencing of SATB1 and β-catenin provided the conclusive evidence for their direct roles in the differentiation of CD4+ cells. Upon siRNA-mediated silencing of SATB1 the expression of GATA-3 was downregulated in T_H2 cells. Overexpression of SATB1 led to a significant increase in the expression of GATA-3 in T_H2, suggesting that SATB1 positively regulates GATA-3 expression (Notani et al., 2010). In summary, Wnt signaling is essential for T_H2 differentiation whereby SATB1 upregulates GATA-3 expression which further enhances IL-4 secretion. $CD4^+$ T cells are receptive to Wnt signals because they produce different Wnts themselves (Notani et al., 2010). The differential sensitivity of T_H cell subtypes to Wnt signaling could be due to the fact that the downstream processes such as stabilization of β-catenin occur prominently in the T_H2 subtype and not T_H1 (Notani et al., 2010). Thus, these evidences clearly argue in favor of requirement of SATB1 and Wnt/β-catenin signaling during T_H cell differentiation.

GATA3 facilitates chromatin remodeling of T_H2 cytokine locus leading to conversion of the *Il4–Il5–Il13* locus to an open conformation, allowing transcription of this locus by transcription factors involved in T_H2-cell differentiation (Avni et al., 2002). The associated specific epigenetic changes include histone modifications upon binding of GATA-3 to its DNA targets were found to be mainly H3K4 and H3K27 methylation (Wei et al., 2011). Another chromatin protein CTCF binds to T_H2 cytokine locus and assists GATA-3 and SATB1 mediated T_H2 commitment (Almeida et al., 2009). Thus, collectively the three regulators namely SATB1, GATA-3 and CTCF could be responsible for orchestrating the coordinated regulation of T_H cell differentiation.

A model for regulation of T_H2 differentiation by SATB1 is illustrated in Figure 3. T_H0 cell is activated and polarized by TCR docking and IL-4 cytokine respectively. In the absence of

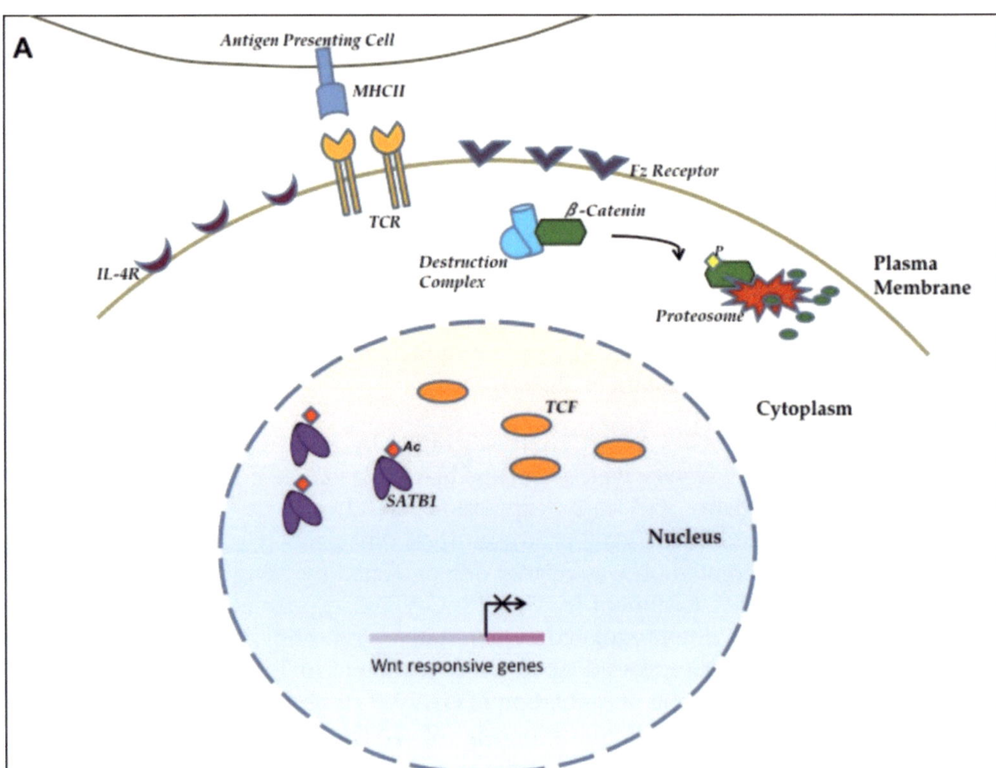

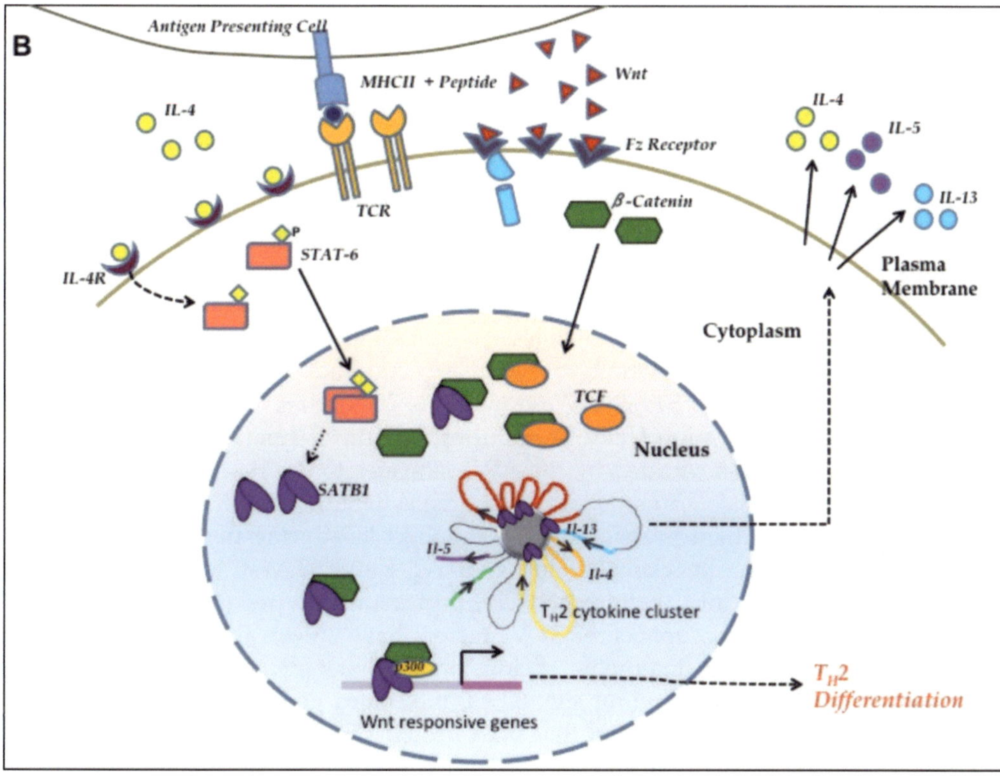

Fig. 3. Model depicting the early events occurring upon Wnt signaling in polarized T_H2 cell and role of SATB1 in this process. In the complex paradigm of T_H2 polarization model there have been several studies suggesting role(s) of different mechanisms and it is now evident that SATB1 plays a major role during this process of T_H2 commitment. **A**, In naïve cells when IL-4 signalling is absent, expression of SATB1 is low and GATA-3 is not upregulated. **B,** Under T_H2 conditions, when a peptide antigen is presented by an antigen presenting cell (APC) to the TCR on T cell surface and IL-4 secreted by the APCs causes the activation of Jak Kinases which phosphorylate STAT-6, which in turn upregulates SATB1 and GATA-3. SATB1 interacts with β-catenin which is translocated to the nucleus in Wnt-dependent manner and this complex regulates *Gata-3* expression. STAT-6, SATB1 and GATA-3 coordinatively regulate *Il-4* expression which is a characteristic cytokine of T_H2 differentiation. However, the role of STAT-6 in regulation of SATB1 as depicted here is speculative.

Wnt signaling, β-catenin is phosporylated by destruction complex and targeted for degradation to proteosomal complex. SATB1 is acetylated and has low DNA-binding affinity in the absence of Wnt signal. Also, in the absence of nuclear β-catenin TCF does not regulate Wnt responsive genes and hence their transcription is suppressed (Figure 3A). Upon Wnt signaling, the destruction complex that sequesters β-catenin does not form and β-catenin is stabilized, which then translocates to nucleus. SATB1 is deacetylated upon Wnt signaling and it then competes with TCF for interaction with β-catenin. Deacetylated SATB1 recruits β-catenin to genomic targets and regulates Wnt-responsive genes resulting into T_H2 differentiation (Notani et al., 2010). SATB1 also binds to T_H2 cytokine locus and upregulates transcription of *Il-4*, *Il-5* and *Il-13* resulting into T_H2 commitment (Figure 3B).

4. Regulation of SATB1 via STAT-6

Signal transducer and activator of transcription (STATs) are important in various biological processes such as development, programed cell death, organogenesis, cell growth regulation and adaptive immunity (Horvath, 2000). Upon appropriate cytokine signaling STAT molecules are phosphorylated by Janus kinases and they form homodimers. The phosphorylated STATs translocate to the nucleus and affect the transcription of their target genes (Schindler and Darnell, 1995). Cytokine signaling mediates the activation of specific STAT molecules and plays an important role during T helper cell differentiation. During the T_H differentiation STAT-4 and STAT-6 play seminal roles during T_H1 and T_H2 differentiation process respectively. IL-12 signaling initiates from binding of IL-12 to the IL-12 receptor, which further associates with protein tyrosine kinases and Jak2. The Jak2 kinase specifically causes the phosphorylation of STAT-4 (Waltford et al., 2004). STAT-4 causes the expression of Interferon γ and transcription factor Tbet during T_H1 differentiation (Thieu et al., 2008, Robertson et al., 2005). IL-4 secreted by the APCs engages to the IL-4 receptor on $CD4^+$ T cells which then recruits Jak 3 kinases and causes the activation of STAT-6 (Witthuhn et al., 1994). STAT-6 regulates the expression of IL-4 and GATA-3 during the T_H2 differentiation (Zhu and Paul, 2008). The knockout models of STAT-4 and STAT-6 have revealed that T cells cannot differentiate into their respective effector phenotypes (Wuster et al., 2000). Genome-wide analysis of occupancy of STAT factors have shown that they preferentially bind to the promoters and intergenic regions in the genome. STAT proteins have a palindromic GAA consensus binding site. STAT molecules generally colocalize with the active histone marks, and it is shown that both proteins SAT4 and SAT6 colocalize with H3K4 trimethylation marks in the genome (Wei et al., 2010). Gene expression studies along with elucidation of the epigenetic marks at key loci using STAT knockout mice have revealed that STAT are important for the maintenance of epigenetic marks on such genes and thus regulation of gene expression.

STAT-6 knockdown caused the downregulation of CRTH2 expression in cells polarised to T_H2 phenotype (Elo et al., 2010). Another study also demonstrated that STAT-6 knockdown resulted in downregulation of SATB1 expression at both RNA and protein level (Ahlfors et al., 2010). Microarray-based gene expression profiling data from different groups using mouse and human models depicted similar results showing downregulation of SATB1 (Wei et al., 2010; Elo et al., 2010). Bsed on these finding, we hypothesize that STAT-6 may directly bind to the SATB1 promoter and mediate activating epigenetic histone modifications leading to the upregulation of SATB1 during T_H2 differentiation. SATB1 in turn causes positive regulation of *Il-4* expression.

Interestingly, two recent studies have implicated Foxp3 in the regulation of SATB1 (Beyer et al. 2011; McInnes et al., 2011). Foxp3 tumor suppressor regulates SATB1 expression in breast epithelial cells and downregulates its expression in miRNA-dependent manner (McInnes et al., 2011). Repression of SATB1 has been also identified as a crucial mechanism for the phenotype and function of T(reg) cells. Foxp3 acts as a transcriptional repressor for the SATB1 locus and indirectly suppresses it through the induction of microRNAs that bound the SATB1 3' untranslated region (Beyer et al., 2011). Thus, elucidation of such regulatory loops will be important steps towards understanding the regulation and in vivo functions of SATB1.

5. Loss of SATB1 function: Sézary syndrome

Adaptive immune response raised against pathogen includes clonal expansion of antigen-specific T cells which are then cleared from the system mainly by activation-induced cell death (AICD), a type of apoptosis (Krammer et al., 2007). Sézary syndrome which is a variant of cutaneous T cell lymphoma results by clonal accumulation of mature T cells originating from skin (Willemze et al., 2005). This accumulation of cells occurs as a result of resistance of cells to AICD (Klemke et al., 2006). The pathogenesis of Sézary Syndrome (SS) is still not very clear. A recent study by Wang et al. (2011) revealed that the deficiency of SATB1 leads to SS. Sézary cells obtained from patients are $CD4^{+}$ $CD7^{-}$ mature memory T cells and show a T_H2 cytokine profile with loss of expression of CD7. Transcription profiling of the Sézary cells from patients and Hut78 (Sézary-derived cell line) revealed that SATB1 was drastically downregulated in these cells as compared to non-Sézary control cells such as Jurkat T cells. Additionally, immunofluorescence staining showed a lowered nuclear localization of SATB1 in of primary Sézary cells as well as in Hut98 cells (Wang et al., 2011). Retroviral transduction mediated restoration of SATB1 in Hut98 cells increased apoptosis in these cells within 4 days without changing their proliferation rate. Subsequently, it was demonstrated that the SATB1 restored cells were sensitized to AICD. The transcriptome analysis of these SATB1 restored cells showed remarkable up-regulation of FASL/CD95L which is a death receptor ligand. Further, 32 out of total 153 (12%) dysregulated genes in Sézary cells were normalized upon SATB1 restoration in these cells (Wang et al., 2011). The increased AICD in SATB1 restored Sézary cells was shown to be induced by FASL via caspase 8-dependent pathway. These studies strongly suggested that SATB1 plays a very important role in pathogenesis of Sézary syndrome and it plays a vital role in regulation of homeostasis of T cells. Sézary cells are known not to respond to radiation therapy as these cells do not have increased proliferation but rather possess resistance to apoptosis. Currently the therapies for SS include upregulation of FASL to sensitize these cells for apoptosis. Restoration of SATB1 in Sézary cells could be a promising new strategy for the treatment of Sézary syndrome. The SS cells would also serve as a knockout model for studying role of SATB1 in human T cell functions.

6. Conclusions

In the field of T cell biology, T_H differentiation is itself a complex phenomenon, one reason being that T_H cell fate is not pre-decided during development in thymus, it is primarily executed upon the encounter of undifferentiated T cell with the antigen in the peripheral immune system. Hence T_H cell polarization leading to final differentiation is a multi-cascade process with several epigenetic changes invoked in response to various signals. In this Chapter we focused on role of SATB1 which is an important global regulator involved in T cell development, maturation and differentiation. We elaborated on the role of SATB1 during T_H cell differentiation which is an important pool of cells for humoral as well as cell mediated immunity. To summarize the findings of various studies, it can be concluded that SATB1 plays an important role at the very early stages of T_H cell differentiation. The studies discussed here suggest that SATB1 represses the chromatin in undifferentiated cells by recruiting repressors to the gene loci. Upon early events of cell polarization such as TCR signal and cytokine secretion by cells, SATB1 immediately responds to even lower level of cytokine signal such as IL-4 by changing the chromatin 'loopscape' of specific loci in T_H2

cells which culminates into synthesis of downstream transcription factors required for further differentiation such as GATA-3. Wnt signaling acts as a booster for the differentiation signal in these cells which brings about changes in chromatin organization via SATB1 as a mediator of Wnt signaling and promotes GATA-3 transcription. In the later stages of differentiation, T_H subtype specific factors such as GATA-3 take over and competitively overcome the SATB1 mediated repression of T_H2 cytokines and in turn upregulate the T_H2 signature cytokines such as IL-5. Thus, SATB1 presumably acts as a regulatory switch at the very early stages of cell polarization and differentiation by repressing various cell type specific genes, however it specifically responds to polarization signal by changing its acetylation status. The indispensible role of SATB1 in T_H cell differentiation is exemplified by diseases such as Eosinophila and Sézary syndrome, the later manifests as a result of SATB1 deficiency.

7. Future perspectives

The role of SATB1 in differentiation of $CD4^+$ T cells has come into the limelight as described in this review. However, the role of SATB1 during earlier events such as thymocyte maturation are not studied in detail and requires further investigation. Since SATB1 is known to regulate genes such as *Thpok* which are important for the lineage commitment process, it is essential to evaluate whether SATB1 plays a direct role during the thymocyte lineage commitment. Findings from recent studies have highlighted the requirement for delineation of molecular mechanisms governing the expression of SATB1 during the process of thymocyte maturation. In the $CD4^+$ T cells, it would be important to study the regulation of SATB1 which might be regulated by an IL-4:STAT6-dependent mechanism as seen during the differentiation of T_H2 cells. It would be also interesting to investigate whether SATB1 plays any role(s) in the differentiation of the other subtypes of $CD4^+$ T cells. Studies elucidating role of miRNAs in the regulation of SATB1 in these various subtypes of T cells would also shed light on the signaling pathways and associated mechanisms regulating the development and differentiation of various subtypes of T cells.

8. Acknowledgements

Work was supported by grants from the Centre of Excellence in Epigenetics program of the Department of Biotechnology, Government of India and IISER Pune. KG is supported by fellowship from the Council of Scientific and Industrial Research, India.

9. References

Ahlfors A, Limaye A, Elo LL, Tuomela S, Burute M, Notani D, Gottimukkala K, Rasool O, Galande S & Lahesmaa R. (2010) SATB1 dictates expression of multiple genes including IL-5 involved in human T helper cell differentiation. *Blood.* 116:1443-1453.

Almeida C, Heath H, Krpic S, Dingjan G, Hamburg J, Bergen I, Nbelen S, Sleutels F, Grosveld F, Galjart N & Hendriks R (2009) Critical role for the transcription regulator CCCTC-Binding factor in the control of Th2 cytokine expression. *J. Immunol.* 182:999-1010.

Alvarez JD, Yasui DH, Niida H, Joh T, Loh DY & Kohwi-Shigematsu T. (2000) The MAR-binding protein SATB1 orchestrates temporal and spatial expression of multiple genes during T-cell development. *Genes Dev.* 14:521-535.

Amsen D, Blander JM, Lee GR, Tanigaki K, Honjo T & Flavell RA. (2004) Instruction of distinct CD4 T helper cell fates by different notch ligands on antigen-presenting cells. Cell. 117:515-526.

Avni O, Lee D, Macian F, Szabo SJ, Glimcher LH & Rao A. (2002) T(H) cell differentiation is accompanied by dynamic changes in histone acetylation of cytokine genes. *Nature Immunol.* 3:643-651

Beyer M, Thabet Y, Müller RU, Sadlon T, Classen S, Lahl K, Basu S, Zhou X, Bailey-Bucktrout SL, Krebs W, Schönfeld EA, Böttcher J, Golovina T, Mayer CT, Hofmann A, Sommer D, Debey-Pascher S, Endl E, Limmer A, Hippen KL, Blazar BR, Balderas R, Quast T, Waha A, Mayer G, Famulok M, Knolle PA, Wickenhauser C, Kolanus W, Schermer B, Bluestone JA, Barry SC, Sparwasser T, Riley JL & Schultze JL. (2011) Repression of the genome organizer SATB1 in regulatory T cells is required for suppressive function and inhibition of effector differentiation. *Nat Immunol.* 12:898-907.

Cai S, Han HJ & Kohwi-Shigematsu T. (2003) Tissue-specific nuclear architecture and gene expression regulated by SATB1. *Nat Genet.* 34:42-51.

Cai S, Lee CC & Kohwi-Shigematsu T. (2006) SATB1 packages densely looped, transcriptionally active chromatin for coordinated expression of cytokine genes. *Nat Genet.* 38:1278:1288.

Campbell HD, Tucker WQ, Hort Y, Martinson ME, Mayo G, Clutterbuck EJ, Sanderson CJ & Young IG. (1987) Molecular cloning, nucleotide sequence, and expression of the gene encoding human eosinophil differentiation factor (interleukin 5). *Proc Natl Acad Sci U S A.* 84:6629–6633.

DiPaolo RJ, Brinster C, Davidson TS, Andersson J, Glass D, Shevach EM. (2007) Autoantigen-specific TGFbeta-induced Foxp3+ regulatory T cells prevent autoimmunity by inhibiting dendritic cells from activating autoreactive T cells. *J Immunol.* 179:4685-4693.

Dong C. (2008) TH17 cells in development: an updated view of their molecular identity and genetic programming. *Nat Rev Immunol.* 8:337-348.

Elo LL, Järvenpää H, Tuomela S, Raghav S, Ahlfors H, Laurila K, Gupta B, Lund RJ, Tahvanainen J, Hawkins RD, Oresic M, Lähdesmäki H, Rasool O, Rao KV, Aittokallio T & Lahesmaa R. (2010) Genome-wide profiling of interleukin-4 and STAT6 transcription factor regulation of human Th2 cell programming. *Immunity.* 32:852-862.

Galande S, Dickinson LA, Mian IS, Sikorska M & Kohwi-Shigematsu T. (2001) SATB1 cleavage by caspase 6 disrupts PDZ domain-mediated dimerization, causing detachment from chromatin early in T-cell apoptosis. *Mol Cell Biol.* 21:5591-5604.

Galande S, Purbey PK, Notani D & Kumar PP. (2007) The third dimension of gene regulation: organization of dynamic chromatin loopscape by SATB1. *Curr Opin Genet Dev.* 17:408-414.

Han HJ, Russo J, Kohwi Y, Kohwi-Shigematsu T. (2008) SATB1 reprogrammes gene expression to promote breast tumour growth and metastasis. Nature. 452:187-93.

Hirota K, Duarte JH, Veldhoen M, Hornsby E, Li Y, Cua DJ, Ahlfors H, Wilhelm C, Tolaini M, Menzel U, Garefalaki A, Potocnik AJ & Stockinger B. (2011) Fate mapping of IL-17 producing T cells in inflammatory responses. *Nat Immunol.* 12:255-263.

Ho IC, Tai TS, Pai SY. (2009) GATA3 and the T-cell lineage: essential functions before and after T-helper-2-cell differentiation. *Nat Rev Immunol.* 9:125-135.

Horvath CM. (2000) STAT proteins and transcriptional responses to extracellular signals. *Trends Biochem Sci.* 10:496-502.

King C, Tangye SG, Mackay CR. (2008) T follicular helper (TFH) cells in normal and dysregulated immune responses. *Annu Rev Immunol.* 26:741-766.

Kitano M, Moriyama S, Ando Y, Hikida M, Mori Y, Kurosaki T & Okada T. (2011) Bcl6 protein expression shapes pre-germinal center B cell dynamics and follicular helper T cell heterogeneity. *Immunity.* 34:961-972.

Klemke CD, Brenner D, Weiss EM, Schmidt M, Leverkus M, Gülow K & Krammer PH. (2009) Lack of T-cell receptor-induced signaling is crucial for CD95 ligand up-regulation and protects cutaneous T-cell lymphoma cells from activation-induced cell death. *Cancer Res.* 69:4175-4183.

Krammer PH, Arnold R & Lavrik IN. (2007) Life and death in peripheral T cells. *Nat Rev Immunol.* 7:532-542.

Kreslavsky T, Gleimer M, Garbe AI & Von Boehmer H. (2010) αβ versus Υδ fate choice: counting the T-cell lineages at the branch point. *Immunol Rev.* 238:169-181.

Kumar PP, Bischof O, Purbey PK, Notani D, Urlaub H, Dejean A & Galande S. (2007) Functional interaction between PML and SATB1 regulates chromatin-loop architecture and transcription of the MHC class I locus. *Nat Cell Biol.* 9:45-56.

Logan CY & Nusse R (2004) The Wnt signaling pathway in development and disease. *Annu Rev Cell Dev Biol.* 20: 781-810.

Lund R, Aittokallio T, Nevalainen O & Lahesmaa R. (2003) Identification of novel genes regulated by IL-12, IL-4 or TGF-β during the early polarization of $CD4^+$ lymphocytes. *J Immunol.* 171:5428-5336.

Lund R, Ahlfors H, Kainonen E, Lahesmaa AM, Dixon C & Lahesmaa R. (2005) Identification of genes involved in the initiation of human Th1 or Th2 cell commitment. *Eur J Immunol.* 35: 3307-3319.

Marrack P & Kappler J. (1997) Positive selection of thymocytes bearing alpha beta T cell receptors. *Curr Opin Immunol.* 9:250-255.

McInnes N, Sadlon TJ, Brown CY, Pederson S, Beyer M, Schultze JL, McColl S, Goodall GJ, Barry SC. (2011) FOXP3 and FOXP3-regulated microRNAs suppress SATB1 in breast cancer cells. Oncogene. doi: 10.1038/onc.2011.293.

Michie AM & Zúñiga-Pflücker JC. (2002) Regulation of thymocyte differentiation: pre-TCR signals and beta-selection. *Semin Immunol.* 14:311-323.

Mosmann TR & Coffman RL. (1987) TH1 and TH2 cells: different patterns of lymphokine secretion lead to different functional properties. *Annu Rev Immunol.* 7:145–173.

Mosmann TR, Cherwinski H, Bond MW, Giedlin MA & Coffman RL. (1986) Two types of murine helper T cell clone. I. Definition according to profiles of lymphokine activities and secreted proteins. *J. Immunol.* 136:2348–574.

Notani D, Gottimukkala KP, Jayani RS, Limaye AS, Damle MV, Mehta S, Purbey PK, Joseph J & Galande S. (2010) Global regulator SATB1 recruits beta-catenin and regulates T(H)2 differentiation in Wnt-dependent manner. *PLoS Biol.* 8(1):e1000296.

Oosterwegel M, Timmerman J, Leiden J & Clevers H. (1992) Expression of GATA-3 during lymphocyte differentiation and mouse embryogenesis. *Dev Immunol.* 3:1-11.

Pancer Z & Cooper MD. (2006) The evolution of adaptive immunity. *Annu Rev Immunol.* 24:497-518.

Pavan Kumar P, Purbey PK, Sinha CK, Notani D, Limaye A, Jayani RS & Galande S. (2006) Phosphorylation of SATB1, a global gene regulator, acts as amolecular switch regulating its transcriptional activity in vivo. *Mol cell.* 22:231-243.

Pavan Kumar P, Purbey PK, Sinha CK, Notani D, Limaye A, Jayani RS, Galande S. (2006) Phosphorylation of SATB1, a global gene regulator, acts as a molecular switch regulating its transcriptional activity in vivo. *Mol Cell.* 22:231-243.

Purbey PK, Singh S, Notani D, Kumar PP, Limaye AS & Galande S. (2009) Acetylation-dependent interaction of SATB1 and CtBP1 mediates transcriptional repression by SATB1. *Mol Cell Biol.* 29:1321-1337.

Rappl G, Muche JM, Abken H & et al. (2001) $CD4^{+}CD7^{-}$ T cells compose the dominant T-cell clone in the peripheral blood of patients with Sezary syndrome. *J Am Acad Dermatol.* 44:456-461.

Robertson MJ, Chang HC, Pelloso D & Kaplan MH (2005) Impaired interferon-gamma production as a consequence of STAT4 deficiency after autologous hematopoietic stem cell transplantation for lymphoma. *Blood.* 106:963-970.

Rothenberg EV, Zhang J & Li L. (2010) Multilayered specification of the T-cell lineage fate. *Immunol Rev.* 238:150-168.

Sakaguchi S, Yamaguchi T, Nomura T & Ono M. (2008) Regulatory T cells and immune tolerance. *Cell.* 133:775-787.

Sanderson CJ. (1988) Interleukin-5: an eosinophil growth and activation factor. *Dev Biol Stand.*69:23–29.

Schindler C & Darnell JE Jr. (1995) Transcriptional responses to polypeptide ligands: the JAK-STAT pathway. *Annu Rev Biochem.* 64:621-651.

Singer A, Adoro S & Park JH. (2008) Lineage fate and intense debate: myths, models and mechanisms of CD4- versus CD8-lineage choice. *Nat Rev Immunol.* 8:788-801.

Singer A. (2002) New prespectives on a developmental dilemma: the kinetic signaling model and the importance of signal duration for the CD4/CD8 lineage decision. *Curr Opin Immunol.* 14:207-215.

Sokolowska-Wojdylo M, Wenzel J, Gaffal E, Steitz J, Roszkiewicz J, Bieber T &Tüting T. (2005) Absence of CD26 expression onskin-homing CLA+ CD4+ T lymphocytes in peripheral blood is a highly sensitive marker for early diagnosis and therapeutic monitoring of patients with Sezary syndrome. *Clin Exp Dermatol.* 30:702-706.

Staudt V, Bothur E, Klein M, Lingnau K, Reuter S, Grebe N, Gerlitzki B, Hoffmann M, Ulges A, Taube C, Dehzad N, Becker M, Stassen M, Steinborn A, Lohoff M, Schild H, Schmitt E & Bopp T. (2010) Interferon-regulatory factor 4 is essential for the developmental program of T helper 9 cells. *Immunity.* 33:192-202.

Surh CD & Sprent J. (1994) T-cell apoptosis detected in situ during positive and negative selection in the thymus. *Nature.* 372:100-103.

Thieu VT, Yu Q, Chang HC, Yeh N, Nguyen ET, Sehra S & Kaplan MH. (2008) Signal transducer and activator of transcription 4 is required for the transcription factor T-bet to promote T helper 1 cell-fate determination. *Immunity.* 29: 679-670.

Wang Y, Su M, Zhou LL, Tu P, Zhang X, Jiang X, Zhou Y. (2011) Deficiency of SATB1 expression in Sezary cells causes apoptosis resistance by regulating FasL/CD95L transcription. *Blood*. 117: 3826-3835.

Watford WT, Hissong BD, Bream JH, Kanno Y, Muul L & O'Shea JJ. (2004) Signaling by IL-12 and IL-23 and the immunoregulatory roles of STAT4. *Immunol Rev*. 202:139-156.

Wei L, Vahedi G, Sun HW, Watford WT, Takatori H, Ramos HL, Takahashi H, Liang J, Gutierrez-Cruz G, Zang C, Peng W, O'Shea JJ & Kanno Y. (2010) Discrete roles of STAT4 and STAT6 transcription factors in tuning epigenetic modifications and transcription during T helper cell differentiation. *Immunity*. 32:840-851.

Willemze R, Jaffe ES, Burg G, Cerroni L, Berti E, Swerdlow SH, Ralfkiaer E, Chimenti S, Diaz-Perez JL, Duncan LM, Grange F, Harris NL, Kempf W, Kerl H, Kurrer M, Knobler R, Pimpinelli N, Sander C, Santucci M, Sterry W, Vermeer MH, Wechsler J, Whittaker S & Meijer CJ. (2005) WHO-EORTC classification for cutaneous lymphomas. *Blood*. 105:3768-3785.

Witthuhn BA, Silvennoinen O, Miura O, Lai KS, Cwik C, Liu ET & Ihle JN. (1994) Involvement of the Jak-3 Janus kinase in signaling by interleukins 2 and 4 in lymphoid and myeloid cells. *Nature*. 370: 153–157.

Yang Q, Jeremiah Bell J & Bhandoola A. (2010) T-cell lineage determination. *Immunol Rev*. 238:12-22.

Yao X, Nie H, Rojas IC, Harriss JV, Maika SD, Gottlieb PD, Rathbun G & Tucker PW. (2010) The L2a element is a mouse CD8 silencer that interacts with MAR-binding proteins SATB1 and CDP. *Mol Immunol*. 48:153-163.

Yasui D, Miyano M, Cai S, Varga-Weisz P & Kohwi-Shigematsu T. (2002) SATB1 targets chromatin remodelling to regulate genes over long distances. *Nature*. 419:641-645.

Yu D, Rao S, Tsai LM, Lee SK, He Y, Sutcliffe EL, Srivastava M, Linterman M, Zheng L, Simpson N, Ellyard JI, Parish IA, Ma CS, Li QJ, Parish CR, Mackay CR & Vinuesa CG. (2009) The transcriptional repressor Bcl-6 directs T follicular helper cell lineage commitment. *Immunity*. 31:457-468.

Yui MA, Feng N & Rothenberg EV. (2010) Fine-scale staging of T cell lineage commitment in adult mouse thymus. *J Immunol*. 185:284-293.

Zhu J & Paul WE. (2008) CD4 T cells: fates, functions and faults. *Blood*. 112:1557-1569

Zhu J, Min B, Hu-Li J, Watson CJ, Grinberg A, Wang Q, Killeen N, Urban JF Jr, Guo L & Paul WE. (2004) Conditional deletion of Gata3 shows its essential function in T_H1-T_H2 responses. *Nat Immunol*. 5:1157-1165.

Zhu J, Yamane H & Paul WE. (2010) Differentiation of effector CD4 T cell populations. *Annu Rev Immunol*. 28:445-489.

Zlotoff DA & Bhandoola A. (2011) Hematopoietic progenitor migration to the adult thymus. *Ann N Y Acad Sci*. 1217:122-138.

8

Neutrophil Chemotaxis and Polarization: When Asymmetry Means Movement

Doris Cerecedo
Laboratorio de Hematobiología, Escuela Nacional de Medicina y Homeopatía, Instituto Politécnico Nacional (IPN), México DF, México

1. Introduction

Neutrophils (also known as polymorphonuclear leukocytes or PMN), the first line of defense against intruding microorganisms, are produced in the bone marrow from stem cells that in turn proliferate and differentiate into mature neutrophils. They play an important role in host defense and contribute to inflammation-related tissue injuries. During inflammation, neutrophils extravasate across the endothelium that lines the blood vessel wall through a multistep process [1, 2], which includes rolling on and subsequent firm adhesion to endothelial cells.

Neutrophil migration through the vascular endothelial layer into lymphoid or inflamed tissues involves a dynamic regulation of cell adhesion in which new adhesions are formed at the cell's leading edge, [3] while filipodia and lamellipodia are generated as exploratory and motile projections and, coordinately, adhesions are released from the trailing edge [4].

For these events, the supply of adhesion molecules to the site of pseudopodial protrusion must be necessarily replenished in order to enable the cell to move forward. There is evidence that the membrane trafficking pathways that recycle adhesion receptors contribute to cell migration [5], which is crucial for polarization and migration in various cell types [6]. Preferential targeting of proteins to the leading or lagging edge of migrating cells is important for polarity and chemotaxis. Asymmetric distribution of proteins has implications beyond polarity and chemotaxis because these same proteins display characteristic localization patterns when cells undergo morphological changes in general. Several proteins have been identified as contributing to cell polarity organization and subsequent inflammatory-cell migration by regulating membrane trafficking. Ly49Q directs the organization of neutrophil polarization as well as neutrophil migration to inflammation sites by regulating membrane raft functions, reorganizing neutrophils in the presence of inflammatory signals, and maintaining neutrophil homeostasis in the absence of such signals [7]. In addition, regulated exocytosis plays a crucial role in conversion of inactive, circulating neutrophils into fully activated cells capable of chemotaxis, phagocytosis, and bacterial killing [8].

Polarity gives cells morphologically and functionally distinct spatial restriction to leading and/or lagging edges by relocating certain proteins or their activities selectively to the poles. Polarization provides cells with morphological, functional, and sensitivity differences to the chemoattractant, altering the way the cell responds to a gradient. Thus, polarization generates a bipolar mechanosensory state with a dynamic leading edge for acquiring new contacts and signals, a stiff mid-body, and a sticky uropod that is dragged along the substrate and stabilizes the cell position in complex environments [9, 10]. Hence, integration of signals generated in both cellular poles leads to a coordinated movement of the leukocyte.

Chemotaxis is conceptually divided into motility, directional sensing, and polarity; however, chemotaxis typically incorporates these features. Many molecules involved in chemotaxis include both lipids and proteins and are localized on the membrane or in the cortex, specifically at either the leading or the lagging edge of polarized cells.

Freely diffusing chemoattractant or soluble molecular cues, known as Damage-associated molecular patterns (DAMP), are liberated from damaged tissue in high abundance. DAMP include Adenosine triphosphate (ATP), bacterial peptides, heat-shock proteins, chromatin, and galectins [11], providing short-lived or pulsatile directional information, in addition to longer-lived cues provided by constitutive or induced tissue-bound chemoattractants [11]. Beyond adhesive migration arrest, local reduction of promigratory signals is achieved by down-modulation of chemoattractant receptors, receptor desensitization, and ligand competition, whereas termination of chemoattractant activity occurs through uptake by neutralizing chemoattractant receptors and/or proteolytic degradation. After ligation, chemoattractant receptors become internalized and are either recycled to the leading edge or stored in vesicles in the uropod, thus limiting the availability of both the chemoattractant and its receptor [12]. The end result is a cascade of activation and adhesion events designed to uptake leukocytes along vessel walls, activate these for them to make stable adhesions, allow them to locomote along the endothelial surface, and to transmigrate across endothelial junctions and through the subendothelial basal lamina, guiding them onto the damage site (Figure 1) [13].

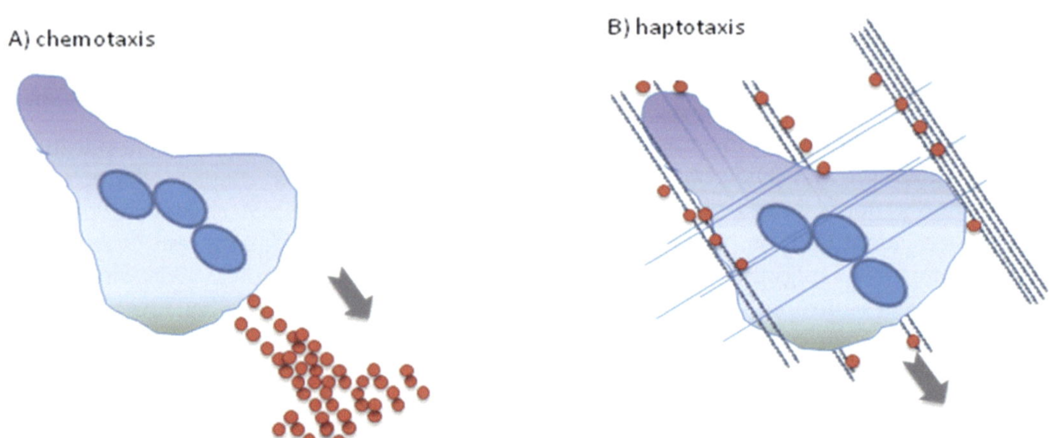

Fig. 1. Type chemotaxis in neutrophils. A) Chemotaxis triggered by soluble diffusing compounds leading to formation of the leading edge. B) Directed-mediated migration toward chemoattractants trapped on tissue structures.

2. Trafficking requirements

Trafficking leukocytes often reduce their migration speed, pause, and polarize toward the bound cell or the tissue structure to execute crucial functions including phagocytosis, cell-to-cell signaling, activation, and the release of cytokines or toxic factors toward an encountered cell.

At least three basic kinetic states govern leukocyte positioning in tissues, including fast migration (5 to 25 μm/min), slow and often locally confined movement (2 to 5 μm), and adhesive arrest, and these rapidly interconvert. Based on these kinetic states, leukocyte accumulation in tissues occurs by means of at least three distinct mechanisms: 1) local engagement of adhesion receptors causes individual leukocytes to stick and become immobilized at a specific spot; 2) degradation of promigratory signals causes cell populations to slow down or stop movement, and 3) loss of exit signals confines cells to a local microenvironment despite ongoing migration [14].

Complete migration arrest is mediated by activation of adhesion receptors on the moving cell followed by attachment to counter-receptors on other cells or on Endothelial cell migration (ECM) structures, leading to an immobilized cell. Within seconds, adhesion overrides ongoing promigratory signals; this is followed by cytoskeletal polarization toward the bound cell or the ECM structure [15].

3. Ensuring tightened adhesion

Endothelial cells (EC) are the critical substrate for leukocyte attachment and motility within the vascular lumen via adhesion molecules such as integrin, ligands whose expression is enhanced on activated ECs, which in turn react to molecules generated during infection and inflammation such as Tumor necrosis factor alpha (TNF- α), interleukin 1β (IL-1 β), and interleukin 17 (IL-17). Expression of these molecules can be further regulated through the cross-talk between EC and leucocytes; binding of PSGL-1 to P-selectin and E-selectin establishes the initial contact between neutrophils and activated ECs. Interaction of EC adhesion molecules (ICAM-1 and VCAM-1) with leukocyte ligands triggers the formation of docking structures or transmigrating cups [16, 17], which embrace adherent leucocytes [18]. Additionally, formation of pro-adhesive sites termed "endothelial adhesive platforms" (EAP) is determined by the existence of pre-formed, tetraspanin-enriched microdomains such as CD9, CD151, and CD81 [19].

Adherent leukocytes may transmigrate at the point of initial arrest, but sometimes rather locomote laterally to preferred sites of Transendothelial cell migration (TECM) [20, 21]; *in vitro* and *in vivo* luminal crawling is dependent on β2 integrins and its blockade appears to increase the incidence of trans- as opposed to paracellular cell migration [21]. The junctional adhesion molecule A (JAM-A), an adhesion molecule expressed on both EC and leukocytes [22], regulate integrin internalization and re-cycling [23].

There are other molecules and mechanisms that have been recently implicated in leukocyte motility; for example, it has been demonstrated both *in vivo* and *in vitro* that platelets enhance neutrophil TECM in inflammation, which is consistent with a mechanistic role for PSGL-1 for this response [24].

4. Neutrophil mobilization

Leukocyte interactions with the endothelial surface trigger cellular and sub-cellular events that initiate and/or facilitate leukocyte passage through the endothelium by interaction of docking structures with cytoskeleton via adaptor proteins such as vinculin, paxilin, and Ezrin, radixin, and moesin (ERM) proteins [18, 25], although Guanosine triphosphate (GTP)ases (RhoG and RhoA) induce actin polymerization leading to the formation of small membrane protrusions called apical cups or docking structures.

Once firm adhesion is established, two routes can be taken for transendothelial migration: the transcellular road, whereby neutrophils penetrate the individual EC, or the paracellular road, by which neutrophils squeeze between EC Figure 2.

A number of molecules at EC junctions actively facilitate leukocyte transmigration via a paracellular route such as Platelet endothelial adhesion molecular-1 (PECAM-1), Intracellular adhesion molecule-2 (ICAM-2), CD99, Endothelial cell-selective adhesion molecules (ESAM), and junctional adhesion molecules (JAM) [22, 26] and, according to *in vivo* and *in vitro* evidence, a sequence of events has been suggested that regulate neutrophil transmigration to EC walls and that include the following: (i) ICAM-1 and ICAM-2 on the luminal surface of EC and within the junction may provide a haptotactic gradient to guide neutrophils to EC junctions via their β2 partners (LFA-1 and MAC-1) [27]; (ii) once within junctions, endothelial-cell JAM-A (through interaction, possibly with LFA-1) [28], facilitates completion of neutrophil passage through the EC layer, and (iii) within the EC junction, homophilic interactions between endothelial and leukocyte PECAM-1 stimulates neutrophils to express the key leukocyte laminin receptor, integrin α6β1, on their surface, which facilitates neutrophil passage through the vascular basement membrane [29-31]. It is also noteworthy that signals from ICAM-1 activate Src and Pyk-2 tyrosine kinases, which phosphorylate VE-Cadherin, destabilizing its bonds and loosening endothelial cell-cell junctions [32].

The transcellular route is taken by some 20% of neutrophils and has been observed in a broad range of tissues including bone marrow, thymus, lymph nodes, pancreas, and the blood brain barrier [33]. Apparently, there is clear evidence for the formation of a transcellular pore requiring membrane fusion and displacement of cytoplasmic organelles during transcellular migration. Vesicular vacuolar organelles (VVO) are enriched at pore-formation sites, apparently providing additional membrane to the area and facilitating the fusion of apical and basal membranes in a process dependent on SNARE-containing membrane fusion complexes [34], and there is increasing evidence for a role for caveolin-1 in determining transendothelial migration route [35].

Carman et al. (2008) [34] have identified *in vitro* and *in vivo* the existence of protrusive podosomes on the basal side of crawling lymphocytes ; these protrusive podosomes appear to identify the cell's thinner peripheral areas rather than the perinuclear region in order to identify a pore formation-permissive site. These dynamic investigatory podosomes can then extend to form invasive podosomes, resembling invadopodia of metastatic tumor cells, which extend down into the EC, bringing the apical and basal membranes into close apposition.

5. Mobilization beyond the endothelium

Beyond the endothelium, migrating cells face two further barriers; the pericyte sheath, and the tough venular Basement membrane (BM) [36, 37]. Neutrophils have the ability to migrate through the pericyte sheath via both para- [38] and transcellular pathways

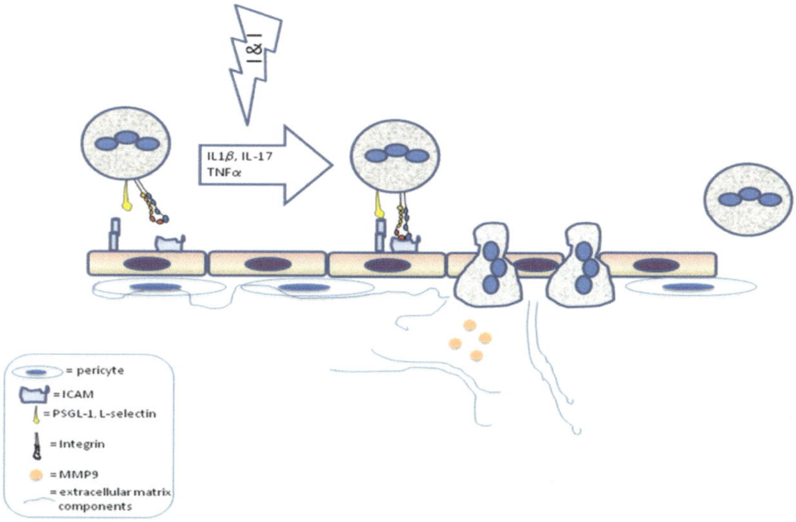

Fig. 2. Hypothetical sequence of events during neutrophil transmigration. Neutrophils are tethered by P- and E-selectin on endothelial cells and PSGL, L-selectin, and CD44 on neutrophils simultaneously participate in neutrophil rolling and activation. Endothelium activation by stimuli such as IL-1β, IL17, TNF-α promote transmigration dependent of molecules such as PECAM-1, ICAM-1, and JAM-A, thus unzipping the tight junctions and restoring themselves while TNF- α promote transmigration via ESAM. Neutrophils take trans- or paracellular routes. Postendothelial cleavage of structural proteins occurs by means of secreted or membrane-anchored matrix metalloproteases (MMPs). Abbreviations: Basement membrane (BM), Endothelial cells (EC), Platelet endothelial cell adhesion molecule (PECAM-1), Intracellular adhesion molecule-1 (ICAM-1), Endothelial cell-selective adhesion molecule (ESAM), Tumor necrosis factor- α (TNF-α) [39].

On the other hand, leukocyte penetration of the vascular BM depends on the vascular bed. Additionally, it has recently been shown that the venular BM contains pre-formed regions with low expression of certain BM components, denominated Low expression regions (LER), which are preferentially utilized by transmigrating neutrophils and monocytes [29, 40]. Alignment of these regions with gaps between adjacent pericytes suggests a key role for these cells in vascular BM generation *in vivo*. Vascular BM architecture depends on the migration of neutrophils, but not monocytes, through the LER remodeling these regions and increasing their size [41, 42], suggesting the involvement of proteases in this response.

6. Neutrophil polarization and migration structures

Neutrophils present in the blood are able to tissue-injury or infection signals by adhering to vascular endothelial cells, then transmigrating across the endothelium through the basement membrane and homing into sites of infection or inflammation.

The following four steps mediate the multiple cycles of attachment and detachment generating neutrophil forward movement during migration: the leading edge protrudes one or several pseudopods by actin flow; protruding membrane and surface receptors interact with the substrate; actomyosin-mediated contraction of the cell body occurs in mid-region, thus the rear of the cell moves forward. Neutrophil migration moves at up to 30 µm/min, lacks strong adhesive interactions to the tissue, and commonly preserves tissue integrity [9].

Receptors such as β2 integrins in neutrophils show discrete relocation toward the tips of ruffles [43]. The mid-region of amoeboid cells contains the nucleus and a relatively immobile cell region that maintains the front-rear axis. The trailing edge contains the highly glycosylated surface receptors CD43 and CD44, adhesion receptors including Intercellular adhesion molecule (ICAM)-1, ICAM-3, β1 integrins, and Ezrin-radixin-moesin adaptor proteins (ERM), as well as GM-1-type cholesterol-rich microdomains [44]. The uropod mediates cell–matrix and cell–cell interactions during migration and has a putative anchoring function [45]. The uropod extends rearward from the nucleus and contains the microtubule-organizing center and rearward-polarized microtubules, the Golgi, and abundant actin-binding ERM proteins. In association with microtubules, mitochondria localize to the rear of the cell that, presumably, due to local ATP delivery to the region of ATP-dependent actomyosin contraction, is required for proper polarization, uropod retraction, and migration [10, 46].

7. Polarization of cytoskeletal and signaling scaffolds

In neutrophils, polarization and migration to chemoattractant gradients such as chemokines and cytokines, lipid mediators, bacterial factors, and Extracellular matrix (ECM) degradation products including collagen, fibronectin, and elastin fragments [47, 48], is known as chemotaxis. After chemokines and chemoattractants bind to the extracellular domains of their cognate G protein-coupled receptor (GPCRs) pseudo- and lamellipodia protrusion are induced. In leukocytes, the majority of GPCRs transmit through the α subunit of Giα. These GPCR include the following: the fMLP (N-formyl-Met-Leu-Phe) receptor and the C5a receptor; chemokine receptors including CCR7, CXCR4, CXCR5, and CCR3; the leukotriene B4 receptor BLT1; sphingosine-1-phosphate receptors 1–4 (S1P1–4), and Lysophosphatidic acid (LPA) receptors 1–3 [49]. All these GPCR mediate promigratory signals but also enhance cell activation. A key GPCR-mediated pathway is signaling through the Phosphatidylinositol-3-kinase (PI(3)K), which contains the p110γ catalytic subunit). PI(3)K-γ is recruited into the inner leaflet of the plasma membrane by the G protein βγ subunit, where it becomes activated and subsequently phosphorylates Phosphatidylinositol phosphates (PIP) and other effectors [50]. PIP serve as docking sites for pleckstrin-homology domain-containing proteins, notably Akt (also known as protein kinase B), which is implicated in inducing actin polymerization and pseudopod protrusion by phosphorylating downstream effectors [51] such as the actin-binding protein girdin [52]. A second pathway linked with PI(3)K activation is induced by ζ-chain-associated receptors, including T cell receptors (TCRs) and receptors FC (FcRs). These receptors signal through tyrosine kinases Lck and Zap-70 to class Ia PI(3)Ks (consisting of p110δ) and activate downstream Akt, as well as the GTPases Rac and Cdc42 [53]. A third, PI(3)K-independent pathway induced by the fMLP receptor in neutrophils leads to the activation of p38 mitogen-associated protein kinase and downstream Rac activation [54, 55]. Ultimately, Rac induces actin polymerization through WAVE (Scar) and Arp2/3. WAVE, a member of the WASP family of actin-binding proteins, mediates actin filament formation [56], while Arp2/3 causes sideward branching of actin filaments. Together, these activities generate interconnected, branched networks [57]. Thus, promigratory signals received at the leading edge generate local Rac activation and actin network protrusion, pushing the plasma membrane outward. Preferential receptor-sensitivity mechanisms at the leading edge are likely diverse and may include local signal- amplification mechanisms [58] and exclusion of counter-regulatory proteins. The mid-region generates actomyosin-based stiffness and contractility, limits lateral protrusions, and thereby maintains a stable, bipolar cortex. The cytoskeletal motor protein myosin II, located in the central and rear regions of leukocytes, promotes actin-filament contraction and limits lateral protrusions. Myosin II cross-links actin filaments in parallel, forming the contractile shell required to hold the extending cell together and propelling the cell nucleus, the most rigid part of the cell, forward [59].

8. Leukocyte movement in different environments and initial migration

Neutrophils are able to migrate along or through 2- or 3- dimensional (2-D or 3-D) surfaces. 2-D Surfaces, such as inner vessel walls, peritoneum, and pleura, require integrin-mediated attachment known as haptokinesis and polarized adhesion through binding of integrins α4β1 and LFA-1 (αLβ2) to their counterparts (VCAM-1 and ICAM-1)(Figure 3A). In contrast, migration in 3-D, ECM environments, which are composed mainly of cellular (lymph node) or fibrillar ECM components, is integrin-independent and cells use weakly adhesive-to-nonadhesive interaction and traction mechanisms that are mediated by actin flow along the confining ECM scaffold structure, contributing to shape change and squeezing [9, 44, 60] (Figure 3B). It is likely that neutrophils adapt to tissue geometry and follow paths of least resistance, a process known as contact guidance (Figure 2).

For passage, the first postendothelial tissue structure and barrier to cells undergoing diapedesis, locally confined cleavage of the structural proteins laminin-10 and type IV collagen, occurs by secreted or membrane-anchored Matrix metalloproteases (MMPs) and serine proteases [61, 62]. Cell-body deformation is coupled with cytoplasmic propulsion and streaming through preexisting or newly formed pores; the deformation and constriction capability of leukocytes is considerable, especially for neutrophils [63].

Interestingly, a recent study showed the existence of venule-wall regions in which laminin-10, collagen IV, and nidogen-2 expression is considerably diminished; neutrophil transmigration enlarges the size of these regions, and their protein content is further reduced, an effect that appears to involve neutrophil-derived serine proteases [40]. Location of proteases at the leukocyte cell surface takes place through two different mechanisms: either by endogenous expression as transmembrane proteins or by binding of extracellular proteases to integral membrane receptors. Integrins are shown to act as anchoring receptors for several proteases including MMPs; such interactions have been detected in caveolae, invadopodia, and at the leading edge of migrating cells, where directed proteolytic activity is required [64]. In this regard, pro-MMP-2 and pro-MMP-9 are bound to αLβ2 and αMβ2 on the surface of activated leukemic cells, and inhibition of these complexes blocks β2 integrin-dependent leukocyte migration [65]. Pro-MMP-9– αMβ2 complexes are primarily localized into intracellular granules of resting neutrophils, but after cellular activation, they are relocalized to the cell surface [66]. Neutrophils secrete laminin, suggesting that leukocyte-derived matrix proteins might also contribute to the transmigration process [67].

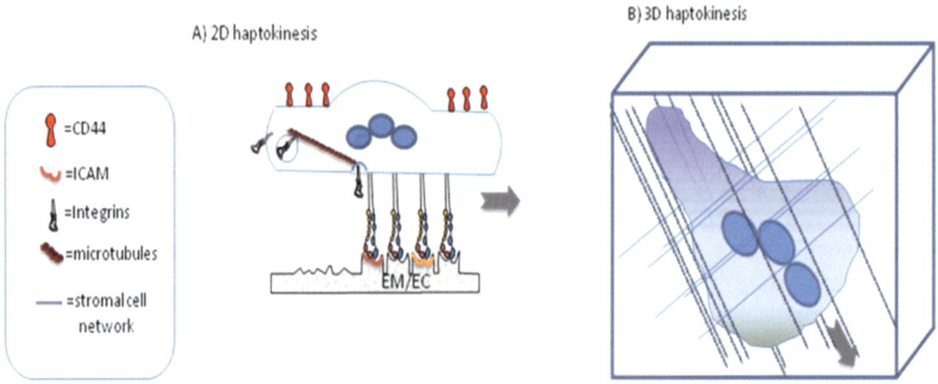

Fig. 3. Type-substrate interaction with neutrophils. A) Two-dimensional integrin-mediated neutrophil migration. *In vivo* 2-D haptokinetic migration is present during crawling on Endothelial cell (EC) or through Extracellular matrix (EM). B) Three-dimensional integrin-independent neutrophil migration. *In vivo,* this occurs through organized tissue structures.

9. Role of cytoskeleton in regulating integrin adhesiveness

Integrins are a superfamily of heterodimeric cell-surface receptors that are found in a broad range of animal species [68]; their main role, as their name implies, is to integrate the cell cytoskeleton with adhesion points of extracellular matrix and cell-surface ligands in order to mediate essential cellular processes such as cell-cell and cell-extracellular matrix interactions, polarization in response to extracellular cues, cell migration, differentiation, survival, and cell-pathogen interactions [69].

In vertebrates, 19 different integrin α subunits and eight different integrin β subunits have been reported, in combination forming about 25 αβ heterodimers [70]. The majority of α/β-subunit combinations can be organized into three fundamental groups based on subunit type (β1, β2, and β3, or αv chains, on the extracellular matrix protein-type recognized, or on the specific adhesion motifs [71] (Table 1).

β1 integrins form the first and largest group of integrins and are ubiquitously distributed in nucleated cells as well as in platelets. β1 Integrins are expressed in bone marrow-derived cells (except for neutrophils), in certain tumor cells, and in muscle development. A second major group of integrins shares either the β3 or the αv subunit (Table 1) and recognizes different ligands from a broad gamma of cell and tissue sources. Integrins with the αv subunit may form dimers with at least five different β chains, including the β1 chain. Subunits αv and β3 recognize Arg-Gly-Asp (RGD) domains present in extracellular matrix proteins.

The third group of integrins shares the β2 integrin chain, whose expression is restricted to leukocytes [72] (Table 1). Receptors such as α4β2, also known as the LFA-1 integrin, determine the capability of leukocytes in endothelial epithelium transmigration and recognize members of the Intercellular adhesion molecule (ICAM) family of adhesion proteins. In contrast, expression of αMβ2 is restricted to monocytes, macrophages, and granulocytes; it recognizes

	Ligands	Motifs	Distribution
β1 integrin			
α1β1	*Co1,Lm*	ND	*EC, SMC, TC, Monos*
α2β1	*Col, Fn, Lm, Echovirus 1*	*DGEA*	*Plt, EC, Fb, SMC, TC, EPC*
α3β1	*Col, Epiligrin, Fn, Lm, Invasin*	*RGD*	*EC, TC, EPC, Fb*
α4β1	Fn, Invasin, VCAM-1	EILDV (Fn) *QIDSPL(VCAM-1)*	TC, Monos, Eos, LC, ER
α5β1	Fn, Invasin	RGD	Fb, EC, Monos, TC, Plt
α6β1	Lm, Invasin	ND	Plts, TC, EC, EPC
α7β1	Lm	ND	Myocytes
α8β1		ND	*SMC*
α9β1	Col, Lm, Tenascin	RGD	EPC, Myocytes
αϖβ1	Fn,Vn	RGD	Fb
αv and β3 integrins			
αvβ1	Fn, Vn	RGD	Fb
αvβ5	Vn, HIV Tat, Adenovirus	RGD	EC, EPC, Fb, Tumors
αvβ6	Fn, Tenascin	RGD	
αvβ3	Vn	RGD	Melanoma
αvβ3	Col, Fib, Fn, Lm Opn, Pn, TSP, Vn	RGD	EC, FB, Monos, SMC, OC
	vWf, HIV Tat, Tenascin, Adenovirus		Plt, Tumors
αIIbβ3	Col, Fib, Fn, TSP, Vn, vWf, *Borrelia*	KQAGDV	Plt, Mega
αRβ3	Fib, Fn, Vn, vWf	RGD	PMN
β2 integrin			
αLβ2	ICAMs (1-3)	ND	TC, BC, LGL, Monos, PMN, Eos
αMβ2	Fib, Fn, Factor X, ICAM-1, iC3b		PMN, Monos, Macros, LGL
αχβ2	Fib, iC3b	GPRP	Monos, Macros, PMN
αΔβ2		ND	TC. Macros
Other integrins			
α6β4	Lm	ND	EC, EPC, Schwann cells
α4β7	Fn, MAdCAM, VCAM-1	EILDV (Fn)	Gut homing, TC
αEβ7	E-Cadherin	ND	Epithelial TC

Table 1. Classification of integrins according to ligand motifs and distribution. Abbreviations: BC = B cells; Col = Collagen; EC = Endothelial cells; Eos = Eosinophils; EPC = Epithelial cells; Fb = Fibroblasts; Fib = Fibrinogen; Fn = Fibronectin; iC3b = inactivated component of complement; Lm = Laminin; LGL = Large granular lymphocytes; Macros = Macrophages; Mega = Megakaryocytes; Monos = Monocytes; OPN = Osteopontin; Plt = Platelets; PMN = Neutrophils or Polymorphonuclear leukocytes; SMC = Smooth muscle cells; TC = T cells; TSP = Thrombospondin; Vn = Vitronectin; vWf = von Willebrand disease. (Modified from [71]).

fibrinogen and inactivated C3b, playing an important role in the phagocytosis of opsonized particles and bacteria [73]. The fourth group of integrins includes three integrins (α6β4, α4β7, and αEβ7); these integrins recognize extracellular matrix components as well as adhesion molecules of the Immunoglobulin superfamily (IgSF). Common integrins expressed on leukocytes and their counterparts are summarized in Table 1.

Association of extended forms of integrins with the cortical cytoskeleton is required to integrate mechanical forces from shear flow and F-actin and to undergo ligand-induced strengthening at endothelial contacts. Key differences between α4 and β2 integrins regarding their increase in cytoskeleton-mediated avidity may occur. The α4 integrins can bind paxillin upon dephosphorylation of Ser988 in their cytoplasmic domain at the sides and rear pole of the cell, whereas PKA-mediated phosphorylation of these integrins is confined to the cell's leading edge. Paxillin regulates α4 integrin function (tethering and firm adhesion) [74], enhancing their migration rate and reducing their spreading, and paxillin–α4 interaction downregulates the formation of focal adhesions, stress fibers, and lamellipodia by triggering activation of different tyrosine kinases, such as Focal adhesion kinase (FAK), Pyk2, Src, and Abl [75, 76]. The α4–paxillin complex inhibits stable lamellipodia by recruiting an ADP-ribosylation factor (Arf)-GTPase-activating protein that decreases Arf activity, thereby inhibiting Rac, and limiting lamellipodia formation to the cell front [77]. Recently, it was discovered that integrins can induce PIP5K1C-90 polarization independently of chemoattractants. This integrin-induced PIP5K1C-90 polarization works together with chemoattractant signaling in regulating neutrophil polarization and directionality *in vitro* and infiltration *in vivo* [78].

It has been described that LFA-1 and Mac-1 may use adapter molecules talin, α-actinin, filamin, and 14-3-3 to anchor to the actin cytoskeleton properly [79, 80]. Regarding subcellular localization, LFA-1 pattern ranges from low- in the lamellipodia to high expression in the uropod. However, it has been reported that high-affinity clustered LFA-1 is restricted to a mid-cell zone, termed the "focal zone", different from focal adhesions and focal contacts. In addition, talin, properly activated by phosphorylation or by phosphatidylinositol-4,5-bisphosphate (PIP2), is essential for formation and stability of the focal zone and for LFA-1-dependent migration [81].

Locomotion can be regulated by integrins because the signals involved in integrin-mediated leukocyte firm adhesion to endothelium are subsequently attenuated to allow leukocyte migration toward an appropriate transmigration site. β2 integrins appear to promote direct locomotion, success in correct positioning at the endothelial junction, and effective diapedesis [82, 83]. Upon interaction with their ligands, integrins activate distinct myosin-contractility effectors, actin-remodeling GTPases, and molecules involved in microtubule-network regulation at motile leukocyte leading and trailing edges [84]. During cell polarization, Cdc42, Myosin light chain kinase (MLCK), Rac, RapL, Rap1, mDia, myosin-IIA, and chemokine receptors are redistributed to the cellular front, participating in exploratory filopodia formation and in lamellipodia extension. In contrast, Rho- and Rho-associated kinase (ROCK) (both involved in trailing- edge retraction), the Microtubule-organizing center (MTOC), and adhesion receptors ICAM-1, ICAM-3, CD44, and CD43 move toward the rear pole [85].

Recently, dystrophin protein-adhesion complex proteins such as short dystrophins, utrophins, and the dystrophin-associated protein complex (α-dystroglycan, α–syntrophin and α–dystrobrevins) form part of actin-based structures such as lamellipodia and uropod, in which their polarized distribution is evident and their feasible role in chemotaxis and migration is strongly suggested [86].

Other proteins with differential distribution appear in Figure 4 and the list is increasing.

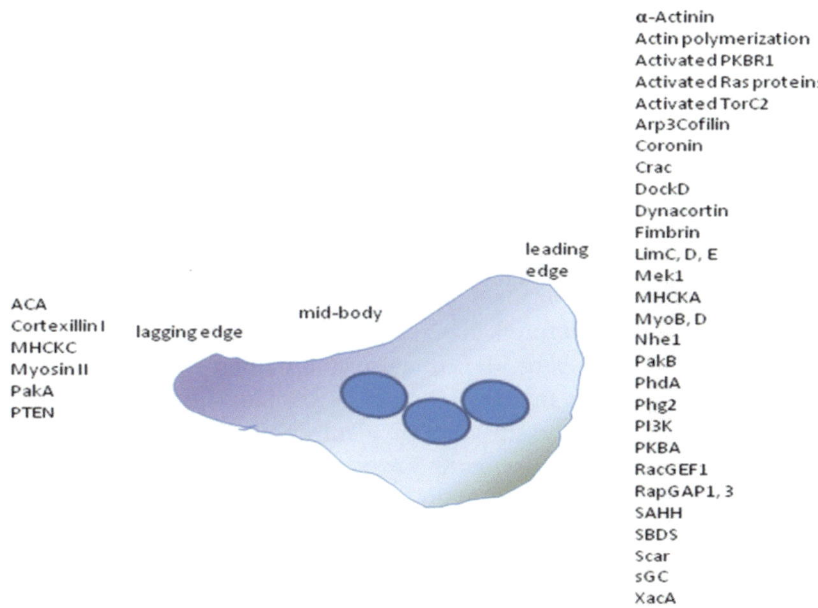

Fig. 4. Neutrophil regions observed after triggered activation and differential protein distribution. Adapted from [87].

10. Conclusions

For exiting the vasculature, leukocytes follow a consecutive sequence of events that starts with the first contact of free-flowing neutrophil to the vascular endothelium followed by leukocyte rolling along the vessel wall. Both events are mediated by specialized receptor ligand pairs consisting of a member of the selectin family of adhesion molecules and specific carbohydrate determinants on selectin ligands. During rolling, leukocytes are in intimate contact with the vascular endothelium, enabling endothelial-bound chemokines to interact with their respective chemokine receptors on the neutrophil surface. Upon binding to the receptor, chemokine receptor-mediated signaling events trigger the activation of β2 integrins. Activated integrins subsequently interact with endothelium-expressed ligands, which lead to a reduction in leukocyte rolling velocity and eventually, to mediate stable adhesion and migration across the blood vessel wall. Following neutrophil spreading and intravascular crawling along the endothelium, tethered neutrophils reach the correct spot for exiting into tissue. Upon neutrophil stimulation, actin, which is one of the major components of the cytoskeleton in neutrophils, is reorganized through reversible cycles of polymerization and depolymerization, thereby comprising the driving motor for the formation of lamellipodia and pseudopodia during migration and phagocytosis. Activated neutrophils become polarized with a contracted tail (uropod) in the rear and F-actin-rich protrusions at the front and start crawling. Actin and the proteins regulating actin polymerization are key players in the establishment of morphological and functional cell polarity. Actin polymerization and membrane ruffling comprise the first events leading to the establishment of chemoattractant-stimulated neutrophil polarization.

Morphological changes imply cytoskeleton redistribution triggered by certain activated pathways which are spatiotemporally coordinated.

Undesrtanding the molecular and cellular interactions that regulate neutrophil transmigration could be of great value to design novel therapeutic strategies directed to promote or suppress an inflammatory response, which may be of potential benefit under physiological or pathological circumstances.

11. References

[1] Luo BH, Carman CV, and Springer TA. Structural basis of integrin regulation and signaling. Annu Rev Immunol. 2007; 25:619-47.

[2] Rose DM, Alon R, and Ginsberg MH. Integrin modulation and signaling in leukocyte adhesion and migration. Immunol Rev. 2007; 218:126-34.

[3] Alcaide P, Auerbach S, and Luscinskas FW. Neutrophil recruitment under shear flow: it's all about endothelial cell rings and gaps. Microcirculation. 2009; 16:43-57.

[4] Woodfin A, Voisin MB, Beyrau M, Colom B, Caille D, Diapouli FM, Nash GB, Chavakis T, Albelda SM, Rainger GE, Meda P, Imhof BA, and Nourshargh S. The junctional adhesion molecule JAM-C regulates polarized transendothelial migration of neutrophils in vivo. Nat Immunol. 2011; 12:761-9.

[5] Veale KJ, Offenhauser C, and Murray RZ. The role of the recycling endosome in regulating lamellipodia formation and macrophage migration. Commun Integr Biol. 2011; 4:44-7.

[6] Pierini LM, Eddy RJ, Fuortes M, Seveau S, Casulo C, and Maxfield FR. Membrane lipid organization is critical for human neutrophil polarization. J Biol Chem. 2003; 278:10831-41.

[7] Sasawatari S, Yoshizaki M, Taya C, Tazawa A, Furuyama-Tanaka K, Yonekawa H, Dohi T, Makrigiannis AP, Sasazuki T, Inaba K, and Toyama-Sorimachi N. The Ly49Q receptor plays a crucial role in neutrophil polarization and migration by regulating raft trafficking. Immunity. 2010; 32:200-13.

[8] Faurschou M and Borregaard N. Neutrophil granules and secretory vesicles in inflammation. Microbes Infect. 2003; 5:1317-27.

[9] Wolf K, Muller R, Borgmann S, Brocker EB, and Friedl P. Amoeboid shape change and contact guidance: T-lymphocyte crawling through fibrillar collagen is independent of matrix remodeling by MMPs and other proteases. Blood. 2003; 102:3262-9.

[10] Friedl P and Brocker EB. The biology of cell locomotion within three-dimensional extracellular matrix. Cell Mol Life Sci. 2000; 57:41-64.

[11] Kono H and Rock KL. How dying cells alert the immune system to danger. Nat Rev Immunol. 2008; 8:279-89.

[12] Servant G, Weiner OD, Neptune ER, Sedat JW, and Bourne HR. Dynamics of a chemoattractant receptor in living neutrophils during chemotaxis. Mol Biol Cell. 1999; 10:1163-78.
[13] Muller WA. Mechanisms of leukocyte transendothelial migration. Annu Rev Pathol. 2011; 6:323-44.
[14] Friedl P and Weigelin B. Interstitial leukocyte migration and immune function. Nat Immunol. 2008; 9:960-9.
[15] Gunzer M, Weishaupt C, Hillmer A, Basoglu Y, Friedl P, Dittmar KE, Kolanus W, Varga G, and Grabbe S. A spectrum of biophysical interaction modes between T cells and different antigen-presenting cells during priming in 3-D collagen and in vivo. Blood. 2004; 104:2801-9.
[16] Carman CV and Springer TA. A transmigratory cup in leukocyte diapedesis both through individual vascular endothelial cells and between them. J Cell Biol. 2004; 167:377-88.
[17] Barreiro O, Yanez-Mo M, Serrador JM, Montoya MC, Vicente-Manzanares M, Tejedor R, Furthmayr H, and Sanchez-Madrid F. Dynamic interaction of VCAM-1 and ICAM-1 with moesin and ezrin in a novel endothelial docking structure for adherent leukocytes. J Cell Biol. 2002; 157:1233-45.
[18] Barreiro O, de la Fuente H, Mittelbrunn M, and Sanchez-Madrid F. Functional insights on the polarized redistribution of leukocyte integrins and their ligands during leukocyte migration and immune interactions. Immunol Rev. 2007; 218:147-64.
[19] Barreiro O, Zamai M, Yanez-Mo M, Tejera E, Lopez-Romero P, Monk PN, Gratton E, Caiolfa VR, and Sanchez-Madrid F. Endothelial adhesion receptors are recruited to adherent leukocytes by inclusion in preformed tetraspanin nanoplatforms. J Cell Biol. 2008; 183:527-42.
[20] Schenkel AR, Mamdouh Z, and Muller WA. Locomotion of monocytes on endothelium is a critical step during extravasation. Nat Immunol. 2004; 5:393-400.
[21] Phillipson M, Heit B, Colarusso P, Liu L, Ballantyne CM, and Kubes P. Intraluminal crawling of neutrophils to emigration sites: a molecularly distinct process from adhesion in the recruitment cascade. J Exp Med. 2006; 203:2569-75.
[22] Ley K, Laudanna C, Cybulsky MI, and Nourshargh S. Getting to the site of inflammation: the leukocyte adhesion cascade updated. Nat Rev Immunol. 2007; 7:678-89.
[23] Cera MR, Fabbri M, Molendini C, Corada M, Orsenigo F, Rehberg M, Reichel CA, Krombach F, Pardi R, and Dejana E. JAM-A promotes neutrophil chemotaxis by controlling integrin internalization and recycling. J Cell Sci. 2009; 122:268-77.
[24] Lam FW, Burns AR, Smith CW, and Rumbaut RE. Platelets enhance neutrophil transendothelial migration via P-selectin glycoprotein ligand-1. Am J Physiol Heart Circ Physiol. 2011; 300:H468-75.
[25] Wittchen ES. Endothelial signaling in paracellular and transcellular leukocyte transmigration. Front Biosci. 2009; 14:2522-45.
[26] Dejana E. Endothelial cell-cell junctions: happy together. Nat Rev Mol Cell Biol. 2004; 5:261-70.

[27] van Buul JD, van Rijssel J, van Alphen FP, van Stalborch AM, Mul EP, and Hordijk PL. ICAM-1 clustering on endothelial cells recruits VCAM-1. J Biomed Biotechnol. 2010:120328.
[28] Wojcikiewicz EP, Koenen RR, Fraemohs L, Minkiewicz J, Azad H, Weber C, and Moy VT. LFA-1 binding destabilizes the JAM-A homophilic interaction during leukocyte transmigration. Biophys J. 2009; 96:285-93.
[29] Voisin MB, Woodfin A, and Nourshargh S. Monocytes and neutrophils exhibit both distinct and common mechanisms in penetrating the vascular basement membrane in vivo. Arterioscler Thromb Vasc Biol. 2009; 29:1193-9.
[30] Woodfin A, Voisin MB, Imhof BA, Dejana E, Engelhardt B, and Nourshargh S. Endothelial cell activation leads to neutrophil transmigration as supported by the sequential roles of ICAM-2, JAM-A, and PECAM-1. Blood. 2009; 113:6246-57.
[31] Dangerfield J, Larbi KY, Huang MT, Dewar A, and Nourshargh S. PECAM-1 (CD31) homophilic interaction up-regulates alpha6beta1 on transmigrated neutrophils in vivo and plays a functional role in the ability of alpha6 integrins to mediate leukocyte migration through the perivascular basement membrane. J Exp Med. 2002; 196:1201-11.
[32] van Buul JD and Hordijk PL. Endothelial signalling by Ig-like cell adhesion molecules. Transfus Clin Biol. 2008; 15:3-6.
[33] Carman CV. Mechanisms for transcellular diapedesis: probing and pathfinding by 'invadosome-like protrusions'. J Cell Sci. 2009; 122:3025-35.
[34] Carman CV, Sage PT, Sciuto TE, de la Fuente MA, Geha RS, Ochs HD, Dvorak HF, Dvorak AM, and Springer TA. Transcellular diapedesis is initiated by invasive podosomes. Immunity. 2007; 26:784-97.
[35] Marmon S, Hinchey J, Oh P, Cammer M, de Almeida CJ, Gunther L, Raine CS, and Lisanti MP. Caveolin-1 expression determines the route of neutrophil extravasation through skin microvasculature. Am J Pathol. 2009; 174:684-92.
[36] Hirschi KK and D'Amore PA. Pericytes in the microvasculature. Cardiovasc Res. 1996; 32:687-98.
[37] Rowe RG and Weiss SJ. Breaching the basement membrane: who, when and how? Trends Cell Biol. 2008; 18:560-74.
[38] Voisin MB, Probstl D, and Nourshargh S. Venular basement membranes ubiquitously express matrix protein low-expression regions: characterization in multiple tissues and remodeling during inflammation. Am J Pathol. 2010; 176:482-95.
[39] Feng D, Nagy JA, Pyne K, Dvorak HF, and Dvorak AM. Neutrophils emigrate from venules by a transendothelial cell pathway in response to FMLP. J Exp Med. 1998; 187:903-15.
[40] Wang S, Voisin MB, Larbi KY, Dangerfield J, Scheiermann C, Tran M, Maxwell PH, Sorokin L, and Nourshargh S. Venular basement membranes contain specific matrix protein low expression regions that act as exit points for emigrating neutrophils. J Exp Med. 2006; 203:1519-32.

[41] Mamdouh Z, Kreitzer GE, and Muller WA. Leukocyte transmigration requires kinesin-mediated microtubule-dependent membrane trafficking from the lateral border recycling compartment. J Exp Med. 2008; 205:951-66.
[42] Reichel CA, Rehberg M, Lerchenberger M, Berberich N, Bihari P, Khandoga AG, Zahler S, and Krombach F. Ccl2 and Ccl3 mediate neutrophil recruitment via induction of protein synthesis and generation of lipid mediators. Arterioscler Thromb Vasc Biol. 2009; 29:1787-93.
[43] Fernandez-Segura E, Garcia JM, and Campos A. Topographic distribution of CD18 integrin on human neutrophils as related to shape changes and movement induced by chemotactic peptide and phorbol esters. Cell Immunol. 1996; 171:120-5.
[44] Friedl P, Entschladen F, Conrad C, Niggemann B, and Zanker KS. CD4+ T lymphocytes migrating in three-dimensional collagen lattices lack focal adhesions and utilize beta1 integrin-independent strategies for polarization, interaction with collagen fibers and locomotion. Eur J Immunol. 1998; 28:2331-43.
[45] Fais S and Malorni W. Leukocyte uropod formation and membrane/cytoskeleton linkage in immune interactions. J Leukoc Biol. 2003; 73:556-63.
[46] Campello S, Lacalle RA, Bettella M, Manes S, Scorrano L, and Viola A. Orchestration of lymphocyte chemotaxis by mitochondrial dynamics. J Exp Med. 2006; 203:2879-86.
[47] Laskin DL, Kimura T, Sakakibara S, Riley DJ, and Berg RA. Chemotactic activity of collagen-like polypeptides for human peripheral blood neutrophils. J Leukoc Biol. 1986; 39:255-66.
[48] Senior RM, Gresham HD, Griffin GL, Brown EJ, and Chung AE. Entactin stimulates neutrophil adhesion and chemotaxis through interactions between its Arg-Gly-Asp (RGD) domain and the leukocyte response integrin. J Clin Invest. 1992; 90:2251-7.
[49] Thelen M and Stein JV. How chemokines invite leukocytes to dance. Nat Immunol. 2008; 9:953-9.
[50] Marone R, Cmiljanovic V, Giese B, and Wymann MP. Targeting phosphoinositide 3-kinase: moving towards therapy. Biochim Biophys Acta. 2008; 1784:159-85.
[51] Stambolic V and Woodgett JR. Functional distinctions of protein kinase B/Akt isoforms defined by their influence on cell migration. Trends Cell Biol. 2006; 16:461-6.
[52] Enomoto A, Murakami H, Asai N, Morone N, Watanabe T, Kawai K, Murakumo Y, Usukura J, Kaibuchi K, and Takahashi M. Akt/PKB regulates actin organization and cell motility via Girdin/APE. Dev Cell. 2005; 9:389-402.
[53] Rommel C, Camps M, and Ji H. PI3K delta and PI3K gamma: partners in crime in inflammation in rheumatoid arthritis and beyond? Nat Rev Immunol. 2007; 7:191-201.
[54] Heit B, Robbins SM, Downey CM, Guan Z, Colarusso P, Miller BJ, Jirik FR, and Kubes P. PTEN functions to 'prioritize' chemotactic cues and prevent 'distraction' in migrating neutrophils. Nat Immunol. 2008; 9:743-52.
[55] Billadeau DD. PTEN gives neutrophils direction. Nat Immunol. 2008; 9:716-8.
[56] Ibarra N, Pollitt A, and Insall RH. Regulation of actin assembly by SCAR/WAVE proteins. Biochem Soc Trans. 2005; 33:1243-6.

[57] Machesky LM, Mullins RD, Higgs HN, Kaiser DA, Blanchoin L, May RC, Hall ME, and Pollard TD. Scar, a WASp-related protein, activates nucleation of actin filaments by the Arp2/3 complex. Proc Natl Acad Sci U S A. 1999; 96:3739-44.
[58] Charest PG and Firtel RA. Feedback signaling controls leading-edge formation during chemotaxis. Curr Opin Genet Dev. 2006; 16:339-47.
[59] Bendix PM, Koenderink GH, Cuvelier D, Dogic Z, Koeleman BN, Brieher WM, Field CM, Mahadevan L, and Weitz DA. A quantitative analysis of contractility in active cytoskeletal protein networks. Biophys J. 2008; 94:3126-36.
[60] Lammermann T, Bader BL, Monkley SJ, Worbs T, Wedlich-Soldner R, Hirsch K, Keller M, Forster R, Critchley DR, Fassler R, and Sixt M. Rapid leukocyte migration by integrin-independent flowing and squeezing. Nature. 2008; 453:51-5.
[61] Monaco S, Sparano V, Gioia M, Sbardella D, Di Pierro D, Marini S, and Coletta M. Enzymatic processing of collagen IV by MMP-2 (gelatinase A) affects neutrophil migration and it is modulated by extracatalytic domains. Protein Sci. 2006; 15:2805-15.
[62] Delclaux C, Delacourt C, D'Ortho MP, Boyer V, Lafuma C, and Harf A. Role of gelatinase B and elastase in human polymorphonuclear neutrophil migration across basement membrane. Am J Respir Cell Mol Biol. 1996; 14:288-95.
[63] Yap B and Kamm RD. Cytoskeletal remodeling and cellular activation during deformation of neutrophils into narrow channels. J Appl Physiol. 2005; 99:2323-30.
[64] Smart EJ, Graf GA, McNiven MA, Sessa WC, Engelman JA, Scherer PE, Okamoto T, and Lisanti MP. Caveolins, liquid-ordered domains, and signal transduction. Mol Cell Biol. 1999; 19:7289-304.
[65] Stefanidakis M and Koivunen E. Cell-surface association between matrix metalloproteinases and integrins: role of the complexes in leukocyte migration and cancer progression. Blood. 2006; 108:1441-50.
[66] Stefanidakis M, Ruohtula T, Borregaard N, Gahmberg CG, and Koivunen E. Intracellular and cell surface localization of a complex between alphaMbeta2 integrin and promatrix metalloproteinase-9 progelatinase in neutrophils. J Immunol. 2004; 172:7060-8.
[67] Wondimu Z, Geberhiwot T, Ingerpuu S, Juronen E, Xie X, Lindbom L, Doi M, Kortesmaa J, Thyboll J, Tryggvason K, Fadeel B, and Patarroyo M. An endothelial laminin isoform, laminin 8 (alpha4beta1gamma1), is secreted by blood neutrophils, promotes neutrophil migration and extravasation, and protects neutrophils from apoptosis. Blood. 2004; 104:1859-66.
[68] Humphries MJ. Integrin structure. Biochem Soc Trans. 2000; 28:311-39.
[69] Hynes RO. Integrins: bidirectional, allosteric signaling machines. Cell. 2002; 110:673-87.
[70] Shimaoka M, Takagi J, and Springer TA. Conformational regulation of integrin structure and function. Annu Rev Biophys Biomol Struct. 2002; 31:485-516.
[71] Gille J and Swerlick RA. Integrins: role in cell adhesion and communication. Ann N Y Acad Sci. 1996; 797:93-106.
[72] Springer TA. Adhesion receptors of the immune system. Nature. 1990; 346:425-34.

[73] Tuffery-Giraud S, Saquet C, Chambert S, Echenne B, Marie Cuisset J, Rivier F, Cossee M, Philippe C, Monnier N, Bieth E, Recan D, Antoinette Voelckel M, Perelman S, Lambert JC, Malcolm S, and Claustres M. The role of muscle biopsy in analysis of the dystrophin gene in Duchenne muscular dystrophy: experience of a national referral centre. Neuromuscul Disord. 2004; 14:650-8.

[74] Han J, Rose DM, Woodside DG, Goldfinger LE, and Ginsberg MH. Integrin alpha 4 beta 1-dependent T cell migration requires both phosphorylation and dephosphorylation of the alpha 4 cytoplasmic domain to regulate the reversible binding of paxillin. J Biol Chem. 2003; 278:34845-53.

[75] Rose DM, Liu S, Woodside DG, Han J, Schlaepfer DD, and Ginsberg MH. Paxillin binding to the alpha 4 integrin subunit stimulates LFA-1 (integrin alpha L beta 2)-dependent T cell migration by augmenting the activation of focal adhesion kinase/proline-rich tyrosine kinase-2. J Immunol. 2003; 170:5912-8.

[76] Cohen-Hillel E, Mintz R, Meshel T, Garty BZ, and Ben-Baruch A. Cell migration to the chemokine CXCL8: paxillin is activated and regulates adhesion and cell motility. Cell Mol Life Sci. 2009; 66:884-99.

[77] Nishiya N, Kiosses WB, Han J, and Ginsberg MH. An alpha4 integrin-paxillin-Arf-GAP complex restricts Rac activation to the leading edge of migrating cells. Nat Cell Biol. 2005; 7:343-52.

[78] Xu W, Wang P, Petri B, Zhang Y, Tang W, Sun L, Kress H, Mann T, Shi Y, Kubes P, and Wu D. Integrin-induced PIP5K1C kinase polarization regulates neutrophil polarization, directionality, and in vivo infiltration. Immunity. 2010; 33:340-50.

[79] Fagerholm SC, Hilden TJ, Nurmi SM, and Gahmberg CG. Specific integrin alpha and beta chain phosphorylations regulate LFA-1 activation through affinity-dependent and -independent mechanisms. J Cell Biol. 2005; 171:705-15.

[80] Pavalko FM and LaRoche SM. Activation of human neutrophils induces an interaction between the integrin beta 2-subunit (CD18) and the actin binding protein alpha-actinin. J Immunol. 1993; 151:3795-807.

[81] Smith A, Carrasco YR, Stanley P, Kieffer N, Batista FD, and Hogg N. A talin-dependent LFA-1 focal zone is formed by rapidly migrating T lymphocytes. J Cell Biol. 2005; 170:141-51.

[82] Springer TA. Traffic signals for lymphocyte recirculation and leukocyte emigration: the multistep paradigm. Cell. 1994; 76:301-14.

[83] Laudanna C, Kim JY, Constantin G, and Butcher E. Rapid leukocyte integrin activation by chemokines. Immunol Rev. 2002; 186:37-46.

[84] Chrzanowska-Wodnicka M and Burridge K. Rho-stimulated contractility drives the formation of stress fibers and focal adhesions. J Cell Biol. 1996; 133:1403-15.

[85] Vicente-Manzanares M and Sanchez-Madrid F. Role of the cytoskeleton during leukocyte responses. Nat Rev Immunol. 2004; 4:110-22.

[86] Cerecedo D, Cisneros B, Gomez P, and Galvan IJ. Distribution of dystrophin- and utrophin-associated protein complexes during activation of human neutrophils. Exp Hematol. 2010; 38:618-628 e3.

[87] Swaney KF, Huang CH, and Devreotes PN. Eukaryotic chemotaxis: a network of signaling pathways controls motility, directional sensing, and polarity. Annu Rev Biophys. 2010; 39:265-89.

9

Intravascular Leukocyte Chemotaxis: The Rules of Attraction

Sara Massena and Mia Phillipson
Department of Medical Cell Biology, Integrative Physiology
Uppsala University
Sweden

1. Introduction

The security system of the body against pathogenic invaders includes leukocytes that efficiently scan the organism. Leukocytes within the vasculature utilize the comprehensive circulatory system to examine the blood vessels of the entire body for signs of *e.g.* bacteria displayed on vascular endothelial cells. Upon infection, a successful immune response is dependent on prompt recruitment of leukocytes from the bloodstream to the afflicted site where they exert their effector functions. A critical aspect of leukocyte recruitment out of vasculature is the chemotactic gradient that guides leukocytes over the blood vessel wall, and further through the extracellular matrix towards the affected site. Leukocyte recruitment is a strictly regulated cascade of events involving different molecular mechanisms. To rapidly and efficiently reach their target, specific interactions between circulating leukocytes and vascular endothelium orchestrates leukocyte activation and guides them already within blood vessels to optimal transmigration sites at endothelial *loci* close to the source of inflammation.

Despite the obvious need for effective leukocyte recruitment to eradicate bacteria and to maintain tissue homeostasis, amplified and dysregulated recruitment of leukocytes is a key factor in diverse disorders including autoimmune diseases and sepsis. For many of these conditions, therapeutic options are limited and unspecific. Understanding the triggering signals, involved molecules and underlying mechanisms by which the body enhances, controls and limits immune responses is therefore critical for the development of novel therapeutic interventions.

In this chapter we summarize leukocyte recruitment during inflammation, highlighting a recent finding, namely intravascular leukocyte chemotaxis.

2. Leukocyte recruitment and chemotaxis

Over the last years, research groups have been dedicating their efforts to delineate the cellular and molecular mechanisms behind leukocyte recruitment using a wide range of *in vivo* imaging techniques (*e.g.* fluorescence intravital microscopy, spinning disk confocal, as well as two-photon confocal microscopy). These techniques, together with genetically altered mice (transgenic or knockout) combined with fluorescently labeled proteins and antibodies, allow detailed examination of leukocyte-endothelial cell interactions, adhesion molecule expression and chemokine distribution. Thereby, an expanded and more detailed version of the leukocyte recruitment cascade was established.

Leukocyte recruitment can be described as a sequential process having at least five distinct events, as depicted in **Figure 1**, induced by upregulation of endothelial adhesion molecules and molecular guidance signals (chemotactic stimuli).

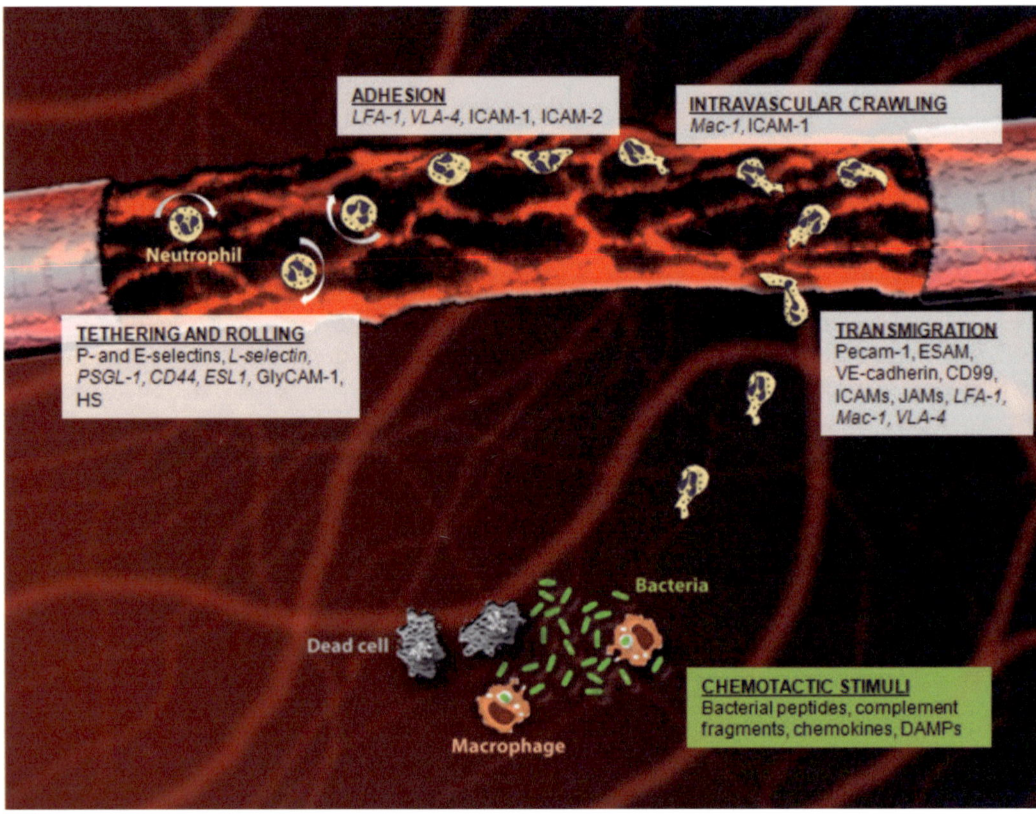

Fig. 1. The leukocyte recruitment cascade. The vessels is stained red by monoclonal antibodies to CD31 conjugated to Alexa Fluor 555, and cartoon neutrophils are added to the phtograph. The white boxes contain involved adhesion molecules, where the ones expressed by neutrophils are written in italics. Illustration adapted with permission from Phillipson M, Kubes P, *Nature Medicine*, 2011.

2.1 Leukocyte tethering and rolling

In order to leave the vasculature at the site of infection, leukocytes have to become marginated, leave the center of the blood stream, and decelerate to come in contact with the vascular endothelium. However, due to the force of blood flow in postcapillary venules (shear rate ~150 to 1600 s^{-1}, depending on flow rate and vessel diameter) collisional contact duration between leukocytes and unstimulated endothelium is brief (*i.e.* <25 ms) (Simon S. I., Goldsmith H. L., 2002). Specific interaction mechanisms between leukocytes and activated endothelium under shear flow are therefore required for leukocyte recruitment to inflammatory foci.

In fact, during inflammation, locally released stimuli (*e.g.* bacterial peptides, complement fragments, chemokines, histamine, and damage-associated molecular patterns) activate endothelial cells in the nearby venules to upregulate adhesion molecules on the plasma membrane which will aid leukocyte tethering, slow rolling and adhesion to the endothelium, leading ultimately to leukocyte transmigration into the tissue.

Selectins are a family of long adhesive molecules, extending from the plasma membrane, which facilitate attachment of circulating leukocytes to the endothelium (Patel K. D. *et al.*, 1995; Kansas G.S., 1996). Increased expression of P- and E-selectin (CD62P and CD62E, respectively) on activated venular endothelium induces leukocyte tethering (Kunkel E. J., Ley K., 1996; Petri B. *et al.*, 2008). While P-selectin is stored in Weibel-Palade bodies within the endothelial cells, E-selectin requires *de novo* synthesis. Once tethered, leukocytes can rapidly release and reengage selectin ligand bonds, resulting in a slow rotational movement along the vessel wall termed rolling (Norman M. U., Kubes P., 2005; Kelly M. *et al.*, 2007; Ley K. *et al.*, 2007). Rolling dynamics is optimized by force-regulated transitions from catch bonds to slip bonds[1], which explains the requirement for a shear threshold to support rolling (McEver R. P., Zhu C., 2010). L-selectin (CD62L), constitutively expressed on leukocytes, participates redundantly with P- and E-selecting, and supports both capture and rolling of leukocytes in blood vessels (Kunkel E. J., Ley K., 1996; Petri B. *et al.*, 2008).

Each of the three selectins binds with different affinity to sialylated and fucosylated oligosaccharides including sialyl Lewis^X (sLe^X) moieties, which are present on multiple glycolipids and glycoproteins on leukocytes and endothelium (McEver R. P., 2001; Simon S. I., Green C. E., 2005; Kelly M. *et al.*, 2007). The best characterized selectin ligand is PSGL-1 (P-selectin glycoprotein ligand-1), a heavily sialylated mucin present on leukocytes and endothelial cells, which can serve as a ligand to P-, E- and L-selectins although it binds P-selectin with the highest affinity (Kansas G. S., 1996). Besides PSGL-1, other ligands have been identified for E-selectin, *e.g.* sialophorin (leukosialin, CD43), hematopoietic cell E-selectin ligand (HCELL, CD44), and E-selectin ligand-1 (ESL1) (Kelly M. *et al.*, 2007; Ley K. *et al.*, 2007). L-selectin can also bind other ligands *e.g.* glycosylation-dependent cell adhesion molecule-1 (GlyCAM-1), mucosal addresin cell adhesion molecule-1 (MAdCAM-1), podocalyxin (CD34), heparan sulfate (HS) and sulphated glycoprotein-200 (Sgp200) (Wang L. *et al.*, 2005).

Rolling along the endothelium provides leukocytes a great opportunity to interact with and be further activated by chemokines or other inflammatory mediators presented on the luminal endothelium.

2.2 Intravascular chemokine presentation to rolling leukocytes

To initiate activation and recruitment of circulating leukocytes to tissue, tissue-derived chemokines need to be presented to rolling leukocytes at the apical endothelium. Within blood vessels, immobilization of chemokines on the endothelium is essential to avoid that they are washed away from the site of inflammation by the blood flow.

---

[1] *Catch bond:* a bond that prolongs its lifetime in response to tensile force; *Slip bond:* a bond that shortens its lifetime in response to tensile force (McEver R. P., Zhu C., 2010).

Heparan sulfate proteoglycans (HSPGs) are proteins bearing covalently attached complex polysaccharide chains that are negatively charged (heparan sulfate, HS), and are found on cell surfaces of most cell types as well as in the extracellular matrix (Bernfield M. *et al.*, 1999, Parish C., 2005). Chemokines and a variety of positively charged proteins bind to HS through specific and/or electrostatic interactions (Lindhal U., Kjellén L., 1991; Lindhal U., 2007). Indeed, interstitially released chemokines were shown to cross the endothelium and to be presented by luminal HSPGs to leukocytes both *in vitro* (Ihrcke N. S. *et al.*, 1993; Parish C., 2005; Wang L. *et al.*, 2005; Lindhal U., 2007) and *in vivo* (Massena S. *et al.*, 2010). Binding of chemokines to endothelial HSPG may promote molecular encounters between rolling leukocytes and chemokines, and thereby further inducing leukocyte activation. Moreover, endothelial HS acts as a ligand for L-selectin aiding neutrophil slow rolling (Wang L. *et al.*, 2005), which increase the propensity for leukocyte-chemokine encounters.

How chemokines originating from the afflicted site or released by tissue leukocytes reach the luminal side of the endothelium in order to be presented by HS to leukocytes is not completely established. However, electron microscopy studies suggested that chemokines bound to HS are transported through the endothelium by transcytosis (Middleton J. *et al.*, 1997) as endothelium exposed to interleukin-8 (IL-8, CXCL8) contained IL-8 within intracellular caveola, while no chemokines were found at endothelial cell junctions. Nevertheless, under the experimental conditions of this study, it is impossible to tell if the intracellular chemokines are being transported through endothelium towards the apical membrane or if they are on their way to lyzosomes for degradation. In addition, soluble chemokines passing through junctions cannot be detected using electron microscopy, as they would be lost during tissue preparation prior to examination.

Edema formation is one of the cardinal signs of inflammation, and is caused by increased vascular permeability and consequent plasma leakage. The primary cause of increased vascular permeability is leakage of plasma through paracellular gaps (Curry F. E., Adamson R. H., 2010; Lindbom L., Kenne E., 2011), which is regulated by the interplay of adhesive forces between adjacent endothelial cells and counter adhesive forces generated by endothelial actomyosin contraction (Mehta D., Malik A. B., 2006). The physiological importance of this event for leukocyte recruitment is debated. It is well documented that increased vascular permeability in presence of inflammatory mediators is accompanied by increased leukocyte adhesion and diapedesis (Curry F.E., Adamson R. H., 1999; Michel C. C., Curry F. E., 1999). Nevertheless, temporal and spatial uncoupling between these two events has also been described. During inflammation, vascular permeability can increase at a faster rate than leukocyte transmigration (Kim M. H. *et al.*, 2009), suggesting that increased vascular permeability precedes leukocyte recruitment. Further, in aseptic wounds, vascular permeability and leukocyte extravasation were shown to be uncoupled (Curry F.E., Adamson R. H., 1999; Kim M. H. *et al.*, 2009). It is generally believed that increased permeability supports chemokine influx into the vessels and one hypothesis is that the increase in vascular permeability during inflammation grants the paracellular transport of chemokines for rapid presentation to intravascular leukocytes, guiding them out to the afflicted area in the tissue. A recent study using intravital spinning-disk confocal microscopy in anesthetized mice revealed that chemokines added extravascularly became accumulated intra-luminally at endothelial cell junctions (Massena S. *et al.*, 2010). High junctional sequestration of chemokines suggests that chemokines are transported either paracellularly into blood vessels or longitudinally on the apical endothelial cell membrane towards junctions after being transcytosed. Further, this observation might simply reflect high concentrations of HS in junctional regions. However, these findings suggest that increased vascular permeability during inflammation does not necessary account for amplified leukocyte extravasation *per se,* but instead might promote cytokine/chemokine transport and thereby induce leukocyte recruitment.

Endothelial cells display extraordinary phenotypic and functional heterogeneity. Endothelial cell structural features such as shape, thickness, molecular characteristics of apical membrane and junctions, as well as the thickness of the luminal glycocalyx are some of the features, which vary across the vascular tree (Van Den Berg B. M. *et al.*, 2003; Aird W. C., 2007). Heparan sulfate is known to display miscellaneous structural features in various tissues and on different cell types (Lindhal U., Li J. P., 2009), which accounts for binding of proteins in a selective fashion. Differences in proteoglycan composition (altered structure of HS epitopes or sequences, and/or expression pattern of different syndecans) might result in different chemokine binding properties, explaining the observed differences in leukocyte recruitment of different organs upon diverse inflammatory stimuli.

2.3 Leukocyte activation and adhesion to the endothelium

After being stimulated by chemokines sequestered on the endothelium, rolling leukocytes adhere to the endothelium by rapid formation of shear-resistant bindings mediated by specialized leukocyte integrins (Rose D. M. *et al.*, 2007). Integrins are noncovalently associated heterodimeric cell surface adhesion molecules consisting of combinations of α and β-molecules. Leukocytes express at least 10 members of the integrin family belonging to the β_1-, β_2- and β_7-subfamilies (Luo B. H. *et al.*, 2007). Leukocyte adhesion molecules relevant for recruitment belong to the β_1- and β_2-integrin families (Ley K. *et al.*, 2007), of which LFA-1 (Lymphocyte function-associated antigen-1, ITGAL, CD11a/CD18, $\alpha_L\beta_2$), Mac-1 (Macrophage antigen-1, ITGAM, CD11b/CD18, $\alpha_M\beta_2$) and VLA-4 (very late antigen-4, CD49d/CD29, $\alpha_4\beta_1$) are the most studied.

Members of the β_1-subfamily (also called VLA integrins) contain the β_1-subunit associated to one of at least six different α subunits (Hemler M. E., 1990). VLA-4 integrin is amply expressed on peripheral blood B-lymphocytes, T-lymphocytes and monocytes (Hemler M. E., 1990). Peripheral blood neutrophils are believed to generally be devoid of cell surface β_1-integrin structures (Hemler M. E., 1990), even though some reports claim that immature neutrophils expressing surface VLA-4 can also be found in circulation (Lund-Johansen F., Terstappen L. W., 1993; Pillay J. *et al.*, 2010).

Most circulating leukocytes express integrins in a low affinity state (Carman C. V., Springer T. A., 2003). Upon binding of chemokines to G-protein-coupled receptors (GPCRs) expressed on leukocytes, a complex intracellular signaling network is triggered within milliseconds (Shamri R. *et al.*, 2005; Ley K. *et al.*, 2007). This induces integrins to undergo an almost instantaneous change in avidity and ligand affinity (Von Andrian U. H. *et. al.*, 1992; Shamri R. *et al.*, 2005; Hyduk S. J., Cybulsky M. I., 2009). Thus, inside-out signaling after chemokine binding to GPCRs shifts the integrins from a resting to an active conformation (Simon S.I., Goldsmith H. L., 2002; Simon S. I., Green C. E., 2005), which is necessary for binding to its ligands expressed on activated endothelial cells (Ley K. *et al.*, 2007).

Differential leukocyte expression levels of integrins and chemokine receptors as well as receptor affinity for chemokines might account for selective arrest and recruitment of leukocyte subtypes. Additionally, chemokine-triggered signaling networks can regulate distinct integrins in specific leukocyte subtypes, contributing for differential leukocyte recruitment.

2.3.1 Neutrophil adhesion

β_2-integrin dependent neutrophil adhesion is fundamental for effective bacterial clearance. In fact, the genetic disorder leukocyte adhesion deficiency I (LAD I) is characterized by a profound defect in leukocyte recruitment and therefore severe immunodeficiency, due to neutrophils failing to adhere to the activated endothelium since the surface levels of β_2-integrins are dramatically reduced or absent (Bunting M. *et al.*, 2002).

It was recently found that binding of the β_2-integrin LFA-1 to intercellular adhesion molecule-1 (ICAM-1, CD54) expressed by endothelial cells, mediates neutrophil firm adhesion to the vascular endothelium under shear flow (Shamri R. *et al.*, 2005; Phillipson M. *et al.*, 2006; Ley K. *et al.*, 2007; Petri B. *et al.*, 2008). LFA-1 is also able to bind to other immunoglobulin superfamily members, ICAM-2 (CD102) and ICAM-3 (CD50), albeit with lower affinity relative to ICAM-1 (De Fougerolles A. R. *et al.*, 1994), in addition to JAM-A (junction adhesion molecule-A).

However, there is some evidence that neutrophils adhere via other adhesion molecules than LFA-1, or by non-adhesion processes such as physical trapping, described to occur in lung capillaries or liver sinusoids (Doerschuk C. M. *et al.*, 1990; Wong J. *et al.*, 1997; Norman M. U., Kubes P., 2005). Indeed, anti-CD18 treatment did not reduce leukocyte recruitment to the lung of rabbits (Doerschuk C. M. *et al.*, 1990), or in the rat liver (Jaeschke H. *et al.*, 1996). In the liver, neutrophils have been reported to adhere via CD44 interacting with sinusoidal hyaluronan (McDonald B. *et al.*, 2008). Furthermore, under systemic inflammatory conditions, such as sepsis, neutrophils have been suggested to adhere to the endothelium via VLA-4 (Ibbotson G. C. *et al.*, 2001). This integrin was also proposed to be involved in neutrophil adhesion in the lung microvasculature (Ibbotson G. C. *et al.*, 2001).

2.3.2 Monocyte adhesion

In contrast to neutrophil adhesion, β_2-integrins seem to play a moderate role in monocyte arrest, since monocytes both adhere and polarize after blockade of β_2-integrins as well as after blockade of ICAM-1 or ICAM-2 *in vitro* (Schenkel A. R. *et al.*, 2004). Instead, β_1-integrins seem to play a more substantial role in monocyte adhesion to the endothelium. In fact, recent mouse models showed that monocytes firmly adhered to endothelium by VLA-4 binding to endothelial VCAM-1 (vascular cell adhesion molecule-1, CD106) (Luscinkas F. W. *et al.*, 1994; Meerschaert J., Furie M. B., 1995; Lee T. D. *et al.*, 2003; Ley K. *et al.*, 2007; Soehnlein O. *et al.*, 2009).

2.3.3 Lymphocyte adhesion

During lymphocyte recruitment to peripheral tissues, LFA-1 is the dominant integrin involved in firm adhesion (Dustin M., Springer T. A., 1989; Shamri R. *et al.*, 2005) by binding to its ligand ICAM-1 (Shamri R. *et al.*, 2005). As described for neutrophils, LFA-1 prevails in a low affinity state on most circulating lymphocytes. Stimulation of lymphocyte-GPCRs rapidly shifts LFA-1 integrin to a high avidity state (Carman C. V., Springer T. A., 2003). This high avidity state of LFA-1 on T-lymphocytes is transient, peaking 5 to 10 minutes after receptor stimulation and returns to the low affinity state by 30 min to 2 hours (Dustin M., Springer T. A., 1989).

T-lymphocytes are not only recruited to tissue, they also home to lymph nodes. *In vitro* studies of T-lymphocyte adhesion to the specialized lymph node endothelium (high endothelial venules, HEV), demonstrated that besides LFA-1, VLA-4 is involved in T-cell adhesion (Faveew C. *et al.*, 2000). Adhesion was reduced by 40-50% upon treatment with inhibiting antibodies to either integrin. Interestingly, the effects of VLA-4 and LFA-1 antibodies were additive, giving >90% inhibition of T-lymphocyte adhesion.

2.4 Intravascular chemotactic gradients and leukocyte crawling

Using time-lapse *in vivo* microscopy, adherent neutrophils and monocytes were recently observed to crawl significant distances within the vessels (Phillipson M. *et al.*, 2006; Auffray C. *et al.*, 2007; Phillipson M. *et al.*, 2009). The crawling neutrophils were searching the endothelium for optimal sites for transmigration, since inhibition of crawling significantly delayed neutrophil transmigration (Phillipson M. *et al.*, 2006; Sumagin R. *et al.*, 2010).

2.4.1 Neutrophil crawling

Intravascular crawling of neutrophils is dependent on the leukocyte β_2-integrin Mac-1 and its ligand ICAM-1 on endothelial cells (Phillipson M. *et al.*, 2006; Sumagin R. *et al.*, 2010). Compared to LFA-1, Mac-1 binds a wider spectrum of ligands, including complement fragment iC3b, fibrinogen, fibronectin, laminin, collagen, myeloperoxidase, elastase, JAM-B and –C to name just a few (Simon S. I., Green C. E., 2005; Kelly M. *et al.*, 2007; Luo B. H. *et al.*, 2007) suggesting that this integrin might have other roles apart from intravascular crawling.

Neutrophil crawling on the stimulated endothelium occurs in two distinct stages. In the initial phase directly following neutrophil adhesion, a mechanotactic signal provided by shear stress induces neutrophil crawling perpendicular to blood flow until an endothelial cell junction is encountered (Phillipson M. *et al.*, 2009). This observation has also been made *in vitro* when adherent neutrophils crawled perpendicular to the direction of flow when shear was applied to the system (Phillipson M. *et al.*, 2009). However, as soon as the crawling neutrophils meet the junction, the shear stress signal is ignored and neutrophils instead begin to follow the junction. Considering that endothelial cells are elongated in the direction of flow, perpendicular crawling generates the greatest probability for a neutrophil to find an endothelial junction in the shortest period of time.

More recently, the existence of an intravascular gradient of chemokines (macrophage inflammatory protein-2, CXCL2 [MIP-2]; keratinocyte-derived chemokine, CXCL1 [KC]) originating from the infection or released by tissue leukocytes on endothelial cells has been described (Massena S. *et al.*, 2010). Indeed, this chemotactic gradient is sequestered on endothelial HS and provides directional cues to crawling neutrophils, which follow this gradient to optimal transmigration sites close to the origin of the infection (Massena S. *et al.*,

2010). However, whether haptotactic gradients can be established by all chemokines remains unclear, since different chemokines have diverse affinity to HS (Lindhal U., Kjellén L., 1991; Lindhal U., 2007).

Directional intravascular crawling along a chemotactic gradient expedites neutrophil recruitment, compared to when no chemokine gradient is formed due to homogenous extravascular chemokine concentrations (Massena S. *et al.*, 2010). Disruption of the chemokine gradient is translated into random crawling and inefficient recruitment of neutrophils which ultimately leads to a decreased ability to clear infections, as seen in *Staphylococcus aureus* infected mice with truncated HS chains (overexpressing heparanase, Massena S. *et al.*, 2010).

2.4.2 Monocyte crawling

Intravascular crawling monocytes have been reported *in vivo* (Auffray C. *et al.*, 2007; Sumagin R. *et al.*, 2010), and crawling on endothelium is critical to reach optimal transmigration sites, as demonstrated *in vitro* (Schenkel A. R. *et al.*, 2004).

Whereas the integrin Mac-1 alone is responsible for crawling of neutrophils, LFA-1 and Mac-1 integrins were in some studies reported to play a redundant role in monocyte crawling via binding to ICAM-1 and ICAM-2 (Schenkel A. R. *et al.*, 2004; Sumagin R. *et al.*, 2010). Blockade of each of these molecules led to a pirouette behavior at the adhesion site (Schenkel A. R. *et al.*, 2004). Nevertheless, monocytes were shown to be able to adhere and polarize.

Recently, a distinct role for each of these integrins on monocyte crawling under different endothelial activation states has been described. Monocytes were shown to crawl long distances on resting endothelium in a patrolling behavior (*i.e.* monitoring healthy tissue) in a LFA-1-dependent manner (Auffray C. *et al.*, 2007; Sumagin R. *et al.*, 2010). However, upon inflammatory stimulation, monocyte crawling became Mac-1-dependent and assumed a neutrophil-like crawling pattern, *i.e.* similar crawling distance and confinement ratio (Sumagin R. *et al.*, 2010). These results have been suggested to correspond to differences between two different monocyte populations rather than to a shift in integrin expression upon inflammatory stimulation.

Two monocyte subsets distinguished by their expression levels of selectins, integrins and chemokine receptors have already been characterized in various mammals (Geissman F. *et al.*, 2003; Gordon S., Taylor P. R., 2005). These phenotypic differences encompass distinct effector functions. A monocyte subset termed "resident" (CX_3CR1^{hi} $CCR2^-$ $Ly6C^-$ in mice; $CD14^{lo}$ $CD16^+$ in humans) is involved in tissue remodeling and wound repair (Gordon S., Taylor P. R., 2005; Auffray C. *et al.*, 2007; Soehnlein O. *et al.*, 2009). In contrast, another monocyte subset denominated "inflammatory" (CX_3CR1^{lo} $CCR2^+$ $Ly6C^+$ in mice; $CD14^{hi}$ $CD16^-$ in humans) is specialized in pro-inflammatory activities such as bacterial phagocytosis, secretion of inflammation-promoting cytokines and reactive species as well as proteolytic activity (Gordon S., Taylor P. R., 2005; Auffray C. *et al.*, 2007; Soehnlein O. *et al.*, 2009). Resident monocytes, express high amounts of LFA-1. In contrast, inflammatory monocytes do not express LFA-1, even though no differences were found for Mac-1 between the two monocyte subsets (Auffray C. *et al.*, 2007).

It is possible that the two subsets of circulating monocytes might use different integrins and display different crawling patterns to achieve the different effector functions.

2.4.3 Lymphocyte crawling

In vitro, adherent T-lymphocytes have been reported to crawl over the luminal surface of the endothelium in a LFA-1-dependent manner (Shulman *et al.*, 2009). LFA-1 is also responsible for T-lymphocyte adhesion, but the distribution of the membrane LFA-1 is altered correlating with changes in cell morphology as soon as the T-lymphocyte starts to migrate (Smith A. *et al.*, 2005). LFA-1 turnover at numerous focal points ensures rapid crawling and resistance to detachment by shear forces (Shulman *et al.*, 2009). Low expression levels of LFA-1 were detected at the leading edge of the cell and high expression level in the non-attached uropod at the rear (Smith A. *et al.*, 2005). Interestingly, LFA-1 in the leading edge was not in a high-affinity state, as detected by use of specific antibodies that recognize LFA-1 in different conformational states (Smith A. *et al.*, 2007). Instead LFA-1 in the leading edge was in an intermediate affinity conformation allowing crawling possibly by weaker interactions with ICAM-1.

Published studies have identified intravascular natural killer T-lymphocytes (NKT cells) with possible sentinel functions for the detection of bacteria in the blood (Geissmann F. *et al.*, 2005; Lee T. D. *et al.*, 2010; Thomas S. Y. *et al.*, 2011). These cells are distinguished by their restricted repertoire of T-cell receptor (TCR) variants that recognize lipids and glycolipids presented by CD1d (Kawano T. *et al.*, 1997; Brossay L. *et al.*, 1998). NKT cells primarily reside and wander within the vasculature of the liver and spleen (Geissmann F. *et al.*, 2005; Bendelac A. *et al.*, 2007) but have also been suggested to accumulate in smaller amounts in the vascular compartment of the lung (Thomas S. Y. *et al.*, 2011). The mechanisms underlying adhesion and crawling of NKT cells are still poorly understood. It has been reported that treatment of mice with blocking antibodies to LFA-1 and ICAM-1 induced rapid detachment of adherent NKT cells from sinusoidal endothelium (Thomas S. Y. *et al.*, 2011). In contrast, blocking VLA-4 or VCAM-1 had no effect. Integrin activation typically relies on inside-out signaling after chemokine binding to GPCRs (Ley K. *et al.*, 2007). However, genetic ablation of CXCR6 (the major chemokine receptor expressed on NKT cells) or treatment with an inhibitor of GPCRs, did not induce detachment of NKT cells from liver microvasculature (Geissmann F. *et al.*, 2005; Lee T. D. *et al.*, 2010). Furthermore, previous studies on NKT cells transferred into CD1d-deficient mice suggested that TCR activation was not a prerequisite for NKT cells sinusoidal adhesion (McNab F. W. *et al.*, 2005; Wei D. G. *et al.*, 2005). Crawling was also unimpeded in mice treated with anti-CD1d antibody (Lee T. D. *et al.*, 2010). Interestingly, upon infection with the blood-borne pathogen *Borrelia burgdorferi* (a spirochete injected intravenously through tick bite), NKT cells were reported to slow their crawling and to accumulate in clusters on Kupffer cells in a GPCRs-dependent way (CXCR3, and CD1d) (Lee T. D. *et al.*, 2010). Kupffer cells are specialized ramified macrophages, which line the walls of liver sinusoids and prevent the dissemination of pathogens via the blood by capturing and engulfing them. Kupffer cells can then present glycolipid antigens via CD1d (Lee T. D. *et al.*, 2010). In the absence of Kupffer or NKT cells, dissemination of *Borrelia burgdorferi* occurred, suggesting a role for NKT cells in vascular surveillance for blood-borne pathogens captured by Kupffer cells (Lee T. D. *et al.*, 2010).

2.5 Diapedesis: Trans- and paracellular routes

Leukocyte diapedesis out of vasculature into affected tissue can occur both between neighboring endothelial cells (paracellularly through junctions) and directly through the endothelium (transcellularly) (Feng D. *et al.*, 1998; Shaw S. K. *et al.*, 2001; Carman C. V., Springer T. A., 2004; Engelhardt B., Wolburg H., 2004; Yang L. *et al.*, 2005; Phillipson M. *et al.*, 2006). The route employed most likely depends on inflammatory stimuli, as well as the type of leukocyte and vascular bed.

Diapedesis has been reported to be mediated by numerous endothelial adhesion molecules expressed in high density at endothelial junctions, such as platelet-endothelial cell adhesion molecule 1 (PECAM-1, CD31), CD99, vascular endothelial-cadherins (VE-cadherins), endothelial cell-selective adhesion molecule (ESAM), ICAM-1 and -2 and JAMs (Luscinskas F. W. *et al.*, 2002; Engelhardt B., Wolburg H., 2004; Yang L. *et al.*, 2005; Ley K. *et al.*, 2007; Lou O. *et al.*, 2007; Petri B. *et al.*, 2008; Woodfin A. *et al.*, 2011). Other molecules involved in leukocyte transmigration are integrins expressed on leukocytes (*e.g.* LFA-1, Mac-1, VLA-4) (Ley K. *et al.*, 2007; Petri B. *et al.*, 2008; Woodfin A. *et al.*, 2011). The specific molecules involved in either of the transmigration pathways remains to be identified.

The different molecules appear to mediate leukocyte transmigration in either a stimulus-specific or leukocyte-specific manner. For example PECAM-1, ICAM-2 and JAM-A mediate leukocyte transmigration in response to interleukin-1β (IL-1β) but not to tumor necrosis factor-alpha (TNF-α) (Wang S. *et al.*, 2006; Ley K. *et al.*, 2007). Direct activation of leukocytes by TNF-α, fMLP (N-formyl-methionyl-leucyl-phenylalanine) or leukotriene-B_4 (LTB_4) appears to bypass the need for these molecules. Studies of activated mouse cremaster muscle and intravital microscopy in mice knocked down for ESAM gene (Ley K. *et al.*, 2007) have shown that ESAM does not show a stimulus-specific role but appears to mediate neutrophil rather than T-lymphocyte transmigration.

Neutrophils have been found to transmigrate predominantly through the paracellular route, *i.e.* between adjacent endothelial cells (Phillipson M. *et al.*, 2006; Woodfin A. *et al.*, 2011). Paracellular transmigration was found to be dependent on the ability for leukocytes to crawl to optimal transmigration sites at the endothelial cell junctions. In Mac-1 deficient mice, due to inhibition of intravascular crawling, transcellular transmigration predominated (Phillipson M. *et al.*, 2006).

Using *in vivo* spinning disk or multi-photon confocal microscopy, profound anatomical changes of the endothelium that facilitated leukocyte extravasation without compromising vascular barrier integrity were observed (Phillipson M. *et al.*, 2008; Petri B. *et al.*, 2011). Docking cup-like structures were formed by endothelial cells (endothelial projections) at the base of the transmigrating neutrophil, which has also been described for T-lymphocytes *in vitro* (Carman C. V., Springer T. A., 2004). The endothelial projections extended towards the top of the neutrophil and eventually formed a dome that surrounded the entire neutrophil, prior to basolateral opening and neutrophil migration further into tissue. If the dome formations were prevented, neutrophil transmigration was delayed (Petri B. *et al.*, 2011), further implicating an active role of endothelium during leukocyte diapedesis, while maintaining the barrier function and vascular permeability.

2.5.1 Migration through the subendothelial basement membrane and pericyte sheet

To overcome the barrier of the blood vessel and finally reach the inflamed tissue, leukocytes also have to transmigrate across the subendothelial basement membrane (BM) surrounding the venular endothelium. This has been shown to occur in areas low in collagen IV, laminin-10 and nidogen-2 (Wang S. *et al.*, 2006). These areas were seen to be closely associated to gaps between pericytes (Wang S. *et al.*, 2006). Interestingly, leukocytes have been observed to initiate transmigration through endothelium at sites superimposing these specific areas. How intravascular crawling leukocytes can detect these areas from the luminal side of the endothelium remains unknown.

2.6 Extravascular crawling

Following leukocyte diapedesis across the vessel wall, further movement in tissue is required in order for the leukocytes to reach the affected site to exert their effector functions. As within the vasculature, leukocyte movement in the tissue is guided by chemotactic gradients leading to the source (Foxman E. F. *et al.*, 1997; Lindbom L., Werr J., 2002). Upon binding to GPCRs on leukocytes, chemoattractants trigger downstream signaling, which translates to cytoskeletal reorganization, polarization and directional locomotion (Friedl P. *et al.*, 2001). Migrating leukocytes thereby adopt a polarized morphology consisting of a leading edge and a tail-like uropod (Friedl P. *et al.*, 2001).

In order to initiate movement, leukocytes have to establish adhesive contacts with the tissue stroma via interactions between the extracellular integrin domains and components of the extracellular matrix (ECM) (Friedl P. *et al.*, 2001; Lindbom L., Werr J., 2002). Stimulation by encountered chemoattractants activates surface integrins and recruits additional integrins from cytoplasmic stores (Diamond M. S., Springer T. A., 1994; Friedl P. *et al.*, 2001). Binding to ECM macromolecules triggers integrin-mediated signals, which regulate further integrin apposition, actin assembly, cell polarity, and migration (Friedl P. *et al.*, 2001).

Accumulating evidence suggests that leukocyte chemotaxis in the ECM is mostly associated with β_1-integrins while a limited role for β_2-integrins is described (Sixt M. *et al.*, 2001). Members of the β_1-family shown to be involved in leukocyte locomotion (Gao J. X., Issekutz A. C., 1997; Werr J. *et al.*, 1998; Sixt M. *et al.*, 2001) show high affinity interactions with proteins of the ECM, including fibronectin, vibronectin, collagen and laminin (Hemler M. E., 1990). Circulating neutrophils are not believed to constitutively express β_1-integrins. However, it has been suggested that upregulation of β_2-integrins by chemotactic stimuli induced an outside-in signaling leading to mobilization of β_1-integrins to the neutrophil surface, in order to prepare recruited neutrophils for subsequent interactions with ECM (Lindbom L., Werr J., 2002). There are also studies demonstrating upregulation of neutrophil surface expression of β_1-integrins in association with emigration from the vasculature (Kubes P. *et al.*, 1995; Werr J. *et al.*, 1998).

Another adhesion molecule involved in extravascular crawling is L-selectin. Indeed, studies using L-selectin-deficient mice revealed no role of L-selectin on leukocyte rolling or adhesion, but transmigration was significantly impaired (Hickey M. J. *et al.*, 2000). Furthermore, leukocytes in L-selectin-deficient mice were unable to respond to directional cues (platelet activating factor [PAF]; KC) in the interstitium (Hickey M. J. *et al.*, 2000). These findings provided strong evidence of an important L-selectin function in leukocyte emigration and extravascular locomotion. Intriguingly, L-selectin expression on emigrated leukocytes is dramatically reduced in comparison to levels on circulating leukocytes (Hickey M. J. *et al.*, 2000). Shedding of L-selectin upon transmigration has been reported both *in vitro* (Smith C. W. *et al.*, 1991; Allport J. R. *et al.*, 1997) and *in vivo* (Jutila M. A. *et al.*, 1989). These results raise the possibility that L-selectin early in the recruitment cascade triggers downstream signals that modulate consecutive transmigration and migration in the interstitium (Hickey M. J. *et al.*, 2000).

Further, integrins bind different components of the tissue stroma and with diverse affinities (Lindbom L., Werr J., 2002). Leukocyte chemotaxis in the tissue is therefore influenced not only by the stimuli encountered but also by the matrix proteins in the tissue.

2.6.1 Prioritazing chemotactic cues

During bacterial infections, the chemotaxing leukocytes are exposed to a cacophony of different chemotactic gradients of diverse origins. Chemoattractants originate from the bacteria themselves (*e.g.* fMLP; lipopolysaccharide [LPS]) or complement fragments bound to bacteria (*e.g.* complement fragment C5a), but also from nearby activated leukocytes and endothelial cells (*e.g.* LTB_4; IL-8) (Foxman E. F. *et al.*, 1997; Heit B. *et al.*, 2008; Muller W. A., 2011). A microenvironment where numerous chemoattractants are encountered requires tightly regulated intracellular mechanisms for leukocytes to readily prioritize between the cues, in order for them to effectively reach the target. Thus, to fulfill their missions, leukocytes need to find the bacteria without being distracted by opposing gradients. A hierarchical relationship between chemotactic factors has developed, and "end-target" chemotactic factors like bacterial products *versus* the "intermediate" chemokines released by activated endothelium or tissue leukocytes have been shown to activate separate signaling pathways in neutrophils (p38-mitogen-activated protein kinase [p38MAPK] and phosphoinositide 3-kinase [PI3K], respectively [Campbell J. J. *et al.*, 1997; Heit B. *et al.*, 2002]). In this way, neutrophils are able to sort signals in the noisy environment of inflammation, and respond to chemotactic cues in a hierarchical manner, preferring "end-target" chemoattractant factors like fMLP and C5a over "intermediate" chemokines like IL-8 (Foxman E. F. *et al.*, 1997). This has been suggested to occur through the p38MAPK pathway inhibiting PI3K through relocalization of phosphatase and tensin homologue (PTEN) on the basolateral cell membrane of the polarized moving cell (Heit B. *et al.*, 2008). However, additional parallel scenarios of how chemotacting leukocytes are directed to their goal have been described (PLA2, cGMP and DOCK2/phosphatic acid). Despite the mentioned advances in understanding how leukocytes find their way in tissue, many issues remain to be deciphered considering the very complex nature of the extravascular environment during infection. Leukocytes will not only encounter bacterial chemoattractants and chemokines, but also cytokines, lipids and complement fragments. Cytokines (IL-1β, TNF-α) are released simultaneously during infection and induce chemokine production. Chemokines and cytokines have been shown to act in concert to direct leukocyte delivery and activation, and chemokines of different families have been demonstrated *in vitro* to synergistically enhance influx of both neutrophils and monocytes (Gouwy M. *et al.*, 2008; Kuscher K. *et al.*, 2009). Further, interplay between lipid chemoattractant LTB_4, the cytokine IL-1β and the chemokine ligands to first CCR1 and later CXCR2 was shown in a model of arthritogenesis (Chou R. C. *et al.*, 2010). This vividly demonstrates that leukocyte recruitment *in vivo*, in contrast to during *in vitro* settings hardly is the result of release of a single chemokine, and that synergistic as well as opposing effects of involved signaling molecules are to be expected to enhance as well as steer the inflammatory response. This interplay needs to be further clarified and the importance of these observations has to be confirmed *in vivo*, to determine therapeutic targets during different inflammatory conditions.

3. Additional stimuli for leukocyte recruitment

Inflammation is closely linked to hypoxia, and numerous leukocytes are detected at sites of tissue ischemia (Eltzschig H. K., Carmeliet P., 2011). Severe hypoxia causes both apoptosis and necrosis of somatic cells, which results in release of various damage-associated danger signals, like DAMPs (danger associated molecular pattern molecules). DAMPs include molecules originating from the cytosol or the nucleus, such as adenosine triphosphate (ATP), formylated peptides from mitochondria, heat shock proteins, chromatin and galectins, that often undergo denaturation when leaving the intracellular milieu, where after they become pro-inflammatory (Kono H., Rock K. L., 2008). Even though most of them are not considered directly chemotactic, they induce leukocyte recruitment by activating tissue macrophages and nearby endothelial cells to secrete pro-inflammatory cytokines (*e.g.* IL-1β) and chemokines (*e.g.* IL-8), in addition to upregulating expression of adhesion molecules on endothelial cells (Muller W. A., 2011). However, fomylated peptides originating from mitochondria were recently found to recruit neutrophils via activation of the fMLP receptor formyl-peptide receptor-1 (McDonald B. *et al.*, 2010; Zhang Q. *et al.*, 2010).

During hypoxia and cell injury, recruited neutrophils are believed to contribute to wound healing processes by clearing the area of debris through phagocytosis. In addition to phagocytosis, leukocytes have recently been acknowledged for their role in angiogenesis and tissue remodeling both during health and disease. Neutrophils produce and store within their granules pro-angiogenic molecules such as VEGF-A (vascular endothelial growth factor-A, [Gaudry M. *et al.*, 1997]) and MMP-9 (matrix metalloproteinase-9, [Ardi V. C. *et al.*, 2007]). VEGF is a key player in blood vessel formation and has a direct chemotactic effect on endothelial cells, while the pro-angiogenic function of MMP-9 is attributed to its ability to digest extra cellular matrix (ECM), which pave way for new vessels as well as release and thereby activate ECM-bound VEGF and other growth factors. The neutrophils are in fact the only cells in the body that release MMP-9 free of its endogenous inhibitor TIMP (tissue inhibitor of metalloproteinase), and are therefore capable of deliver highly active MMP-9 to sites of angiogenesis (Ardi V. C. *et al.*, 2007). The pro-angiogenic capacity of neutrophils has been demonstrated in a corneal injury model, where the number of infiltrated neutrophils positively correlated to angiogenesis and VEGF levels (Gong Y., Koh D. R., 2010). Neutrophil depletion significantly impaired tissue healing in this model, as well as the release of VEGF. Further, neutrophils recruited to islets of Langerhans transplanted to striated muscle were recently shown to be crucial for revascularization to occur, as transplantation of islets to neutropenic mice resulted in complete inhibition of islets revascularization (Christoffersson G. *et al.*, 2010). Neutrophils were shown to accumulate at sites for islet engraftment and were specifically localized at the newly formed vessels, as demonstrated in **Figure 2**.

Monocytes have also been shown to have pro-angiogenic properties. For instance, tissue healing following myocardial infarction requires sequential mobilization of the two

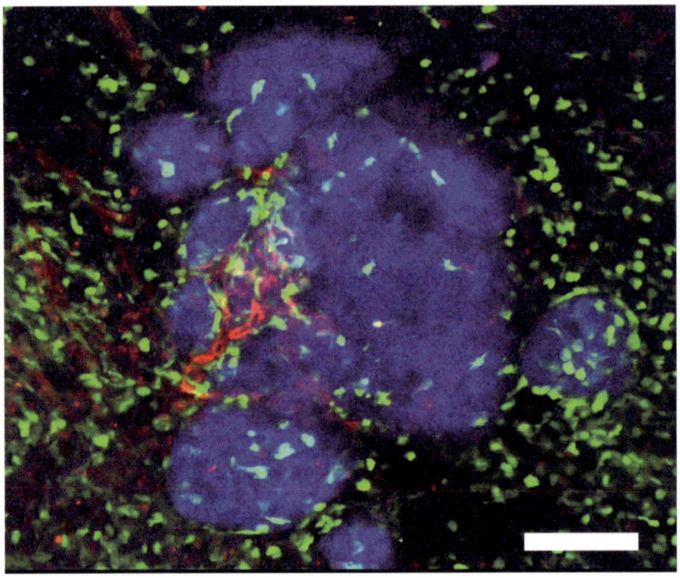

Fig. 2. Isolated pancreatic islets (blue) transplanted to muscle causes Gr1+ cell (green) accumulation (courtesy of G. Christoffersson). Blood vessels are stained with anti-CD31 (red). Scale bar equals 100 μm.

described monocyte subsets which exhibit opposing phenotypes (Nahrendorf M. *et al.*, 2007). Recruited "inflammatory" monocytes exhibit proteolytic activity and inflammatory functions, whereas monocytes of the "resident" subtype contribute to angiogenesis and have attenuated inflammatory properties (Nahrendorf M. *et al.*, 2007).

In the field of tumor biology, it is known that the ability of tumors to create an immunomodulating microenvironment to escape cytotoxic immune cells and to allow for angiogenesis is central for tumor growth. Different factors have been shown to skew tumor-associated leukocytes including neutrophils and macrophages from a pro-inflammatory, anti-tumorigenic to a pro-tumorigenic, pro-angiogenic phenotype (Fridlender Z. G. *et al.*, 2009; Hanahan D., Weinberg R. A., 2011; Rolny C. *et al.*, 2011). Indeed, the angiogenic switch in islet dysplasia and tumors in the RIP1-Tag2 transgenic mouse model of pancreatic cancer was mediated by tumor-infiltrated MMP-9 expressing neutrophils (Nozawa H. *et al.*, 2006).

The identity of these pro-angiogenic leukocytes is currently being investigated, and whether circulating subpopulations with pro-angiogenic and anti-inflammatory properties exist, or if they attain their phenotype giving the stimuli, are under debate. Myeloid-derived suppressor cells (MDSCs) are a heterogenic population that increases in numbers in the spleen and bone marrow of tumor bearing mice, and consists of monocyte and neutrophil subsets with potent ability of suppressing immune functions such as T-lymphocyte activation (Bronte V. *et al.*, 2000). In mice, they express CD11b and Gr-1, where the GR-1^{hi} CD11b^{+} corresponds to immature and mature neutrophil subpopulations while the Gr-1^{int} CD11b^{+} to the monocyte subset (Peranzoni E. *et al.*, 2010; Youn J. I., Gabrilovich D. I., 2010). How other surface markers differ from the classical pro-inflammatory neutrophils or monocytes are not completely established, but the roles of neutrophils during restitution and angiogenesis described above might indeed involve the neutrophil subset of MDSC.

Further characterization of the identities of leukocytes involved in tissue restitution and angiogenesis, and even more importantly their functions during these situations, is of great relevance.

4. Therapeutic interventions

A variety of disorders are associated with leukocyte activation and infiltration. Asthma (Fanta C. H., 2009; Broide D. H. *et al.*, 2011; Minnicozzi M. *et al.*, 2011); emphysema (Martinez F. J. *et al.*, 2011); atherosclerosis (Ross R., 1999; Hansson G., 2005); inflammatory bowel disease (Khor B. *et al.*, 2011); rheumatoid arthritis (Olsen N. J., Stein C. M., 2004; O'Dell J. R., 2004; Scott D. L., Kingsley G. H., 2006); multiple sclerosis (Frohman E. M. *et al.*, 2006); sepsis (Hotchkiss R. S., Karl I. E., 2003); and allograft rejection after transplantation (Savasta M., Lentini S., 2011; Arias M. *et al.*, 2011), are just some examples of this broad spectrum. Although many details remain to be delineated, the consensus is that the over-exuberant, maladaptive and/or uncontrolled inflammation is in the pathogenesis of these conditions and leads to tissue injury.

Over the past few years, pharmacotherapeutic advances have been made, with most therapeutic options focusing on means to prevent leukocyte activation and recruitment. Anti-adhesion therapies directed against different adhesion molecules have been evaluated. However, despite positive data from animal studies, many of the integrin antagonists have failed in clinical trials or are associated with severe side effects (Rutgeerts P. *et al.*, 2009; Fontoura P., 2010; Del Zoppo G. J., 2010).

A new approach for reducing leukocyte recruitment to tissue was recently described in mice (Maiguel D. *et al.*, 2011). This study was based upon a nearly 20-year-old observation for eosinophils, which, in response to activating antibodies trapping VLA-4-integrin in a high-avidity state, were able to adhere but not migrate (Kuijpers T. W. *et al.*, 1993). Accordingly, the recent study screened for selective small-molecule Mac-1 agonists, named leukadherins. These agonists caused increased intravascular adhesion, but not transmigration of neutrophils, resulting in reduced leukocyte recruitment in experimental models of acute peritonitis and nephritis. Integrin clustering or outside-in signaling were not induced by binding of the agonist, which might account for the lack of detectable vascular injury, even though the effects on tissue blood flow by the increased number of intravascular adherent neutrophils remains to be studied. These observations are all very intriguing, even though further experimental evaluation of this course of action is required.

5. Conclusion

Leukocyte recruitment is a hallmark event in acute and chronic inflammation. Tightly regulated activation of circulating leukocytes and intravascular leukocyte guidance by the establishment of chemokine gradients within blood vessels is fundamental for leukocytes to efficiently transmigrate to the inflamed tissue, where they finally exert their effector functions. Specific interactions between transmigrating leukocytes and the activated vascular endothelium orchestrate profound anatomical changes of the endothelium which facilitate leukocyte extravasation while maintaining the barrier function and vascular permeability. Targeting intravascular leukocyte chemotaxis and the gating property of the endothelium would limit leukocyte transmigration and/ or vascular permeability during detrimental inflammation. Understanding the underlying mechanisms behind these processes might therefore contribute for the development of novel therapeutic interventions.

6. Acknowledgements

The authors would like to acknowledge Gustaf Christoffersson who kindly supplied the image presented as Figure 2.

This work was supported by grants from the Swedish Medical Research Council, the Royal Swedish Academy of Sciences, Magnus Bergvalls Foundation, the Swedish Society for Medical Research, the Swedish Diabetes Foundation, Lars Hiertas Foundation, Harald and Greta Jeanssons Foundation, Åke Wibergs Foundation, and the Wallenberg Foundation.

7. References

Aird W. C. Phenotypic heterogeneity of the endothelium: II. Representative vascular beds. Circ. Res. (2007); 100 (2): 174-190.

Allport J. R., Ding H. T., Ager A., Steeber D. A., Tedder T. F., Luscinskas F. W. L-selectin shedding does not regulate human neutrophil attachment, rolling, or transmigration across human vascular endothelium *in vitro*. J. Immunol. (1997); 158 (9): 4365-4372.

Ardi V. C., Kupriyanova T. A., Deryugina E. I., Quingly J. P. Human neutrophils uniquely release TIMP-free MMP-9 to provide a potent catalytic stimulator of angiogenesis. Proc. Natl. Acad. Sci. U. S. A. (2007); 104 (51): 20262-20267.

Arias M., Serón D., Moreso F., Bestard O., Praga M. Chronic renal allograft damage: existing challenges. Transplantation (2011); 91 (9 Suppl): S4-S5.

Auffray C., Fogg D., Garfa M., Elain G., Join-Lambert O., Kayal S., Sarnacki S., Cumano A., Lauvau G., Geissmann F. Monitoring blood vessels and tissues by a population of monocytes with patrolling behavior. Science (2007); 317 (5838): 666-670.

Bendelac A., Savage P. B., Teyton L. The biology of NKT cells. Annu. Rev. Immunol. (2007); 25: 297-336.

Bernfield M., Götte M., Park P. W., Reizes O., Fitzgerald M. L., Lincecum J., Zako M. Functions of cell surface heparan sulfate proteoglycans. Annu. Rev. Biochem. (1999); 68: 729-777.

Broide D. H., Finkelman F. Bochner B. S., Rothenberg M. E. Advances in mechanisms of asthma, and immunology in 2010. J. Allergy Clin. Immunol. (2011); 127 (3): 689-695.

Bronte V., Apolloni E., Cabrelle A., Ronca R., Serafini P., Zamboni P., Restifo N. P., Zanovello P. Identification of a CD11b(+)/Gr-1(+)/CD31(+) myeloid progenitor capable of activating or suppressing CD8(+) T cells. Blood (2000); 96 (12): 3838-3846.

Brossay L., Chioda M., Burdin N., Koezuka Y., Casorati G., Dellabona P., Kronenberg M. CD1d-mediated recognition of an alpha-galactosylceramide by natural killer T cells is highly conserved through mammalian evolution. J. Exp. Med. (1998); 188 (8): 1521-1528.

Bunting M., Harris E. S., McIntyre T. M., Prescott S. M., Zimmerman G. A. Leukocyte adhesion deficiency syndromes: adhesion and tethering defects involving beta 2 integrins and selectin ligands. Curr. Opin. Hematol. (2002); 9 (1): 30-35.

Campbell J. J., Foxman E. F., Butcher E. C. Chemoattractant receptor cross talk as a regulatory mechanism in leukocyte adhesion and migration. Eur. J. Immunol. (1997); 27 (10): 2571-2578.

Carman C. V., Springer T.A. Integrin avidity regulation: are changes in affinity and conformation underemphasized? Curr. Opin. Cell Biol. (2003); 15 (5): 547-556.

Carman C. V., Springer T.A. A transmigratory cup in leukocyte diapedesis both through individual vascular endothelial cells and between them. J. Cell Biol. (2004); 167 (2): 377-388.

Chou R. C., Kim N. D., Sadik C. D., Seung E., Lan Y., Byrne M. H., Haribabu B., Iwakura Y., Luster A. D. Lipid-cytokine-chemokine cascade drives neutrophil recruitment in a murine model of inflammatory arthritis. Immunity (2010); 33 (2): 266-278.

Christoffersson G., Henriksnäs J., Johansson L., Rolny C., Ahlström H., Caballero-Corbalan J., Segersvärd R., Permert J., Korsgren O., Carlsson P. O., Phillipson M. Clinical and experimental pancreatic islet transplantation to striated muscle: establishment of a vascular system similar to that in native islets. Diabetes (2010); 59 (10): 2569-2578.

Curry F. R., Adamson R. H. Transendothelial pathways in venular microvessels exposed to agents which increase permeability: the gaps in our knowledge. Microcirculation (1999); 6(1): 3-5.

Curry F. R., Adamson R. H. Vascular permeability modulation at the cell, microvessel, or whole organ level: towards closing gaps in our knowledge. Cardiovasc. Res. (2010); 87 (2): 218-229.

De Fougerolles A. R., Qin X., Springer T. A. Characterization of the function of intercellular adhesion molecule (ICAM)-3 and comparison with ICAM-1 and ICAM-2 in immune responses. J. Exp. Med. (1994); 179 (2): 619-629.

Del Zoppo G. J. Acute anti-inflammatory approaches to ischemic stroke. Ann. N. Y. Acad. Sci. (2010); 1207: 143-148.

Diamond M. S., Springer T. A. The dynamic regulation of integrin adhesiveness. Curr. Biol. (1994); 4 (6): 506-517.

Doerschuk C. M., Winn R. K., Coxson H. O., Harlan J. M. CD18-dependent and independent mechanisms of neutrophil emigration in the pulmonary and systemic microcirculation of rabbits. J. Immunol. (1990); 144 (6): 2327-2333.

Dustin M. L., Springer T. A. T-cell receptor cross-linking transiently stimulates adhesiveness through LFA-1. Nature (1989); 341 (6243): 619-624.

Eltzschig H. K., Carmeliet P. Hypoxia and inflammation. N. Engl. J. Med. (2011); 364 (7); 656-665.

Engelhardt B., Wolburg H. Mini-review: Transendothelial migration of leukocytes: through the front door or around the sides of the house? Eur. J. Immunol. (2004); 34 (11): 2955-2963.

Fanta C. H. Asthma. N. Engl. J. Med. (2009); 360 (10): 1002-1014.

Faveew C., Di Mauro M. E., Price A. A., Ager A. Roles of alpha(4) integrins/ VCAM-1 and LFA-1/ ICAM-1 in the binding and transendothelial migration of T lymphocytes and T lymphoblasts across high endothelial venules. Int. Immunol. (2000); 12 (3): 241-251.

Feng D., Nagy J. A., Pyne K., Dvorak H. F., Dvorak A. M. Neutrophils emigrate from venules by transendothelial cell pathway in response to FMLP. J. Exp. Med. (1998); 187 (6): 903-915.

Friedl P., Borgmann S., Bröcker E. B. Amoeboid leukocyte crawling through extracellular matrix: lessons from the Dictyostelium paradigm of cell movement. J. Leukoc. Biol. (2001); 70 (4): 491-509.

Frohman E. M., Racke M. K., Raine C. S. Multiple Sclerosis - The plaque and its pathogenesis. N. Engl. J. Med. (2006); 354 (9): 942-955.

Fontoura P. Monoclonal antibody therapy in multiple sclerosis: Paradigm shifts and emerging challenges. MAbs. (2010); 2 (6): 670-681.

Foxman E. F., Campbell J. J., Butcher E. C. Multistep navigation and the combinatorial control of leukocyte chemotaxis. J. Cell Biol. (1997); 139 (5): 1349-1360.

Fridlender Z. G., Sun J., Kim S., Kapoor V., Cheng G., Ling L., Worthen G. S., Albelda S. M. Polarization of tumor-associated neutrophil phenotype by TGF-beta: "N1" *versus* "N2" TAN. Cancer Cell (2009); 16 (3): 183-194.

Gao J. X., Issekutz A. C. The beta 1 integrin, very late activation antigen-4 on human neutrophils can contribute to neutrophil migration through connective tissue fibroblast barriers. Immunology (1997); 90 (3): 448-454.

Gaudry M., Brégerie O., Andrieu V., El Benna J., Pocidalo M. A., Hakim J. Intracellular pool of vascular endothelial growth factor in human neutrophils. Blood (1997); 90 (10): 4153-4161.

Gouwy M., Struyf S., Noppen S., Schutyser E., Springael J. Y., Parmentier M., Proost P., Van Damme J. Synergy between coproduced CC and CXC chemokines in monocyte chemotaxis through receptor-mediated events. Mol. Pharmacol. (2008); 74 (2): 485-495.

Geissmann F., Cameron T. O., Sidobre S., Manlongat N., Kronenberg M., Briskin M. J., Dustin M. L., Littman D. R. Intravascular immune surveillance by CXCR6+ NKT cells patrolling liver sinusoids. PLoS Biol. (2005); 3 (4): e113.

Geissmann F., Jung S., Littman D. R. Blood monocytes consist of two principal subsets with distinct migratory properties. Immunity (2003); 19 (1): 71-82.

Gong Y., Koh D. R. Neutrophils promote inflammatory angiogenesis via release of preformed VEGF in an *in vivo* corneal model. Cell Tissue Res. (2010); 339 (2): 437-448.

Gordon S., Taylor P. R. Monocyte and macrophage heterogeneity. Nat. Rev. Immunol. (2005); 5 (12): 953-964.

Hanahan D., Weinberg R. A. Hallmarks of cancer: the next generation. Cell (2011); 144 (5): 646-674.

Hansson G. K. Inflammation, Atherosclerosis, and Coronary Artery Disease. N. Engl. J. Med. (2005); 352 (16): 1685-1695.

Heit B., Robbins S. M., Downey C. M., Guan Z., Colarusso P., Miller B. J., Jirik F. R., Kubes P. PTEN functions to 'prioritize' chemotactic cues and prevent 'distraction' in migrating neutrophils. Nat. Immunol. (2008); 9: 716-718.

Heit B., Tavener S., Raharjo E., Kubes P. An intracellular signaling hierarchy determines direction of migration in opposing chemotactic gradients. J. Cell. Biol. (2002); 159 (1): 91-102.

Hemler M. E. VLA proteins in the integrin family: structures, functions, and their role on leukocytes. Annu. Rev. Immunol. (1990); 8: 365-400.

Hickey M. J., Forster M., Mitchell D., Kaur J., De Caigny C., Kubes P. L-selectin facilitates emigration and extravascular locomotion of leukocytes during acute inflammatory responses *in vivo*. J. Immunol. (2000); 165 (12): 7164-7170.

Hotchkiss R. S., Karl I. E. The Pathophysiology and Treatment of Sepsis. N. Engl. J. Med. (2003); 348 (2): 138-150.

Hyduk S. J., Cybulsky M. I. Role of alpha4beta1 integrins in chemokine-induced monocyte arreest under conditions of shear stress. Microcirculation (2009); 16 (1): 17-30.

Ibbotson G. C., Doig C., Kaur J., Gill V., Ostrovsky L., Fairhead T., Kubes P. Functional alpha4-integrin: a newly identified pathway of neutrophil recruitment in critically septic patients. Nat. Med. (2001); 7 (4): 465-470.

Ihrcke N. S., Wrenshall L. E., Lindman B. J., Platt J. L. Role of heparan sulfate in immune system-blood vessel interactions. Immunol. Today (1993); 14: 500-505.

Jaeschke H., Farhood A., Fisher M. A., Smith C. W. Sequestration of neutrophils in the hepatic vasculature during endotoxemia is independent of beta 2 integrins and intercellular adhesion molecule-1. Shock (1996); 6 (5): 351-356.

Jutila M. A., Rott L., Berg E. L., Butcher E. C. Function and regulation of the neutrophil MEL-14 antigen *in vivo*: comparison with LFA-1 and MAC-1. J. Immunol. (1989); 143 (10): 3318-3324.

Kansas G. S. Selectins and their ligands: current concepts and controversies. Blood (1996); 88 (9): 3259-3287.

Kawano T., Cui J., Koezuka Y., Toura I., Kaneko Y., Motoki K., Ueno H., Nakagawa R., Sato H., Kondo E., Koseki H., Taniguchi M. CD1d-restricted and TCR-mediated activation of valpha14 NKT cells by glycosylceramides. Science (1997); 278 (5343): 1626-1629.

Kelly M., Hwang J. M., Kubes P. Modulating leukocyte recruitment in inflammation. J. Allergy Clin. Immmunol. (2007); 120 (1): 3-10.

Kenne E., Lindbom L. Imaging inflammatory plasma leakage *in vivo*. Thromb. Haemost. (2011); 105 (5): 783-789.

Kim M. H., Curry F. R., Simon S. I. Dynamics of neutrophil extravasation and vascular permeability are uncoupled during aseptic cutaneous wounding. Am. J. Physiol. Cell Physiol. (2009); 296 (4): C848-856.

Kono H., Rock K. L. How dying cells alert the immune system to danger. Nat. Rev. Immunol. (2008); 8 (4): 279-289.

Kubes P., Niu X. F., Smith C. W., Kehrli M. E. Jr., Reinhardt P. H., Woodman R. C. A novel β_1-dependent adhesion pathway on neutrophils: a mechanism invoked by dihydrocytochalasin B or endothelial transmigration. FASEB J. (1995); 9 (11): 1103-1111.

Kuijpers T. W., Mul E. P., Blom M., Kovach N. L., Gaeta F. C., Tollefson V., Elices M. J., Harlan J. M. Freezing adhesion molecules in a state of high-avidity binding blocks eosinophil migration. J. Exp. Med. (1993); 178 (1): 279-284.

Kunkel E. J., Ley K. Distinct phenotype of E-selectin-deficient mice. E-selectin is required for slow rolling *in vivo*. Circ. Res. (1996); 79 (6); 1196-1204.

Kuscher K., Danelon G., Paoletti S., Stefano L., Schiraldi M., Petkovic V., Locati M., Gerber B. O., Uguccioni M. Synergy-inducing chemokines enhance CCR2 ligand activities on monocytes. Eur. J. Immunol. (2009); 39 (4): 1118-1128.

Lee T. D., Gonzalez M. L., Kumar P., Grammas P., Pereira H. A. CAP37, a neutrophil-derived inflammatory mediator, augments leukocyte adhesion to endothelial monolayers. Microvasc. Res. (2003); 66 (1): 38-48.

Ley K., Laudanna C., Cybulsky M. I., Nourshargh S. Getting to the site of inflammation: the leukocyte adhesion cascade updated. Nat. Rev. Immunol. (2007); 7 (9): 678-689.

Lindbom L., Werr J. Integrin-dependent neutrophil migration in extravascular tissue. Semin. Immunol. (2002); 14 (2): 115-121.

Lindhal U. Heparan sulfate-protein interactions: a concept for drug design? Thromb. Haemost. (2007); 98 (1): 109-115.

Lindhal U., Kjellén L. Heparin or heparan sulfate: what is the difference? Thromb. Haemost. (1991); 66 (1): 44-48.

Lindahl U., Li J. P. Interactions between heparan sulfate and proteins-design and functional implications. Int. Rev. Cell Mol. Biol. (2009); 276: 105-159.

Lou O., Alcaide P., Luscinskas F. W., Muller W. A. CD99 is a key mediator of the transendothelial migration of neutrohils. J. Immunol. (2007); 178 (2): 1136-1143.

Lund-Johansen F., Terstappen L. W. Differential surface expression of cell adhesion molecules during granulocyte maturation. J. Leukoc. Biol. (1993); 54 (1): 47-55.

Luo B. H., Carman C. V., Springer T. A. Structural basis of integrin regulation and signaling. Annu. Rev. Immunol (2007); 25: 619-647.

Luscinskas F. W., Kansas G. S., Ding H., Pizcueta P., Schleiffenbaum B. E., Tedder T. F., Gimbrone M. A. Jr. Monocyte rolling, arrest and spreading on IL-4-activated vascular endothelium under flow is mediated via sequential action of L-selectin, beta 1-integrins, and beta 2-integrins. J. Cell Biol. (1994); 125 (6): 1417-1427.

Luscinskas F. W., Ma S., Nusrat A., Parkos C. A., Shaw S. K. Leukocyte transendothelial migration: a junctional affair. Semin. Immunol. (2002); 14 (2): 105-113.

Maiguel D., Faridi M. H., Wei C., Kuwano Y., Balla K. M., Hernandez D., Barth C. J., Lugo G., Donnelly M., Nayer A., Moita L. F., Schürer S., Traver D., Ruiz P., Vazquez-Padron R. I., Ley K., Reiser J., Gupta V. Small Molecule-Mediated Activation of the Integrin CD11b/CD18 Reduces Inflammatory Disease. Sci. Signal. (2011); 4 (189): ra57.

Martinez F. J., Donohue J. F., Rennard S. I. The future of chronic obstructive pulmonary disease treatment - difficulties of and barriers to drug development. Lancet (2011); 378: 1027-1037.

Massena S., Christoffersson G., Hjertström E., Zcharia E., Vlodavsky I., Ausmees N., Rolny C., Li J. P., Phillipson M. A chemotactic gradient sequestered on endothelial heparan sulfate induces directional intraluminal crawling of neutrophils. Blood (2010); 116 (11): 1924-1931.

McDonald B., McAvoy E. F., Lam F., Gill V., de la Motte C., Savani R. C., Kubes P. Interaction of CD44 and hyaluronan is the dominant mechanism for neutrophil sequestration in inflamed liver sinusoids. J. Exp. Med. (2008); 205 (4): 915-927.

McDonald B., Pittman K., Menezes G. B., Hirota S. A., Slaba I., Waterhouse C. C., Beck P. L., Muruve D. A., Kubes P. Intravascular danger signals guide neutrophils to sites of sterile inflammation. Science (2010); 330 (6002): 362-366.

McEver R. P. Adhesive interactions of leukocytes, platelets, and the vessel wall during hemostasis and inflammation. Thromb. Haemost. (2001); 86 (3): 746-756.

McEver R. P., Zhu C. Rolling Cell Adhesion. Annu. Rev. Cell Dev. Biol. (2010); 26: 363-396.

McNab F. W., Berzins S. P., Pellicci D. G., Kyparissoudis K., Field K., Smyth M. J., Godfrey D. I. The influence of CD1d in postselection NKT cell maturation and homeostasis. J. Immunol. (2005); 175 (6): 3762-3768.

Meerschaert J., Furie M. B. The adhesion molecules used by monocytes for migration across the endothelium include CD11a/CD18, CD11b/CD18, and VLA-4 on monocytes and ICAM-1, VCAM-1, and other ligands on endothelium. J. Immunol (1995); 154 (8): 4099-4112.

Mehta D., Malik A. B. Signaling mechanisms regulating endothelial permeability. Physiol. Rev. (2006); 86 (1): 279-367.

Michel C. C., Curry F. E. Microvascular permeability. Physiol. Rev. (1999); 79 (3): 703-761.

Middleton J., Neil S., Wintle J., Clark-Lewis I., Moore H., Lam C., Auer M., Hub E., Rot A. Transcytosis and surface presentation of IL-8 by venular endothelial cells. Cell (1997); 91: 385-395.

Minnicozzi M., Sawyer R. T., Fenton M. J. Innate immunity in allergic disease. Immunol Rev. (2011); 242 (1): 106-127.

Muller W. A. Sorting the signals from the signals in the noisy environment of inflammation. Sci. Signal. (2011); 4 (170): pe23.

Nahrendorf M., Swirski F. K., Aikawa E., Stangenberg L., Wurdinger T., Figueiredo J. L., Libby P., Weissleder R., Pittet M. J..The healing myocardium sequentially mobilizes two monocyte subsets with divergent and complementary functions. J. Exp. Med. (2007); 204 (12): 3037-3047.

Norman M. U., Kubes P. Therapeutic intervention in inflammatory diseases: a time and place for anti-adhesion therapy. Microcirculation (2005); 12 (1): 91-98.

Nozawa H., Chiu C., Hanahan D. Infiltrating neutrophils mediate the initial angiogenic switch in a mouse model of multistage carcinogenesis. PNAS (2006); 103 (33): 12493-12498.

O'Dell J. R. Therapeutic targets for rheumatoid arthritis. N. Engl. J. Med. (2004); 350 (25): 2591-2602.

Olsen N. J., Stein C. M. New drugs for rheumatoid arthritis. N. Engl. J. Med. (2004); 350 (21): 2167-2179.

Parish C. Heparan sulfate and inflammation. Nat. Immunol. (2005); 6 (9): 861-862.

Patel K. D., Nollert M. U., McEver R. P. P-selectin must extend a sufficient length from the plasma membrane to mediate rolling of neutrophils. J. Cell. Biol. (1995); 131: 1893-1902.

Peranzoni E., Zilio S., Marigo I., Dolcetti L., Zanovello P., Mandruzzato S., Bronte V. Myeloid-derived suppressor cell heterogeneity and subset definition. Curr. Opin. Immunol. (2010); 22 (2): 238-244.

Petri B., Kaur J., Long E. M., Li H., Parsons S. A., Butz S., Phillipson M., Vestweber D., Patel K. D., Robbins S. M., Kubes P. Blood (2011); 117 (3): 942-952.

Petri B., Phillipson M., Kubes P. The physiology of leukocyte recruitment: an *in vivo* perspective. J. Immunol. (2008); 180 (10): 6439-6446.

Phillipson M., Heit B., Colarusso P., Liu L., Ballantyne C. M., Kubes P. Intraluminal crawling of neutrophils to emigration sites: a molecularly distinct process from adhesion in the recruitment cascade. J. Exp. Med. (2006); 203 (12): 2569-2575.

Phillipson M., Heit B., Parsons S. A., Petri B., Mullaly S. C., Colarusso P., Gower R. M., Neely G., Simon S. I., Kubes P. Vav1 is essential for mechanotactic crawling and migration of neutrophils out of the inflamed microvasculature. J. Immunol. (2009); 182 (11): 6870-6878.

Phillipson M., Kaur J., Colarusso P., Ballantyne C. M., Kubes P. Endothelial domes encapsulate adherent neutrophils and minimize increases in vascular permeability in paracellular and transcellular emigration. PLoS One (2008); 3: e1649.

Phillipson M., Kubes P. The neutrophil in vascular inflammation. Nat. Med. (2011); 17 (11): 1381-1390.

Pillay J., Ramakers B. P., Kamp V. M., Loi A. L., Lam S. W., Hietbrink F., Leenen L. P., Tool A. T. Pickkers P., Koenderman L. Functional heterogeneity and differential priming of circulating neutrophils in human experimental endotoxemia. J. Leukoc. Biol. (2010); 88 (1): 211-220.

Rolny C., Mazzone M., Tugues S., Laoui D., Johansson I., Coulon C., Squadrito M. L., Segura I., Li X., Knevels E., Costa S., Vinckier S., Dresselaer T., Åkerud P., De Mol M., Salomäki H., Phillipson M., Wyns S., Larsson E., Buysschaert I., Botling J., Himmelreich U., Van Ginderachter J. A., De Palma M., Dewerchin M., Claesson-Welsh L., Carmeliet P. HRG inhibits tumor growth and metastasis by inducing macrophage polarization and vessel normalization through downregulation of PIGF. Cancer Cell (2011); 19 (1): 31-44.

Rose D. M., Alon R., Ginsberg M. H. Integrin modulation and signaling in leukocyte adhesion and migration. Immunol. Rev. (2007); 218: 126-134.

Ross R. Atherosclerosis - An Inflammatory Disease. N. Engl. J. Med. (1999); 340 (2): 115-126.

Rutgeerts P.,Vermeire S., Van Assche G. Biological therapies for inflammatory bowel diseases. Gastroenterology (2009); 136 (4): 1182-1197.

Savasta M., Lentini S. Immunology insights into cardiac allograft rejection. Rev. Cardiovasc. Med. (2011); 12 (2): e68-76.

Schenkel A. R., Mamdouh Z., Muller W. A. Locomotion of monocytes on endothelium is a critical step during extravasation. Nat. Immunol. (2004); 5: 393-400.

Scott D. L., Kingsley G. H. Tumor necrosis factor inhibitors for rheumatoid arthritis. N. Engl. J. Med. (2006); 355 (7): 704-712.

Shamri R., Grabovsky V., Gauguet J. M., Feigelson S., Manevich E., Kolanus W., Robinson M. K., Stauton D. E., Andrian U. H., Alon R. Lymphocyte arrest requires instantaneous induction of an extended LFA-1 conformation mediated by endothelium-bound chemokines. Nat. Immunol. (2005); 6 (5): 497-506.

Shaw S. K., Bamba P. S., Perkins B. N., Luscinskas F. W. Real-time imaging of vascular endothelial-cadherin during leukocyte transmigration across endothelium. J. Immunol. (2001); 164 (4): 2323-2330.

Shulman Z., Shinder V., Klein E., Grabovsky V., Yeger O., Geron E., Montresor A., Bolomini-Vittori M., Feigelson S. W., Kirchhausen T., Laudanna C., Shakhar G., Alon R. Lymphocyte crawling and transendothelial migration require chemokine triggering of high-affinity LFA-1 integrin. Immunity (2009); 30 (3): 384-396.

Simon S. I., Goldsmith H. L. Leukocyte adhesion dynamics under in shear flow. Ann. Biomed. Eng. (2002); 30 (3): 315-332.

Simon S. I., Green C. E. Molecular mechanisms and dynamics of leukocyte recruitment during inflammation. Annu. Rev. Biomed. Eng. (2005); 7: 151-185.

Sixt M., Hallmann R., Wendler O., Scharffetter-Kochanek K., Sorokin L. M. Cell adhesion and migration properties of beta 2-integrin negative polymorphonuclear granulocytes on defined extracellular matrix molecules. Relevance for leukocyte extravasation. J. Biol. Chem. (2001); 276 (22): 18878-18887.

Smith A., Carrasco Y. R., Stanley P., Kieffer N., Batista F. D., Hogg N. A talin-dependent LFA-1 focal zone is formed by rapidly migrating T lymphocytes. J. Cell. Biol. (2005); 170 (1): 141-151.

Smith A., Stanley P., Jones K., Svensson L., McDowall A., Hogg N. The role of the integrin LFA-1 in T-lymphocyte migration. Immunol. Rev. (2007); 218: 135-146.

Smith C. W., Kishimoto T. K., Abbassi O., Hughes B., Rothlein R., McIntire L. V., Butcher E., Anderson D. C. Chemotactic factors regulate lectin adhesion molecule 1 (LECAM-1)-dependent neutrophil adhesion to cytokine-stimulated endothelial cells *in vitro*. J. Clin. Invest. (1991); 87 (2): 609-618.

Soehnlein O., Lindbom L., Weber C. Mechanisms underlying neutrophil-mediated monocyte recruitment. Blood (2009); 114 (21): 4613-4623.

Sumagin R., Prizant H., Lomakina E., Waugh R. E., Sarelius I. H. LFA-1 and Mac-1 define characteristically different intraluminal crawling and emigration patterns for monocytes and neutrophils in situ. J. Immunol. (2010); 185 (11): 7057-7066.

Van Den Berg B. M., Vink H., Spaan J. A. The endothelial glycocalyx protects against myocardial edema. Circ. Res. (2003); 92 (6): 592-594.

Von Andrian U. H., Hansell P., Chambers J. D., Berger E. M., Torres Filho I., Butcher E. C., Arfors K. E. L-selectin function is required for beta-2-integrin-mediated neutrophil adhesion at physiological shear rates *in vivo*. Am. J. Physiol. (1992); 263: H1034-1044.

Wang L., Fuster M., Sriramarao P., Esko J. D. Endothelial heparan sulfate deficiency impairs L-selectin- and chemokine-mediated neutrophil trafficking during inflammatory responses. Nat. Immunol. (2005); 6: 902-910.

Wang S., Voisin M. B., Larbi K. Y., Dangerfield J., Scheiermann C., Tran M., Maxwell P. H., Sorokin L., Nourshargh S. Venular basement membranes contain specific matrix protein low expression regions that act as exit points for emigrating neutrophils. J. Exp. Med. (2006); 203 (6): 1519-1532.

Wei D. G., Lee H., Park S. H., Beaudoin L., Teyton L., Lehuen A., Bendelac A. Expansion and long-range differentiation of the NKT cell lineage in mice expressing CD1d exclusively on cortical thymocytes. J. Exp. Med. (2005); 202 (2): 239-248.

Werr J., Xie X., Hedqvist P., Ruoslahti E., Lindbom L. Beta1 integrins are critically involved in neutrophil locomotion in extravascular tissue *In vivo*. J. Exp. Med. (1998); 187 (12): 2091-2096.

Wong J., Johnston B., Lee S. S., Bullard D. C., Smith C. W., Beaudet A. L., Kubes P. A minimal role for selectins in the recruitment of leukocytes into the inflamed liver microvasculature. J. Clin. Invest. (1997); 99 (11): 2782-2790.

Woodfin A., Voisin M. B., Beyrau M., Colom B., Caille D., Diapouli F. M., Nash G. B., Chevakis T., Albelda S. M., Rainger G. E., Meda P., Imhof B. A., Nourshargh S. The junctional adhesion molecule JAM-C regulates polarized transendothelial migration of neutrophils *in vivo*. Nat. Immunol. (2011); 12 (8): 761-769.

Yang L., Froio R. M., Sciuto T. E., Dvorak A. M., Alon R., Luscinskas F. W. ICAM-1 regulates neutrophil adhesion and transcellular migration of TNF-alpha-activated vascular endothelium under flow. Blood (2005); 106 (2): 584-592.

Youn J. I., Gabrilovich D. I. The biology of myeloid-derived suppressor cells: the blessing and the curse of morphological and functional heterogeneity. Eur. J. Immunol. (2010); 40 (11): 2969-2975.

Zhang Q., Raoof M., Chen Y., Sumi Y., Sursal T., Junger W., Brohi K., Itagaki K., Hauser C. J. Circulating mitochondrial DAMPs cause inflammatory responses to injury. Nature (2010); 464 (7285): 104-107.

10

Membrane Trafficking and Endothelial-Cell Dynamics During Angiogenesis

Ajit Tiwari, Jae-Joon Jung, Shivangi M. Inamdar and Amit Choudhury
Department of Anatomy and Cell Biology, University of Iowa, Iowa City
USA

1. Introduction

The formation of new blood vessels, or neovascularization, involves multiple processes, including cell proliferation and migration, cell-cell and cell-matrix adhesion, and tube morphogenesis. Neovascularization can occur through one of two events: vasculogenesis, the *de novo* formation of blood vessels from angioblasts; or angiogenesis, the extension of new vessels from a pre-existing vasculature. Among these, angiogenesis in particular is relevant throughout life; its dysregulation has been causally related to several disorders that involve malignancy, inflammation, and ischemia. Angiogenesis is thought to depend on a set of signaling proteins – including certain kinases, integrins and vascular endothelial growth factor receptor-2 (VEGFR2) – that are enriched in specific plasma membrane domains. Both physiological and pathological angiogenesis rely on intracellular trafficking, a process that governs signaling by such proteins, as well as cell motility.

In this chapter, we discuss our current understanding of angiogenesis from the perspective of trafficking of the membrane components that are responsible for endothelial-cell (EC) dynamics.

2. Angiogenesis: Mechanism and importance

The vascular system carries out a variety of functions vital to vertebrates. It delivers oxygen and nutrients to tissues and organs. It is required for waste disposal, including the detoxification of toxic metabolites in the liver and their excretion through kidney. It is needed for the onset of immune responses against pathogens, since it transports immune cells to the site of infection and/or inflammation. Finally, its constituent vessels produce instructive signals for organogenesis.

Blood vessels are the main component of the vascular system and comprise: an EC monolayer that lines the vessel lumen, vascular smooth muscle cells that surround the EC monolayer, and a basement membrane that covers the vascular tube (**Figure 1**). The larger vessels, arteries and veins are stabilized by a thick layer of vascular smooth muscle cells, whereas the medium-sized vessels are supported by mural cells, for example pericytes (Gerhardt and Betsholtz, 2003).

The vascular system is among the earliest organ systems to develop in embryos; it first emerges when haemangioblast progenitors proliferate, migrate and differentiate into

ECs and form a primitive vascular plexus. The formation of new blood vessels, or neovascularization, then occurs either through vasculogenesis or angiogenesis, as mentioned above.

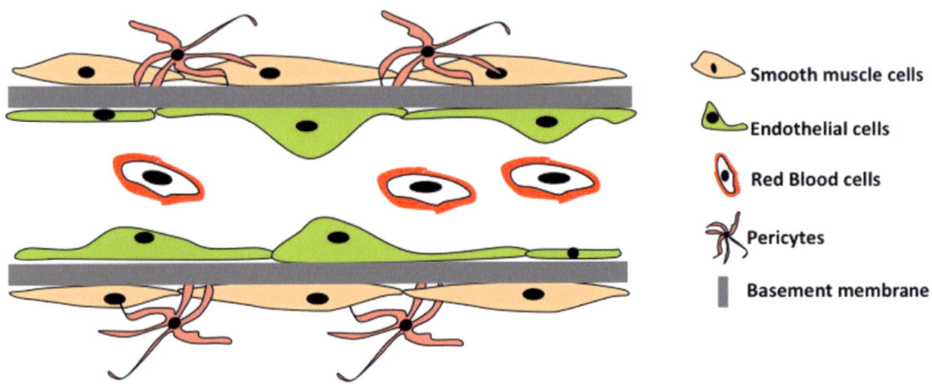

Fig. 1. Schematic representation of a mature blood vessel. Endothelial cells at the luminal side line tubular blood vessel. The smooth muscle cells and the pericytes that remain in contact with the endothelial cell lining through the basement membrane strengthen this tubular structure.

2.1 Vasculogenesis

Vasculogenesis, defined as *de novo* formation of blood vessels from precursor cells, starts with differentiation of precursor cells (angioblasts) into ECs and a primitive vascular network. In the first phase of vasculogenesis (during gastrulation), the splanchnic mesoderm gives rise to hemangioblasts, which are presumed to be the common progenitors of ECs and blood cells (Baron, 2001; Choi, 2002), and subsequently the outer cells of the blood island differentiate into angioblasts. In the second phase, angioblasts differentiate into ECs. In the third and final phase, the ECs participate in tube formation, giving rise to the primitive vascular plexus (**Figure 2**). Growth factor, fibroblast growth factor 2 (FGF2) generates hemangioblasts from the mesoderm, whereas vascular endothelial growth factor (VEGF) and its receptor, VEGFR, cooperate in hemangioblast generation and tube formation, and Angiopoietin-1 (Ang-1) regulates the connection between ECs and pericytes (Hiratsuka, 2011).

2.2 Angiogenesis

Angiogenesis, the establishment of new vessels from a pre-existing vasculature, starts with stimulation of ECs that line the luminal surface of blood vessels. The process of angiogenesis can be classified into two types: "sprouting" and "nonsprouting" (Risau, 1997). Sprouting angiogenesis refers to a process that entails proteolytic degradation of the extracellular matrix, the migration and proliferation of cells, the formation of a lumen, and maturation of ECs into functional capillaries. Specifically, ECs in pre-existing vessels respond to activation by a stimulatory molecule supplied by neighboring cells (e.g. VEGF), by producing a protease that degrades the surrounding basement membrane, to facilitate EC migration towards stimulatory signal. The sprout is comprised of a growth-arrested leading tip cell and proliferating stalk cells (Gerhardt et al., 2003). The tips cells are migratory and extend long filopodia that guide the sprouts towards the stimulus. Subsequently, the sprout anastomoses with other newly formed vessels to allow circulation. The basement membrane reassembles pericytes and gets recruited to newly formed vessels (**Figure 2**). Sprouting angiogenesis occurs during yolk sac and embryo development, and later during brain development (Scappaticci, 2002). Non-sprouting angiogenesis is a process that occurs by invagination involving EC proliferation within a vessel, and results in an enlarged lumen that can be split by transcapillary or by the fusion and splitting of capillaries. Non-sprouting angiogenesis occurs mainly during development of the lung and heart (Scappaticci, 2002). Both sprouting and non-sprouting angiogenesis contribute to vessel formation in the adult, via a process known as "adult vasculogenesis". This process is thought to rely on endothelial progenitor cells (EPCs) that originate from the bone marrow. While circulating in the blood, EPCs are incorporated into vessels at the site of angiogenesis (Caplice and Doyle, 2005).

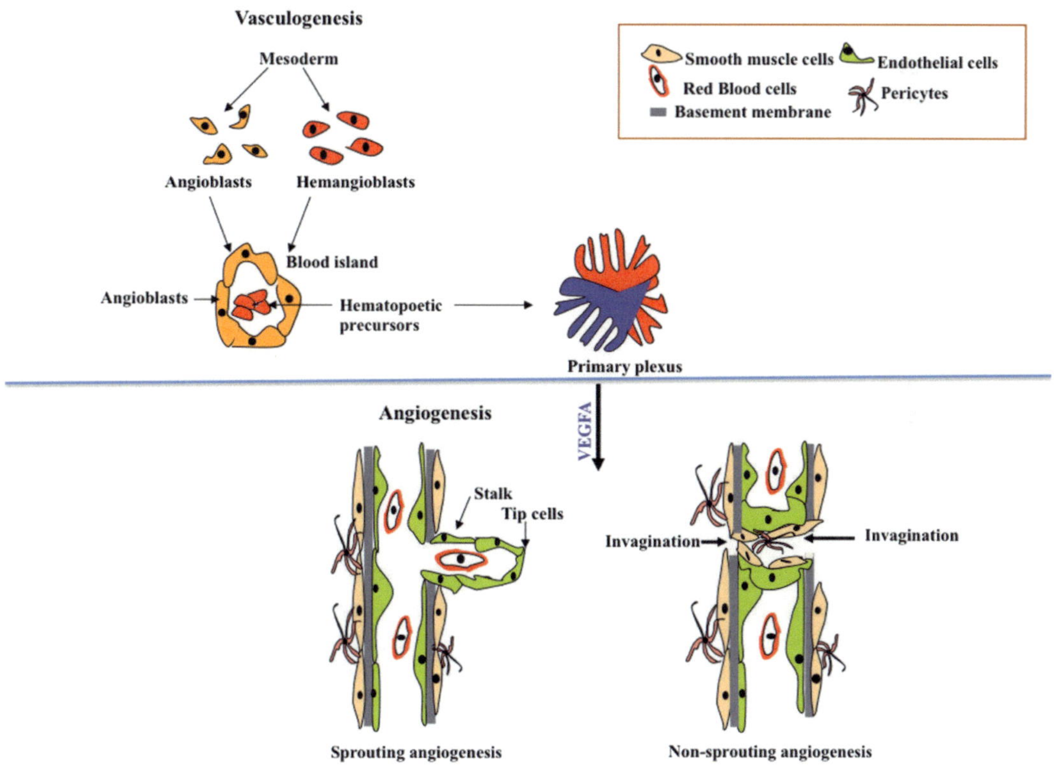

Fig. 2. Schematic outline of vasculogenesis (above) and angiogenesis (below). Both sprouting and non-sprouting mechanism of angiogenesis are shown.

2.3 Pathological angiogenesis

The process of angiogenesis is highly regulated in healthy adults and occurs only rarely, for example during ovulation and the endometrial growth that is central to the menstrual cycle. Angiogenesis is also required for wound healing, and ceases once this process is completed.

Since vessels nourish nearly every organ of the body the strict limitation of angiogenesis to such contexts is essential; deviation from normal vessel growth - in either direction - leads to fatal disease. Excess angiogenesis is characteristic of conditions such as retinopathy, rheumatoid arthritis, psoriasis and tumor growth (Folkman, 1995), and insufficient angiogenesis is a feature of ischemic heart and limb disease, stroke and gastrointestinal ulcers (Carmeliet and Jain, 2000).

The process of angiogenesis plays a crucial role in cancer metastasis - the major cause of mortality in cancer patients. In tumor diseases, angiogenesis is stimulated by the secretion of signaling molecules, e.g. VEGFA, by either the tumor cells themselves or tumor-infiltrating macrophages. In most cancers, tumor angiogenesis is crucial for disease progression, as it supplies the tumor cells with nutrients and oxygen, enabling them to survive and spread (Folkman, 2002). Notably, tumor-supporting vessels tend to be disorganized and leaky; thus vessel function is suboptimal and angiogenesis is further stimulated by hypoxia-driven expression of VEGFA in the tumor tissue. These findings have stimulated great interest in targeting tumor vessels as a means of developing novel cancer therapies. Indeed, intensive research efforts toward this end have revealed that, in patients with metastatic colorectal cancer, supplementing chemotherapy with a neutralizing antibody against VEGFA (Avastin/Bevacizumab) results in significantly improved survival (McCarthy, 2003).

Angiogenesis can also be regulated by microRNA (miRNA) (Wang and Olson, 2009). MicroRNA is a class of highly conserved, single stranded, non-coding small RNAs influencing gene expression by inhibiting translation of protein from mRNA or by promoting the degradation of mRNA (Bartel, 2004; Kim, 2005). The direct evidence of miRNA importance in angiogenesis was provided by observation of defective vascular remodeling during developmental angiogenesis in hypomorphic mouse line with EC-specific deletion of Dicer, one of key enzymes involved in miRNA generation (Otsuka et al., 2008; Yang et al., 2005). Endothelial cell primarily express miRNA-221/222, miRNA-21, the Let-7 family, the miR-17-92 cluster, the miRNA-23-24 cluster, and miRNA-126 (Harris et al., 2008; Kuehbacher et al., 2007; Suarez et al., 2007). miRNA-210 which gets activated upon hypoxia is an important regulator of EC survival, migration and differentiation during angiogenesis (Fasanaro et al., 2008). miRNA-210 overexpression under normoxic conditions stimulates angiogenesis and VEGF-induced cell migration whereas its blockade by anti-mRNA inhibits tube formation stimulated by hypoxia (Fasanaro et al., 2008). miRNA-210 may play an important role in pathological angiogenesis since hypoxia is associated with tumor development and organ ischemia. miRNA-21 and miRNA-31 are the other pro-angiogenic miRNAs which are upregulated in various various cancers to stimulate invasion and metastasis in cancer (Tsai et al., 2009).

3. Ligands and receptors in angiogenesis

At the molecular level, the initiation of vascular development is dependent on a number of cell-surface receptors and their respective ligands. Upon binding to a wide range of peptide growth factors, members of the receptor tyrosine kinase (RTK) family of transmembrane proteins transduce proliferative and morphogenic signals, thereby fine-tuning the orchestration of vascular remodeling and angiogenic processes. Although angiogenesis is controlled by a wide range of extracellular signals, the most potent pro-angiogenic signaling is initiated by binding of VEGF (vascular endothelial growth factor) to EC-resident VEGF receptors (VEGFRs) like VEGFR1 [Flt (Fms-like tyrosine kinase)-1], VEGFR2 [Flk-1 (fetal liver kinase 1)/KDR (kinase insert domain receptor)] and VEGFR3 (Flt-4) (Zachary, 2003).

Remodeling from existing vessels during angiogenesis is governed by VEGF-mediated EC proliferation, and their sprouting from points of loose contact between capillaries and the extracellular matrix. The nascent capillary network then matures through the actions of TGF-β and platelet-derived growth factor (PDGF). The arterial and venous ECs within the final primary capillary express Ephrin B2 and its receptor EphB4, respectively, in their cell membranes; this enables correct fusion between arterial and venous vessels.

3.1 The VEGF-VEGFR system coordinates the process of angiogenesis

3.1.1 VEGF

The VEGF family is a branch of the PDGF/VEGF supergene family and its members have a homodimeric structure (Ferrara and Davis-Smyth, 1997). The VEGF family consists of five related growth factors: VEGFA, VEGFB, VEGFC, VEGFD and PlGF (placental growth factor). Although VEGFs are homodimeric polypeptides, naturally occurring heterodimers have also been reported (DiSalvo et al., 1995). VEGFA, which was also isolated as vascular permeability factor (VPF), is alternatively spliced to generate VEGFA121, VEGFA145, VEGFA165 and VEGFA189 (the numbers indicate final residue in each polypeptide in humans). Alternative splicing and processing regulates ligand binding to VEGF receptors, heparan sulfate and neuropilins (NRPs) (Grunewald et al., 2010). VEGFA165 and VEGFA189 bind to both heparan sulfate and NRP1. VEGFA plays an important role in the proliferation and migration of ECs, and also acts on monocytes and macrophages, neurons, cancer cells, and kidney epithelial cells. VEGFA is known to be regulated by hypoxia-inducible factor (HIF) (Germain et al., 2010), an event that leads to increased expression during embryonic development and wound healing, and also in the context of cancer. VEGFA produced by most parenchymal cells, act in paracrine manner on adjacent ECs to regulate signaling by the VEGF receptors. Autocrine VEGFA is essential for EC survival (Lee et al., 2007), and is consistent with their requirement for complete development of the vasculature in mice; both homozygosity and heterozygosity for knockout of the VEGFA gene result in embryonic lethality characterized by incomplete development of the vasculature (Carmeliet et al., 1996; Ferrara et al., 1996). The biological activity of VEGF is manifested after it binds to VEGF receptors, which are of 3 different types in human, and bind VEGF with distinct affinities.

3.2 VEGF receptors

Orthologs of each of the VEGF receptor tyrosine kinases (VEGFRs) - namely VEGFR1, VEGFR2 and VEGFR3 - have been identified in humans, mice and other mammals. Structurally, the VEGFRs have a common organization consisting of: an extracellular, ligand-binding domain that features 7 immunoglobulin (Ig)–like loops, a transmembrane domain; a juxtamembrane domain; a split kinase domain and a C-terminal tail **(Figure 3)**. Structurally, the VEGFRs are distantly related to the PDGFRs, which have five extracellular Ig-like domains (Matthews et al., 1991; Terman et al., 1991). All three VEGFRs undergo alternative splicing to generate more than one receptor form. The truncated form of VEGFR1, known as soluble VEGFR1 (sVEGR1, sFlt-1) (Kendall and Thomas, 1993), is implicated as causative agent in preeclampsia, a major disorder that can occur during pregnancy (Levine et al., 2004). A naturally occurring soluble form of VEGFR2 has also been described; it could potentially arise as a result of alternative splicing or through proteolytic processing (Ebos et al., 2004). In humans, alternative splicing of VEGFR3 generates two isoforms with distinct C-terminal tails (Hughes, 2001).

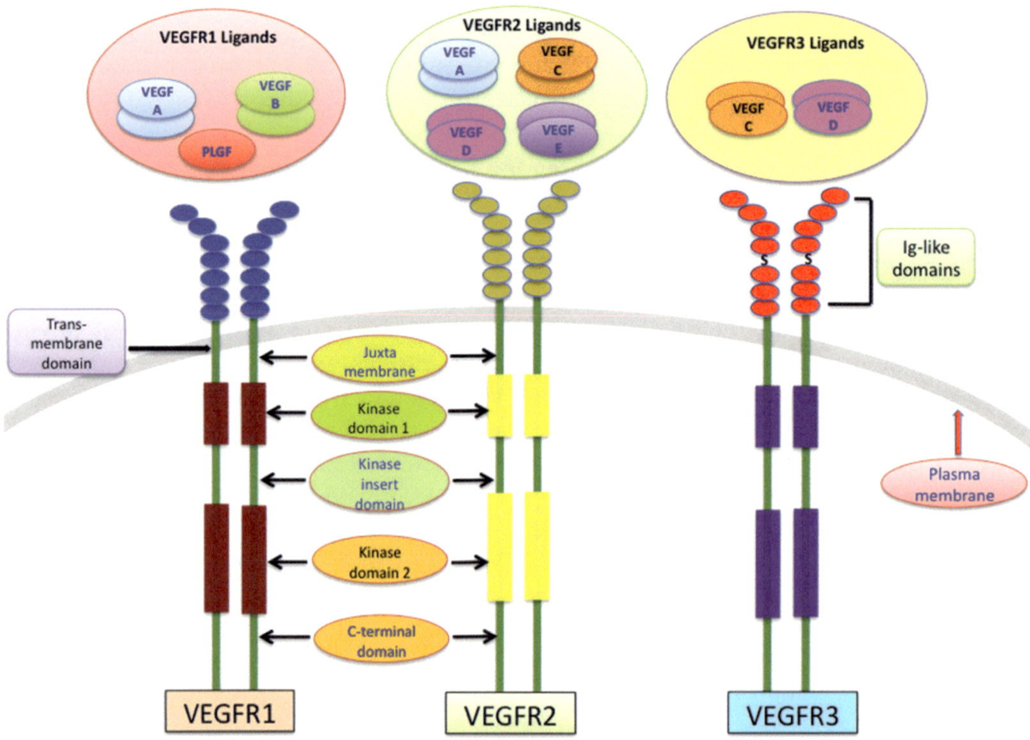

Fig. 3. VEGF receptors and their ligands. Schematic presentation of VEGF receptors (VEGFR1, VEGFR2 and VEGFR3). The signaling domain of all three receptors is present within cytosol. The Ig-like domains of VEGFRs are involved in VEGF binding, shown in elliptical structures that are present extracellularly. More than one kind of VEGF can bind to one receptor with different affinities.

3.2.1 VEGFR1

VEGFR1 (also known as Flt1 in mouse) is a glycoprotein of 150-184 kDa (de Vries et al., 1992; Shibuya et al., 1990) that gets activated upon binding of VEGFA, VEGFB and PLGF. VEGFR1 is expressed in vascular ECs at relatively high levels, throughout development and in the adult (Peters et al., 1993). It is also expressed in various other cell types such as monocytes, macrophages, human trophoblasts, renal mesangial cells, vascular smooth muscle cells, dendritic cells and a variety of human tumor-cell types (Barleon et al., 1996; Dikov et al., 2005; Sawano et al., 2001).

Alternative splicing of VEGFR1 generates soluble VEGFR1 (sVEGFR1), which is abundantly expressed in the placenta. Although the affinity of VEGFR1 for VEGFA is greater than that of VEGFR2, VEGFR1 transduces only weak signals for EC and pericyte growth and survival, as well as for macrophage migration (Barleon et al., 1996; Nomura et al., 1995). In response to ligand binding, VEGFR1 undergoes autophosphorylation at various tyrosines within the intracellular domain (TYRs1169, 1213, 1242, 1327, 1333) (Ito et al., 1998; Sawano et al., 1997). Phosphorylation of TYR1169 allows binding and activation of phospholipase C (PLC)γ1, which regulates EC proliferation via the mitogen-activated protein kinase (MAPK) pathway (Sawano et al., 1997). Tyr1213 binds a variety of SH2-containing proteins, including PLCγ, growth-factor-receptor bound protein (GRB) 2, non-catalytic region of tyrosine kinase adaptor protein (Nck) and SH2-domain-containing protein tyrosine phosphatase 2 (SHP-2) (Igarashi et al., 1998; Ito et al., 1998). Tyr1309 is however phosphorylated in response to PLGF but not VEGF (Autiero et al., 2003) (**Figure 4**). Although the exact role of VEGFR1

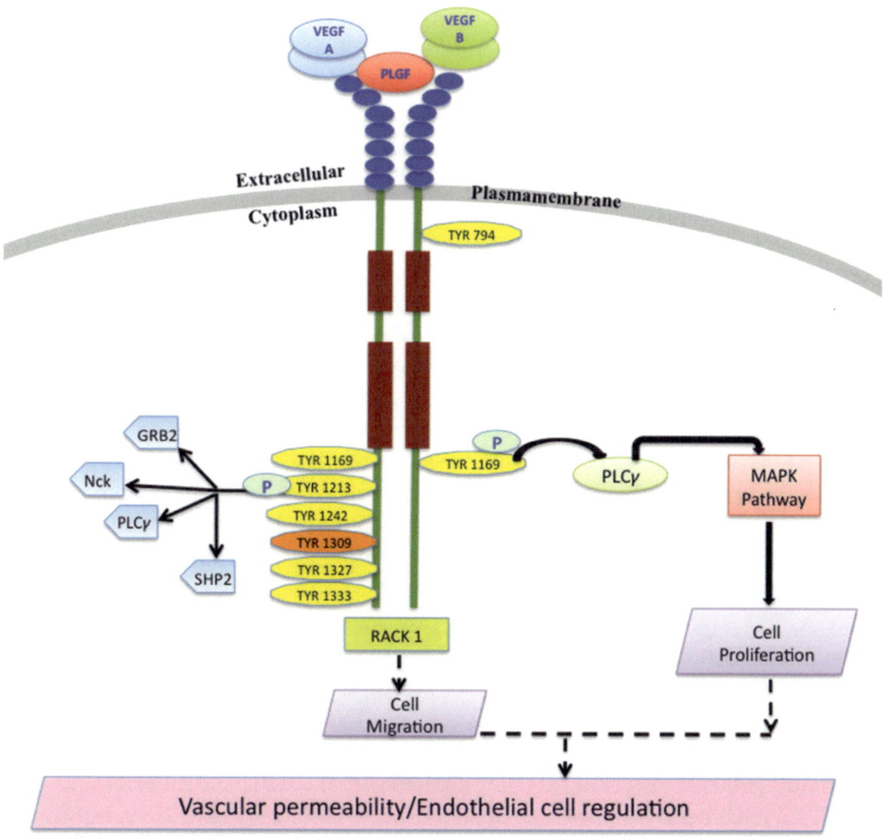

Fig. 4. VEGFR1 tyrosine phosphorylation and signaling. Schematic presentation of intracellular dimerized VEGFR1. VEGFA/VEGFB binding induces tyrosine phosphorylation of VEGFR1 at different tyrosine (TYR) positions shown in yellow ellipses. PLGF binding stimulates phosphorylation at TYR1309 shown in orange ellipse. Signaling molecules (shown within boxes) binds to certain phosphorylated tyrosine residues (circled P) and activates downstream signaling events leading to specific physiological outcome (shown in purple boxes) required for vascular permeability and endothelial cell regulation. PLCγ, phospholipase C-γ; MAPK, mitogen-activated protein; RACK1, receptor for activated C-kinase 1; SHP2, SH2-domain-containing protein tyrosine phosphatase 2.

remains a subject of debate, studies using VEGFR1-neutralizing antibodies have implicated this receptor in actin reorganization within, and the migration of ECs (Kanno et al., 2000), and suggested that receptor for activated C-kinase 1 (RACK1) is its downstream effector in this context (Wang et al., 2011). VEGFR1-dependent activation of PI3K/Akt may play a role in EC differentiation and organization (Huang et al., 2001) **(Figure 4)**. Under *in vitro* conditions, VEGFR1 and VEGFR2 are known to form heterodimers on cells co-expressing these receptors (Huang et al., 2001), so it is believed that VEGFR1 can regulate EC functions via cross-talk with VEGFR2, through dimerization as a result of VEGFA binding to both. Binding of PLGF can also lead to crosstalk between VEGFR2 and VEGFR1 through transphosphorylation, leading to sensitization of VEGFR2 subsequent to activation by VEGFA (Autiero et al., 2003). Soluble VEGFR1 (sVEGFR1, sFlt1) can negatively influence vascular development, either by sequestering VEGFA from signaling receptors or by forming non-functional heterodimers with VEGFR2 (Kendall et al., 1994). Although, VEGFR1 and sVEGFR1 are considered VEGF decoys that control signaling by VEGFR1 and the formation of angiogenic sprouts (Kappas et al., 2008), the importance of VEGFR1 in angiogenesis is demonstrated by the fact that the VEGR1 null (*vegfr1*$^{-/-}$) mouse dies at embryonic day 9, due to increased proliferation of ECs, disorganization and dysfunction of the vascular system (Fong et al., 1995).

3.2.2 VEGFR2

VEGFR2 (also known as KDR or Flk-1) is generally accepted to be the main receptor tyrosine kinase responsible for transducing the angiogenic activities of VEGFA, a factor that stimulates vascular-cell survival/growth and promotes angiogenesis. VEGFR2 knockout results in embryonic lethality due to deficiencies in vasculogenesis and hematopoiesis (Shalaby et al., 1995). VEGFR2 is highly expressed in vascular endothelial progenitors during early embryogenesis and generates a variety of angiogenic signals, not only for the proliferation of ECs but also their migration and morphogenesis, and as such has an important role in vascular tube formation. VEGFR2 expression is upregulated under conditions that trigger pathological angiogenesis, such as in tumors (reviewed in (Matsumoto and Claesson-Welsh, 2001). The binding of VEGF to VEGFR2 leads to receptor dimerization and promotes EC differentiation, proliferation, migration and vascular-tube formation. Both homo- and heterodimerization occurs following the trans-phosphorylation of tyrosine in the receptor intracellular domain. The major phosphorylation sites on VEGFR2 are TYR951 (in the kinase-insert domain), TYR1054 and TYR1059 (within the kinase domain), and TYR1175 and TYR1214 (in the C-terminal domain) (Matsumoto et al., 2005; (Takahashi et al., 2001). Additional phosphorylation sites on VEGFR2 have been identified at postions 1223, 1305, 1309 and 1319, but their function remains to be established (Matsumoto et al., 2005). Although TYR801 within the juxtamembrane can be phosphorylated when the intracellular portion of VEGFR2 is tested in isolation (Solowiej et al., 2009), its phosphorylation in the context of the intact protein has not yet been demonstrated. Phosphorylation at TYR951, within the kinase-insert domain, leads to binding and tyrosine phosphorylation of the SH2-domain–containing signaling molecule T-cell specific adapter (TSAd)(Matsumoto et al., 2005). TSAd, which is equipped with Src Homology 2 (SH2) and protein tyrosine binding (PTB) domains, in turn associates with the cytoplasmic tyrosine kinase Src, thereby regulating actin stress fiber organization and the migratory responses of ECs to VEGFA (**Figure 5**). Phosphorylation at TYR1054 and TYR1059, both of which are located within the kinase domain activation loop (Kendall et al., 1999), is preceded by autophosphorylation at TYR801 (Solowiej et al., 2009). Phosphorylation at TYR1059 induces Src binding, which in turn phosphorylates TYR1175 of VEGFR2, as well as residues within downstream signal transducers, such as the actin binding protein IQ-motif-contaning GTPase-activating protein 1 (IQGAP1), which is implicated in the regulation of cell-cell contacts, proliferation and migration (Meyer et al., 2008; Yamaoka-Tojo et al., 2006).

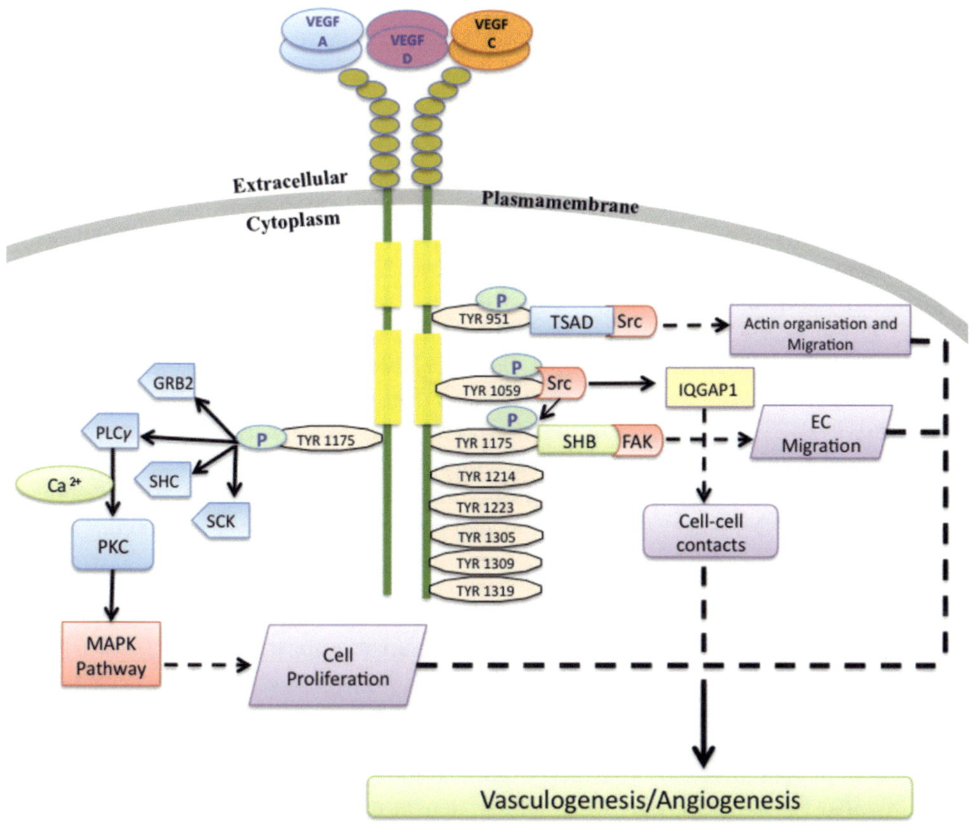

Fig. 5. VEGFR2 tyrosine phosphorylation and signaling. Schematic presentation of dimerized VEGFR2. VEGFA/VEGFB/VEGFC binding induces tyrosine phosphorylation of VEGFR2 at different tyrosine (TYR) positions shown in ellipses. Signaling molecules (shown within boxes) binds to certain phosphorylated TYR residues (circled P) and activates network of downstream signaling events required for variety of physiological outcomes (shown in purple boxes) essential during vasculogenesis and angiogenesis.

Phosphorylation at TYR1175 is required for the binding of PLCγ, which mediates activation of the mitogen-activated protein kinase (MAPK)/extracellular-signal-regulated kinase-1/2 (ERK1/2) cascade and the proliferation of ECs (Takahashi et al., 2001). Binding of PLCγ stimulates the protein kinase C (PKC) pathway, leading to inositol triphosphate generation and calcium mobilization. In addition to interacting with PLCγ, phosphorylated TYR1175 binds to the SH2-domain-containing adaptor protein B (SHB) and Src homology and collagen homology (Sck/SHC) (Holmqvist et al., 2004; Warner et al., 2000). SHB binds to Tyrosine-phosphorylated focal adhesion kinase (FAK) in VEGF-treated cells (Abu-Ghazaleh et al., 2001) and thereby contributes to EC attachment and migration (Holmqvist et al., 2003). The binding of SHC to TYR1175-phosphorylated VEGFR2 is believed to control Ras activation and mitogenicity in response to VEGF (Meadows et al., 2001).

3.2.3 VEGFR3

VEGFR3, also denoted Flt4, is a protein with a molecular weight of around 195 kDa, and becomes activated when bound to VEGFC or VEGFD. VEGFR3 is an essential protein; its inactivation results in embryonic death at E9.5, due to abnormal remodeling of the primary vascular plexus (Dumont et al., 1998). Although VEGFR3 plays a role in vascular development in the early embryo, its expression is later largely confined to ECs of the lymphatic system (Kaipainen et al., 1995). The exception is when its expression is induced in vascular ECs during active phases of angiogenesis, for example in the tumor vasculature or the endothelial tip cells of angiogenic sprouts in the retina (Tammela et al., 2008). VEGFR3 has five tyrosine phosphorylation sites - at positions 1230, 1231, 1265, 1337 and 1363 in the C-terminal tail (Dixelius et al., 2003) - that are activated and phosphorylated upon binding of VEGFC or VEGFD. TYR1337 when phosphorylated is known to bind to Shc and Grb2 to initiate signaling by the MAPK pathway. Both TYR1063 and TYR1068, which are located within the kinase activation domain, are crucial for kinase activity. Phosphorylation of TYR1230 and TYR1231 creates a docking site for SHC–GBR2, which promotes signaling by the ERK1/2 and PI3K/Akt pathways **(Figure 6)**. Phosphorylated TYR1063 has been shown to interact with adaptor protein C10 regulator of kinase (CRK I/II), which activates the c-Jun N-terminal kinase (JNK) pathway to promote cell survival (Salameh et al., 2005).

3.2.4 Neuropilins (NRP)

The cell-surface glycoprotein neuropilin is a transmembrane protein with a small cytoplasmic tail that lacks intrinsic catalytic function (Fujisawa et al., 1997). The neuropilin homolog NRP1 is expressed in arteries, whereas NRP2, is expressed in the venous and lymphatic vessels (Yuan et al., 2002). NRP1 was originally identified as a receptor for the collapsin/semaphorin family of neuronal guidance molecule (Chen et al., 1997). Later it was reported to also be expressed in ECs, where it acts as a coreceptor for VEGFA164 and VEGFA165 in mice and humans, respectively (Miao et al., 1999; Soker et al., 1998). NRP1 modulates VEGFR signaling, leading to enhanced survival and migration of ECs *in vitro* (Favier et al., 2006). NRP1 has also been implicated in VEGFR2-mediated vascular permeability (Becker et al., 2005) and VEGFA-induced vessel sprouting and branching (Kawamura et al., 2008). Although the exact influence of NRP1 on VEGFA mediated VEGFR2 signaling remains to be deciphered, the importance of NRP1 in angiogenesis was established by the fact that overexpression or deletion of NRP1 in mice leads to embryonic lethality and vascular abnormalities (Kawasaki et al., 1999). Neuropilin is also expressed in tumors and is believed to enhance tumor angiogenesis (Miao et al., 2000); it probably does so by stabilizing VEGF/VEGFR signaling on adjacent cell in trans.

3.3 Role of the extracellular matrix (ECM) in endothelial-cell interactions during angiogenesis

The angiogenic process is influenced not only by ligand/receptor systems, but also overall composition of extracellular matrix (ECM) surrounding the vasculature. Indeed, the ECM

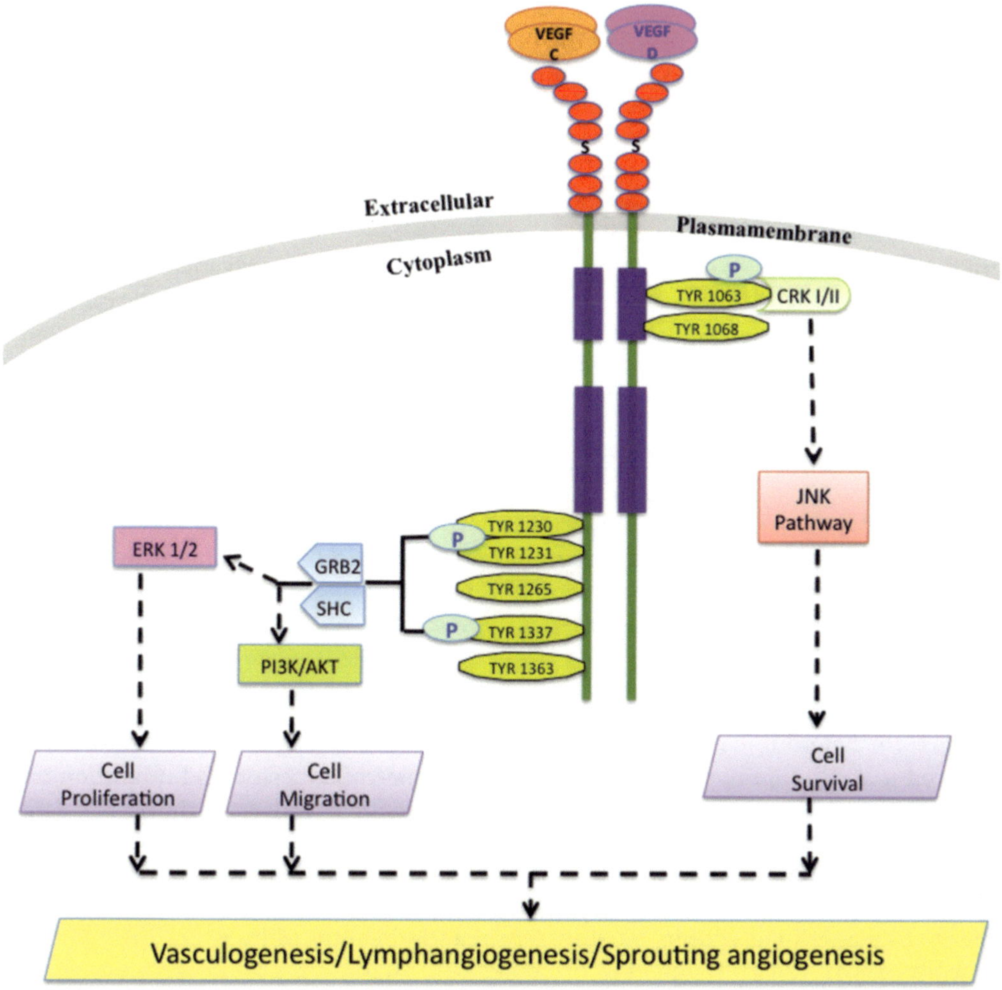

Fig. 6. VEGFR3 tyrosine phosphorylation and signaling. Schematic presentation of intracellular dimerized VEGFR3. VEGFC/VEGFD binding induces tyrosine phosphorylation of VEGFR3 at different tyrosine (TYR) positions shown in green ellipses. Signaling molecules (shown within boxes) binds to certain phosphorylated tyrosine residues (circled P) and activates network of downstream signaling events required for variety of physiological outcomes (shown in purple boxes) essential during vasculogenesis and angiogenesis

provides an essential connection between ECs and the surrounding tissues and affect angiogenesis either positively or negatively (Nyberg et al., 2005). ECs are attached to a basement membrane (BM), which forms a continuous coat around the vessels. The main components of the vascular BM are type IV collagen, laminins, fibronectin, heparan-sulphate proteoglycans and nidogens. The BM provides structural support to the ECs (Kalluri, 2003), and interaction of ECs with components in the BM is important for maintaining integrity of the vessel wall (Hallmann et al., 2005). When ECs are exposed to angiogenic growth factors such as VEGFA, several kind of matrix-degrading enzymes, such as matrix metalloproteinases, dissolve the BM. Matrix-degrading enzymes are produced by ECs and stromal cells, as well as by tumor and inflammatory cells (Egeblad and Werb, 2002). Endothelial sprouting is activated not only by growth factors, but also signals from the matrix proteins. Degradation of the BM reveals so-called cryptic sites that can activate the angiogenic properties of ECs. As the BM is degraded and vascular permeability increases, the blood-clotting protein fibrinogen leaks out of the vessels and polymerizes into a fibrin gel (Iivanainen et al., 2003). Constituents of the degraded BM, fibrin, and EC-produced extracellular matrix (ECM) components then form a provisional matrix that ECs invade with guidance from both growth factors and matrix proteins. Once through the provisional matrix, the endothelial sprout further invades the interstitial matrix, which is composed of many proteins including fibrillar collagens (such as collagen I) and fibronectin. These proteins may also promote angiogenesis, collagen I for example, has pro-angoigenic effects (Davis and Senger, 2005; Senger et al., 2002). The signals from the ECM are transmitted by cell-surface expressed adhesion receptors called integrins, which bind to different ECM proteins in a specific manner (Stupack and Cheresh, 2004). In conjunction with the fusion of newly formed vessel sprouts to allow perfusion, the BM reassembles and pericytes are recruited to the vessel. ECs recruit pericytes by secreting PDGF, which binds to the PDGFβ-receptor expressed on pericytes; this process is crucial for vessel stabilization, and lack of pericyte engagement causes remodelling defects and leaky vessels (Uemura et al., 2002)

3.4 Role of Integrin in endothelial-cell dynamics during angiogenesis

Integrins are heterodimeric transmembrane glycoproteins consisting of non-covalently associated α and β subunits, and they promote cell-matrix adhesion and migration on the surrounding ECM. Integrins have no intrinsic enzymatic or kinase activity, but activate signaling pathways by co-clustering with kinases and adaptor proteins in a focal adhesion complex comprising: protein kinases such as FAK and Src; adaptor proteins such as Shc; signaling intermediates such as GTPases of the Rho family; and actin-binding cytoskeletal proteins such as talin, α-actinin, paxillin, tensin and vinculin (Mitra et al., 2005; Mitra and Schlaepfer, 2006). Integrin signaling promotes cell migration, proliferation and survival (Avraamides et al., 2008). Eighteen α and eight β subunits can associate to form 24 unique integrin heterodimers. EC integrins that regulate cell growth, survival and migration during angiogenesis include heterodimers α1β1, α2β1, α4β1, α5β1, α6β1, α6β4, α9β1, αvβ3 and αvβ5 (Avraamides et al., 2008). Integrin αvβ3 (a receptor for RGD-containing ECM proteins such as vitronectin, fibronectin, fibrinogen and osteopontin) was the first αv integrin shown to regulate EC survival and migration during angiogenesis. The expresssion of αvβ3 integrin on resting ECs is negligible, but is upregulated by the presence of angiogenic growth factors such as bFGF, TNFα and IL8 (Brooks et al., 1994). Integrin αvβ3 also regulate pathological angiogenesis during processes such as wound healing. The VEGFR2–αvβ3-integrin association is important for full VEGFR2 signaling activity, for activation of p38MAPK and FAK, and for the recruitment of actin-binding vinculin as needed to initiate EC migration (Mahabeleshwar et al., 2008). The ligation of endothelial αvβ3 integrin has also been shown to activate FAK, Src, and other kinases, resulting in cell proliferation, differentiation and migration (Eliceiri et al., 2002). Whereas αvβ3 dimers initiate angiogenesis in response to bFGF and TNFα, the related integrin αvβ5 is required for TNFα- and VEGF-mediated angiogenesis (Friedlander et al., 1995). β1 integrin, which pairs with variety of α integrin subunits, plays an important role in angiogenesis. Mice with EC-specific deletion of β1 integrin die during embryonic stages due to severe vascular defects (Tanjore et al., 2008). Matrix-bound VEGF induces the formation of a complex between VEGFR2 and β1 integrin, which leads to prolonged phosphorylation of VEGFR2 at TYR 1214 and association of β1 integrin with focal adhesions (Chen et al., 2010).

Fibronectin secreted by ECs is a key ECM component. It is deposited by ECs during normal and tumor angiogenesis (Clark et al., 1982; Kim et al., 2000). Fibronectin interacts with integrins such as α5β1, αvβ5 and αvβ3 (Plow et al., 2000). During embryonic vascular development, as well as during tumor angiogenesis, the ECM protein fibronectin serves as an adhesive support and signals through α5β1 integrin to regulate the spreading, migration and contractility of ECs (Francis et al., 2002). Although the expression of α5β1 in quiescent endothelium is low, it is upregulated by exposure to a subset of angiogenic stimuli including bFGF, IL8 and the ECM protein (Kim et al., 2000). Integrin α5β1 promotes EC migration and survival in *in vivo* and *in vitro* models of angiogenesis by suppressing the activity of protein kinase A (PKA) (Kim et al., 2000b(Kim et al., 2002). Further, our recent study has demonstrated that integrin α5β1 recycling is essential for EC adhesion and migration on fibronectin (Tiwari et al., 2011), a process required during angiogenesis. Integrin α5β1 promotes the formation of focal adhesions and signaling through FAK (Schlaepfer and Hunter, 1998), which is required for EC migration (Mitra et al., 2005). The reduction in EC surface associated adhesion through integrin α5β1 in the context of impaired recycling leads to further reduction in total and activated FAK (Tiwari et al., 2011). During embryogenesis, integrin α5 is required for the development of early blood vessels and other tissues, as revealed by the fact that α5 integrin-deficient mice exhibit a mesodermal defect and are embryonic lethal (Yang et al., 1993). Integrin α4β1, another fibronectin receptor, affects the adhesion and extravasation of lymphocytes by binding to VCAM1, a member of the immunoglobulin superfamily, that is expressed on inflamed ECs. Deletion of integrin α4 in a mouse model leads to defects in plancentation, heart development and coronary artery development, and thus to embryonic lethality (Yang et al., 1995). Integrin α4β1 promotes adhesion of the endothelium to VCAM1-expressing vascular smooth muscle cells during blood vessel formation (Garmy-Susini et al., 2005). Integrin α4β1–VCAM1 facilitates cell-cell attachment between ECs expressing the pericyte chemoattractant PDGF and pericytes expressing VEGF, in response to growth and survival signals that emanate from each cell type during angiogenesis (Garmy-Susini et al., 2005). Integrin α9β1 is another fibronectin-binding integrin known to have role in angiogenesis (Vlahakis et al., 2007). Although structurally similar to integrin α4β1, integrin α9β1 can bind to a number of ECM proteins and cell-surface receptors including tenascin C, thrombospondin, osteopontin, fibronectin, VCAM1 and other ligands (Liao et al., 2002; Marcinkiewicz et al., 2000; Staniszewska et al., 2007). α4β1 binds only to VEGF, and promotes VEGFA-induced angiogenesis. β1 integrin, which pairs with variety of alpha integrin subunits, plays a key role in angiogenesis. Mice with an EC-specific deletion of β1 integrin die at embryonic stages due to a severe vascular defect (Tanjore et al., 2008). Matrix-bound VEGF induces the formation of complex between VEGFR2 and β1 integrin, which leads to prolonged phosphorylation of VEGFR2 at TYR 1214 and to an association of β1 integrin with focal adhesions (Chen et al., 2010).

4. Membrane trafficking

Membrane trafficking is an active process that relocates proteins from one region of a cell to another, and contributes to the regulation of cell migration (Ulrich and Heisenberg, 2009). Signaling by the membrane-resident proteins/receptors is regulated by their availability at the cell surface or correct locations that are controlled by membrane trafficking events. The trafficking of membrane receptors and their signaling are intertwined: trafficking itself affects signal transduction, and signaling by RTKs regulates the trafficking machinery (Sorkin and von Zastrow, 2009). The secretory and endocytic pathways, which are made up of a network of membrane-bound compartments, modify newly synthesized proteins, deliver them to their appropriate locations, and regulate the uptake and turnover of those that are targeted to the cell surface. Trafficking accomplishes the specific and regulated transfer of molecules between distinct membrane-enclosed organelles. The transport process involves the budding of vesicular or tubular carriers from donor membranes, followed by their delivery to specific acceptor membranes. Budding requires the formation of cargo-laden vesicles or tubules at a donor compartment, and also the involvement of (i) specific coat proteins like COPI or COPII; (ii) adaptor proteins such as clathrin, AP-1, 2, 3; and (iii) membrane-deforming proteins like Bar-family proteins (Doherty and McMahon, 2009). The cargo-containing donor vesicle then docks to the acceptor compartment with the help of rab GTPases and a tether. Finally, fusion of the donor and acceptor membranes for the delivery of the cargo is accomplished with the help of N-ethylmaleimide-sensitive factor (NSF)-attachment protein receptor (SNARE) protein complexes (Jahn and Scheller, 2006; Sudhof and Rothman, 2009).

4.1 Biosynthetic/secretory pathway

After being synthesized in the cytoplasm, new proteins are translocated to the endoplasmic reticulum (ER) (Lee et al., 2004) and then move to Golgi via membranous vesicles. After moving through the cis and medial cisternae of the Golgi, the ER-derived cargoes move to trans-Golgi cisternae, where the proteins destined for secretion or presentation on the PM are packed into secretory vesicle that subsequently fuse with the PM (Emr et al., 2009). The Golgi apparatus is the major sorting compartment of the cell; its cargo is sorted not only to the PM for presentation or secretion, but also to endosomes and lysosomes, or back to the ER (Emr et al., 2009).

4.2 Endocytic and exocytic pathways

The endocytic pathway regulates internalization and recycling of proteins internalized from the PM, through a variety of mechanisms, to early and/or late endosomes. Depending on the receptor type and the particular requirements of a particular cell, protein from the endosomes are either sorted to the lysosome, a major degradation site for both internalized and cellular proteins, or recycled back to the PM (Doherty and McMahon, 2009).

Efficient protein trafficking within endomembrane system is further regulated by cross-talk between the two pathways. Endosomal and lysosomal proteins that maintain their integrity and functionality shuttle from the ER, via the Golgi, to endosomes and lysosomes (Ghosh et al., 2003). In polarized cells, movement of the proteins from one side of the cell to the other, via the transcytotic pathway, involves both the biosynthetic/secretory and the endo/exocytic routes (Tuma and Hubbard, 2003). Thus, the membrane trafficking events control the cell communication network connected with signaling events, determining not only the intensity and duration, but also the final biological outcome.

The membrane trafficking process is also important for the signaling activities required for cell survival and migration during the normal physiological response, as well as for those that take place during angiogenesis. In ECs, modulation of receptor tyrosine activity through endocytosis and vesicle trafficking affects downstream targets such as endothelial nitric oxide synthase (eNOS) and VE-cadherin. Further, activation of RTKs results in the dissolution of EC–specific adhesion through endocytosis of VE-cadherin, thereby promoting cell migration and vascular permeability (Mukherjee et al., 2006). Directional cell migration requires the trafficking of adhesion and growth factor receptors including VEGFR2, which is involved with angiogenesis (Lanahan et al., 2010). The angiogenic signals generated in response to VEGFR2 receptor activation are highly regulated by sorting pathways during intracellular trafficking (Manickam et al., 2011). VEGFR2 signaling is regulated by a broad range of angiogenic regulators that in turn regulates receptor trafficking through the endosomal system (Manickam et al., 2011; Scott and Mellor, 2009). Rab GTPases regulate key events in VEGFR2 trafficking between the PM, early endosomes and late endosomes (Bruns et al., 2009). In addition, the Golgi (which is the central hub for membrane trafficking across the mammalian cell) coordinates the cell-surface expression of VEGFR2 by regulating the secretory transport of newly synthesized VEGFR2 (Manickam et al., 2011).

4.3 Endocytic trafficking of VEGFR2

Resting ECs have two pools of VEGFR2: a stable cell-surface pool that can form a complex with VE-cadherin at cell-cell junctions and does not undergo rapid internalization (Lampugnani et al., 2006), and a pool that continuously cycles between the surface and sorting endosomes and is independent of VEGF binding (Gampel et al., 2006). The VEGFR2 is associated with the caveolin-containing and cholesterol-enriched membrane microdomain (Labrecque et al., 2003). Binding of VEGF to extracellular domain of VEGFR2 triggers internalization of receptor subsequent to its dimerization and phosphorylation at TYR1054 and TYR1059. Upon activation, VEGFR2 dissociates from caveolin and transported to endosomes (Salikhova et al., 2008). Multiple modes of VEGFR2 internalization exist, since VEGF-stimulated endocytosis of VEGFR2 is clathrin-dependent (Lampugnani et al., 2006), and VEGFR2 is known to be translocated to perinuclear caveosomes through caveolar endocytosis (Bauer et al., 2005; Labrecque et al., 2003). Thus, the intracellular distribution of VEGFR2 depends on VEGF stimulation. Endosomal trafficking and the signaling of VEGFR2 is dependent on the Rab5a protein, a Ras-related small GTPase associated with early endosomes (Jopling et al., 2009). Depletion of Rab5a enhances VEGFR2 tyrosine phosphorylation and MAPK signaling, whereas overexpression of a Rab5a GTPase-deficient (constitutively active mutant, Q79L) causes VEGFR2 accumulation within endosomes (Jopling et al., 2009). Rab7a GTPase regulates VEGFR2 trafficking from early to late endosomes. Rab7a depletion is inhibitory whereas Rab5a depletion is stimulatory for EC migration (Jopling et al., 2009). VEGF stimulation also can increase the rate of VEGFR2 recycling from sorting endosomes. The vesicles containing VEGFR2 /Src complex traffic to a late endosomal compartment after a longer duration (30 mins) of VEGF stimulation (Gampel et al., 2006). Since Src is an important downstream target of VEGFR2 in an angiogenesis and vascular permeability pathway (Zachary, 2003), it is believed that recycling of VEGFR2/Src to the PM would sensitize pro-angiogenic signals. VEGF stimulation direct VEGFR2 from sorting endosomes to late endosomes finally directs it toward lysosomes for degradation (Gampel et al., 2006).

Regulation of VEGFR2 degradation is important for angiogenesis since VEGFR2 down-regulation controls the sensitivity of ECs to VEGF stimulation. Reports of VEGFR2 degradation upon VEGF stimulation are varied. One study suggests that VEGFR2 degradation is complete upon VEGF A stimulation (Ewan et al., 2006), whereas another study revealed degradation of only 30-40% of the total receptor population (Gampel et al., 2006). Degradation of activated VEGFR2 is promoted by its ubiquitination by c-Cbl, a protein that forms a complex with phospholipase Cγ1 (PLCγ1), a mediator of VEGFR2 signaling (Singh et al., 2007). VEGFR2 trafficking can also be regulated by the co-receptors such as VEGFR1 and NRP1, which can interact with VEGFR2. VEGFR1 is ubiquitylated upon VEGF stimulation and recruits Cbl (Kobayashi et al., 2004). As discussed above, VEGFR1 forms a heterodimer with VEGFR2 upon VEGF binding, so that the decision for sorting of VEGFR2 along a degradative pathway could be influenced by VEGFR1. NRP1, one of the other VEGFR2 co-receptors, which forms a complex with VEGFR2 upon VEGF binding, could stabilize VEGFR2 on the EC surface since loss of NRP1 increases the degradation of VEGFR2 upon VEGF stimulation (Holmes and Zachary, 2008).

4.4 Secretory transport of VEGFR2

Although the endocytic transport of VEGFR2 has been characterized in detail, the reports on secretory transport, i.e transport of newly synthesized VEGFR2, are scant. The Golgi apparatus regulates the trafficking of newly synthesized VEGFR2, since the Golgi receives newly synthesized proteins and lipids from the endoplasmic reticulum (ER), the central organelle in which trafficking-route decisions are made. Recently, studies from our group demonstrated that a significant amount of VEGFR2 is present in the Golgi apparatus, and that VEGF mobilizes this pool from the Golgi compartment (Manickam et al., 2011). The post-Golgi trafficking of cargo occurs in vesicular fashion, where the cargo-loaded vesicles bud from Golgi, delivering the cargoes to their target destinations by membrane fusion events. Membrane fusion steps in eukaryotic cells require SNAREs (Chen and Scheller, 2001; Hong, 2005). The SNAREs are classified into 2 major groups based on the presence of a glutamine (Q SNAREs or t-SNAREs) or an arginine (R SNAREs or v-SNAREs) in the center of the SNARE motif. The trans-Golgi network- and endosome-localized t-SNARE syntaxin 6 (STX6), but not syntaxin 10 and syntaxin 16, regulates secretory transport of VEGFR2 as well as VEGF-induced angiogenic processes (Manickam et al., 2011). Earlier studies demonstrated that STX6 participates in post-Golgi transport of components of membrane microdomains to the PM (Choudhury et al., 2006). Inhibition of STX6 either by loss-of-function approaches, applying an siRNAs against *STX6* or by expressing the inhibitory, cytosolic domains of STX6 interferes with trafficking of Golgi-resident pool of VEGFR2 and targets it to lysosomes for degradation in human ECs, as described in model **(Figure 7).** Further, inhibition of STX6 in cell culture reduced VEGF-induced cell proliferation, cell migration, and vascular tube formation (Manickam et al., 2011). Thus, the t-SNARE STX6 plays a crucial role in maintaining cellular VEGFR2 levels and, subsequently, in physiological processes associated with VEGF-mediated angiogenesis.

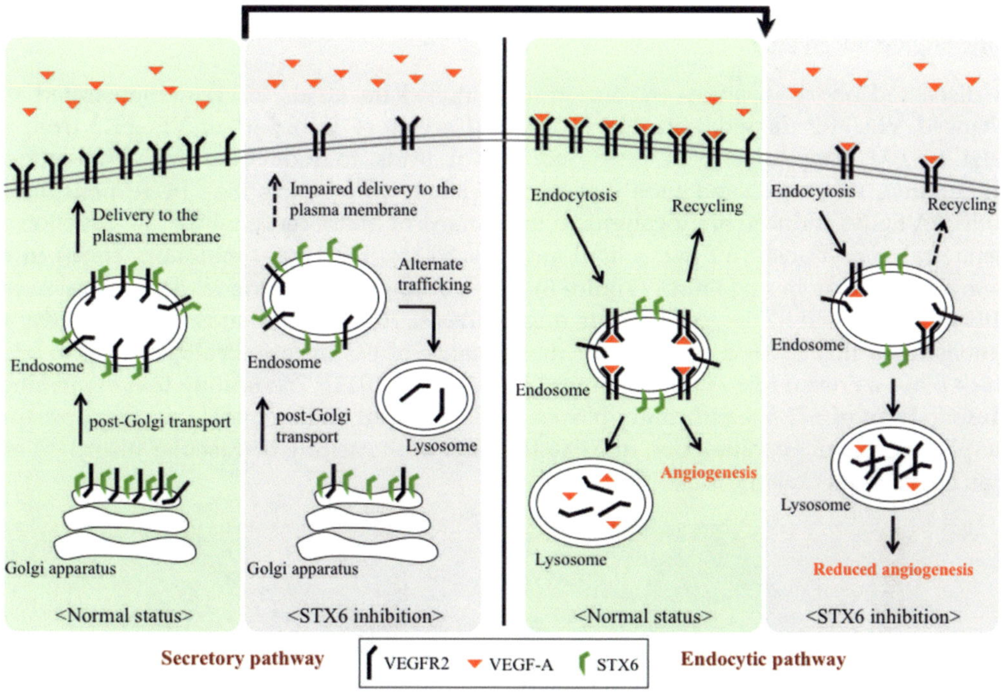

Fig. 7. Schematic summary of VEGFR2 trafficking. In endothelial cells, VEGFR2 is enriched in the plasma membrane, endosomes and Golgi apparatus. These VEGFR2 pools are maintained by endocytic and secretory transport pathways. The subcellular localization of VEGFR2 is essential for VEGF mediated signaling and angiogenesis, and is regulated by syntaxin 6, which colocalizes with VEGFR2 at the Golgi apparatus and endosomes. When syntaxin 6 function is inhibited, the cellular pool of VEGFR2 is depleted as a consequence of enhanced degradation in lysosomes. Syntaxin 6 contributes to trafficking of VEGFR2 from the Golgi and/or endosomes and the maintenance of proper levels of this receptor in different subcellular compartments required for efficient receptor signaling and angiogenesis. (Modified from Manickam et al., 2011. Blood *117*, 1425-1435. © the American Society of Hematology.)

4.5 VEGFR2 trafficking and angiogenesis

The process of angiogenesis is regulated by the response of VEGFR2 to VEGF binding. The availability of VEGFR2 at the PM may directly control the signaling response of ECs to VEGF for the onset of pro-angiogenic events. Thus, the trafficking mechanisms, such as secretory transport, recycling or degradation that affects the surface level VEGFR2, would determine the response of ECs to VEGF during angiogenesis. The EC-surface proteins that stabilize VEGFR2 at the plasma membrane contribute to the VEGF-driven cellular response during angiogenesis. A reduction in the engagement of VE-cadherin with ECs present in the stable vasculature leads to a reduction in surface levels of VEGFR2, thus reducing the sensitivity of ECs to VEGF (Lampugnani et al., 2006). The trafficking of VEGF receptors becomes more important under pathological conditions such as wound healing or ischemic heart disease, which may require rapid recycling and/or secretory transport of VEGF receptors to the surface, ensuring continuous activation of the VEGF/VEGFR pathway to guide angiogenic events.

As discussed above, a study by our group (Manickam et al., 2011) demonstrated that enhanced VEGFR2 degradation due to reduced secretory transport of VEGFR2 from the Golgi to PM (due to lack of functional STX6) leads to reductions in VEGF-induced proliferation, migration, and tube formation. Such *in vitro* effects may be responsible for reduced VEGFA-induced angiogenesis in the context of interference with STX6 function via adenoviral gene transfer of cytosolic domain of STX6 (STX6-cyto, inhibitory form) in ear angiogenesis assay in nude mice **(Figure 8).** This ear angiogenesis model demonstrated that trafficking of VEGFR2 is essential for angiogenesis. Also, in our most recent study, we demonstrated that STX6 is essential for maintenance of EC surface-localized integrin α5β1, which plays a crucial role in angiogenesis (Tiwari et al., 2011). The finding that expressing a cytosolic form of STX6 significantly blocks VEGF-induced angiogenesis raises the prospect that pharmacologic manipulation of STX6 function in the setting of vascular disorders may be an effective therapeutic tool.

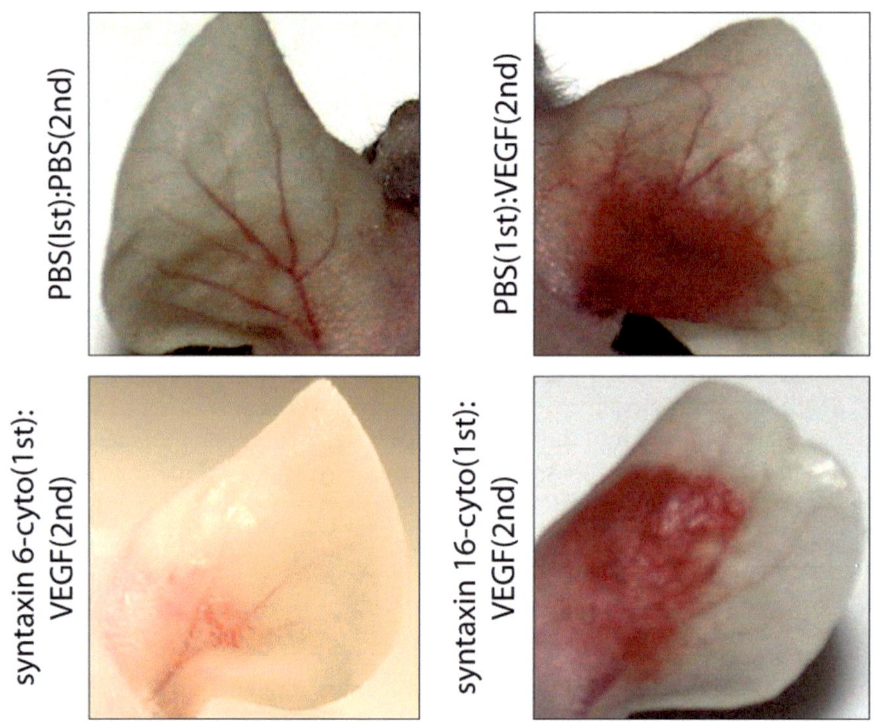

Fig. 8. Mice Ear Angiogenesis Assay: Representative images showing gross appearance of angiogenesis in mock, syntaxin 6-cyto- or syntaxin 16-cyto-injected mouse ears, 5 days before adenovirus expressing VEGF164 (Ad-VEGF164) administration. Nude mice (Nu/Nu strain) were given 2 injections under anesthesia. The first set of injections (1st) was PBS, syntaxin 6-cyto, or syntaxin 16-cyto. The second (2nd) was PBS or Ad-VEGF164, and given 2 days later at the site of first injection. At 7 days after the first set of injections, animals were euthanized and the ears were photographed. (from Manickam et al., 2011. Blood *117*, 1425-1435. © the American Society of Hematology).

5. Conclusions

Angiogenesis is regulated by VEGF-stimulated sensitization of the VEGF receptor and subsequent signaling events that are required during this process. Intracellular trafficking of VEGFR2 controls the VEGF signals that govern angiogenesis. Deciphering the mechanism underlying this trafficking and the roles of mediators in the transport of other VEGF receptors, as well as identifying other angiogenic components that play a role in the formation of new vessels, may provide better insight into angiogenesis. Syntaxin 6-regulated membrane trafficking events control outside-in signaling via the haptotactic and chemotactic mechanisms that regulate integrin α5β1-mediated EC movement on fibronectin and VEGF-mediated VEGFR2 signaling- important components of the angiogenic process (Manickam et al., 2011; Tiwari et al., 2011). A great deal has been deciphered about angiogenesis-related signaling pathways, but a detailed investigation of the intracellular and membrane trafficking of molecules associated directly or indirectly with angiogenesis would add to our knowledge of the angiogenic process, as well as help us to design therapeutic strategies for pathological angiogenesis therapeutic strategies for pathological angiogenesis.

6. Acknowledgement

Supported by grant from National Institutes of Health, National Heart, Lung, and Blood Institute (HL089599 to AC).

7. References

Abu-Ghazaleh, R., Kabir, J., Jia, H., Lobo, M., and Zachary, I. (2001). Src mediates stimulation by vascular endothelial growth factor of the phosphorylation of focal adhesion kinase at tyrosine 861, and migration and anti-apoptosis in endothelial cells. Biochem J *360*, 255-264.

Autiero, M., Waltenberger, J., Communi, D., Kranz, A., Moons, L., Lambrechts, D., Kroll, J., Plaisance, S., De Mol, M., Bono, F., *et al.* (2003). Role of PlGF in the intra- and intermolecular cross talk between the VEGF receptors Flt1 and Flk1. Nat Med *9*, 936-943.

Avraamides, C.J., Garmy-Susini, B., and Varner, J.A. (2008). Integrins in angiogenesis and lymphangiogenesis. Nat Rev Cancer *8*, 604-617.

Barleon, B., Sozzani, S., Zhou, D., Weich, H.A., Mantovani, A., and Marme, D. (1996). Migration of human monocytes in response to vascular endothelial growth factor (VEGF) is mediated via the VEGF receptor flt-1. Blood *87*, 3336-3343.

Baron, M. (2001). Induction of embryonic hematopoietic and endothelial stem/progenitor cells by hedgehog-mediated signals. Differentiation *68*, 175-185.

Bartel, D.P. (2004). MicroRNAs: genomics, biogenesis, mechanism, and function. Cell *116*, 281-297.

Bauer, P.M., Yu, J., Chen, Y., Hickey, R., Bernatchez, P.N., Looft-Wilson, R., Huang, Y., Giordano, F., Stan, R.V., and Sessa, W.C. (2005). Endothelial-specific expression of caveolin-1 impairs microvascular permeability and angiogenesis. Proc Natl Acad Sci U S A *102*, 204-209.

Becker, P.M., Waltenberger, J., Yachechko, R., Mirzapoiazova, T., Sham, J.S., Lee, C.G., Elias, J.A., and Verin, A.D. (2005). Neuropilin-1 regulates vascular endothelial growth factor-mediated endothelial permeability. Circ Res *96*, 1257-1265.

Bruns, A.F., Bao, L., Walker, J.H., and Ponnambalam, S. (2009). VEGF-A-stimulated signalling in endothelial cells via a dual receptor tyrosine kinase system is dependent on co-ordinated trafficking and proteolysis. Biochem Soc Trans *37*, 1193-1197.

Caplice, N.M., and Doyle, B. (2005). Vascular progenitor cells: origin and mechanisms of mobilization, differentiation, integration, and vasculogenesis. Stem Cells Dev *14*, 122-139.

Carmeliet, P., Ferreira, V., Breier, G., Pollefeyt, S., Kieckens, L., Gertsenstein, M., Fahrig, M., Vandenhoeck, A., Harpal, K., Eberhardt, C., *et al.* (1996). Abnormal blood vessel development and lethality in embryos lacking a single VEGF allele. Nature *380*, 435-439.

Carmeliet, P., and Jain, R.K. (2000). Angiogenesis in cancer and other diseases. Nature *407*, 249-257.

Chen, H., Chedotal, A., He, Z., Goodman, C.S., and Tessier-Lavigne, M. (1997). Neuropilin-2, a novel member of the neuropilin family, is a high affinity receptor for the semaphorins Sema E and Sema IV but not Sema III. Neuron *19*, 547-559.

Chen, Y.A., and Scheller, R.H. (2001). SNARE-mediated membrane fusion. Nat Rev Mol Cell Biol *2*, 98-106.

Choi, K. (2002). The hemangioblast: a common progenitor of hematopoietic and endothelial cells. J Hematother Stem Cell Res *11*, 91-101.

Choudhury, A., Marks, D.L., Proctor, K.M., Gould, G.W., and Pagano, R.E. (2006). Regulation of caveolar endocytosis by syntaxin 6-dependent delivery of membrane components to the cell surface. Nat Cell Biol *8*, 317-328.

Clark, R.A., DellaPelle, P., Manseau, E., Lanigan, J.M., Dvorak, H.F., and Colvin, R.B. (1982). Blood vessel fibronectin increases in conjunction with endothelial cell proliferation and capillary ingrowth during wound healing. J Invest Dermatol *79*, 269-276.

Davis, G.E., and Senger, D.R. (2005). Endothelial extracellular matrix: biosynthesis, remodeling, and functions during vascular morphogenesis and neovessel stabilization. Circ Res *97*, 1093-1107.

de Vries, C., Escobedo, J.A., Ueno, H., Houck, K., Ferrara, N., and Williams, L.T. (1992). The fms-like tyrosine kinase, a receptor for vascular endothelial growth factor. Science *255*, 989-991.

Dikov, M.M., Ohm, J.E., Ray, N., Tchekneva, E.E., Burlison, J., Moghanaki, D., Nadaf, S., and Carbone, D.P. (2005). Differential roles of vascular endothelial growth factor receptors 1 and 2 in dendritic cell differentiation. J Immunol *174*, 215-222.

DiSalvo, J., Bayne, M.L., Conn, G., Kwok, P.W., Trivedi, P.G., Soderman, D.D., Palisi, T.M., Sullivan, K.A., and Thomas, K.A. (1995). Purification and characterization of a naturally occurring vascular endothelial growth factor.placenta growth factor heterodimer. J Biol Chem *270*, 7717-7723.

Dixelius, J., Makinen, T., Wirzenius, M., Karkkainen, M.J., Wernstedt, C., Alitalo, K., and Claesson-Welsh, L. (2003). Ligand-induced vascular endothelial growth factor receptor-3 (VEGFR-3) heterodimerization with VEGFR-2 in primary lymphatic endothelial cells regulates tyrosine phosphorylation sites. J Biol Chem *278*, 40973-40979.

Doherty, G.J., and McMahon, H.T. (2009). Mechanisms of endocytosis. Annu Rev Biochem *78*, 857-902.

Dumont, D.J., Jussila, L., Taipale, J., Lymboussaki, A., Mustonen, T., Pajusola, K., Breitman, M., and Alitalo, K. (1998). Cardiovascular failure in mouse embryos deficient in VEGF receptor-3. Science *282*, 946-949.

Ebos, J.M., Bocci, G., Man, S., Thorpe, P.E., Hicklin, D.J., Zhou, D., Jia, X., and Kerbel, R.S. (2004). A naturally occurring soluble form of vascular endothelial growth factor receptor 2 detected in mouse and human plasma. Mol Cancer Res *2*, 315-326.

Egeblad, M., and Werb, Z. (2002). New functions for the matrix metalloproteinases in cancer progression. Nat Rev Cancer *2*, 161-174.

Eliceiri, B.P., Puente, X.S., Hood, J.D., Stupack, D.G., Schlaepfer, D.D., Huang, X.Z., Sheppard, D., and Cheresh, D.A. (2002). Src-mediated coupling of focal adhesion kinase to integrin alpha(v)beta5 in vascular endothelial growth factor signaling. J Cell Biol *157*, 149-160.

Emr, S., Glick, B.S., Linstedt, A.D., Lippincott-Schwartz, J., Luini, A., Malhotra, V., Marsh, B.J., Nakano, A., Pfeffer, S.R., Rabouille, C., *et al.* (2009). Journeys through the Golgi--taking stock in a new era. J Cell Biol *187*, 449-453.

Ewan, L.C., Jopling, H.M., Jia, H., Mittar, S., Bagherzadeh, A., Howell, G.J., Walker, J.H., Zachary, I.C., and Ponnambalam, S. (2006). Intrinsic tyrosine kinase activity is required for vascular endothelial growth factor receptor 2 ubiquitination, sorting and degradation in endothelial cells. Traffic *7*, 1270-1282.

Fasanaro, P., D'Alessandra, Y., Di Stefano, V., Melchionna, R., Romani, S., Pompilio, G., Capogrossi, M.C., and Martelli, F. (2008). MicroRNA-210 modulates endothelial cell response to hypoxia and inhibits the receptor tyrosine kinase ligand Ephrin-A3. J Biol Chem *283*, 15878-15883.

Favier, B., Alam, A., Barron, P., Bonnin, J., Laboudie, P., Fons, P., Mandron, M., Herault, J.P., Neufeld, G., Savi, P., *et al.* (2006). Neuropilin-2 interacts with VEGFR-2 and VEGFR-3 and promotes human endothelial cell survival and migration. Blood *108*, 1243-1250.

Ferrara, N., Carver-Moore, K., Chen, H., Dowd, M., Lu, L., O'Shea, K.S., Powell-Braxton, L., Hillan, K.J., and Moore, M.W. (1996). Heterozygous embryonic lethality induced by targeted inactivation of the VEGF gene. Nature *380*, 439-442.

Ferrara, N., and Davis-Smyth, T. (1997). The biology of vascular endothelial growth factor. Endocr Rev *18*, 4-25.

Folkman, J. (1995). Angiogenesis in cancer, vascular, rheumatoid and other disease. Nat Med *1*, 27-31.

Folkman, J. (2002). Role of angiogenesis in tumor growth and metastasis. Semin Oncol *29*, 15-18.

Fong, G.H., Rossant, J., Gertsenstein, M., and Breitman, M.L. (1995). Role of the Flt-1 receptor tyrosine kinase in regulating the assembly of vascular endothelium. Nature *376*, 66-70.

Francis, S.E., Goh, K.L., Hodivala-Dilke, K., Bader, B.L., Stark, M., Davidson, D., and Hynes, R.O. (2002). Central roles of alpha5beta1 integrin and fibronectin in vascular development in mouse embryos and embryoid bodies. Arterioscler Thromb Vasc Biol *22*, 927-933.

Friedlander, M., Brooks, P.C., Shaffer, R.W., Kincaid, C.M., Varner, J.A., and Cheresh, D.A. (1995). Definition of two angiogenic pathways by distinct alpha v integrins. Science *270*, 1500-1502.

Fujisawa, H., Kitsukawa, T., Kawakami, A., Takagi, S., Shimizu, M., and Hirata, T. (1997). Roles of a neuronal cell-surface molecule, neuropilin, in nerve fiber fasciculation and guidance. Cell Tissue Res *290*, 465-470.

Gampel, A., Moss, L., Jones, M.C., Brunton, V., Norman, J.C., and Mellor, H. (2006). VEGF regulates the mobilization of VEGFR2/KDR from an intracellular endothelial storage compartment. Blood *108*, 2624-2631.

Garmy-Susini, B., Jin, H., Zhu, Y., Sung, R.J., Hwang, R., and Varner, J. (2005). Integrin alpha4beta1-VCAM-1-mediated adhesion between endothelial and mural cells is required for blood vessel maturation. J Clin Invest *115*, 1542-1551.

Gerhardt, H., and Betsholtz, C. (2003). Endothelial-pericyte interactions in angiogenesis. Cell Tissue Res *314*, 15-23.

Gerhardt, H., Golding, M., Fruttiger, M., Ruhrberg, C., Lundkvist, A., Abramsson, A., Jeltsch, M., Mitchell, C., Alitalo, K., Shima, D., *et al.* (2003). VEGF guides angiogenic sprouting utilizing endothelial tip cell filopodia. J Cell Biol *161*, 1163-1177.

Germain, S., Monnot, C., Muller, L., and Eichmann, A. (2010). Hypoxia-driven angiogenesis: role of tip cells and extracellular matrix scaffolding. Curr Opin Hematol *17*, 245-251.

Ghosh, P., Dahms, N.M., and Kornfeld, S. (2003). Mannose 6-phosphate receptors: new twists in the tale. Nat Rev Mol Cell Biol *4*, 202-212.

Grunewald, F.S., Prota, A.E., Giese, A., and Ballmer-Hofer, K. (2010). Structure-function analysis of VEGF receptor activation and the role of coreceptors in angiogenic signaling. Biochim Biophys Acta *1804*, 567-580.

Hallmann, R., Horn, N., Selg, M., Wendler, O., Pausch, F., and Sorokin, L.M. (2005). Expression and function of laminins in the embryonic and mature vasculature. Physiol Rev *85*, 979-1000.

Harris, T.A., Yamakuchi, M., Ferlito, M., Mendell, J.T., and Lowenstein, C.J. (2008). MicroRNA-126 regulates endothelial expression of vascular cell adhesion molecule 1. Proc Natl Acad Sci U S A *105*, 1516-1521.

Hiratsuka, S. (2011). Vasculogenensis, angiogenesis and special features of tumor blood vessels. Front Biosci *16*, 1413-1427.

Holmes, D.I., and Zachary, I.C. (2008). Vascular endothelial growth factor regulates stanniocalcin-1 expression via neuropilin-1-dependent regulation of KDR and synergism with fibroblast growth factor-2. Cell Signal *20*, 569-579.

Holmqvist, K., Cross, M., Riley, D., and Welsh, M. (2003). The Shb adaptor protein causes Src-dependent cell spreading and activation of focal adhesion kinase in murine brain endothelial cells. Cell Signal *15*, 171-179.

Holmqvist, K., Cross, M.J., Rolny, C., Hagerkvist, R., Rahimi, N., Matsumoto, T., Claesson-Welsh, L., and Welsh, M. (2004). The adaptor protein shb binds to tyrosine 1175 in vascular endothelial growth factor (VEGF) receptor-2 and regulates VEGF-dependent cellular migration. J Biol Chem *279*, 22267-22275.

Hong, W. (2005). SNAREs and traffic. Biochim Biophys Acta *1744*, 493-517.

Huang, K., Andersson, C., Roomans, G.M., Ito, N., and Claesson-Welsh, L. (2001). Signaling properties of VEGF receptor-1 and -2 homo- and heterodimers. Int J Biochem Cell Biol *33*, 315-324.

Hughes, D.C. (2001). Alternative splicing of the human VEGFGR-3/FLT4 gene as a consequence of an integrated human endogenous retrovirus. J Mol Evol *53*, 77-79.

Igarashi, K., Isohara, T., Kato, T., Shigeta, K., Yamano, T., and Uno, I. (1998). Tyrosine 1213 of Flt-1 is a major binding site of Nck and SHP-2. Biochem Biophys Res Commun *246*, 95-99.

Iivanainen, E., Kahari, V.M., Heino, J., and Elenius, K. (2003). Endothelial cell-matrix interactions. Microsc Res Tech *60*, 13-22.

Ito, N., Wernstedt, C., Engstrom, U., and Claesson-Welsh, L. (1998). Identification of vascular endothelial growth factor receptor-1 tyrosine phosphorylation sites and binding of SH2 domain-containing molecules. J Biol Chem *273*, 23410-23418.

Jahn, R., and Scheller, R.H. (2006). SNAREs--engines for membrane fusion. Nat Rev Mol Cell Biol *7*, 631-643.

Jopling, H.M., Odell, A.F., Hooper, N.M., Zachary, I.C., Walker, J.H., and Ponnambalam, S. (2009). Rab GTPase regulation of VEGFR2 trafficking and signaling in endothelial cells. Arterioscler Thromb Vasc Biol *29*, 1119-1124.

Kaipainen, A., Korhonen, J., Mustonen, T., van Hinsbergh, V.W., Fang, G.H., Dumont, D., Breitman, M., and Alitalo, K. (1995). Expression of the fms-like tyrosine kinase 4 gene becomes restricted to lymphatic endothelium during development. Proc Natl Acad Sci U S A *92*, 3566-3570.

Kalluri, R. (2003). Basement membranes: structure, assembly and role in tumour angiogenesis. Nat Rev Cancer *3*, 422-433.

Kanno, S., Oda, N., Abe, M., Terai, Y., Ito, M., Shitara, K., Tabayashi, K., Shibuya, M., and Sato, Y. (2000). Roles of two VEGF receptors, Flt-1 and KDR, in the signal transduction of VEGF effects in human vascular endothelial cells. Oncogene *19*, 2138-2146.

Kappas, N.C., Zeng, G., Chappell, J.C., Kearney, J.B., Hazarika, S., Kallianos, K.G., Patterson, C., Annex, B.H., and Bautch, V.L. (2008). The VEGF receptor Flt-1 spatially modulates Flk-1 signaling and blood vessel branching. J Cell Biol *181*, 847-858.

Kawamura, H., Li, X., Goishi, K., van Meeteren, L.A., Jakobsson, L., Cebe-Suarez, S., Shimizu, A., Edholm, D., Ballmer-Hofer, K., Kjellen, L., *et al.* (2008). Neuropilin-1 in regulation of VEGF-induced activation of p38MAPK and endothelial cell organization. Blood *112*, 3638-3649.

Kawasaki, T., Kitsukawa, T., Bekku, Y., Matsuda, Y., Sanbo, M., Yagi, T., and Fujisawa, H. (1999). A requirement for neuropilin-1 in embryonic vessel formation. Development *126*, 4895-4902.

Kendall, R.L., Rutledge, R.Z., Mao, X., Tebben, A.J., Hungate, R.W., and Thomas, K.A. (1999). Vascular endothelial growth factor receptor KDR tyrosine kinase activity is increased by autophosphorylation of two activation loop tyrosine residues. J Biol Chem *274*, 6453-6460.

Kendall, R.L., and Thomas, K.A. (1993). Inhibition of vascular endothelial cell growth factor activity by an endogenously encoded soluble receptor. Proc Natl Acad Sci U S A *90*, 10705-10709.

Kendall, R.L., Wang, G., DiSalvo, J., and Thomas, K.A. (1994). Specificity of vascular endothelial cell growth factor receptor ligand binding domains. Biochem Biophys Res Commun *201*, 326-330.

Kim, S., Bakre, M., Yin, H., and Varner, J.A. (2002). Inhibition of endothelial cell survival and angiogenesis by protein kinase A. J Clin Invest *110*, 933-941.

Kim, S., Bell, K., Mousa, S.A., and Varner, J.A. (2000). Regulation of angiogenesis in vivo by ligation of integrin alpha5beta1 with the central cell-binding domain of fibronectin. Am J Pathol *156*, 1345-1362.

Kim, V.N. (2005). MicroRNA biogenesis: coordinated cropping and dicing. Nat Rev Mol Cell Biol *6*, 376-385.

Kobayashi, S., Sawano, A., Nojima, Y., Shibuya, M., and Maru, Y. (2004). The c-Cbl/CD2AP complex regulates VEGF-induced endocytosis and degradation of Flt-1 (VEGFR-1). FASEB J *18*, 929-931.

Kuehbacher, A., Urbich, C., Zeiher, A.M., and Dimmeler, S. (2007). Role of Dicer and Drosha for endothelial microRNA expression and angiogenesis. Circ Res *101*, 59-68.

Labrecque, L., Royal, I., Surprenant, D.S., Patterson, C., Gingras, D., and Beliveau, R. (2003). Regulation of vascular endothelial growth factor receptor-2 activity by caveolin-1 and plasma membrane cholesterol. Mol Biol Cell *14*, 334-347.

Lampugnani, M.G., Orsenigo, F., Gagliani, M.C., Tacchetti, C., and Dejana, E. (2006). Vascular endothelial cadherin controls VEGFR-2 internalization and signaling from intracellular compartments. J Cell Biol *174*, 593-604.

Lanahan, A.A., Hermans, K., Claes, F., Kerley-Hamilton, J.S., Zhuang, Z.W., Giordano, F.J., Carmeliet, P., and Simons, M. (2010). VEGF receptor 2 endocytic trafficking regulates arterial morphogenesis. Dev Cell *18*, 713-724.

Lee, M.C., Miller, E.A., Goldberg, J., Orci, L., and Schekman, R. (2004). Bi-directional protein transport between the ER and Golgi. Annu Rev Cell Dev Biol *20*, 87-123.

Lee, S., Chen, T.T., Barber, C.L., Jordan, M.C., Murdock, J., Desai, S., Ferrara, N., Nagy, A., Roos, K.P., and Iruela-Arispe, M.L. (2007). Autocrine VEGF signaling is required for vascular homeostasis. Cell *130*, 691-703.

Levine, R.J., Maynard, S.E., Qian, C., Lim, K.H., England, L.J., Yu, K.F., Schisterman, E.F., Thadhani, R., Sachs, B.P., Epstein, F.H., *et al.* (2004). Circulating angiogenic factors and the risk of preeclampsia. N Engl J Med *350*, 672-683.

Liao, Y.F., Gotwals, P.J., Koteliansky, V.E., Sheppard, D., and Van De Water, L. (2002). The EIIIA segment of fibronectin is a ligand for integrins alpha 9beta 1 and alpha 4beta 1 providing a novel mechanism for regulating cell adhesion by alternative splicing. J Biol Chem *277*, 14467-14474.

Mahabeleshwar, G.H., Chen, J., Feng, W., Somanath, P.R., Razorenova, O.V., and Byzova, T.V. (2008). Integrin affinity modulation in angiogenesis. Cell Cycle *7*, 335-347.

Manickam, V., Tiwari, A., Jung, J.J., Bhattacharya, R., Goel, A., Mukhopadhyay, D., and Choudhury, A. (2011). Regulation of vascular endothelial growth factor receptor 2 trafficking and angiogenesis by Golgi localized t-SNARE syntaxin 6. Blood *117*, 1425-1435.

Marcinkiewicz, C., Taooka, Y., Yokosaki, Y., Calvete, J.J., Marcinkiewicz, M.M., Lobb, R.R., Niewiarowski, S., and Sheppard, D. (2000). Inhibitory effects of MLDG-containing heterodimeric disintegrins reveal distinct structural requirements for interaction of the integrin alpha 9beta 1 with VCAM-1, tenascin-C, and osteopontin. J Biol Chem *275*, 31930-31937.

Matsumoto, T., Bohman, S., Dixelius, J., Berge, T., Dimberg, A., Magnusson, P., Wang, L., Wikner, C., Qi, J.H., Wernstedt, C., *et al.* (2005). VEGF receptor-2 Y951 signaling and a role for the adapter molecule TSAd in tumor angiogenesis. EMBO J *24*, 2342-2353.

Matsumoto, T., and Claesson-Welsh, L. (2001). VEGF receptor signal transduction. Sci STKE *2001*, re21.

Matthews, W., Jordan, C.T., Gavin, M., Jenkins, N.A., Copeland, N.G., and Lemischka, I.R. (1991). A receptor tyrosine kinase cDNA isolated from a population of enriched primitive hematopoietic cells and exhibiting close genetic linkage to c-kit. Proc Natl Acad Sci U S A *88*, 9026-9030.

McCarthy, M. (2003). Antiangiogenesis drug promising for metastatic colorectal cancer. Lancet *361*, 1959.

Meadows, K.N., Bryant, P., and Pumiglia, K. (2001). Vascular endothelial growth factor induction of the angiogenic phenotype requires Ras activation. J Biol Chem *276*, 49289-49298.

Meyer, R.D., Sacks, D.B., and Rahimi, N. (2008). IQGAP1-dependent signaling pathway regulates endothelial cell proliferation and angiogenesis. PLoS One *3*, e3848.

Miao, H.Q., Lee, P., Lin, H., Soker, S., and Klagsbrun, M. (2000). Neuropilin-1 expression by tumor cells promotes tumor angiogenesis and progression. FASEB J *14*, 2532-2539.

Miao, H.Q., Soker, S., Feiner, L., Alonso, J.L., Raper, J.A., and Klagsbrun, M. (1999). Neuropilin-1 mediates collapsin-1/semaphorin III inhibition of endothelial cell motility: functional competition of collapsin-1 and vascular endothelial growth factor-165. J Cell Biol *146*, 233-242.

Mitra, S.K., Hanson, D.A., and Schlaepfer, D.D. (2005). Focal adhesion kinase: in command and control of cell motility. Nat Rev Mol Cell Biol *6*, 56-68.

Mitra, S.K., and Schlaepfer, D.D. (2006). Integrin-regulated FAK-Src signaling in normal and cancer cells. Curr Opin Cell Biol *18*, 516-523.

Mukherjee, S., Tessema, M., and Wandinger-Ness, A. (2006). Vesicular trafficking of tyrosine kinase receptors and associated proteins in the regulation of signaling and vascular function. Circ Res *98*, 743-756.

Nomura, M., Yamagishi, S., Harada, S., Hayashi, Y., Yamashima, T., Yamashita, J., and Yamamoto, H. (1995). Possible participation of autocrine and paracrine vascular endothelial growth factors in hypoxia-induced proliferation of endothelial cells and pericytes. J Biol Chem *270*, 28316-28324.

Nyberg, P., Xie, L., and Kalluri, R. (2005). Endogenous inhibitors of angiogenesis. Cancer Res *65*, 3967-3979.

Otsuka, M., Zheng, M., Hayashi, M., Lee, J.D., Yoshino, O., Lin, S., and Han, J. (2008). Impaired microRNA processing causes corpus luteum insufficiency and infertility in mice. J Clin Invest *118*, 1944-1954.

Peters, K.G., De Vries, C., and Williams, L.T. (1993). Vascular endothelial growth factor receptor expression during embryogenesis and tissue repair suggests a role in endothelial differentiation and blood vessel growth. Proc Natl Acad Sci U S A *90*, 8915-8919.

Risau, W. (1997). Mechanisms of angiogenesis. Nature *386*, 671-674.

Salameh, A., Galvagni, F., Bardelli, M., Bussolino, F., and Oliviero, S. (2005). Direct recruitment of CRK and GRB2 to VEGFR-3 induces proliferation, migration, and survival of endothelial cells through the activation of ERK, AKT, and JNK pathways. Blood *106*, 3423-3431.

Salikhova, A., Wang, L., Lanahan, A.A., Liu, M., Simons, M., Leenders, W.P., Mukhopadhyay, D., and Horowitz, A. (2008). Vascular endothelial growth factor and semaphorin induce neuropilin-1 endocytosis via separate pathways. Circ Res *103*, e71-79.

Sawano, A., Iwai, S., Sakurai, Y., Ito, M., Shitara, K., Nakahata, T., and Shibuya, M. (2001). Flt-1, vascular endothelial growth factor receptor 1, is a novel cell surface marker for the lineage of monocyte-macrophages in humans. Blood *97*, 785-791.

Sawano, A., Takahashi, T., Yamaguchi, S., and Shibuya, M. (1997). The phosphorylated 1169-tyrosine containing region of flt-1 kinase (VEGFR-1) is a major binding site for PLCgamma. Biochem Biophys Res Commun *238*, 487-491.

Scappaticci, F.A. (2002). Mechanisms and future directions for angiogenesis-based cancer therapies. J Clin Oncol *20*, 3906-3927.

Schlaepfer, D.D., and Hunter, T. (1998). Integrin signalling and tyrosine phosphorylation: just the FAKs? Trends Cell Biol *8*, 151-157.

Scott, A., and Mellor, H. (2009). VEGF receptor trafficking in angiogenesis. Biochem Soc Trans *37*, 1184-1188.

Senger, D.R., Perruzzi, C.A., Streit, M., Koteliansky, V.E., de Fougerolles, A.R., and Detmar, M. (2002). The alpha(1)beta(1) and alpha(2)beta(1) integrins provide critical support for vascular endothelial growth factor signaling, endothelial cell migration, and tumor angiogenesis. Am J Pathol *160*, 195-204.

Shalaby, F., Rossant, J., Yamaguchi, T.P., Gertsenstein, M., Wu, X.F., Breitman, M.L., and Schuh, A.C. (1995). Failure of blood-island formation and vasculogenesis in Flk-1-deficient mice. Nature *376*, 62-66.

Shibuya, M., Yamaguchi, S., Yamane, A., Ikeda, T., Tojo, A., Matsushime, H., and Sato, M. (1990). Nucleotide sequence and expression of a novel human receptor-type tyrosine kinase gene (flt) closely related to the fms family. Oncogene *5*, 519-524.

Singh, A.J., Meyer, R.D., Navruzbekov, G., Shelke, R., Duan, L., Band, H., Leeman, S.E., and Rahimi, N. (2007). A critical role for the E3-ligase activity of c-Cbl in VEGFR-2-mediated PLCgamma1 activation and angiogenesis. Proc Natl Acad Sci U S A *104*, 5413-5418.

Soker, S., Takashima, S., Miao, H.Q., Neufeld, G., and Klagsbrun, M. (1998). Neuropilin-1 is expressed by endothelial and tumor cells as an isoform-specific receptor for vascular endothelial growth factor. Cell *92*, 735-745.

Solowiej, J., Bergqvist, S., McTigue, M.A., Marrone, T., Quenzer, T., Cobbs, M., Ryan, K., Kania, R.S., Diehl, W., and Murray, B.W. (2009). Characterizing the effects of the juxtamembrane domain on vascular endothelial growth factor receptor-2 enzymatic activity, autophosphorylation, and inhibition by axitinib. Biochemistry *48*, 7019-7031.

Sorkin, A., and von Zastrow, M. (2009). Endocytosis and signalling: intertwining molecular networks. Nat Rev Mol Cell Biol *10*, 609-622.

Staniszewska, I., Zaveri, S., Del Valle, L., Oliva, I., Rothman, V.L., Croul, S.E., Roberts, D.D., Mosher, D.F., Tuszynski, G.P., and Marcinkiewicz, C. (2007). Interaction of alpha9beta1 integrin with thrombospondin-1 promotes angiogenesis. Circ Res *100*, 1308-1316.

Stupack, D.G., and Cheresh, D.A. (2004). Integrins and angiogenesis. Curr Top Dev Biol *64*, 207-238.

Suarez, Y., Fernandez-Hernando, C., Pober, J.S., and Sessa, W.C. (2007). Dicer dependent microRNAs regulate gene expression and functions in human endothelial cells. Circ Res *100*, 1164-1173.

Sudhof, T.C., and Rothman, J.E. (2009). Membrane fusion: grappling with SNARE and SM proteins. Science *323*, 474-477.

Takahashi, T., Yamaguchi, S., Chida, K., and Shibuya, M. (2001). A single autophosphorylation site on KDR/Flk-1 is essential for VEGF-A-dependent activation of PLC-gamma and DNA synthesis in vascular endothelial cells. EMBO J *20*, 2768-2778.

Tammela, T., Zarkada, G., Wallgard, E., Murtomaki, A., Suchting, S., Wirzenius, M., Waltari, M., Hellstrom, M., Schomber, T., Peltonen, R., *et al.* (2008). Blocking VEGFR-3 suppresses angiogenic sprouting and vascular network formation. Nature *454*, 656-660.

Tanjore, H., Zeisberg, E.M., Gerami-Naini, B., and Kalluri, R. (2008). Beta1 integrin expression on endothelial cells is required for angiogenesis but not for vasculogenesis. Dev Dyn *237*, 75-82.

Terman, B.I., Carrion, M.E., Kovacs, E., Rasmussen, B.A., Eddy, R.L., and Shows, T.B. (1991). Identification of a new endothelial cell growth factor receptor tyrosine kinase. Oncogene *6*, 1677-1683.

Tiwari, A., Jung, J.J., Inamdar, S.M., Brown, C.O., Goel, A., and Choudhury, A. (2011). Endothelial cell migration on fibronectin is regulated by syntaxin 6-mediated {alpha}5{beta}1 integrin recycling. J Biol Chem.

Tuma, P.L., and Hubbard, A.L. (2003). Transcytosis: crossing cellular barriers. Physiol Rev *83*, 871-932.

Uemura, A., Ogawa, M., Hirashima, M., Fujiwara, T., Koyama, S., Takagi, H., Honda, Y., Wiegand, S.J., Yancopoulos, G.D., and Nishikawa, S. (2002). Recombinant angiopoietin-1 restores higher-order architecture of growing blood vessels in mice in the absence of mural cells. J Clin Invest *110*, 1619-1628.

Vlahakis, N.E., Young, B.A., Atakilit, A., Hawkridge, A.E., Issaka, R.B., Boudreau, N., and Sheppard, D. (2007). Integrin alpha9beta1 directly binds to vascular endothelial growth factor (VEGF)-A and contributes to VEGF-A-induced angiogenesis. J Biol Chem *282*, 15187-15196.

Wang, F., Yamauchi, M., Muramatsu, M., Osawa, T., Tsuchida, R., and Shibuya, M. (2011). RACK1 regulates VEGF/Flt1-mediated cell migration via activation of a PI3K/Akt pathway. J Biol Chem *286*, 9097-9106.

Wang, S., and Olson, E.N. (2009). AngiomiRs--key regulators of angiogenesis. Curr Opin Genet Dev *19*, 205-211.

Warner, A.J., Lopez-Dee, J., Knight, E.L., Feramisco, J.R., and Prigent, S.A. (2000). The Shc-related adaptor protein, Sck, forms a complex with the vascular-endothelial-growth-factor receptor KDR in transfected cells. Biochem J *347*, 501-509.

Yamaoka-Tojo, M., Tojo, T., Kim, H.W., Hilenski, L., Patrushev, N.A., Zhang, L., Fukai, T., and Ushio-Fukai, M. (2006). IQGAP1 mediates VE-cadherin-based cell-cell contacts and VEGF signaling at adherence junctions linked to angiogenesis. Arterioscler Thromb Vasc Biol *26*, 1991-1997.

Yang, J.T., Rayburn, H., and Hynes, R.O. (1993). Embryonic mesodermal defects in alpha 5 integrin-deficient mice. Development *119*, 1093-1105.

Yang, J.T., Rayburn, H., and Hynes, R.O. (1995). Cell adhesion events mediated by alpha 4 integrins are essential in placental and cardiac development. Development *121*, 549-560.

Yang, W.J., Yang, D.D., Na, S., Sandusky, G.E., Zhang, Q., and Zhao, G. (2005). Dicer is required for embryonic angiogenesis during mouse development. J Biol Chem *280*, 9330-9335.

Yuan, L., Moyon, D., Pardanaud, L., Breant, C., Karkkainen, M.J., Alitalo, K., and Eichmann, A. (2002). Abnormal lymphatic vessel development in neuropilin 2 mutant mice. Development *129*, 4797-4806.

Zachary, I. (2003). VEGF signalling: integration and multi-tasking in endothelial cell biology. Biochem Soc Trans *31*, 1171-1177.

Part 2

Hematological Pathologies

11

Translational Control in Myeloid Disease

Nirmalee Abayasekara and Arati Khanna-Gupta
Brigham and Women's Hospital,
Harvard Medical School, Boston, MA,
USA

1. Introduction

Over the years a wealth of information on the role played by transcription factors in myeloid biology has contributed to our understanding of both normal and abnormal myeloid development. However, the regulation of mRNA translation in myeloid cell maturation has, in comparison, been a neglected area of study. A better understanding of the translational control of myeloid gene expression will undoubtedly provide important insights into both normal and abnormal myeloid maturation. This chapter summarizes our current understanding of the regulation of myeloid gene expression at the mRNA translational level and delineates levels of disruption in myeloid disease, with an emphasis on leukemias.

2. Myeloid differentiation and neutrophil development

During hematopoiesis, granulocytes and monocytes arise from a common progenitor cell in the bone marrow and differentiate in response to cytokines and transcription factors ultimately giving rise to mature neutrophils and monocytes in the circulation. The granulocyte progenitor cells pass through several identifiable maturational stages, during which they acquire the morphologic appearance and granule contents that characterize the mature granulocyte(Rev in(Berliner, 1998)). The earliest identifiable granulocyte precursor is the myeloblast, which is characterized by very few granules, little cytoplasm and a prominent nucleolus. Transition to the promyelocyte stage is associated with the acquisition of primary granules. Primary granules are found in both granulocytes and monocytes and contain many of the proteins necessary for intracellular microbicidal activity (Bainton, 1975). The transition to the myelocyte stage is associated with the acquisition of secondary or "specific" granules(Bainton, 1971). Myelocytes further mature to give rise to bands and mature neutrophils. The appearance of secondary granules and their content proteins, provides a unique marker of commitment to terminal neutrophil differentiation (reviewed in (Borregaard *et al.*, 2001)). Several lines of evidence from our laboratory have established that the expression of the secondary granule protein (SGP) genes, which are functionally diverse and physically unlinked, is coordinately regulated at the level of mRNA transcription (reviewed in(Berliner, 1998)). Absence of SGP gene expression is a consistent abnormality in Myelodysplastic syndrome (MDS) and acute myeloid leukemia (AML).

2.1 Transcriptional control of myeloid maturation

Maturation of myeloid progenitor cells into specialized blood cells that play a vital role in innate immunity, is regulated by a well-orchestrated interplay of transcription factors (Tenen, 2003). Recent studies have delineated transcription factors that contribute to the process of maturation. These include a category of factors termed "master regulators" of lineage development and include PU.1, and CCAAT enhancer-binding protein-α (C/EBPα) (Tenen, 2003). These factors not only promote lineage-specific gene expression but also suppress alternative lineage pathways. For example, Laslo et al (Laslo *et al.*, 2006) elegantly demonstrated that cell fate determination is dependent upon subtle changes in expression levels of transcription factors, which regulate differential lineage maturation. Levels of PU.1 expression are increased by Egr-1/Nab-2 in developing monocytes/macrophages; while Egr-1 simultaneously represses the expression of the neutrophil specific Gfi-1 transcription factor (see below), thereby repressing the neutrophil development program.

2.1.1 C/EBPα

C/EBPα has been recognized to be a master regulator of the granulopoietic developmental program. It is expressed at high levels throughout myeloid differentiation (Tsukada *et al.*, 2011). C/EBPα binds to the promoters of multiple myeloid-specific genes, thereby regulating gene expression at many different stages of myeloid maturation. C/EBPα$^{-/-}$ mice die perinatally due to defects in gluconeogenesis that result in fatal hypoglycemia, and demonstrate an early block in the differentiation of granulocytes without affecting either monocyte/macrophage maturation or the differentiation of other hematopoietic lineages. The expression of C/EBPα is associated with growth arrest and differentiation of granulocyte precursor cells. This block in proliferation is thought to occur via the interaction of C/EBPα with cyclin-dependent protein kinases (cdk2 and cdk4), resulting in a block in cell proliferation. In addition, C/EBPα inhibits E2F-dependent transcription, which also contributes to inhibition of cell proliferation and induction of differentiation associated with C/EBPα-induced granulopoiesis (Timchenko *et al.*, 1997; Timchenko *et al.*, 1999)

2.1.2 PU.1

A second master myeloid regulator PU.1, is a member of the Ets family of transcription factors and is expressed in both B cells and monocyte/macrophages (Chen *et al.*, 1995). PU.1 is also expressed at lower levels in granulocytes and eosinophils as well as in CD34^{+} hematopoietic progenitor cells. High levels of PU.1 expression in fetal livers of mice preferentially directs monocyte/macrophage development, whereas low levels of PU.1 result in B-cell development (DeKoter and Singh, 2000). Studies have revealed that downregulation of c-Jun, a coactivator of PU.1, by C/EBPα is necessary for granulocytic maturation and is the mechanism through which C/EBPα blocks macrophage development (Rangatia *et al.*, 2002). Gene knockout studies of PU.1 in mice resulted in perinatal lethality accompanied by the absence of mature monocytes/macrophages, B cells as well as and delayed and reduced granulopoiesis (Scott *et al.*, 1994). Following *in vitro* differentiation, embryonic stem (ES) cells derived from PU.1$^{-/-}$ blastocysts fail to express mature myeloid cell markers, suggesting that PU.1 is not essential for the initial events associated with myeloid lineage commitment but is necessary for the later stages of development.

2.1.3 Growth Factor Independence-1 (Gfi-1)

Gfi-1 is a highly conserved transcriptional repressor that encodes a 55kD nuclear proto-oncogene that is composed of six zinc finger domains at the carboxy terminus and a N-terminal SNAG or repression domain (rev in (van der Meer *et al.*, 2010). Gfi-1 is expressed at high levels in the thymus and bone marrow, while its paralog Gfi1B, is expressed in the bone marrow and spleen. An essential role of Gfi-1 in neutrophil differentiation became apparent following reports of gene disruption in mice (Hock *et al.*, 2003). Gfi1-null mice are severely neutropenic and eventually succumb to bacterial infections. These mice lack mature neutrophils and their granulocyte precursors are unable to differentiate into mature neutrophils and also lack expression of specific granule proteins (SGPs). In addition, Gfi-1–/– bone marrow expresses atypical $Gr1^{+}Mac1^{+}$ myeloid precursor cells that appear to have characteristics of both granulocyte and macrophage precursors. These observations confirm a critical role for Gfi-1 in the neutrophil maturation program. Work from our laboratory has shown that Gfi-1 synergizes with another member of the CCAAT enhancer binding protein family of transcription factors, C/EBPε to transactivate the promoters of late myeloid genes. This synergy is lost in a patient with specific granule deficiency (SGD), who has a heterozygous substitution mutation in the C/EBPε gene as well as decreased levels of Gfi-1 in the bone marrow (Khanna-Gupta *et al.*, 2007). Heterozygous dominant negative mutations in the Gfi-1 gene have been described in two patients with severe congenital neutropenia (SCN) (Person *et al.*, 2003), thus emphasizing the role of Gfi-1 in the neutrophil maturation pathway.

Over the years a great deal of information pertaining to the transcriptional regulation of myeloid development has become available and has aided in our understanding of the process of granulopoiesis and how it goes awry in myeloid leukemias. In contrast, as outlined below, the role of mRNA translation in the process of normal myeloid development is only just beginning to be understood (rev in (Khanna-Gupta, 2011))

3. An overview of the process of mRNA translation in eukaryotic cells

Eukaryotic protein synthesis involves the coordinated interplay of hundreds of macromolecules such as mRNAs, tRNAs, activating enzymes, protein factors and ribosomes. Ribosomes are the protein synthetic factories upon which protein synthesis proceeds and are composed of a large (60S) and a small (40S) subunit. Each of these subunits is composed of two-thirds RNA and one-third protein. Protein synthesis occurs on the ribosome in three phases: translation initiation, elongation and termination. Regulation of gene expression takes place primarily at the initiation stage which therefore is the rate-limiting step in protein synthesis. The delicate balance of events leading to protein expression is critical for cellular growth, proliferation, differentiation and apoptosis (Rev in (Van Der Kelen *et al.*, 2009)). In eukaryotes, translation initiation factors (eIFs) play a crucial role in the dissociation of 40S and 60S ribosomal subunits thus enabling recruitment of mRNA and initiator tRNAs to the 40S subunit followed by interaction with the 60S subunit resulting in the reformation of the 80S ribosome allowing for elongation and termination of the polypeptide chain to ensue (rev in (Van Der Kelen *et al.*, 2009)).

3.1 Control of translation initiation

The first step in the translation of mRNA in eukaryotic cells begins with the binding of the 40S small ribosomal subunit to the 5′ end of the mRNA to be translated in the process of 5′

cap-dependent translation. Cap-binding protein eukaryotic initiation factor 4E (eIF4E) recognizes and binds to the m^7GpppN cap (where m is a methyl group and N any nucleotide) structure at the 5'end of the mRNA to be translated. Under normal physiologic conditions, eIF4E strongly associates with 4E-binding proteins (4E-BPs) thus preventing eIF4E from initiating protein synthesis, this represents the first rate limiting step in the process of protein synthesis. This inhibition is overcome by the phosphorylation of 4E-BPs via signal transduction pathways (involving PI3K and mTOR among others, see below) that are regulated by growth factors and nutrient status of the cell, thus causing 4E-BPs to be phosphorylated and to dissociate from eIF4E (Figure 1). This enables a competing adapter molecule eIF4G, to bind to eIF4E. eIF4G then recruits the ATP-dependent RNA helicase eIF4A (eIF4E, 4G and 4A are collectively referred to as eIF4F in the literature), the ubiquitously expressed cofactor eIF4B as well as eIF3, a multisubunit initiation factor, all of which bind to the 5' cap region of the mRNA, thus setting the stage for mRNA translation to begin (rev in(Sonenberg and AG., 2009)).

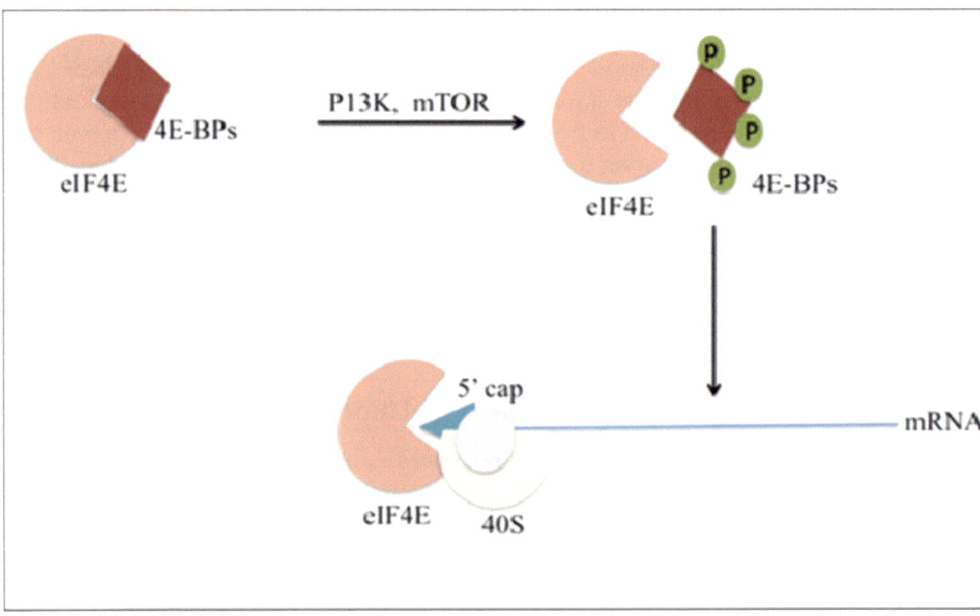

Fig. 1. Under basal conditions eIF4E is tightly bound to 4E-BPs. When cells are under stress or nutrient deprived, Phosphorylation of 4E-BPs is triggered by P13K (Phospho-inositol Kinase) and mTOR, which causes the 4E-BPs to be phosphorylated and/or to have reduced affinity for eIF4E. eIF4E is now free to bind eIF4G to initiate mRNA translation.

Translation initiation however requires the small ribosomal subunit 40S to be complexed with the so called ternary complex before it associates with the mRNA (Figure 2). The assembly of the ternary complex, consisting of the G protein eIF2B, eIF2, the initiator tRNA, $tRNAi^{met}$ and GTP, is the second rate-limiting step in mRNA translation. Recognition of the first AUG codon in the mRNA to be translated followed by initiation of protein synthesis is dependent on this process. Upon recognition of the first in-frame AUG, eIF2-GTP is hydrolyzed and the resulting eIF2-GDP is restored to eIF2-GTP by the guanine-nucleotide-exchange factor known as eIF2B to continue another round of translation initiation (Figure

2). This process is inbibited when the α subunit (S51 residue) of eIF2 is phosphorylated. This is brought about by the activation of a number of eIF2α kinases which are activated under conditions of cellular stress and aid in the reduction of protein synthesis until the stressful circumstance has passed (Figure 2). If stress remains unabated, apoptosis ensues. EIF2α kinases include the Heme-regulated inhibitor kinase (HRI), RNA-dependent protein kinase (PKR), PKR-like endoplasmic-reticulum kinase (PERK) and mGCN2(mammalian general control non-derepressing) (rev in (Raven and AE., 2008) and (Chen, 2007) and references therein). Since phosphorylated eIF2α has a higher affinity for eIF2B than eIF2α, phosphorylation of even a small percentage of eIF2α can lead to a reduction in protein synthesis. Phosphorylation of eIF2α can be reversed upon removal of the phosphate group by specific phosphatases thus restoring the cell to homeostasis (Harding *et al.*, 2009).

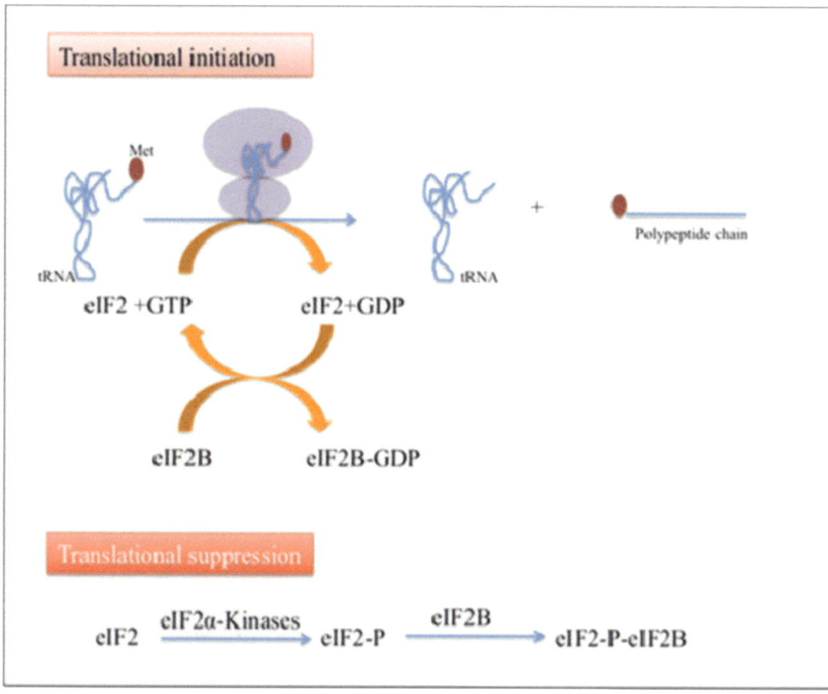

Fig. 2. During initiation, a GTP molecule is hydrolyzed to GDP which is then recycled by eIF2B, making eIF2α-GTP available for the continuation of the synthesis cycle. However, under cellular stress conditions, alterations in nutrient status, growth factors, mitogens and inducers of differentiation a variety of a eIF2α kinases are activated which causes the phosphorylation of eIF2α which has an increased affinity towards eIF2B. This traps available eIF2α and eIF2B resulting in a block in protein synthesis.

Formation of the 43S preinitiation complex occurs once the ternary complex binds to the 40S subunit complexed with eIF3 and eIF1A. The pre-initiation complex further associates with the mRNA through eIF3 and eIF4G, thus forming the 48S initiation complex. mRNA scanning begins when the 40S subunit moves along the mRNA in a 5′ to 3′ direction. Upon encountering the first in-frame translation initiation codon AUG, a codon (mRNA) - anticodon (tRNA) recognition is established resulting in the dissociation of initiation factors from the 40S subunit. This enables the binding of the 60S subunit resulting in the assembly of the functional ribosome (80S) and for peptide elongation to proceed.

The 3′ end of the mRNA together with a number of the initiation factors ensure the stabilization of ribosome-mRNA interaction. Poly (A) tail and polyA binding protein (PABP) interact with eIF4G to form a pseudo-circular mRNA. This structure is thought to reduce the translational error rate as translation from intact RNAs alone would be permitted. This mRNA configuration also gives the initiation factors the necessary spatial proximity that ensures efficient dissociation and re-association capabilities to permit another round of protein synthesis to occur.

3.2 The mTOR pathway

mTOR (mammalian/mechanistic target of rapamycin) is involved in an evolutionarily conserved pathway that is critical for cellular responses to environmental cues. mTOR is a serine/threonine protein kinase belonging to the phospho inositide 3-kinase (PI3K)-related protein kinases (PIKK) family of protein kinases, which consists of a protein complex that enable organisms to cope with metabolic, environmental and genetic stresses (rev in (Sengupta *et al.*, 2010)). Mammalian TOR forms two structurally and functionally distinct multiprotein complexes, mTORC1: in which mTOR is complexed with Raptor (the regulatory protein of mTOR), LST8 (also called GβL) and PRAS40 (proline-rich Akt/PKB substrate 40kDa), and mTORC2, harboring both LST8 and Rictor (rapamycin-insensitive companion of mTOR). Only mTORC1 is responsive to the inhibitory effects of the antibiotic rapamycin (Figure 3) (Wullschieger *et al.*, 2006). When activated, mTORC1 functions to regulate protein synthetic pathways in response to nutritional, environmental and growth factor mediated signals. The TCS1 and TCS2 (tuberous sclerosis 1 and 2) proteins form a tumor suppressor complex that transmits signals to mTORC1 by regulating the activation of Rheb (Ras homolog enriched in brain; a GTP-GDP exchange protein). The TCS1 and TSC2 complex regulates the GTP-loading state of Rheb. GTP-bound Rheb interacts with mTORC1 and renders it active. The two major targets of mTOR are the 4E-BPs (see Figure 1) and the 40S ribosomal protein S6 kinase (S6K1), both important components of the translational machinery (Figure 3).

Upon activation, mTORC1 regulates the phosphorylation/activation of p70 S6 kinase (S6K1) and the phosphorylation/deactivation of 4E-BP1(Platanias, 2005). Activation of S6 kinase modulates ribosome biogenesis through the activation of ribosomal protein S6 (rpS6)(Lee-Fruman *et al.*, 1999) (Figure 3). S6K1 also phosphorylates eIF2B, SKAR (S6K1 Aly/REF-like target) and eukaryotic elongation factor 2 kinase, thus affecting both the initiation and elongation stages of mRNA translation.

As described above, hypo-phosphorylation of the 4E-BPs increases their affinity for eIF4E, thus blocking the interaction of eIF4G and eIF4A thereby hampering translation initiation of mRNA from proceeding (Figure 1). However, phosphorylation of the 4E-BPs by activation of the mTORC1 signaling pathway (Figure 3) results in lowered affinity of these proteins for eIF4E, thus allowing for the formation of the competing eIF4E-eIF4G-eIF4A (eIF4F)-mRNA complex that permits mRNA translation to proceed(Gingras *et al.*, 2001). Thus inhibition of mTORC1 activity results in the down regulation of the activity of several components of the translational machinery resulting in a block in cell proliferation and eventually to cell death.

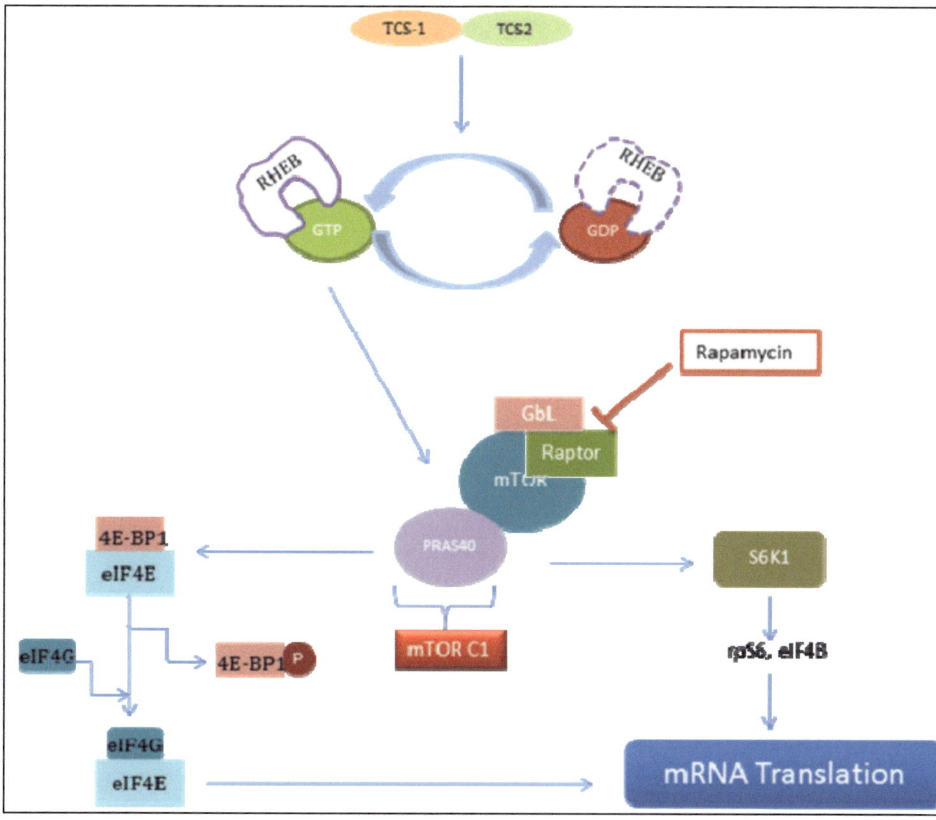

Fig. 3. mTOR pathway. See text for details

4. Translation control in Myeloid cells

While the general principles of mRNA translation hold in myeloid cells, it has been shown that when *4E-BP1* and *4E-BP2* genes were knocked out in mice an impairment of myelopoiesis was observed with no obvious effect on thymocyte maturation(Olson *et al.*, 2008). An increase in the number of immature granulocytic precursors and a decrease in the numbers of mature granulocytes was observed in these mice compared to their wild type littermates. Other studies have shown that expression of the 4E-BPs is significantly increased during granulopoiesis(Grolleau *et al.*, 1999). It was thus concluded that 4E-BP1 and 4E-BP2 play an important role in the early phases of granulo-monocytic differentiation thereby highlighting a critical role for translation initiation during granulopoiesis. It should be noted that 4E-BP1 has been shown to be constitutively phosphorylated in both chronic myeloid leukemia (CML) and in acute myeloid leukemia (AML) due to the constitutive activation of mTOR and Bcr-Abl in CML(Ly *et al.*, 2003) and PI3K-Akt in AML(Xu *et al.*, 2003).

4.1 Translational defects in myeloid leukemias

Activation of aberrant transcriptional and signaling pathways leading to enhanced survival and proliferation of leukemic progenitors is a hallmark of acute myeloid leukemia (AML)

(Scholl *et al.*, 2008; Tenen, 2003). The recent past has seen marked changes for the better in our understanding of the biology underlying AML. Based on these advances, targeting overactive signaling pathways in transformed cells has become an active area of research with the ultimate goal of finding molecules that specifically target only the transformed cell.

4.1.1 mTOR

The mTOR pathway has been shown to be activated in a number of cancers including AML (rev in (Tamburini *et al.*, 2009a)). In fact, mTORC1 has been shown to be activated in over 90% of primary AML samples (Tamburini *et al.*, 2009b). There has thus been a great effort to demonstrate the efficacy and use of Rapalogs, a class of drugs that include the mTORC1 inhibitor Rapamycin (see Figure 3) and RAD001, as anti-cancer agents. However, despite the anticipated cell death that blocking the mTORC1 pathway should result in, it has been demonstrated that the anti-leukemic effects of rapalogs are merely cytostatic. This is likely due to the fact that mTORC1 inhibition by rapalogs results in the activation of a number of feedback loops involving leukemogenic kinases such as P13K and ERK, thus limiting the anti-leukemic effects of this class of drugs.(Wang *et al.*, 2008)

4.1.2 Oncogenic mRNAs

The translation efficiencies of different mRNAs are dependent partly on the structural complexity of their 5'UTR (untranslated region). mRNAs with simple or short 5'UTRs, such as in the actin mRNA, are translated with high efficiency even in untransformed cells. However, mRNAs harboring long and complex 5'UTRs are generally translated with low efficiency and are referred to as "weak" mRNAs because of weak interactions with the eIF4F translation initiation complex (see above). In transformed cells on the other hand, this interaction improves due to the increased activity of eIF4F leading to increased translation of the weak mRNAs. It is noteworthy that a number of these weak mRNAs have oncogenic potential because they encode proteins involved in cell cycle regulation (e.g. cyclin D1) DNA replication (ornithine decarboxylase) and other pathways (c-myc, VEGF, Bcl-2, survin), all of which contribute to cell survival and proliferation. Expression of such mRNAs is regulated at the translational level and their overexpression likely contributes to the transformation process in AML ((Tamburini *et al.*, 2009a) and references therein). Since these "oncogenic" mRNAs have been found to be more sensitive to translation inhibition, there has been an effort to identify compounds that block mRNA translation. An example of such a compound is 4EGI-1 which is a 4E-BP1 mimetic and potently blocks the interaction of eIF4E and eIF4G during translation initiation (see above). 4EGI-1 has been shown to abrogate the expression of c-Myc and Bcl-x_L, both proteins with oncogenic potential. Additionally, this compound has shown therapeutic potential as it induces selective apoptosis in AML blast while allowing normal CD34+ hematopoietic progenitors to survive (Tamburini *et al.*, 2009b).

Overexpression of the initiation factor eIF4E has been described in primary cells derived from M4/M5 AML compared to bone marrow mononuclear cells (Topisirovic *et al.*, 2003). EIF4E expression has been known to increase protein synthesis and to transform cells (Wendel *et al.*, 2007). It should be noted that the antiviral compound ribavarin has been shown to inhibit the activity of eIF4E (Kentsis *et al.*, 2004). In a small study involving 11 M4/M5 AML patients who were given ribavarin, three patients responded with one in complete remission and two in partial remission (Assouline *et al.*, 2009). This study demonstrates that blocking the translational engine could prove to be a very important tool in the development of future AML therapeutics.

5. Translational control of the myeloid master regulator C/EBPα

C/EBPα is the founding member of a family of basic region/leucine zipper (bzip) transcription factors many of which contribute to granulopoiesis and are regulated at the translation level. (Rev in(Fuchs, 2007; Koschmieder *et al.*, 2009; Muller and Pabst, 2006; Schuster and Porse, 2006)). For the sake of simplicity only the translational control of the master myeloid regulator C/EBPα will be discussed here.

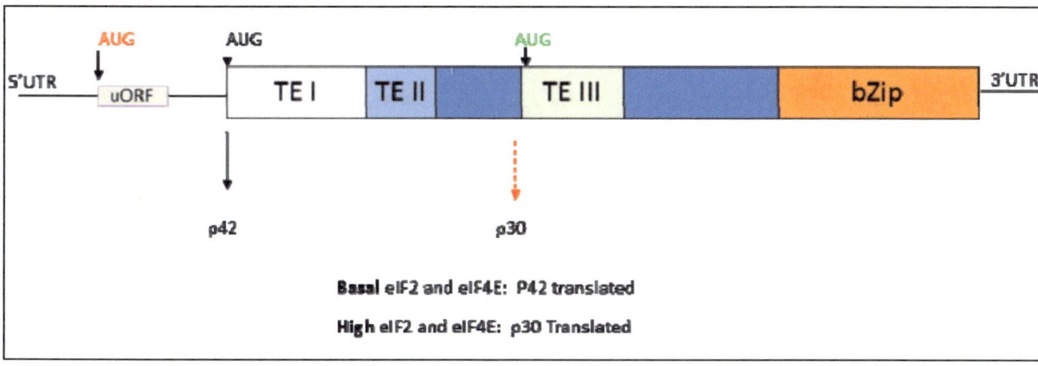

Fig. 4. Structure of the C/EBPα mRNA. TE I, II and III are activation domains. bZip is the basic leucine-zipper DNA binding domain.

Profound hematopoietic abnormalities have been reported for mice in which C/EBPα is ablated(Zhang *et al.*, 1997). The C/EBPα gene is intronless and generates two isoforms as a result of the differential utilization of alternate translation start codons. The resultant p42kD (full length) and p30kD (truncated) C/EBPα proteins differ from each other at the N-terminus, which is shorter in the p30kD protein (Figure 4). Translational control of C/EBPα-isoform expression occurs via a conserved cis-regulatory uORF (upstream open reading frame) in the 5'UTR (untranslated region) that is out of frame with the coding region of C/EBPα and is thought to be responsive to the activities of the translation initiation factors eIF4E and eIF2 (Figure 4 and see above). Thus, an increase in the activity of eIF2 or eIF4E, results in the increase in expression of the shorter p30 isoform (rev in(Calkhoven *et al.*, 2000)). An uORF monitors the site of translation initiation by sensing the activity of the eIF2 and eIF4E. When levels of these factors are high, the out-of-frame uORF (Figure 4, red AUG) is translated, but termination of its translation very close to the translational start site (black AUG) for p42 is thought to prevent reinitiation at the p42 AUG. Instead, ribosomes continue to scan and reinitiate at a downstream AUG (Figure 4, green AUG), resulting in the expression of C/EBPα p30. In contrast, under basal conditions, when levels of the initiation factors are relatively low, most ribosomes do not initiate translation at the uORF but instead initiate translation at the p42 AUG by a process involving "leaky ribosome scanning", resulting in translation of the full length C/EBPα p42 isoform(Calkhoven *et al.*, 2000). This mechanism of translational control appears to be conserved among key regulatory proteins which govern differentiation and proliferation (rev in (Khanna-Gupta, 2011)).

High levels of expression of the p30 C/EBPα protein have been shown to interfere with the DNA binding ability of the full length p42 C/EBPα, thus inhibiting transactivation of key granulocytic target genes in a dominant-negative manner (Pabst *et al.*, 2001), In addition, p30 transactivates the expression of a distinct subset of target genes different from that of the full length p42 C/EBPα thereby altering their expression (Geletu *et al.*, 2007). Mice engineered to express only the p30 C/EBPα isoform resulted in the development of AML with complete penetrance (Kirstetter *et al.*, 2008). Thus changes in the ratio of p42:p30 isoforms of C/EBPα play a critical role in contributing to AML(Fu *et al.*, 2010).

Suppression of C/EBPα translation has also been observed in the leukemic blasts of patients with CML (chronic myelogenous leukemia). This occurs via an RNA binding protein, hnRNP-E2, which binds to the uORF of the C/EBPα mRNA, thereby inhibiting translation. Expression of hnRNP-E2 is thought to be upregulated by the activity of the oncogenic BCR-ABL fusion protein in CML patients, and downregulation of hnRNP-E2 by the BCR-ABL inhibitor Imatinib results in restoration of C/EBPα protein expression and granulocytic differentiation of the CML blasts(Perrotti *et al.*, 2002).

6. Role of microRNAs in translation control

6.1 General principles

MicroRNAs (miRNAs) are 18-24 nucleotides long non-coding RNAs that regulate eukaryotic gene expression influencing cellular functions as diverse as cell proliferation, differentiation and apoptosis. miRNAs are non-coding RNAs which silence target genes post-transcriptionally by binding to complementary sequences in the 3'UTR (untranslated region) of the target mRNA resulting in either mRNA degradation or translation repression (rev in (Ambros, 2004)). More than 100 miRNAs are expressed in the hematopoieteic compartment (rev in (Gazzar and McCall, 2011)). MiRNAs are encoded in the genome and are initially transcribed by RNA polymerase II as long primary transcripts referred to as primary miRNAs (pri-miRNAs). These hairpin transcripts are recognized and processed by RNase III enzymes called Drosha and DGCR8 into 60-80 nucleotide intermediates called precursor miRNAs (pre-miRNAs) which are then exported to the cytoplasm by Exportin 5 where a second ribonuclease termed Dicer cleaves the pre-miRNAs to generate double stranded 18-24 nucleotide long miRNAs. One strand of the miRNA is next destroyed and the remaining strand, the guide strand, is then incorporated into the RNA-induced silencing complex or RISC, a large protein complex that also contains the Argonaute 2 or mRNA cleaving proteins. The miRNA guides the RISC complex to target complementary regions in the 3'UTRs of mRNAs, leading to repression of translation or destabilization of the mRNA by deadenylation. (rev in (Manikandan *et al.*, 2008)). In mammalian cells, 6-8 nucleotides of the miRNA (known as the seed region) base pair with the cognate recognition sequence in the 3'UTR of the target mRNA. In general, a perfectly matched sequence between the seed region and mRNA target results in degradation of the mRNA target. An imperfect match however, results in translation repression (rev in (Gazzar and McCall, 2011)). MiRNAs are thought to repress translation by blocking translation initiation of the target mRNA (Filipowicz *et al.*, 2008).

6.2 miRNAs in myeloid biology

An increasing body of evidence implicates miRNA activity in mediating both normal and abmormal myelopoiesis (rev in (Pelosi *et al.*, 2009) and (Gazzar and McCall, 2011)).

Granulocytes arise from the GMPs (granulocyte monocyte progenitors) which are capable of developing into granulocytes or monocytes as a result of cytokines and thus transcription factor activation (Dahl R *et al.*, 2003). MiRNAs have been shown to activate or be activated by myeloid specific transcription factors such as PU.1, C/EBPα and Gfi-1. Mir-223, for example, is thought to be a direct target of C/EBPα and its expression increases during granulopoiesis. C/EBPα is a master regulator of granulopoiesis (Tenen, 2003). Complete loss of mir-223 in mice results in the expansion of granulocyte precursor cells resulting from a cell autonomous increase in the number of granulocytic progenitors (Johnnidis *et al.*, 2008). In contrast, overexpression of mir-223 in acute promyelocytic leukemia (APL) cells results in an enhanced capacity for granulocytic differentiation (Fazi *et al.*, 2005). Mir-223 is thus thought to be a positive regulator of granulopoietic differentiation. It has also been shown that mir-223 targets E2F1, a master cell cycle regulator, by inhibiting translation of its mRNA. Thus, granulopoiesis appears to be regulated by a C/EBPα–miR-223–E2F1 axis, where miR-223 functions as a key regulator of myeloid cell proliferation associated with E2F1 in a negative feedback loop(Pulikkan *et al.*, 2010).

In a recent study, Eiring et al demonstrated a new "decoy" role for miRNAs involving the master reugator C/EBPα. They showed that mir-328 is down regulated in myeloid cells of chronic myelogenous leukemia (CML) patients in blast crisis. Restoration of mir-328 expression however rekindles differentiation in the CML blast cells by a mechanism involving the simultaneous interaction of mir-328 with the C/EBPα translational inhibitor hnRNP-E2 (see above), as well as with the mRNA for PIM1, a survival factor. Since, the interaction with hnRNP-E2 occurs independently of mir-328's seed sequence, this miRNA acts as a "sink" for hnRNA-E2 binding allowing for the release of C/EBPα mRNA from the negative effects of hnRNA-E2-mediated translational inhibition. Thus mir-328 appears to control cell fate by its ability to base pair with the 3'UTR of target mRNAs (PIM1) as well as by acting as a decoy for hnRNP binding resulting in the release of C/EBPα from translational inhibition, thereby altering cell fate(Eiring *et al.*, 2010).

Gfi-1 (growth factor independence-1), a transcriptional repressor that promotes granulocytic differention, has been shown to regulate the expression of mir-196b (Velu *et al.*, 2009). The expression of mir-196b is high in the common myeloid progenitors (CMPs) which can differentiate either along the granulocytic or monocytic lineages. Gfi-1 has been shown to bind to the promoter of mir-196b thereby repressing its expression and promoting granulopoiesis. Additionally, overexpression of mir-196b was shown to block granulopoieis, confirming the importance of low level expression of this miRNA in contributing to granulopoietic maturation (Hock *et al.*, 2003) .

PU.1, a master transcriptional regulator of monocyte/macrophage differentiation, regulates the expression of mir-424, which in turn inhibits the expression of the transcription factor NFI-A. Mir-424 expression has been shown to promote monocyte/macrophage differentiation. Thus the two primary transcriptional determinants of myeloid differentiation, PU.1 and C/EBPα, both involve the activity of microRNAs for lineage maturation (Rosa *et al.*, 2007). Thus, miRNAs and myeloid specific transcription factors play a critical role in lineage maturation pathways by forming lineage-specific regulatory loops (rev in (Gazzar and McCall, 2011)), which if disrupted can lead to the development of leukemias.

Numerous studies have analyzed the expression of miRNAs in acute myeloid leukemias and the resulting miR signatures generated have proved to be helpful in classifying sub-types of AML and hence the choice of treatment options to be used, as well as in determining the efficacy of targeted therapies against AML. For example, Pelosi et al analyzed the expression of 12 selected granulocytic signature miRNAs and the impact of all *trans*-retinoic acid (ATRA)-based therapy in a cohort of acute promyelocytic leukemia (APL) patients (Pelosi *et al.*, 2009). APL is a subtype of acute leukemia and is characterized by the accumulation of promyelocytes as a result of a chromosomal translocation, most commonly involving the retinoic acid alpha receptor and the PML gene in a t(15;17) configuration. APL patients respond well to treatment with retinoic acid, a vitamin A derivative. The authors demonstrated using a quantitative real time PCR approach, that 9 miRNAs were overexpressed while three (mir-107, -342 and Let-7c) were downregulated in the blasts of APL patients, compared to normal promyelocytes. They showed in addition, that patients successfully treated with ATRA showed down regulation of mir-181b and upregulation of mir-15b, -16,-107, -223, -342 and let-7c. Thus, a small subset of miRNAs appeared to be differentially regulated in APL and could be modulated by treatment with ATRA. This approach is fast becoming a paradigm in diagnosing and determining the efficacy of treatment regimens used in acute myeloid leukemias.

7. Concluding remarks and perspectives

Inspite of the fact that there has been a surge of interest in the role of mRNA translational regulation in mediating gene expression in myeloid cells in recent times, a great deal of work has yet to be done. A general interest in this subject derives its source from the fact that cellular pathways commonly deregulated in AML including cell cycle progression, proliferation and differentiation are mechanistically tied to mRNA translation. For example, several upstream (AKT, TSC1/2) and downstream (eIF4E) mediators of the mTORC1 pathway are either mutated or activated in AML. Although there has been an intense search for therapeutic strategies targeting the mTOR pathway in myeloid cells, much work is yet to be done to gain a fundamental understanding of the role of the key players that contribute to translation initiation and control in normal and abnormal myeloid cells.

8. References

Ambros V (2004). The functions of animal microRNAs. *Nature* 431: 350-55.

Assouline S, Culjkovic B, Cocolakis E, Rousseau C, Beslu N, Amri A *et al* (2009). Molecular targeting of the oncogene eIF4E in AML: a proof-of-principle clinical trial with ribavarin. *Blood* 114: 257-60.

Bainton D (1975). Neutrophil granules. *Br. J Hematol* 29: 19.

Bainton D, Ullyot, JL, Farquhar, MG (1971). The development of the neutrophil secondary granule. *J Exp Med* 134: 907.

Berliner N (1998). Molecular biology of neutrophil differentiation. *Curr Opin Hematol* 5: 49-53.

Borregaard N, Theilgaard-Monch K, Sorensen O, Cowland J (2001). Regulation of human neutrophil granule protein expression. *Curr. Opin. Hematol* 8: 23-27.

Calkhoven C, Müller C, A. L (2000). Translational control of C/EBPalpha and C/EBPbeta isoform expression. *Gene Dev* 14: 1920-32.

Chen HM, Zhang P, Voso MT, Hohaus S, Gonzalez DA, Glass CK *et al* (1995). Neutrophils and monocytes express high levels of PU.1 (Spi-1) but not Spi-B. *Blood* 85: 2918-28.

Chen J (2007). Regulation of protein synthesis by the heme-regulated eIF2 kinase: relevance to anemias. *Blood* 109: 2693-2699.

Dahl R, Walsh JC, Lancki D, Laslo P, Iyer SR, Singh H *et al* (2003). Regulation of macrophage and neutrophil cell fates by the PU.1:C/EBPalpha ratio and granulocyte colony-stimulating factor.

DeKoter RP, Singh H (2000). Regulation of B- lymphocyte and macrophage development by graded expression of PU.1. *Science* 288: 1439-41.

Eiring A, Harb JG, Neviani P, Garton C, Oaks JJ, Spizzo R *et al* (2010). miR-328 functions as an RNA decoy to modulate hnRNP E2 regulation of mRNA translation in leukemic blasts. *Cell* 140: 652-65.

Fazi F, Rosa A, Fatica A, Gelmetti V, De Marchis ML, Nervi C *et al* (2005). Aminicircuitry comprised of microRNA-223 and transcription factors NFI-A and C/EBPalpha regulates human granulopoiesis. *Cell* 123: 819-31.

Filipowicz A, Bhattacharyya S, Sonenberg N (2008). Mechanisms of post transcriptional regulation by microRNAs: are the answers in sight? *Nat Rev Genet* 9: 102-114.

Fu C-T, Zhu K-Y, Mi J-Q, Liu Y, ST M, Fu Y-F *et al* (2010). An evolutionarily conserved PTEN-C/EBPα-CTNNA1 axis controls myeloid development and transformation. *Blood* ePublication April 6th.

Fuchs O (2007). Growth-inhibiting activity of transcription factor C/EBPa, its role in hematopoiesis and its tumour suppressor or oncogenic properties in leukaemias. *Folia Biologica (Praha)* 53: 97-108.

Gazzar M, McCall C (2011). MicroRNAs regulatory network in myeloid lineage development and differentiation: regulators of the regulators. *Immunology Cell Biol*: 1-7.

Geletu M, Balkhi M, Peer Zada A, Christopeit M, J, Pulikkan J, Trivedi A *et al* (2007). Target proteins of C/EBPalphap30 in AML: C/EBPalphap30 enhances sumoylation of C/EBPalphap42 via up-regulation of Ubc9. *Blood* 110: 3301-9.

Gingras A-C, Raught B, Sonenberg N (2001). Regulation of translation initiation by FRAP/mTOR. *Gene Dev* 15: 807-26.

Grolleau A, Sonenberg N, J W, L B (1999). Differential regulation of 4E-BP1 and 4E-BP2, two repressors of translation initiation, during human myeloid cell differentiation. *J Immunol.* 162: 3491-7.

Harding H, Zhang Y, D S, JJ C, RJ K, D R (2009). Ppp1r15 gene knockout reveals an essential role for translation initiation factor 2 alpha (eIf2a) dephosphorylation in mammalian delvelopment. *Proc Natl Acad Sci USA* 106: 1832-37.

Hock H, Hamblen M, Rooke H, Traver D, Bronson R, Cameron S *et al* (2003). Intrinsic requirement for zinc finger transcription factor Gfi-1 in neutrophil differentiation. *Immunity* 18: 109-120.

Johnnidis J, Harris MH, Wheeler RT, Stehling-Sun S, Lam MH, Kirak O *et al* (2008). Regulation of progenitor cell proliferation and granulocyte function by microRNA-223. *Nature* 451: 1125-29.

Kentsis A, Topisirovic I, Culjkovic B, Shao L, Borden K (2004). Ribavarin supresses eIF4E-mediated oncogenic transfornation by physical mimicry of the 7-methyl guanosine mRNA cap. *Proc Natl Acad Sci USA* 101: 18105-10.

Khanna-Gupta A (2011). Regulation and deregulation of mRNA translation during myeloid maturation. *Exp Hematol* 39: 133-41.

Khanna-Gupta A, Sun H, Zibello T, Lee H, Dahl R, Boxer L *et al* (2007). Growth factor independence-1 (Gfi-1) plays a role in mediating specific granule deficiency (SGD) in a patient lacking a gene-inactivating mutation in the C/EBPepsilon gene. *Blood* 15;109.: 4181-90.

Kirstetter P, Schuster MB, Bereshchenko O, Moore S, Dvinge H, Kurz E *et al* (2008). Modeling of C/EBPalpha mutant acute myeloid leukemia reveals a common expression signature of committed myeloid leukemia-initiating cells. *Cancer Cell* 13: 299-310.

Koschmieder S, Halmos B, Levantini E, DG. T (2009). Dysregulation of the C/EBPalpha differentiation pathway in human cancer. *J.Clin. Oncol.* 27: 619-28.

Laslo P, Spooner CJ, Warmflash A, Lancki DW, Lee HJ, Sciammas R *et al* (2006). Multilineage transcriptional priming and determination of alternate hematopoietic cell fates. *Cell* 126.

Lee-Fruman K, CJ K, J L, N T, J B (1999). Characterization of S6K2, a novel kinase homologous to S6K1. *Oncogene* 18: 5108-114.

Ly C, Arechiga AF, Melo JV, Walsh CM, Ong CM (2003) Bcr-Abl kinase modulates translation regulators ribosomal protein S6 and 4E-BP1 in chronic myelogenous leukemia via the mammalian targtet of rapamycin. Cancer Res. 63, 5716-22

Manikandan J, Aarthi JJ, Kumar SD, PN P (2008). Oncomirs: The potential role of non-coding microRNAs in understanding cancer. *Bioinformation* 8: 330-4.

Muller B, Pabst T (2006). C/EBPα and the pathophysiology of acute myeloid leukemia. *Curr Opin Hematol* 13: 7-14.

Olson K, GC B, F P, Sonenberg N, L B (2008). Impaired myelopoiesis in mice lacking the repressors of translation initiation, 4E-BP1 and 4E-BP2. *Immunology* 128: e379-e384.

Pabst T, Muller B, Zhang P (2001). Dominant negative mutations of CEBPA encoding CCAAT/enhancer binding protein-α (C/EBPα), in acute myeloid leukemia. *Nat Genet* 27: 263-270.

Pelosi E, Labbaye C, U. T (2009). MicroRNAs in normal and malignant myelopoiesis. *Lukemia Res* 33: 1584-93.

Perrotti D, Cesi V, Trotta R, Guerzoni C, Santilli G, Campbell K *et al* (2002). BCR-ABL suppresses C/EBPalpha expression through inhibitory action of hnRNP E2. *Nat Genet.* 30: 48-58.

Person R, Li F, Duan Z, Benson K, Wechsler J, Papadaki H *et al* (2003). Mutations in protooncogene Gfi1 cause human neutropenia and target ELA2. *Nat. Genet.* 34: 308-312.

Platanias L (2005). Mechaisms of type-1 and type-II interferon-mediated signaling. *Nat Rev Immunol* 5: 375-86.

Pulikkan J, Dengler V, Peramangalam PS, Peer Zada AA, Müller-Tidow C, Bohlander SK *et al* (2010). Cell-cycle regulator E2F1 and microRNA-223 comprise an autoregulatory negative feedback loop in acute myeloid leukemia. *Blood* 115: 1768-78.

Rangatia J, Vangala R, Treiber N, Zhang P, Radomska H, Tenen D *et al* (2002). Downregulation of c-Jun expression by transcription factor C/EBPalpha is critical for granulocytic lineage commitment. *Mol. Cell.Biol* 22: 8681-94.

Raven J, AE. K (2008). PERK and PKR: old kinases learn new tricks. *Cell Cycle* 7: 1146-50.

Rosa A, Ballarino M, Sorrentino A, Sthandier O, De Angelis F, Marchioni M *et al* (2007). The interplay between the master transcription factor PU1 and mir-424 regulates human monocyte/macrophage differentiation. *Proc Natl Acad Sci USA* 104: 19849-54.

Scholl C, Gilliland D, Frohling S (2008). Deregulation of signaling pathways in acute myeloid leukemia. *Semin Oncol* 35: 336-45.

Schuster M, Porse B (2006). C/EBPa: a tumour suppressor in multiple tissues? *Biochim. Biophys. Acta* 1766: 88-103.

Scott EW, Simon MC, Anastasi J, Singh H (1994). Requirement of transcription factor PU.1 in the development of multiple hematopoietic lineages. *Science* 265: 1573-1577.

Sengupta S, Peterson T, Sabatini D (2010). Regulation of the mTOR Complex 1 Pathway by Nutrients, Growth Factors, and Stress. *Mol Cell* 40: 310-22.

Sonenberg N and Hinnebucsh AG (2009) Regulation of translation initiation in eukaryotes: mechanisms and biological targets. Cell 136, 731-45.

Tamburini J, Green A, Chapuis N, Bardet V, Lacombe C, Mayeux P *et al* (2009a). Targeting translation in acute myeloid leukemia. A new paradigm for therapy. *Cell Cycle* 23: 3893-99.

Tamburini J, Green AS, Bardet V, Chapuis N, Park S, Willems L *et al* (2009b). Protein synthesis is resistant to rapamycin and constitutes a promising therapeutic target in acute myeloid leukemia. *Blood* 114.

Tenen D (2003). Disruption of differentiation in human cancer: AML shows the way. *Nature Rev: Cancer* 3: 89-101.

Timchenko N, Harris T, Wilde M, al. e (1997). CCAAT/enhancer binding protein alpha regulates p21 protein and hepatocyte proliferation in newborn mice. *Mol Cell Biol* 17: 7353-61.

Timchenko N, Wilde M, Darlington G (1999). C/EBPalpha regulates formation of S-phase-specific E2F-p107 complexes in livers of newborn mice. *Mol Cell Biol* 19: 2936-45.

Topisirovic I, Guzman ML, McConnell MJ, Licht JD, Culjkovic B, Neering SJ *et al* (2003). Aberrant eukaryotic translation initiation factor 4E-dependent mRNA transport impedes hematopoietic differentiation and contributes to leukemogenesis. *Mol Cell Biol* 23: 8992-9002.

Tsukada J, Yoshida Y, Kominato Y, Auron P (2011). The CCAAT/enhancer (C/EBP) family of basic-leucine zipper (bZIP) transcription factors is a multifaceted highly regulated system for gene regulation. *Cytokine* 54: 6-19.

Van Der Kelen K, Beyaert R, Inzé D, L. DV (2009). Translational control of eukaryotic gene expression. *Crit Rev Biochem Mol Biol.* 44: 143-68.

van der Meer L, Jansen JH, BA. vdR (2010). Gfi1 and Gfi1b: key regulators of hematopoiesis. . *Leukemia* 24: 1834-43.

Velu C, Baktula AM, HL. G (2009). Gfi1 regulates miR-21 and miR-196b to control myelopoiesis. *Blood* 113: 4720-8. .

Wang X, Hawk N, Yue P, Kauh J, Ramalingam S, Fu H *et al* (2008). mTOR inhibition induced paradoxical activation of survival signalling pathways enhances mTOR inhibitors' anti-cancer efficacy. *Cancer Biol and Therapy* 7: 1952-58.

Wendel H, Silva R, Malina A, Mills J, Zhu H, Ueda T *et al* (2007). Dissecting eIF4E action in tumorigenesis. *Genes and Dev* 21: 3232-37.

Wullschieger S, Loewith R, Hall M (2006). TOR signaling in growth and metabolism. *Cell* 124: 471-84.

Xu Q, Simpson SE, Scialla TJ, Bagg A, Carroll M. (2003) Survival of Acute Myeloid Leukemia cells requires PI3 kinase activation. Blood, 102, 972-80.

Zhang P, Iwama A, Datta MW, Darlington GJ, Link DC, Tenen DG. (1997). *39th Annual Meeting of the American Society of Hematology, San Diego, California, USA, December, Vol. 90.*

12

Molecular Mechanisms in Philadelphia Negative Myeloproliferative Neoplasia

Ciro Roberto Rinaldi[1], Ana Crisan[1] and Paola Rinaldi[2]
[1]*Department of Haematology – United Lincolnshire Hospital NHS Trust – Boston*
[2]*University Federico II and CEINGE Biotecnologie Avanzate – Naples*
[1]*UK*
[2]*Italy*

1. Introduction

The myeloproliferative neoplasia (MPNs) are a spectrum of clonal disorders of the hematopoietic system. The distinct clinical manifestations are dictated by the primary cell type affected, and thus chronic myeloid leukemia (CML) is a proliferation of mature granulocytes, polycythemia vera (PV) is an expansion or red blood cells, essential thrombocythemia (ET) results in an increase of platelets, etc.. The natural history of MPNs is generally chronic in nature, and patients come to medical attention either by coincidence (abnormal blood findings during routine exam) or by signs and symptoms related to the expansion of the hematopoetic system (e.g., an enlarged spleen). Common to most MPNs is a small but finite risk of disease evolution to an acute leukemia, where hematopoetic development is blocked at an early stage of differentiation, leading to the accumulation of poorly functioning myeloid blasts at an expensive of critical depletion of normal white blood cells and platelets, leading to morbidity and mortality from infections and bleeding complications. If they do not progress to an acute leukemia, the natural history of MPNs often results in fibrosis of the bone marrow, migration of hematopoesis to other organs (spleen and liver), and eventual complications of this secondary organ involvement, as well as from decreased normal blood counts from marrow fibrosis. A unifying theme in the pathogenesis of MPNs is the activation of tyrosine kinases. The "poster child" is CML, where the BCR-ABL translocation is found in all cases; the fusion BCR-ABL activates proliferative and antiapoptotic pathways; and most importantly, inhibition by tyrosine kinase inhibitors (TKIs) can markedly reverse the natural history of the disease. The molecular lesions responsible for PV, ET, and myelofibrosis (MF) were unknown until relatively recently. From 2005, a flurry of reports found that a point mutation in JAK2, resulting in a valine for phenylalanine substitution at codon 617 (JAK2V617F), occurred at a high prevalence in these disorders. The mutation was found in roughly half of MF and ET cases and nearly all PV cases. Constitutive activation of JAK2 activates STAT and MAPK proliferative signaling pathways, leading to transformation of hematopoetic progenitors. Curiously, not all hematopoetic stem cells in cases with the JAK2V617F harbor the mutation. Moreover, the data suggested a differential dosage effect in the different diseases. Whereas in most cases the JAK2V617F is heterozygous with a normal JAK2 allele, in many cases of

PV the mutation is homozygous through the process of acquired uniparental disomy. Curiously, in vitro cultures of PV cases will often show homozygous JAK2V617F erythroid colonies, whereas similar colonies from ET patients are heterozygous for the mutation. There has been a substantial body of work attempting to study the effects of the JAK2V617F in mouse models. Early reports focused on a bone marrow transplantation model, where mouse bone marrow cells harboring exogenous JAK2-V617F were transplanted into irradiated mice. These models produced a syndrome of what appeared mostly like PV, but most failed to completely recapitulate the spectrum of leukocytosis, thrombocytosis, and myelofibrosis found in human disease. Transgeneic models followed, which again produced a spectrum of MPN disorders, with a suggestion of phenotype relating to the JAK2V617F expression levels. Very recently, several groups have created knockin systems placing a conditionally inducible JAK2V617F allele under control of the endogenous JAK2 promoter. This allows for control of the JAK2V617F expression in only hematopoetic tissues, getting one closer to replicating the disease experience of the human patient. Marty et al. found that the heterozygous expression of JAK2V617F produced a PV-like syndrome, not like human where heterozygousity is more often associated with ET. However, Akada et al. demonstrated that both heterozygous and homozygous JAK2V617F caused a PV syndrome, with a demonstration of a dose effect, as indicated by the fact that homozygous expressors had a greater manifestation of elevated blood counts and spleen size, compared to those mice with lower levels of JAK2V617F. In addition, Li et al. have produced a very provocative study in which a human JAK2V617F knockin was created. This model produced a transplantable disease with some features of both ET and PV. Of interest is the finding that affected mice had reduced numbers of primitive hematopoetic cells that had evidence of impaired normal function (cell cycling, apoptosis, and DNA damage). Moreover, competitive marrow transplantation showed impaired hematopoetic stem cell function. Recently, Mullally and colleagues used a conditional JAK2V617F expression model to yield physiological levels of the mutated allele. The phenotype in the mice resembled much of the cellular biology and clinical features of human PV, and it was serially transplantable with great efficiency. Separation of the bone marrow into immature Lineage- SCA-1+ c-Kit+ (LSK) and more mature myeloid erythroid progenitor (MEP) and granulocytic monocytic progenitor (GMP) subpopulations demonstrated that the "MPN-initiating" JAK2V617F cell capable of transplantation resided in the LSK population, but not in the committed myeloid MEP or GMP progenitors. Surprisingly, several studies showed that mutant cells in the LSK compartment were quite similar to wildtype cells in regard to cell cycle status, STAT signaling, and gene expression (though JAK2V617F cells showed enrichment of the erthyroid, myeloid, and megakaryocytic differentiation pathways). Similar to the Li et al. paper, competitive transplantation experiments showed that mutant cells had at best a minor competitive edge compared to wild-type, and a small number of mutated cells nonetheless causes a PV phenotype. Lastly, the authors demonstrated that the MPN initiating cell was not killed by JAK2 inhibition. Mice treated with the inhibitor had a dramatic decrease in spleen size and a reduction of erthyroid precursors in the marrow, but LSK cells from treated mice were able to cause the PV phenotype in subsequently transplanted mice. These studies in total offer an increased understanding of the MPN that may usher in a new era of therapy, much like what occurred in the study of CML. Similar to CML, these studies suggest the initiating cell resides in the primitive compartment but is genetically and phenotypically quite similar to its normal complement. Like CML, mutated cells in the stem cell compartment appear resistant to kinase inhibition. However, as we move toward better therapies for MPN, these findings have implications in the feasibility of ''stem cell'' therapy, because there may not be a large therapeutic window to selectively kill MPN ''stem cells.'' In addition, a limitation of murine systems is that however eloquent, they are still only models of human disease. For example, human MPN may well have additional genetic lesions contributing to initiation and progression, and mouse models cannot easily recapitulate this complexity. In this regard it is interesting that several other mutations have recently been discovered in MPN (e.g., TET2, ASXL1, IDH1, and IDH2); TET2 mutations have been found in JAK2V617F-positive and -negative clones from the same patient, suggesting that TET2 mutations may be a relatively early event in MPN. Moreover, if tumor initiation and progression is influenced by interactions with a host's innate immunological system, then disease in the mouse model might be expected to be very different than in humans. Nonetheless, the work presented by Mullally and others are quite significant, and provide us with powerful tools to better understand disease and test new agents of therapy.However, it should be noted that some mutations might possess more than one mechanism of action, for example, *JAK2*V617F results in dysregulation of kinase signaling but might also have an epigenetic effect. Recently, Dawson et al.identified a novel nuclear role of JAK2 in the phosphorylation of Tyr 41 of histone H3 leading to chromatin displacement of HP1a. The authors suggested that the inability of HP1a to regulate chromatin could reduce the potential tumor suppressive functions of HP1a resulting in erratic mitotic recombination and transcription deregulation of several JAK2-regulated genes such as *LMO2*. These results were confirmed in hematopoietic cell lines and in the CD34+ cells collected from the peripheral blood of one PMF patient with JAK2V617F mutation. Our group defined the subcellular localization of JAK2 in total BM cells and in sorted cell populations collected from MPN (ET, PV, PMF) patients with the JAK2V617F mutation or from MPN patients with wild type (wt) JAK2. We find that in contrast to cells with normal JAK2 in which the protein is detected predominantly in the cytoplasm, JAK2 is mostly nuclear in V617F-positive CD34+ cells. However, this nuclear localization is no longer observed in V617F-positive differentiated cells. After expressing JAK2V617F in K562 cells, we observe a similar preferential accumulation of JAK2 in the nucleus in contrast to untrasfected- and wt JAK2-expressing cells in which the protein is found in the cytoplasm. The mutated-JAK2 nuclear translocation is mainly reverted by the addiction of the JAK2 inhibitor AG490.

1.1 Functional hallmarks of myeloid progenitors in myeloproliferative neoplasms

The BCR-ABL-negative myeloproliferative diseases, which include polycythemia vera (PV), essential thrombocythemia (ET) and primary myelofibrosis (PMF), were recently renamed myeloproliferative neoplasms (MPNs).[1] PV, ET and PMF are disorders of hematopoietic stem cells (HSCs) and early myeloid progenitors,[2, 3] where myeloid progenitors are hypersensitive and/or independent of cytokines for survival, proliferation and differentiation. For instance, the majority of PV patients harbor erythropoietin (Epo)-independent erythroid colonies.[4] Several intracellular anti-apoptotic pathways and molecules, such as STAT3, Akt or BclXL, are activated/induced constitutively in such MPN myeloid progenitors,[5, 6, 7] along with hypersensitivity to insulin-like growth factor 1 (IGF-1), granulocyte macrophage colony-stimulating factor, interleukin 3 (IL-3), granulocyte colony-stimulating factor (G-CSF) or thrombopoietin (Tpo).[8,9, 10, 11] Unlike many malignancies, where the INK4a locus is inactivated, erythroid progenitors from PV patients exhibit increased expression of the INK4a/ARF locus.[12]

1.2 Mutations involved in PV, ET and PMF

The acquired somatic *JAK2* V617F mutation is harbored by the majority of PV patients and by more than 50% of ET and PMF patients.[13, 14, 15, 16, 17]Subsequent identification of exon 12 mutants of *JAK2* in a minority of PV patients gave a molecular lesion to virtually all PV cases.[18] Sequencing of the gene coding for the Tpo receptor (TpoR/c-Mpl) identified mutations in the juxtamembrane tryptophan residue W515 (W515L and W515K) in a low percentage of PMF and ET patients, the majority of which are *JAK2* V617F-negative.[19, 20] The W515 residue of TpoR is required to maintain the receptor inactive in the absence of ligand.[21] All these mutations lead to constitutively active JAK–STAT pathway, especially JAK2, STAT5, STAT3, MAP kinase ERK1,2 and Akt.[13, 16, 21]Advancement over the past 3 years in the MPN research field has raised several major questions, such as: (i) What are the molecular bases for the significant differences in the *in vivo* phenotypes induced by *JAK2* V617F and TpoR W515L? (ii) How can a unique somatic mutation, *JAK2* V617F, be involved in the induction of three different diseases ET, PV or PMF? (iii) What mechanisms are responsible for the evolution of MPNs toward acute myeloid leukemia? (iv) What are the effects of *JAK2* V617F and of the other JAK2 and TpoR mutants at the level of HSC? and (v) What preceding and subsequent (to *JAK2* V617F) genetic events contribute to myeloproliferative diseases?Answers to these questions have begun to emerge. Gene dosage, as initially suggested by genotype/phenotype studies in patient cells,[22] by retroviral bone marrow reconstitution studies[23] and most recently probed in transgenic mice,[24]could be critically involved in inducing one or the other of the MPN phenotypes. It is fascinating that progenitors homozygous for the *JAK2* V617F mutation occur in almost all PV patients, but very rarely in ET patients.[25, 26] Although this can be seen as an argument in favor of the gene dosage hypothesis, other preceding or subsequent genetic changes might have an important function. Interestingly, host-modifying influences might have a major part in establishing the disease phenotype.[27] A screen for genetic variation within the genes coding for EpoR, TpoR, G-CSF receptor (G-CSFR) and JAK2 led to the discovery of three JAK2 single nucleotide polymorphisms that were significantly but reciprocally associated with PV and ET, but not with PMF. Three additional JAK2 single nucleotide polymorphisms were uniquely associated with PV. Such single nucleotide polymorphisms, although not in the coding region of the genes, might affect the levels of gene transcription, regulation by other factors or possibly expression of other genes.

1.3 Unknown effects of JAK2 V617F signaling in HSCs

JAK2 V617F mutation was detected at the HSC and the common myeloid/lymphoid progenitor levels, it skews the HSC differential potential toward the erythroid lineage and gives a selective proliferative advantage to myeloid lineages.[28, 29] The HSC compartment of PV and PMF patients was found to contain *JAK2* V617F-positive long-term, multipotent and self-renewing cells, with a much higher proportion of mutated HSCs in PMF than in PV.[30] It is not clear at this moment whether *JAK2* V617F profoundly affects the biology of HSCs[30] or whether it only gives a strong selection advantage past the HSC stage. A certain degree of heterogeneity exists between HSC subsets.[31] HSCs exist in niches, some near osteoblasts and others near endothelial cells. Exactly where and in which HSC subset the *JAK2* V617F mutation initially occurs might have a major impact on the subsequent disease phenotype.The *JAK2* V617F mutation was present in 30–40% of splanchnic venous thrombosis patients (Budd–Chiari syndrome and portal vein thrombosis).[32, 33,34, 35] A 'special' stem cell with hematopoietic/endothelial potential was suggested to be at the origin of splanchnic venous thrombosis, and it might harbor *JAK2*V617F.[36] A recent case report described a human allogeneic transplantation with*JAK2* V617F-positive cells from such a splanchnic venous thrombosis donor (with one episode of *JAK2* V617F-positive splanchnic venous thrombosis), but no MPN, to her HLA-matched sister with high-risk myelodysplastic syndrome (RAEB2).[37]The recipient exhibited a *JAK2* V617F burden similar to the donor immediately after transplant, but this burden decreased over time, and 7 years later, the recipient continues to be in remission and to exhibit low levels of *JAK2* V617F positivity.[37] These data suggest that, indeed, the *JAK2* V617F mutation can occur in an HSC, but at least in the transplantation setting, this HSC has no proliferative advantage. A considerable amount of data suggests that in addition to the presence of the*JAK2* V617F mutation, preceding or subsequent genetic events might be necessary for developing the MPN disease. First, in certain MPN patients, the clonality of expanded myeloid progenitors is found to be larger than the *JAK2* V617F clone, with the acquisition of *JAK2* V617F being a late genetic event.[38] Second, acute myeloid leukemia cases developed in*JAK2* V617F-positive patients can occur with leukemic blasts not harboring *JAK2*V617F.[39] Third, Epo-independent colonies might not always harbor the *JAK2*mutation in patients with the *JAK2* V617F mutation.[40] Such preceding or subsequent events could be associated differently with the three diseases, namely ET, PV and PMF.

1.4 The signaling space

Molecular cell biology textbooks list eight major signaling pathways that control gene expression that are linked to eight classes of cell surface receptors: cytokine receptors, receptor tyrosine kinases, receptors for transforming growth factor (TGF)-β, Wnt, Hedgehog, tumor necrosis factor (TNF)-α, Notch (Delta) and G-protein-coupled receptors.[41] Nuclear and corticoid receptor pathways, as well as integrin signaling, complete the picture of intracellular cell signaling. In several paperit has been well described that aberrant signaling occurs in MPNs through some of the listed pathways, such as cytokine receptors, receptor tyrosine kinases, TGF-β and TNF-α. It is not clear whether aberrant signaling in MPNs is simply due to the constitutive nature of signaling induced by mutated JAK2 or TpoR, or whether specific cross-talk events occur to other pathways that might confer specificity to JAK2 V617F versus JAK2 signaling. It is important to recognize from the outset that the experimental systems used by signal transduction research, such as phosphorylation studies, co-immunoprecipitation, gene expression and determination of protein localization, may not be able to identify subtle relative changes, such as kinetics and amplitude differences, between signals engaging generic pathways that are redundantly triggered by many stimuli. Such subtle quantitative differences might, however, be crucial for the disease phenotypes *in vivo*. That is the reason why genetics, *in vivo* models, results obtained with inhibitors and data derived from primary cells, must be taken into account to draw a picture describing aberrant signaling in MPNs.

1.5 Constitutive signaling and kinase activity of JAK2 V617F

The mammalian genome codes for four Janus kinases (JAKs), JAK1, JAK2, JAK3 and Tyk2. On the basis of homology, JAKs share seven JAK homology domains (JH), denoted as JH1–JH7. From the C to the N terminus, JH1 represents the kinase domain, JH2 the pseudokinase domain, JH3 and JH4 contain an SH2-like domain and linker regions, whereas JH5–JH7 contain a FERM (band 4.1, ezrin, radixin, moesin) domain[42, 43] (Figure 1).

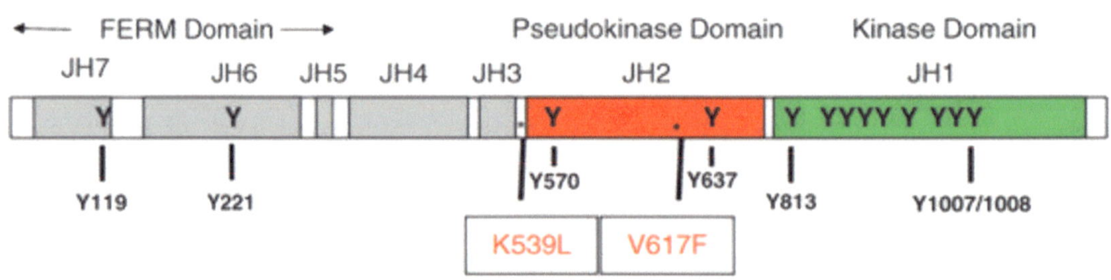

Fig. 1. Schematic illustration of Janus kinase (JAK)2 and the different JAK homology (JH) domains. The V617F mutation occurs in the pseudokinase domain rendering the kinase domain constitutively active. Exon 12 mutations, such as K539L, occur in the linker region between the JH3 and JH2 domains. Tyrosine residues that can be phosphorylated are depicted by their single letter. See text for details.

JAKs have been proposed to have a bipartite structure and the N terminus is required for binding to receptors, chaperoning and stabilizing them at the surface,[44, 45, 46, 47] whereas the kinase domain is absolutely crucial for signaling. The pseudokinase domain precedes the kinase domain, and because of sequence differences at key residues required for catalysis, it cannot transfer phosphate and thus is catalytically inactive.[42]Nevertheless, the pseudokinase domain is structurally required for the response of JAKs to cytokine receptor activation and for inhibiting the basal activity of the kinase domain.[48, 49] The V617F mutation occurs in the pseudokinase domain, leading to constitutive activation of the kinase domain (Figure 1). Although no X-ray crystal structure of full-length JAK2 exists, modeling has suggested that the pseudokinase domain of JAK2 maintains the kinase domain inactive in the basal state.[50] Thus, the V617F mutation is expected to relieve the inhibitory effect of JH2 on JH1 and to lead to basal kinase activity. The homologous V617F mutations in JAK1 and Tyk2 also lead to constitutive activation,[51] which strongly supports this model. Activating mutations in the pseudokinase domain of JAK1 at the homologous V658 position or at neighboring residues have been reported in 20% of patients with T-acute lymphoblastic leukemia.[52, 53] In transiently transfected JAK2-deficient cells, such as the γ-2A human fibrosarcoma cell line,[54] JAK2 V617F expression leads to constitutive activation of STAT5 and STAT3 signaling. In such transient transfection experiments, JAK2 V617F is constitutively tyrosine phosphorylated at the activation loop Y1007. Co-transfection of wild-type JAK2 reduces signaling by JAK2 V617F, presumably due to competition for an interaction partner, such as a cytokine receptor,[13] but does not prevent constitutive phosphorylation of JAK2 V617F.[16]To investigate the catalytic activity of JAK2 V617F mutation, kinase assays have been performed on GST fusion proteins. In COS7 overexpression conditions, when compared with wild-type JAK2, the JAK2 V617F mutated protein exhibits enhanced basal kinase activity on a reporter GST fusion protein containing the sequence of the activation loop of JAK2 containing tyrosine (Y) 1007.[17, 55] The kinase activity was clearly increased, but it appeared to be weak. In stably transfected Ba/F3 cells, JAK2 V617F also exhibits enhanced kinase activity on the same Y1007-containing GST fusion protein, but the levels of activation were also small (C Pecquet *et al.*, unpublished results). This is very different from BCR-ABL or other fusion proteins such as TEL-JAK2, where the kinase domain alone is oligomerized and activated by a fused exogenous oligomeric domain. In contrast, the kinase domain of JAK2 V617F is expected to maintain most of the negative regulatory intramolecular interactions that normally limit kinase domain activation.

1.6 JAK2 V617F and cytokine receptors

The FERM domain of JAKs is responsible for appending JAKs to cytokine receptors. Cytokine receptors contain in the cytosolic juxtamembrane region a proline-rich sequence, usually PxxPxP, denoted as Box 1, located 10–15 amino acid residues downstream of the TM domain, and further down 50–60 amino acid residues downstream of the TM domain, a sequence composed of hydrophobic and charged residues denoted as Box 2.[56]JAK2 binds to the region of EpoR that encompasses cytosolic residues of Box 1, Box 2 and also most of the residues between these boxes.[44, 56]Interaction between JAK2 and EpoR or TpoR is disrupted by a point mutation (Y114A) in the FERM domain.[47] Expression of the double-mutant JAK2 V617F Y114A in Ba/F3-EpoR cells did not lead to constitutive signaling through STAT5 or to autonomous growth,[57] suggesting that the V617F mutation does not suffice for activation in the absence of the assembly between the JAK2 V617F and a cytokine receptor. It can be noted that members of the JAK family are localized to membranes through recruitment by cytokine receptors, whereas mutations such as Y114A lead to cytosolic localization.[58] Furthermore, a mutation in the pseudokinase domain of JAK2 was identified (Y613 to glutamic acid, Y613E), which promotes constitutive activation only when JAK2 is in complex with the EpoR.[59] This result suggests that in the absence of an association with a cytokine receptor, JAK2 is locked into an inactive state and that receptor binding through the FERM domain is important for activation.[59]Another argument supporting the notion that binding to a cytokine receptor is important for the activity of the V617F mutant arises from the lack of activation of JH2–JH1 fusion proteins where the V617F mutation was introduced in the JH2 sequence.[60] The low basal activity of JH1 was shown to be suppressed by fusion with JH2.[49, 61] However, the presence of the FERM–SH2 domains is required for the activation effect exerted by the V617F mutation. JAK2 is crucial for signaling by EpoR[62] and TpoR,[63, 64] participates in signaling by G-CSFR[65, 66] (Figure 2) and also mediates signaling by the IL-3/IL-5/granulocyte macrophage colony-stimulating factor family of cytokines, as well as by several type-II cytokine receptors, such as interferon-γ receptor 2[67]. Given that MPNs mainly affect the erythroid, the megakaryocytic and the granulocyte lineages, as stated before, complexes between JAK2 V617F and EpoR, TpoR and G-CSFR may explain cytokine hypersensitivity and independence in these diseases (Figure 2).

(i)

(ii)

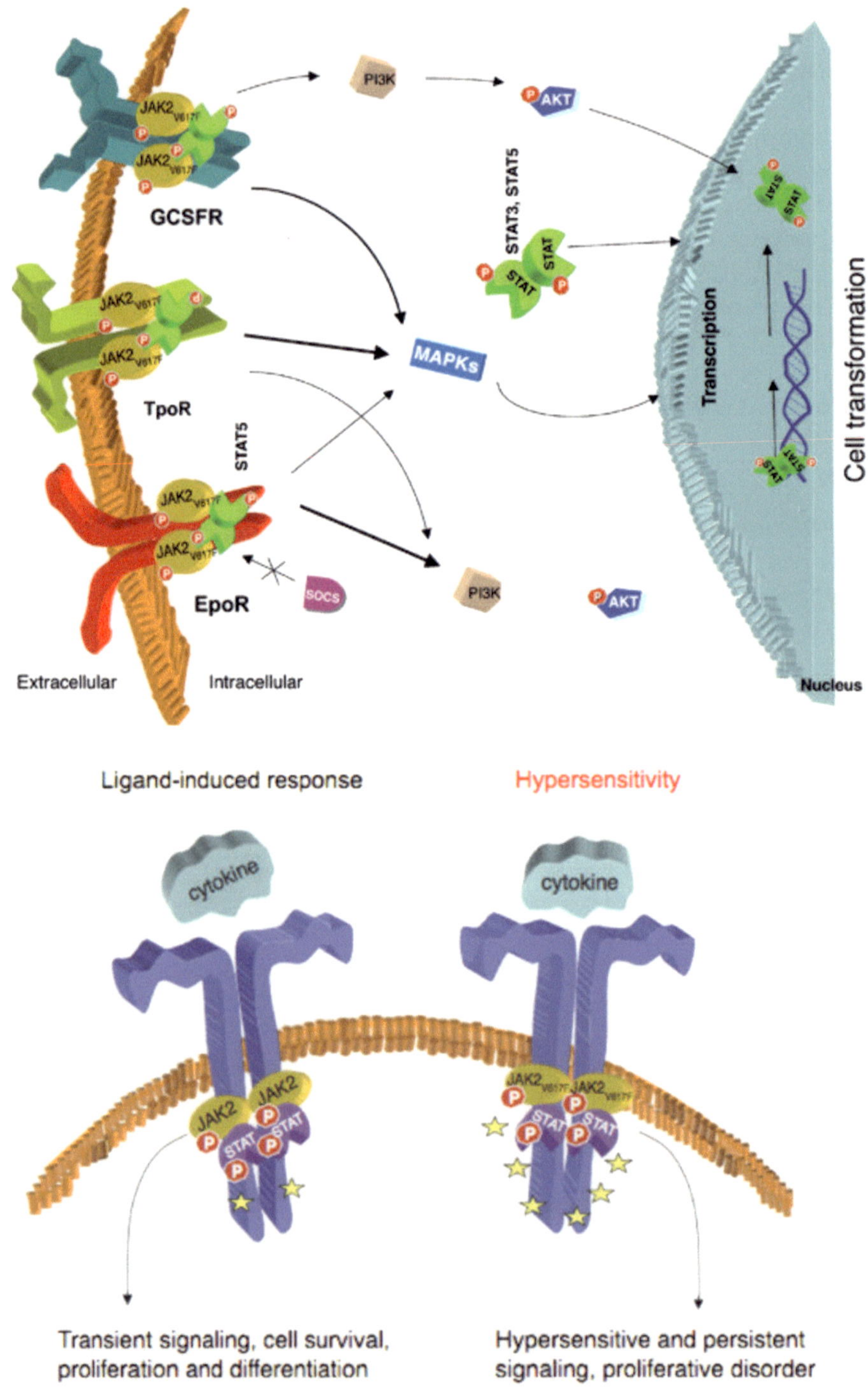

Fig. 2. Model of constitutive (ligand-independent) signaling induced by JAK2 V617F through erythropoietin receptor (EpoR), thrombopoietin receptor (TpoR) and granulocyte

colony-stimulating factor receptor (G-CSFR). (i) Janus kinase 2 (JAK2) is the main JAK used by EpoR and TpoR, but JAK1 is also used physiologically by G-CSFR. Primarily, EpoR and TpoR are expected to be bound by JAK2 V617F, whereas G-CSFR is expected to be in complex with JAK2 V617F at high JAK2 V617F levels, i.e., in homozygous *JAK2* V617F situations. Scaffolding of JAK2 V617F on the cytosolic tails of cytokine receptors leads to the enhanced activation of JAK2 V617F and downstream signaling through STATs, MAP kinase, PI-3-kinase (PI3K) and Akt. SOCS proteins are expected to engage both EpoR and activated wild-type JAK2, leading and down-modulation of JAK2 activity; the EpoR–JAK2 V617F complex appears to escape the down-modulation activity of SOCS3. (ii) Cytokine receptors that are in complex with JAK2 V617F are hypersensitive to their ligands for signaling. Cytokine binding to receptors coupled to wild-type JAK2 induce transient physiologic signals, leading to survival, proliferation and differentiation of myeloid progenitors. In contrast, receptors coupled to JAK2 V617F respond to lower levels of ligand, and are constitutively signaling after ligand withdrawal. It is not known whether dimeric receptor complexes, where one monomer is coupled to JAK2 V617F and the other to wild-type JAK2, are also hypersensitive to ligand or constitutively active.

1.7 EpoR and MPNs

EpoR functions as a preformed dimer on the cell surface, which upon cytokine binding undergoes a conformational change that triggers the activation of the receptor pre-bound JAK2.[68, 69] This involves a rotation of the receptor monomers within the dimer,[70] which is transmitted to JAK2 by switch residues, that is W258 in the juxtamembrane domain of EpoR.[69] Current data suggest that JAK2 V617F can scaffold on the cytosolic domain of EpoR and induce Epo-independent signaling, possibly by phosphorylating key cytosolic tyrosine residues on EpoR, which leads to strong STAT5 activation.[71]Early on after the identification of *JAK2* V617F, the need for a co-expressed type I dimeric cytokine receptor for constitutive signaling by JAK2 V617F provoked a controversy, which in the end led to a model of how dimeric receptors might actually promote JAK2 V617F activation. One study by Levine *et al.*[16] reported that JAK2 V617F readily induced autonomous growth in Ba/F3 cells engineered to express the EpoR (Ba/F3 EpoR cells), but not in parental Ba/F3 cells. In contrast, the study by James *et al.*[13] had shown that JAK2 V617F could induce autonomous growth in both Ba/F3 EpoR and parental Ba/F3 cells. This controversy (also described in Ihle and Gilliland[72]) was solved by carefully assaying the levels of JAK2 V617F transduction: at low levels, co-expression of a type I cytokine receptor was necessary for autonomous growth, whereas at higher levels JAK2 V617F alone induced autonomous growth, most likely by binding to an endogenous cytokine receptor, such as the IL-3-receptor β-subunit.[60] It is not clear whether other receptors—besides dimeric type I—could also promote signaling by low levels of transduced JAK2 V617F (Figure 2(ii)). Nevertheless, given that EpoR is a dimer in the absence of ligand, an insightful model was proposed by Harvey Lodish. In it, dimerization of JAK2 V617F by such a receptor is considered necessary for the activation of JAK2 V617F signaling, and the subtle V617F mutation promotes kinase activation when JAK2 is scaffolded on an inactive receptor dimer (Figure 2(i)).[71] Given that in MPNs the three lineages affected are controlled by the three type I dimeric cytokine receptors, EpoR, TpoR and G-CSFR, the model that JAK2 V617F mainly functions as a transforming kinase in association with these receptors is very plausible. EpoR signals mainly by JAK2–STAT5 and PI-3-kinase/Akt (Figure 2(i)) pathways. It is a weak activator of MAP kinase and of STAT3,[73] as it does not contain a consensus site for STAT3 binding, whereas several phosphorylated tyrosine residues (Y343, Y401, Y429 and Y431) can bind STAT5 and are required for maximal STAT5 activation.[74, 75] A consequence of STAT5 activation is induction of the anti-apoptotic BclXL protein expression,[76] which is constitutively expressed in PV erythroid progenitors.[7] The connection of EpoR with the PI-3-kinase pathway is accomplished by specific tyrosine residues, that is Y479, which appears to bind the regulatory subunit p85.[77, 78] PI-3-kinase and Akt activations are critically involved in erythroid differentiation,[79] possibly by the involvement of the transcription factor Forkhead family, FKHRL1.[80] Another mechanism appears to be the phosphorylation of S310 of GATA1.[81] Thus, scaffolding of an activated JAK2 to EpoR is predicted to activate the JAK2-STAT5 and PI-3-kinase/Akt pathways and stimulate proliferation and differentiation of erythroid progenitors.

1.8 EpoR and exon 12 JAK2 mutations

Patients with exon 12 *JAK2* mutations, such as JAK2 K539L, exhibit an erythrocytosis phenotype, without pathology changes to megakaryocytes typical for MPNs.[18] Unlike the uniqueness of the point mutation that generates JAK2 V617F, several deletions and insertions were noted in the case of exon 12 mutations.[18, 82] An attractive hypothesis is that exon 12 mutants of JAK2 favor interaction with EpoR over TpoR or G-CSFR, although a mechanistic basis for such a preference has yet to be found. Modeling of JAK2 suggests that the K539L falls in a loop in the linker region between the SH2 and the JH2 domain (Figure 1), which would be placed in space quite close to the loop represented by β4–β5 where V617 is located.

1.9 TpoR and MPNs

TpoR is coupled to and activates both JAK2 and Tyk2,[64, 83, 84] which appear to have comparable affinities for the receptor juxtamembrane domain and to promote cell surface traffic of the receptor to a similar extent.[47] However, JAK2 is much more effective than Tyk2 in transmitting the signals of the receptor.[47,64] TpoR activates JAK2, STAT5 and PI-3-kinase/Akt,[85] but in contrast to EpoR, it is a very strong activator of Shc, of the MAP kinase pathway and of STAT3 (Figure 2(i)).[83, 86, 87, 88, 89, 90] It is interesting that the first consequence of expressing the JAK2 V617F (at lower than physiologic levels in the transgenic model) mutation is to promote platelet formation.[24] Bipotential megakaryocyte-erythroid progenitors appear to be stimulated to engage on the platelet formation by STAT3 activation, whereas STAT5 activation favors erythroid differentiation programs.[91] STAT5 emerged as a critical factor for lineage commitment between erythroid and megakaryocytic cell fates. Depletion of STAT5 from CD34(+) cells in the presence of Tpo and stem cell factor favors megakaryocytic differentiation at the expense of erythroid differentiation.[91] Overexpression of an activated form of STAT5 impaired megakaryocyte development favoring erythroid differentiation at the expense of megakaryocyte differentiation.[91] Thus, at low levels of expression, JAK2 V617F might only activate STAT3, which might suffice for platelet formation. At higher expression levels, coupling to both TpoR and EpoR will lead to STAT5 activation, and this would favor the erythroid program. It is not clear at this point whether the PV phenotype is exclusively the result of EpoR activation or whether the pathologic activation of TpoR might also contribute to the PV phenotype. It is interesting to note that overexpression of TpoR in certain animal models led to an expansion of the erythroid compartment.[92]The SH2 and PH (pleckstrin homology domain) adapter protein Lnk was shown to not only bind to phosphorylated tyrosine residues of both TpoR and EpoR but also to exert a negative role on signaling by these receptors.[93, 94] It is not known whether the defects in this negative regulatory mechanism are operating in MPNs. Co-expression of JAK2 V617F and TpoR in Ba/F3 cells leads to down-modulation of TpoR, most likely due to internalization and down-modulation seen after excessive activation of cytokine receptors (J Staerk, C Pecquet, C Diaconu and SN Constantinescu, unpublished observations). This is consistent with early studies that have identified a maturation defect and down-modulation of cell surface TpoR in platelets and megakaryocytes from MPN patients.[95] More recently, an inverse correlation was reported between the burden of *JAK2* V617F and the levels of cell surface TpoR on platelets.[96] Although these results suggest that JAK2 V617F may contribute to the down-modulation of TpoR, several patients with MPNs in the absence of JAK2 V617F also exhibited down-modulated TpoR. Such down-modulation is not seen for EpoR. TpoR is a long-lived receptor at the cell surface[47] and recycles,[97] which is not the case for EpoR. Further experiments are necessary to follow up on the original observation of TpoR down-modulation in MPNs, which may be due to traffic alterations, excessive internalization and degradation or decreased protein synthesis. Several mutations in Mpl induce myeloid malignancies. A mutation in the transmembrane domain of Mpl, S505N, constitutively activates the receptor[98]and has been discovered in familial ET.[99] The S505N mutation in the transmembrane domain is expected to promote constitutive activation due to polar interactions between the asparagines that replace the natural serine. As stated earlier, mutations in Mpl at W515 induce severe MPNs with myeloprofibrosis.[19, 20] W515 mutations activate constitutive signaling by the receptor because W515 belongs to an amphipathic juxtamembrane helix (RWQFP in the human receptor), which is required for maintaining the un-liganded receptor in the inactive state. Another activating mutation was recently described for TpoR, where a threonine residue in the extracellular juxtamembrane region (located symmetrically from the W515 mutation on the N-terminal side of the transmembrane domain) is mutated to alanine (T487A) in a non-Down's syndrome childhood acute megakaryocytic leukemia.[100] In bone marrow transplantation assays, this Mpl T487A also induces a severe myeloproliferative disease, close to the phenotype induced by TpoR W515L.[100] Juxtamembrane mutations such as W515L/K or T487A may not only promote active dimeric conformations, but they could also induce receptor conformational changes by changing crossing angles between receptor monomers, whereas the S505N highly polar mutation in the transmembrane domain is predicted to stabilize an active dimeric conformation of the receptor. It will be interesting to test side by side in bone marrow transplantation experiments the effects of S505N, W515L and T487A mutations and to assess whether indeed the phenotype of the TpoR S505N mutation would be milder.

1.10 G-CSFR and MPNs

Bone marrow transplanted mice with HSCs expressing JAK2 V617F present not only an MPN phenotype, with low Epo, as predicted, but also with low G-CSF serum levels, suggesting that constitutive activation of G-CSFR occurs in these mice.[101]G-CSFR uses both JAK1 and JAK2 for signaling.[65, 66] JAK2 V617F may affect G-CSFR signaling with less efficiency than for EpoR and TpoR, as JAK1 may be the key JAK for G-CSFR. This is perhaps the reason why the granulocytic lineage is affected to a lower extent in MPNs, when compared with the erythroid and megakaryocytic lineages, especially at low levels of JAK2

V617F. Activation of the G-CSFR JAK2 V617F complexes may lead to enhanced numbers of granulocytes, constitutive activation of granulocytes (with release of enzymes) as well as interactions with platelets, which would contribute to thrombotic complications. It is not clear whether leukocytosis, which is seen in certain MPN patients and which appears to be associated with certain complications or evolution toward leukemia,[102] may be due to the pathologic activation of G-CSFR by JAK2 V617F. Granulocytes from patients with MPNs presented altered gene expression promoted by JAK2 V617F expression and confirmed a recapitulation of cytokine receptor signaling, resembling profiles of granulocytes activated by G-CSF.[103]Similar to TpoR, G-CSFR activates STAT3 and MAP kinase pathways, in addition to the JAK2–STAT5 and PI-3–kinase/Akt pathways. It can be noted that for this receptor, a very delicate balance has been identified between the activation of STAT3, required for differentiation and inducing a stop in cell growth (necessary for differentiation), and STAT5, which promotes proliferation.[102] Binding of SOCS3 through its SH2 domain to a phosphorylated tyrosine residue in the receptor's cytosolic end specifically downregulates STAT5 signaling. Deletion of the cytosolic region, which contains the binding site for SOCS3, leads to enhanced STAT5-to-STAT3 signaling ratio,[102] and this is associated with evolution toward acute myeloid leukemia of patients with severe congenital neutropenia. G-CSFR activation might synergize with other mechanisms and promote the mobilization of CD34(+) stem cells and progenitors from the bone marrow to the periphery. Interestingly, an increased number of circulating CD34(+) cells in MPN patients has been observed, and they exhibit granulocyte activation patterns similar to those induced by the administration of G-CSF.[104] The release of CD34(+) cells is generally due to a combination of increased levels of proteases[105] and especially due to the downregulation of the CXCR4 receptor on CD34(+) cells.[106] An altered SDF-1/CXCR4 axis was demonstrated in PMF patients with CD34(+) cells in the periphery.[107] These findings are supported by the rapid mobilization of CD34(+) cells with AMD3100, a CXCR4 antagonist.[108]

1.11 Tyrosine phosphorylation pattern of JAK2 V617F

JAK2 V617F is constitutively tyrosine phosphorylated. However, besides Y1007 in the activation loop, which is crucial for activation,[109] it is not known whether other phosphorylated tyrosines overlap with those phosphorylated in the wild-type JAK2. It can be noted that, JAK2 contains multiple tyrosine residues, of which at least 14 can be phosphorylated[110] (Figure 1). Some of these tyrosine residues exert positive (Y221) and other negative (Y119, Y570) effects on signaling by JAK2.[111, 112, 113] Y813 is a recruitment site for SH2-containing proteins,[114] such as SH2B, which can promote homodimerization of JAK2.[115] In theory, the constitutive activation of JAK2 V617F might promote a different pattern of phosphorylated tyrosines from that of wild-type JAK2.

1.12 STAT activation and MPNs

A hallmark of MPNs is constitutive or hypersensitive activation of the STAT family of transcription factors in myeloid precursors. As mentioned, the expressions of JAK2 V617F, TpoR mutants or exon 12 JAK2 mutants lead to constitutive STAT5 and STAT3 activation in various systems.[18, 116] As a function of the MPN disease type, one or the other of the STATs was suggested to be predominantly activated by JAK2 V617F. For example, in myelofibrosis, JAK2 V617F expression in neutrophils is associated with the activation of STAT3 but apparently not with that of STAT5.[117] In another study, in bone marrow biopsies and irrespective of JAK2 V617F, PV patients exhibited high STAT5 and STAT3 phosphorylation and ET patients exhibited high STAT3, but low STAT5 phosphorylation, whereas myelofibrosis patients exhibited low STAT5 and STAT3 phosphorylation.[118] Thus, constitutive activation of the STAT5/STAT3 signaling appears to be a major determinant of MPNs, irrespective of the particular JAK2 or receptor mutation. Furthermore, STAT3 activation by IL-6 has been shown in a murine model system to hold the potential to experimentally induce MPN. Mice homozygous for a knockin mutation in the IL-6 receptor gp130 (gp130(Y757F/Y757F)), which leads to gp130-dependent hyperactivation of STAT1 and STAT3 develop myeloproliferative diseases with splenomegaly, lymphadenopathy and thrombocytosis. gp130(Y757F/Y757F) is hyperactive owing to impaired recruitment of negative regulators such as SOCS3 and the SHP2 phosphatase.[119,120] The hematological phenotype disappeared when the knockin mice were crossed with heterozygous Stat3(+/-) mice.[121] Thus, the threshold of STAT3 signaling elicited by IL-6 family cytokines may have an important function in the myeloid lineage and may contribute to the development of MPN.

1.13 SOCS3 and JAK2 V617F

Suppressors of cytokine signaling (SOCS) proteins negatively regulate cytokine receptors and JAK-STAT signaling. There are eight members of the SOCS/CIS (cytokine-inducible SH2-domain-containing protein) family, namely SOCS1-SOCS7 and CIS. Each SOCS molecule contains a divergent N-terminal domain, a central SH2 domain, and a C-terminal 40 amino acid domain known as the SOCS box.[122] CIS/SOCS proteins are supposed to function as E3 ubiquitin ligases and target proteins bound to the SOCS N terminus, such as active JAKs, as well as themselves for proteasome-mediated degradation.[122] SOCS1 and SOCS3 can also inhibit the catalytic activity of JAK proteins directly, as they contain a kinase inhibitory region (KIR) that targets the activation loop of JAK proteins. SOCS proteins bind receptors and then target the activation loop of JAKs for inhibition by KIR and SH2 interactions.[122]SOCS3 is known to strongly down-modulate EpoR signaling.[123] JAK2 V617F appears not to be downregulated by SOCS3, possibly due to continuous phosphorylation of SOCS3, which can impair its E3 ligase activity.[124] Constitutive tyrosine phosphorylation of SOCS3 was also reported in peripheral blood mononuclear cells derived from patients homozygous for the JAK2 V617F mutant.[124] Taken together, a model was proposed in which JAK2 V617F may escape physiologic SOCS regulation by hyperphosphorylating SOCS3. It would be important to also determine whether exon 12 mutants of JAK2 are able to overcome down-modulation by SOCS3.Furthermore, one of the two tyrosine residues in the C terminus of SOCS3 that become phosphorylated upon ligand-activated cytokine receptors interacts with the Ras inhibitor p120 RasGAP.[125] This leads, in the case of IL-2 signaling, to sustained ERK activation, whereas the JAK-STAT pathway is down-modulated.[125]Whether part of the sustained ERK activation detected in cells transformed by JAK2 V617F may involve complexes of degradation-resistant SOCS3 and p120 RasGAP is yet to be determined.

1.14 Other JAK2 mutations activate JAK2

Substitution of pseudokinase domain residue V617 by large non-polar amino acids causes activation of JAK2.[126] Saturation mutagenesis at position 617 of JAK2 showed that, in addition to V617F, four other JAK2 mutants, V617W, V617M, V617I and V617L, were able to induce cytokine independence and constitutive downstream signaling. However, only V617W induced a level of constitutive activation comparable with V617F, and like V617F it was able to stabilize tyrosine-phosphorylated SOCS3.[126] Also, the V617W mutant induced a myeloproliferative disease in bone-marrow-reconstituted mice, mainly characterized by erythrocytosis and megakaryocytic proliferation. Although JAK2 V617W would predictably be pathogenic in humans, the substitution of the Val codon, GTC, by TTG, the codon for Trp, would require three base pair changes, which makes it unlikely to occur. Therefore, codon usage and resistance to SOCS3-induced down-modulation are two mechanisms that might explain the uniqueness of JAK2 V617F in MPNs.

2. Animal models of MPNs

2.1 JAK2 mutants

Mouse bone marrow reconstitution experiments with HSCs retrovirally transduced with JAK2 V617F resulted in strain-dependent myeloproliferative disease phenotypes. In these models, JAK2 V617F is expressed at ~10-fold higher than endogenous levels. In C57Bl6 mice, JAK2 V617F induces erythrocytosis, and in some animals myelofibrosis, although most reconstituted mice remain alive several months, and in some the erythrocytosis regresses; in Balb/c mice, the phenotype is more severe with erythrocytosis being followed by myelofibrosis.[13, 23, 127] Only very rarely, at low transduction levels, was a thrombocytosis phenotype observed, which, together with initial studies on primary patient cells,[22] led to the suggestion that gene dosage may be important for a particular phenotype to develop.[23] This hypothesis has been supported by studies in transgenic mice in which the expression of the JAK2 V617F was carefully regulated.[24] When JAK2 V617F levels were lower than endogenous JAK2 levels, an ET phenotype was obtained. When levels of JAK2 V617F were similar to those of endogenous wild-type JAK2, a PV-like phenotype was developed. Interestingly, upon development of the PV phenotype, a selection for higher levels of JAK2 V617F occurs, up to 5- to 6-fold higher than the endogenous JAK2 levels, which is not the case for the ET phenotype.[24] This indicates positive selection for JAK2 V617F expression in PV progenitors, a phenomenon that can be detected in stably transfected Ba/F3 cells.[51] In addition overexpression of several non-mutated JAK proteins, including JAK2, was shown to promote hematopoietic transformation to cytokine independence.[128]The phenotype induced by exon 12 mutants of JAK2 is more restricted to erythrocytosis, without the abnormal megakaryocyte clusters seen in the classical MPNs.[18] These *in vivo* data indicate that a difference must exist between signaling by JAK2 V617F and exon 12 JAK2 mutants.

2.2 Mpl (TpoR) mutants

The phenotype induced by TpoR W515L is different than that induced by JAK2 mutants, in that it is much more severe, with initial myeloproliferation, marked thrombocytosis, splenomegaly and myelofibrosis, and is established within 20–30 days after reconstitution.[19] At least one other mutation at W515 was identified in patients with PMF and ET, that is W515K.[20] W515 is located in an amphipathic motif (RWQFP) at the junction between the transmembrane and cytosolic domains. This motif is required to maintain the un-liganded TpoR in an inactive state. Given that a W515A mutation is also active,[21] it is not surprising that such different residues (Leu and Lys) are found in active TpoR mutants. We predict that other W515 mutations will be found in patients, as the loss of a Trp (W) residue is responsible for activation. The striking difference in severity and histopathology between the phenotypes induced by JAK2 V617F and Mpl 515 mutants is hard to understand when standard phosphorylation studies are performed on cell lines, such as Ba/F3 cells, where the same redundant pathways are activated by both JAK2 V617F and Mpl 515 mutants. Interestingly, deletion of the amphipathic motif (Δ5TpoR) that contains W515 or the mutation of either the lysine K514 (R514 in the human receptor) or the W515 in this motif to alanine leads to constitutive JAK2 and STAT activation and colony formation in primary cells and hypersensitivity to Tpo.[21] In hematopoietic cells transformed by Δ5TpoR (amphipathic motif deleted) or TpoR W515A, we noted enhanced STAT5 and MAP kinase activation in the absence of Tpo, and high levels of activation of STAT5, STAT3 and MAP kinase pathways on Tpo treatment.[21] Such TpoR mutants do not down-modulate cell surface levels of TpoR,[21] unlike TpoR in complex with JAK2 V617F, which is down-modulated (J Staerk *et al.*, unpublished observations). It is therefore tempting to speculate that prolonged activation of MAP kinase and STAT3 might be a distinct feature of TpoR W515 mutants, whereas JAK2 V617F, which couples not only to TpoR but also to other cytokine receptors expressed in myeloid progenitors, would generate a weaker or different signal. Taken together, these data suggest that some level of signaling specificity must exist, which would make the excessive activation of TpoR through JAK2 V617F qualitatively different from that induced by W515 mutations. Understanding this difference at the signaling level will be of utmost importance.

2.3 JAK2 inhibitors

Since 2005, mutations that directly or indirectly led to deregulated activation of non-receptor tyrosine kinase (TK) Janus activated kinase 2 (JAK2) have been implicated in the pathogenesis of MPN. These mutations activate the JAK2–signal transducer and activator of transcription (STAT) intracellular signaling pathways, which lead to increased cellular proliferation and resistance to apoptosis. These discoveries spurred the development of molecularly targeted agents (JAK2 inhibitors) as therapy for MPNs.

In clinical development, JAK2 inhibitors exhibit differential inhibitory activity against the JAK family members, and some exhibit effects on other receptor kinases and therefore are not selective forJAK2 TK. For example, INCB018424 inhibits JAK1, whereas CEP-701 and TG101348 inhibit FLT3. JAK2 inhibitors are small molecules that act by competing with adenosine triphosphate for the adenosine triphosphate–binding catalytic site in the TK domain. The V617F mutation locates outside the TK domain of JAK2. Therefore, the current JAK2 inhibitors target both wild-type and mutated JAK2 indiscriminately. This could explain why these drugs are active in patients with both wild-type and mutated JAK2. However, targeting the wild-type JAK2 is expected to lead to myelosuppression as a result of the exquisite signalling through JAK2 of thrombopoietin and erythropoietin receptors in normal hematopoiesis. This probably explains the reported therapy-related anaemia and thrombocytopenia observed with JAK2 inhibitors in clinical trials.

Previous research demonstrated that JAK2-deficiency is embryonically fatal in mice due to a lack of erythropoiesis. As a consequence, no in vivo JAK2 knock out animal model exists, which makes the biological characterization of JAK2 more difficult. siRNA knock down models may be useful for this purpose, but for the time being, they cannot be considered as therapeutic agents. JAK2 antagonists, however, could be used efficiently for analyzing the possible therapeutic benefit of JAK2 inhibition in hematologic malignancies and myeloproliferative disorders.

On the other hand, only a small number of JAK2 inhibitors have been reported in the literature so far. AG490 possesses significant JAK2 inhibition, for that reason it has been used extensively as a research tool. AG490 blocks leukemic cell growth significantly both in vitro and in vivo.[16] On the other hand, this compound lacks sufficient target specificity, therefore the interpretation of results obtained with AG490 may not be limited to JAK2 inhibition. Several other non-specific JAK2 inhibitors have already been reported in the literature (LFM-A13,21 INCB20,22 WP106623 and SD-100824). Since off-target effects may cause serious immune-modulative or proliferative side effects, specific JAK2 inhibition is highly desirable.

One molecule, TG101209, was able to inhibit proliferation of both JAK2 V617F- and TpoR W515L/K-expressing hematopoietic cells.[130] It may be recalled that TpoR W515-mutated proteins are expected to constitutively activate the wild-type JAK2.

TG101348, a nano-molar JAK2 inhibitor, was highly specific for JAK2 as evidenced by a 300-fold selectivity over JAK3. TG101348, was effective in a murine model of MPN induced by JAK2 V617F131 and inhibited the engraftment of JAK2 V617F-positive HSCs and myeloid progenitors in a bioluminescent xenogeneic transplantation assay.[132] Importantly, the inhibitor decreased GATA1 expression and phosphorylation of GATA1 at S310 and, as expected, STAT5 activation. These signaling events might be associated with erythroid-skewing of JAK2 V617F-positive progenitor differentiation, as phosphorylation at GATA1 S310 was shown to be important for erythroid differentiation.[81] GATA1 is absolutely required for erythroid and megakaryocyte formation.[133, 134] Although both EpoR and GATA1 are crucial for erythroid differentiation, this phosphorylation event, which depends on PI-3-kinase and Akt,81 appears to be the only one described where a direct EpoR downstream signal affects GATA1.

An experimental JAK2 inhibitor has been shown to be well tolerated and to produce a significant reduction in disease burden and durable clinical benefit in patients with myelofibrosis reports a study. [161] Currently there are no FDA approved treatments for myelofibrosis. Common treatments of the malignancy, which is associated with anaemia and splenomegaly, are palliative and do not alter the natural course of the disease. Median survival ranges from less than two years to greater than 15 years. Patients with myelofibrosis frequently harbour JAK-STAT activating mutations that are sensitive to TG101348, a selective small-molecule JAK2 inhibitor. It is estimated that JAK2 mutations occur in approximately 50 % of patients. Last September researchers reported positive results from a trial testing the experimental agent INCBO18424, (which inhibits JAK1 as well as JAK2) in patients with advanced myelofibrosis. In the current phase 1 study, Ayalew Tefferi and colleagues from the Mayo Clinic enrolled 59 patients, including 28 who took part in the dose-escalating phase. A substantial portion of patients experienced improvements in primary symptoms including splenomegaly, leukocytosis, thrombocytosis, and constitutional symptoms. There was also evidence for significant reductions in genomic disease burden, indicating the potential for disease-modifying activity. Although the drug was generally well tolerated, it caused anaemia in some patients, especially at higher doses.

A follow-up study is planned to see whether adjusting the dose will allow patients to achieve the benefits without the anaemia. In an accompanying editorial Srdan Verstovsek from the University of Texas MD Anderson Cancer Center wrote, "The development of JAK2 inhibitors has ushered in a new era of targeted therapies for Philadelphia-negative MPNs. These drugs do not eradicate the malignant clone, but they provide significant clinical benefit. Given that the current clinical management of patients with MF is largely palliative and minimally effective, significant improvements in two of the three most important clinical manifestations of MF (splenomegaly and systemic symptoms) seen with JAK2 inhibitors is significant therapeutic progress." Long term results, he added, are required to determine the full potential of JAK2 inhibitors in myelofibrosis and to determine whether they will have an impact on survival.

3. Cross-talk: JAK2 V617F and other pathways

3.1 JAK2 V617F and other tyrosine kinases

Tyrosine kinase receptors have been suggested to contribute to the pathogenesis of PV. In patients with PV, circulating erythroid progenitor cells are hypersensitive to IGF-1 and this effect requires the IGF-1 receptor.[10, 135]Expression of JAK2 V617F in Ba/F3 cells renders the cells responsive to IGF-1 at doses where parental Ba/F3 cells are unresponsive.[51] After selection for autonomous growth, these Ba/F3 JAK2 V617F cells acquire the ability to respond to IGF-1 by further tyrosine phosphorylation of the mutant JAK2 and of STAT5 and STAT3. Which adaptor/signaling protein mediates this cross-talk is not clear, but it might be relevant for the hypersensitivity of PV erythroid progenitors to IGF-1.

Treatment with imatinib, an inhibitor of the Abl, c-KIT and PDGF receptor kinase, leads to minimal responses in PV, but nevertheless some rare patients achieve remission and a decrease in the *JAK2* V617F allele burden.[136] Imatinib exerts a dose-dependent growth inhibitory effect on factor dependent cell paterson (FDCP) cells expressing JAK2 V617F, most likely by interrupting the cross-talk between JAK2 V617F and c-KIT.[137] Thus, this study predicts that in PV patients where imatinib exerts benefic effects, pathologic signaling occurs through c-KIT.Src tyrosine kinases have also been suggested to contribute to signaling by EpoR.[138] However, Src kinases were dispensable for the polycythemia phenotype induced by JAK2 V617F, as shown by bone marrow reconstitution studies in mice deficient for Lyn, Fyn or Fgr kinases.[139]

3.2 JAK2 V617F and TNF-α

In BALB/c mice reconstituted with HSCs transduced for the expression of JAK2 V617F, the PV-like phenotype is associated with increased serum levels of TNF-α.[101] TNF-α might be required for suppressing normal hematopoiesis, and in this manner it might favor the mutated clone. Reconstitution experiments in TNF-α knockout mice supported the notion that TNF-α might be required for the establishment of the MPN phenotype and for clonal dominance (Bumm TGP, VanDyke J, Loriaux M, Gendron C, Wood LG, Druker BJ, Deininger MW. TNF-α plays a crucial role in the JAK2-V617F-induced myeloproliferative disorder. *Blood*2007; 110. American Society of Hematology 2007 Abstract 675). Further studies will be required to firmly establish whether TNF signaling may contribute to clonal dominance. Erythroblasts from JAK2 V617F-positive PV patients show increased death receptor resistance, which may give them a proliferative advantage over the non-mutated erythroblasts.[101, 140] This effect was mediated by incomplete caspase-mediated cleavage of the erythroid transcription factor GATA-1, which in normal erythroblasts is completely degraded on CD95 stimulation.

3.3 MPNs and TGF-β

An increase of TGF-β expression in circulating megakaryocytic cells and platelets was demonstrated in PMF.[141] Fibroblasts participating in myelofibrosis were shown to be polyclonal, as opposed to the hematopoietic progenitors, thus suggesting that myelofibrosis is a reactive process.[141]In myelofibrosis induced by excessive levels of Tpo,[142] severe spleen fibrosis was seen only in wild-type mice but not in homozygous TGF-β1 null (TGF-β1 (-/-)) mice.[143] Studies using peripheral CD34(+) cells cultured in medium with Tpo and stem cell factor concluded that PMF is a consequence of an increased ability of PMF CD34(+) progenitor cells to generate megakaryocytes and a decreased rate of megakaryocyte apoptosis, which lead to high levels of megakaryocyte-produced TGF-β.[144] In other models with hyperactive JAK–STAT signaling, such as knock-in with a mutant hyperactive gp130 receptor, the activation of the JAK–STAT pathway led to the expression of the inhibitory Smad7, which prevents the anti-proliferative effect of TGF-β.[145] A pathway linking Tpo, GATA-1 and TGF-βin the development of myelofibrosis was invoked, given that mice expressing low levels of the transcription factor GATA-1 also develop myelofibrosis.[146]

3.4 JAK2 V617F and chromatin

Studies in *Drosophila melanogaster* show that persistent activation of D-STAT by mutated D-JAK leads to chromatin effects and gene induction other than the normal targets of D-STAT, with counteracting heterochromatic gene silencing.[147]A genome-wide survey of genes required for JAK/STAT activity identified a WD40/bromodomain protein *Drosophila* homolog of BRWD3,[148] a gene that is disrupted in human B-cell leukemia patients. Whether any histone acetylase, deacetylase, methyl-transferase or other proteins containing bromo-, chromo- or chromoshadow domains are direct targets of JAK2 V617F is not clear. Recently, encouraging results were obtained with an HDAC (histone deacetylase) inhibitor, which seems to target only *JAK2* V617F-positive cells among primary myeloid progenitors from PV patients.[149] Thus, like other cancers,[150] MPNs might also show restriction of fate options through hypermethylation. This notion is supported by the different effects of sequential treatment with the DNA methyltransferase inhibitor, decitabine, followed by the histone deacetylase inhibitor, trichostatin A (TSA), on normal CD34(+) versus PMF CD34(+) cells. In the former, the treatment led to the expansion of cells, whereas in the latter the total number of CD34(+) cells and hematopoietic cells was reduced.[151]Furthermore, promoter de-methylation appears to be at least partially at the basis of the dysregulated expression of the polycythemia rubra vera-1 (PRV-1) protein,[152] which is a key marker of PV.[153] Finally, hypermethylation of the SOCS1 promoter was reported approximately in 15% of MPN patients irrespective of *JAK2* V617F positivity.[154] SOCS1 promoter methylation may contribute to growth factor hypersensitivity, as SOCS1 appears to maintain the ability to down-modulate JAK2 V617F signaling.[124] Recently, Dawson et al.[155]identified a novel nuclear role of JAK2 in the phosphorylation of Tyr 41 of histone H3 leading to chromatin displacement of HP1a. The authors suggested that the inability of HP1a to regulate chromatin could reduce the potential tumor suppressive functions of HP1a resulting in erratic mitotic recombination and transcription deregulation of several JAK2-regulated genes such as *LMO2*[155,156]. These results were confirmed in hematopoietic cell lines and in the CD34+ cells collected from the peripheral blood of one PMF patient with JAK2V617F mutation. In this work we define the subcellular localization of JAK2 in total BM cells and in sorted cell populations collected from MPN (ET, PV, PMF) patients with the JAK2V617F mutation or from MPN patients with wild type (wt) JAK2. We find that in contrast to cells with normal JAK2 in which the protein is detected predominantly in the cytoplasm, JAK2 is mostly nuclear in V617F-positive CD34+ cells. However, this nuclear localization is no longer observed in V617F-positive differentiated cells. After expressing JAK2V617F in K562 cells, we observe a similar preferential accumulation of JAK2 in the nucleus in contrast to untrasfected- and wt JAK2-expressing cells in which the protein is found in the cytoplasm. The mutated-JAK2 nuclear translocation is mainly reverted by the addiction of the JAK2 inhibitor AG490.

4. Methods

4.1 Cell cultures

K562 were grown in RPMI 1640 medium (Sigma-Aldrich), supplemented with 10% fetal bovine serum (FBS), 1% penicillin/streptomycin, and 1% glutamine. The cells were maintained at 37 C and 5% CO2. Transfection was performed by AMAXA electroporation in accordance with the manufacturer's instructions. Stable cell lines were obtained by puromycin selection (3μg/ml). Leptomycine B was added to a final concentration of 1 uM and the cells were harvested after 24 h of incubation. The differentiation of K562 cells was obtained by culturing the cells with 10 nMol PMA.

4.2 Plasmids

pMSCV-puro-JAK2 and pMSCV-puro-JAK2V617F were kindly provided by Dr. J. Cools.

4.3 Confocal immunofluorescence (CFI) microscopy

The BM fractions of CD34+, CD15+, CD41+, CD71+ cells and the K562 cells were washed once in PBS before cytocentrifugation onto polylysine-coated microscope slides. The cells were fixed for 5 min in methanol at room temperature and 5 min in acetone at -20 C. After stepwise incubation with a primary antibody and a secondary fluorescent antibody, the cells were stained with DAPI and mounted with glycerol. Confocal laser images were captured with a laser scanning microscope LSM 510 META microscope equipped with a 403 oil-immersion lens.

4.4 Patients

BM aspirates and PB samples were obtained from 15 patients newly diagnosed with MPN according to the WHO criteria. Ten of the patients (ET n=4, PV n=3, PMF n=3) had the V617F mutation. The remaining 5 patients (PMF n= 2, ET n=3) had a normal JAK2. Informed consent for the study was obtained from all patients in accordance with the Declaration of

Helsinki. The study was conducted according to the guidelines of the Italian ethics committee.

4.5 Cell sorting

Mononucleated cells were isolated by Ficoll centrifugation. After erythrocyte lyses, 10 million BM (or PB) cells were labelled by incubation with the antibodies CD15-APC, CD41-FITC, CD71-PerCP, CD34-Pe (BD Biosciences, San Jose, CA), analyzed, and sorted with a fluorescence-activated cell sorter FACSAria (BD Biosciences) using FACS Diva software (BD Biosciences) according to the manufacturer's recommendations.

4.6 ASO-PCR and RT-PCR

The JAK2V617F mutation was identified by ASO-PCR as previously described[13-15]. Briefly, total RNA was isolated with the TRIzol reagent (Invitrogen) and cDNA was synthesised with the First Strand cDNA Synthesis kit (MBI Fermentas). Syber Green RQ-PCR was performed as previously described[155]. Quantitative values were obtained from the threshold cycle number (Ct) by subtracting the average Ct of the target gene from that of GAPDH and expressed as $2^{-\Delta Ct}$.

4.7 Cell fractionation and immunoblotting

Cytoplasmic and nuclear fractions were prepared using nuclei isolation KIT by Sigma-Aldrich according to the manufacturer's instructions. Equal amounts of cytoplasmic or nuclear fractions or total cell extracts were separated by SDS–PAGE, transferred to nitrocellulose and probed with relevant antibodies.

4.8 JAK2 inhibitor and antibodies

AG490 was provided by Invivogen. To establish the best experimental condition, the cells were cultured for 3 hours with 2 different concentrations of the inhibitor (12.5 uM and 25 uM). The following antibodies were used at the stated dilutions: anti-JAK2 antibodies (D2E12 no. 3230; Cell Signaling Technology), p-JAK2 (tyr1007/tyr1008)-R and p-JAK2 (tyr1007/tyr1008) (Santa Cruz), anti-b-tubulin (T5201; Sigma-Aldrich), anti-laminin A (Sigma-Aldrich); western blot 1:1000. Alex Fluor-488-conjugated IgG (Invitrogen) immunofluorescence 1:250.

4.9 Apoptotic rate

K562 cells were stained with propidium iodide and annexin V before and after 3 h incubation with AG490. Cell cycle parameters were assessed by FACS analysis using FACSCanto II flow cytometer (Becton Dickinson, San Jose, CA, USA).

4.10 Statistical analysis

Student *t* test was used to evaluate individual differences between means. $P \leq 0.05$ was considered significant.

5. Results and discussion

5.1 V617FJAK2 goes into the nucleus of JAK2 mutated K562

To determine whether the V617F mutation affects the sub-cellular localization of JAK2, we used CIF microscopy to analyze K562 cells stably transfected with pMSCV-puroJAK2V617F or pMSCV-puroJAK2. The results (Figure 3A) confirm the nuclear and cytoplasmic localization of JAK2 in K562 as reported by Dawson et al[155]. However, we consistently observed a much stronger nuclear signal in the cells expressing JAK2V617F than in those carrying wt JAK2, suggesting that the mutation leads to a nuclear accumulation of JAK2V617F. By CIF, this accumulation can be seen as a diffused nuclear pattern (Figure 3A top, upper and middle panels) or as nuclear spots (Figure 3A top, lower panel). This altered sub-cellular distribution was not affected by the addition of the nuclear export inhibitor leptomycin B (data not shown) and was confirmed by Western blot analysis of K562 cells (Figure 3A, bottom panels).

5.2 Preferential nuclear JAK2 in V617FJAK2 positive CD34+ but not in differentiated erythroid, granulocytic or megakaryocytic cells

To determine whether there is a preferential nuclear translocation of JAK2V617F *in vivo*, we analyzed by CIF microscopy the BM cells of 10 JAK2V617F-positive MPN patients (ET n=4, PV n=3, PMF n=3, allele burden median: 56%, 70%, 72% respectively) and of 5 MPN patients with wt JAK2 (PMF n= 2, ET n=3). We did not observe a significant signal in the nucleus of cells with wt JAK2 (Figure 3B). In contrast, we found a strong nuclear signal in 3%-5% of total BM mononucleated cells in 10 of 10 JAK2V617F-positive patients, suggesting that, unlike the wt JAK2, JAK2V617F has a predominantly nuclear homing. To identify the phenotype of these cells, we used fluorescence activated cell sorting (FACS) to isolate CD34+, CD15+, CD41+ and CD71+ fractions from the BM of three JAK2V617F-positive MPN patients (1 ET, 1 PV, 1 early PMF). We found nuclear JAK2 only in the fraction containing the CD34+ positive cells (Figure 3C, left panels). It should be noted that in these patients the CD34+ cells correspond to approximately 3% to 5% of total BM mononucleated cells. The nuclear localization of JAK2V617F was confirmed by WB analysis (Figure 3C, right panels). However, no predominant nuclear signal was detected in differentiated granulocytic, megakaryocytic and erythroid cells obtained from the patients (n=15) (Figure 3D). Similar results were obtained with PB cells (data not shown). The relocation of the mutated JAK2 to the cytoplasm was confirmed in K562 cells after their differentiation with PMA (Figure 4A). However, the relocation was not complete as observed for the primary BM cells and nuclear JAK2 was still observed. We believe that this is due to the nature of K562 cells, which are BCR-ABL-positive CML cells, and to the difficulty to obtain their terminal differentiation in vitro.

5.3 The JAK2 inhibitor AG490 relocate JAK2 in cytoplasm

To determine whether an alteration of JAK2 activity could interfere with the nuclear localization of JAK2, we incubated K562 cells expressing JAK2V617F or JAK2 with the selective JAK2 inhibitor AG490[158-160]. After 3 h of incubation at the IC50 dose of 25 uM, CIF images showed a relocalization of JAK2V617F to the cytoplasm in the vast majority of K562 cells (Figure 4B). Analyses with annexin V and propidium iodide did not reveal any significant change in the apoptotic rate of V617F-positive and wt-K562 cells.

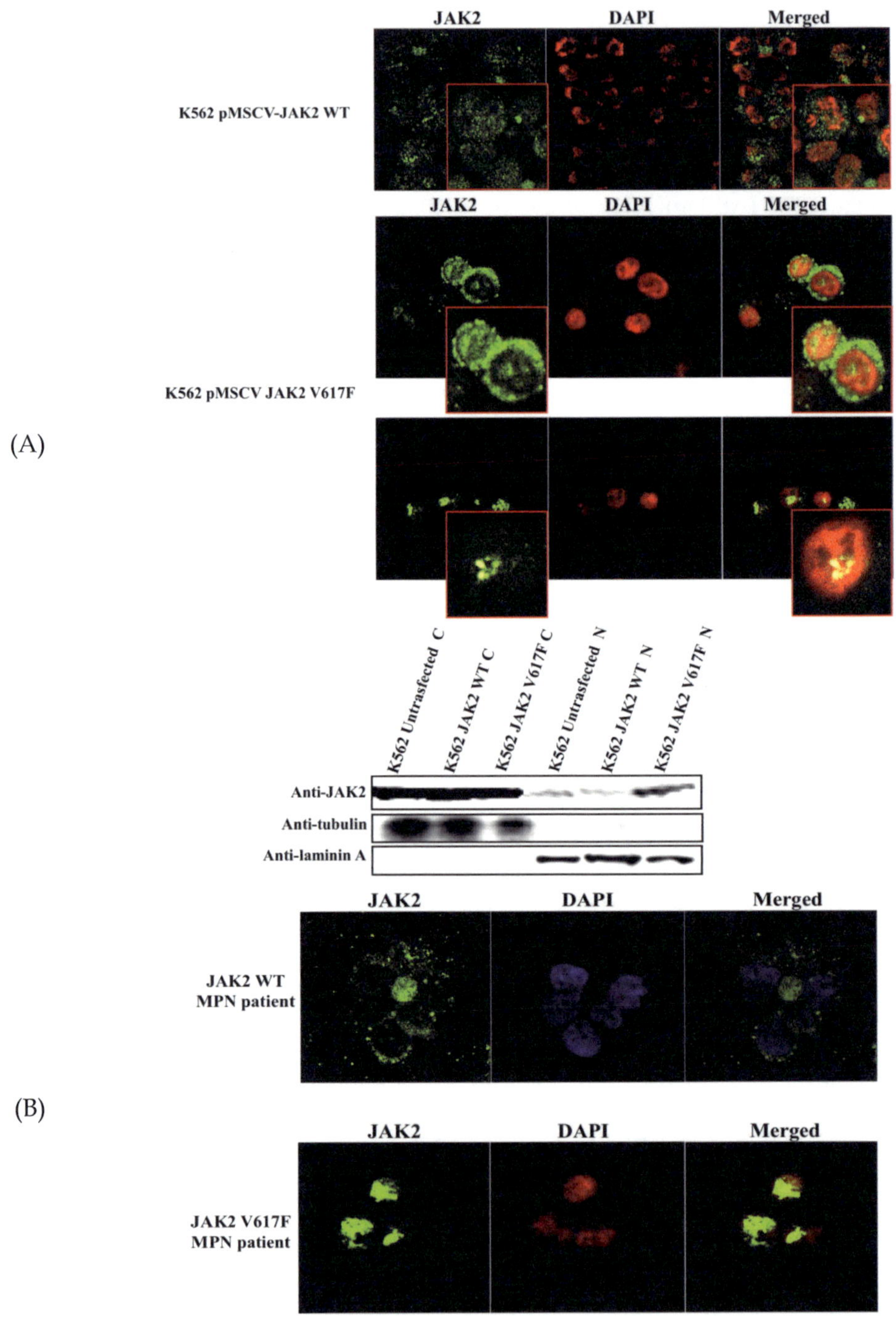

Fig. 3. V617F mutation favors nuclear translocation of JAK2 in K562 and early CD34+ progenitors isolated from BM of MPN patients. This translocation is not observed in differentiated cells.(A) CIF microscopy images of K562 cells stably transfected with pMSCV-JAK2 (upper panels) or pMSCV-JAK2V617F (middle and lower panels) and Western

blotting of cytoplasmic (C) and nuclear (N) fractions confirm that JAK2V617F is more abundant than JAK2 in K562 nuclei. (B)CIF images of BM cells from an MPN patient with wt JAK2 (upper panels) and an MPN patient with JAK2V617F (lower panels) confirm a nuclear increase of the mutated protein.

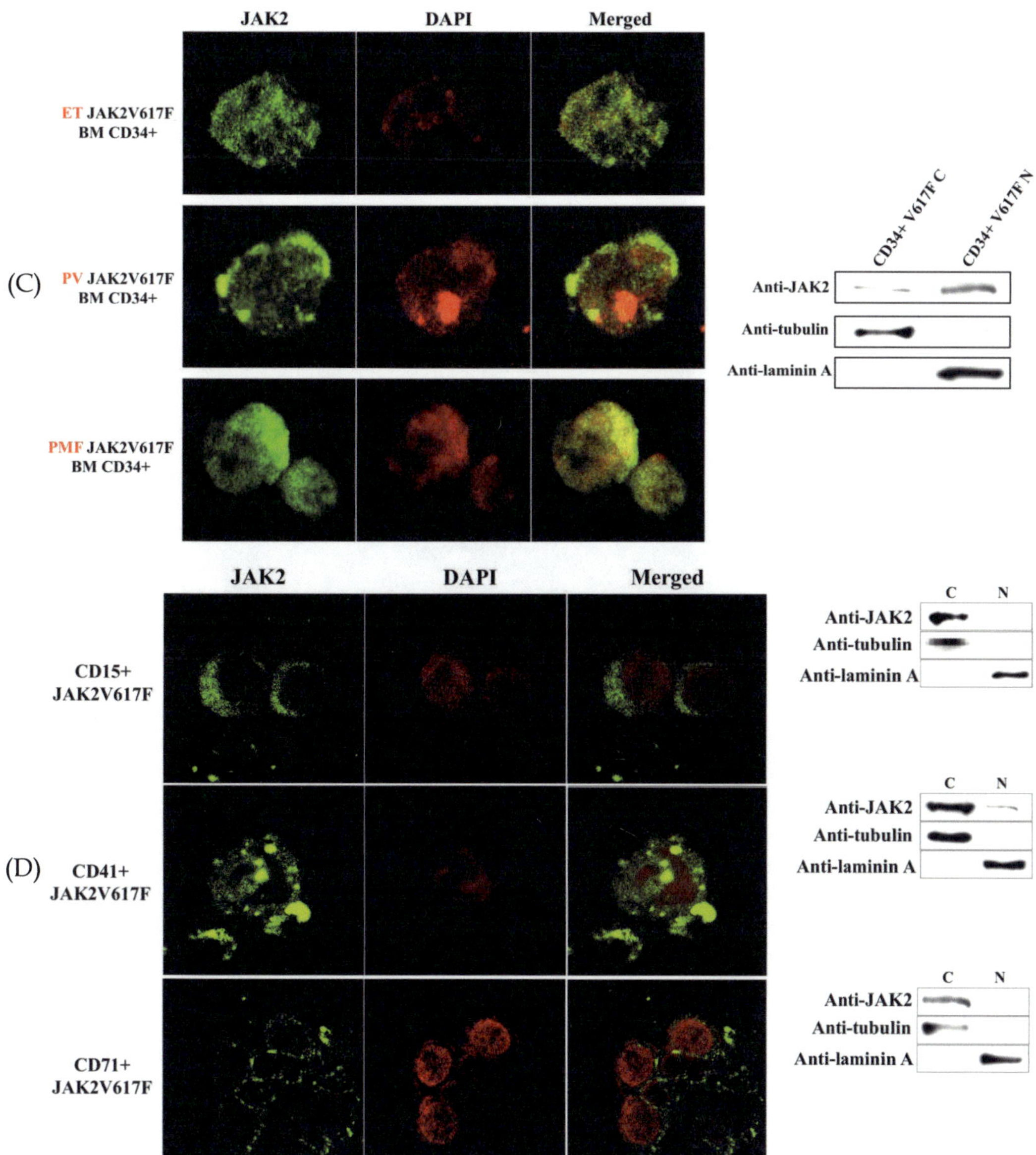

Fig. 3. V617F mutation favors nuclear translocation of JAK2 in K562 and early CD34+ progenitors isolated from BM of MPN patients. This translocation is not observed in differentiated cells.(C) Confocal IF demonstrates a predominantly nuclear accumulation of JAK2V617F in CD34+ cells isolated from BM of 1 ET, 1 PV and 1 earlyPMF (left panels) and Western blotting of cytoplasmic (C) and nuclear (N) extracts (right panel) confirm the data.

(D) Confocal IF images of CD15+, CD41+, CD71+ cells isolated from a JAK2V617F–positive MPN patient (PV, JAK2 allele burden 71%) and Western blotting of cytoplasmic (C) and nuclear (N) extracts (right panel). DAPI, 4,6-diamidino-2-phenylindole; Anti-JAK2, Cell Signaling monoclonal antibody; Anti-Tubulin and Anti-Laminin A, Sigma-Aldrich monoclonal antibodies.

5.4 V617F JAK2 up-regulates LMO2 and AG490 restores its level.

By QRT-PCR we show that the V617F mutation strongly up-regulates the expression of *LMO2* in K562 and in CD34+ cells (Figure 4C, left panels). The link between *LMO2* expression and JAK2 inhibition has been reported previously[156,157]. In our assay, the addition of AG490 progressively and completely restore*LMO2* levels in V617F expressing K562 (Figure 4C, right panels).

(A)

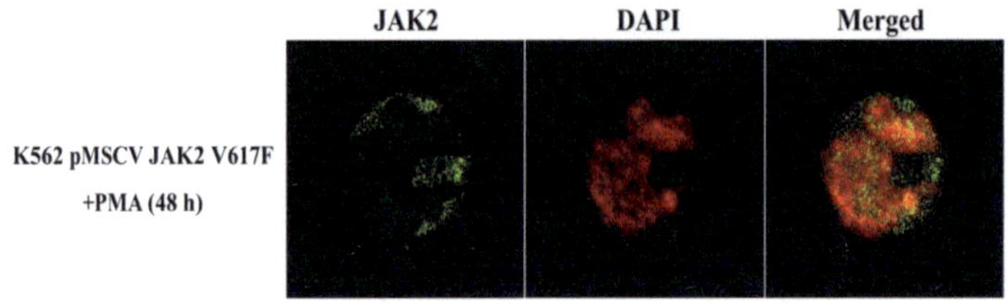

(B)

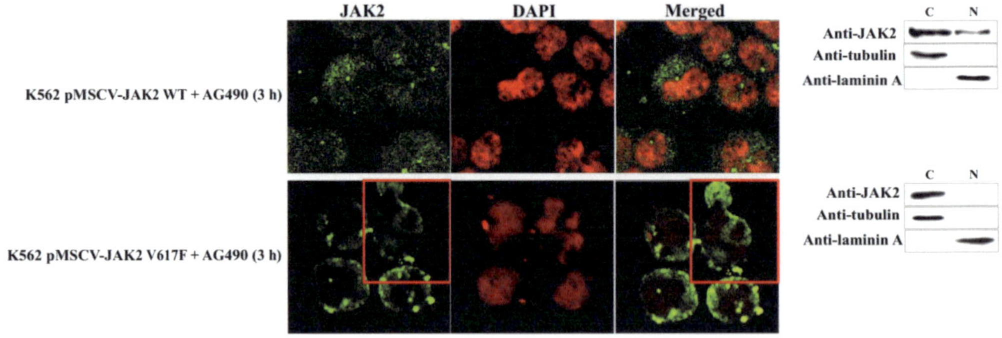

(C)

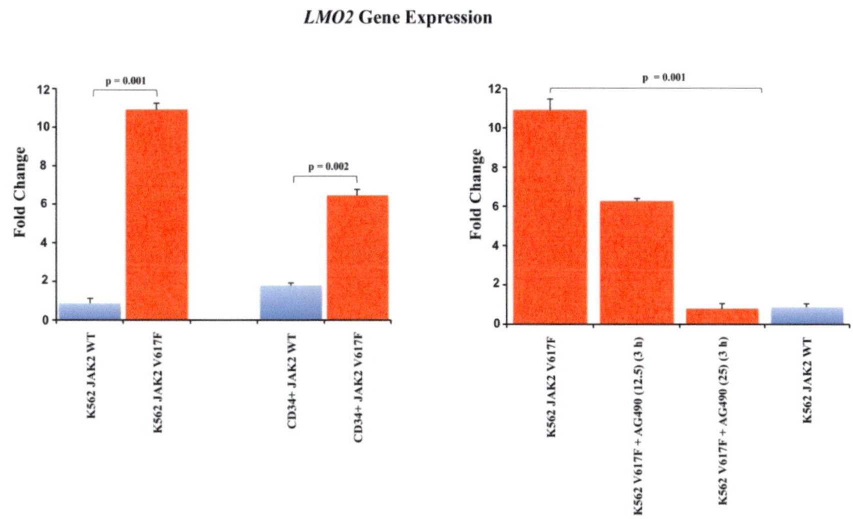

Fig. 4. V617F mutation causes up-regulation of *LMO2*. The JAK2 inhibitor AG490 replaces JAK2 into cytoplasm and restores LMO2 levels.(A) Confocal IF images show the redistribution of JAK2 and the replacement in the cytoplasm in V617F expressing K562 after PMA differentiation (B) Confocal IF images show the redistribution of JAK2 and the replacement in the cytoplasm in the vast majority of V617F expressing K562 (bottom panels) but not in wt cells (top panels) after AG490 incubation. (C) Quantitative RT-PCR revels that V617F mutation strongly up-regulates *LMO2* expression in K562 and in CD34+ cells (left panels). The addiction of AG490 progressively and completely restore*LMO2* levels in V617F expressing K562 (right panels). DAPI, 4,6-diamidino-2-phenylindole; Anti-JAK2, Cell Signaling monoclonal antibody.

6. Conclusions

Where do the major advances towards understanding the precise molecular bases of MPNs lead us? One striking observation is the key role played by various tyrosine kinases, constitutively activated either by balanced translocations or deletions generating fusion oncoproteins, or by activating point mutations. These mechanisms seem to be the molecular hallmark of MPNs, although there are probably alternative mechanisms directly involving cytokine receptors, adaptor proteins or transcription factors. All the molecular defects identified in MPNs to date confer proliferation and survival advantages on transformed cells, which retain the capacity to differentiate into mature cells. Differentiation may be disrupted by additional events, such as transcription factor deregulation, as frequently observed in acute myeloid leukaemia. *KIT* mutations and *FLT3* abnormalities are frequently found in cases of acute myeloid leukaemia. However, these molecular defects are now considered to be secondary events.

Strikingly, the diverse mutants and fusion proteins with constitutive tyrosine kinase activity each appear to stimulate a specific lineage. For example, PDGFR fusion proteins induce eosinophil differentiation, FGFR fusion proteins induce lymphoid malignancies, and

JAK2V617F mostly expands the erythroid compartment, whereas translocations involving the JAK2 kinase domain promote lymphoid proliferation as well. Thus, constitutive signalling via these different kinases is likely to result in effects on specific differentiation programs. Uncovering the molecular details of this specificity remains a major challenge, particularly as similar signalling molecules (*i.e.* STAT5, STAT3, RAS/MAPK, PI3K/AKT and others) are constitutively activated by all oncogenic fusion proteins.

Although the discovery of the JAK2V617F allele and the subsequent discovery of JAK2 exon 12 mutations and MPLW515L/K alleles have provided crucial insights into the genetic basis of PV, ET and PMF, many questions remain regarding the molecular pathogenesis of these MPNs. The activating mutations that cause JAK2 and MPL-negative MPN are not known, and the inherited and acquired alleles that can cooperate with JAK2V617F remain to be identified. In addition, the predominance of the JAK2V617F allele is surprising given that JAK2 exon 12 mutations, as well as activating JAK2 alleles identified in AML (JAK2T875N and JAK2ΔIREED), have similar in vitro and in vivo effects as JAK2V617F. The different JAK2 alleles might differentially interact with different cytokine receptor scaffolds, activate different signalling pathways, and/or be differentially affected by negative-feedback mechanisms; structural insight and additional in vitro and in vivo studies are needed to elucidate differences between JAK2V617F and the other activating JAK2 alleles. Another important question relates to the effects of JAK2V617F gene dosage on signalling and on phenotype. In vitro studies do not conclusively show whether the co-expression of wildtype JAK2 with JAK2V617F alters the signalling and/or transforming properties of the JAK2V617F kinase, and although retroviral models allow for an assessment of the in vivo effects of JAK2V617F expression, they do not provide the appropriate genetic context to investigate the importance of JAK2V617F gene dosage. Subsequent studies using more accurate genetic models will enable the delineation of the differential effects of JAK2V617F heterozygosity and homozygosity on signalling and on phenotype. Moreover, the role of the JAK2V617F allele in three distinct disorders of the myeloid lineage is not known, and the ability of different activated tyrosine kinases (for example, BCR-ABL and FIP1L1–PDGFRA) to cause distinct MPN remains to be delineated.

Dawson et al. identified a previously unrecognized nuclear role for JAK2 in the phosphorylation of the tyrosine 41 of the histone H3 with the exclusion of HP1a from chromatin and resulting in a disregulation of several JAK2-regulated genes such as LMO2 in haematopoietic cell lines and in one case on peripheral CD34+ cells from a JAK2V617F mutated PMF patient.

Our data corroborate recently published results of a nuclear localization of JAK2 in hematopoietic cells and they also extend these findings by showing that in all subtypes of MPN patients JAK2V617F accumulates in the nucleus of progenitor CD34+ cells while it remains mostly in the cytoplasm of their differentiated progeny. The chromatin alterations due to the preferential accumulation of JAK2V617F in the nucleus correlates with a significant increase in LMO2 expression in cell lines and in sorted CD34+ cells. The selective JAK2 inhibitor AG490 is able to revert nuclear JAK2 and normalize LMO2 levels in vitro, suggesting how the block in JAK2 nuclear translocation could be a new treatment strategy for JAK2 mutated patients. A question that remains to be answered is why mutated JAK2 is found only in the cytoplasm of the differentiated cells. MPN are clonal disorders arising in a pluripotent hematopoietic stem cell and it is well known that the constitutive activation of

JAK2 provides a sustained growth and survival advantage to the hematopoietic mutated stem cell clones. Signaling by the mutated kinase utilizes normal pathways, and normal or mutated JAK2 regulate EPO, TPO, and GCS-F response during differentiation, though they are probably not necessary to the differentiated cell. The signals that are required for the translocation of normal and mutated JAK2 to the nucleus are unknown. It is possible that the activation of the kinase by phosphorylation could be the first one of a number of modifications that control nuclear translocation, similarly to what happens to the STAT proteins. If this is true, then it is also possible that as the cell undergoes differentiaition these modifications are shut off, leaving mutated JAK2 predominantly in the cytoplasm.

7. Acknowledgements

The Authors thank Prof. Anthony R. Green (Cambridge Institute for Medical Research and Department of Haematology, University of Cambridge, Cambridge, United Kingdom) for his kind contribution and suggestions.

8. References

[1] Tefferi A, Gangat N, Wolanskyj AP, Schwager S, Pardanani A, Lasho TL *et al*. 20+ Year without leukemic or fibrotic transformation in essential thrombocythemia or polycythemia vera: predictors at diagnosis. *Eur J Haematol* 2008; 80: 386–390.

[2] Damashek W. Some speculations on the myeloproliferative syndromes.*Blood* 1951; 6: 372–375.

[3] Adamson JW. Analysis of haemopoiesis: the use of cell markers and *in vitro* culture techniques in studies of clonal haemopathies in man. *Clin Haematol* 1984; 13: 489–502.

[4] Prchal JF, Axelrad AA. Bone-marrow responses in polycythemia vera. *N Engl J Med* 1974; 290: 1382.

[5] Roder S, Steimle C, Meinhardt G, Pahl HL. STAT3 is constitutively active in some patients with polycythemia rubra vera. *Exp Hematol* 2001; 29: 694–702.

[6] Dai C, Chung IJ, Krantz SB. Increased erythropoiesis in polycythemia vera is associated with increased erythroid progenitor proliferation and increased phosphorylation of Akt/PKB. *Exp Hematol* 2005; 33: 152–158.

[7] Silva M, Richard C, Benito A, Sanz C, Olalla I, Fernandez-Luna JL. Expression of Bcl-x in erythroid precursors from patients with polycythemia vera. *N Engl J Med* 1998; 338: 564–571.

[8] Dai CH, Krantz SB, Dessypris EN, Means Jr RT, Horn ST, Gilbert HS. Polycythemia vera. II. Hypersensitivity of bone marrow erythroid, granulocyte-macrophage, and megakaryocyte progenitor cells to interleukin-3 and granulocyte gmacrophage colony-stimulating factor.*Blood* 1992; 80: 891–899.

[9] Dai CH, Krantz SB, Green WF, Gilbert HS. Polycythaemia vera. III. Burst-forming units-erythroid (BFU-E) response to stem cell factor and c-kit receptor expression. *Br J Haematol* 1994; 86: 12–21.

[10] Correa PN, Eskinazi D, Axelrad AA. Circulating erythroid progenitors in polycythemia vera are hypersensitive to insulin-like growth factor-1 *in vitro*: studies in an improved serum-free medium. *Blood* 1994; 83: 99–112.

[11] Axelrad AA, Eskinazi D, Correa PN, Amato D. Hypersensitivity of circulating progenitor cells to megakaryocyte growth and development factor (PEG-rHu MGDF) in essential thrombocythemia. *Blood* 2000; 96: 3310-3321.

[12] Dai C, Krantz SB. Increased expression of the INK4a/ARF locus in polycythemia vera. *Blood* 2001; 97: 3424-3432.

[13] James C, Ugo V, Le Couedic JP, Staerk J, Delhommeau F, Lacout C *et al.* A unique clonal JAK2 mutation leading to constitutive signalling causes polycythaemia vera. *Nature* 2005; 434: 1144-1148.

[14] Baxter EJ, Scott LM, Campbell PJ, East C, Fourouclas N, Swanton S *et al.* Acquired mutation of the tyrosine kinase JAK2 in human myeloproliferative disorders. *Lancet* 2005; 365: 1054-1061.

[15] Kralovics R, Passamonti F, Buser AS, Teo SS, Tiedt R, Passweg JR *et al.* A gain-of-function mutation of JAK2 in myeloproliferative disorders. *N Engl J Med* 2005; 352: 1779-1790.

[16] Levine RL, Wadleigh M, Cools J, Ebert BL, Wernig G, Huntly BJ *et al.* Activating mutation in the tyrosine kinase JAK2 in polycythemia vera, essential thrombocythemia, and myeloid metaplasia with myelofibrosis.*Cancer Cell* 2005; 7: 387-397.

[17] Zhao R, Xing S, Li Z, Fu X, Li Q, Krantz SB *et al.* Identification of an acquired JAK2 mutation in polycythemia vera. *J Biol Chem* 2005; 280: 22788-22792.

[18] Scott LM, Tong W, Levine RL, Scott MA, Beer PA, Stratton MR *et al.* JAK2 exon 12 mutations in polycythemia vera and idiopathic erythrocytosis. *N Engl J Med* 2007; 356: 459-468.

[19] Pikman Y, Lee BH, Mercher T, McDowell E, Ebert BL, Gozo M *et al.* MPLW515L is a novel somatic activating mutation in myelofibrosis with myeloid metaplasia. *PLoS Med* 2006; 3: e270.

[20] Pardanani AD, Levine RL, Lasho T, Pikman Y, Mesa RA, Wadleigh M *et al.* MPL515 mutations in myeloproliferative and other myeloid disorders: a study of 1182 patients. *Blood* 2006; 108: 3472-3476.

[21] Staerk J, Lacout C, Smith SO, Vainchenker W, Constantinescu SN. An amphipathic motif at the transmembrane-cytoplasmic junction prevents autonomous activation of the thrombopoietin receptor. *Blood* 2006; 107: 1864-1871.

[22] Campbell PJ, Scott LM, Buck G, Wheatley K, East CL, Marsden JT *et al.* Definition of subtypes of essential thrombocythaemia and relation to polycythaemia vera based on JAK2 V617F mutation status: a prospective study. *Lancet* 2005; 366: 1945-1953.

[23] Lacout C, Pisani DF, Tulliez M, Moreau Gachelin F, Vainchenker W, Villeval JL. JAK2V617F expression in murine hematopoietic cells leads to MPD mimicking human PV with secondary myelofibrosis. *Blood* 2006; 108: 1652-1660.

[24] Tiedt R, Hao-Shen H, Sobas MA, Looser R, Dirnhofer S, Schwaller J *et al.* Ratio of mutant JAK2-V617F to wild-type Jak2 determines the MPD phenotypes in transgenic mice. *Blood* 2008; 111: 3931-3940.

[25] Scott LM, Scott MA, Campbell PJ, Green AR. Progenitors homozygous for the V617F mutation occur in most patients with polycythemia vera, but not essential thrombocythemia. *Blood* 2006; 108: 2435-2437.

[26] Dupont S, Masse A, James C, Teyssandier I, Lecluse Y, Larbret F *et al.* The JAK2 617V>F mutation triggers erythropoietin hypersensitivity and terminal erythroid amplification in primary cells from patients with polycythemia vera. *Blood* 2007; 110: 1013–1021.

[27] Pardanani A, Fridley BL, Lasho TL, Gilliland DG, Tefferi A. Host genetic variation contributes to phenotypic diversity in myeloproliferative disorders. *Blood* 2008; 111: 2785–2789.

[28] Jamieson CH, Gotlib J, Durocher JA, Chao MP, Mariappan MR, Lay M *et al.* The JAK2 V617F mutation occurs in hematopoietic stem cells in polycythemia vera and predisposes toward erythroid differentiation. *Proc Natl Acad Sci USA* 2006; 103: 6224–6229.

[29] Delhommeau F, Dupont S, Tonetti C, Masse A, Godin I, Le Couedic JP *et al.* Evidence that the JAK2 G1849T (V617F) mutation occurs in a lymphomyeloid progenitor in polycythemia vera and idiopathic myelofibrosis. *Blood* 2007; 109: 71–77.

[30] James C, Mazurier F, Dupont S, Chaligne R, Lamrissi-Garcia I, Tulliez M *et al.* The hematopoietic stem cell compartment of JAK2V617F positive myeloproliferative disorders is a reflection of disease heterogeneity. *Blood*2008; e-pub ahead of print 8 July 2008; doi:10.1182/blood-2008-02-137877.

[31] Sieburg HB, Cho RH, Dykstra B, Uchida N, Eaves CJ, Muller-Sieburg CE. The hematopoietic stem compartment consists of a limited number of discrete stem cell subsets. *Blood* 2006; 107: 2311–2316.

[32] Pardanani A, Lasho TL, Schwager S, Finke C, Hussein K, Pruthi RK *et al.* JAK2V617F prevalence and allele burden in non-splanchnic venous thrombosis in the absence of overt myeloproliferative disorder. *Leukemia*2007; 21: 1828–1829.

[33] Pardanani A, Lasho TL, Hussein K, Schwager SM, Finke CM, Pruthi RK *et al.* JAK2V617F mutation screening as part of the hypercoagulable work-up in the absence of splanchnic venous thrombosis or overt myeloproliferative neoplasm: assessment of value in a series of 664 consecutive patients.*Mayo Clin Proc* 2008; 83: 457–459.

[34] Kiladjian JJ, Cervantes F, Leebeek FW, Marzac C, Cassinat B, Chevret S *et al.* The impact of JAK2 and MPL mutations on diagnosis and prognosis of splanchnic vein thrombosis. A report on 241 cases. *Blood* 2008; 111: 4922–4929.

[35] Patel RK, Lea NC, Heneghan MA, Westwood NB, Milojkovic D, Thanigaikumar M *et al.* Prevalence of the activating JAK2 tyrosine kinase mutation V617F in the Budd-Chiari syndrome. *Gastroenterology* 2006; 130: 2031–2038.

[36] Leibundgut EO, Horn MP, Brunold C, Pfanner-Meyer B, Marti D, Hirsiger H*et al.* Hematopoietic and endothelial progenitor cell trafficking in patients with myeloproliferative diseases. *Hematologica* 2006; 91: 1467–1474.

[37] Van Pelt K, Nollet F, Selleslag D, Knoops L, Constantinescu SN, Criel A *et al.* The JAK2V617F mutation can occur in a hematopoietic stem cell that exhibits no proliferative advantage: a case of human allogeneic transplantation. *Blood* 2008; 112: 921–922.

[38] Kralovics R, Teo SS, Li S, Theocharides A, Buser AS, Tichelli A *et al.* Acquisition of the V617F mutation of JAK2 is a late genetic event in a subset of patients with myeloproliferative disorders. *Blood* 2006; 108: 1377–1380.

[39] Theocharides A, Boissinot M, Girodon F, Garand R, Teo SS, Lippert E *et al*. Leukemic blasts in transformed JAK2-V617F-positive myeloproliferative disorders are frequently negative for the JAK2-V617F mutation. *Blood*2007; 110: 375–379.

[40] Nussenzveig RH, Swierczek SI, Jelinek J, Gaikwad A, Liu E, Verstovsek S *et al*. Polycythemia vera is not initiated by JAK2V617F mutation. *Exp Hematol*2007; 35: 32–38.

[41] Lodish HF, Berk A, Kaiser CA, Krieger M, Scott MP, Bretscher A *et al*.*Molecular Cell Biology, Chapter 16 Cell Signaling II: Signaling Pathways that Control Gene Activity*, 6th edn. WH Freeman and Company: New York, NY, 2007, pp 666–667.

[42] Wilks AF, Harpur AG, Kurban RR, Ralph SJ, Zurcher G, Ziemiecki A. Two novel protein-tyrosine kinases, each with a second phosphotransferase-related catalytic domain, define a new class of protein kinase. *Mol Cell Biol*1991; 11: 2057–2065.

[43] Girault JA, Labesse G, Mornon JP, Callebaut I. The N-termini of FAK and JAKs contain divergent band 4.1 domains. *Trends Biochem Sci* 1999; 24: 54–57.

[44] Huang LJ, Constantinescu SN, Lodish HF. The N-terminal domain of Janus kinase 2 is required for Golgi processing and cell surface expression of erythropoietin receptor. *Mol Cell* 2001; 8: 1327–1338.

[45] Radtke S, Hermanns HM, Haan C, Schmitz-Van De Leur H, Gascan H, Heinrich PC *et al*. Novel role for Janus kinase 1 in the regulation of oncostatin M receptor surface expression. *J Biol Chem* 2002; 10: 10.

[46] Ragimbeau J, Dondi E, Alcover A, Eid P, Uze G, Pellegrini S. The tyrosine kinase Tyk2 controls IFNAR1 cell surface expression. *EMBO J* 2003; 22: 537–547.

[47] Royer Y, Staerk J, Costuleanu M, Courtoy PJ, Constantinescu SN. Janus kinases affect thrombopoietin receptor cell surface localization and stability. *J Biol Chem* 2005; 280: 27251–27261.

[48] Yeh TC, Dondi E, Uze G, Pellegrini S. A dual role for the kinase-like domain of the tyrosine kinase Tyk2 in interferon-alpha signaling. *Proc Natl Acad Sci USA* 2000; 97: 8991–8996.

[49] Saharinen P, Silvennoinen O. The pseudokinase domain is required for suppression of basal activity of Jak2 and Jak3 tyrosine kinases and for cytokine-inducible activation of signal transduction. *J Biol Chem* 2002; 277: 47954–47963.

[50] Lindauer K, Loerting T, Liedl KR, Kroemer RT. Prediction of the structure of human Janus kinase 2 (JAK2) comprising the two carboxy-terminal domains reveals a mechanism for autoregulation. *Protein Eng* 2001; 14: 27–37.

[51] Staerk J, Kallin A, Demoulin J-B, Vainchenker W, Constantinescu SN. JAK1 and Tyk2 activation by the homologous polycythemia vera JAK2 V617F mutation: cross-talk with IGF1 receptor. *J Biol Chem* 2005; 280: 41893–41899.

[52] Jeong EG, Kim MS, Nam HK, Min CK, Lee S, Chung YJ *et al*. Somatic mutations of JAK1 and JAK3 in acute leukemias and solid cancers. *Clin Cancer Res* 2008; 14: 3716–3721.

[53] Flex E, Petrangeli V, Stella L, Chiaretti S, Hornakova T, Knoops L *et al*. Somatically acquired JAK1 mutations in adult acute lymphoblastic leukemia. *J Exp Med* 2008; 205: 751–758.

[54] Kohlhuber F, Rogers NC, Watling D, Feng J, Guschin D, Briscoe J *et al*. A JAK1/JAK2 chimera can sustain alpha and gamma interferon responses. *Mol Cell Biol* 1997; 17: 695–706.

[55] Li Z, Xu M, Xing S, Ho WT, Ishii T, Li Q *et al.* Erlotinib effectively inhibits JAK2V617F activity and polycythemia vera cell growth. *J Biol Chem* 2007;282: 3428–3432.
[56] Miura O, Cleveland JL, Ihle JN. Inactivation of erythropoietin receptor function by point mutations in a region having homology with other cytokine receptors. *Mol Cell Biol* 1993; 13: 1788–1795.
[57] Wernig G, Gonneville JR, Crowley BJ, Rodrigues MS, Reddy MM, Hudon HE*et al.* The Jak2V617F oncogene associated with myeloproliferative diseases requires a functional FERM domain for transformation and for expression of the Myc and Pim proto-oncogenes. *Blood* 2008; 111: 3751–3759.
[58] Behrmann I, Smyczek T, Heinrich PC, Schmitz-Van de Leur H, Komyod W, Giese B *et al.* Janus kinase (Jak) subcellular localization revisited: the exclusive membrane localization of endogenous Janus kinase 1 by cytokine receptor interaction uncovers the Jak.receptor complex to be equivalent to a receptor tyrosine kinase. *J Biol Chem* 2004; 279: 35486–35493.
[59] Funakoshi-Tago M, Pelletier S, Moritake H, Parganas E, Ihle JN. Jak2 FERM domain interaction with the erythropoietin receptor regulates Jak2 kinase activity. *Mol Cell Biol* 2008; 28: 1792–1801.
[60] Lu X, Huang LJ, Lodish HF. Dimerization by a cytokine receptor is necessary for constitutive activation of JAK2V617F. *J Biol Chem* 2008; 283: 5258–5266.
[61] Saharinen P, Takaluoma K, Silvennoinen O. Regulation of the Jak2 tyrosine kinase by its pseudokinase domain. *Mol Cell Biol* 2000; 20: 3387–3395.
[62] Witthuhn BA, Quelle FW, Silvennoinen O, Yi T, Tang B, Miura O *et al.* JAK2 associates with the erythropoietin receptor and is tyrosine phosphorylated and activated following stimulation with erythropoietin. *Cell* 1993; 74: 227–236.
[63] Tortolani PJ, Johnston JA, Bacon CM, McVicar DW, Shimosaka A, Linnekin D*et al.* Thrombopoietin induces tyrosine phosphorylation and activation of the Janus kinase, JAK2. *Blood* 1995; 85: 3444–3451.
[64] Drachman JG, Millett KM, Kaushansky K. Thrombopoietin signal transduction requires functional JAK2, not TYK2. *J Biol Chem* 1999; 274: 13480–13484.
[65] Shimoda K, Feng J, Murakami H, Nagata S, Watling D, Rogers NC *et al.* Jak1 plays an essential role for receptor phosphorylation and Stat activation in response to granulocyte colony-stimulating factor. *Blood* 1997;90: 597–604.
[66] Touw IP, van de Geijn GJ. Granulocyte colony-stimulating factor and its receptor in normal myeloid cell development, leukemia and related blood cell disorders. *Front Biosci* 2007; 12: 800–815.
[67] Watowich SS, Wu H, Socolovsky M, Klingmuller U, Constantinescu SN, Lodish HF. Cytokine receptor signal transduction and the control of hematopoietic cell development. *Annu Rev Cell Dev Biol* 1996; 12: 91–128.
[68] Constantinescu SN, Keren T, Socolovsky M, Nam H, Henis YI, Lodish HF. Ligand-independent oligomerization of cell-surface erythropoietin receptor is mediated by the transmembrane domain. *Proc Natl Acad Sci USA* 2001;98: 4379–4384.
[69] Constantinescu SN, Huang LJ, Nam H, Lodish HF. The erythropoietin receptor cytosolic juxtamembrane domain contains an essential, precisely oriented, hydrophobic motif. *Mol Cell* 2001; 7: 377–385.

[70] Seubert N, Royer Y, Staerk J, Kubatzky KF, Moucadel V, Krishnakumar S *et al.* Active and inactive orientations of the transmembrane and cytosolic domains of the erythropoietin receptor dimer. *Mol Cell* 2003; 12: 1239–1250.

[71] Lu X, Levine R, Tong W, Wernig G, Pikman Y, Zarnegar S *et al.* Expression of a homodimeric type I cytokine receptor is required for JAK2V617F-mediated transformation. *Proc Natl Acad Sci USA* 2005; 102: 18962–18967.

[72] Ihle JN, Gilliland DG. Jak2: normal function and role in hematopoietic disorders. *Curr Opin Genet Dev* 2007; 17: 8–14.

[73] Kirito K, Nakajima K, Watanabe T, Uchida M, Tanaka M, Ozawa K *et al.* Identification of the human erythropoietin receptor region required for Stat1 and Stat3 activation. *Blood* 2002; 99: 102–110.

[74] Gobert S, Chretien S, Gouilleux F, Muller O, Pallard C, Dusanter-Fourt I *et al.* Identification of tyrosine residues within the intracellular domain of the erythropoietin receptor crucial for STAT5 activation. *EMBO J* 1996; 15: 2434–2441.

[75] Klingmuller U, Bergelson S, Hsiao JG, Lodish HF. Multiple tyrosine residues in the cytosolic domain of the erythropoietin receptor promote activation of STAT5. *Proc Natl Acad Sci USA* 1996; 93: 8324–8328.

[76] Socolovsky M, Fallon AE, Wang S, Brugnara C, Lodish HF. Fetal anemia and apoptosis of red cell progenitors in Stat5a-/-5b-/- mice: a direct role for Stat5 in Bcl-X(L) induction. *Cell* 1999; 98: 181–191.

[77] Klingmuller U, Wu H, Hsiao JG, Toker A, Duckworth BC, Cantley LC *et al.* Identification of a novel pathway important for proliferation and differentiation of primary erythroid progenitors. *Proc Natl Acad Sci USA*1997; 94: 3016–3021.

[78] Damen JE, Cutler RL, Jiao H, Yi T, Krystal G. Phosphorylation of tyrosine 503 in the erythropoietin receptor (EpR) is essential for binding the P85 subunit of phosphatidylinositol (PI) 3-kinase and for EpR-associated PI 3-kinase activity. *J Biol Chem* 1995; 270: 23402–23408.

[79] Bao H, Jacobs-Helber SM, Lawson AE, Penta K, Wickrema A, Sawyer ST. Protein kinase B (c-Akt), phosphatidylinositol 3-kinase, and STAT5 are activated by erythropoietin (EPO) in HCD57 erythroid cells but are constitutively active in an EPO-independent, apoptosis-resistant subclone (HCD57-SREI cells). *Blood* 1999; 93: 3757–3773.

[80] Kashii Y, Uchida M, Kirito K, Tanaka M, Nishijima K, Toshima M *et al.* A member of Forkhead family transcription factor, FKHRL1, is one of the downstream molecules of phosphatidylinositol 3-kinase–Akt activation pathway in erythropoietin signal transduction. *Blood* 2000; 96: 941–949.

[81] Zhao W, Kitidis C, Fleming MD, Lodish HF, Ghaffari S. Erythropoietin stimulates phosphorylation and activation of GATA-1 via the PI3-kinase/AKT signaling pathway. *Blood* 2006; 107: 907–915.

[82] Butcher CM, Hahn U, To LB, Gecz J, Wilkins EJ, Scott HS *et al.* Two novel JAK2 exon 12 mutations in JAK2V617F-negative polycythaemia vera patients. *Leukemia* 2008; 22: 870–873.

[83] Miyakawa Y, Oda A, Druker BJ, Kato T, Miyazaki H, Handa M *et al.* Recombinant thrombopoietin induces rapid protein tyrosine phosphorylation of Janus kinase 2 and Shc in human blood platelets. *Blood* 1995; 86: 23–27.

[84] Sattler M, Durstin MA, Frank DA, Okuda K, Kaushansky K, Salgia R *et al.* The thrombopoietin receptor c-MPL activates JAK2 and TYK2 tyrosine kinases. *Exp Hematol* 1995; 23: 1040–1048.
[85] Miyakawa Y, Rojnuckarin P, Habib T, Kaushansky K. Thrombopoietin induces phosphoinositol 3-kinase activation through SHP2, Gab, and insulin receptor substrate proteins in BAF3 cells and primary murine megakaryocytes. *J Biol Chem* 2001; 276: 2494–2502.
[86] Drachman JG, Griffin JD, Kaushansky K. The c-Mpl ligand (thrombopoietin) stimulates tyrosine phosphorylation of Jak2, Shc, and c-Mpl. *J Biol Chem*1995; 270: 4979–4982.
[87] Miyakawa Y, Oda A, Druker BJ, Miyazaki H, Handa M, Ohashi H *et al.* Thrombopoietin induces tyrosine phosphorylation of Stat3 and Stat5 in human blood platelets. *Blood* 1996; 87: 439–446.
[88] Drachman JG, Kaushansky K. Dissecting the thrombopoietin receptor: functional elements of the Mpl cytoplasmic domain. *Proc Natl Acad Sci USA*1997; 94: 2350–2355.
[89] Rouyez MC, Boucheron C, Gisselbrecht S, Dusanter-Fourt I, Porteu F. Control of thrombopoietin-induced megakaryocytic differentiation by the mitogen-activated protein kinase pathway. *Mol Cell Biol* 1997; 17: 4991–5000.
[90] Filippi MD, Porteu F, Le Pesteur F, Schiavon V, Millot GA, Vainchenker W *et al.* Requirement for mitogen-activated protein kinase activation in the response of embryonic stem cell-derived hematopoietic cells to thrombopoietin *in vitro*. *Blood* 2002; 99: 1174–1182.
[91] Olthof SG, Fatrai S, Drayer AL, Tyl MR, Vellenga E, Schuringa JJ. Downregulation of STAT5 in CD34+ cells promotes megakaryocytic development while activation of STAT5 drives erythropoiesis. *Stem Cells*2008; 26: 1732–1742.
[92] Cocault L, Bouscary D, Le Bousse Kerdiles C, Clay D, Picard F, Gisselbrecht S *et al.* Ectopic expression of murine TPO receptor (c-mpl) in mice is pathogenic and induces erythroblastic proliferation. *Blood* 1996; 88: 1656–1665.
[93] Tong W, Lodish HF. Lnk inhibits Tpo-mpl signaling and Tpo-mediated megakaryocytopoiesis. *J Exp Med* 2004; 200: 569–580.
[94] Tong W, Zhang J, Lodish HF. Lnk inhibits erythropoiesis and Epo-dependent JAK2 activation and downstream signaling pathways. *Blood* 2005; 105: 4604–4612.
[95] Moliterno AR, Spivak JL. Posttranslational processing of the thrombopoietin receptor is impaired in polycythemia vera. *Blood* 1999; 94: 2555–2561.
[96] Moliterno AR, Williams DM, Rogers O, Spivak JL. Molecular mimicry in the chronic myeloproliferative disorders: reciprocity between quantitative JAK2 V617F and Mpl expression. *Blood* 2006; 108: 3913–3915.
[97] Dahlen DD, Broudy VC, Drachman JG. Internalization of the thrombopoietin receptor is regulated by 2 cytoplasmic motifs. *Blood* 2003; 102: 102–108.
[98] Onishi M, Mui AL, Morikawa Y, Cho L, Kinoshita S, Nolan GP *et al.* Identification of an oncogenic form of the thrombopoietin receptor MPL using retrovirus-mediated gene transfer. *Blood* 1996; 88: 1399–1406.
[99] Ding J, Komatsu H, Wakita A, Kato-Uranishi M, Ito M, Satoh A *et al.* Familial essential thrombocythemia associated with a dominant-positive activating mutation of the c-

MPL gene, which encodes for the receptor for thrombopoietin. *Blood* 2004; 103: 4198–4200.

[100] Malinge S, Ragu C, Della-Valle V, Pisani D, Constantinescu SN, Perez C *et al.* Activating mutations in human acute megakaryoblastic leukemia. *Blood*2008.

[101] Bumm TG, Elsea C, Corbin AS, Loriaux M, Sherbenou D, Wood L *et al.* Characterization of murine JAK2V617F-positive myeloproliferative disease.*Cancer Res* 2006; 66: 11156–11165.

[102] Gangat N, Strand J, Li CY, Wu W, Pardanani A, Tefferi A. Leucocytosis in polycythaemia vera predicts both inferior survival and leukaemic transformation. *Br J Haematol* 2007; 138: 354–358.

[103] Kralovics R, Teo SS, Buser AS, Brutsche M, Tiedt R, Tichelli A *et al.* Altered gene expression in myeloproliferative disorders correlates with activation of signaling by the V617F mutation of Jak2. *Blood* 2005; 106: 3374–3376.

[104] Passamonti F, Rumi E, Pietra D, Della Porta MG, Boveri E, Pascutto C *et al.* Relation between JAK2 (V617F) mutation status, granulocyte activation, and constitutive mobilization of CD34+ cells into peripheral blood in myeloproliferative disorders. *Blood* 2006; 107: 3676–3682.

[105] Xu M, Bruno E, Chao J, Huang S, Finazzi G, Fruchtman SM *et al.* Constitutive mobilization of CD34+ cells into the peripheral blood in idiopathic myelofibrosis may be due to the action of a number of proteases. *Blood* 2005; 105: 4508–4515.

[106] Rosti V, Massa M, Vannucchi AM, Bergamaschi G, Campanelli R, Pecci A *et al.* The expression of CXCR4 is down-regulated on the CD34+ cells of patients with myelofibrosis with myeloid metaplasia. *Blood Cells Mol Dis*2007; 38: 280–286.

[107] Migliaccio AR, Martelli F, Verrucci M, Migliaccio G, Vannucchi AM, Ni H *et al.* Altered SDF-1/CXCR4 axis in patients with primary myelofibrosis and in the Gata1 low mouse model of the disease. *Exp Hematol* 2008; 36: 158–171.

[108] Broxmeyer HE, Orschell CM, Clapp DW, Hangoc G, Cooper S, Plett PA *et al.* Rapid mobilization of murine and human hematopoietic stem and progenitor cells with AMD3100, a CXCR4 antagonist. *J Exp Med* 2005; 201: 1307–1318.

[109] Feng J, Witthuhn BA, Matsuda T, Kohlhuber F, Kerr IM, Ihle JN. Activation of Jak2 catalytic activity requires phosphorylation of Y1007 in the kinase activation loop. *Mol Cell Biol* 1997; 17: 2497–2501.

[110] Matsuda T, Feng J, Witthuhn BA, Sekine Y, Ihle JN. Determination of the transphosphorylation sites of Jak2 kinase. *Biochem Biophys Res Commun*2004; 325: 586–594.

[111] Argetsinger LS, Kouadio JL, Steen H, Stensballe A, Jensen ON, Carter-Su C. Autophosphorylation of JAK2 on tyrosines 221 and 570 regulates its activity. *Mol Cell Biol* 2004; 24: 4955–4967.

[112] Feener EP, Rosario F, Dunn SL, Stancheva Z, Myers Jr MG. Tyrosine phosphorylation of Jak2 in the JH2 domain inhibits cytokine signaling. *Mol Cell Biol* 2004; 24: 4968–4978.

[113] Funakoshi-Tago M, Pelletier S, Matsuda T, Parganas E, Ihle JN. Receptor specific downregulation of cytokine signaling by autophosphorylation in the FERM domain of Jak2. *EMBO J* 2006; 25: 4763–4772.

[114] Kurzer JH, Argetsinger LS, Zhou YJ, Kouadio JL, O'Shea JJ, Carter-Su C. Tyrosine 813 is a site of JAK2 autophosphorylation critical for activation of JAK2 by SH2-B beta. *Mol Cell Biol* 2004; 24: 4557–4570.

[115] Nishi M, Werner ED, Oh BC, Frantz JD, Dhe-Paganon S, Hansen L *et al.* Kinase activation through dimerization by human SH2-B. *Mol Cell Biol*2005; 25: 2607–2621.

[116] Vainchenker W, Constantinescu SN. A unique activating mutation in JAK2 is at the origin of polycythemia vera and allows a new classification of myeloproliferative diseases. *Hematology Am Soc Hematol Educ Program*2005; 2005: 195–200.

[117] Mesa RA, Tefferi A, Lasho TS, Loegering D, McClure RF, Powell HL *et al.* Janus kinase 2 (V617F) mutation status, signal transducer and activator of transcription-3 phosphorylation and impaired neutrophil apoptosis in myelofibrosis with myeloid metaplasia. *Leukemia* 2006; 20: 1800–1808.

[118] Teofili L, Martini M, Cenci T, Petrucci G, Torti L, Storti S *et al.* Different STAT-3 and STAT-5 phosphorylation discriminates among Ph-negative chronic myeloproliferative diseases and is independent of the V617F JAK-2 mutation. *Blood* 2007; 110: 354–359.

[119] Nicholson SE, De Souza D, Fabri LJ, Corbin J, Willson TA, Zhang JG *et al.* Suppressor of cytokine signaling-3 preferentially binds to the SHP-2-binding site on the shared cytokine receptor subunit gp130. *Proc Natl Acad Sci USA* 2000; 97: 6493–6498.

[120] Schmitz J, Weissenbach M, Haan S, Heinrich PC, Schaper F. SOCS3 exerts its inhibitory function on interleukin-6 signal transduction through the SHP2 recruitment site of gp130. *J Biol Chem* 2000; 275: 12848–12856.

[121] Jenkins BJ, Roberts AW, Najdovska M, Grail D, Ernst M. The threshold of gp130-dependent STAT3 signaling is critical for normal regulation of hematopoiesis. *Blood* 2005; 105: 3512–3520.

[122] Yoshimura A, Naka T, Kubo M. SOCS proteins, cytokine signalling and immune regulation. *Nat Rev Immunol* 2007; 7: 454–465.

[123] Hortner M, Nielsch U, Mayr LM, Heinrich PC, Haan S. A new high affinity binding site for suppressor of cytokine signaling-3 on the erythropoietin receptor. *Eur J Biochem* 2002; 269: 2516–2526.

[124] Hookham MB, Elliott J, Suessmuth Y, Staerk J, Ward AC, Vainchenker W *et al.* The myeloproliferative disorder-associated JAK2 V617F mutant escapes negative regulation by suppressor of cytokine signaling 3. *Blood* 2007;109: 4924–4929.

[125] Cacalano NA, Sanden D, Johnston JA. Tyrosine-phosphorylated SOCS-3 inhibits STAT activation but binds to p120 RasGAP and activates Ras. *Nat Cell Biol* 2001; 3: 460–465.

[126] Dusa A, Staerk J, Elliott J, Pecquet C, Poirel HA, Johnston JA *et al.* Substitution of pseudokinase domain residue V617 by large non-polar amino acids causes activation of JAK2. *J Biol Chem* 2008; 283: 12941–12948.

[127] Wernig G, Mercher T, Okabe R, Levine RL, Lee BH, Gilliland DG. Expression of Jak2V617F causes a polycythemia vera-like disease with associated myelofibrosis in a murine bone marrow transplant model. *Blood* 2006;107: 4274–4281.

[128] Knoops L, Hornakova T, Royer Y, Constantinescu SN, Renauld JC. JAK kinases overexpression promotes *in vitro* cell transformation. *Oncogene*2008; 27: 1511–1519.

[129] Ugo V, Marzac C, Teyssandier I, Larbret F, Lecluse Y, Debili N *et al.* Multiple signaling pathways are involved in erythropoietin-independent differentiation of erythroid progenitors in polycythemia vera. *Exp Hematol*2004; 32: 179–187.

[130] Pardanani A, Hood J, Lasho T, Levine RL, Martin MB, Noronha G *et al.* TG101209, a small molecule JAK2-selective kinase inhibitor potently inhibits myeloproliferative disorder-associated JAK2V617F and MPLW515L/K mutations. *Leukemia* 2007; 21: 1658–1668.

[131] Wernig G, Kharas MG, Okabe R, Moore SA, Leeman DS, Cullen DE *et al.* Efficacy of TG101348, a selective JAK2 inhibitor, in treatment of a murine model of JAK2V617F-induced polycythemia vera. *Cancer Cell* 2008; 13: 311–320.

[132] Geron I, Abrahamsson AE, Barroga CF, Kavalerchik E, Gotlib J, Hood JD *et al.* Selective inhibition of JAK2-driven erythroid differentiation of polycythemia vera progenitors. *Cancer Cell* 2008; 13: 321–330.

[133] Weiss MJ, Orkin SH. GATA transcription factors: key regulators of hematopoiesis. *Exp Hematol* 1995; 23: 99–107.

[134] Cantor AB, Orkin SH. Transcriptional regulation of erythropoiesis: an affair involving multiple partners. *Oncogene* 2002; 21: 3368–3376.

[135] Mirza AM, Correa PN, Axelrad AA. Increased basal and induced tyrosine phosphorylation of the insulin-like growth factor I receptor beta subunit in circulating mononuclear cells of patients with polycythemia vera. *Blood*1995; 86: 877–882.

[136] Jones AV, Silver RT, Waghorn K, Curtis C, Kreil S, Zoi K *et al.* Minimal molecular response in polycythemia vera patients treated with imatinib or interferon alpha. *Blood* 2006; 107: 3339–3341.

[137] Gaikwad A, Verstovsek S, Yoon D, Chang KT, Manshouri T, Nussenzveig R*et al.* Imatinib effect on growth and signal transduction in polycythemia vera. *Exp Hematol* 2007; 35: 931–938.

[138] Chin H, Arai A, Wakao H, Kamiyama R, Miyasaka N, Miura O. Lyn physically associates with the erythropoietin receptor and may play a role in activation of the Stat5 pathway. *Blood* 1998; 91: 3734–3745.

[139] Zaleskas VM, Krause DS, Lazarides K, Patel N, Hu Y, Li S *et al.* Molecular pathogenesis and therapy of polycythemia induced in mice by JAK2 V617F.*PLoS ONE* 2006; 1: e18.

[140] Zeuner A, Pedini F, Signore M, Ruscio G, Messina C, Tafuri A *et al.* Increased death receptor resistance and FLIPshort expression in polycythemia vera erythroid precursor cells. *Blood* 2006; 107: 3495–3502.

[141] Le Bousse-Kerdilès MC, Martyré MC. Involvement of the fibrogenic cytokines, TGF-beta and bFGF, in the pathogenesis of idiopathic myelofibrosis. *Pathol Biol (Paris)* 2001; 49: 153–157.

[142] Villeval JL, Cohen-Solal K, Tulliez M, Giraudier S, Guichard J, Burstein SA*et al.* High thrombopoietin production by hematopoietic cells induces a fatal myeloproliferative syndrome in mice. *Blood* 1997; 90: 4369–4383.

[143] Chagraoui H, Komura E, Tulliez M, Giraudier S, Vainchenker W, Wendling F. Prominent role of TGF-beta 1 in thrombopoietin-induced myelofibrosis in mice. *Blood* 2002; 100: 3495–3503.

[144] Ciurea SO, Merchant D, Mahmud N, Ishii T, Zhao Y, Hu W *et al.* Pivotal contributions of megakaryocytes to the biology of idiopathic myelofibrosis.*Blood* 2007; 110: 986–993.

[145] Jenkins BJ, Grail D, Nheu T, Najdovska M, Wang B, Waring P *et al.* Hyperactivation of Stat3 in gp130 mutant mice promotes gastric hyperproliferation and desensitizes TGF-beta signaling. *Nat Med* 2005; 11: 845–852.

[146] Vannucchi AM, Bianchi L, Paoletti F, Pancrazzi A, Torre E, Nishikawa M *et al.* A pathobiologic pathway linking thrombopoietin, GATA-1, and TGF-beta1 in the development of myelofibrosis. *Blood* 2005; 105: 3493–3501.

[147] Shi S, Calhoun HC, Xia F, Li J, Le L, Li WX. JAK signaling globally counteracts heterochromatic gene silencing. *Nat Genet* 2006; 38: 1071–1076.

[148] Muller P, Kuttenkeuler D, Gesellchen V, Zeidler MP, Boutros M. Identification of JAK/STAT signalling components by genome-wide RNA interference. *Nature* 2005; 436: 871–875.

[149] Guerini V, Barbui V, Spinelli O, Salvi A, Dellacasa C, Carobbio A *et al.* The histone deacetylase inhibitor ITF2357 selectively targets cells bearing mutated JAK2(V617F). *Leukemia* 2008; 22: 740–747.

[150] Schuebel KE, Chen W, Cope L, Glockner SC, Suzuki H, Yi JM *et al.* Comparing the DNA hypermethylome with gene mutations in human colorectal cancer. *PLoS Genet* 2007; 3: 1709–1723.

[151] Shi J, Zhao Y, Ishii T, Hu W, Sozer S, Zhang W *et al.* Effects of chromatin-modifying agents on CD34+ cells from patients with idiopathic myelofibrosis. *Cancer Res* 2007; 67: 6417–6424.

[152] Jelinek J, Li J, Mnjoyan Z, Issa JP, Prchal JT, Afshar-Kharghan V. Epigenetic control of PRV-1 expression on neutrophils. *Exp Hematol* 2007; 35: 1677–1683.

[153] Temerinac S, Klippel S, Strunck E, Roder S, Lubbert M, Lange W *et al.* Cloning of PRV-1, a novel member of the uPAR receptor superfamily, which is overexpressed in polycythemia rubra vera. *Blood* 2000; 95: 2569–2576.

[154] Jost E, do ON, Dahl E, Maintz CE, Jousten P, Habets L *et al.* Epigenetic alterations complement mutation of JAK2 tyrosine kinase in patients with BCR/ABL-negative myeloproliferative disorders. *Leukemia* 2007; 21: 505–510.

[155] Dawson MA, Bannister AJ, Gottgens B, et al. JAK2 phosphorylates histone H3Y41 and excludes HP1alpha from chromatin. Nature. 2009;461(7265):819-22.

[156] McCormack, M. P. & Rabbitts, T. H. Activation of the T-cell oncogene LMO2 after gene therapy for X-linked severe combined immunodeficiency. N Engl J Med. 2004;350:913–922.

[157] Yoshihiro Y, Warren AJ, Dobson C, Foster A, Pannel R, Rabbits TH. The T cell leukemia LIM protein Lmo2 is necessary for adult mouse hematopoiesis. Proc Natl Acad Sci USA. 1998; 95:3890–3895.

[158] Ma AC, Ward AC, Liang R, Leung AY. The role of jak2a in zebrafish hematopoiesis. Blood. 2007;110:1824–1830.

[159] Seo IA, Lee HK, Shin YK, Lee SH, et al. Janus Kinase 2 Inhibitor AG490 Inhibits the STAT3 Signaling Pathway by Suppressing Protein Translation of gp130. Korean J Physiol Pharmacol. 2009;13(2):131-138.

[160] Tsuchiya Y, Takahashi N, Yoshizaki T, et al. A Jak2 inhibitor, AG490, reverses lipin-1 suppression by TNF-alpha in 3T3-L1 adipocytes. Biochem Biophys Res Commun. 2009;382(2):348-352.

[161] A Pardanani, J Gotlib, C Jamieson, et al Safety and efficacy of TG101348, a selective JAK2 inhibitor, in myelofibrosis *Journal of Clinical Oncology* (2011)

13

Physiological and Pathological Aspects of Human NK Cells

Chiara Vitale[1], Renato Zambello[2], Mirna Balsamo[3], Maria Cristina Mingari[1,4] and Massimo Vitale[4]

[1]*DI.ME.S. Università di Genova, Genova*

[2]*Padova University School of Medicine, Department of Clinical and Experimental Medicine, Hematology and Clinical Immunology Branch – Padova*

[3]*Istituto G. Gaslini – Genova*

[4]*IRCCS A.O.U. S.Martino-IST Istituto Nazionale per la Ricerca sul Cancro, S.C. Immunologia - Genova*

Italy

1. Introduction

Natural Killer (NK) cells were first defined, more than 30 years ago, on the basis of their unique capability of killing spontaneously different targets including tumor and virus-infected cells. Thus, since their first discovery, NK cells came across as a potential attractive tool for the implementation of immuno-therapeutic strategies for different diseases. Accordingly, besides the plethora of studies aimed at investigating their functional and phenotypic properties, considerable efforts have also been spent in the past several years to understand how these cells could be generated and how their functions could be regulated and/or manipulated. At the same time further attention has been paid on their alteration in vivo and their potential role in the occurrence of NK cell-based hematological malignancies.

2. NK cells: From a function to a multifaceted population

2.1 The discovery of NK cells

NK cells were originally identified on a functional basis. In the middle '70s, it was discovered that healthy individuals could display selective cytotoxic activity against tumor or virally infected cells and that this activity was hidden within the circulating lymphocyte population (West et al., 1977; Santoli et al., 1978). This implied the presence in the Peripheral Blood (PB) of a lymphocyte subset capable of killing different targets without previous sensitization. These cells, that for their functional properties were termed 'Natural Killer', were then characterized morphologically as Large Granular Lymphocytes (LGL) by virtue of their size and cytolytic granule content. Finally, in the late '80s, NK cells were more precisely defined with the $CD3^-CD56^+CD16^+$ surface immuno-phenotype. This also allowed the identification of the CD16/FcγRIII as the receptor responsible for the Antibody-Dependent Cell Cytotoxicity (ADCC) function shown by NK cells (Lanier et al., 1986; Trinchieri, 1989). In the same period, the circulating NK cell population, which represented approximately 10-15% of PB lymphocytes, was further split into CD56^{bright}CD16$^{dim/neg}$ and CD56^{dim}CD16^{bright} cell subsets, expressing respectively low and high cytolytic properties. In the following 10 years great efforts were done to widen the list of NK cell markers and to define the surface receptors responsible for the regulation of NK cell cytotoxicity. Finally, in the last decade it was discovered that NK cells could exert different regulatory functions, and many studies were oriented to the definition of novel NK cell subsets involved in such unexpected functional features.

2.2 The regulation of NK cell function: Activating and inhibitory receptors

Once NK cells could be physically identified and isolated, the goal was to understand how these cells could work; and the first questions were: "How can a single NK cell kill different targets?" and "how do NK cells recognize and spare self normal cells?" The answer to these questions was indicated by Karre in his "missing self hypothesis". He postulated that NK cells could sense the absence (or reduction) of self MHC class I molecules (MHC-I) during cell-to-cell interaction: the missing recognition of self would allow NK cells to kill the targets, while recognition of self MHC-I would inhibit their cytolytic activity (Ljunggren & Karre, 1990). This would explain how NK cells could kill tumor or virus infected cells, which frequently undergo surface MHC-I down-regulation, and spare self non-pathogenic cells, equipped with appropriate levels MHC-I. The hypothesis was then confirmed, and the inhibitory MHC-I-specific receptors responsible for the recognition of Self were identified. In humans, major HLA-I-specific inhibitory receptors are represented by the C-type lectin CD94/NKG2A dimer that recognizes the non-classical HLA-E alleles, and the Killer Ig-like Receptors (KIR). The CD94/NKG2A encoding genes are located in the NK Receptor complex on chromosome 12, while the KIR locus is located in the Leukocyte Receptor Complex in Chromosome 19. The KIRs constitute a family of strictly homologous proteins characterized by the presence of two or three extracytoplasmic Ig-like domains (KIR2D or KIR3D) and a long cytoplasmic tail (KIR2DL or KIR3DL) containing Immuno Tyrosine-based Inhibitory Motifs (ITIMs) for the inhibitory signal transduction. Each KIR recognizes a specific epitope common to a defined group of HLA-I alleles. In particular, KIR2DL1 recognizes the Lys80 containing C2 epitope, that is shared by a group of HLA-C alleles; KIR2DL2/L3 recognize the Asn80 containing C1 epitope, that is shared by the remaining alleles of the locus HLA-C; KIR3DL1 recognizes the Ile/Thr80 containing HLA-Bw4 epitope, that is common to certain HLA-A and HLA-B alleles, while KIR3DL2 recognizes certain HLA-A alleles (Biassoni et al., 2001; Parham, 2005). Interestingly, KIR3DL2 has also been recently shown to bind microbial nucleic acids at the cell surface and to shuttle them to TLR9 in the endosome, suggesting for certain KIR a novel (or rather an ancient) function as pathogen sensors (Sivori et al., 2010). The HLA-I-specific inhibitory receptors are clonally distributed within the NK cell population of each individual. Most NK cells express one or more receptors and at least one that recognize an autologous HLA-I allele. Recently, a KIR$^-$ NKG2A$^-$ NK cell subset has been described in different donors. These cells, however, appeared to be poorly functional. This suggested that the expression and the engagement of inhibitory receptors during maturation of NK cells could dictate the acquisition of their cytolytic potential (Licensing theory) (Anfossi et al., 2006). The KIR family also includes activating KIRs. These are homologous to their inhibitory counterparts, but display a short cytoplasmic tail (KIR2DS or KIR3DS), lack ITIMs and associate an ITAM-bearing molecule (DAP12) to transduce activating signals. Similarly, also for NKG2A, does exist a short-tailed activating counterpart, termed NKG2C. The meaning of these receptors is poorly known. It has been hypothesized that they may recognize HLA-I molecules loaded with viral or tumor peptides, or, with low affinity, normal HLA-I molecules. In this latter case, when target cells selectively down-regulate HLA alleles, recognized by inhibitory KIR, the engagement of activating KIR may result in NK cell activation. The simultaneous expression of activating and inhibitory KIRs may therefore represent a strategy whereby NK cells can recognize and kill pathologic cells uniquely by detecting changes in their HLA alleles repertoire. At present, however, binding to HLA-I molecules has been formally demonstrated only for KIR2DS1 and NKG2C.

NK cells are also equipped with a large array of non-HLA-specific triggering receptors and co-receptors, whose engagement by specific Ligands expressed on target cells induces NK cell cytotoxicity and cytokine release (Moretta A. et al., 2001; Vivier et al., 2011). The group of NK-triggering receptors is largely heterogeneous: it encompasses molecules either structurally unrelated or belonging to different molecular families. At variance with KIRs, triggering receptors are expressed by virtually all NK cells and, in most cases, by different lymphocyte subsets or monocytes. The activating receptor Ligands till now identified, appear to be over-expressed in one or more of the following cases: tumor transformation, viral infection, cell stress or activation. Consistently, most of the activating receptors have been shown to be variably involved in the recognition and killing of virus infected and/or tumor cells. Two members of CD2 family: 2B4 (CD244) and NTBA, which recognize CD48 and NTBA respectively, have been involved in the clearance of EBV-infected cells. NKp80 and NKG2D, two Killer cell Lectin Receptors (KLR) encoded in the NK gene Complex on human chromosome 12, recognize molecules that can be expressed on tumor and/or virus infected cells. NKp80 recognizes AICL (encoded in the same NK gene complex) that is expressed on activated monocytes, but it can be also expressed on malignant myeloid cells (Welte et al., 2006). NKG2D recognizes MHC-I-related stress-inducible molecules of the MIC and ULBP families, that can be up-regulated on virus infected or tumor cells. Three receptors, that are expressed on cytotoxic lymphocytes (both NK and T cells), DNAM-1 (CD226), TACTILE (CD96) and CRTAM, recognize members of the Nectin/Nectin-Like (NecL) family (Fuchs & Colonna, 2006). In particular DNAM-1, that is the most highly espressed on NK cells, recognizes Nectin2 (CD112) and NecL5 (CD155 - poliovirus receptor) (Bottino et al., 2003). Nectin/NecL molecules are involved in the formation of various types of cell-to-cell junctions, especially in epithelial cells, neurons or fibroblasts. Nectins 1 and 2, and NecL5 can also serve as viral entry receptors. These molecules, however, are frequently up-regulated in tumor cells of different histotypes. In addition, CMV infection can alter NecL5-Nectin3 intercellular interaction: in this case NecL5 would be exposed outside the cellular junction and allow DNAM-1 recognition.

While all the above-mentioned activating receptors are expressed by different leukocyte subsets, NKp30, NKp46 and NKp44 triggering receptors are restricted to NK cells. NKp44 and NKp46 are involved in the recognition of both viral antigens (as the influenza virus HA) (Mandelboim et al., 2001) and ligands expressed by tumor cells. NKp30 recognizes B7H6 and BAT-3 (Brandt et al., 2009; Pogge von Strandmann et al., 2007). B7H6 is a member of the B7 family (which includes ligands for stimulatory/inhibitory T cell co-receptors CD28/CTLA4). B7H6 is poorly expressed on normal cells, while it is up-regulated in different tumor cell lines. BAT-3 is a nuclear factor released in exosomes by tumor cells and Dendritic Cells (DC) in response to stress/activation stimuli. The tumor ligands for NKp46 and NKp44 remain still undefined. The NKp30, NKp46 and NKp44 receptors are structurally and genetically unrelated. NKp46 encoding gene is located within the Leukocyte Receptor Complex in Chromosome 19, while the NKp30 and NKp44 encoding genes are located in separated regions in chromosome 6. However, for their expression pattern, restricted to NK cells, and their impressive capability of triggering NK cell cytotoxicity against an extremely wide range of tumor cell lines, they were grouped and collectively termed Natural Cytotoxicity Receptors (NCRs).

Among the triggering receptors, NKp30, NKp46, NKp44, NKG2D and DNAM-1 are indispensable for the NK-mediated recognition and killing of tumor cells. Different studies have demonstrated how their blockade, impairment of function, or expression failure, heavily compromise the efficacy of NK cells in killing tumor cells in vitro, or in containing tumor growth in animal models (Bottino et al., 2004; Iguchi-Manaka et al., 2008; Guerra et al., 2008; Halfteck et al., 2009). Notably, NK cells can significantly improve their functional capabilities in response to various cytokines including type I IFN, IL-2, IL-15, IL-12 and IL-18. In this context, exposure to IL-2, IL-15 and IL-12 can indeed induce up-regulation of NCRs, NKG2D and DNAM-1. In particular major effect is exerted on NKp44 that is not expressed at all on resting NK cells (Biron et al., 1999; Moretta A. et al., 2001; Della Chiesa et al., 2006; Balsamo et al., 2009; Vivier et al., 2011).

Thus, NK cells by their inhibitory and activating receptors can sense the altered expression of both protective self HLA-I molecules and a large array of pathogenic markers, and on this basis can discriminate which cells have to be killed.

The fact that, at variance with activating receptors, the inhibitory HLA-specific receptors are clonally distributed, allows the generation of a repertoire of NK cell subsets capable of sensing alteration of even single HLA-alleles. Importantly, this phenomenon is the basis for the exploitation of alloreactive NK cell subsets in aplo-identical Hematopoietic Stem Cell Transplanation (HSCT) in hematological malignancies (see section 2.4).

2.3 Multiple NK cell subsets and functions

Besides their involvement in direct pathogen clearance, NK cells are also implied in the regulation of the immune responses. Indeed they can produce and respond to various cytokines, functionally interact with different immune cell types and participate at regulation of T cell functions, in particular at Th1/Th2 polarization (Cooper et al., 2001; Moretta A. et al., 2005; Scordamaglia et al., 2008).

Up today several NK cell types, with distinct phenotype, function and anatomical location have been described (Table 1).

The $CD56^{bright}CD16^{dim/neg}KIR^{-}NKG2A^{+}$ NK cells are characterized by low granule content and low cytolytic activity but produce large amounts of cytokines, in particular IFN-γ. These cells cover 5-10% of circulating NK cells but represent the large majority of NK cells in Lymph Nodes (L.N.). At these sites, upon interaction with maturing DC, $CD56^{bright}$ NK cells can proliferate and produce IFN-γ, thus favoring Th1 response (Fehniger et al., 2003; Ferlazzo & Munz 2004).

The classical $CD56^{dim}CD16^{bright}$ NK cells (approx. 90% of circulating NK cells) are highly cytotoxic, and also produce cytokines, in particular IFN-γ and TNF-α and, to a lesser extent, chemokines, such as MIP-1β. These cells may migrate to peripheral tissues driven by chemokines and type I IFNs. Indeed, CD56^{dim}CD16^{bright} NK cells express receptors (CXCR1 ChemR23 and CX_3CR1) specific for chemokines (CXCL8, Chemerin and CX_3CL1 respectively) that are usually produced during inflammatory events by Macrophages, Neutrophils, DC and Endothelial cells (Moretta A. et al., 2005; Della Chiesa et al., 2006b; Parolini et al., 2007). In addition they also express GPR56, a molecule that would function as receptor for Extra Cellular Matrix components (Della Chiesa et al., 2010). In inflamed tissues, different viral or bacterial products (i.e. PAMPs - Pathogen Associated Molecular Patterns) may either directly activate NK cells (which express TLR6 and TLR9 PAMP receptors) or induce DC, plasmacytoid DC (pDC), M1 type Macrophages, to produce cytokines capable of activating NK cells. At these sites, CD56^{dim}CD16^{bright} NK cells can physically interact with immature DC (iDC) and, by the engagement of NKp30 and DNAM-1, they can release TNF-α and HMGB1 and promote DC maturation. Once activated, NK cells, by using the same receptors (NKp30 and DNAM-1), can also kill iDCs (and spare mature DC - mDC). As compared to mDC, iDC express lower HLA-I levels, and are not "protected" from activated NK cells. This phenomenon may represent either a mechanism to eliminate those DC that have not properly undergone maturation or a signal to terminate the response and avoid chronic inflammation (Zitvogel et al., 2002; Moretta A. et al., 2005).

Recently, a novel CD56^{+}NKp44^{+} NK cell type was described in MALT (tonsils and Peyer patches), and was called NK22, by virtue of its ability to produce IL-22 in response to IL-23 (Colonna, 2009). IL-22 is a IL-10 family cytokine with anti-bacterial effects, as it maintains epithelial-cell barrier function in the gut thus contrasting bacterial dissemination. The meaning of NK22 cells, as well as their ontogenesis, are not fully understood, nevertheless these cells may play an important role in constraining inflammation and in defense against bacterial infection in the mucosa.

A unique NK cell subset expressing the phenotype CD56^{bright}CD16$^{dim/neg}$KIR^{+}NKG2A^{+}, populates decidua in the first trimester of pregnancy (Moffet-King, 2002; Hanna et al., 2006). These cells display peculiar functional features: they express the NCRs but are poorly cytolytic; rather, the engagement of NKp30 and NKp44 would induce them to produce a defined pattern of chemokines and pro-angiogenic factors (see Table 1). These factors would favor trophoblast migration and decidua vascularization, ensuring an appropriate placenta and fetus development. Decidual NK (dNK) cells may also have a role in the induction of tolerance at the maternal/fetal interface. dNK cells, by producing IFN-γ, would induce expression of IDO in decidual myelomonocytic cells. In turn IDO, together with TGF-β, would favor induction and proliferation of Tregs. Interestingly, unlike PB NK cells (see section 2.4), dNK cells are resistant to the inhibition of the IDO-induced Trp-catabolite, L-kynurenine. This resistance implies that dNK cells can maintain production of IFN-γ and sustain the tolerogenic pathway over time (Vacca et al., 2010).

It has been recently proposed that the CD56^{bright}CD16$^{dim/neg}$KIR^{-}NKG2A^{++} cells could undergo further differentiation through different stages (Bjorkstrom et al., 2010; Lopez-Verges et al., 2010). The relatively immature and poorly cytotoxic CD56^{bright}CD16$^{dim/neg}$KIR^{-}NKG2A^{++} cells, would progressively increase the expression of cytolytic granules, CD16, KIRs and CD57, down-regulate NKG2A, and modify the kinetics of IFN-γ release. In line with this hypothesis, four phenotypically distinct NK cell populations, possibly representing sequential stages of this differentiation process, have been identified within circulating pool:

$CD56^{bright}CD16^{dim/neg}CD57^{-}KIR^{-}NKG2A^{++}perforin^{+/-}$, $CD56^{dim}CD16^{dim}CD57^{-}KIR^{-}NKG2A^{++}perforin^{+}$, $CD56^{dim}CD16^{bright}CD57^{+/-}KIR^{+}NKG2A^{+}perforin^{++}$, $CD56^{dim}CD16^{bright}CD57^{+}KIR^{+}NKG2A^{-}perforin^{+++}$.

Interestingly, along these putative differentiation steps NK cells would also progressively lose CCR7 and CD62L expression and acquire the fraktalkine receptor CX_3CR1, thus skewing their initial homing capabilities to L.N., towards inflamed Peripheral Tissues (Juelke et al., 2010; Hamann et al., 2011). This latter point should not be disregarded, especially in view of the future perspective of selecting appropriate NK cell subsets for cancer immunotherapy.

NK cell subpopulation (phenotype)	Anatomical/ tissue localization	Functional features
$CD3^{-}CD56^{bright}CD16^{dim/neg}$ $KIR^{-}NKG2A^{++}$ $CCR7^{++}CD62L^{++}$ $CD57^{-}$	Lymph Nodes 5-10% PB NK cells	Differentiation towards KIR+ cells Cytokines production (IFN-γ TNF-α) mDC-induced prolif. and IFN-γ prod. (promote Th1 polarization)
$CD3^{-}CD56^{dim}CD16^{bright}$ KIR^{+}/KIR^{-} $NKG2A^{+}/NKG2A^{-}$ $CCR7^{-}CD62L^{+/-}$ $ChemR23^{+}CX3CR3^{+}$ $GPR56^{+}$	90% PB NK cells inflamed periph. tissues?	Cytotoxicity Cytokines production (IFN-γ TNF-α) Induction of DC maturation
$CD56^{-}CD161^{+}$	5-10% PB NK cells	Produce type2 cytokines (IL-5 IL-13) Low cytotox. Expanded in HIV patients
$CD3^{-}CD56^{bright}CD16^{dim}$ KIR^{+}	Decidua (1st. trimester pregnancy)	Low cytotox. $IFN\text{-}\gamma^{+}$ $IL\text{-}8^{++}$ $IP\text{-}10^{+}$ $VEGF^{+}$ Regulatory interactions with Trophoblasts (Placenta development) Decidua vascularization Induction of Tregs
$CD3^{-}CD56^{+}NKp44^{+}$	MALT	$IL\text{-}22^{+}$ / mucosal immunity
$CD3^{-}CD56^{+}CD16^{+/-}$ KIR^{+}	Liver	Cytotoxicity

Table 1. Surface phenotype, anatomical localization and function of different NK cell subsets

2.4 Role of NK cells in the control of tumors

The impressive advances obtained in the last 15-20 years in the knowledge of the mechanism of action of NK cells and of their regulation, have been fuelled by the evident therapeutic potential that these cells have shown since their first discovery. However, although the efficacy of NK cells in containing tumors in vivo has been demonstrated in different animal models (Kim et al., 2000; Smyth et al., 2000; Guerra et al., 2008; Halftech et al., 2009), the way to develop effective NK-based immunotherapy has been elusive for many years and only very recently it yielded promising results.

After the initial attempts by Rosenberg's group (Rosenberg et al., 1985), several trials had been done to set protocols for the adoptive transfer of ex-vivo activated autologous NK cell populations or for the use of different cytokines to elicit NK cell responses in vivo (Sutlu & Alici, 2009). The advantages of these approaches, however, appeared minimal: both because of the technical limits in expanding ex vivo large bulk populations (as repeated infusions were necessary to overcome the short life-span of transferred mature NK cells), and because of the putative adverse effects induced by IL-2 in vivo (such as the possible expansion of $CD25^+$ Tregs or the induction the AICD) (Ghiringhelli et al., 2005; Rodella et al., 2001). In addition, another possible limitation could be that tumor cells could retain sufficient HLA-I expression to protect themselves from autologous NK cell attack. A turning point in the definition of efficient NK-based immunotherapeutic strategies against cancer, was represented by the study by Velardi and co-workers, primarily aimed at the evaluation of the clinical outcome of aplo-identical HSCT in Acute Myeloid Leukemia (AML) (Ruggeri et al., 2002). In this study the authors suggested that, in the presence of HLA/KIR mismatch (i.e. recipient and donor expressing different HLA-I alleles that are recognized by different KIRs), NK cells that developed from donor's progenitors could play an active role in reducing both the risk of leukemia relapse and even the Graft versus Host Disease (GvHD). This implied that heterologous NK cells could develop in the conditioned host, and kill Leukemic blasts more efficiently than autologous NK cells could do. Further studies by different groups have led to the current hypothesis that in the host, heterologous NK cell population expressing KIRs specific for donor's and not for recipient's HLA-I alleles can develop and be educated (licensed) by the donor's bone marrow cells, thus acquiring efficient killing capabilities towards host (allogeneic) malignant cells or activated leukocytes (Pende et al., 2009; Cooley et al., 2010; Haas et al., 2011; L. Moretta et al., 2011). The functional capabilities of allogeneic NK cells would also explain the reduction of GvHD observed in patients undergoing HLA/KIR mismatched HSCT, as, besides the elimination of heterologous Leukemic blasts (Graft-versus-Leukemia - GvL - effect), donor's NK cells would also be involved in the killing of those host's DC capable of priming donor's T cells. Interestingly, this alloreactive NK cell population may persist (and exert the its beneficial effect) for years (Pende et al., 2009; Haas et al., 2011) without causing apparent detrimental clinical signs ascribable to NK cell activity.

The above studies open new perspectives for the exploitation of NK cells in immunotherapy. In this context, different trials have been designed for the treatment of hematological malignancies, and in some cases also for solid tumors (Miller et al., 2005; Terme et al., 2008; Sutlu & Alici, 2009). Several problems, however, still remain to be solved. For example the fact that immature, not fully competent, NK cells may predominate (and persist) in circulation during (and after) the recipient immunological reconstitution (Nguyen et al., 2005) with negative effects on the anti-tumor activity and surveillance against viruses. Another problem regards a general negative effect that malignancies may exert on NK cell functions. In this context, different studies have reported a down-regulation of activating receptors in circulating NK cells from tumor patients (Sanchez et al., 2010; Le Maux-Chansac et al., 2005; Fregni et al., 2011). Moreover , in solid tumors, the tumor microenvironment may play an additional negative role by contrasting both the responses and the infiltration capabilities of the immune effector cells (Albertsson et al., 2003). In this context, different studies have indicated that in some tumors, infiltrating NK cells may be rare or poorly functional (Albertsson et al., 2003; Carrega et al., 2009; Platonova et al., 2011). At the tumor site several stromal components, induced by aberrant tumor-driven inflammation, can contribute to NK cell down-regulation (Mantovani et al., 2008). Tregs, by the release of TGF-β, may suppress NK cell functions (Zimmer et al., 2008). The induction of M2 macrophages may reduce the macrophage-mediated NK cell activation (as this effect is prominently sustained by M1 macrophages) (Bellora et al., 2010). Also the Tumor Associated Fibroblasts (TAF) may contrast NK cells in their anti-tumor activity. Indeed, fibroblasts derived from melanoma lesions were found to inhibit, by mean of cell-to-cell contact and PGE_2 release, the IL-2-driven up-regulation of NKp44, DNAM-1 and NKp30 on NK cells (Balsamo et al., 2009). Finally, even the tumor cells can induce down-modulation of activating NK receptors. Several tumor cell lines constitutively express IDO, an enzyme involved in the Trp catabolism. The IDO-induced Trp catabolite Kynurenine has been shown to down-regulate NKp46 and NKG2D (Della Chiesa et al., 2006). In addition, tumor cells can also induce down-regulation of NKG2D or DNAM-1 on NK cells by the release of soluble NKG2D-Ligands (Doubrovina et al., 2003) or by the prolonged engagement of DNAM-1 in cell-to-cell contact (Carlsten et al., 2009)

3. Human Natural Killer cell development

3.1 In vitro NK cell development

3.1.1 Acquisition of NK cell receptors and function

Most of information available on human NK cell development came from in vitro studies of NK cell differentiation from $CD34^+$ Hematopoietic Stem Cells (HSC) or $CD34^{+/-}CD45RA^+$ early lymphoid precursors. These cells can be isolated from different sources such as fetal liver, Bone Marrow (BM), Thymus, PB and Umbilical Cord Blood (UCB) and stimulated with IL-2 or IL-15, in the presence or in the absence of feeder cells, to obtain NK cell differentiation (Freud & Caligiuri , 2006). In the 90s' it was shown that it was possible to obtain $CD3^-CD56^+$ $CD94/NKG2A^+$ cytolytic NK cells from either $CD34^-CD45RA^+CD7^+CD1a^-$ early thymic precursors (Mingari et al., a1991,b1997; Lanier et al., 1992; Sanchez et al., 1994) or $CD34^+$HSC isolated from BM or UCB (Miller et al., 1994; Lotzova et al., 1993).

Currently, optimal culturing conditions require the simultaneous presence of different cytokines: Stem Cell Factor (SCF), FMS-Like Tyrosine Kynase Ligand (Flt3-L), IL-7, IL-15 and IL-21.

During in vitro differentiation the development of NK cells proceeds through a step-by-step process (figure 1) (Freud& Caligiuri, 2006). Freshly isolated HSC precursors already express CD117 and Flt3, which are the SCF and Flt3-L receptors, respectively, and play an important role for their proliferation and survival before any cell lineage commitment takes place . The first cell markers that would suggest a NK-lymphoid commitment are the IL-2/IL-15 receptors CD122, CD132 and the IL-7 α-chain receptor (CD127). These receptors play an important role in transducing proliferation and differentiation signals upon interaction with the appropriate cytokines (IL-15 and IL-7 respectively). However, in humans, these markers are rarely detectable on ex-vivo isolated $CD34^+CD45RA^+$ precursors, while they can be detected on small fractions of precursor after first days of culture (Freud& Caligiuri, 2006).

The first surface cell marker that clearly identify NK cell precursors is CD161 (Bennet et al., 1996). It can be detected on small percentages of $CD3^-CD56^-CD117^+$cells, which already express CD244 co-receptor: the acquisition of NKp44 activating receptor and CD56 represents the following differentiation step. Next, the expression of the NKp46, NKG2D and DNAM-1 activating receptors and of CD94/NKG2A inhibitory receptor occurs. The acquisition of CD16 and KIRs can be hardly observed in vitro (Mingari et al., 1997; Miller et al., 2001; Sivori et al., 2002). These receptors are typical of functionally differentiated circulating NK cells: their acquisition by small percentages of cell precursors undergoing differentiation, appears after long term cultures in the presence of IL-21, a pro-inflammatory cytokine (Sivori et al., 2003). On the other hand, the early expression of NKp44 may be related to the fact that recombinant IL-15, present in the culture, rapidly activates NKp44 gene transcription. Hence, NKp44 transcription could be differently regulated from that of the other activating receptors.

This sequential process of cell marker acquisition identifies NK cell precursor intermediates with different functional properties (Freud & Caligiuri, 2006; Grzywacz et al., 2006). Early NK cell precursors $CD117^+CD161^+CD244^+CD56^{+/-}$ $NKp44^{+/-}$ are not cytolytic but can secrete cytokines such as GM-CSF and IL-13. These cells lack the expression of all the other activating receptors and inhibitory receptors. The next stage of in vitro NK cell differentiation correlates with the definitive acquisition of CD56 and of NKp44 ($CD117^+CD161^+$ $CD244^+CD56^+NKp44^+$): these precursors can be defined as immature NK cells (iNK). Immature NK cells secrete large amounts of CXCL8 and low amounts of IL-22 while they do not produce IFN-γ (Freud & Caligiuri, 2006; Vitale et al., 2008; Tang et al., 2011). The production of CXCL8 could have a role in the modulation of hematopoietic cell lineage commitment. In particular, CXCL8 inhibits myelopoiesis (Youn et al., 2000) and, thus, might favour NK cell differentiation. On the other hand, iNK cells are not cytotoxic. Indeed they have not acquired yet cytolytic granules in their cytoplasm, important NK activating receptors (i.e. NKp46), and the adhesion molecule LFA-1, that strongly contribute to the activation of cytolytic machinery (Bryceson et al., 2006).

The acquisition of a weak cytolytic activity correlates with the expression of NKp46 activating receptor and LFA-1; however, at this stage of development, the NKp46-mediated cytotoxicity against susceptible cell targets may be inhibited by the CD244 co-receptor, that acts as inhibitory receptor on these iNK cells. CD244 works as an activating co-receptor on mature NK cells thanks to the recruitment of an intra-cytoplasmic adaptor molecule SAP. However, on $CD117^{+/-}CD161^+$ $CD244^+CD56^+NKp46^{+/-}CD94/NKG2A^-LFA\text{-}1^{+/-}$ iNK cells SAP it is not synthetized yet, leading to inhibitory rather than activating function of CD244 (Moretta et al., 2001; Sivori et al., a2002, b2003; Vitale et al., 2008).

The full acquisition of cell functions typical of mature NK cells, such as IFN-γ secretion and cytolytic activity, correlates with the surface bright expression of NKp46, the expression of NKG2D and DNAM-1 activating receptors, CD94/NKG2A inhibitory receptor and of LFA-1 molecule. At this stage, SAP starts to be synthesized, and CD244 acquires a co-stimulatory activity. These cells are defined as $CD56^{bright}$ NK cells since they are very similar to $CD56^{bright}$ $CD94/NKG2A^+CD16^-KIR^-$ NK cells present in the PB. Notably, differentiation is a continuous process and cells may not be synchronized in their maturation status: hence, a certain heterogeneity of the different cell subsets may be observed.

Altogether these experimental evidences indicate that NK cell development is tightly regulated and that evolution had particularly tuned the acquisition of cytolytic activity. NK cells, to become cytotoxic, must express at least the NKp46 activating receptor and the LFA-1 adhesion molecule. Simultaneously, they have to loose the inhibitory activity of CD244 co-receptor. The ability to control NK cytotoxicity by inhibitory CD244 could be a "safe" mechanism, important in the interactions between NK cell precursors and other hematopoietic cells. CD244 ligand is the CD48 molecule, which is expressed by different types of leucocytes and hematopoietic precursors (Cannons et al., 2011). On the other hand, iNK cells secrete a peculiar pattern of cytokines, such as IL-22 and CXCL8, involved in inflammatory process, defence against bacteria, neo-angiogenesis and modulation of haematopoiesis. Hence, iNK cells might exert important crosstalk with other cells present in microenvironment where their differentiation takes place.

3.2 Factors that modulate NK cell differentiation

Hematopoietic cell lineage commitment depends on a wide variety of factors. Genetic components dictate the initial commitment but the milieu that surrounds lineage precursors may have a key role in the fate of these cells. The balance between specific transcription factors and the appropriate cytokines and hormones can change the commitment of intermediate lymphoid precursors, inducing their switch towards alternative lineages (Laiosa et al., 2006; Doulatov et al., 2010). In this context, in vitro analysis have shown that NK cells can share intermediate precursors not only among lymphoid cells but also with dendritic cells and myeloid cells (Miller et al., 1999; Marquez et al., 1998; Perez et al., 2003; Vitale et al., 2008; Grzywacz et al., 2011).

3.2.1 Cytokines

Cytokines are important factors that modulate NK cell differentiation. SCF and Flt3-L have a role in the first days of in vitro development because they induce HSC to enter into the cell cycle, and sustain precursor proliferation and survival (Yu et al., 1998). Then, IL-7 supports the lymphoid lineage commitment, since this cytokine is involved in T cell homeostasis and lymphoid differentiation (Ma A. et al., 2006). However, it is IL-15 that plays a key role in NK cell differentiation, through the interaction with IL-2/IL-15 common β and γ chains receptors (CD122 and CD132, respectively). Indeed, IL-15 has been shown to be critical in the terminal differentiation of $CD117^{+/-}CD161^{+}CD56^{+}$ iNK towards mature NK cells (Mrozek et al., 1995; Freud & Caligiuri, 2006). In murine models, NK cell deficiencies are more pronounced in mice lacking IL-15 or its receptors, than in mice lacking IL-2 or IL-7 related products (Di Santo et al., 1990; Giliani et al., 2005; Kennedy et al., 2000). In vitro assays revealed that high dose soluble IL-15 binds to its receptors and promote NK cell differentiation but, in vivo, IL-15 is primarily detectable complexed to its IL-15 Receptor α (IL15-Rα) present on accessory (stromal) cells (Dubois et al., 2002). IL-15/IL15-Rα complex would then present the cytokine *in trans* to $CD122^{+}CD132^{+}$ cells, meaning that also stromal cells could exert an important role in the terminal differentiation of iNK cells (Miller et al., 1994; Briard et al., 2002; Vacca et al., 2011). Finally, IL-21 have been shown to increase the proportions of $CD56^{+}KIR^{+}$ cells undergoing in vitro differentiation (Sivori et al., 2003).

3.2.2 Transcription factors

In vitro and in vivo studies using mice with loss-of-function mutation helped to clarify the role of many transcription factors (TFs) involved in NK cell commitment, proliferation and maturation. Some of them, like the E proteins, orchestrate a lymphoid-biased cellular context versus myeloid compartment (de Pooter et al., 2010) but must be down-regulated to allow NK cell differentiation (Boos et al., 2007). Other TFs are important both in the NK cell and T cell commitment, such as Notch-1 or Id2 (Benne et al., 2009; Boos et al., 2007). Id2 is an helix loop helix TF, able to modulate the activation the E protein E2A, and have been shown to exert a prominent role in NK cell commitment. Recently, other two TF have been suggested to induce definitive early NK cell commitment: a High Mobility Group protein, called TOX, and a basic leucin zipper, E4PB4 (also known as NFIL3)(Aliahmad et al., 2010; Gascoyne et al., 2009; Kamizono et al., 2009). It has been shown that IL-15 activates E4PB4 that, in turn, would activate Id2 transcription, leading to a definitive NK cell commitment and expansion of NK cell precursors. In humans, E4BP4 and Id2 expression can be observed either in ex-vivo-isolated early committed $CD34^{+/-}CD122^{+}CD127^{+}$ NK cell precursors either in in vitro-derived $CD117^{+/-}CD161^{+}CD56^{+}LFA\text{-}1^{-}NKG2A^{-}$ iNK cells (Hughes et al., 2010; Vacca at al., 2011). On the other hand, TOX would influence the activation of T-bet, a TF that correlates with the acquisition of cytolytic activity and the ability to produce IFN-γ by more differentiated $CD161^{+}CD56^{+}LFA\text{-}1^{+}$ $NKp46^{+}$ $CD94/NKG2A^{+}$ NK cells (Yun et al., 2011).

Expression of others TFs appears to correlate with the different stages of NK cell differentiation. RORC correlates with the secretion of IL-22 by iNK cells (Tang et al., 2011) while the expression of EOMES (a T-box TF), similar to T-bet, correlates with IFN-γ production by more differentiated NK cells (Glimcher et al., 2004).

3.2.3 Corticosteroids

In the last years the studies on in vitro NK cell development offered new important clues on NK cell lineage commitment and on the factors that may modulate this process.

The attempt to improve models of in vitro NK cell differentiation, induced many groups to test additional factors, besides cytokines, that could favour in vitro NK cell differentiation: in particular, stromal cells and/or corticosteroids. These new protocols revealed an unexpected function for glucocorticoids, which were already known to exert a modulatory effect on T cell development (Jondal et al., 2004). Studies with Hydrocortisone (HC) showed that it was possible to obtain NK cells from the in vitro culture of $CD33^{+}CD14^{+/-}$ myeloid progenitors isolated from UCB (Perez et al., 2003). These results suggested that, in cord blood, it was possible to switch the differentiation of monocyte precursors towards NK cells. We obtained similar results with Methylprednisolone (MePDN). This corticosteroid is commonly used as first line of treatment for acute GvHD after allogeneic HSCT. Our hypothesis was that MePDN could inhibit not only mature NK cell proliferation and functions but also the in vitro NK cell differentiation. Surprisingly, our results showed that pharmacological concentrations of MePDN accelerated NK cell differentiation and were able to induce myeloid precursors to switch their differentiation towards $CD161^{+}CD56^{+}NKp44^{+}$ iNK cells (Vitale et al., 2008). More recently, Grwaycz et al., with an elegant in vitro experiment, provided evidence that HC, in combination with a stromal cell line, induce differentiation of $CD33^{+}CD13^{+}CD115^{+/-}$ myelomonocytic precursors into cytolytic $CD56^{+}NKp46^{+}CD94/NKG2A^{+}KIR^{+/-}CD16^{+/-}$ NK cells (Grwaycz et al., 2011).

These results offer important clues to better clarify some major issues that have been discussed in the last years.

The first one is related to the hematopoietic cell lineage commitment. Current models of haematopoiesis suggest that HSC may commit early to the erythroid/platelet lineages or to leukocyte lineages. However, once committed to the leukocyte lineage, hematopoietic precursors would retain a high plasticity. Thus, the choice to terminally differentiate towards myeloid or lymphoid lineages would then depend on the role of lineage-specific transcription factors and on a permissive milieu (Doulatov et al., 2010). This would be of particular interest for NK cells, which are the only lymphocytes assigned to natural immunity compartment and that appear to be the connection ring with acquired immunity.

The second issue regards the role of NK cells after HSCT and their use in immunotherapy to obtain GvL reaction. The possibility that myeloid precursors, in the presence of corticosteroids, could generate more rapidly functional NK cells offers important clues also in the clinical settings (Vitale et al., 2008; Grwaycz et al., 2011). It is conceivable that NK

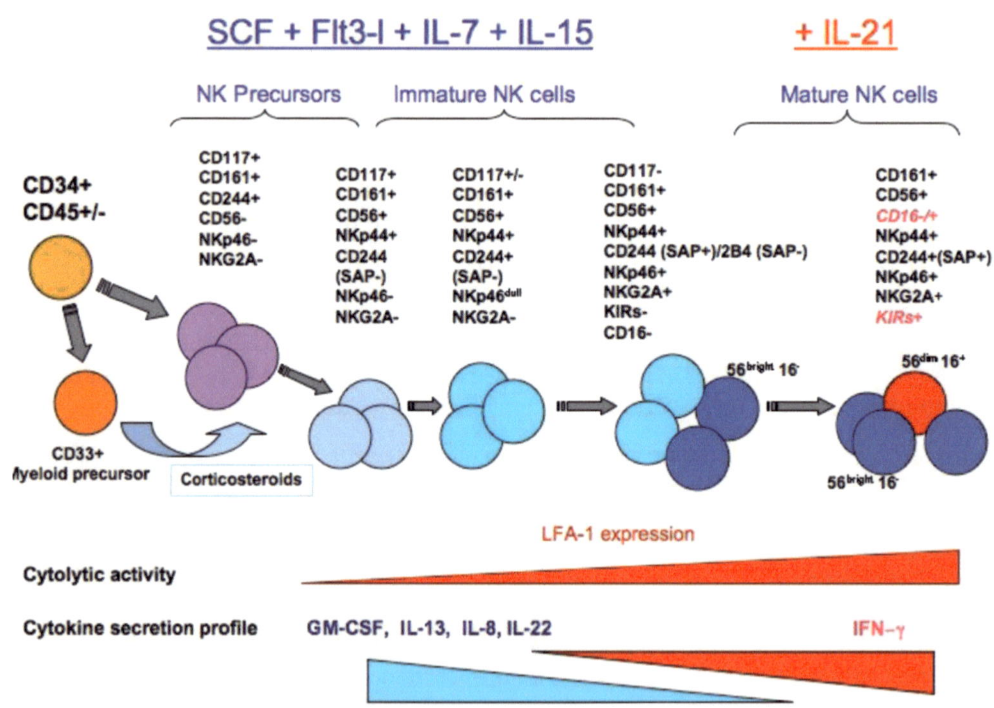

Fig. 1. Acquisition kinetic of receptors and functions by NK cells undergoing in vitro cell development.
Three main precursor subsets may be identified along different time intervals of culture: NK cell precursors, immature NK cells and more differentiated $CD56^{bright}$ NK cells. The appearance of $CD56^{dim}CD16^{+}KIR^{+}$ NK cells (red cell) is a late and rare event and is more achievable in the presence of IL-21. Stages of differentiation are endowed with a peculiar surface phenotype and functions. In particular the acquisition of cytolytic activity correlates with the expression of LFA-1, activating receptors and the production of IFN-γ, while high secretion of IL-8 correlates with the immature NK cell stage.

cells, present in high percentages in peripheral blood of patients at the earliest time intervals after HCST, may derive, at least in part, from myeloid precursors. Importantly, this maturation could not occur wholly in BM but also in PB and other sites. This is the third important issue that have been matter of debate of the last years: the site of in vivo human NK cell development and maturation.

3.3 In vivo NK cell development and maturation

NK cells were generally believed to differentiate into the BM from $CD34^+$ hematopoietic stem cells (Freud & Caligiuri, 2006). However, NK cell developmental intermediates were detectable in vivo neither in the BM nor in thymus. The possibility to observe in vivo any different NK cell developmental stages detectable in vitro, came from analysis of lymphocyte recovery in patients undergoing allogeneic HSCT. Analysis of PB of these patients revealed that, in some of them, the first waves of lymphocytes recovering at early time after transplant (2-3 weeks) are mostly NK cells. These lymphocytes are characterized by the $CD56^{bright}$ $CD16^-$ $CD94/NKG2A^+KIR^-$ phenotype and a dull expression of NCRs, while $CD56^{dim}CD16^+CD94/NKG2A^+KIR^+$ NK cells can be detected later, (4-8 weeks after transplant). (Vitale et al., 2000; Shilling et al., 2003; Vitale et al., 2004).

3.3.1 Sites of in vivo NK cell development: Stages of NK cell differentiation

The finding that in vitro models of NK cell differentiation led to the generation of $CD56^{bright}$ $CD16^-$ NK cells, supported the hypothesis that, in vivo, this subset could be a precursor reservoir, able to promptly differentiate towards more cytotoxic $CD56^{dim}CD16^+$ upon specific stimuli. However, experimental evidences that support this hypothesis have been acquired only recently. Freud and co-workers discovered that $CD45RA^+CD117^-$ and $CD34^+CD45^+CD117^+CD161^{+/-}$ cells were enriched in Secondary Lymphoid Tissue (SLT), particularly in lymphnodes and tonsils. Importantly, these precursors were able to generate selectively NK cells upon culture in the presence of appropriate cytokines. They defined these cells as pro-NK and pre-NK cells respectively. Further analysis revealed that in SLT, it was possible to detect and isolate four different subsets of NK cell precursors representing different stages of NK cell differentiation (Freud et al., a2005, b2006).

Stage 1: $CD34^+CD45RA^+CD117^-CD161^-$ pro-NK cells; stage 2: $CD34^+CD45RA^+CD117^+CD161^{+/-}$ pre-NK cells; stage 3: $CD34^-CD117^+CD161^+CD56^{+/-}NKp46^-CD94/NKG2A^-KIR^-CD16^-$ immature NK cells; stage 4: $CD117^{+/-}CD161^+CD56^+NKp46^+CD94/NKG2A^+KIR^{+/-}CD16^-$, defined as $CD56^{bright}$ NK cells. Further analysis suggested that also the expression of CD122 and CD127 could help to identify stage 1/2 of pre-NK cell precursors. These discoveries confirmed for the first time that in vitro models of NK cell differentiation may have in vivo similar counterpart. Indeed, the above stages 2, 3 and 4 remind the differentiation steps observed in vitro (Freud & Caligiuri et al., 2006; Caligiuri, 2008). This discovery suggests that hematopoietic precursors could migrate from BM to SLT and generate NK cells in organs far from the BM. It is possible that at least a fraction of $CD56^{bright}$ NK cells present in SLT could differentiate from these precursors upon interaction with DC and other cells capable of presenting membrane-bound IL-15.

As mentioned above a particular subset of NK cells has been found to be enriched in tonsils and gut-mucosa associated tissue: these cells are $CD56^{+/-}NKp46^{+/-}NKp44^+NKG2A^-$ and produce IL-22. Their development appears to be independent from IL-15. However, whether these cells may represent a new subset of NK cells (called NK22 cells) or simply immature NK cells with peculiar in vivo functions is still a matter of debate (Colonna, 2009).

In conclusion, BM microenvironment may provide a fundamental support for the early stages of NK cell differentiation but peripheral tissues, in particular SLT, could provide a unique cell-to-cell interactions and cytokines to induce the terminal NK cell differentiation.

Surface markers	STAGE 1: Pro-NK	STAGE 2: Pre-NK	STAGE 3: iNK	STAGE 4: CD56 bright	STAGE 5: CD56dim CD16+
CD34	+	+	-	-	-
CD45RA	+/-	+/-	(+)/-	+/(-)	+/(-)
CD117	-	+	+	+/-	-
CD122	-	-	-	+/-	+
CD127	dull	dull	+	+/-	-
CD161	-	+/-	+	+	+
CD244	+	+	+	+	+
CD56	-	(+)/-	+/-	+	+
NKp44	-	-	+/(-)	(+)/-	(+)/-
NKp46	-	-	-	+	+
NKG2A	-	-	-	+	+/-
KIR	-	-	-	(+)/-	+/-
CD16	-	-	-	-	-

Table 2. Expression of surface markers by NK cell precursor intermediates isolated in SLT, according to model proposed by Freud and co. Legend: +/- variable expression; (+)/- majority of cells negative; +/(-) majority of cells positive; dull= weak expression

3.3.2 Other sites of in vivo NK cell development

The next step was to verify the possibility that NK-committed cell precursors could be isolated in other peripheral tissues, where peculiar NK cell subsets were enriched. Indeed NK-committed precursors were found in gut, endometrium and placenta (Chinen at al., 2007; Male et al., 2010; Vacca et al., 2011). In all these districts there is a high concentration of CD56^{bright} NK cells characterized by immune-regulatory activity. In particular, NK cells present in human decidua (dNK) during the first trimester of pregnancy display a peculiar phenotype (CD56^{bright}CD16^{-}NKG2A^{+}KIR$^{-/+}$) and exert peculiar functions. For long time dNK cells were supposed to derive from PB NK cells undergone phenotypic and functional modifications upon interaction with decidual microenvironment. Recently, different experimental evidences suggested that dNK cells could derive from NK precursors already present in endometrium or in decidua, able to promptly differentiate upon stimuli given by the onset of pregnancy (Male et al., 2010; Vacca et al., 2011). In particular, it has been shown that NK cell lineage-committed CD34^{+}CD127^{+}CD122^{+} cells expressing E4BP4 and Id2 TFs are present in human decidua (dCD34^{+}) during the first trimester of pregnancy. They can undergo in vitro differentiation into functional CD56^{bright}CD16^{-} NK cells in the presence of suitable cytokines. More importantly, they could also differentiate without exogenous cytokines when co-cultured with decidual stromal cells (dSC), able to express endogenous membrane-bound IL-15. These results suggest that interaction between CD34+ cell and decidual stromal cells would be sufficient to promote in situ NK cell differentiation.

3.3.3 The stage five of human NK cell differentiation: $CD56^{dim}$ $CD16^{+}CD94/NKG2A^{+/-}$ KIR^{+} NK cells

As already discussed, several evidences suggest that $CD56^{dim}$ NK cells may derive from $CD56^{bright}$ NK cells. After HSCT the first wave of NK cells is represented by $CD56^{bright}CD16^{-}CD94/NKG2A^{+}KIR^{-}$ cells while $CD56^{dim}CD16^{+}CD94/NKG2A^{+/-}KIR^{+}$ cells appear later. Importantly, $CD56^{bright}$ display longer telomeres than $CD56^{dim}$ NK cells. Moreover, different phenotypically defined NK cell subsets have been recently proposed as functional intermediates between the $CD56^{bright}$ and $CD56^{dim}$ cell types (see section 2.3) (Romagnani et al., 2007; Juelke et al., 2010).

However, in in vitro assay, it is almost impossible to observe significant expansions of KIR^{+} NK cells from any type $CD34^{+}$ cell precursors. Similar problems must be related to our inability to fully recreate the in vivo milieu in in vitro assay. $CD56^{dim}$ may acquire their surface phenotype and functional properties upon peripheral tissues/blood microenvironment stimuli. However, signals that drive the differentiation of $CD56^{dim}$ NK cells, both during normal homeostasis and infections, remain still elusive. Recent studies provided evidence that $CD56^{dim}$ cells change their phenotypic properties and continue to differentiate throughout their lifespan. The loss of expression of NKG2A, the acquisition of KIRs and CD57 would allow the identification of sequential steps of cell maturation accompanied by a progressive decline of cell proliferation and of responsiveness to cytokine stimulation. In particular, CD16 and KIR would be acquired at late stages of peripheral blood NK cell maturation (Björkström et al., 2010; Lopez-Vergès et al., 2010). Since the acquisition of KIR repertoire in each single NK cell is a stochastic process, related to the KIR genotype and polymorphism, it is important to understand how NK cells may be educated to avoid auto-reactivity. They should acquire appropriate KIR able to prevent them from killing healthy self-cells. However, in PB of normal donors, it is possible to detect NK cells expressing KIR mismatched for self HLA-I ligands or not expressing any HLA-I inhibitory receptor at all. These cells could represent a danger as they would not recognize self HLA-I on self normal cells. As above mentioned, however, it has been recently proposed that during their development only those NK cells expressing inhibitory receptors specific for self HLA-I ligands would acquire full functional competence, while cells that fail to express such receptors (i.e. potentially autoreactive NK cells) would retain a state of hypo-responsiveness. It has to be noted, however, that the question on how such licensing/educational process could actually occur in vivo is still matter of debate (Parham, 2006; Vivier et al., 2011).

The interest for NK cells and their clinical application for the control of leukemic relapse after allogeneic HSCT is enormously increased in the last years: hence, it is mandatory trying to clarify the epigenetic factors that regulate KIR acquisition and functions, because their expression pattern on allogeneic donor NK cells play a crucial role in the eradication of recipient's leukemia (Moretta et al., 2011).

4. Classification of NK cell disorders

The World Health Organization (WHO) classification of tumors of hematopoietic and lymphoid tissues encompasses four distinct entities, two of which are provisional: 1) NK cell lymphoblastic leukemia/lymphoma (*provisional*) (Borowitz et al., 2008); 2) Chronic Lymphoproliferative Disorder of NK cells (*provisional*) (Villamor et al., 2008); 3) Aggressive NK cell leukemia (Chan et al., 2008a); and 4) Extranodal NK/T-cell lymphoma, nasal type (Chan et al., 2008b). In addition, on the basis of morphology, immuno-phenotype, functional NK cell activity, and expression of cytotoxic molecules, NK cell neoplasms can be divided into immature and mature categories (Jaffe, 1996).

In recent years rare cases of lymphoblastic lymphomas/leukemia arising from immature NK cells has been reported, although the lack of suitable markers for immature NK cells mentioned above makes it difficult to distinguish NK-cell lymphoblastic lymphoma (LBL) from precursor T-cell LBL. It is also worth mentioning that the plasticity of hematopoietic-cell lineage seems greater than previously thought, and relations between phenotypically dissimilar neoplastic disorders are being reassessed. In contrast, it is believed that chronic lymphoproliferative disorder of NK cells, aggressive NK cell leukemia and extranodal NK cell lymphoma, nasal type, originate from mature NK cells (Chan et al., 2008a and b). Relevant biological features of NK cell neoplasms are summarized in Table 3.

	NK cell lymphoblastic leukemia/ lymphoma	Extranodal NK/T-cell lymphoma, nasal type	Aggressive NK cell leukemia	Chronic Lymphoproliferative Disorder of NK cells
Age	Pediatric	Middle-aged adult	Young to Middle aged adult	Adults (6th decade)
Geographic distribution	Worldwide	Asia	Asia	Worldwide
Cell origin	Immature NK cell	Mature NK cell	Mature NK cell	Mature NK cell
Relevant phenotype	sCD3-CD4-CD13-CD33- CD16-CD7+ CD2+CD56+CD3e+	CD2+sCD3-cCD3e+CD56+CD16- CD57-Granzyme B+ Perforin+TIA1+	sCD3-cCD3e±CD56+CD16± CD57-, CD94+	CD3-CD8±CD16+CD56+CD57+ KIRs±CD94/NKG2A± Granzyme B+Perforin+
Relevant cytogenetic aberrations	Complex karyotype	Deletion 6q	Deletion 6q Complex Karyotype	Usually Normal Karyotype
EBV association	No	Yes	Yes	No
Clinical course	Aggressive	Aggressive	Very Aggressive	Indolent
Prognosis	Poor	Poor	Poor	Good

Table 3. Clinical and Biological features of NK cell neoplasms

4.1 Immature NK cell neoplasms

4.1.1 NK cell lymphoblastic leukemia/lymphoma, provisional

A considerable confusion has been generated in the literature concerning this type of disorder, mostly due to the definition of NK cell leukemia on the basis of expression of CD56 antigen. This is indeed the most important and sensitive NK marker; unfortunately, CD56 is not specific for NK cells and can be also expressed in AML and ALL and blastic plasmacytoid dendritic cell neoplasms (BPDCN). On the other hand it may not be expressed by immature NK cells. NK cell lymphoblastic leukemia/lymphoma can be considered in cases showing blastic morphology, expressing CD56, TdT, immature T associated markers such as CD7 and CD2, and cytoplasmic CD3ε, but lacking the expression of surface CD3, CD19, CD20, CD13, CD33, and MPO (Liang & Graam, 2008). These patients frequently presented with leukemia and lymphadenopathy without skin involvement and were negative for EBV. TCR and/or Ig genes were in germline configuration in all cases in which the tests were performed. Outcomes of these patients were absolutely unfavourable. The immature morphology with NK cell-associated phenotype and genotype suggests that these tumours represent the true precursor NK cell neoplasms.

Some well characterized cases of NK precursor tumours with lymphomatous presentation that expressed CD94 1A transcripts have been reported (Lin et al., 2005). CD94 1A, a distal promoter of the CD94 molecule, is activated only by IL-15 (Lopez-Botet et al., 1997). Lin et al., recently reported that CD94 1A is the predominant form found in immature NK cells and it is expressed in TCR^- lymphoblastic leukemia (NK lineage LBL) but not in TCR^+ LBL (T lineage LBL) (Lin et al., 2005). By studying 21 patients with LBL and, on the basis of the expression of CD94 1A transcripts and the lack of TCR, the above investigators identified 7 patients with LBL of immature NK cell origin (CD94 $1A^+$, TCR^-). It is noteworthy that those NK-LBLs occurred in young patients and had better outcomes as compared with patients who had T-LBL (CD94 $1A^-$, TCR^+); none of the tumours was positive for CD56 (Lin et al., 2005). Thus, the use of CD94 1A associated with TCR appears to be more suitable than CD56 for identifying an immature NK cell neoplasm.

A standard treatment protocol for immature NK cell neoplasms has not been established mainly because of the rarity of these cases. Current chemotherapy strategies for non-Hodgkin's lymphoma or acute lymphoblastic leukemia (ALL) were the most commonly used. However, the overall outcomes were dismal and HSCT represents the only effective therapy to achieve a complete remission (Lin et al., 2005).

4.2 Mature NK cell neoplasms

4.2.1 Extranodal NK/T cell lymphoma, nasal type

The WHO classification encompasses both nasal NK/T cell lymphoma and extra-nasal NK/T cell lymphoma in the same category (Chan et al., 2008a). They share the same histology, even though these lymphomas may have different clinical manifestations, treatment approaches, and prognoses (Oshimi, 2007). Although most cases are genuine NK cell neoplasms, the term "NK/T" rather than "NK" is used because this entity also includes cytotoxic T cell neoplasms (Sozumiya et al., 1994). Nasal and extra-nasal NK/T cell lymphoma are invariably associated with EBV and have a ethnic predisposition, being more prevalent in Asia, Mexico, and Central and South America (Chan et al., 2008b; Kwong, 2005) and rare in Western Countries, the Middle East and Africa.

Nasal NK/T cell lymphomas refer to tumours that occur in the nose and the upper aero digestive tract (Oshimi, 2007; Cheung et al., 1998). They are the most common type among primary lymphomas of the nasal cavity (Cheung et al., 1998). The site of disease is primarily in the midline and includes the nasal cavity in more than 80% of cases. The tumour is locally invasive and might infiltrate surrounding tissues and organs, such as oropharynx, palate, orbits, till the appearance of the characteristic mid-facial destructive lesions, the so called "lethal midline granuloma" (Cheung et al., 1998). Common symptoms include nasal discharge, nasal obstruction, purulent rhinorrhea, epitasis and local swelling of the nasal bridge. The tumours may be destructive, leading to the highly characteristic midline perforation.

Extra-nasal NK/T cell lymphomas represent the counterpart of nasal NK/T cell lymphomas and involve any other part of the body. Males are predominantly affected, and the median age of presentation is the fifth decade. Primary sites of involvement include the skin, gastrointestinal tract, salivary glands, spleen, and testis (Chan et al., 1997). Patients with extra-nasal NK/T cell lymphoma more likely exhibit an advanced stage of disease with significantly higher general involvement, high levels of lactate dehydrogenise and a significantly decrease of haemoglobin and platelet count as compared with patients who have nasal NK/T cell lymphoma (Chan et al., 1997). The histological features are similar, regardless of the involved sites. Mucosal sites often show ulceration. A diffuse infiltrate of lymphoid cells is found in association with tissue necrosis and coagulation, although in some cases infiltrating cells lack atypical morphology, resulting in misdiagnosis as chronic inflammation. An angiocentric and angiodestructive growth pattern with associated fibrinoid changes in the blood vessels is frequently observed. In most patients, the neoplastic cells are characterized by the $CD45^+$ surface (s)$CD3^-$ cytoplasm (c)$CD3\varepsilon^+$ $CD56^+$ phenotype and lack myeloid and B lymphoid markers. Proliferating cells are also positive for cytotoxic granules, granzyme B, perforin, TIA. Rarely cells express CD30 and CD7, while CD56 negative cases have also been reported. Association with EBV can be demonstrated in nearly all patients (Harabuchi et al., 1990). Using *in situ* hybridization technique, EBV-encoded RNA can be found in neoplastic cells and Southern Blot analysis can detect monoclonal proliferation of EBV. Analyses of the terminal repeat region of the EBV genome indicates that the virus is in a clonal episomal form. Other than providing an indirect proof of the clonal nature of the lymphoid proliferation, this finding suggests that the EBV might play an etiologic role in mature NK cell neoplasms (Minarovitz, 1994). A defect in immune surveillance for EBV infection is demonstrated by the high frequency of 30-base pair deletions of the LMP1 gene in EBV-infected Asians. In addition, amino acid changes in the sequence coding HLA-A2- restricted CTL epitopes of the LMP1 and LMP2 genes, and low frequency of HLA-A*0201 in NK/T cell lymphoma patients have been reported (Kanno et al., 2000; Harabuchi et al., 2009). Genetic alterations have been detected in the tumour suppression genes and several oncogenes enabling tumour cells to proliferate and resist apoptosis. Mutations of *p53* have been demonstrated, with variable frequencies (24 to 60%). Mutation of *c-kit* can also be frequently demonstrated, as far as *Fas* gene mutations (Hoshida et al., 2003; Shen et al., 2002). The most common cytogenetic aberration is deletion of 6q. A recent microarray study showed that several genes associated with vascular biology, EBV induced genes, and *PDGFRa* gene are over-expressed, pointing to the deregulation of the tumor suppressor HACE1 in the frequently deleted 6q21 region (Huang et al., 2010). Moreover, in NK/T cell lymphoma, gene signatures related to angiogenesis, genotoxic stress and proliferation, and signaling pathways (TGF-β, Notch and Wnt), were significantly enriched as compared to IL2-activated normal NK cells. Interestingly, NK/T lymphoma cells of NK lineage have a very similar molecular profile to that of NK/T-cell or peripheral T-cell lymphoma of γδ-T cell lineage (Iqbal et al., 2010).

The clinical outcome of patients with nasal NK cell lymphoma is variable. Most observational studies have consistently demonstrated that radiotherapy is superior to chemotherapy alone in patients with stage I/II disease (Sakata et al., 1997). Some patients with early-stage disease are cured by radiation therapy. It has been demonstrated that radiotherapy, either as initial treatment or as part of the chemotherapy regimen, is the single most important key to a successful outcome (Ribrag et al., 2001). However, some patients with early-stage disease have early local or systemic recurrences and die of disease. For patients with stage III/IV disease, chemotherapy is the treatment of choice (Kwong, 2005). In several published series, the median survival of patients with advanced-stage disease was approximately 12 months. Extra-nasal NK cell lymphomas are clinically aggressive, the response to therapy is poor, and most patients die within 6 months after diagnosis. The long-term remission rate with allogeneic HSCT is less than 10% (Cheung et al., 1998).

4.2.2 Aggressive NK cell leukemia

First described by Fernandez et al., (Fernandez et al., 1986), aggressive NK cell leukemia (ANKL) is a systemic disease, more common in Asians than in Caucasians (Chan et al., 2008a), which is characterized by the presence of neoplastic NK cells in the peripheral blood, bone marrow, liver and spleen and by a rapidly progressive clinical course with poor prognosis. There is an equal sex incidence in men and women. The disease typically affects young to middle-aged adults with a median age in the third decade. At presentation, patients usually are very compromised with systemic symptoms, liver dysfunction, and hepato-splenomegaly sometimes accompanied by systemic lymphoadenopathy. In contrast to extra-nodal NK cell lymphoma, skin lesions are uncommon. The clinical progression is devastating despite treatment, and most patients survive for only days to weeks. Disseminated intravascular coagulation and hemophagocytic syndrome are often seen during the course of disease (Oshimi, 2007). In tissue sections, the neoplastic infiltrate is diffuse and destructive with lymphoid cell population usually appearing monomorphous (Siu, Chan & Kwong, 2002). Morphologically, leukemic cells are slightly larger than normal LGLs (Oshimi, 2007). There is an ample amount of pale or slightly basophilic cytoplasm that contains fine or coarse azurophilic granules. These cells are $sCD3^{-}cCD3\varepsilon^{+}CD56^{+}CD16^{+}$ (75% of cases), $CD57^{-}$ $CD94^{+}$ with a germ line configuration of β and γ genes of TCR. The chemokine system plays a critical role in the tumor cell diffusion, leading to the fulminant clinical courses. Serum levels of soluble FasL, IL-8, MIP-1α, and MIP-1β are significantly elevated in ANKL patients and proliferating cells are highly positive for Fas, IL-8, RANTES, MIP-1α, and MIP-1β (Makishima et al., 2007). Although clonal EBV is found in tumour cells in most patients and EBV is considered to be the etiological agent (Oshimi, 2007), little is known about the mechanisms through which EBV infection triggers clonal proliferation of NK cells. A defective T cell and NK cell response to EBV infection may play a role in the development of this disorder. However up to 10% of cases have been shown to be EBV-negative (Suzuki et al., 2004).

Several chromosomal abnormalities have been reported. In particular, the finding of abnormalities involving del(6q) in aggressive NK cell leukemia and in extranodal NK/T lymphoma provides a biological link between these two diseases (Wong, Chan & Kwong, 1997). A recent array-based comparative genomic hybridization study on 27 NK cell lymphoma/leukemia cases, classified into two disease groups based on the World Health Organization Classification (10 ANKL cases and 17 extranodal NK/T lymphomas, nasal type), showed recurrent gain of 1q and loss of 7p15.1–p22.3 and 17p13.1 in ANKL (Nakashima et al., 2005). The same study also demonstrated clear genetic differences between aggressive NK cell leukemia and extranodal NK/T cell lymphoma, suggesting that these are two separate entities (Nakashima et al., 2005).

Aggressive NK cell leukemia is a catastrophic disease with an almost uniform mortality. A few patients have a clinical response with conventional chemotherapy (Kwong, 2005), although the response is typically transient and survival is measured in days to weeks. Allogeneic HSCT results in short-term remission in a few patients (Kwong, 2005). Taking together, big efforts for the recognition of new therapeutical targets and for development of new experimental protocols are urgently required to address the issue of ANKL therapy. As a matter of fact, recent data in a murine model have reported impressive response by targeting of survivin by nanoliposomal ceramide (Liu et al., 2010).

4.2.3 Chronic lymphoproliferative disorder of NK cells (provisional)

The chronic lymphoproliferative disorders of NK cells (CLPD-NK) are included among the novelties of the current WHO classification (Villamor et al., 2008). These rare and heterogeneous disorders are characterized by a chronic expansion of mature appearing NK cells (usually more than 2,000/μl) in peripheral blood for more than 6 months (Loughran, 1993; Semenzato et al., 1987; Tefferi et al., 1994; Semenzato et al., 1997; Oshimi, 1996), without a clearly identified cause (Figure 2). Patients are usually adults with a mean age of 60 years without gender and racial predisposition (Pandolfi et al., 1990). In recent years several studies have been published focusing on the pathogenetic mechanisms of this disease (Zambello & Semenzato, 2009; Loughran et al., 1997; Zambello et al., 2003; Hodge et al., 2009; Gattazzo et al., 2010; Epling-Burnette et al., 2008). NK cell activation in response to an unknown stimulus, likely of viral origin, is postulated to play a role in the initial steps of CLPD-NK by selecting NK clones (Zambello & Semenzato, 2009). No prototypical HTLV infection was demonstrated in these patients. However, the evidence that sera from a series of patients from Europe and USA reacted with the recombinant HTLV env protein p21E, suggests that exposure to a protein containing homology to BA21 may be important in the pathogenesis of this lymphoproliferative disorder (Loughran et al., 1997). In contrast with other mature NK cell neoplasms, EBV is not usually detected within affected lymphocytes (Zambello & Semenzato, 2009). It is believed that BM, which is frequently involved in CLPD-NK patients, represents the setting where the putative inciting antigen could reside. In this compartment, DCs may represent the target of infection (Zambello et al., 2005). Bone marrow biopsies demonstrated a topographic distribution of DCs and NK cells that indicates a close contact between the two cell types (Zambello et al., 2005). Patients' NK cells also showed a reduced capability of promoting Mo-DC maturation and of killing iDC (Balsamo et al., 2009). These findings could be explained, at least in part, by the low expression levels of NKp30 activating receptor, usually involved in the molecular interactions occurring between NK cells and DC. It is suggested that impairment of DC killing capabilities detected in patients' NK-GLs may allow an accumulation of DC that, at certain sites, may sustain the chronic proliferation of NK cells themselves. DCs are also likely to represent the source of IL-15 that is crucial in the mechanisms sustaining the maintenance of NK proliferation. IL-15 has been found to mediate its activity by interfering with Bcl-2 family members, and more specifically by modulating Bid expression (Hodge et al., 2009). Hodge et al., demonstrated that CLPD-NK cells express low levels of Bid, that are reversed by blockade of IL-15 signaling (Hodge et al., 2009). Bid is also increased following bortezomib (Velcade/PS341) treatment and this effect is coordinate with increased susceptibility to Fas- or TRAIL- independent apoptosis. In fact, bortezomib increased cell surface expression of DR4, a TRAIL death receptor decoy. The inability of death receptors to account for the apoptosis may be explained by the putative role of Bid in DNA damage and repair. It is possible that elevation of Bid expression in CLPD-NK cells promotes S phase cell cycle block and death (Hodge et al., 2009).

A genetic susceptibility for this disease has been suggested and has been related to the detection of type B *KIR gene* repertoire which is characterized by a high number of activating genes (Zambello & Semenzato, 2009). In fact, a restricted pattern of KIR expression has usually been reported in these patients. A typical feature is the preferential expression of the KIR activating receptor isoforms and this pattern correlates with a reduced expression of other activating receptors, such as NCRs (Zambello et al., 2003). Together with a bias towards activating KIR expression, a deep silencing of inhibitory KIR through increased gene methylation has been recently demonstrated by our group (Gattazzo et al., 2010). More specifically, we showed the complete lack of KIR3DL1 expression in most analyzed patients, being the receptor expressed in 13% of patients as compared to 90% of controls ($p<0.01$). Interestingly, the results of methylation patterns of *KIR3DL1* promoter showed a significantly higher methylation status (0.76 ± 0.12 SD) in the patients with respect to the healthy subjects (0.49 ± 0.10 SD, $p<0.01$). These data suggest that together with the increased expression of activating receptors, the lack of the inhibitory signal could also play a role in the pathogenesis of disease (Gattazzo et al., 2010). Recent data on the pathogenesis of CLPD-NK are summarized in Figure 2.

Biochemical studies on the mechanisms sustaining the growth of NK cells in these patients have demonstrated a role of RAS farnesil transferase (Epling-Burnette et al., 2008), with clinical implications (see below). Pathological NK cells express CD16 and usually low levels of CD56 and CD57. As expected, cells express TIA1, granzyme and perforins, which correlate with the cytotoxic potential of these cells. CD94 is expressed at high density on patients' NK cells, frequently associated with the inhibitory subunit NKG2A, although, in a relevant number of cases, the dimer CD94/NKG2C has been reported (Zambello & Semenzato, 2003). Patients' NK cells express functional β and γ chains of IL-2/IL-15 receptor, which are strictly related to the role of these cytokines in the pathogenesis of disease (Zambello & Semenzato, 2009).

Most patients are asymptomatic, and the disease has a chronic indolent clinical course, similar to that reported for patients with T-LGL leukemia (Loughran, 1993; Semenzato et al., 1987; Tefferi et al., 1994; Semenzato et al., 1997; Oshimi 1996). In some cases this disorder is associated with other conditions, including pure red cell aplasia, vasculitic syndromes, solid and hematologic tumors, splenectomy, neuropathy and autoimmune disorders (Loughran,

1993; Semenzato et al., 1987; Tefferi et al., 1994; Semenzato et al., 1997; Oshimi, 1996). Recently, in patients with chronic myelogenous leukaemia, the association has been reported between treatment with dasatinib and the development of CLPD-NK. It has been suggested that the development of CLPD-NK might contribute on the control of Ph positive leukemic cells proliferation (Kim et al., 2009). Systemic symptoms, such as cytopenia (mostly neutropenia and anemia), are rare. Lymphoadenopathy, hepatomegaly, splenomegaly and cutaneous lesions are uncommon. Occasionally, patients present a slow progressive increase of peripheral blood NK cells and organ involvement. Several cases with a spontaneous complete remission have been reported (Zambello & Semenzato, 2009). Cytologically, the circulating cells show typical granular lymphocyte morphology, with moderate amount of pale cytoplasm that contains ≥ 3 azurophilic granules. Bone marrow biopsy is characterized by interstitial infiltration of cells with small nuclei and pale cytoplasm, which are difficult to recognize without the help of immunohistochemical techniques. Cytogenetic is normal in most cases (Zambello & Semenzato, 2009) and the germ line configuration of TCR is demonstrated, as expected for normal NK cells. Since clonality of proliferating cells is difficult to detect in these patients, the analysis of restriction fragment length polymorphism (RLFP) has been used as an indirect marker to demonstrate the clonality in some but not all patients. In rare case, in which EBV can be demonstrated in plasmid form within NK cells, the clonality of cells might be easily examined by Southern Blot analysis using probes recognizing the EBV terminal repeats (Kawa-Ha et al., 1989). Patients with CLPD-NK usually have an indolent clinical course and respond to immunosuppressive therapy with low doses of methotrexate (usually 10 mg/m^2/week) or of cyclophosphamide (50 or 100 mg/day) or cyclosporin (3-5 mg/kg/day) with or without inclusion of low doses of steroids (Lamy & Loughran, 2011).

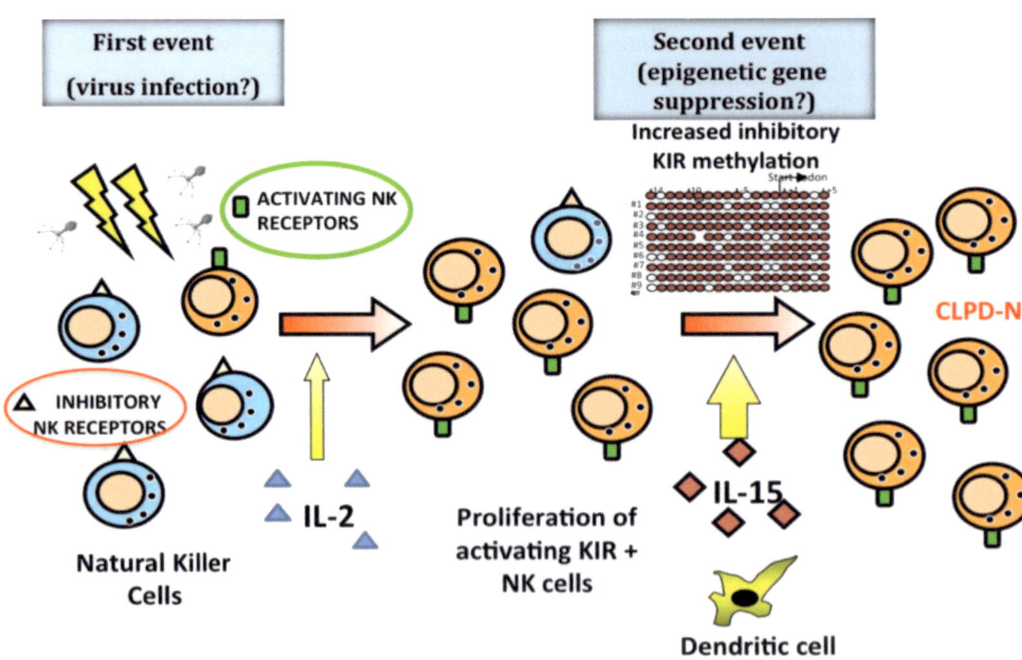

Fig. 2. Possible mechanisms of CLPD-NK pathogenesis.

5. Conclusions

NK cells are bone marrow–derived granular lymphocytes that have a key role in the recognition and in the killing of tumor- or virus-infected cells. The identification of a large array of surface NK receptors capable of transducing inhibitory or activating signals, let to explain how their effector functions could be regulated.

In recent years, it has also been shown that NK cells may play a role in the regulation of the immune response. This has been based on the finding that NK cells were able to functionally interact with different cells of the innate immune system including DCs, pDCs and macrophages. Besides the well known $CD56^{dim}CD16^{+}$ cytotoxic PB NK cells, different NK cell subsets located in specific tissue/organ compartments have been shown to exert various, alternative, regulatory functions. NK cells homing in SLT promote Th1 polarization. Conversely, decidual NK cells favour Treg expansion and play an important role in tissue remodelling and neo-angiogenesis process. In MALT, NK22 cells may support immune defence against bacteria invasion by their peculiar cytokine and chemokine secreting profile.

Whether the above described different NK cell subsets may derive from the same lineage or from different ones, is still a matter of debate. Studies on NK cell development may help to clarify the possible lineage relationship between the different NK cell subsets. In vitro models of NK cell development helped to define phenotypically and functionally different maturation stages that were, at least in part, confirmed by in vivo analysis. For example, the $CD56^{bright}CD16^{-}CD94/NKG2A^{+}KIR^{-}$ subset, that is largely represented at the end on in vitro development, represents the first wave of lymphocytes appearing in PB at early time intervals after HSCT. NK cells originate from $CD34^{+}$ hematopoietic precursors but several experimental evidences suggest that the NK cell development and terminal maturation does not occur wholly in the BM. Other secondary lymphoid organs, including L.N. and MALT, as well as decidua, may represent sites where NK cell development occurs. This suggest how defined subsets of NK cells may differentiate in peculiar tissues and point the attention on the role of the microenvironment in such a process. The full characterization of the genetic and epigenetic factors that may contribute to determine the type of NK cell that will develop is still in process and it will be important also to better define mechanisms leading to NK cell malignant transformation.

It is hopeful that investigation on NK cell neoplasm pathogenesis could lead to identify molecular targets and discovery of more efficient and less toxic treatments. The elucidation of pathways by which EBV transform NK cells might help to identify new molecular targets. Furthermore, the mechanisms of resistance to therapy, including alteration of apoptosis pathways should be deeply characterized. Thus, the definition the NK neoplasm patho-physiology and the identification of possible biological targets may help to improve therapeutical approaches.

6. References

Albertsson PA, Basse PH, Hokland M, Goldfarb RH, Nagelkerke JF, Nannmark U, Kuppen PJ. (2003) NK cells and the tumour microenvironment: implications for NK-cell function and anti-tumour activity. *Trends Immunol.* 24:603-609.

Aliahmad P, de la Torre B, Kaye J. (2010). Shared dependence on the DNA-binding factor TOX for the development of lymphoid tissue-inducer cell and NK cell lineages. *Nat Immunol* 11: 945-52

Anfossi N, André P, Guia S, Falk CS, Roetynck S, Stewart CA, Breso V, Frassati C, Reviron D, Middleton D, Romagné F, Ugolini S, Vivier E. (2006) Human NK cell education by inhibitory receptors for MHC class I. *Immunity*. 25:331-342.

Balsamo M, Scordamaglia F, Pietra G, Manzini C, Cantoni C, Boitano M, Queirolo P, Vermi W, Facchetti F, Moretta A, Moretta L, Mingari MC and Vitale M. (2009) Melanoma-associated fibroblasts modulate NK cell phenotype and antitumor cytotoxicity. *Proc Natl Acad Sci U S A*. 106:20847-20852

Balsamo M., Zambello R., Teramo A., Pedrazzi M., Sparatore B., Scordamaglia F., Pende D., Mingari M.C., Moretta L., Moretta A., Semenzato G. and Vitale M. (2009) Analysis of NK cell/DC interaction in NK-type Lymphoproliferative Disease of Granular Lymphocytes (LDGL): role of DNAM-1 and NKp30. *Exp. Hematol.* 37:1167-1175

Bellora F, Castriconi R, Dondero A, Reggiardo G, Moretta L, Mantovani A, Moretta A, Bottino C. (2010) The interaction of human natural killer cells with either unpolarized or polarized macrophages results in different functional outcomes. *Proc Natl Acad Sci U S A*. 107:21659-21664.

Benne C, Lelievre JD, Balbo M, Henry A, Sakano S, Levy Y. (2009). Notch increases T/NK potential of human hematopoietic progenitors and inhibits B cell differentiation at a pro-B stage. *Stem Cells* 27: 1676-85

Bennett IM, Zatsepina O, Zamai L, Azzoni L, Mikheeva T, Perussia B. (1996). Definition of a natural killer NKR-P1A+/CD56-/CD16- functionally immature human NK cell subset that differentiates in vitro in the presence of interleukin 12. *J Exp Med* 184: 1845-56

Biassoni R, Cantoni C, Pende D, Sivori S, Parolini S, Vitale M, Bottino C, Moretta A. (2001) Human natural killer cell receptors and co-receptors. *Immunol Rev.* 181:203-214.

Biron CA, Nguyen KB, Pien GC, Cousens LP and Salazar-Mather P. (1999) Natural Killer cells in antiviral defense: function and regulation by innate cytokines. *Annu Rev Immunol.* 17:189-220.

Bjorkstrom NK, Riese P, Heuts F, Andersson S, Fauriat C, Ivarsson MA, Bjorklund AT, Flodstrom-Tullberg M, Michaelsson J, Rottenberg ME, Guzman CA, Ljunggren HG, Malmberg KJ. (2010). Expression patterns of NKG2A, KIR, and CD57 define a process of CD56dim NK-cell differentiation uncoupled from NK-cell education. *Blood* 116: 3853-64

Boos MD, Yokota Y, Eberl G, Kee BL. (2007). Mature natural killer cell and lymphoid tissue-inducing cell development requires Id2-mediated suppression of E protein activity. *J Exp Med* 204: 1119-30

Borowitz M.J., Béné M.C., Harris N.L., Porwit A., Matutes E. Acute leukemias of ambigous lineage. *In*: Swerdlow S.H., Campo E., Harris N.L., Jaffe E.J., Pileri S.A., Stein H., Thiele J., Vardiman J. eds. (2008) WHO *Classification of Tumours of Haematopoietic and Lymphoid Tissues*. IARC Lyon: 155.

Bottino C, Castriconi R, Pende D, Rivera P, Nanni M, Carnemolla B, Cantoni C, Grassi J, Marcenaro S, Reymond N, Vitale M, Moretta L, Lopez M, Moretta A. (2003) Identification of PVR (CD155) and Nectin-2 (CD112) as cell surface ligands for the human DNAM-1 (CD226) activating molecule. *J Exp Med.* 198:557-567.

Bottino, C., L. Moretta, D. Pende, M. Vitale, and A. Moretta. (2004) Learning how to discriminate between friends and enemies, a lesson from Natural Killer cells. *Mol. Immunol.* 41: 569-575.

Brandt CS, Baratin M, Yi EC, Kennedy J, Gao Z, Fox B, Haldeman B, Ostrander CD, Kaifu T, Chabannon C, Moretta A, West R, Xu W, Vivier E, Levin SD. (2009) The B7 family member B7-H6 is a tumor cell ligand for the activating natural killer cell receptor NKp30 in humans. *J Exp Med.* 206:1495-1503.

Briard D, Brouty-Boye D, Azzarone B, Jasmin C. (2002). Fibroblasts from human spleen regulate NK cell differentiation from blood CD34(+) progenitors via cell surface IL-15. *J Immunol* 168: 4326-32

Bryceson YT, March ME, Ljunggren HG, Long EO. (2006). Activation, coactivation, and costimulation of resting human natural killer cells. *Immunol Rev* 214: 73-91

Caligiuri MA. (2008). Human natural killer cells. *Blood* 112: 461-9

Cannons JL, Tangye SG, Schwartzberg PL. (2011). SLAM family receptors and SAP adaptors in immunity. *Annu Rev Immunol* 29: 665-705

Carlsten M, Norell H, Bryceson YT, Poschke I, Schedvins K, Ljunggren HG, Kiessling R, Malmberg KJ. (2009) Primary human tumor cells expressing CD155 impair tumor targeting by down-regulating DNAM-1 on NK cells. *J Immunol.* 183:4921-4930.

Carrega P, Morandi B, Costa R, Frumanto G, Forte G, Altavilla G, Ratto G.B., Mingari M.C., Moretta L., Ferlazzo G.. (2008) Natural killer cells infiltrating human nonsmall-cell lung cancer are enriched in CD56 bright CD16(-) cells and display an impaired capability to kill tumor cells. *Cancer* 112:863-875.

Chan J.K., Sin V.C., Wong K.F., et al., (1997) Nonnasal lymphoma expressing the natural killer cell marker CD56: a clinicopathologic study of 49 cases of an uncommon aggressive neoplasm. *Blood* 89: 4501-4514.

Chan J.K.C., Jaffe E.S., Ralfkiaer E., Ko Y.K. Aggressive NK-leukemia. *In*: Swerdlow S.H., Campo E., Harris N.L., Jaffe E.J., Pileri S.A., Stein H., Thiele J., Vardiman J. eds. (2008a) *WHO Classification of Tumours of Haematopoietic and Lymphoid Tissues.* IARC Lyon 276-277.

Chan J.K.C., Quintanilla-Martinez N.L., Ferry J.A., Peh S.C. Extranodal NK/T-cell lymphoma, nasal type. *In*: Swerdlow S.H., Campo E., Harris N.L., Jaffe E.J., Pileri S.A., Stein H., Thiele J., Vardiman J. eds. (2008b) *WHO Classification of Tumours of Haematopoietic and Lymphoid Tissues.* IARC Lyon 285-288.

Cheung M.M., Chan J.K., Lau W.H., et al., (1998) Primary non-Hodgkin's lymphoma of the nose and nasopharynx: clinical features, tumor immunophenotype, and treatment outcome in 113 patients. *Journal of Clinical Oncology* 16: 70-77.

Chinen H, Matsuoka K, Sato T, Kamada N, Okamoto S, Hisamatsu T, Kobayashi T, Hasegawa H, Sugita A, Kinjo F, Fujita J, Hibi T. (2007). Lamina propria c-kit+ immune precursors reside in human adult intestine and differentiate into natural killer cells. *Gastroenterology* 133: 559-73

Colonna M. 2009. Interleukin-22-producing natural killer cells and lymphoid tissue inducer-like cells in mucosal immunity. *Immunity* 31: 15-23

Cooley S, Weisdorf DJ, Guethlein LA, Klein JP, Wang T, Le CT, Marsh SG, Geraghty D, Spellman S, Haagenson MD, Ladner M, Trachtenberg E, Parham P, Miller JS. (2010) Donor selection for natural killer cell receptor genes leads to superior survival after unrelated transplantation for acute myelogenous leukemia. *Blood.* 116:2411-2419.

Cooper MA, Fehniger TA and Caligiuri MA. (2001) The biology of human natural killer-cell subsets. *Trends Immunol*. 22:633-640.

de Pooter RF, Kee BL. (2010). E proteins and the regulation of early lymphocyte development. *Immunol Rev* 238: 93-109

Della Chiesa M, Carlomagno S, Frumento G, Balsamo M, Cantoni C, Conte R, Moretta L, Moretta A and Vitale M. (2006a) The tryptophan catabolite L-kynurenine inhibits the surface expression of NKp46- and NKG2D-activating receptors and regulates NK-cell function. *Blood*. 108:4118-4125.

Della Chiesa M, Romagnani C, Thiel A, Moretta L, Moretta A. (2006b) Multidirectional interactions are bridging human NK cells with plasmacytoid and monocyte-derived dendritic cells during innate immune responses. *Blood*. 108:3851-3858.

Della Chiesa M, Falco M, Parolini S, Bellora F, Petretto A, Romeo E, Balsamo M, Gambarotti M, Scordamaglia F, Tabellini G, Facchetti F, Vermi W, Bottino C, Moretta A and Vitale M. (2010) GPR56 as a novel marker identifying the $CD56^{dull}$ $CD16^{+}$ NK cell subset both in Blood Stream and Inflamed Peripheral Tissues. *Int. Immunol.* 22:91-100

DiSanto JP, Keever CA, Small TN, Nicols GL, O'Reilly RJ, Flomenberg N. (1990). Absence of interleukin 2 production in a severe combined immunodeficiency disease syndrome with T cells. *J Exp Med* 171: 1697-704

Doubrovina ES, Doubrovin MM, Vider E, Sisson RB, O'Reilly RJ, Dupont B, Vyas YM. (2003) Evasion from NK cell immunity by MHC class I chain-related molecules expressing colon adenocarcinoma. *J Immunol*.171:6891-6899.

Doulatov S, Notta F, Eppert K, Nguyen LT, Ohashi PS, Dick JE. (2010). Revised map of the human progenitor hierarchy shows the origin of macrophages and dendritic cells in early lymphoid development. *Nat Immunol* 11: 585-93

Dubois S, Mariner J, Waldmann TA, Tagaya Y. (2002). IL-15Ralpha recycles and presents IL-15 In trans to neighboring cells. *Immunity* 17: 537-47

Epling-Burnette P.K., Sokol L., Chen X., Bai F., Zhou J. et al., (2008) Clinical improvement by farnesyltransferase inhibition in NK large granular lymphocyte leukemia associated with imbalanced NK receptor signaling. *Blood* 112: 4694-4698.

Fehniger TA, Cooper MA, Nuovo GJ, Cella M, Facchetti F, Colonna M, Caligiuri MA. (2003) CD56bright natural killer cells are present in human lymph nodes and are activated by T cell-derived IL-2: a potential new link between adaptive and innate immunity. *Blood*. 101:3052-3057.

Ferlazzo G, Munz C. (2004) NK cell compartments and their activation by dendritic cells. *J. Immunol*. 172:1333-1339.

Fernandez L.A., Pope B., Lee C., Zayed E. (b1986) Aggressive natural killer cell leukemia in an adult with establishment of an NK line. *Blood* 67: 925-930.

Fregni G, Perier A, Pittari G, Jacobelli S, Sastre X, Gervois N, Allard M, Bercovici N, Avril MF, Caignard A. (2011) Unique functional status of natural killer cells in metastatic stage IV melanoma patients and its modulation by chemotherapy. *Clin Cancer Res*. 17:2628-2637.

Freud AG, Becknell B, Roychowdhury S, Mao HC, Ferketich AK, Nuovo GJ, Hughes TL, Marburger TB, Sung J, Baiocchi RA, Guimond M, Caligiuri MA. (2005). A human CD34(+) subset resides in lymph nodes and differentiates into $CD56^{bright}$ natural killer cells. *Immunity* 22: 295-304

Freud AG, Yokohama A, Becknell B, Lee MT, Mao HC, Ferketich AK, Caligiuri MA. (2006). Evidence for discrete stages of human natural killer cell differentiation in vivo. *J Exp Med* 203: 1033-43

Freud AG, Caligiuri MA. (2006). Human natural killer cell development. *Immunol Rev* 214: 56-72

Fuchs A. & Colonna M. (2006) The role of NK cell recognition of nectin and nectin-like proteins in tumor immunosurveillance. *Seminars in Cancer Biology*. 16:359-366.

Gascoyne DM, Long E, Veiga-Fernandes H, de Boer J, Williams O, Seddon B, Coles M, Kioussis D, Brady HJ. (2009). The basic leucine zipper transcription factor E4BP4 is essential for natural killer cell development. *Nat Immunol* 10: 1118-24

Gattazzo C., Teramo A., Miorin M., Scquizzato E., Cabrelle A., Balsamo M et al., (2010) Lack of expression of inhibitory KIR3DL1 receptor in patients with natural killer cell-type lymphoproliferative disease of granular lymphocytes. *Haematologica* 95:1722-1729.

Ghiringhelli F, Ménard C, Terme M, Flament C, Taieb J, Chaput N, Puig PE, Novault S, Escudier B, Vivier E, Lecesne A, Robert C, Blay JY, Bernard J, Caillat-Zucman S, Freitas A, Tursz T, Wagner-Ballon O, Capron C, Vainchencker W, Martin F, Zitvogel L. (2005) CD4+CD25+ regulatory T cells inhibit natural killer cell functions in a transforming growth factor-beta-dependent manner. *J Exp Med*. 202:1075-1085.

Giliani S, Mori L, de Saint Basile G, Le Deist F, Rodriguez-Perez C, Forino C, Mazzolari E, Dupuis S, Elhasid R, Kessel A, Galambrun C, Gil J, Fischer A, Etzioni A, Notarangelo LD. (2005). Interleukin-7 receptor alpha (IL-7Rα) deficiency: cellular and molecular bases. Analysis of clinical, immunological, and molecular features in 16 novel patients. *Immunol Rev* 203: 110-26

Glimcher LH, Townsend MJ, Sullivan BM, Lord GM. (2004). Recent developments in the transcriptional regulation of cytolytic effector cells. *Nat Rev Immunol* 4: 900-11

Grzywacz B, Kataria N, Sikora M, Oostendorp RA, Dzierzak EA, Blazar BR, Miller JS, Verneris MR. (2006). Coordinated acquisition of inhibitory and activating receptors and functional properties by developing human natural killer cells. *Blood* 108: 3824-33

Grzywacz B, Kataria N, Blazar BR, Miller JS, Verneris MR. (2011). Natural killer-cell differentiation by myeloid progenitors. *Blood* 117: 3548-58

Guerra N, Tan YX, Joncker NT, Choy A, Gallardo F, Xiong N, Knoblaugh S, Cado D, Greenberg NM, Raulet DH. (2008) NKG2D-deficient mice are defective in tumor surveillance in models of spontaneous malignancy. *Immunity*. 28:571-580.

Haas P, Loiseau P, Tamouza R, Cayuela JM, Moins-Teisserenc H, Busson M, Henry G, Falk CS, Charron D, Socié G, Toubert A, Dulphy N. (2011) NK-cell education is shaped by donor HLA genotype after unrelated allogeneic hematopoietic stem cell transplantation. *Blood*. 117:1021-1029.

Halfteck, G. G., M. Elboim, C. Gur, H. Achdout, H. Ghadially, and O. Mandelboim. (2009) Enhanced in vivo growth of lymphoma tumors in the absence of the NK-activating receptor NKp46/NCR1. *J. Immunol*. 182:2221-2230.

Hamann I, Unterwalder N, Cardona AE, Meisel C, Zipp F, Ransohoff RM, Infante-Duarte C. (2011) Analyses of phenotypic and functional characteristics of CX3CR1-expressing natural killer cells. *Immunology*. 133:62-73.

Hanna J, Goldman-Wohl D, Hamani Y, Avraham I, Greenfield C, Natanson-Yaron S, Prus D, Cohen-Daniel L, Arnon TI, Manaster I, Gazit R, Yutkin V, Benharroch D, Porgador

A, Keshet E, Yagel S and Mandelboim O. (2006) Decidual NK cells regulate key developmental processes at the human fetal-maternal interface. *Nat Med.* 12:1065-1074.

Harabuchi Y., Takahara M., Kishibe K., Moriai S., Nagato T., Ishii H. (2009) Nasal natural killer (NK)/T-cell lymphoma: clinical, histological, virological, and genetic features. *International Journal of Clinical Oncology* 14:181–190.

Harabuchi Y., Yamanaka N., Kataura N., Imai S., Kinoshita T., et al., (1990) Epstein-Barr virus in nasal T-cell lymphomas in patients with lethal midline granuloma. *Lancet* 335: 128-130.

Hodge D.L., Yang J., Buschman M.D., Schaughency P.M., Dang H. et al., (2009). Interleukin-15 enhances proteasomal degradation of Bid in normal lymphocytes: implications for large granular lymphocyte leukemias.*Cancer Res.* ;69:3986-94.

Hoshida Y., Hongyo T., Jia X., He Y., Hasui K., Dong Z., et al., (2003). Analysis of p53, K-ras, c-kit, and beta-catenin gene mutations insinonasal NK/T cell lymphoma in northeast district of China. *Cancer Sci.*94:297–301.

Huang Y., de Reynie`s A., de Leval L., Ghazi B., Martin-Garcia N., Travert M., et al., (2010) Gene expression profiling identifies emerging oncogenic pathways operating in extranodal NK/T-cell lymphoma,nasal type. *Blood* 115:1226–37.

Hughes T, Becknell B, Freud AG, McClory S, Briercheck E, Yu J, Mao C, Giovenzana C, Nuovo G, Wei L, Zhang X, Gavrilin MA, Wewers MD, Caligiuri MA. (2010). Interleukin-1beta selectively expands and sustains interleukin-22+ immature human natural killer cells in secondary lymphoid tissue. *Immunity* 32: 803-14

Iguchi-Manaka A, Kai H, Yamashita Y, Shibata K, Tahara-Hanaoka S, Honda S, Yasui T, Kikutani H, Shibuya K, Shibuya A. (2008) Accelerated tumor growth in mice deficient in DNAM-1 receptor. *J Exp Med.* 205:2959-2964.

Iqbal J., Weisenburger D.D., Chowdhury A., Tsai M.Y, Srivastava G., Greiner T.C., et al., (2010) The International Peripheral T-cell Lymphoma Project. Natural killer cell lymphoma shares strikingly similar molecular features with a group of non hepatosplenic γδ T-cell lymphoma and is highly sensitive to a novel aurora kinase a inhibitor in vitro. *Leukemia* 25: 348-358

Jaffe E.S. (1996) Classification of natural killer (NK) cell and NK-like T cell malignancies. *Blood* 87: 1207-1210.

Jondal M, Pazirandeh A, Okret S. (2004). Different roles for glucocorticoids in thymocyte homeostasis? *Trends Immunol* 25: 595-600

Juelke K, Killig M, Luetke-Eversloh M, Parente E, Gruen J, Morandi B, Ferlazzo G, Thiel A, Schmitt-Knosalla I, Romagnani C. (2010). CD62L expression identifies a unique subset of polyfunctional CD56dim NK cells. *Blood* 116: 1299-307

Kamizono S, Duncan GS, Seidel MG, Morimoto A, Hamada K, Grosveld G, Akashi K, Lind EF, Haight JP, Ohashi PS, Look AT, Mak TW. (2009). Nfil3/E4bp4 is required for the development and maturation of NK cells in vivo. *J Exp Med* 206: 2977-86

Kanno H, Kojya S, Li T, Ohsawa M, Nakatsuka S, Miyaguchi M, et al., (2000) Low frequency of HLA-A*0201 allele in patients with Epstein–Barr virus-positive nasal lymphomas with polymorphic reticulosis morphology. *Int J Cancer* ;87:195–9.

Kawa-Ha K., Ishihara S., Ninomiya T., Yumura-Yagi K., Hara J., et al., (1989) CD3-negative lymphoproliferative disease of granular lymphocytes containing Epstein-Barr viral DNA. *Journal of Clinical Investigation* 84: 51-55.

Kennedy MK, Glaccum M, Brown SN, Butz EA, Viney JL, Embers M, Matsuki N, Charrier K, Sedger L, Willis CR, Brasel K, Morrissey PJ, Stocking K, Schuh JC, Joyce S, Peschon JJ. (2000). Reversible defects in natural killer and memory CD8 T cell lineages in interleukin 15-deficient mice. *J Exp Med* 191: 771-80

Kim DH, Kamel-Reid S., Chang H., Sutherland R., et al., (2009) Natural Killer or natural killer/T cell lineage large granular lymphocytosis associated with dasatinib therapy for Philadelphia chromosome positive leukemia. *Haematologica* 94: 135-9.

Kim S, Iizuka K, Aguila HL, Weissman IL, Yokoyama WM. (2000) In vivo natural killer cell activities revealed by natural killer cell-deficient mice. *Proc Natl Acad Sci U S A.* 97:2731-2736.

Kwong YL, Chan AC, Liang R, et al., (1997) CD56+ NK lymphomas: clinicopathological features and prognosis. *Br J Haematol* 97: 821-829.

Kwong YL (2005) Natural killer-cell malignancies: diagnosis and treatment. *Leukemia* 19: 2186-2194

Laiosa CV, Stadtfeld M, Graf T. (2006). Determinants of lymphoid-myeloid lineage diversification. *Annu Rev Immunol* 24: 705-38

Lamy T., Loughran T.P. Jr. (2011) How we treat LGL leukemia. *Blood* 117:2764-74.

Lanier LL, Le AM, Civin CI, Loken MR, Phillips JH. (1986) The relationship of CD16 (Leu-11) and Leu-19 (NKH-1) antigen expression on human peripheral blood NK cells and cytotoxic T lymphocytes. *J Immunol.* 136:4480-4486.

Lanier LL, Spits H, Phillips JH. (1992). The developmental relationship between NK cells and T cells. *Immunol Today* 13: 392-5

Le Maux Chansac B, Moretta A, Vergnon I, Opolon P, Lécluse Y, Grunenwald D, Kubin M, Soria JC, Chouaib S, Mami-Chouaib F. (2005) NK cells infiltrating a MHC class I-deficient lung adenocarcinoma display impaired cytotoxic activity toward autologous tumor cells associated with altered NK cell-triggering receptors. *J Immunol.* 175:5790-5798.

Liang X., Graam G.K. (2008) Natural Killer cell neoplasms. *Cancer* 112:1425-1436.

Lin C.W., Liu T.Y., Chen S.U., et al., (2005) CD94 1A transcripts characterize lymphoblastic lymphoma/leukemia of immature natural killer cell origin with distinct clinical features. *Blood* 106: 3567-3574.

Liu X., Ryland L., Yang J., Liao A., Aliaga C., Watts R., Tan S.F., et al., (2010) Targeting of survivin by nanoliposomal ceramide induces complete remission in a rat model of NK-LGL leukemia. *Blood* 116:4192-201.

Ljunggren HG, Kärre K. (1990) In search of the 'missing self': MHC molecules and NK cell recognition. *Immunol Today.* 11(7):237-244.

Lopez-Botet M., Perez-Villar J.J., Carreterro M., et al., (1997) Structure and function of the CD94 C-type lectin receptor complex involved in recognition of HLA class I molecules. *Immmunology Reviews* 155: 165-174.

Lopez-Verges S, Milush JM, Pandey S, York VA, Arakawa-Hoyt J, Pircher H, Norris PJ, Nixon DF, Lanier LL. (2010). CD57 defines a functionally distinct population of mature NK cells in the human CD56dimCD16+ NK-cell subset. *Blood* 116: 3865-74

Lotzova E, Savary CA. (1993). Human natural killer cell development from bone marrow progenitors: analysis of phenotype, cytotoxicity and growth. *Nat Immun* 12: 209-17

Loughran T.P. Jr, Hadlock K.G., Yang Q., Perzova R., Zambello R. et al., (1997) Seroreactivity to an envelope protein of human T-cell leukemia/lymphoma virus in patients with

CD3- (natural killer) lymphoproliferative disease of granular lymphocytes. *Blood* 90:1977-1981.

Loughran T.P., Jr. (1993) Clonal diseases of large granular lymphocytes. *Blood* 82:1-14.

Ma A, Koka R, Burkett P. (2006). Diverse functions of IL-2, IL-15, and IL-7 in lymphoid homeostasis. *Annu Rev Immunol* 24: 657-79

Makishima H., Ito T., Momose K., Nakazawa H., Shimodaira S., Kamijo Y., et al., (2007) Chemokine system and tissue infiltration in aggressive NK-cell leukemia. *Leukemia Research* 31:1237–45.

Male V, Hughes T, McClory S, Colucci F, Caligiuri MA, Moffett A. (2010). Immature NK cells, capable of producing IL-22, are present in human uterine mucosa. *J Immunol* 185: 3913-8

Mandelboim O, Lieberman N, Lev M, Paul L, Arnon TI, Bushkin Y, Davis DM, Strominger JL, Yewdell JW, Porgador A. (2001) Recognition of haemagglutinins on virus-infected cells by NKp46 activates lysis by human NK cells. *Nature.* 409:1055-1060.

Mantovani A, Allavena P, Sica A, Balkwill F. (2008) Cancer-related inflammation. *Nature* 454:436-444.

Marquez C, Trigueros C, Franco JM, Ramiro AR, Carrasco YR, Lopez-Botet M, Toribio ML. (1998). Identification of a common developmental pathway for thymic natural killer cells and dendritic cells. *Blood* 91: 2760-71

Miller JS, Alley KA, McGlave P. (1994). Differentiation of natural killer (NK) cells from human primitive marrow progenitors in a stroma-based long-term culture system: identification of a CD34+7+ NK progenitor. *Blood* 83: 2594-601

Miller JS, McCullar V, Punzel M, Lemischka IR, Moore KA. (1999). Single adult human CD34(+)/Lin-/CD38(-) progenitors give rise to natural killer cells, B-lineage cells, dendritic cells, and myeloid cells. *Blood* 93: 96-106

Miller JS, McCullar V. (2001). Human natural killer cells with polyclonal lectin and immunoglobulinlike receptors develop from single hematopoietic stem cells with preferential expression of NKG2A and KIR2DL2/L3/S2. *Blood* 98: 705-13

Miller JS, Soignier Y, Panoskaltsis-Mortari A, McNearney SA, Yun GH, Fautsch SK, McKenna D, Le C, Defor TE, Burns LJ, Orchard PJ, Blazar BR, Wagner JE, Slungaard A, Weisdorf DJ, Okazaki IJ, McGlave PB. (2005) Successful adoptive transfer and in vivo expansion of human haploidentical NK cells in patients with cancer. *Blood.* 105:3051-3057.

Minarovits J., Hu L.F., Imai S., et al., (1994) Clonality, expression and methylation patterns of the EBV genomes in lethal midline granulomas classified as peripheral angiocentric T-cell lymphomas. *Journal Genetic Virology* 75: 77-84.

Mingari MC, Poggi A, Biassoni R, Bellomo R, Ciccone E, Pella N, Morelli L, Verdiani S, Moretta A, Moretta L. (1991). In vitro proliferation and cloning of CD3- CD16+ cells from human thymocyte precursors. *J Exp Med* 174: 21-6

Mingari MC, Vitale C, Cantoni C, Bellomo R, Ponte M, Schiavetti F, Bertone S, Moretta A, Moretta L. (1997). Interleukin-15-induced maturation of human natural killer cells from early thymic precursors: selective expression of CD94/NKG2-A as the only HLA class I-specific inhibitory receptor. *Eur J Immunol* 27: 1374-80

Moffett-King A. (2002). Natural killer cells and pregnancy. *Nat Rev Immunol* 2: 656-63

Moretta A, Bottino C, Vitale M, Pende D, Cantoni C, Mingari MC, Biassoni R, Moretta L. (2001). Activating receptors and coreceptors involved in human natural killer cell-mediated cytolysis. *Annu Rev Immunol* 19: 197-223

Moretta A., Marcenaro E., Sivori S., Della Chiesa M., Vitale M. and Moretta L. (2005) Early liaisons between cells of the innate immune system in inflamed peripheral tissues. *Trends Immunol.* 26:668-675.

Moretta L, Locatelli F, Pende D, Marcenaro E, Mingari MC, Moretta A. (2011) Killer Ig-like receptor-mediated control of natural killer cell alloreactivity in haploidentical hematopoietic stem cell transplantation. *Blood.* 117(3):764-771.

Mrozek E, Anderson P, Caligiuri MA. (1996). Role of interleukin-15 in the development of human CD56+ natural killer cells from CD34+ hematopoietic progenitor cells. *Blood* 87: 2632-40

Nakashima Y., Tagawa H., Suzuki R., Karman S., Karube K., et al., (2005) Genoma-wide array-based comparative genomic hybridization of natural killer cell lymphoma/leukemia: different genomic alteration pattern of aggressive NK-leukemia and extranodal NK/T cell lymphoma, nasal type. *Genes Chromosomes Cancer* 44: 247-255.

Nguyen S, Dhedin N, Vernant JP, Kuentz M, Al Jijakli A, Rouas-Freiss N, Carosella ED, Boudifa A, Debré P, Vieillard V. (2005) NK-cell reconstitution after haploidentical hematopoietic stem-cell transplantations: immaturity of NK cells and inhibitory effect of NKG2A override GvL effect. *Blood.* 105:4135-4142.

Oshimi K. (1996) Lymphoproliferative disorders of natural killer cells. *International Journal of Hematology* 63: 279-290.

Oshimi K. (2007) Progress in undestanding and managing natural killer cell-malignancies. *British Journal of Haematology* 139:532-544.

Pandolfi F., Loughran T.P.Jr, Starkebaum G., et al., (1990) Clinical course and prognosis of the lymphoproliferative disease of granular lymphocytes. A multicenter study. *Cancer* 65:341-348.

Parham P. (2005) MHC class I molecules and KIRs in human history, health and survival. *Nat Rev Immunol.* 5:201-214.

Parham P. (2006). Taking license with natural killer cell maturation and repertoire development. *Immunol Rev* 214: 155-60

Parolini S, Santoro A, Marcenaro E, Luini W, Massardi L, Facchetti F, Communi D, Parmentier M, Majorana A, Sironi M, Tabellini G, Moretta A, Sozzani S. (2007) The role of chemerin in the colocalization of NK and dendritic cell subsets into inflamed tissues. *Blood.* 109:3625-3632.

Pende D, Marcenaro S, Falco M, Martini S, Bernardo ME, Montagna D, Romeo E, Cognet C, Martinetti M, Maccario R, Mingari MC, Vivier E, Moretta L, Locatelli F, Moretta A. (2009) Anti-leukemia activity of alloreactive NK cells in KIR ligand-mismatched haploidentical HSCT for pediatric patients: evaluation of the functional role of activating KIR and redefinition of inhibitory KIR specificity. *Blood.* 113:3119-3129.

Perez SA, Sotiropoulou PA, Gkika DG, Mahaira LG, Niarchos DK, Gritzapis AD, Kavalakis YG, Antsaklis AI, Baxevanis CN, Papamichail M. (2003). A novel myeloid-like NK cell progenitor in human umbilical cord blood. *Blood* 101: 3444-50

Platonova S, Cherfils-Vicini J, Damotte D, Crozet L, Vieillard V, Validire P, André P, Dieu-Nosjean MC, Alifano M, Régnard JF, Fridman WH, Sautès-Fridman C, Cremer I. (2011) Profound coordinated alterations of intratumoral NK cell phenotype and function in lung carcinoma. *Cancer Res.* 71:5412-5422.

Pogge von Strandmann E, Simhadri VR, von Tresckow B, Sasse S, Reiners KS, Hansen HP, Rothe A, Böll B, Simhadri VL, Borchmann P, McKinnon PJ, Hallek M, Engert A.

(2007) Human leukocyte antigen-B-associated transcript 3 is released from tumor cells and engages the NKp30 receptor on natural killer cells. *Immunity.* 27:965-974.

Ribrag V., Ell Hajj M., Janot F., et al., (2001) Early locoregional high-dose radiotherapy is associated with long-term disease control in localized primary angiocentric lymphoma of the nose and nasopharynx *Leukemia* 15: 1123-1126.

Rodella L, Zamai L, Rezzani R, Artico M, Peri G, Falconi M, Facchini A, Pelusi G, Vitale M. (2001) Interleukin 2 and interleukin 15 differentially predispose natural killer cells to apoptosis mediated by endothelial and tumour cells. *Br J Haematol.* 115:442-450.

Romagnani C, Juelke K, Falco M, Morandi B, D'Agostino A, Costa R, Ratto G, Forte G, Carrega P, Lui G, Conte R, Strowig T, Moretta A, Munz C, Thiel A, Moretta L, Ferlazzo G. (2007). $CD56^{bright}CD16^{-}$ killer Ig-like receptor- NK cells display longer telomeres and acquire features of CD56dim NK cells upon activation. *J Immunol* 178: 4947-55

Rosenberg SA, Lotze MT, Muul LM, Leitman S, Chang AE, Ettinghausen SE, Matory YL, Skibber JM, Shiloni E, Vetto JT, Seipp C.A., R.N., Simpson C., and Reichert C.M. (1985) Observations on the systemic administration of autologous lymphokine-activated killer cells and recombinant interleukin-2 to patients with metastatic cancer. *N Engl J Med.* 313:1485-1492

Ruggeri L, Capanni M, Urbani E, Perruccio K, Shlomchik WD, Tosti A, Posati S, Rogaia D, Frassoni F, Aversa F, Martelli MF, Velardi A. (2002) Effectiveness of donor natural killer cell alloreactivity in mismatched hematopoietic transplants. *Science.* 295:2097-2100.

Sakata K., Hareyama M., Ohuchi A., et al., (1997) Treatment of lethal midline granuloma type nasal T-cell lymphoma. *Acta Oncologica* 36: 307-311.

Sanchez CJ, Le Treut T, Boehrer A, Knoblauch B, Imbert J, Olive D, Costello RT. (2011) Natural killer cells and malignant haemopathies: a model for the interaction of cancer with innate immunity. *Cancer Immunol Immunother.* 60:1-13.

Sanchez MJ, Muench MO, Roncarolo MG, Lanier LL, Phillips JH. (1994). Identification of a common T/natural killer cell progenitor in human fetal thymus. *J Exp Med* 180: 569-76

Santoli D., G. Trinchieri and F.S. Lief (1978) Cell-mediated cytotoxicity against virus-infected terget cells in humans. I. Characterization of the effector lymphocyte. *J. Immunol.* 121:526-531.

Scordamaglia F, Balsamo M, Scordamaglia A, Moretta A, Mingari MC, Canonica GW, Moretta L, and Vitale M. (2008) Perturbations of natural killer cell regulatory functions in respiratory allergic diseases. *J Allergy Clin Immunol.* 121: 479-485.

Semenzato G., Pandolfi F., Chisesi T., et al., (1987) The lymphoproliferative disease of granular lymphocytes. A heterogeneous disorder ranging from indolent to aggressive conditions. *Cancer* 60: 2971-2978.

Semenzato G., Zambello R., Starkebaum G., Oshimi K, Loughran T.P., Jr. (1997) The lymphoproliferative disease of granular lymphocytes: updated criteria for diagnosis. *Blood* 89: 256-260.

Shen L, Liang ACT, Lu L, Au WY, Kwong YL, Liang RHS, et al., (2002) Frequent deletion of Fas gene sequences encoding death and transmembrane domains in nasal natural killer/T-cell lymphoma. *Am J Pathol.* 161:2123–31.

Shilling HG, McQueen KL, Cheng NW, Shizuru JA, Negrin RS, Parham P. (2003). Reconstitution of NK cell receptor repertoire following HLA-matched hematopoietic cell transplantation. *Blood* 101: 3730-40

Siu L.L.P., Chan J.K.C., Kwong Y.L. (2002) Natural killer cell malignancies: clinicopathologic and molecular features. *Histol Histopathol* 17: 539-554.

Sivori S, Cantoni C, Parolini S, Marcenaro E, Conte R, Moretta L, Moretta A. (2003). IL-21 induces both rapid maturation of human CD34+ cell precursors towards NK cells and acquisition of surface killer Ig-like receptors. *Eur J Immunol* 33:3439-47

Sivori S, Falco M, Carlomagno S, Romeo E, Soldani C, Bensussan A, Viola A, Moretta L, Moretta A. (2010) A novel KIR-associated function: evidence that CpG DNA uptake and shuttling to early endosomes is mediated by KIR3DL2. *Blood.* 116:1637-1647.

Sivori S, Falco M, Marcenaro E, Parolini S, Biassoni R, Bottino C, Moretta L, Moretta A. (2002). Early expression of triggering receptors and regulatory role of 2B4 in human natural killer cell precursors undergoing in vitro differentiation. *Proc Natl Acad Sci U S A* 99: 4526-31

Smyth MJ, Thia KY, Street SE, Cretney E, Trapani JA, Taniguchi M, Kawano T, Pelikan SB, Crowe NY, Godfrey DI. (2000) Differential tumor surveillance by natural killer (NK) and NKT cells. *J Exp Med.* 191:661-668.

Sozumiya J., Takeshita M., Kimura N., Kikuchi M., Uchida T., et al., (1994) Expression of adult and fetal natural killer cell markers in sinunasal lymphomas. *Blood* 83: 2255-2260.

Sutlu T, Alici E. (2009) Natural killer cell-based immunotherapy in cancer: current insights and future prospects. *J Intern Med.* 266:154-181.

Suzuki R., Suzumiya J., Nakamura S., Aoki S., Notoya A., Ozaki S. (2004) NK-cell Tumor Study Group, et al., Aggressive natural killer-cell leukemia revisited: large granular lymphocyte leukemia of cytotoxic NK cells. *Leukemia* 18(4):763–70.

Tang Q, Ahn YO, Southern P, Blazar BR, Miller JS, Verneris MR. (2011). Development of IL-22-producing NK lineage cells from umbilical cord blood hematopoietic stem cells in the absence of secondary lymphoid tissue. *Blood* 117: 4052-5

Tefferi A., Li C.Y., Witzig T.E., Dhodapkar M.V., Okuno S.H., Phyliky R.L. (1994) Chronic natural killer cell lymphocytosis: a descriptive clinical study. *Blood* 84: 2721-2725.

Terme M, Ullrich E, Delahaye NF, Chaput N, Zitvogel L. (2008) Natural killer cell-directed therapies: moving from unexpected results to successful strategies. *Nat Immunol.* 9:486-494.

Trinchieri G. (1989) Biology of natural killer cells. *Adv Immunol.* 47:187-376

Vacca P, Cantoni C, Vitale M, Prato C, Canegallo F, Fenoglio D, Ragni N, Moretta L, Mingari MC. (2010) The crosstalk between decidual NK and CD14+ myelomonocytic cells results in induction of Tregs and immunosuppression. *Proc Natl Acad Sci U S A.* 107:11918-11923

Vacca P, Vitale C, Montaldo E, Conte R, Cantoni C, Fulcheri E, Darretta V, Moretta L, Mingari MC. (2011). CD34+ hematopoietic precursors are present in human decidua and differentiate into natural killer cells upon interaction with stromal cells. *Proc Natl Acad Sci U S A* 108: 2402-7

Villamor N., Morice W.G., Chan W.C., Foucar K. Chronic lymphoproliferative disorders of NK cells. In: Swerdlow S.H., Campo E., Harris N.L., Jaffe E.J., Pileri S.A., Stein H., Thiele J., Vardiman J. eds. (2008) *WHO Classification of Tumours of Haematopoietic and Lymphoid Tissues.* IARC Lyon 274-275.

Vitale C, Chiossone L, Morreale G, Lanino E, Cottalasso F, Moretti S, Dini G, Moretta L, Mingari MC. (2004). Analysis of the activating receptors and cytolytic function of human natural killer cells undergoing in vivo differentiation after allogeneic bone marrow transplantation. *Eur J Immunol* 34: 455-60

Vitale C, Cottalasso F, Montaldo E, Moretta L, Mingari MC. (2008). Methylprednisolone induces preferential and rapid differentiation of CD34+ cord blood precursors toward NK cells. *Int Immunol* 20: 565-75

Vitale C, Pitto A, Benvenuto F, Ponte M, Bellomo R, Frassoni F, Mingari MC, Bacigalupo A, Moretta L. (2000). Phenotypic and functional analysis of the HLA-class I-specific inhibitory receptors of natural killer cells isolated from peripheral blood of patients undergoing bone marrow transplantation from matched unrelated donors. *Hematol J* 1: 136-44

Vivier E, Raulet DH, Moretta A, Caligiuri MA, Zitvogel L, Lanier LL, Yokoyama WM, Ugolini S. (2011). Innate or adaptive immunity? The example of natural killer cells. *Science.* 331: 44-49

Vivier E, Tomasello E, Baratin M, Walzer T, Ugolini S. (2008) Functions of natural killer cells. *Nat Immunol.* 9:503-510.

Welte S, Kuttruff S, Waldhauer I, Steinle A. (2006) Mutual activation of natural killer cells and monocytes mediated by NKp80-AICL interaction. *Nat Immunol.* 7:1334-42.

West W. H., G.B. Cannon, H.D. Kay, G.D. Bonnard, and R.B. Herberman (1977) Natural Cytotoxic Reactivity of human lymphocytes against a myeloid cell line: characterization of effector cells. *J. Immunol.* 118: 355-361.

Wong K.F., Chan J.K., Kwong Y.L. (1997) Identification of del (6)(q21q25) as a recurring chromosomal abnormality in putative NK cell lymphoma/leukemia. *British Journal of Haematology* 98: 922-926.

Youn BS, Mantel C, Broxmeyer HE. (2000). Chemokines, chemokine receptors and hematopoiesis. *Immunol Rev* 177: 150-74

Yu H, Fehniger TA, Fuchshuber P, Thiel KS, Vivier E, Carson WE, Caligiuri MA. (1998). Flt3 ligand promotes the generation of a distinct CD34(+) human natural killer cell progenitor that responds to interleukin-15. *Blood* 92: 3647-57

Yun S, Lee SH, Yoon SR, Kim MS, Piao ZH, Myung PK, Kim TD, Jung H, Choi I. (2011). TOX regulates the differentiation of human natural killer cells from hematopoietic stem cells in vitro. *Immunol Lett* 136: 29-36

Zambello R., Berno T., Cannas G., Baesso I., Binotto G., Bonoldi E, Bevilacqua P, Miorin M, Facco M, Trentin L, Agostini C, and Semenzato G. (2005) Phenotypic and functional analyses of dendritic cells in patients with lymphoproliferative disease of granular lymphocytes (LDGL). *Blood* 102: 1797-1805.

Zambello R., Falco M., Della Chiesa M., Trentin L., Carollo D., Castriconi R, Cannas G, Carlomagno S, Cabrelle A, Lamy T, Agostini C, Moretta A, and Vitale M. (2003) Expression and function of KIR and natural cytotoxicity receptors in NK-type lymphoproliferative disease of granular lymphocytes. *Blood* 102:1797-1805

Zambello R., Semenzato G. (2003) Natural killer receptors in patients with lymphoproliferative diseases of granular lymphocytes. *Sem Hematol.* 40: 201-212.

Zambello R., Semenzato G. (2009) Large granular lymphocyte disorders: new etiopathogenetic clues as a rationale for innovative therapeutic approaches. *Haematologica* 94:1341-5.

Zimmer J, Andrès E, Hentges F. (2008) NK cells and Treg cells: a fascinating dance cheek to cheek. *Eur J Immunol.* 38:2942-2945.

Zitvogel L, Dendritic and Natural Killer Cells cooperate in the Control/Switch of innate immunity. (2002) *J. Exp. Med.* 195:9-14.

14

Stratification of Patients with Follicular Lymphoma

Hasan A. Abd El-Ghaffar et al.*
Clinical Pathology Department, Faculty of Medicine, Mansoura University, Mansoura
Oncology Center, Mansoura University, Mansoura
Egypt

1. Introduction

Follicular lymphoma (FL) is an indolent lymphoid neoplasm that is derived from mutated germinal center B cells and exhibits a nodular or follicular histologic pattern. It is typically composed of a mixture of small, cleaved follicle center cells referred to as centrocytes and large noncleaved follicular center cells referred to as centroblasts. FL accounts for about 20 % of all lymphomas with the highest incidence in the USA and Western Europe. In Asia and in the developing countries the incidence is much lower [1].

2. The cell of origin of follicular lymphoma

The current theory that tumors are derived from mutated stem cells called cancer stem cells was suggested because stem cells and some cancer cells share self-renewal and differentiation capacities [2-4]. Although this hypothesis was postulated in early reports [5-7],definite proof of their existence came from recent studies in leukemia, where among the complete tumor cell population only a small subset of cells could initiate, regenerate and maintain the leukemia after transplantation into immunocompromised mice [8,9].Using similar functional approaches, a variety of cancer stem cells have been identified in an increasing number of epithelial tumors, including breast, prostate, pancreatic and head and neck carcinomas [10].Despite these outstanding discoveries in leukemias and solid tumors, the existence of lymphoma-originating cells with stem cell properties that may similarly generate lymphoma upon mutation remains a controversial and largely unexplored issue [11]. Recently, it has been proposed that commited lymphoid progenitors/precursor cells with an active V-D-J recombination program are the initiating cells of follicular lymphoma when targeted by immunoglobulin-gene translocations in the bone marrow. However, these pre-malignant lymphoma initiating cells cannot drive complete malignant transformation,

* Sameh Shamaa[2,4], Nadia Attwan[3], Tarek E. Selim[1], Nashwa K. Abosamra[1,4], Dalia Salem[1,4], Sherin M. Abd El-Aziz[1,4] and Layla M. Tharwat[1,4]
[1]*Clinical Pathology Department, Faculty of Medicine, Mansoura University, Mansoura, Egypt*
[2]*Internal Medicine Department, Faculty of Medicine, Mansoura University, Mansoura, Egypt*
[3]*Pathology Department, Faculty of Medicine, Mansoura University, Mansoura, Egypt*
[4]*Oncology Center, Mansoura University, Mansoura, Egypt*

requiring additional cooperating mutations in specific stem cell programs to be converted into the lymphoma originating cells able to generate and sustain lymphoma development [12].

3. Clinical aspects of follicular lymphoma

Signs and Symptom

Follicular lymphoma mainly affects older adults. The average age at diagnosis is about 55. Men and women are nearly equally affected. Follicular lymphoma is a slow-growing disease with minor warning signs that often go unnoticed for a long time before it is diagnosed. The disease is often advanced before a diagnosis is made. Most individuals are diagnosed in stage III or IV. However, even in advanced stages there is no immediate threat to life. The disease has a "waxing and waning" course, meaning that it flares up and regresses a number of times over years.

The first sign of the condition is often a painless swelling in the neck, armpit or groin that is caused by enlarged lymph nodes. However the majority of patients initially present with disseminated disease that follows a relatively indolent clinical course. Patients with follicular lymphoma typically present with superficial lymph nodes of small to medium size. All common superficial territories can be involved by the disease.

In some patients, the first symptoms are more insidious and related to the slow growth of lymph nodes in deep areas, usually in the infradiaphragmatic territories such as the retroperitoneum, the mesenteric, or the iliac areas. In those cases, patients may complain of atypical symptoms while the tumor bulk can be important, with single or confluent lymph nodes. Primary mediastinal involvement is uncommon, as well as isolated splenic enlargement[13]. Other symptoms may include loss of appetite and tiredness. The general status of the patient is usually preserved, Some people have night sweats, unexplained high temperatures and weight loss. These are known as B symptoms. Others have an altered performance status.

Primary involvement of extranodal areas is also very uncommon[14]. The bone marrow is involved in 50% to 60% of the cases. Follicular lymphoma can arise in the gastrointestinal (GI) tract, predominantly in the duodenum or the small intestine, [15,16]. where it can eventually represent the unique site of disease. Lymphoma infiltration may be unifocal or multifocal[13]. The new World Health Organization–European Organization for Research on Treatment of Cancer (WHO-EORTC) cutaneous lymphoma classification recognizes an entity called "primary cutaneous follicle center cell lymphoma" that includes what was previously known as "cutaneous follicular lymphoma variant" in the WHO classification. [17]. Other follicular lymphomas that may be considered as peculiar entities with a distinct behavior are those involving the testis [18] and the rare cases of follicular lymphoma encountered in children [19].

Follicular lymphoma is characterised by response to treatment with disease-free or asymptomatic disease intervals, alternating with recurrence/progression and may transform to aggressive lymphoma at a rate of around 3% per year [13]. This feature is usually—but not systematically—associated with a poor outcome [20].The clinical factors associated with the risk of transformation (as well as the biology underlying this phenomenon) are not fully characterized. Some reports indicated that early treatment and achievement of a complete response after the first-line therapy were associated with a lower risk of transformation in patients with follicular lymphoma [21].

4. Clinical prognostic factors

Several prognostic parameters for follicular lymphomas were identified in the last two decades, that led to the development of some prognostic indexes. The International Prognostic Index developed for aggressive lymphomas was also found to be able of predicting the outcome for patients with follicular lymphoma, but the proportion of patients in the higher-risk categories was usually limited. [13]

The first prognostic system specific to follicular lymphoma was developed by the Italian Lymphoma Intergroup (ILI) in the late 1990s [22]. Currently, the Follicular Lymphoma International Prognostic Index (FLIPI) [23] is deemed to be more applicable across a range of clinical settings . Both systems were developed prior to the introduction of monoclonal antibody therapy, which has profoundly changed the treatment and outcome of follicular lymphoma [24]. Hence, the FLIPI-2 was recently developed, in a prospective series of patients needing treatment, using parameters which were not previously amenable to retrospective analysis, and may represent a promising new tool for the identification of follicular lymphoma patients with different risk profiles in the era of immunochemotherapy [25].

The description of the Follicular Lymphoma International Prognostic Index (FLIPI) represents an important step in identifying patient subgroups with predictable outcome and comparing the results of clinical trials. Analyses of gene expression profiles or constitutive gene variations may also provide additional insights for prognostication in the near future. Furthermore, these data underline the complex interactions between the tumor cells and their microenvironment; recent attempts to translate these findings with immunohistochemical studies remain unable to robustly predict patient outcome. The therapeutic strategies in follicular lymphoma have been transformed by monoclonal antibodies, used alone or in combination with chemotherapy. Treatment options should be adapted to the clinical features at diagnosis and appear to be able to modify the overall survival of some subgroups of patients. Further efforts may focus on strategies that can alter the natural history of this disease [13].

5. Treatment

There is a general consensus that the natural history of advanced stages of low-grade or indolent lymphoma has not changed for the last 30 years. Patients with advanced stages of indolent non-Hodgkin's lymphoma have been treated for many years with various approaches, including deferred initial therapy (watch and wait), single-agent alkylating agents, radiation therapy, combination chemotherapy, and autologous stem-cell transplantation. Unfortunately, it has been impossible to demonstrate that the long-term prognosis for these patients has significantly changed with any these treatment options [26].

The decision to start first-line treatment depends not only on the stage but also on the symptoms of the disease [27].According to The Swiss Group for Clinical Cancer Research

(SAKK) trials at least one of the following signs is present in order to start treatment: B symptoms; symptomatic enlarged lymph nodes or spleen; steady, clinically significant progression of lymphadenopathy, splenomegaly or other follicular lymphoma lesions documented by a 50% increase in size over a period of at least 6 months; involvement of at least 3 nodal sites (>3 cm), bulky disease (>7 cm), haemoglobin <10g/dL, and platelets <100 x 10^9/L due to bone marrow infiltration or splenomegaly [28].

Inspite of encouraging early results [29],there is still no solid data to confirm that early treatment with rituximab significantly delays the need for new therapy,and whether this approach may alter the natural history of the disease and there is also conflicting results Whether early treatment of follicular lymphoma is associated with a decreased risk of transformation [27].

Horning [30],reported the results of sequential treatment studies conducted at Stanford University from 1960 to 1991. Median survival times have ranged from 7 to 10 years, and the OS for each group of studies was overlapping. Indolent lymphoma is generally considered incurable because no plateau in the survival curve has been demonstrable. However, the development of monoclonal antibodies (MoAbs) has revolutionized the treatment of patients with follicular lymphoma [26].

Many trials utilizing different protocols of combination chemotherapy plus rituximab,eg. CVP [31], CHOP [32,33] concluded that OS for patients with follicular lymphoma has improved over time and that the choice of initial therapy may matter. Sacchi et al [34],concluded that FFS and OS have significantly improved in advanced-stage follicular lymphoma patients treated on GISL(Gruppo Italiano Studio Linfomi) protocols during the last 18 years. These improvements are related to evolving front-line and salvage therapies, particularly the introduction of rituximab in combination with chemotherapy

For patients needing therapy, most patients are treated with chemotherapy plus rituximab, which has improved response rates, duration of response, and overall survival. Randomized studies have shown additional benefit for maintenance rituximab both following chemotherapy-rituximab and single agent rituximab [35]. Rituximab maintenance for up to 2 years has a favorable side effect profile and, based on a systematic meta-analysis, substantially prolongs PFS and OS in relapsed disease even after antibody-containing induction in patients who have not received antibody as first-line therapy [36].

Stem cell transplantation (SCT) including both autologous and allogeneic SCT or experimental agent therapy is considered for recurrent disease [35].

In the small proportion of patients with limited non-bulky stages I–II, radiotherapy (involved or extended field, 30–36 Gy) is the preferred treatment having a curative potential [37]. However, In selected cases a watchful waiting may be discussed to avoid the side effects of radiation [38]. Radioimmunotherapy or chlorambucil plus rituximab remains an alternative in patients with low risk profile or contraindications for a more intensive chemoimmunotherapy [39,40].

Therfore, the therapeutic strategies in follicular lymphoma have been transformed by monoclonal antibodies, used alone or in combination with chemotherapy. Treatment options should be adapted to the clinical features at diagnosis and appear to be able to modify the overall survival of some subgroups of patients. Further efforts may focus on strategies that can alter the natural history of this disease [13].

6. Cytomorphology of follicular lymphoma

Follicular NHLs are characterized by a follicular growth pattern , but a diffuse area may also be present. The follicles of follicular lymphoma were more closely packed together, more monotonous in size and shape, and frequently lacked an obvious mantle zone [41].

These follicles contained a comparatively monomorphic cellular phenotype, mostly of centrocytes (small cells with cleaved nuclei) and occasional centroblasts (large cells with multilobated nuclei and multiple nucleoli). Mitotic figures were fewer than in reactive follicular hyperplasia (RFH) and tingible body macrophages were sparse or absent. Polykaryocytes were not observed in RFH or follicular lymphoma and sclerosis was only focally present to a minimal degree [42].

The distinction of FL from RFH is essential, as the latter represents a benign condition [43].A number of morphological features are of value in making this distinction; in particular, a low density of follicles per unit area, The follicles are separated by wide interfollicular areas with prominent mantle zones. The variably sized follicles were composed of a polymorphic population of lymphocytes, dendritic cells, and tingible body macrophages that imparted a"starry sky" pattern. Mitotic figures were conspicuous. The presence of polarity within follicles and the lack of a monomorphic appearance within the follicles all favor RFH [42].

7. Immunophenotype

Being a mature B-cell lymphoma, FL express a large spectrum of B-cell markers, such as CD20, CD19, CD22, CD79a, and Pax5[1] [44].

FL cells express antigens of the germinal center including CD10 and Bcl-6. Most cases of FL express Bcl-2 protein which is highly correlated with the presence of the t(14;18) but may be expressed in cases with a clonal karyotype lacking the t(14;18) [45].

The follicles of RFH and follicular lymphoma stained positively for the B cell marker CD20 which highlight the difference in the width of the interfollicular region between the follicles. In RFH, T cells were predominantly located in the interfollicular zones but also lightly percolated throughout the center of the follicles, demonstrated by T cell marker CD3. CD5 stained T cells are in a nearly identical pattern. T cells stained positively for CD3 and CD5 in follicular lymphoma located within the interfollicular zones. The latter also displaying a more prominent spillover of CD20-positive cells than in RFH [42].

Follicles in both RFH and follicular lymphoma were positive for BCL-6. BCL-2 staining revealed that the follicular centers in RFH were negative and those in follicular lymphoma were positive. CD10 staining was positive for both RFH and follicular lymphoma but showed a greater interfollicular staining in follicular lymphoma [41].

Some cases of both RFH and follicular lymphoma manifested a vague follicular architecture that is difficult to detect. In these cases, CD23, a dendritic cell marker, outlined the follicles of RFH more clearly by disclosing a scaffolding or a cluster of interconnecting cells with elongated cytoplasmic processes. Follicular lymphoma manifested the same pattern of CD23 staining. Ki-67, a marker for cellular proliferation, showed dense positivity that was polarized (unevenly distributed or centered at one edge of the follicle) within RFH follicles. In contrast, follicular lymphoma demonstrated a more diffuse, evenly distributed staining pattern within the follicular centers. Polyclonality was evident in RFH, with in situ hybridization revealing roughly equal populations of both kappa and lambda light chains. In follicular lymphoma rare cells stained positive for kappa or lambda [42].

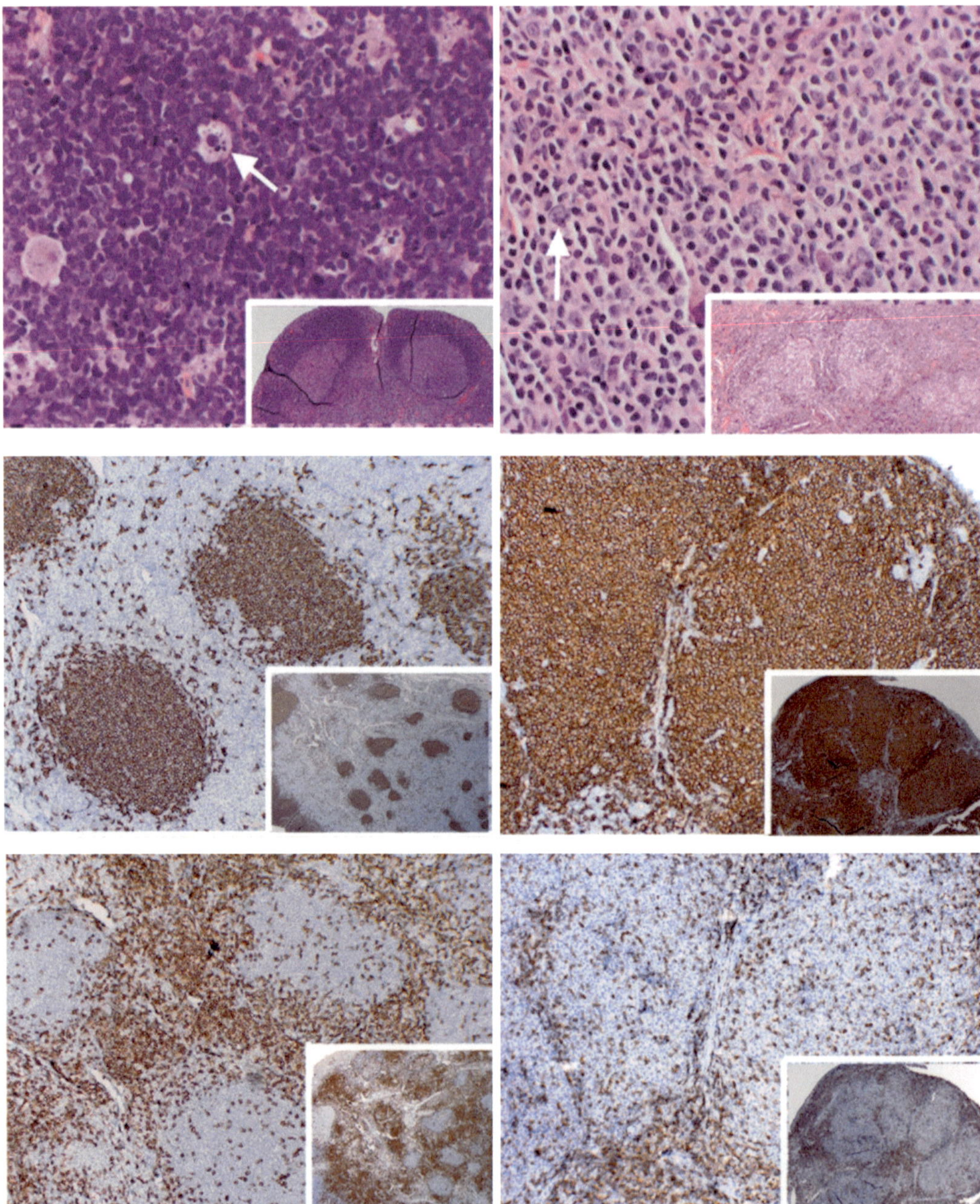

Fig. 1. Histopathological and immunohistochemical characterization of reactive lymphoid hyperplasia and follicular lymphoma.(Top left) Hematoxylin-eosin staining demonstrates follicles in reactive lymphoid hyperplasia (RLH) (inset). The follicles are composed of small

cells with mitotic figures and tingible body macrophages (arrow). (Top right) Hematoxylin-eosin-stainedsection of follicular lymphoma shows mostly small centrocytes with cleaved nuclei and an occasional centroblast (arrow) with a large nucleus and peripheral nucleoli. Inset shows the closer, less well-defined arrangement of several follicles. (Middle left) CD20 stains B cells within the follicles of RLH. The inset indicates the substantial width of the interfollicular zones. (Middle right) CD20 also stains the B cells in the follicles of follicular lymphoma; the close arrangement of the follicles can again be appreciated in the inset.(Bottom left) CD3 stains T cells in the interfollicular zones (inset); the T cells can also be seen percolating throughout the folliclesof RLH. (Bottom right) Follicular lymphoma manifests nearly identical CD3 staining, with CD3_ cells prominent in the interfollicular zones (inset) as well as scattered within the follicles. (Top left and top right, hematoxylin-eosin, 400, insets, 25;Middle left through Bottom right, immunoperoxidase reactions, diaminobenzidine chromogen, 200, insets 25) [42].

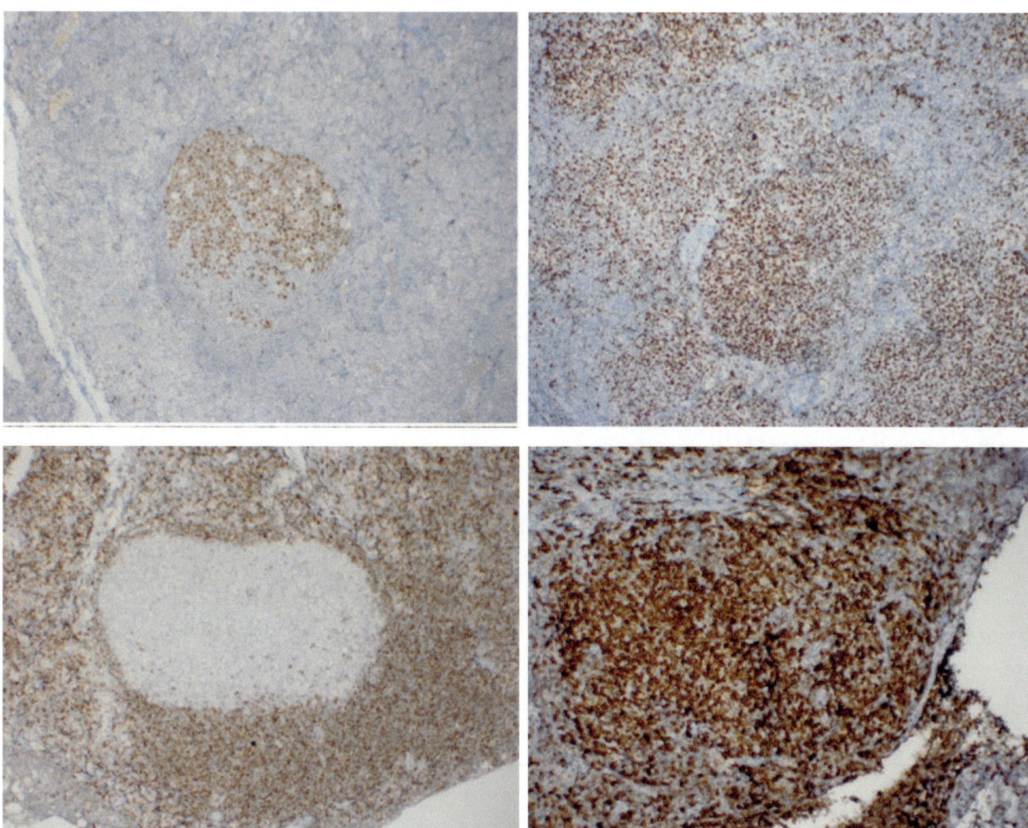

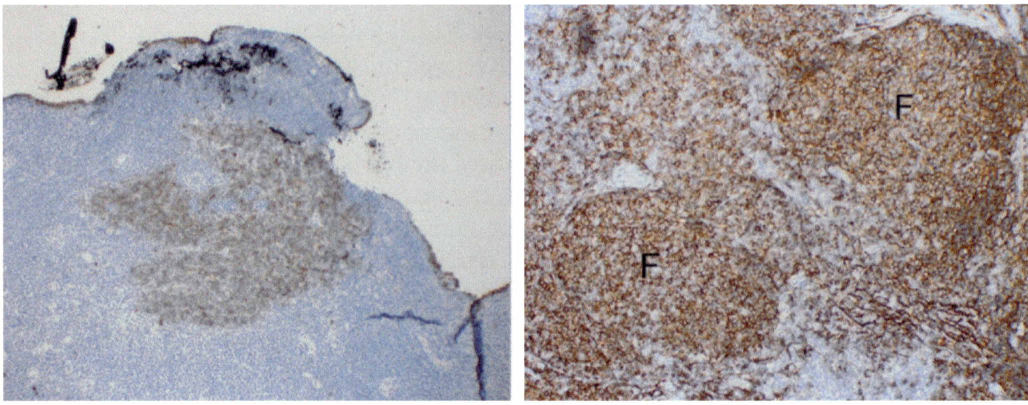

Fig. 2. Immunohistochemical characterization of reactive lymphoid hyperplasia and follicular lymphoma. (Top left) BCL-6stains B cells within follicles of reactive lymphoid hyperplasia (RLH). (Top right) Follicles of follicular lymphoma are also positivefor BCL-6. (Middle left) The follicles of RLH are negative for BCL-2. (Middle right) Follicles of follicular lymphoma are positivefor BCL-2. (Bottom left) Follicles in RLH are positive for CD10. (Bottom right) Follicles (F) of follicular lymphoma are also positive for CD10 but with more interfollicular staining than RLH. (Immunoperoxidase reactions, diaminobenzidine chromogen,200) [42].

8. Follicular lymphoma—How many grades?

The grading of FL was the subject of spirited discussion, both among the authors and the participants in the Clinical Advisory Committee. FL has traditionally been graded according to the proportion of centroblasts and into three Grades, 1-3 as detailed:

World Health Organization classification of follicular lymphoma (FL).

Follicular Lymphoma: Grading & Variants

Grade 1: 0–5 centroblasts/HPF
Grade 2: 6–15 centroblasts/HPF
Grade 3: > 15 centroblasts/HPF

3a: > 15 centroblasts, but centrocytes are still present
3b: centroblasts form solid sheets with no residual centrocytes [46].

Variants:

Primary cutaneous follicle center lymphoma
Pediatric follicle center lymphoma
Intestinal follicle center lymphoma
Diffuse follicle center lymphoma
Grade 1, 0–5 centroblasts/HPF
Grade 2, 6–15centroblasts/HPF[43]

Pediatric FL lacking an association with the t(14;18). Primary cutaneous follicle center lymphoma (PCFCL) may contain a high proportion of large B-cells including large

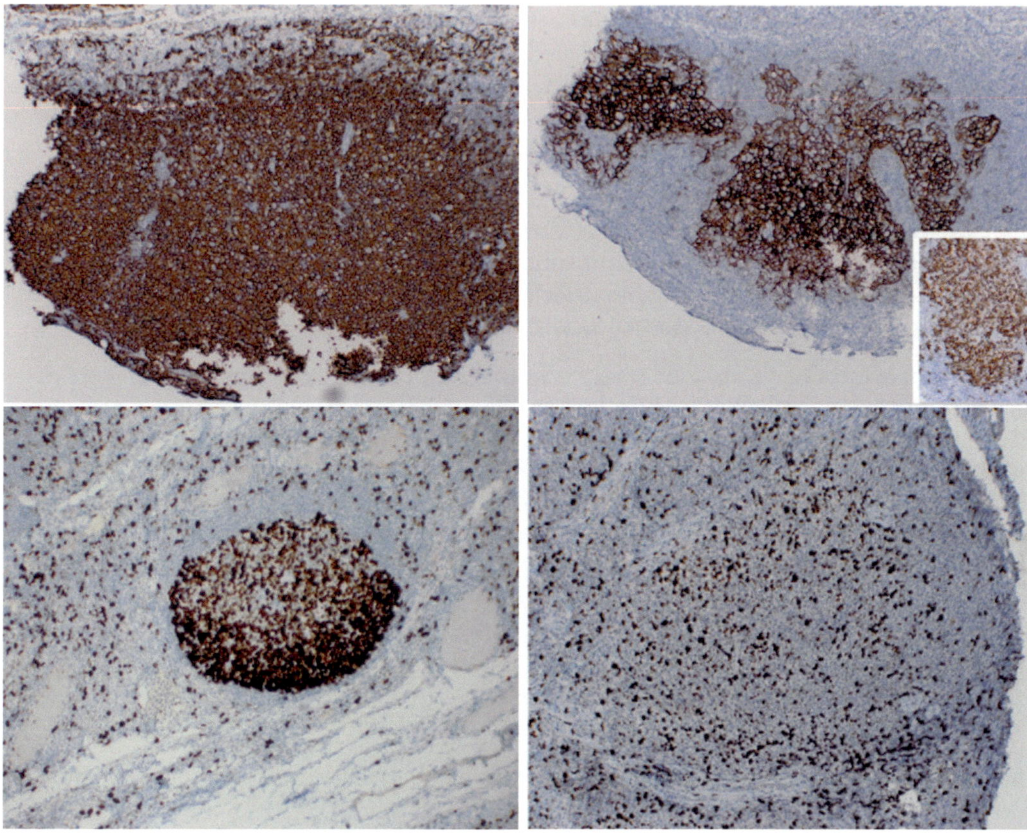

Fig. 3. Further immunohistochemical characterization of reactive lymphoid hyperplasia (RLH) and follicular lymphoma. (Topleft) CD20 densely stains this region of RLH without obvious follicular architecture. (Top right) CD23 highlights the dendritic cell scaffolding of the follicles in an adjacent section. The inset shows a similar dendritic architecture broughtout by CD23 in follicular lymphoma. (Bottom left) Ki-67 stains cells within follicles of RLH in an uneven distribution; staining is crescentic and more dense at the bottom of the follicle. (Bottom right) Follicular cells in follicular lymphoma are more evenly and diffusely positive for Ki-67.(Immunoperoxidase reactions, diaminobenzidine chromogen, 200, inset, 25) [42].

centrocytes and centroblasts. Evidence of the t(14;18) is uncommon and most cases are BCL2 negative. Dissemination beyond the skin is rare, and the prognosis is usually excellent [47].

However, most studies have shown poor interobserver and intraobserver reproducibility. Moreover, the clinical significance of the separation of Grades 1 and 2 has been questioned, with minimal differences seen in long term outcome. Thus, the 2008 WHO classification lumps cases with few centroblasts as "FL Grade 1-2 (low grade)" and does not require or recommend further separation. FL Grade 3 is divided into Grades 3A and 3B, based on the absence of centrocytes in the latter category. Several studies have identified biological differences between these two subtypes, with most cases of FL Grade 3B being more closely related to DLBCL at the molecular level [47].

However, in clinical practice the separation of Grades 3A and 3B can be challenging. Diffuse areas in any Grade 3 FL should be designated as DLBCL (with FL) and are more commonly observed in Grade 3B. Further studies are likely to lead to more precise delineation of the Grade 3 cases truly belonging within FL and those representing an intrafollicular variant of the GCB (germinal center B cell) type of DLBCL.

The presence of diffuse areas within a FL appears to confer more aggressive clinical behavior. In addition, unusual cytological variants can be encountered that are not included in the World Health Organization classification, including cases with large centrocytes and others with small centroblasts; in some cases the latter may resemble the cytomorphology of Burkitt lymphoma and may be associated with MYC oncogene translocations [43].

A truly diffuse form of FL may be rarely encountered, but on closer inspection, most cases demonstrate vaguely follicular architecture that is underappreciated without the routine use of immunostains for follicular dendritic cells. When a diagnosis of true diffuse follicle center lymphoma is considered, the pathologist is encouraged to demonstrate co-expression of CD10 and Bcl-6 as well as presumptive evidence of the t(14;18). Approximately 10% of FL cases reveal the presence of a zone of cells resembling marginal zone B cells, immediately surrounding neoplastic follicles. Importantly, a residual benign mantle zone is not seen, helping to distinguish FL from a marginal zone lymphoma. The area of marginal zone differentiation within a FL takes on a distinct morphology with cells having moderate amount of pale cytoplasm; moreover, the immunophenotype is also different, with downregulation of CD10 and Bcl-6 expression by cells within the marginal zone compartment [48].

Unresolved issues in FL pathology remain and to some extent contribute to problems with reproducibility. Diffuse areas in FL are often not identified, due to underutilization of follicular dendritic cell stains. Similarly, follicular areas in suspected de novo DLBCL are underappreciated. Variability in the cytology of cells within follicles contributes to inconsistent reporting of FL grade. Follicular dendritic are commonly misidentified as centroblasts, resulting in higher grade and, in general, there is poor interobserver reproducibility for the counting of centroblasts. All of these factors lead to inconsistencies in the diagnosis and grading of FL biopsies, and to some extent raise questions regarding the validity of grading and clinical decision making based on grade [43].

Finally, a rare form of FL may be seen referred to as "in-situ" FL. In these uncommon cases, scattered malignant follicles are identified within lymph nodes revealing mostly benign features. The malignant follicles show typically more monomorphic germinal centres (GCs). GCs involved in intrafollicular neoplasia/in situ follicular lymphoma are composed mainly of centrocytes with no evident atypia. A feature of these centres is the relative absence of macrophages with tingible bodies and the absence of polarization into light and dark zones. The paucity of large centroblasts reflects their low proliferation rate in insitu FLs. Intrafollicular neoplasia/in situ follicular lymphoma is characterized by strong co-expression of Bcl-2 and CD10 in the involved GCs [49].

9. Fine needle aspiration cytology

FNA is a useful tool for staging as well as evaluating recurrences in lymph nodes and extra nodal sites without subjecting patients to multiple excisional biopsies. Transformation can occur in some lymph nodes while low-grade lymphoma persists in others. An advantage of FNA is the ability to sample multiple lymph nodes, whereas open biopsy of different anatomic sites is not feasible

Grading FL is based on the proportion of centroblasts in neoplastic follicles; therefore, the ability to identify the various cellular components in a fine-needle aspirate is the first essential step to the grading process. In Papanicolaou stained preparations, centrocytes or cleaved follicular center cells are small to medium-sized cells with angulated, elongated, twisted, or cleaved nuclei with inconspicuous nucleoli and scant, pale cytoplasm.

Centroblasts are at least two times larger than a lymphocyte and usually are round or oval but occasionally have indented, irregular, or even lobulated nuclei. There is a narrow rim of cytoplasm, often basophilic to amphophilic. A large and central nucleolus with chromatin clearing around it is characteristic of immunoblasts. In more typical centroblasts, the chromatin generally is vesicular with one to three prominent, often peripherally located nucleoli. The cells also may be hyperchromatic. Centroblasts tend to be more fragile and, in some preparations, may not be preserved well [50].

It is important not to confuse centroblasts with follicular dendritic reticulum cells, which tend to aggregate within the center of the neoplastic follicles. Although dendritic cells have nuclei that are similar in size to centroblasts, the nuclei of dendritic cells are somewhat coffee bean-shaped with one side typically flattened and with fine, smooth nuclear membranes. The cytoplasm is indistinct, not basophilic, in contrast to that of centroblasts. In Papanicolaou-stained preparations, the chromatin is pale gray and finely granular with small, central, eosinophilic nucleoli. The cytoplasm of dendritic cells form long, dendritic processes that can be appreciated in cell blocks by IHC staining for CD21. Large cleaved cells also must be distinguished from centroblasts. Although there is an overlap in size with centroblasts, large centrocytes are more irregular in shape and lack the prominent nucleoli and chromatin pattern of centroblasts [50]

When it comes to differentiating individual cells, cytologic preparations are superior to hematoxylin and eosin-stained histologic sections, although cytologic preparations typically are less informative about architecture.

Cell blocks are complimentary to smears and provide additional architectural clues. The FNA process often aspirates intact follicular structures that can be appreciated in the cell block. The presence of intact follicles may be proven by special stains on sections of the cell block [50].

10. Grade versus pattern

All three grades of lymphoma can have varying proportions of follicular and diffuse areas. Grade 1 and 2 FL generally have a predominantly follicular pattern. Because they are better differentiated, they have retained the ability to recapitulate follicles [51].

Grade 3 FL occurs less frequently than Grade 1 and 2 FL, and a pure follicular pattern in Grade 3 FL is even more unusual. In Grade 3 FL, the presence of diffuse areas is more common, and most (but not all) studies show that this finding is associated with a worse prognosis.

In Grade 1 and 2 FL, there is conflicting evidence regarding whether the presence of large, diffuse areas or the degree of nodularity may alter prognosis significantly.

SO the WHO classification system recommends estimating the proportion of follicular and diffuse components in the pathology report

- Follicular (75% follicular),
- Follicular and diffuse (25–75% follicular),
- Minimally follicular (25% follicular).

Note, however, that the proportion of centroblasts within the neoplastic follicles is what determines the grade of a FL, not the degree of nodularity. Furthermore, the grade of FL, in combination with other clinical factors,ultimately is what influences treatment decisions [50].

11. Cytogenetics of follicular lymphoma

The t(14;18)(q32;q21) chromosome translocation represents the defining cytogenetic hallmark of FL and is encountered in 80%-90% of cases. Its molecular consequence is the juxtaposition of the B-cell lymphoma/leukemia 2 (BCL2) proto-oncogene with enhancer sequences of the immunoglobulin heavy chain gene (IGH) promoter region, thereby deregulating its expression and resulting in an overexpression of the BCL2 protein in the neoplastic follicles [52,53]. However, 10–15% of cases do not harbor the t(14;18)(q32;q21) and in these t(14;18)-negative cases, other mechanisms are thought to be involved in the pathogenesis [54]. Moreover, t(14;18)- positive B cells can be identified in the blood and lymphoid tissues of healthy individuals, and the number of t(14;18)-positive cells is influenced by gender, personal lifestyle and exposure to toxic substances [55].

The BCL2 proto oncogene, a potent anti-apoptotic molecule, is expressed in resting B cells in the perifollicular mantle zone and in post-follicular B cells, thereby promoting long-lived follicular precursor and memory B cells. Germinal center B cells, however, physiologically lack BCL2 expression and undergo apoptosis unless they are selected by specific antigens that drive them into processes termed somatic hypermutation and class switching. Due to the lack of BCL2 expression, amongst other factors, the large bulk of B-cells entering the GC microenvironment will be removed by apoptosis. The constitutive overexpression of BCL2 in germinal center B cells inferred by the t(14;18)(q32;q21) leads to an accumulation of inappropriately rescued B cells with a prolonged life span, allowing for the development of additional genetic hits to occur, that are required for the establishment of overt FL . Variant translocations of the t(14;18), such as the t(2;18) or t(18;22), juxtapose BCL2 to the loci of the immunoglobulin light chains (k,l) and, likewise, result in inappropriate and sustained BCL2 expression in GC B cells [56].

The occurrence of the t(14;18) in a pre-FL B cell can be viewed as a first hit in a multistep process that results in the clonal dysregulation of cell cycle control and apoptosis of the tumor cells. During process of lymphomagenesis, a number of additional genetic or epigenetic events occur in a non-random fashion that lead to overt FL .For example, constitutive expression of activation-induced cytidine deaminase (AID) in the GC environment in B cells overexpressing BCL2 may propagate continuous somatic hypermutation and class switch recombination activity that results in increased genomic instability. This may, in turn, foster the occurrence of secondary oncogenic hits and, finally, result in the malignant transformation to overt FL [57].

Cong and co-workers[58],described the phenomenon of what they termed follicular lymphoma in situ in otherwise reactive, hyperplastic lymph nodes possibly representing the morphological equivalent of early, pre-invasive FL.

12. Secondary chromosomal aberrations in follicular lymphoma

A number of secondary chromosomal alterations have been described in FL including: structural and numerical changes. The complexity of the secondary alterations correlates with the grade - the higher the grade, the more complex aberrations are usually encountered [59].

It has long been recognized that these alterations occur in a non-random fashion. Partial trisomies of chromosomes 1q, 7, 8 and 18q, and deletions in 1p and 6q have been described as the most common secondary alterations, and deletions in the long arm of chromosomes 1 and 6 and in the short arm of chromosome 17 have been associated with a worse prognosis [60]. Some of these alterations may occur early in the course of the disease, whereas others might represent late genetic events. In addition, some of the alterations are mutually exclusive, while alterations of other chromosomal regions frequently appear together possibly leading to a coordinated deregulation of genetic pathways [61].

Some of the secondary chromosomal alterations may cancel the effect of the t(14;18) that initially forms a low-grade neoplasia with a follicular growth pattern and subsequently enable the transformation to highgrade lymphoma. This process has been associated with three distinct secondary genetic alterations in FL that have a profound impact on the biological program and the clinical course in FL. These include an additional introduction of a t(8;14)/MYC rearrangement in the tumor cells [62], the inactivation of TP53 by mutation and deletion and, finally, the inactivation of p16, frequently occurring by biallelic deletion [63].

The occurrence of a secondary MYC rearrangement in FL deserves particular attention, because these cases frequently demonstrate a Burkitt-like appearance and may be detectable by virtue of this specific morphology in combination with an overexpression of the BCL2 protein caused by the t(14;18) that is usually not encountered in classical Burkitt's lymphomas. Some studies suggest that the detection of TP53 mutations in primary diagnostic specimens of FL without signs of transformation also characterizes a patient subgroup with worse prognosis [64].

13. BCL2-negative follicular lymphoma

From recent studies t(14;18)-negative FLs belong to the biologic spectrum of FL, but show distinct genetic features as well as gene expression and immunohistochemical profiles that differ from their t(14;18)-positive counterparts [65]. The t(14;18)-negative FL appears to harbor genetic rearrangements of the BCL6 gene in 3q27[66] or trisomy 3 [67] whereas others show BCL2 expression on the immunohistochemical level despite the lack of the t(14;18)[68]. Moreover, increased expression of IRF4/MUM1, a protein associated with plasma cell differentiation has been described in FL without BCL2 rearrangement [69].

14. Molecular genetics of follicular lymphoma

Immunoglobulin heavy and light chains are rearranged in FL with the variable region genes showing extensive and ongoing somatic hypermutation [70, 71]. As a result of these mutations in the CDR-regions, PCR primer annealing may be hampered and depending on the primers used, immunoglobulin-PCR may not yield monoclonal products in a proportion of FL cases (10-40%). Multiplex PCR reactions using BIOMED-2 expanded primer sets detect closer to 90% of complete *IGH* (VH-JH) gene rearrangements, and clonality detection approximates 100% when primers detecting incomplete *IGH* (DH-JH) and light chain gene rearrangements are included [72].

For amplification of complete *IGH* (VH-JH) gene rearrangement, BIOMED-2 developed three sets of VH primers corresponding to the three VH FR regions (FR1, FR2, and FR3). Each set of primers consisted of six or seven oligonucleotides capable of annealing to their corresponding VH segments (VH1–VH7) with no mismatches for most VH segments. These VH primer sets were used in conjunction with a single JH consensus primer. The JH primer is fluorescently labeled to allow the detection of PCR products by Gene Scanning [73].

For incomplete *IGH* (DH-JH) rearrangements, seven family-specific DH primers were designed based on the high degree of homology within each DH family in combination with the consensus JH primer. Primers were designed such that crossannealing to other DH family segments would be minimal or preferably absent [73].

Six family-specific Vk primers were designed by van Dongen et al [73], to recognize the various Vk gene segments of the seven Vk families. The family-specific Vk primers were designed to be used in combination with either a set of two Jk primers or a Kde primer.A single consensus primer recognizing both Vλ1 and Vλ2 gene segments, as well as a Vλ3 primer, were designed by van Dongen et al [73], in combination to a single consensus primer for the Jλ1, Jλ2, and Jλ3 gene segments.

The *t(14;18)* and *BCL2* gene rearrangements is one of the best characterized recurrent cytogenetic abnormalities in peripheral B-cell lymphoproliferative disease[74] . FL is genetically characterized by this translocation which is present in up to 90% of the grade 1-2 FL cases [75,76] but the proportion depends on the technique used [77, 78, 79]. BCL2 rearrangements are much less frequent in grade 3B FL [80]. As a consequence of the translocation, the *BCL2* gene (anti-apoptotic) from 18q21 is placed under the control of the strong enhancers of the *IGH* locus resulting in the deregulation of its normal pattern of expression [81,82]. The *BCL2/IGH* rearrangement is found in the PB of 25-75% of healthy donors, and also in reactive nodes, particularly if using sensitive nested or RT-PCR assays [83,84,85]. A recent study suggests that rather than being naive B-cells, these *BCL2*-rearranged cells are memory B-cells [86].

There is no single gold standard detection strategy for the *t(14;18)*, and a combination of cytogenetics and southern blotting have been generally used [87,88]. Interphase FISH detection strategies offer an applicable alternative that have the potential to pick up more translocations [89]. For molecular diagnostic laboratories PCR-based detection strategies offer rapid results, are generally applicable, and can be used for residual disease monitoring. However, the primers commonly used have not been designed to take into account recent information on the molecular anatomy of the breakpoints. As a consequence when compared to gold standard approaches, PCR-based techniques only detect up to 60% of translocations, which seriously impairs the diagnostic capability of PCR. However, BIOMED-2 primers have been developed using three multiplex tubes for detection of MBR-JH, 3'MBR- JH, and mcr-JH to maximize the detection of t(14;18) [73].). These data are supported by previous report from our molecular hematology laboratory. We found that FISH was superior to PCR in the detection of t(14'18) (q32'q21)-IGH-BCL-2 in formalin-fixed, paraffin-embedded tissue samples. Moreover, strong correlations between the FLIPI score and each of interphase FISH and CD10 expression were demonstrated [90].

Molecular profiling of many types of lymphoma using RQ-PCR and cDNA microarray has been used to predict survival by many researchers [91-94]. Genes involved in cell cycle control and DNA synthesis and metabolism (e.g. CXCL12, which is involved in signaling transduction and NEK2, which is involved in mitotic regulation, and MAPK1) are significantly up-regulated in the aggressive phase of FL[3]. MYC, as a known oncogene, and MYC-target genes (SFRS7, LDHA, MTHFD1, NME1, MSH2, and CKS2) are upregulated on transformation and may be implicated as a direct transforming factor [95-102].On the other hand, there is higher density of the T-cell infiltrate in low-grade FL as compared to high-grade disease and this is reflected by several T cell–related genes (CD3, CD2, CD69). However, genes related to T-cell and macrophage activation including several chemokine receptors (CCR1, CCL3, CCL5, CCL8, AKAP12, ILF3, GEM) are significantly upregulated on transformation, suggesting an important biologic role. Notably, specific antagonists to several of the above-mentioned chemokine receptors are available and offer an attractive possibility for therapeutic interventions [103].

15. Proposed algorithm for stratification of follicular lymphoma

The National Comprehensive Cancer Network(NCCN) has recently launched an algorithm for stratification of follicular lymphoma (Figure 4).

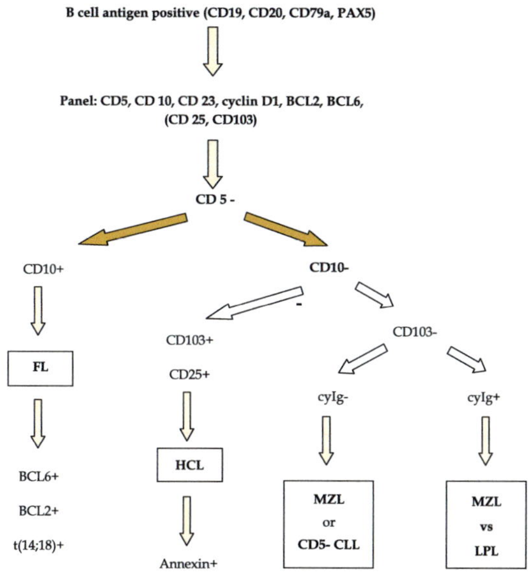

Fig. 4. Proposed algorithm for stratification of follicular lymphoma (NCCN)

16. References

[1] Anderson JR, Armitage JO, Weisenburger DD (1998): Epidemiology of the non-Hodgkin's lymphomas: distributions of the major subtypes differ by geographic locations. Non-Hodgkin's Lymphoma Classification Project. Ann Oncol9: 717-720.

[2] Reya T, Morrison SJ, Clarke MF, Weissman IL. Stem cells, cancer, and cancer stem cells.Nature. 2001;414(6859):105-11.

[3] Pardal R, Molofsky AV, He S, Morrison SJ.Stem cell self-renewal and cancer cell proliferation are regulated by common networks that balance the activation of proto-oncogenes and tumor suppressors. Cold Spring Harb Symp Quant Biol. 2005;70:177-85.

[4] Clarke MF, Fuller M. Stem cells and cancer(2006): two faces of eve. Cell (6):1111-5.

[5] Bruce WR, Van Der Gaag H (1963): A Quantitative assay for the number of murine lymphoma cells capable of proliferation in vivo. Nature. 199:79-80.

[6] Park CH, Bergsagel DE, McCulloch EA (1971).Mouse myeloma tumor stem cells: a primary cell culture assay. J Natl Cancer Inst.46(2):411-22.

[7] Hamburger AW, Salmon SE (1977): Primary bioassay of human tumor stem cells. Science.1977;197(4302):461-3.

[8] Lapidot T, Sirard C, Vormoor J, Murdoch B,Hoang T, Caceres-Cortes J, et al.(1994): A cell initiating human acute myeloid leukaemia after transplantation into SCID mice.Nature. 367(6464):645-8.

[9] Bonnet D, Dick JE (1997): Human acute myeloid leukemia is organized as a hierarchy that originates from a primitive hematopoietic cell. Nat Med.3(7):730-7.

[10] Al-Hajj M, Clarke MF (2004): Self-renewal and solid tumor stem cells. Oncogene.23(43):7274-82.

[11] Boman BM, Wicha MS (2008): Cancer stem cells:a step toward the cure. J Clin Oncol.26(17):2795-9.

[12] Martinez-Climent JA, Fontan L, Gascoyne RD, Siebert R, and Prosper F.(2010): Lymphoma stem cells: enough evidence to support their existence? Haematologica. 95:293-302.

[13] Salles GA (2007):Clinical Features, Prognosis and Treatment of Follicular Lymphoma. *Hematology* 216-25.

[14] Goodlad JR, MacPherson S, Jackson R, Batstone P, White J (2004):Extranodal follicular lymphoma: a clinicopathological and genetic analysis of 15 cases arising at non-cutaneous extranodal sites. Histopathology.44:268–276.

[15] Damaj G, Verkarre V, Delmer A, et al (2003): Primary follicular lymphoma of the gastrointestinal tract: a study of 25 cases and a literature review. Ann Oncol.14:623–629.

[16] Poggi MM, Cong PJ, Coleman CN, Jaffe ES (2002): Low-grade follicular lymphoma of the small intestine. J Clin Gastroenterol.34:155–159.

[17] Willemze R, Jaffe ES, Burg G, et al (2005): WHO-EORTC classification for cutaneous lymphomas. Blood.;105:3768–3785.

[18] Bacon CM, Ye H, Diss TC, et al (2007): Primary follicular lymphoma of the testis and epididymis in adults. Am J Surg Pathol. 31:1050–1058.

[19] Lorsbach RB, Shay-Seymore D, Moore J, et al (2002): Clinicopathologic analysis of follicular lymphoma occurring in children. Blood. 99:1959–1964.

[20] Yuen AR, Kamel OW, Halpern J, Horning SJ (1995): Long-term survival after histologic transformation of low-grade follicular lymphoma. J Clin Oncol. 13:1726–1733.
[21] Montoto S, Davies AJ, Matthews J, et al (2007): Risk and clinical implications of transformation of follicular lymphoma to diffuse large B-cell lymphoma. J Clin Oncol. 25:2426–2433.
[22] Federico M, Vitolo U, Zinzani PL, et al (2000): Prognosis of follicular lymphoma: a predictive model based on a retrospective analysis of 987 cases. Intergruppo Italiano Linfomi. Blood.95:783–9.
[23] Solal-Celigny P, Roy P, Colombat P, et al (2004): Follicular lymphoma international prognostic index. Blood. 104:1258–65.
[24] Conconi A, Motta M, Bertoni F, et al (2010): Patterns of survival of follicular lymphomas at a single institution through three decades. Leuk Lymphoma. 51:1028–34.
[25] Federico M, Bellei M, Marcheselli L, et al (2009): Follicular lymphoma international prognostic index 2: a new prognostic index for follicular lymphoma developed by the international follicular lymphoma prognostic factor project. J Clin Oncol. 27:4555–62 .
[26] Fisher R. , LeBlanc M. , Press O , Maloney D., Unger J, Miller T.(2005):New Treatment Options Have Changed the Survival of Patients With Follicular Lymphoma. JCO , 23 (33); 8447-8452
[27] Hitz F, Kettere N, Lohri A, Mey U, Pederiva S, Renner C, Taverna C, Hatmann A, Yeow K, Bodis S, Zucca E (2011):Diagnosis and treatment of follicular lymphoma Swiss Med Wkly. 141:w13247.
[28] Martinelli G, Hsu Schmitz SF, Utiger U, et al (2010): Long-Term Follow-Up of Patients With Follicular Lymphoma Receiving Single-Agent Rituximab at Two Different Schedules in Trial SAKK 35/98. J Clin Oncol. 28:4480–4.
[29] Ardeshna KM, Smith P, Qian W, et al (2010): An Intergroup Randomised Trial of Rituximab Versus a Watch and Wait Strategy In Patients with Stage II, III, IV, Asymptomatic, Non-Bulky Follicular Lymphoma (Grades 1, 2 and 3a). A Preliminary Analysis. Blood, ASH Annual Meeting Abstracts 116:Abstract 6.
[30] Horning SJ (1993): Natural history of and therapy for the indolent non-Hodgkin's lymphomas. Semin Oncol.20:75-88, (suppl 5.(
[31] Marcus R, Solal-Celigny P, Imrie K, et al (2006): Rituximab plus CVP improves survival in previously untreated patients with advanced follicular non-Hodgkin's lymphoma [abstract]. Blood. 108:481a
[32] Maloney DG, Press OW, Braziel RM, et al (2001): A phase II trial of chop followed by rituximab chimeric monoclonal anti-CD20 antibody for treatment of newly diagnosed follicular non-Hodgkin's lymphoma: SWOG 9800. Blood, 98:843a.
[33] Czuczman MS, Weaver R, Alkuzweny B, et al (2004): Prolonged clinical and molecular remission in patients with low-grade or follicular non-Hodgkin's lymphoma treated with rituximab plus CHOP chemotherapy: 9-Year follow-up. J Clin Oncol , 22:4711-4716
[34] Sacchi S,Pozzi S,Marcheselli L, Bari A,Stefano (2007): Introduction of rituximab in front-line and salvage therapies has improved outcome of advanced-stage follicular lymphoma patients. Cancer Volume 109, Issue 10, 2077–2082,

[35] Freedman A (2011): update on diagnosis and management. . Am. J. Hematol. 86:769-775, 2011.
[36] Vidal L, Gafter-Gvili A, Leibovici L, et al (2009) : Rituximab maintenance for the treatment of patients with follicular lymphoma: systematic review and meta-analysis of randomized trials. *J Natl Cancer Inst*;101:248-255.
[37] MacManus PM, Hoppe RT (1996): Is radiotherapy curative for stage I and II low grade follicular lymphoma? Results of a long term follow-up study of patients treated at Stanford University. *J Clin Oncol*;14:1282-1290.
[38] Advani R, Rosenberg SA, Horning SJ(2004): Stage I and II follicular non-Hodgkin's lymphoma: long-term follow-up of no initial therapy. *J Clin Oncol*;22:1454-1459.
[39] Kaminski MS, Tuck M, Estes J, et al (2005): ^{131}I-Tositumomab therapy as initial treatment for follicular lymphoma. *N Engl J Med*;352:441-449.
[40] Martinelli G, Schmitz SF, Utiger U, et al (2010): *Long-term follow-up of patients with follicular lymphoma receiving single-agent rituximab at two different schedules in trial SAKK 35/98 J Clin Oncol*;28:4480-4484.
[41] Hayashi D., Lee J.C., Devenney-Cakir B., Zaim S., Ounadjela S., Solal-Celigny P., Juweid M., Guermazi A (2010): Follicular non-Hodgkin's lymphoma. Clinical Radiology, (65): 408–420.
[42] Stacy R.C., Jakobiec F. A., Schoenfield L., Singh A. D (2010): Unifocal and Multifocal Reactive Lymphoid Hyperplasia vs Follicular Lymphoma of the Ocular Adnexa. American Journal of Ophthalmology. (150), NO. 3, 412-426.
[43] Winter J. N., Gascoyne R. D., Van Besien K (2004): Low-Grade Lymphoma. Hematology, 203-220.
[44] Klapper W (2011): Pathobiology and diagnosis of follicular lymphoma. Semin Diagn Pathol.28(2):146-60. Review
[45] Vitolo U., Ferreri A.J., Montoto S (2008): Follicular lymphoma. Crit Rev Oncol Hematol. Jun;66(3):248-61.
[46] Samsi S., Lozanski G., Shana'ah A., Krishanmurthy A. K., Gurcan M.N(2010): Detection of Follicles from IHC Stained Slides of Follicular Lymphoma Using Iterative Watersh.Trans Biomed Eng. October; 57(10): 2609–2612.
[47] Jaffe E.S (2009): The 2008 WHO classification of lymphomas: implications for clinical practice and translationalresearch, Hematology, 523-531.
[48] Gradowski J. F., Jaffe E. S., Warnke R. A., Pittaluga S., Surti U., Gole L. A., Swerdlow S. H (2010): Follicular lymphomas with plasmacytic differentiation include two subtypes . Modern Pathology. (23), 71–79.
[49] Montes-Moreno S., Garcı´a O. A., Santiago-Ruiz G., Ferreira J. A., Garcı´a J. F., Pinilla A. P (2010): Intrafollicular neoplasia in situ follicular lymphoma: review of a series of 13 cases., Histopathology, 56, 652–664.
[50] Young N. A (2006): Grading Follicular Lymphoma on Fine-Needle Aspiration Specimens—A Practical Approach (cancer cytopathology), Vol 108 no1
[51] Lejeune M, Álvaro T (2009): Clinicobiological, prognostic and therapeutic implications of the tumor microenvironment in follicular lymphoma. Haematologica, January; 94(1): 16–21.
[52] Bakhshi A, Jensen JP, Goldman P, Wright JJ, McBride OW, Epstein AL, Korsmeyer SJ (1985): Cloning the chromosomal breakpoint of t(14;18) human lymphomas:

clustering around JH on chromosome 14 and near a transcriptional unit on 18. Cell 41:899-906.
[53] Tsujimoto Y, Gorham J, Cossman J, Jaffe E, Croce CM (1985): The t(14;18) chromosome translocations involved in B-cell neoplasms result from mistakes in VDJ joining. Science; 229:1390-3.
[54] Keni Gu, Kai Fu, Smrati Jain, Zhongfen Liu, Javeed Iqbal, Min Li, Warren G Sanger, Dennis D Weisenburger, Timothy C Greiner, Patricia Aoun, Bhavana J Dave and Wing C Chan (2009): t(14;18)-negative follicular lymphomas are associated with a high frequency of BCL6 rearrangement at the alternative breakpoint region. Modern Pathology ; 22: 1251–1257.
[55] de Jong D (2005):. Molecular pathogenesis of follicular lymphoma: a cross talk of genetic and immunologic factors. J Clin Oncol;23:6358-63.
[56] German Ott and Andreas Rosenwald (2008): Molecular pathogenesis of follicular lymphoma. Haematologica; 93:1773-6.
[57] Pasqualucci L, Bhagat G, Jankovic M, Compagno M, Smith P, Muramatsu M, et al (2008): AID is required for germinal centerderived lymphomagenesis. Nat Genet; 40:108-12.
[58] Cong P, Raffeld M, Teruya-Feldstein J, Sorbara L, Pittaluga S, Jaffe ES (2002): In situ localization of follicular lymphoma: description and analysis by laser capture microdissection. Blood;99:3376-82.
[59] Ott G, Katzenberger T, Lohr A, Kindelberger S, Rudiger T, Wilhelm M, et al (2002): Cytomorphologic, immunohistochemical, and cytogenetic profiles of follicular lymphoma: 2 types of follicular lymphoma grade 3. Blood;99:3806- 12.
[60] Cheung KJ, Shah SP, Steidl C, Johnson N, Relander T, Telenius A, et al (2008): Genome-wide profiling of follicular lymphoma by array comparative genomic hybridization reveals prognostically significant DNA copy number imbalances. Blood.
[61] Hoglund M, Sehn L, Connors JM, Gascoyne RD, Siebert R, Sall T, et al (2004): Identification of cytogenetic subgroups and karyotypic pathways of clonal evolution in follicular lymphomas. Genes Chromosomes Cancer;39:195-204.
[62] Macpherson N, Lesack D, Klasa R, Horsman D, Connors JM, Barnett M, Gascoyne RD (1999):. Small noncleaved, non- Burkitt's (Burkit-Like) lymphoma: cytogenetics predict outcome and reflect clinical presentation. J Clin Oncol;17:1558-67.
[63] Elenitoba-Johnson KS, Gascoyne RD, Lim MS, Chhanabai M, Jaffe ES, Raffeld M (1998): Homozygous deletions at chromosome 9p21 involving p16 and p15 are associated with histologic progression in follicle center lymphoma. Blood;91:4677-85.
[64] O'Shea D, O'Riain C, Taylor C, Waters R, Carlotti E, Macdougall F, et al (2008): The presence of TP53 mutation at diagnosis of follicular lymphoma identifies a high-risk group of patients with shortened time to disease progression and a poorer overall survival. Blood;112:3126-9.
[65] Ellen Leich,Itziar Salaverria, Silvia Bea, Andreas Zettl, George Wright, Victor Moreno,Randy D. Gascoyne,Wing-Chung Chan,Rita M. Braziel,Lisa M. Rimsza, Dennis D. Weisenburger, Jan Delabie, Elaine S. Jaffe,Andrew Lister, Jude Fitzgibbon,Louis M. Staudt, Elena M. Hartmann,Hans-Konrad Mueller-Hermelink,Elias Campo,German Ott, and Andreas Rosenwald (2009): Follicular lymphomas with and without translocation t(14;18) differ in gene expression profiles and genetic alterations. Blood. 114: 826-834.

[66] Guo Y, Karube K, Kawano R, et al (2007): Bcl2-negative follicular lymphomas frequently have Bcl6 translocation and/or Bcl6 or p53 expression. Pathol Int.;57:148-152.
[67] Tagawa H, Karube K, Guo Y, et al (2007): Trisomy 3 is a specific genomic aberration of t(14;18) negative follicular lymphoma. Leukemia.;21:2549-2551.
[68] Horsman DE, Okamoto I, Ludkovski O, et al (2003): Follicular lymphoma lacking the t(14;18)(q32;q21): identification of two disease subtypes. Br J Haematol.;120:424-433.
[69] Karube K, Guo Y, Suzumiya J, et al (2007): CD10- MUM1- follicular lymphoma lacks BCL2 gene translocation and shows characteristic biologic and clinical features. Blood.;109:3076-3079.
[70] Cleary ML, Meeker TC, Levy S, Lee E, Trela M, Sklar J, Levy R(1986): clustering of extensive somatic mutations in the variable region of an immunoglobulin heavy chain gene from a human B cell lymphoma. Cell 44:97-106.
[71] Ottensmeier cCH,Thompesett AR, Zhu D,Wikins BS,Sweetenham JW,Stevenson FK,.(1998):Analysis of VH genes in follicular and diffuse lymphoma shows ongoing somatic mutation and multiple isotype transcriptsin early disease with changes during disease progression.Blood.91:4292-4299.
[72] Evans PA,PottC,GroenenPJ , SallesG, Davi F,Berger F,Garcia JF, Van Krieken JH, Pales S, Kluin P,Schuuring E et al.(2007):Significantly improved PCR based clonality testing in B cell malignancies by use of multiple immunoglobulin gene targets.Report of the Biomed -2 Concerted Action BHM4-CT983936.leukemia 21:207-214.
[73] van Dongen JJM, Langerak AW, Bruggemann M, Evans PAS, Hummel , Lavender FL, Delabesse E, Davi F, Schuuring E , Garcia-Sanz R, van Krieken JHJM, Droese J, Gonzalez D, Bastard C, White HE, Spaargaren M, Gonzalez M, Parreira A, Smith JL, Morgan GJ, Kneba M and Macintyre EA (2003):Design and standardization of PCR primers and protocols for detection of clonal immunoglobulin and T-cell receptor gene recombinations in suspect lymphoproliferations: Report of the BIOMED-2 Concerted Action BMH4-CT98-3936. Leukemia 17, 2257–2317.
[74] Fukuhara S, Rowley JD, Variakojis D, Golomb HM (1979): Chromosome abnormalities in poorly differentiated lymphocytic lymphoma. Cancer Res; 39: 3119–3128.
[75] Score J,CurtisC,Waghorn K,Stadler M,Jotterand M,Grand FH, Cross NC (2006): Identification of a novel imatinib responsive KIF5B-PDGFRA fusion gene following PDGFRA overexpression in patients with hyperoesinophilia .Leukemia 20:827-832.
[76] Rowley JD (1988):Chromosome studies in the hodgiken lymphomas:the role of t (14;18) translocation .J Clin Oncol6:919-925.
[77] Aster JC,Longtine JA (2002):Detection of BCL2 rearrangements in follicular lymphoma.Am J Path 160:759-763.
[78] Montolo S,Lopez Guillermo A,Colomer D, Esteve J, Bosh F, Ferrer A, Villamor N, Moreno C, Campo E, Montserrat E (2003): Incidence and clinical significance of bcl2/IgH rearrangements in follicular lymphoma.Leuk Lymphoma 44:71-76.
[79] Vaandrager JW,Schuuring E,RaapT,Phillipo K,Kleiverda K,Kluin P.2000. Interphase FISH detection of BCL2 rearrangement in follicular lymphoma using breakpoint flanking probes.Genes Chromosomes Cancer.27:85-94.
[80] Ott G, Katzenberger T,Lohr A,Kendelberger S, Rudgier T,Wihelm M, Kalla J, Rosenwald A, Muller JG ,Ott MM, Muller Hermlink HK

(2002):Cytomorphologic,immunohistochemical and cytogenetic profiles of follicular lymphoma :2 types of follicular lymphoma grade 3>Blood99:3806-3812.

[81] Bakhshi A, Jensen JP, Goldman P, Wright JJ, McBride OW, Epstein AL et al (1985): Cloning the chromosomal breakpoint of t(14;18) human lymphomas: clustering around JH on chromosome 14 and near a transcriptional unit on 18. Cell; 41: 899–906.

[82] Cleary ML, Sklar J (1985): Nucleotide sequence of a t(14;18) chromosomal breakpoint in follicular lymphoma and demonstration of a breakpoint-cluster region near a transcriptionally active locus on chromosome 18. Proc Natl Acad Sci USA; 82: 7439–7443.

[83] Rouland S,Lebality P, Roussel G,Briand M,Cappellen D,Pottier D,Hardouin A,Troussard X,Bastard C, Henery-Amar M,Gauduchon P(2003):BCL2/JH translocation in peripheral blood lymphocytes of unexposed individuals :lack of seasonal variations in frequency and molecular features.Int J Cancer 104:695-698.

[84] Schmitt C,Balogh B,Grudt A, Buchulotz C, Leo A,Benner A, Hensel M,Ho AD,Leo A(2006):The bcl2/IGH rearrangement in a population of 204 healthy individuals :occurance ,age,and gender distribution ,breakpoints and detection method validity.Leuk Res 30:745-750.

[85] Summers KE, Goff LK, Wilson AG, Gupta RK , Lister TA, Fitzgibbon J (2001): Frequency of BCL2/IgH rearrangement in Normal individuals :implications for the monitoring of disease in patients with follicular lymphoma .JClin Oncol 19 :420-424.

[86] Rouland S , Navaro JM, Grenot P, Milili M,Agopian J, Montpellier B, Gauduchon P, lebailly P, Sciff C,Nadel B (200):Follicular lymphoma like B cells in healthy individuals:a novel intermediate step in early lymphomagenesis .JExp Med 203:2425-2431.

[87] Pezzella F, Ralfkiaer E, Gatter KC, Mason DY (1990): The 14;18 translocation in European cases of follicular lymphoma: comparison of Southern blotting and the polymerase chain reaction. Br J Haematol; 76: 58–64.

[88] Turner GE, Ross FM, Krajewski AS (1995): Detection of t(14;18) in British follicular lymphoma using cytogenetics, Southern blotting and the polymerase chain reaction. Br J Haematol; 89: 223–225.

[89] Vaandrager JW, Schuuring E, Raap T, Philippo K, Kleiverda K, Kluin P (2000): Interphase FISH detection of BCL2 rearrangement in follicular lymphoma using breakpoint-?anking probes. Genes Chromosomes Cancer; 27: 85–94.

[90] Deghiedy H, Fouda M, Shahin D,shamaa S, El-Bedewy A, Abd El-Ghaffar H (2007): Diagnostic and prognostic utility of t(14;18) in follicular lymphoma. Acta Hematol. 118:231-236.

[91] Alizadeh AA, Eisen MB, Davis RE, Lossos IS, Rosenwald A, Boldrick JC, Sabet H, Tran T, Yu X, Powell JI, Yang L, Marti GE, Moore T, Hudson J Jr, Lu L, Lewis DB, Tibshirani R, Sherlock G, Chan WC, Greiner TC, Weisenburger DD, Armitage JO, Warnke R, Levy R, Wilson W, Grever MR, Byrd JC, Botstein D, Brown PO, Staudt LM (2000): Distinct types of diffuse large B-cell lymphoma identified by gene expression profiling. Nature.;403:503-511.

[92] Husson H, th G. Carideo EG, Neuberg D, Schultze J, Munoz O, Marks PW, Donovan JW, C. Chillemi AC, O'Connell P and Freedman AS (2002): Gene expression

profiling of follicular lymphoma and normal germinal center B cells using cDNA arrays. Blood, 99: 282-289

[93] 93 Rosenwald A, Wright G, Chan WC, Connors JM, Campo E, Fisher RI, Gascoyne RD, Muller-Hermelink HK, Smeland EB, Giltnane JM, Hurt EM, Zhao H, Averett L, Yang L, Wilson WH, Jaffe ES, Simon R, Klausner RD, Powell J, Duffey PL, Longo DL, Greiner TC, Weisenburger DD, Sanger WG, Dave BJ, Lynch JC, Vose J, Armitage JO, Montserrat E, López-Guillermo A, Grogan TM, Miller TP, LeBlanc M, Ott G, Kvaloy S, Delabie J, Holte H, Krajci P, Stokke T, Staudt LM (2002):. The use of molecular profiling to predict survival after chemotherapy for diffuse large-B-cell lymphoma. N Engl J Med.;346:1937-1947.

[94] Shipp MA, Ross KN, Tamayo P, Weng AP, Kutok JL, Aguiar RC, Gaasenbeek M, Angelo M, Reich M, Pinkus GS, Ray TS, Koval MA, Last KW, Norton A, Lister TA, Mesirov J, Neuberg DS, Lander ES, Aster JC, Golub TR (2002): Diffuse large B-cell lymphoma outcome prediction by gene-expression profiling and supervised machine learning. Nat Med.;8:68-74.

[95] Glas AM, Kersten MJ, Delahaye LJMJ, Witteveen AT, Kibbelaar RE, Velds A, Wessels LFA, Joosten P, Kerkhoven RM, Bernards R, van Krieken JHJM, Kluin PM, van't Veer LJ and de Jong D (2005): Gene expression profiling in follicular lymphoma to assess clinical aggressiveness and to guide the choice of treatment. Blood, 105: 301-307.

[96] Husson H, Carideo EG, Neuberg D, et al (2002): Gene expression profiling of follicular lymphoma and normal germinal center B cells using cDNA arrays. Blood.;99:282-289.

[97] de Vos S, Hofmann WK, Grogan TM, et al (2003): Gene expression profile of serial samples of transformed B-cell lymphomas. Lab Invest.;83:271-285.

[98] Elenitoba-Johnson KS, Jenson SD, Abbott RT, et al (2003):Involvement of multiple signaling pathways in follicular lymphoma transformation: p38-mitogen-activated protein kinase as a target for therapy. Proc Natl Acad Sci U S A.;100:7259-7264.

[99] Lossos IS, Alizadeh AA, Diehn M, et al (2002): Transformation of follicular lymphoma to diffuse large-cell lymphoma: alternative patterns with increased or decreased expression of c-myc and its regulated genes. Proc Natl Acad Sci U S A.;99:8886-8891.

[100] Adida C, Haioun C, Gaulard P, et al (2000): Prognostic signifcance of survivin expression in diffuse large B-cell lymphomas. Blood.;96:1921-1925.

[101] Akasaka T, Akasaka H, Ueda C, et al (2000): Molecular and clinical features of non-Burkitt's, diffuse large-cell lymphoma of B-cell type associated with the c-MYC/immunoglobulin heavy-chain fusion gene. J Clin Oncol.;18:510-518.

[102] Menssen A, Hermeking H (2002): Characterization of the c-MYC-regulated transcriptome by SAGE: identifcation and analysis of c-MYC target genes. Proc Natl Acad Sci U S A.;99:6274-6279.

[103] Homey B, Muller A, Zlotnik A (2002): Chemokines: agents for the immunotherapy of cancer? Nat Rev Immunol.;2:175-184).

15

MicroRNA Expression in Follicular Lymphoma

Charles H. Lawrie
[1]*Biodonostia Institute, San Sebastián*
[2]*IKERBASQUE, Basque Foundation for Science, Bilbao*
[3]*Nuffield Department of Clinical Laboratory Sciences, University of Oxford,*
[1,2]*Spain*
[3]*UK*

1. Introduction

Lymphoma is the fifth most common cancer type in the Western world, accounting for approximately 12,000 cases per annum in the UK alone. Moreover the occurrence of this type of cancer has been increasing. The age-adjusted incidence of non-Hodgkin's lymphoma (NHL) in the US for example has increased 74% between 1976 and 2001 (SEER 2005). Follicular lymphoma (FL) is the most common form of low grade B-cell lymphoma (75-80% of all cases) representing about a third of all NHL cases in the US, and a quarter of all cases in Europe (Anderson et al. 1998). FL is characterised by the presence of the t(14;18) translocation in 90% of patients associated with up-regulation of the anti-apoptotic protein BCL2. Whilst FL tumours are chemo-sensitive, the disease is essentially incurable, with patients following a relapsing-remitting clinical course, typically experiencing several episodes of disease before eventually becoming refractory to treatment.

Although indolent, with a median overall survival (OS) of ~10 years, about 30% of FL patients undergo high-grade transformation to an aggressive lymphoma that is histologically indistinguishable from diffuse large B-cell lympohoma (DLBCL). Transformed FL (tFL) patients have a particularly poor outcome with a median survival of <14 months (Wrench et al. 2010). The molecular basis of FL transformation is only poorly understood and importantly to date there are no reliable biomarkers that can identify FL patients at risk of transformation. In this chapter we will review the experimental evidence for the involvement of microRNAs in the pathology of FL with particular focus on the transformation process.

2. Follicular lymphoma

FL is a neoplasm of follicle center B cells (centrocytes) characterized by a (partially) follicular growth pattern. FL tumor cells are believed to arise from normal germinal centre–associated (GC) B cells as they express the same antigen profile as GC B cells (i.e. CD19, CD20, CD10, BCL6, and membrane-bound IgM or IgG), share many morphological features of normal GC cells, and are found within a follicular architecture embedded in a network of T cells and follicular dendritic cells. In contrast to normal GC cells however, FL tumour cells are characterised by the presence of t(14:18) translocation resulting in expression of the anti-apoptotic molecule BCL2. This translocation is detectable in approximately 75% of cases by traditional karyotyping techniques but in over 90% of cases measured by polymerase chain reaction (PCR) (Tsujimoto et al. 1985). Although considered to be an essential feature of FL pathology, this genetic insult appears not to be in itself sufficient to cause FL as *BCL2* transgenic mice do not readily develop lymphoma (McDonnell & Korsmeyer 1991; Strasser et al. 1993). Furthermore, the t(14;18) translocation is not an uncommon finding in normal B cells, being detectable in over 50% of healthy individuals (Roulland et al. 2006). Therefore, whilst the presence of t(14:18) is highly suggestive of FL, it is by no means diagnostic, and indeed may be found in other apparently unrelated cases of NHL including 15-30% of DLBCL cases (Iqbal et al. 2004). Furthermore about 5% of FL cases lack the t(14:18) translocation instead being characterised by a BCL6 translocation t(3;14) and displaying an almost exclusive centroblastic morphology (Jaffe et al. 2001).

FL predominantly affects adults with a median age of 59 years and a male:female ratio of 1:1.7 (Anderson et al. 1998). Most FL patients already have widespread disease at time of presentation, predominantly in the lymph nodes, but FL may also involve the spleen, bone marrow, and peripheral blood and occasionally extra-nodal sites such as the gastro-intestinal tract or skin. Patients may be asymptomatic with slowly progressive lymphadenopathy or present with symptomatic complications of advancing tumour growth that require treatment. In nearly all survival studies, despite initial responsiveness to treatment, most patients relapse, and will eventually die of their disease.

2.1 Histological transformation of FL tumors

A percentage of FL patients (10-60% depending on the study) will eventually undergo high grade transformation from indolent FL to a much more aggressive tumor that is histologically indistinguishable from DLBCL, and is associated with a much poorer prognostic outcome. A recent study of 325 patients (median follow-up 15 years) found the risk of transformation to be 28% (Montoto et al. 2007). Despite the use of high dose therapy for transformed FL (tFL) cases, response rates are still lower than histologically equivalent *de novo* cases of DLBCL with a median survival of just 1.2 years. The molecular mechanisms behind this phenomenon, however, are very poorly understood and consequently the identification of at-risk patients, who might benefit from up-front high dose treatment modalities, remains one of the greatest challenges facing onco-hematologists today.

Lossos *et al* identified 671 genes that were aberrantly expressed in at least three of twelve paired biopsy samples which fell into two distinct groups; those that had *c-myc* and its target genes up-regulated and those where these genes were down-regulated (Lossos et al. 2002). Another study of five paired samples identified 36 up-regulated and 66 down-regulated genes, seven of which were common with the study of Lossos *et al* (de Vos et al. 2003). Sixty-seven and 46 genes were found to be up-regulated and down-regulated respectively in a series of eleven paired samples analyzed by Elenitoba-Johnson *et al* (Elenitoba-Johnson et al. 2003). Up-regulation of p38BMAPK was confirmed immunohistochemically as it was detected in DLBCL cases but not FL or normal GC cells. Davies *et al* examined the gene expression profile of twenty paired lymphoma samples taken pre- and post-transformation (Davies et al. 2007). They found that transformation proceeded by at least two molecular pathways; one characterized by a cell proliferation signature that was associated with recurrent oncogenic abnormalities and a decrease in T cell and follicular dendritic cell genes, while the other group showed no increase in proliferation genes and followed an as yet undetermined route. In contrast a gene expression study of non-paired patients (24 FL patients who underwent transformation, 22 FL patients without transformation (after 7 years) and 24 DLBCL patients who had previously transformed from FL) found that gene expression was too heterogeneous to reliably predict transformation (Glas et al. 2007). They did however report a correlation by immunohistochemistry with the spatial distribution to neoplastic follicles and the activation of $CD4^+$ T cells and specifically T-helper 1 cells (P>0.05). They did not find any correlation with other infiltrating cell populations including $CD68^+$ macrophages or regulatory T cells.

Additionally, genomic alterations have been demonstrated to be associated with transformation of FL. The acquisition of novel mutations in PIM-1, PAX-5, RhoH/TTF and c-MYC genes, due to aberrant somatic hypermutation, was found in 5/9 cases that had undergone transformation (Rossi et al. 2006). Genomic aberrations were found to be more common in transformed cases of DLBCL than non-transformed FL and the alterations -6q16-21 and +7pter-q22 were only found in transformed DLBCL but not in follicular lymphoma whereas -4q13-21 was more common in transformed than *de novo* DLBCL (Berglund et al. 2007).

However, despite intensive research the molecular basis for transformation in FL patients remains largely unknown. Recently, ourselves and others, have raised the possibility that microRNAs may be important factors in both FL transformation and antecedent FL lymphogenesis (Roehle et al. 2008; Lawrie et al. 2009).

3. MicroRNAs

MicroRNAs are a recently discovered class of naturally occurring short non-coding RNA molecules that regulate eukaryotic gene expression post-transcriptionally. There are now more than 900 human microRNAs that have been identified through cloning and/or sequence analysis (miRBase- (Griffiths-Jones et al. 2006)), and it is believed some 60% of all human genes are a target for microRNA regulation (Friedman et al. 2009). MicroRNAs have been shown to play key regulatory roles in virtually every aspect of biology including developmental timing, cell differentiation, apoptosis, cell proliferation, metabolism organ development, and hematopoiesis (Kim 2005). The potential importance of microRNAs in cancer is implied by the finding that the majority of human microRNAs are located at cancer-associated genomic regions (Calin et al. 2004), and there is now overwhelming evidence that dysfunctional expression of microRNAs is a common, if not ubiquitous, feature of cancer in general and lymphoid malignancy in particular (Lawrie 2008; Iorio & Croce 2009).

Despite the fundamental role that microRNAs appear to play in biology, these molecules were unknown to the scientific world until 1993 when *lin-4*, a *C. elegans* developmental regulator was identified (Lee et al. 1993; Wightman et al. 1993). The significance of this finding was not however realised until seven years later when another worm microRNA, *let-7* was discovered (Reinhart et al. 2000). Unlike *lin-4*, the sequence of *let-7* was found to be highly conserved in almost all organisms (Pasquinelli et al. 2000). It was soon realised that similar sequences were scattered throughout eukaryotic genomes that were first called microRNAs in 2001 (Lee & Ambros 2001).

3.1 MicroRNA biosynthesis and function

The majority of human microRNAs are encoded within introns of coding or non-coding mRNAs whilst others are located exgenically, within the exons of non-coding mRNAs or within the 3′UTR sequence of mRNA (Rodriguez et al. 2004). MicroRNAs are transcribed as 5′-capped large polyadenylated transcripts (pri-microRNA) primarily in a Pol II-dependent manner (Figure 1), although the involvement of Pol-III transcription has also been postulated for microRNAs encoded within Alu repeat sequences (Borchert et al. 2006). Approximately 40% of human microRNAs are co-transcribed as clusters encoding up to eight distinct microRNA sequences in a single pri-microRNA transcript (Altuvia et al. 2005; Hertel et al. 2006). Pri-microRNAs are cleaved within the nucleus by Drosha, an RNaseIII-type nuclease, to form 60-70 nucleotide hairpin structures (pre-microRNA). Drosha by itself possesses little enzymatic activity and requires the cofactor DiGeorge syndrome critical region 8 gene (DGCR8) in humans (Pasha in *Drosophila*) to form the so-called microprocessor complex (Yeom et al. 2006). Once produced, the pre-microRNAs are

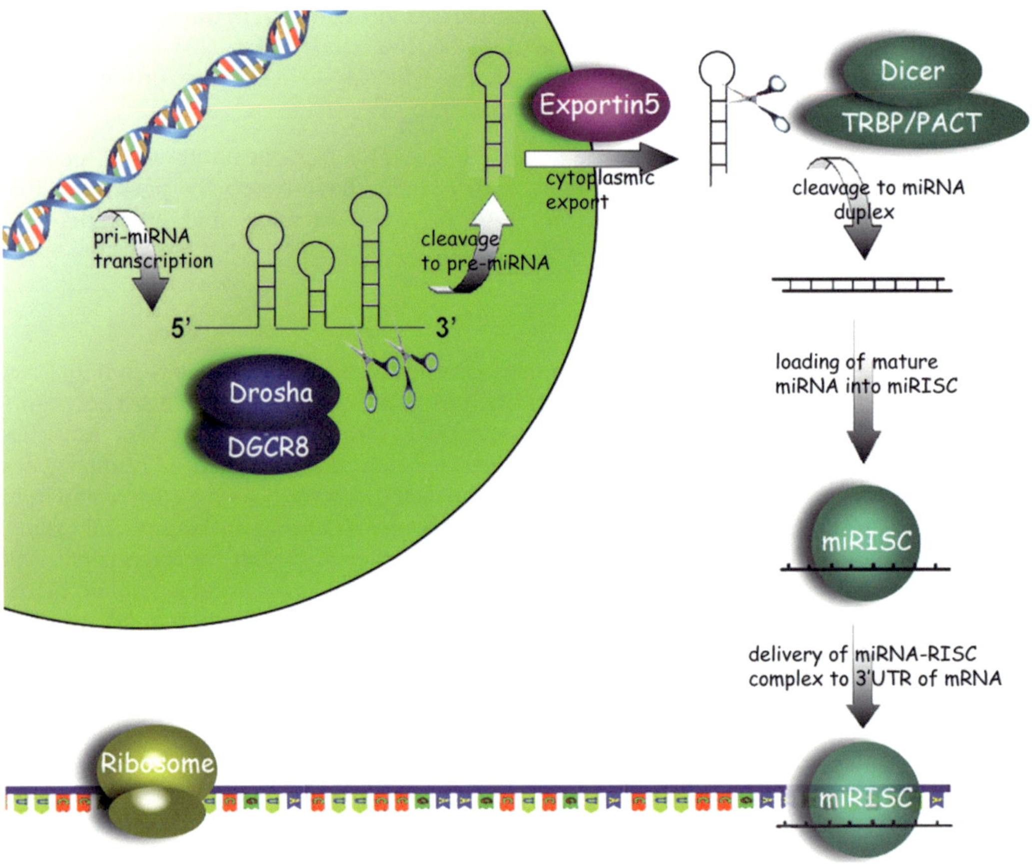

Fig. 1. **Schematic diagram of microRNA biosynthesis and function in animal cells.** Pri-microRNA precursor is transcribed in Pol-II dependent manner and then cleaved by microprocessor complex (Drosha/DGCR8) to form hairpin-structure pre-microRNA. Pre-microRNAs are exported from the nucleus by exportin-5 in a RAN-GTP dependent manner where they are cleaved into an asymmetric duplex by action of Dicer and accessory proteins. The mature microRNA is loaded into the miRISC complex which binds to cognate 3′UTR sequence of target mRNA resulting in either degradation of mRNA, or to blockage of translation without mRNA degradation.

exported from the nucleus to the cytoplasm by Exportin5 in a Ran-GTP dependent manner (Zeng 2006). The cytoplasmic pre-microRNA is further cleaved to form an asymmetric duplex intermediate (microRNA: microRNA*) by Dicer, another RNaseIII-type enzyme. Similar to Drosha, cofactors such as TRBP and PACT (in humans) are necessary for Dicer activity (Lee et al. 2006). The microRNA: microRNA* duplex is in turn loaded into the miRISC complex in which Argonaut (Ago) proteins appear to be the key effector molecules. The strand that becomes the active mature microRNA appears to be dependent upon which has the lowest free energy 5′ end and is retained by the miRISC complex whilst the other strand is usually degraded by an unknown nuclease (Khvorova et al. 2003; Schwarz et al. 2003).

The loaded miRISC is guided by the mature microRNA sequence (19-24 nucleotide) to partially complementary sequences within the 3′UTR (and probably coding sequences and 5′UTR as well) of the target mRNA, leading to inhibition of translation, transcript degradation, or both (Lawrie 2007; Lytle et al. 2007). Although repression of translation without mRNA degradation was originally believed to be the *modus operandi* of animal microRNAs, the situation appears to be more complex than previously thought, as there is now compelling evidence that microRNAs also effect transcriptional levels through de-adenylation and/or degradation (Giraldez et al. 2006) and may even positively affect translation in some instances (Vasudevan et al. 2007). How translational repression occurs remains unclear. It has been suggested that mRNA bound to the microRNA-miRISC complex may be sequestered away from the translational machinery in P-bodies that additionally act in concert with enzymes to remove the 5′-cap hence preventing translation (Liu et al. 2005; Sen & Blau 2005). Alternatively it has been suggested that microRNAs may prevent recognition of the 5′cap by translation factors (Pillai et al. 2005).

4. MicroRNA expression in FL

The following experimental details were taken in part from previously published research (Lawrie, CH et al., 2009). The only other study, as far we are aware, that considers microRNA expression in FL, was by Roehle *et al* which although it included 46 FL samples, only measured levels of 153 microRNA probes (compared with 464 microRNA probes in this study), and did not consider FL transformation (Roehle et al. 2008).

4.1 Materials and methods

4.1.1 Patient material

Formalin-fixed paraffin-embedded (FFPE) biopsy samples from 98 patients were obtained from the Pathology Department of the John Radcliffe Hospital, Oxford, UK. Eighty patients were diagnosed histologically and clinically as having DLBCL; 64 *de novo* (DLBCL-de novo) and 16 transformed cases with previously diagnosed FL (DLBCL-t). Of the 18 cases of FL used in this study, seven subsequently underwent high grade transformation (FL-t) with a median time to transformation of 24 months (range 10-96 months) from initial diagnosis. The remaining 11 FL cases (FL-nt) had no recorded transformation events (median follow-up time 60 months; range 52-132 months). The FL-t and DLBCL-t samples were not paired. All FL cases were grade 1 or 2 at time of original diagnosis. All samples were collected at time of initial diagnosis (i.e. prior to treatment) with the exception of DLBCL-t cases. Samples had >80% of tumor cells as determined by hematoxylin and eosin staining (not shown). Relevant ethical permission was obtained for the use of all samples.

4.1.2 RNA purification and microarray analysis

Total RNA was purified from four x 20 µm FFPE sections using the Recoverall kit from Ambion (Huntington, UK) in accordance with the manufacturers' instructions. RNA (3 µg) were labeled and hybridized to µRNA microarrays as previously described (Lawrie et al. 2008) using tonsillar material (pooled from twelve healthy individuals) as a common reference in a dye-balanced design.

Image analysis was carried out with BlueFuse software (BlueGnome, Cambridge, UK). Raw image data were global median-normalized within arrays and normalized between arrays using the LIMMA package (Smyth & Speed 2003). The normalized log ratios (average of four replicates per probe) were used for subsequent analysis in Genespring 7.2 (Agilent Technologies, CA, US). ANOVA analysis was used to identify microRNAs differentially expressed between sample types and *P* values were adjusted using the Benjamini-Hodgberg correction method. Differentially expressed genes were tested for their ability to predict sample class using the leave-one-out cross-validation support vector machine (SVM) function in Genespring.

4.2 Results & discussion

4.2.1 MicroRNA expression is distinct between DLBCL and FL

In order to investigate differences in microRNA expression between FL and DLBCL samples, and because *de novo* and transformed DLBCL are indistinguishable histologically, we initially compared expression in all DLBCL cases (n = 80) with that of all FL cases (n = 18). Thirty microRNAs were found to be differentially expressed ($P < 0.05$) (Table 1). Expression values of these microRNAs correctly predicted 95/97 (98%) of cases as DLBCL or FL by SVM, and clustered the cases distinctly (Fig. 2A).

The study by Roehle *et al* identified 10 microRNAs that were differentially expressed between FL and DLBCL cases (Roehle et al. 2008). Only two of these microRNAs (*miR-150* and *miR-135a*) were found to be differentially expressed ($P < 0.05$) in our patient cohort, although another two microRNAs, *miR-92* and *miR-125b*, had *P* values of < 0.1. These 10 microRNAs correctly predicted 74/97 (76%) of cases according to diagnosis.

Roehle's study, however, compared *de novo* cases of DLBCL with FL cases that did not undergo subsequent transformation. Therefore, in order to compare the data directly we used the same sample types (64 DLBCL-de novo and 11 FL-nt cases) to re-analyze the data. This resulted in 26 differentially expressed ($P < 0.05$) microRNAs (Table 2), 14 of which were also present in the previous list (Table 1). These microRNAs correctly predicted 73/75 (97%) of cases in this cohort (c.f. 60/75 (80%) with the 10 microRNA signature (Roehle et al. 2008)) and 92/97 (95%) of cases in the extended cohort. Again, the two sets of samples were found to cluster distinctly using the 26-microRNA signature (Fig. 2B).

microRNA	*P* value	Up	Fold change
hsa-miR-200c	8.20E-08	DLBCL	9.39
hsa-miR-518a	1.23E-03	DLBCL	3.15
hsa-miR-638	8.05E-04	DLBCL	3.09
hsa-miR-205	4.36E-02	DLBCL	2.85
hsa-miR-223	1.42E-02	DLBCL	2.75
hsa-miR-573	2.79E-02	DLBCL	2.35
hsa-miR-135b	3.83E-02	DLBCL	1.63
hsa-miR-133a	8.65E-03	DLBCL	1.38
hsa-miR-135a	3.72E-02	DLBCL	1.38
hsa-miR-451	3.67E-03	DLBCL	1.38
hsa-miR-27b	2.12E-06	DLBCL	1.21
hsa-miR-27a	4.62E-07	DLBCL	1.13
hsa-miR-18b	1.03E-02	DLBCL	0.93
hsa-miR-199b	3.23E-03	DLBCL	0.83
hsa-miR-19a	1.20E-02	DLBCL	0.80
hsa-miR-210	1.10E-02	DLBCL	0.75
hsa-miR-19b	7.60E-04	DLBCL	0.75
hsa-miR-99a	9.00E-05	DLBCL	0.72
hsa-miR-100	1.07E-02	DLBCL	0.51
hsa-miR-361	3.57E-02	FL	0.58
hsa-miR-29c	3.07E-02	FL	0.63
hsa-miR-26a	8.85E-03	FL	0.73
hsa-miR-29b	4.22E-03	FL	0.76
hsa-miR-26b	5.50E-03	FL	1.04
hsa-miR-655	4.76E-02	FL	2.32
hsa-miR-10b	3.10E-02	FL	2.38
hsa-miR-634	1.19E-02	FL	2.41
hsa-miR-593	3.30E-02	FL	2.43
hsa-miR-28	1.47E-02	FL	2.49
hsa-miR-150	1.45E-03	FL	3.37

Table 1. MicroRNAs differentially expressed ($P < 0.05$) between DLBCL (DLBCL-de novo and DLBCL-t) and FL (FL-nt and FL-t) diagnoses.

microRNA	*P* value	Up	Fold change
hsa-miR-200c	4.58E-06	DLBCL	10.03
hsa-miR-638	5.30E-04	DLBCL	3.31
hsa-miR-518a	3.85E-02	DLBCL	2.88
hsa-miR-199a	1.57E-02	DLBCL	2.67
hsa-miR-93	3.74E-02	DLBCL	2.64
hsa-miR-22	1.94E-02	DLBCL	2.46
hsa-miR-34a	3.92E-02	DLBCL	2.39
hsa-miR-362	4.68E-02	DLBCL	2.30
hsa-miR-206	3.93E-02	DLBCL	1.73
hsa-miR-451	3.23E-03	DLBCL	1.49
hsa-miR-636	8.55E-03	DLBCL	1.17
hsa-miR-92	4.05E-02	DLBCL	1.08
hsa-miR-27b	6.85E-04	DLBCL	1.04
hsa-miR-199b	1.15E-04	DLBCL	1.03
hsa-miR-27a	4.03E-04	DLBCL	0.97
hsa-miR-24	2.04E-02	DLBCL	0.75
hsa-miR-106a	1.16E-02	DLBCL	0.73
hsa-miR-20a	2.62E-02	DLBCL	0.67
hsa-miR-19b	4.95E-03	DLBCL	0.64
hsa-miR-99a	9.55E-03	DLBCL	0.56
hsa-miR-18b	3.27E-02	DLBCL	0.54
hsa-miR-100	1.95E-02	DLBCL	0.43
hsa-miR-26b	1.88E-02	FL	1.42
hsa-miR-217	2.84E-02	FL	2.44
hsa-miR-634	9.50E-04	FL	2.54
hsa-miR-150	4.55E-02	FL	3.46

Table 2. MicroRNAs differentially expressed ($P < 0.05$) between *de novo* DLBCL and non-transforming FL cases. Members of the *miR-17-92* cluster (and homologous clusters) are depicted in bold type.

Interestingly, six of the microRNAs that were identified as being up-regulated in DLBCL-*de novo* cases compared to FL-nt are encoded by the *miR-17-92* and/or homologous clusters (average fold-increase of 1.05 (range 0.54-2.64)) (He et al. 2005). The other four microRNAs encoded by these clusters, *miR-17-5p, miR-19a, miR-25* and *miR-106b,* had *P* values of 0.067, 0.087, 0.064 and 0.391 respectively. The *miR-17-92* cluster is encoded at the 13q31 locus, a region commonly amplified in lymphomas and ectopic expression of *miR-17-92* greatly accelerated lymphogenesis in a murine model (He et al. 2005). Moreover, direct binding of the c-myc protein up-regulates *miR*-17-92 expression (O'Donnell et al. 2005) and over-expression of c-myc has been demonstrated in the majority (66.6%) of DLBCL cases (Aref et al. 2004), which has also been associated with poorer outcome (Pagnano et al. 2001). An increased level of this cluster in DLBCL compared to FL is consistent with a more aggressive clinical phenotype of DLBCL.

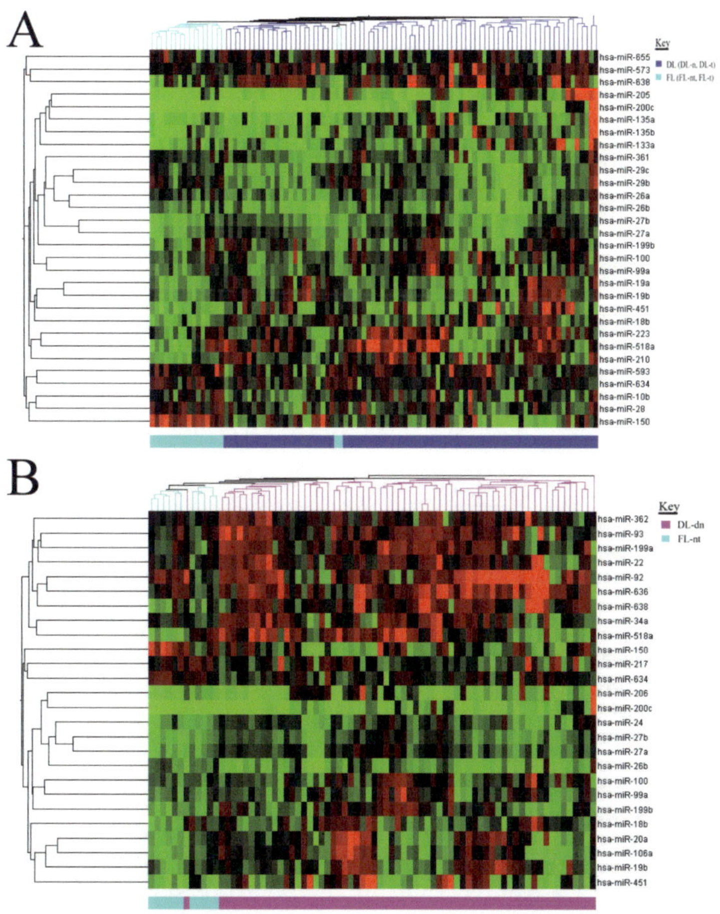

Fig. 2. **Cluster analysis of microRNAs differentially expressed between FL and DLBCL.** (A) All DLBCL cases (n = 80) and FL cases (n = 18). (B) Only *de novo* cases (DLBCL-de novo (n = 64)) and cases of FL that did not undergo transformation (FL-nt (n = 11)). Reproduced from (Lawrie et al. 2009).

4.2.2 Histological transformation of FL is associated with changes in microRNA expression

To investigate whether changes in microRNA expression were associated with transformation we first looked at differences between *de novo* (DLBCL-de novo (n = 64) and transformed (DLBCL-t (n = 16)) cases of DLBCL. Fourteen microRNAs (Table 3) were found to be differentially expressed ($P < 0.05$). These microRNAs correctly predicted transformation status in 73/80 (91%) of samples. Only one of these was up-regulated in DLBCL-t (*miR-491*). Four of the microRNAs down-regulated in DLBCL-t are encoded by the *miR-17-92* cluster suggesting an involvement of the cluster in high grade transformation. An alternative explanation is that because the cluster was also found to be down-regulated in FL compared with DLBCL-de novo (Table 2), the expression pattern of these microRNAs in DLBCL-t cases reflects that of antecedent FL. This latter hypothesis is consistent with gene expression profile studies that found that DLBCL-t cases were more closely related to FL than DLBCL-de novo cases (Lossos et al. 2002).

microRNA	***P* value**	**Up**	**Fold change**
hsa-miR-491	2.11E-02	trans	2.54
hsa-miR-27a	3.90E-02	*de novo*	0.47
hsa-miR-19b	3.77E-03	*de novo*	0.60
hsa-miR-25	3.84E-02	*de novo*	0.67
hsa-miR-18a	1.24E-02	*de novo*	0.72
hsa-miR-636	2.73E-02	*de novo*	1.06
hsa-miR-92	1.94E-02	*de novo*	1.14
hsa-miR-621	2.29E-02	*de novo*	1.98
hsa-miR-526c	2.44E-02	*de novo*	2.38
hsa-miR-766	2.75E-02	*de novo*	2.58
hsa-miR-299-5p	4.76E-02	*de novo*	2.61
hsa-miR-380-3p	5.94E-03	*de novo*	2.65
hsa-miR-129	2.98E-02	*de novo*	2.70
hsa-miR-588	9.05E-03	*de novo*	2.80

Table 3. MicroRNAs differentially expressed ($P < 0.05$) between DLBCL-de novo and DLBCL-t cases.

Next we compared FL cases that subsequently underwent high grade transformation (FL-t (n = 7)) with cases that did not (FL-nt (n = 11)). Six microRNAs were differentially expressed ($P < 0.05$) between these two groups (Table 4), whose expression levels correctly predicted 16/18 (89%) of cases.

microRNA	***P* value**	**Up**	
hsa-miR-223	1.43E-03	FL-nt	1.51
hsa-miR-217	5.56E-03	FL-nt	2.56
hsa-miR-222	1.41E-02	FL-t	1.26
hsa-let-7i	2.09E-02	FL-t	2.45
hsa-miR-221	2.34E-02	FL-t	3.14
hsa-let-7b	2.46E-02	FL-t	3.18

Table 4. MicroRNAs differentially expressed ($P < 0.05$) between FL cases that subsequently underwent high grade transformation (FL-t) and those that did not (FL-nt). Median follow-up time 60 months (range 52-132 months).

Let-7b, let-7i, miR-221 and *miR-222* were up-regulated in FL-t whilst *miR-223* and *miR-217* were down-regulated (Fig. 3). Members of the *let-7* family have been shown to target c-myc expression in Burkitt lymphoma (Sampson et al. 2007) and decreased c-myc expression has been associated with high grade transformation of FL to DLBCL (Lossos et al. 2002). Interestingly, up-regulated microRNAs *miR-221* and *miR-222* target the tumor suppressor molecule p27(Kip1) (le Sage et al. 2007) whilst down-regulated *miR-223* has been shown to target Stathmin, a known oncogene (Alli et al. 2007). Although the number of cases in this analysis was small, and requires further validation, these data open up the exciting possibility that microRNA expression could be used to predict FL patients at risk of transformation that could benefit from an up-front aggressive therapy regimen.

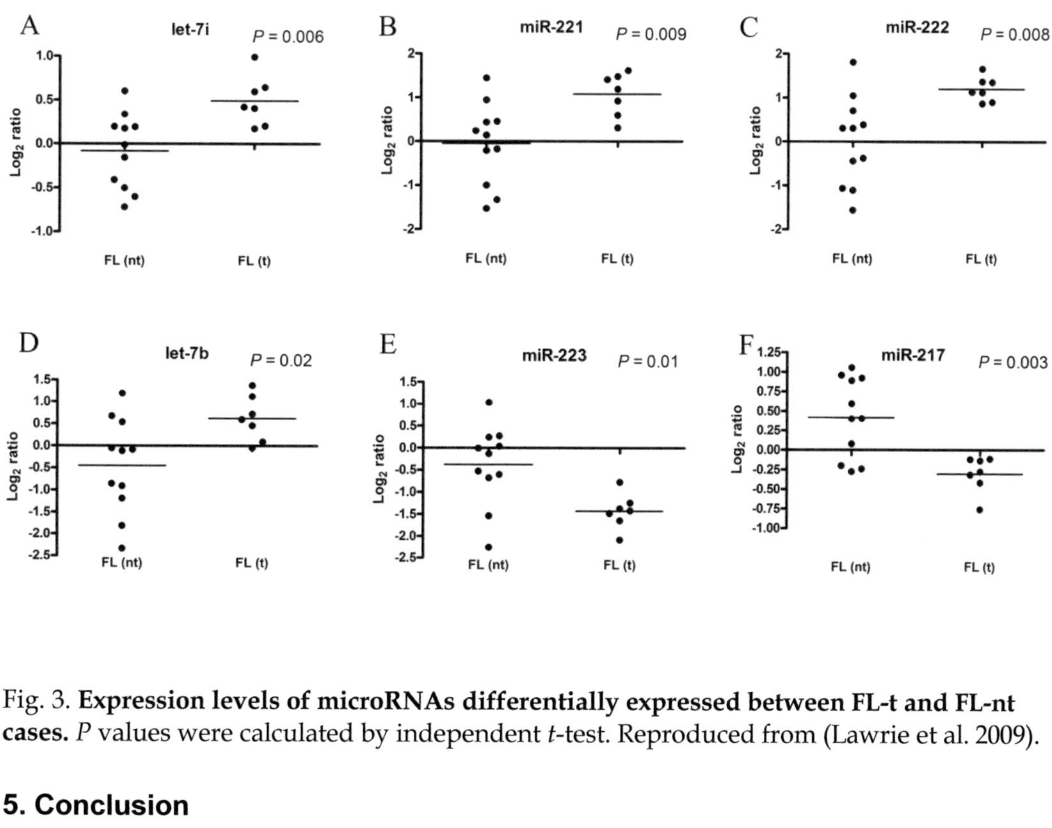

Fig. 3. **Expression levels of microRNAs differentially expressed between FL-t and FL-nt cases.** *P* values were calculated by independent *t*-test. Reproduced from (Lawrie et al. 2009).

5. Conclusion

In this chapter we have discussed some of the clinico-scientific issues pertaining to follicular lymphoma and the role that microRNAs may play in both its pathogenesis and in particular histological high grade transformation. As is outlined in this article there are in fact only two pieces of research published to date that have investigated microRNA expression in FL, and hence some caution should be applied when drawing conclusions about the role/potential of specific microRNAs in this disease, as clearly much more research is required. Nonetheless, these studies do present some interesting insights and offer the tantalizing possibility that microRNAs may deliver novel biomarkers that can identify FL patients at risk of transformation where other molecular techniques have failed.

6. Acknowledgments

CHL and his research are supported by grants from Ikerbasque- the Basque Foundation for Science and the Julian Starmer-Smith Memorial Fund.

7. References

Alli, E, Yang, JM & Hait, WN (2007). Silencing of stathmin induces tumor-suppressor function in breast cancer cell lines harboring mutant p53. *Oncogene*, 26(7), pp.1003-1012.

Altuvia, Y, Landgraf, P, Lithwick, G, Elefant, N, Pfeffer, S, Aravin, A, Brownstein, MJ, Tuschl, T & Margalit, H (2005). Clustering and conservation patterns of human microRNAs. *Nucleic Acids Res*, 33(8), pp.2697-2706.

Anderson, JR, Armitage, JO & Weisenburger, DD (1998). Epidemiology of the non-Hodgkin's lymphomas: distributions of the major subtypes differ by geographic locations. Non-Hodgkin's Lymphoma Classification Project. *Ann Oncol*, 9(7), pp.717-720.

Aref, S, Mabed, M, Zalata, K, Sakrana, M & El Askalany, H (2004). The interplay between c-Myc oncogene expression and circulating vascular endothelial growth factor (sVEGF), its antagonist receptor, soluble Flt-1 in diffuse large B cell lymphoma (DLBCL): relationship to patient outcome. *Leuk Lymphoma*, 45(3), pp.499-506.

Berglund, M, Enblad, G, Thunberg, U, Amini, RM, Sundstrom, C, Roos, G, Erlanson, M, Rosenquist, R, Larsson, C & Lagercrantz, S (2007). Genomic imbalances during transformation from follicular lymphoma to diffuse large B-cell lymphoma. *Mod Pathol*, 20(1), pp.63-75.

Borchert, GM, Lanier, W & Davidson, BL (2006). RNA polymerase III transcribes human microRNAs. *Nat Struct Mol Biol*, 13(12), pp.1097-1101.

Calin, GA, Sevignani, C, Dumitru, CD, Hyslop, T, Noch, E, Yendamuri, S, Shimizu, M, Rattan, S, Bullrich, F, Negrini, M & Croce, CM (2004). Human microRNA genes are frequently located at fragile sites and genomic regions involved in cancers. *Proc Natl Acad Sci U S A*, 101(9), pp.2999-3004.

Davies, AJ, Rosenwald, A, Wright, G, Lee, A, Last, KW, Weisenburger, DD, Chan, WC, Delabie, J, Braziel, RM, Campo, E, Gascoyne, RD, Jaffe, ES, Muller-Hermelink, K, Ott, G, Calaminici, M, Norton, AJ, Goff, LK, Fitzgibbon, J, Staudt, LM & Andrew Lister, T (2007). Transformation of follicular lymphoma to diffuse large B-cell lymphoma proceeds by distinct oncogenic mechanisms. *Br J Haematol*, 136(2), pp.286-293.

de Vos, S, Hofmann, WK, Grogan, TM, Krug, U, Schrage, M, Miller, TP, Braun, JG, Wachsman, W, Koeffler, HP & Said, JW (2003). Gene expression profile of serial samples of transformed B-cell lymphomas. *Lab Invest*, 83(2), pp.271-285.

Elenitoba-Johnson, KS, Jenson, SD, Abbott, RT, Palais, RA, Bohling, SD, Lin, Z, Tripp, S, Shami, PJ, Wang, LY, Coupland, RW, Buckstein, R, Perez-Ordonez, B, Perkins, SL, Dube, ID & Lim, MS (2003). Involvement of multiple signaling pathways in follicular lymphoma transformation: p38-mitogen-activated protein kinase as a target for therapy. *Proc Natl Acad Sci U S A*, 100(12), pp.7259-7264.

Friedman, RC, Farh, KK, Burge, CB & Bartel, DP (2009). Most mammalian mRNAs are conserved targets of microRNAs. *Genome Res*, 19(1), pp.92-105.

Giraldez, AJ, Mishima, Y, Rihel, J, Grocock, RJ, Van Dongen, S, Inoue, K, Enright, AJ & Schier, AF (2006). Zebrafish MiR-430 promotes deadenylation and clearance of maternal mRNAs. *Science*, 312(5770), pp.75-79.

Glas, AM, Knoops, L, Delahaye, L, Kersten, MJ, Kibbelaar, RE, Wessels, LA, van Laar, R, van Krieken, JH, Baars, JW, Raemaekers, J, Kluin, PM, van't Veer, LJ & de Jong, D (2007). Gene-expression and immunohistochemical study of specific T-cell subsets and accessory cell types in the transformation and prognosis of follicular lymphoma. *J Clin Oncol*, 25(4), pp.390-398.

Griffiths-Jones, S, Grocock, RJ, van Dongen, S, Bateman, A & Enright, AJ (2006). miRBase: microRNA sequences, targets and gene nomenclature. *Nucleic Acids Res*, 34(Database issue), pp.D140-144.

He, L, Thomson, JM, Hemann, MT, Hernando-Monge, E, Mu, D, Goodson, S, Powers, S, Cordon-Cardo, C, Lowe, SW, Hannon, GJ & Hammond, SM (2005). A microRNA polycistron as a potential human oncogene. *Nature*, 435(7043), pp.828-833.

Hertel, J, Lindemeyer, M, Missal, K, Fried, C, Tanzer, A, Flamm, C, Hofacker, IL & Stadler, PF (2006). The expansion of the metazoan microRNA repertoire. *BMC Genomics*, 7, pp.25.

Iorio, MV & Croce, CM (2009). MicroRNAs in cancer: small molecules with a huge impact. *J Clin Oncol*, 27(34), pp.5848-5856.

Iqbal, J, Sanger, WG, Horsman, DE, Rosenwald, A, Pickering, DL, Dave, B, Dave, S, Xiao, L, Cao, K, Zhu, Q, Sherman, S, Hans, CP, Weisenburger, DD, Greiner, TC, Gascoyne, RD, Ott, G, Muller-Hermelink, HK, Delabie, J, Braziel, RM, Jaffe, ES, Campo, E, Lynch, JC, Connors, JM, Vose, JM, Armitage, JO, Grogan, TM, Staudt, LM & Chan, WC (2004). BCL2 translocation defines a unique tumor subset within the germinal center B-cell-like diffuse large B-cell lymphoma. *Am J Pathol*, 165(1), pp.159-166.

Jaffe, ES, Harris, NL, Stein, H & Vardiman, J, Eds. (2001). World Health Organisation (WHO) Classification of Tumours-Pathology & Genetics-Tumours of Haematopoietic and Lymphoid Tissues. Lyon, IARC Press (International Agency for Research on Cancer).

Khvorova, A, Reynolds, A & Jayasena, SD (2003). Functional siRNAs and miRNAs exhibit strand bias. *Cell*, 115(2), pp.209-216.

Kim, VN (2005). MicroRNA biogenesis: coordinated cropping and dicing. *Nat Rev Mol Cell Biol*, 6(5), pp.376-385.

Lawrie, CH (2007). MicroRNAs and haematology: small molecules, big function. *Br J Haematol*, 137(6), pp.503-512.

Lawrie, CH (2008). microRNA expression in lymphoid malignancies: new hope for diagnosis and therapy? *J Cell Mol Med*, 12(5A), pp.1432-1444.

Lawrie, CH, Chi, J, Taylor, S, Tramonti, D, Ballabio, E, Palazzo, S, Saunders, NJ, Pezzella, F, Boultwood, J, Wainscoat, JS & Hatton, CS (2009). Expression of microRNAs in diffuse large B cell lymphoma is associated with immunophenotype, survival and transformation from follicular lymphoma. *J Cell Mol Med*, 13(7), pp.1248-1260.

Lawrie, CH, Saunders, NJ, Soneji, S, Palazzo, S, Dunlop, HM, Cooper, CD, Brown, PJ, Troussard, X, Mossafa, H, Enver, T, Pezzella, F, Boultwood, J, Wainscoat, JS & Hatton, CS (2008). MicroRNA expression in lymphocyte development and malignancy. *Leukemia*, 22(7), pp.1440-1446.

le Sage, C, Nagel, R, Egan, DA, Schrier, M, Mesman, E, Mangiola, A, Anile, C, Maira, G, Mercatelli, N, Ciafre, SA, Farace, MG & Agami, R (2007). Regulation of the p27(Kip1) tumor suppressor by miR-221 and miR-222 promotes cancer cell proliferation. *Embo J*, 26(15), pp.3699-3708.

Lee, RC & Ambros, V (2001). An extensive class of small RNAs in Caenorhabditis elegans. *Science*, 294(5543), pp.862-864.

Lee, RC, Feinbaum, RL & Ambros, V (1993). The C. elegans heterochronic gene lin-4 encodes small RNAs with antisense complementarity to lin-14. *Cell*, 75(5), pp.843-854.

Lee, Y, Hur, I, Park, SY, Kim, YK, Suh, MR & Kim, VN (2006). The role of PACT in the RNA silencing pathway. *Embo J*, 25(3), pp.522-532.

Liu, J, Valencia-Sanchez, MA, Hannon, GJ & Parker, R (2005). MicroRNA-dependent localization of targeted mRNAs to mammalian P-bodies. *Nat Cell Biol*, 7(7), pp.719-723.

Lossos, IS, Alizadeh, AA, Diehn, M, Warnke, R, Thorstenson, Y, Oefner, PJ, Brown, PO, Botstein, D & Levy, R (2002). Transformation of follicular lymphoma to diffuse large-cell lymphoma: alternative patterns with increased or decreased expression of c-myc and its regulated genes. *Proc Natl Acad Sci U S A*, 99(13), pp.8886-8891.

Lytle, JR, Yario, TA & Steitz, JA (2007). Target mRNAs are repressed as efficiently by microRNA-binding sites in the 5' UTR as in the 3' UTR. *Proc Natl Acad Sci U S A*, 104(23), pp.9667-9672.

McDonnell, TJ & Korsmeyer, SJ (1991). Progression from lymphoid hyperplasia to high-grade malignant lymphoma in mice transgenic for the t(14; 18). *Nature*, 349(6306), pp.254-256.

Montoto, S, Davies, AJ, Matthews, J, Calaminici, M, Norton, AJ, Amess, J, Vinnicombe, S, Waters, R, Rohatiner, AZ & Lister, TA (2007). Risk and clinical implications of transformation of follicular lymphoma to diffuse large B-cell lymphoma. *J Clin Oncol*, 25(17), pp.2426-2433.

O'Donnell, KA, Wentzel, EA, Zeller, KI, Dang, CV & Mendell, JT (2005). c-Myc-regulated microRNAs modulate E2F1 expression. *Nature*, 435(7043), pp.839-843.

Pagnano, KB, Vassallo, J, Lorand-Metze, I, Costa, FF & Saad, ST (2001). p53, Mdm2, and c-Myc overexpression is associated with a poor prognosis in aggressive non-Hodgkin's lymphomas. *Am J Hematol*, 67(2), pp.84-92.

Pasquinelli, AE, Reinhart, BJ, Slack, F, Martindale, MQ, Kuroda, MI, Maller, B, Hayward, DC, Ball, EE, Degnan, B, Muller, P, Spring, J, Srinivasan, A, Fishman, M, Finnerty, J, Corbo, J, Levine, M, Leahy, P, Davidson, E & Ruvkun, G (2000). Conservation of the sequence and temporal expression of let-7 heterochronic regulatory RNA. *Nature*, 408(6808), pp.86-89.

Pillai, RS, Bhattacharyya, SN, Artus, CG, Zoller, T, Cougot, N, Basyuk, E, Bertrand, E & Filipowicz, W (2005). Inhibition of translational initiation by Let-7 MicroRNA in human cells. *Science*, 309(5740), pp.1573-1576.

Reinhart, BJ, Slack, FJ, Basson, M, Pasquinelli, AE, Bettinger, JC, Rougvie, AE, Horvitz, HR & Ruvkun, G (2000). The 21-nucleotide let-7 RNA regulates developmental timing in Caenorhabditis elegans. *Nature*, 403(6772), pp.901-906.

Rodriguez, A, Griffiths-Jones, S, Ashurst, JL & Bradley, A (2004). Identification of mammalian microRNA host genes and transcription units. *Genome Res*, 14(10A), pp.1902-1910.

Roehle, A, Hoefig, KP, Repsilber, D, Thorns, C, Ziepert, M, Wesche, KO, Thiere, M, Loeffler, M, Klapper, W, Pfreundschuh, M, Matolcsy, A, Bernd, HW, Reiniger, L, Merz, H & Feller, AC (2008). MicroRNA signatures characterize diffuse large B-cell lymphomas and follicular lymphomas. *Br J Haematol*, 142(5), pp.732-744.

Rossi, D, Berra, E, Cerri, M, Deambrogi, C, Barbieri, C, Franceschetti, S, Lunghi, M, Conconi, A, Paulli, M, Matolcsy, A, Pasqualucci, L, Capello, D & Gaidano, G (2006). Aberrant somatic hypermutation in transformation of follicular lymphoma and chronic lymphocytic leukemia to diffuse large B-cell lymphoma. *Haematologica*, 91(10), pp.1405-1409.

Roulland, S, Navarro, JM, Grenot, P, Milili, M, Agopian, J, Montpellier, B, Gauduchon, P, Lebailly, P, Schiff, C & Nadel, B (2006). Follicular lymphoma-like B cells in healthy individuals: a novel intermediate step in early lymphomagenesis. *J Exp Med*, 203(11), pp.2425-2431.

Sampson, VB, Rong, NH, Han, J, Yang, Q, Aris, V, Soteropoulos, P, Petrelli, NJ, Dunn, SP & Krueger, LJ (2007). MicroRNA let-7a down-regulates MYC and reverts MYC-induced growth in Burkitt lymphoma cells. *Cancer Res*, 67(20), pp.9762-9770.

Schwarz, DS, Hutvagner, G, Du, T, Xu, Z, Aronin, N & Zamore, PD (2003). Asymmetry in the assembly of the RNAi enzyme complex. *Cell*, 115(2), pp.199-208.

SEER (2005). Cancer Statistics Review, 1975-2002. *National Cancer Institute.*

Sen, GL & Blau, HM (2005). Argonaute 2/RISC resides in sites of mammalian mRNA decay known as cytoplasmic bodies. *Nat Cell Biol*, 7(6), pp.633-636.

Smyth, GK & Speed, T (2003). Normalization of cDNA microarray data. *Methods*, 31(4), pp.265-273.

Strasser, A, Harris, AW & Cory, S (1993). E mu-bcl-2 transgene facilitates spontaneous transformation of early pre-B and immunoglobulin-secreting cells but not T cells. *Oncogene*, 8(1), pp.1-9.

Tsujimoto, Y, Cossman, J, Jaffe, E & Croce, CM (1985). Involvement of the bcl-2 gene in human follicular lymphoma. *Science*, 228(4706), pp.1440-1443.

Vasudevan, S, Tong, Y & Steitz, JA (2007). Switching from repression to activation: microRNAs can up-regulate translation. *Science*, 318(5858), pp.1931-1934.

Wightman, B, Ha, I & Ruvkun, G (1993). Posttranscriptional regulation of the heterochronic gene lin-14 by lin-4 mediates temporal pattern formation in C. elegans. *Cell*, 75(5), pp.855-862.

Wrench, D, Montoto, S & Fitzgibbon, J (2010). Molecular signatures in the diagnosis and management of follicular lymphoma. *Current Opinion in Hematology*, 17(4), pp.333-340.

Yeom, KH, Lee, Y, Han, J, Suh, MR & Kim, VN (2006). Characterization of DGCR8/Pasha, the essential cofactor for Drosha in primary miRNA processing. *Nucleic Acids Res*, 34(16), pp.4622-4629.

Zeng, Y (2006). Principles of micro-RNA production and maturation. *Oncogene*, 25(46), pp.6156-6162.

16

Epstein-Barr Virus-Encoded miRNAs in Epstein-Barr Virus-Related Malignancy

Jun Lu[1,*], Bidisha Chanda[2,*] and Ai Kotani[1,*]
[1]*Tokai University Institute of Innovative Science and Technology*
[2]*University of Tokyo Institute of Medical Science*
Japan

1. Introduction

In 1958, Denis Burkitt described B cell lymphomas in 2- to 14-year-old African children from malaria-endemic areas.[1] In 1964, Michael Anthony Epstein and Yvonne Barr found that immortalized B lymphocyte cell lines derived from these tumors spontaneously released a herpesvirus.[2] Thus, Epstein-Barr virus (EBV) was discovered by examining electron micrographs of cells cultured from Burkitt's lymphoma; its unusual geographic distribution indicated a viral etiology. It was Gertrud and Werner Henle who demonstrated that EBV is ubiquitous in the human population.[3] Far from having a restricted distribution, EBV, a member of the γ-herpesvirus family, was found to be widespread in all human populations and to persist in the vast majority of individuals as a lifelong, asymptomatic infection of B lymphocytes. Therefore, EBV is usually the cause of clinically inconspicuous infections, although it can cause infectious mononucleosis. The most severe, albeit rare, result of EBV infection is malignant transformation and the development of cancer in various forms, including Burkitt's lymphoma and nasopharyngeal carcinoma, the latter of which is one of the most common cancers in China.[4] The link between EBV and "endemic" Burkitt's lymphoma proved constant and became the first of an unexpectedly wide range of associations discovered between this virus and tumors.[5] As a ubiquitous human pathogen, EBV is responsible for several lymphoid malignancies, including a subset of Burkitt's lymphoma, acquired Immune deficiency syndrome (AIDS)-associated lymphoma, Hodgkin's lymphoma, post-transplant lymphoma, age-associated B cell lymphoma, and peripheral T and NK cell lymphomas.[6,7]

1.1 EBV infection

The primary site of EBV infection is the oropharyngeal cavity.[8] Children and teenagers are often infected after oral contact, hence the nickname "kissing disease". Like other herpesviruses, infection with EBV can exhibit two distinct patterns, or states, of gene expression. During acute (lytic) EBV infection, the virus sequentially expresses its entire repertoire of genes. In this lytic state, linear, double-stranded viral genomes are produced and packaged into virions that spread infection from cell to cell. Shortly after the initial

* These authors equally contributed to this work.

infection, EBV enters into a latent state, whereupon only select "latent" genes are expressed, thereby evading host immune surveillance mechanisms, and establishing a lifelong, persistent infection in the host.[9] During latency, only a few viral genes are transcribed, no viral progeny are produced, and infected cells are protected from apoptotic stimuli and, in some circumstances, driven to proliferate. Based on serology, about 95% of the world's adult population is infected with EBV, and following primary infection, hosts remain lifelong carriers of the virus.[10] In developed countries, exposure to EBV occurs relatively late; only 50–70% of adolescents and young adults are EBV seropositive. About 30% of seronegative individuals will later develop infectious mononucleosis as a result of primary EBV infection. This disease is characterized by fever, pharyngitis, generalized lymphadenopathy, splenomegaly, intense asthenia, hyper-lymphocytosis (>50%) with atypical lymphocytes, and elevated transaminase levels. In developing countries, EBV antibodies are acquired early in life and the disease is mostly asymptomatic.

1.2 EBV-related cancer

EBV has been etiologically linked to a variety of human cancers, such as Burkitt's lymphoma, nasopharyngeal carcinoma (NPC), Hodgkin's disease, and more recently with sporadic cases of gastric adenocarcinoma and invasive breast carcinoma.[11,12] Nearly 100% of NPC tumors, 90% of Burkitt's lymphoma tumors of African origin, and 40–60% of Hodgkin's and non-Hodgkin's lymphomas contain EBV episomes. Clonality of the EBV genome has been confirmed in these tumors, suggesting that the tumors arose from a single EBV-infected cell, and that EBV infection is a very early, if not causal, event. EBV is also commonly associated with lymphoproliferative diseases in patients with congenital or acquired immunodeficiencies. Examples include X-linked lymphoproliferative syndrome, human immunodeficiency virus (HIV)-related non-Hodgkin's lymphoma, and perhaps most importantly post-transplantation lymphoproliferative disease.[5]

Burkitt's lymphoma is a malignant tumor associated with EBV that is endemic to central parts of Africa and New Guinea with an annual incidence of 6–7 cases per 100,000 and a peak incidence in children of 6 or 7 years of age. The epidemiological involvement of EBV in Burkitt's lymphoma was first suspected due to the presence of the EBV viral genome in tumor cells and elevated antibody titers against EBV viral capsid antigen in cancer patients. The highest prevalence of Burkitt's lymphoma occurs in the "lymphoma belt," a region that extends from West Africa to East Africa, between the 10th degree north and 10th degree south of the equator, and continues south along the eastern coast of Africa. This area is characterized by high temperature and humidity, which is likely the reason why an association between malaria and Burkitt's lymphoma was once suspected. In African countries within the lymphoma belt, such as Uganda, the association of Burkitt's lymphoma with EBV is very strong (97%), whereas it is less so elsewhere (e.g., 85% in Algeria and 10–15% in France and the USA). (World Health Organization, WHO)

NPC incidence rates are less than 1 per 100,000 in most populations, except for those in southern China, where an annual incidence of more than 20 cases per 100,000 is reported.[4] Isolated northern populations, such as Eskimos and Greenlanders, also have high incidences. Moderate incidences occur in North Africa, Israel, Kuwait, the Sudan, and parts of Kenya and Uganda. Men are twice as likely to develop NPC as women. The rate of incidence generally increases at ages 20–50 years. In the USA, Chinese-Americans comprise the majority of NPC patients, along with workers exposed to fumes, smoke, and chemicals, implicating a role for chemical carcinogenesis. Studies assessing nutrition and diets have demonstrated an association between eating highly salted foods and NPC. Vitamin C deficiency at a young age may also be a contributing factor. Finally, a study of human leukocyte antigen (HLA) haplotypes revealed a genetically distinct subpopulation in southern China, with an increased frequency of haplotype A-2/B-Sin-2, which may account for the higher disease incidence in that area. (WHO)

1.3 Cytotoxic T lymphocyte therapy for EBV-related cancer

EBV, together with human herpesvirus (HHV)-8 (also known as Kaposi sarcoma-associated virus), belongs to the genus *Lymphocryptovirus* in the subfamily Gammaherpesvirinae of the family Herpesviridae. These are complex, enveloped, DNA viruses, which multiply in the nucleus of the host cell. EBV infects resting human B lymphocytes and epithelial cells, multiplies in the latter, and establishes latent infection in memory B lymphocytes. Thus, infected individuals may produce virions, carry virus-specific cytotoxic T lymphocytes (CTLs), produce EBV-specific antibodies, and yet harbor latently infected memory B cells. EBV-infected individuals maintain the latent EBV genome as an episome that expresses only part of its genetic information, including EBV nuclear antigens (EBNA)-1 (a latent DNA replication factor), EBNA-2 (a transcriptional activator), and EBNA-3A and -3C (involved in the establishment of latency). Also expressed are latent membrane protein (LMP)-1 and LMP-2, which play major roles in the maintenance of latency and escape from the host immune response. Latently infected cells do not express the B7 coactivator receptor and, therefore, are not targeted by CTLs. When peripheral blood from an infected individual is cultured, latently infected B cells replicate and become immortalized lymphoblasts that can be indefinitely propagated in the laboratory.[13]

In a previous study, CTL therapy was proven to be safe and effective as a treatment for patients with EBV-related cancers, and was found to enable the complete remission of patients who failed all previous standard treatments. The first clinical trials using EBV-specific CTLs tested their utility for both prophylaxis and treatment of post-transplant lymphoproliferative diseases arising in stem cell transplant or solid organ transplant recipients.[5]

Nucleoside analogs, such as acyclovir (ACV) and ganciclovir (GCV), are often used as antiviral drugs against acute EBV and other herpesvirus infections.[14] The virally encoded thymidine kinase enzyme converts these analogs into their phosphate forms, which, after conversion into their triphosphate form by host kinases, are then incorporated into newly synthesized DNA, leading to the premature termination of DNA synthesis and apoptosis of the infected cell. The EBV thymidine kinase, however, is only expressed during lytic replication of the virus. Because EBV maintains a latent state of replication in all EBV-associated malignancies, nucleoside analog drugs have very limited, or no, cytopathic effect on virus-infected cells. Novel therapeutic approaches to target EBV-infected tumor cells, which include inducing lytic replication of EBV followed by treatment with nucleoside analogs, have been proposed.

Arginine butyrate induces the expression of the viral thymidine kinase gene in EBV-positive, immunoblastic, non-Hodgkin's lymphoma cell lines and lymphoblastic cell lines (LCLs) and acts synergistically with GCV to inhibit cell proliferation and decrease cell viability.[15] Various other agents have also been used to induce lytic replication of the EBV genome. For example, treatment of EBV-positive lymphoblastoid cells, or primary central nervous system lymphoma, with γ-irradiation promotes GCV-susceptibility of target cells.[15] Other studies successfully used 5-azacytidine, gemcitabine, doxorubicin, or a combination of anti-CD20 monoclonal antibody (Rituximab) and dexamethasone to induce lytic-phase gene expression and sensitize EBV-infected tumor cells to GCV or other nucleoside analogs.[15]

Butyric acid, a short-chain fatty acid, and its derivatives have been experimentally employed in attempts to treat leukemias and other diseases. Butyrate induces the expression of certain EBV lytic proteins, including the thymidine kinase enzyme, from latent EBV-infected cells.[16] The inhibitory effect of butyrate on histone deacetylase (HDAC) is required for this effect. In previous clinical studies, systemic administration of arginine butyrate was used to induce expression of the latent EBV thymidine kinase in the tumors of patients with EBV-positive post-transplantation lymphoproliferative disease or non-Hodgkin's lymphomas, followed by treatment with GCV.[16,17]

Bortezomib, a proteasome inhibitor, also activates EBV lytic gene expression.[18] Bortezomib leads to increased levels of CCAAT/enhancer-binding protein β (C/EBPβ) in a variety of tumor cell lines.[18] C/EBPβ activates the promoter of the EBV lytic switch gene *ZTA* (BZLF1). Bortezomib treatment leads to increased binding of C/EBPβ to sites within the *ZTA* promoter. Knockdown of C/EBPβ inhibits bortezomib activation of EBV lytic gene expression.[18] Bortezomib also induces the unfolded protein response (UPR). Thapsigargin, an inducer of the UPR that does not interfere with proteasome function, also induces EBV lytic gene expression.[18,19] The effect of thapsigargin on EBV lytic gene expression is also inhibited upon C/EBPβ knock-down.[18] Therefore, C/EBPβ mediates the activation of EBV lytic gene expression associated with bortezomib and thapsigargin.[18]

Pretreatment of naturally infected EBV tumor cell lines (from Burkitt's lymphoma and gastric carcinoma) with bortezomib activates viral gene expression.[20] Marked changes in tumor growth are also achieved in naturally infected Kaposi's sarcoma herpesvirus tumors after pretreatment with bortezomib.[20] Bortezomib-induced, enzyme-targeted radiation therapy illustrates the potential of pharmacological modulation of tumor gene expression for targeted radiotherapy.

There is increasing interest in the pharmacologic activation of lytic viral gene expression in tumors. Several therapeutic strategies requiring activation of EBV lytic genes for tumor cell lysis have been described, but concerns have been raised about the possible adverse effects of viral gene activation patients treated with pharmacologic activators.

2. EBV-encoded miRNA

2.1 miRNA

Micro (mi)RNAs are small, non-coding, single-stranded RNAs of approximately 21 to 25 nucleotides (nt) in length. They post-transcriptionally regulate mRNA expression in animals and plants and are transcribed from the non-coding regions of genes in all multi-cellular organisms and certain viruses and are often phylogenetically conserved across species.[21,22] EBV was the first human virus found to encode miRNA.[23] EBV encodes 44 viral miRNAs and a small RNA. EBV-encoded miRNAs are located within the *BHRF1* and BamHI A rightward transcript (*BART*) loci of the EBV genome. The BHRF1 cluster of miRNAs includes BHRF1-1, BHRF1-2, BHRF1-3, and BHRF1-4.[22-24] The other EBV-encoded miRNAs are encoded by BART cluster 1 and BART cluster 2, except miR-BART2, which is expressed from a sight outside of the BART clusters.[22-25] miRNAs bind to the 3′ untranslated region (UTR) of mRNA and interfere with their translation, leading to downregulated protein expression levels. EBV-encoded miRNAs have been found in various EBV-associated carcinomas and lymphomas, such as NPC, gastric carcinoma, diffuse large B cell lymphoma, nasal NK/T cell lymphoma, and Hodgkin's lymphoma.[23,26] Viral miRNAs play vital roles in immunogenesis, host cell survival and proliferation, differentiation, lymphomagenesis, and regulation of viral infection and latency.[23,27-29]

2.2 EBV miRNA-mediated regulation of viral infection states

During lytic infection, EBV genomes are amplified into 1000 copies per cell with the help of replication proteins.[30] EBV expresses six replication proteins, the most important of which are BZLF1 and BALF5. BALF5 is a catalytic DNA polymerase encoded by the *balf5* gene during lytic infection;[30] it is not present in latent infection. This DNA polymerase is a single-stranded DNA binding protein, which functions within viral replication factories in the nucleus, likely generating replication forks on the replicating EBV genome. EBV-encoded miR-BART2 is expressed at low levels during latency, prevents aberrant expression of BALF5 mRNA, and prevents inadvertent viral replication.[31] The sequence of miR-BART2 is perfectly complementary to the 3′UTR of BALF5 mRNA. Therefore, miR-BART2 serves as an inhibitor of viral DNA replication through the degradation of BALF5 mRNA. The miRNA-guided cleavage of mRNA requires an association with Ago2,[32] which is a member of the Argonuate family of proteins and a part of the RNA-induced silencing complex (RISC). Upon its association with Ago2, miR-BART2 guides the sequence-specific cleavage of BALF5 mRNA. This miR-BART2-guided cleavage is substantially reduced after induction of the lytic cycle in EBV-infected cells.[31] The amount of miR-BART2 is reduced during lytic infection, and this causes a de-repression of BALF5 protein expression.[31] However, it is unclear whether the miR-BART2-mediated regulation of viral replication is fully controlled by BALF5 protein or not.

Another regulator of the shift from EBV latency to lytic infection is miR-BART6, which itself is regulated by RNA editing.[33] Editing of the wild-type primary (pri)-miR-BART6 sequence dramatically reduces the loading of miR-BART6-5p onto RISC, without affecting the processing of precursor (pre) or mature miRNAs.[33] Editing of pri-miRNA might affect the selection and loading of the guide strand onto RISC.[34] miR-BART6-5p silences Dicer through multiple target sites located in the 3′UTR of Dicer mRNA, but miR-BART6-3p is unable to perform this function.[33]

In EBV-infected human cells, Dicer protein levels are substantially reduced by miR-BART6-5p,[33] suggesting that miR-BART6-5p may indirectly regulate the biogenesis of all miRNAs. It may even affect the latency of EBV by modulating the expression of viral proteins, including EBNA2, LMP1, RTA, and ZTA. EBNA2 is required for the transition from the less immunologically confrontational type I or type II latency to the more immunity-stimulating type III latency, which occurs through the upregulation of all latent EBV genes and the transformation of infected B lymphocytes.[35,36] However, EBNA2 deficiency is observed in type I and type II latency.[35,36] Low-level expression of LMP1 is also observed in type II latency, but is absent in type I. LMP1 controls the NF-κB signaling pathway and the growth and apoptosis of host cells. RTA and ZTA proteins initiate lytic infection of EBV. Thus, it is clear that miR-BART6-5p regulates EBV infection and latency by suppressing RTA and ZTA protein expression. To modulate protein expression, miR-BART6-5p downregulates viral promoters, such as Cp and Wp, which are characteristic of type III latency, and reduces transcriptional activity via its silencing effect on Dicer. Mutation and adenosine-to-inosine (A-to-I) editing are adaptive mechanisms that antagonize miR-BART6 activities and affect the latent state of viral infection.[33] Therefore, we conclude that miR-BART6-5p, and its mutant or edited versions, are critical for the establishment and maintenance of latent EBV infection.

2.3 EBV miRNA-mediated host cell survival

The miR-BART5 miRNA promotes host cell survival by regulating the p53 upregulated modulator of apoptosis (PUMA) protein.[37] PUMA is an apoptotic protein belonging to the "BH3-only" group of the Bcl-2 family and is encoded by the *BBC3* gene.[38-40] PUMA is regulated by the tumor suppressor p53 and is involved in both p53-mediated and non-mediated apoptosis via independent signaling pathways. PUMA is an important downstream regulator of p53, both of which are master regulators of host cell growth and apoptosis. PUMA function is downregulated or absent in cancer cells, but the absence of PUMA activity alone is not sufficient for the spontaneous formation of malignancies.[41-45] PUMA has four isoforms (i.e., α, β, γ, and δ), which share the same 3'UTR.[39] Only PUMA-α and PUMA-β have pro-apoptotic activity. The PUMA 3'UTR sequence is perfectly complementary to miR-BART5. Thus, binding of miR-BART5 and the PUMA 3'UTR suppresses the expression of the pro-apoptotic protein. PUMA-β protein expression is also reduced by pre-miR-BART5.[37] Abundant expression of miR-BART5 in NPC cells is correlated with significant downregulation of PUMA in 60% of NPC tissues.[37] By this mechanism, miR-BART5 induces anti-apoptotic activity in NPC cells, EBV-infected gastric carcinoma cells, and EBV-infected epithelial cells.[37] Therefore, miR-BART5 may be a good target for anti-cancer therapy in EBV-infected cancer cells.

LMP1 is a viral protein expressed during the type III latency period of EBV infection.[35,36] LMP1 promotes cell growth, resistance to serum deprivation-induced apoptosis, and phenotypic changes in epithelial cells and B cell transformation. It activates the NF-κB, JNK, JAK/STAT, p38/MAP, and RAS/MAPK pathways and regulates host gene expression.[5] NF-κB transcription factors influence proliferation, apoptosis, oncogenesis, and inflammation.[46] Low levels of LMP1 activate NF-κB, but with increasing amounts of LMP1, NF-κB activation reaches a plateau, after which small increases in LMP1 reduces NF-κB activity.[47] Thus, a threshold level of LMP1 can maintain peak NF-κB activity. LMP1 regulates the level of NF-κB activity by modulating the UPR pathway and autophagy. *BARTI* cluster miRNAs negatively regulate LMP1 expression, limiting inappropriately high levels, thereby preventing apoptosis that would otherwise result from LMP1-mediated changes in the UPR. Such *BART1* cluster miRNAs include BART16, BART17-5p, and BART1-5p, which target sites within the 3'UTR of LMP1 mRNA.[47] These miRNAs regulate LMP1 expression at the post-transcriptional level, regulating NF-κB-mediated gene expression. Therefore, the negative regulation of LMP1 expression by *BART1* cluster miRNAs may affect EBV-associated cancer development by balancing the effect of LMP1 on cellular proliferation.

BHRF1 is a latent protein expressed in growth-transformed cells that contributes to virus-associated lymphomagenesis.[48] miR-BHRF1 downregulates this protein, modulates cell transformation,[49] and promotes B cell proliferation after EBV infection. EBV-infected B cells lacking miR-BHRF1 progress less efficiently into the cell cycle and eventually die by apoptosis.[49] miR-BHRF1 is constitutively expressed in LCLs.[49] Without miR-BHRF1, the proportion of G1/G0 cells increases while the numbers of S-phase cells decreases,[49] indicating a definite role of miR-BHRF1 in the control of proliferation of latently infected cells. miR-BHRF1 acts at a stage of the EBV life cycle when multiple EBV-encoded oncogenes become activated.

2.4 EBV-encoded miRNAs regulate immune evasion

Major histocompatibility complex (MHC) class I polypeptide-related sequence B (MICB) protein is a ligand for the NKG2D type II receptor, which is a stress-induced immune molecule.[50,51] B cells and endothelial cells, which are targets of EBV, both express this protein. Binding of MICB activates NK, CD8$^+$ $\alpha\beta$, and $\gamma\delta$ T cells.[52] MICB is upregulated at the cell surface due to various insults, such as viral infection, tumor transformation, heat shock, and DNA damage. Thus, it would be beneficial for a virus to downregulate the expression of this protein ligand to avoid immune detection. Previous studies have shown that downregulated MICB expression leads to reduced lysis of infected cells by NK cells.[53] EBV-expressed miR-BART2-5p has potential binding sites in the MICB mRNA 3′UTR.[54] EBV downregulates MICB via miR-BART2-5p, resulting in decreased NK cell-mediated lysis, to avoid detection by immune cells.

miR-BHLF1-1 is expressed from the 5′UTR, and miR-BHLF1-2 and miR-BHLF1-3 are expressed from the 3′UTR, of the *bhrf1* gene in EBV-infected cells.[28] miR-BHLF1-3 is markedly elevated in EBV-infected, type III latent cell lines[28] and is also detected in EBV-positive primary effusion lymphoma and AIDS-related diffuse large B cell lymphoma.[28] BHRF1 miRNA is characteristic of EBV type III latent infections.[55] EBV miR-BHRF1-3 regulates host immunity by downregulating the interferon (IFN)-inducible T cell attracting chemokine (I-TAC; also known as CXCL-11). CXCL-11/I-TAC belongs to the CXC family of chemokines, and both IFN-β and IFN-γ strongly induce its transcription.[56] CXCL-11/I-TAC promotes cell-mediated immunity by attracting activated T cells. The 3′UTR of CXCL-11/I-TAC mRNA is 100% complementary to the sequence of miR-BART1-3 and, therefore, serves as a target of miR-BART1-3. miR-BART1-3 inversely regulates the expression of CXCL-11/I-TAC; the anti-sense sequence of miR-BART1-3 has the reverse effect.[23] miR-BART1-3 significantly reduces the expression of CXCL-11/I-TAC at both the mRNA and protein levels.[28] Thus, as cellular chemokines can be targets of viral miRNA, EBV-mediated regulation of antigen processing and presentation, and the downregulation of CTL cytokine networks, may occur through such a mechanism.

2.5 Small nucleolar RNAs encoded by the EBV genome

A small nucleolar (sno)RNA, named v-snoRNA1, has been identified within the EBV genome in EBV-infected B lymphocytes.[57] snoRNAs, 60–300 nt in length, guide nucleotide modifications of ribosomal (r)RNAs, i.e., 2′O-ribose methylation or pseudouridylation, that are located in subnuclear compartments.[58,59] snoRNAs are subdivided into the C/D box and H/ACA box classes. The majority of snoRNAs located within introns of protein-encoding genes are processed by splicing, followed by endo- and exonucleolytic cleavage.[60-62] However, some of them are orphan snoRNAs that lack rRNA or small modulatory (sm)RNA targets. v-snoRNA is processed into 24 nt long miRNAs, which then target the 3'UTR of viral DNA polymerase mRNA.

The *v-snoRNA1* gene is located within the *BART* sense stand of the EBV genome.[57] Both v-snoRNA1 and miR-BART2 arise from the same intron. Although v-snoRNA1 is an integral part of the EBV latent transcription program, it is highly expressed during lytic infection. The 3'UTR of the BHLF5 mRNA is fully complementary to v-snoRNA1, so v-snoRNA1 binds and cleaves BALF5 mRNA, enabling its exonucleolytic degradation.[57] It is unclear whether v-snoRNA1 serves an important function during the viral life cycle.

3. Editing and mutation of EBV-encoded miRNAs

Recently widespread RNA-DNA differences in the human transcriptome were found. It also occurs to miRNAs including EBV-encoded miRNAs.[63]

3.1 RNA editing

RNA editing is carried out by enzymes that target mRNA post-transcriptionally, such as adenosine deaminases that act on RNA (ADARs, which convert adenosine to inosine, which is subsequently recognized by translation machinery as a guanosine, i.e., A-to-G mutation) and apolipoprotein B mRNA-editing enzyme catalytic polypeptide-like (APOBEC) proteins, which convert cytidine to uridine (i.e., C-to-U mutation). Editing of pri-miR-142, the primary transcript form of miR-142 that is expressed in hematopoietic tissues, results in suppression of its processing by Drosha.[64] The mutated pri-miR-142 is degraded by Tudor-SN, a component of RISC and also a ribonuclease that is specific to inosine-containing double-stranded (ds)RNAs. Mature miR-142 is substantially upregulated in ADAR1- or ADAR2-null mice,[64] demonstrating that RNA editing helps control miRNA biogenesis. Kawahara et al. found that primary transcripts of certain miRNA genes are subject to RNA editing that converts adenosine to inosine. By way of ADAR, tissue-specific A-to-I editing of miR-376 cluster transcripts lead to the predominant expression of edited miR-376 isoform RNAs. One highly edited site is located in the middle of the 5'-proximal "seed" region of miR-376 critical for its hybridization to its targets, providing evidence that the mutated miR-376 specifically targets a set of genes that is different than those targeted by wild-type miR-376.[65] Mutated miR-376 represses phosphoribosyl pyrophosphate synthetase 1, an enzyme involved in the uric-acid synthesis pathway.

Iizasa et al. reported that the primary transcripts of four EBV miRNAs, including miR-BART6, are subject to A-to-I editing. Moreover, it was demonstrated that editing of pri-miR-BART6, as well as mutations of miR-BART6, found in latently EBV-infected cells prevented its loading onto functionally active RISC.[33] As mentioned, miR-BART6 targets Dicer and affects the latent state of EBV viral infection. Therefore, regulation of miR-BART6 expression and function through A-to-I editing may be critical for the establishment or maintenance of latent EBV infection.

3.2 Mutation of the EBV genome affects encoded miRNAs

Sequence variation in the EBV genome has been extensively studied for a long time; in particular, *BLRF1* and other genes have been reported to have sequence variation in EBV-infected cancer patients.[66] Mechanistic analysis of this sequence variability has recently been reported by Suspène et al.[67] Human APOBEC3 cytidine deaminases target and edit single-stranded DNA, which can be of viral, mitochondrial, or nuclear origin. Retroviral genomes, such those of HIV, deficient in the *vif* gene, and hepatitis B virus, are particularly vulnerable.

The genomes of DNA viruses, such as herpesviruses, are also subject to editing. This is the case for herpes simplex virus type 1 (HSV-1), at least in tissue culture, where APOBEC3C (A3C) overexpression reduces viral titers and the particle/plaque forming unit (PFU) ratio by approximately 10-fold. A3A, A3G, and activation-induced cytidine deaminase (AICDA) can edit what is thought to be a small fraction of HSV genome in an experimental setting without seriously impacting viral titers. Hyper-editing was found to occur in HSV genomes recovered from four of eight uncultured buccal lesions, but the phenomenon was not restricted to HSV; hyper-mutated EBV genomes were readily recovered from four of five established cell lines, indicating that episomes are also vulnerable to editing [67]. These findings suggest that the widely expressed A3C cytidine deaminase can function as a restriction factor for some human herpesviruses.

Other studies reported sequence variation in BART miRNAs.[68] The significance of these mutations and their effect on miRNA processing, as well as the mechanism of mutation, whether it is mediated by A3C, members of other APOBEC families, or other mechanisms, have yet to be determined.

4. Regulation of EBV-encoded miRNA processing

4.1 Processing of miRNAs under normal versus cancerous conditions

The mechanism of miRNA biosynthesis involves sequential endonucleolytic cleavages mediated by two RNase III enzymes, Drosha and Dicer (Fig.1). Following transcription by RNA pol II, Drosha processes the primary miRNA transcript (pri-miRNA) into a 60-100 nt hairpin structure, termed the precursor miRNA (pre-miRNA), in the nucleus (Fig. 1). Following cleavage by Drosha, the pre-miRNA is transported out of the nucleus through an interaction with Exportin-5 and Ran-GTP. Then, the pre-miRNA undergoes further processing catalyzed by Dicer (Fig. 1). This cleavage event gives rise to an approximately 22 nt dsRNA product containing the mature miRNA guide strand and the miRNA* passenger strand (Fig. 1). Then, the mature miRNA guide strand is loaded onto the RISC, while the passenger strand is degraded (Fig. 1).

Although substantial progress has been made in understanding the basic mechanism of miRNA biogenesis, less is known about the mechanisms that regulate miRNA biogenesis and how these systems might be deregulated during oncogenesis. Several studies have reported that various regulatory mechanisms of miRNA biosynthesis are potentially involved in carcinogenesis.[69]

The tumor suppressor protein p53 was recently found to modulate miRNA processing through its association with p68 and Drosha.[70,71] Under conditions of DNA damage, several miRNAs, such as miR-143 and miR-16, are post-transcriptionally induced. This process requires p53, as p53-null HCT116 cells do not induce miRNAs in response to DNA damage.[72] Co-immunoprecipitation studies have indicated that p53 is present in a complex with both Drosha and p68, and the addition of p53 to *in vitro* pri-miRNA processing assays enhances the activity of Drosha. Interestingly, several p53 mutant-containing cells that are linked to oncogenesis have low post-transcriptional miRNA expression.[72]

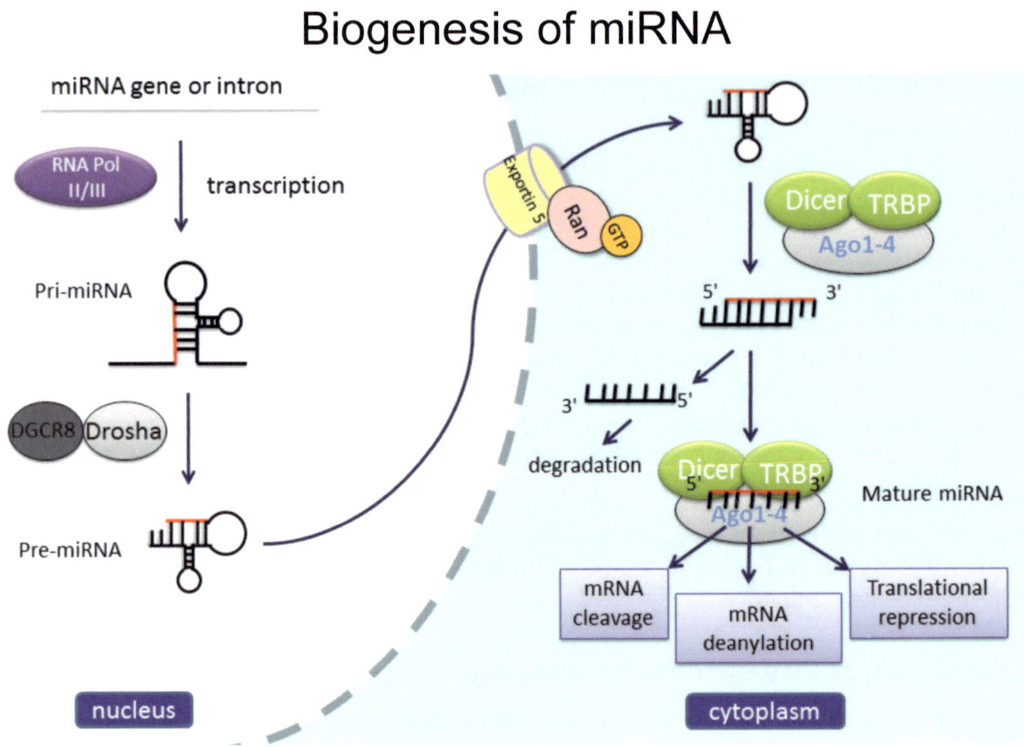

Fig. 1. Processing machinery of miRNA
miRNA genes are transcribed by RNA polymerase II or III into long primary (pri) miRNA transcripts, processed by the nuclear nuclease Drosha into ~60 bp hairpins termed precursor (pre) miRNAs, and further cleaved in the cytosol by the Dicer nuclease into mature miRNAs. Mature miRNAs are then incorporated into the multiprotein RNA-induced silencing complex (RISC), exerting post-transcriptional repression of target mRNAs, either by inducing mRNA cleavage, mRNA degradation or blocking mRNA translation.

4.2 Processing of EBV-encoded miRNAs

For EBV-encoded miRNAs, several regulatory processes have been reported[68]. Almost all of the EBV-encoded miRNAs originate from one of three sequence clusters. Two of the three clusters of miRNAs are made from the BARTs, a set of alternatively spliced transcripts that are highly abundant in NPC, but have not been shown to produce a detectable protein. Edwards et al. investigated the mechanism of BART-derived miRNA processing by comparing the processed miRNAs with the original BART transcript and residual transcripts after processing.[68] First, they showed that residual pieces of the intron sequence were detectable in the nucleus of cells that express the miRNAs. Characterization of these residual pieces indicated that the miRNAs were produced from one large initial transcript prior to splicing and that a specific spliced form of the transcript favored the production of miRNAs. Second, they found that miR-BART12 is not detected at all, even though the primary transcript is abundant. Third, pre-miR-BART5 could be detected in all cell lines and tumors tested, despite low or undetectable expression of the mature miR-BART5, indicating that the processing of pre-miR-BART5 was inhibited.

	function	target viral	Host target	
BLHF1-1	transformation	BFLF2	LILRB-5,E2F1,p53,CBFA2T2	BHRF1
BLHF1-2	transformation	BFLF2	PIK3R1	BHRF1
BLHF1-3	transformation	BFLF2	CXCL11,PRF1,TGIF,NSEP1	BHRF1
BART1-5p	Cancer development	LMP1	CXCL12	BART Cluster1
BART2-5p	viral replication	BALF5、LMP1	MIC B, Bim	
BART3		LMP1	IPO7, Bim	BART Cluster1
BART4		LMP1	Bim	BART Cluster1
BART5	Host cell survival	LMP1	PUMA, Bim	BART Cluster1
BART6	maintain viral latency	LMP1	Dicer, Bim	BART Cluster1
BART7		LMP1	Bim	BART Cluster2
BART8				BART Cluster2
BART9				BART Cluster2
BART10				BART Cluster2
BART11				BART Cluster2
BART12				BART Cluster2
BART13				BART Cluster2
BART14				BART Cluster2
BART15				BART Cluster1
BART16	Cancer development	LMP1	TOMM22	BART Cluster1
BART17	Cancer development	LMP1		BART Cluster1
BART18				BART Cluster2
BART19				BART Cluster2
BART20				BART Cluster2
BART21				BART Cluster2
BART22		LMP2		BART Cluster2

Table 1.

Amoroso et al. reported that the levels of the different BART miRNAs vary up to 50-fold within a given cell line.[73] However, this variation cannot be explained by differential miRNA turnover, as all EBV miRNAs appear to be remarkably stable, suggesting that miRNA maturation is a key step in regulating steady-state levels of EBV miRNAs. Future studies should further investigate the mechanism of miRNA transcript processing in EBV-infected cells, highlighting any differences between the three types of latent infections.

5. Secretory EBV-encoded miRNAs

5.1 Secretory miRNAs

Cellular and viral miRNAs control gene expression by repressing the translation of mRNAs into protein, a process that is tightly regulated in healthy cells, but is deregulated in cancerous and virus-infected cells. Curiously, miRNAs are not strictly intracellular, but are also secreted through the release of small vesicles called exosomes and, therefore, exist extracellularly in the peripheral blood and in cell culture media.[74] It has been suggested that exosome-associated miRNAs play a role in intercellular communication [74], although concrete evidence for this has been lacking. The dynamics of miRNA secretion via exosomes and the proposed transfer mechanisms remain poorly understood. In addition, it is unclear whether miRNAs are secreted in physiologically relevant amounts.

5.2 Existence of secretory EBV-encoded miRNAs

Pegtel et al. were the first to show that exosomes deliver viral miRNAs to non-infected cells.[75] They used EBV B95.8-immortalized LCLs and demonstrated that exosomes contained

BHRF1 miRNAs, which could target the *CXCL11/ITAC* gene in nearby uninfected cells. Furthermore, they showed that non-B cells in EBV-infected patients with elevated viral loads contained EBV miRNAs, demonstrating that exosomes apparently transfer miRNAs *in vivo* to uninfected cells. These findings were confirmed by two studies that demonstrated the release of exosomes from NPC cells. Gourzones et al. showed that EBV miR-BARTs present within exosomes can be detected in the serum of mice xenografted with human NPC cells and that the sera of NPC patients also contain BART miRNAs.[76]

6. Concluding remarks

EBV-related cancers are generally difficult to cure. Despite extensive studies based on well-known concepts and methods, the molecular basis by which EBV mediates tumorigenesis and eludes immunosurveillance remains unclear. Mouse models of EBV-mediated lymphoproliferative disease have recently revealed that EBV infection of B cells is necessary, but not sufficient, for tumorigenesis, as all peripheral mononuclear cells are needed to generate tumors in these mice.[77] Immune cells are also indispensable for EBV-mediated tumorigenesis . The relationship between these cells and EBV-infected cells with regard to tumorigenesis remains unclear. Moreover, the mechanism of drug resistance, which causes poor prognosis of EBV-related tumors, has not yet been elucidated. Therefore, it is important to study the tumor biology of EBV-related tumors from a fresh perspective, such as EBV-encoded miRNAs.

7. References

[1] Burkitt D. A sarcoma involving the jaws in African children. Br J Surg. 1958;46:218-223.
[2] Epstein MA, Achong BG, Barr YM. Virus Particles in Cultured Lymphoblasts from Burkitt's Lymphoma. Lancet. 1964;1:702-703.
[3] Henle G, Henle W. Immunofluorescence in cells derived from Burkitt's lymphoma. J Bacteriol. 1966;91:1248-1256.
[4] Fang W, Li X, Jiang Q, et al. Transcriptional patterns, biomarkers and pathways characterizing nasopharyngeal carcinoma of Southern China. J Transl Med. 2008;6:32.
[5] Young LS, Rickinson AB. Epstein-Barr virus: 40 years on. Nat Rev Cancer. 2004;4:757-768.
[6] Parkin DM, Bray F, Ferlay J, Pisani P. Global cancer statistics, 2002. CA Cancer J Clin. 2005;55:74-108.
[7] Parkin DM. The global health burden of infection-associated cancers in the year 2002. Int J Cancer. 2006;118:3030-3044.
[8] Borza CM, Hutt-Fletcher LM. Alternate replication in B cells and epithelial cells switches tropism of Epstein-Barr virus. Nat Med. 2002;8:594-599.
[9] Ghosh SK, Forman LW, Akinsheye I, Perrine SP, Faller DV. Short, discontinuous exposure to butyrate effectively sensitizes latently EBV-infected lymphoma cells to nucleoside analogue antiviral agents. Blood Cells Mol Dis. 2007;38:57-65.
[10] Thorley-Lawson DA. Epstein-Barr virus: exploiting the immune system. Nat Rev Immunol. 2001;1:75-82.
[11] Thorley-Lawson DA, Allday MJ. The curious case of the tumour virus: 50 years of Burkitt's lymphoma. Nat Rev Microbiol. 2008;6:913-924.

[12] Deyrup AT. Epstein-Barr virus-associated epithelial and mesenchymal neoplasms. Hum Pathol. 2008;39:473-483.

[13] Murray RJ, Kurilla MG, Brooks JM, et al. Identification of target antigens for the human cytotoxic T cell response to Epstein-Barr virus (EBV): implications for the immune control of EBV-positive malignancies. J Exp Med. 1992;176:157-168.

[14] Crumpacker CS. Ganciclovir. N Engl J Med. 1996;335:721-729.

[15] Jones K, Nourse J, Corbett G, Gandhi MK. Sodium valproate in combination with ganciclovir induces lysis of EBV-infected lymphoma cells without impairing EBV-specific T-cell immunity. Int J Lab Hematol;32:e169-174.

[16] He Y, Cai S, Zhang G, Li X, Pan L, Du J. Interfering with cellular signaling pathways enhances sensitization to combined sodium butyrate and GCV treatment in EBV-positive tumor cells. Virus Res. 2008;135:175-180.

[17] Westphal EM, Blackstock W, Feng W, Israel B, Kenney SC. Activation of lytic Epstein-Barr virus (EBV) infection by radiation and sodium butyrate in vitro and in vivo: a potential method for treating EBV-positive malignancies. Cancer Res. 2000;60:5781-5788.

[18] Shirley CM, Chen J, Shamay M, et al. Bortezomib induction of C/EBPbeta mediates Epstein-Barr virus lytic activation in Burkitt lymphoma. Blood. 2011;117:6297-6303.

[19] Taylor GM, Raghuwanshi SK, Rowe DT, Wadowsky R, Rosendorff A. ER-stress causes Epstein-Barr virus lytic replication. Blood. 2011.

[20] Fu DX, Tanhehco Y, Chen J, et al. Bortezomib-induced enzyme-targeted radiation therapy in herpesvirus-associated tumors. Nat Med. 2008;14:1118-1122.

[21] Wang X, Gu J, Zhang MQ, Li Y. Identification of phylogenetically conserved microRNA cis-regulatory elements across 12 Drosophila species. Bioinformatics. 2008;24:165-171.

[22] Chen K, Rajewsky N. The evolution of gene regulation by transcription factors and microRNAs. Nat Rev Genet. 2007;8:93-103.

[23] Pfeffer S, Zavolan M, Grasser FA, et al. Identification of virus-encoded microRNAs. Science. 2004;304:734-736.

[24] Grundhoff A, Sullivan CS, Ganem D. A combined computational and microarray-based approach identifies novel microRNAs encoded by human gamma-herpesviruses. RNA. 2006;12:733-750.

[25] Griffiths-Jones S, Grocock RJ, van Dongen S, Bateman A, Enright AJ. miRBase: microRNA sequences, targets and gene nomenclature. Nucleic Acids Res. 2006;34:D140-144.

[26] Kim do N, Chae HS, Oh ST, et al. Expression of viral microRNAs in Epstein-Barr virus-associated gastric carcinoma. J Virol. 2007;81:1033-1036.

[27] Rana TM. Illuminating the silence: understanding the structure and function of small RNAs. Nat Rev Mol Cell Biol. 2007;8:23-36.

[28] Xia T, O'Hara A, Araujo I, et al. EBV microRNAs in primary lymphomas and targeting of CXCL-11 by ebv-mir-BHRF1-3. Cancer Res. 2008;68:1436-1442.

[29] Barth S, Meister G, Grasser FA. EBV-encoded miRNAs. Biochim Biophys Acta. 2011.

[30] Tsurumi T, Daikoku T, Kurachi R, Nishiyama Y. Functional interaction between Epstein-Barr virus DNA polymerase catalytic subunit and its accessory subunit in vitro. J Virol. 1993;67:7648-7653.

[31] Barth S, Pfuhl T, Mamiani A, et al. Epstein-Barr virus-encoded microRNA miR-BART2 down-regulates the viral DNA polymerase BALF5. Nucleic Acids Res. 2008;36:666-675.

[32] Meister G, Landthaler M, Patkaniowska A, Dorsett Y, Teng G, Tuschl T. Human Argonaute2 mediates RNA cleavage targeted by miRNAs and siRNAs. Mol Cell. 2004;15:185-197.

[33] Iizasa H, Wulff BE, Alla NR, et al. Editing of Epstein-Barr virus-encoded BART6 microRNAs controls their dicer targeting and consequently affects viral latency. J Biol Chem. 2010;285:33358-33370.

[34] Khvorova A, Reynolds A, Jayasena SD. Functional siRNAs and miRNAs exhibit strand bias. Cell. 2003;115:209-216.

[35] Hislop AD, Taylor GS, Sauce D, Rickinson AB. Cellular responses to viral infection in humans: lessons from Epstein-Barr virus. Annu Rev Immunol. 2007;25:587-617.

[36] Pagano JS, Blaser M, Buendia MA, et al. Infectious agents and cancer: criteria for a causal relation. Semin Cancer Biol. 2004;14:453-471.

[37] Choy EY, Siu KL, Kok KH, et al. An Epstein-Barr virus-encoded microRNA targets PUMA to promote host cell survival. J Exp Med. 2008;205:2551-2560.

[38] Han J, Flemington C, Houghton AB, et al. Expression of bbc3, a pro-apoptotic BH3-only gene, is regulated by diverse cell death and survival signals. Proc Natl Acad Sci U S A. 2001;98:11318-11323.

[39] Nakano K, Vousden KH. PUMA, a novel proapoptotic gene, is induced by p53. Mol Cell. 2001;7:683-694.

[40] Yu J, Zhang L, Hwang PM, Kinzler KW, Vogelstein B. PUMA induces the rapid apoptosis of colorectal cancer cells. Mol Cell. 2001;7:673-682.

[41] Jeffers JR, Parganas E, Lee Y, et al. Puma is an essential mediator of p53-dependent and -independent apoptotic pathways. Cancer Cell. 2003;4:321-328.

[42] Villunger A, Michalak EM, Coultas L, et al. p53- and drug-induced apoptotic responses mediated by BH3-only proteins puma and noxa. Science. 2003;302:1036-1038.

[43] Hemann MT, Zilfou JT, Zhao Z, Burgess DJ, Hannon GJ, Lowe SW. Suppression of tumorigenesis by the p53 target PUMA. Proc Natl Acad Sci U S A. 2004;101:9333-9338.

[44] Erlacher M, Labi V, Manzl C, et al. Puma cooperates with Bim, the rate-limiting BH3-only protein in cell death during lymphocyte development, in apoptosis induction. J Exp Med. 2006;203:2939-2951.

[45] Nelson DA, Tan TT, Rabson AB, Anderson D, Degenhardt K, White E. Hypoxia and defective apoptosis drive genomic instability and tumorigenesis. Genes Dev. 2004;18:2095-2107.

[46] Rayet B, Gelinas C. Aberrant rel/nfkb genes and activity in human cancer. Oncogene. 1999;18:6938-6947.

[47] Lo AK, To KF, Lo KW, et al. Modulation of LMP1 protein expression by EBV-encoded microRNAs. Proc Natl Acad Sci U S A. 2007;104:16164-16169.

[48] Kelly GL, Long HM, Stylianou J, et al. An Epstein-Barr virus anti-apoptotic protein constitutively expressed in transformed cells and implicated in burkitt lymphomagenesis: the Wp/BHRF1 link. PLoS Pathog. 2009;5:e1000341.

[49] Seto E, Moosmann A, Gromminger S, Walz N, Grundhoff A, Hammerschmidt W. Micro RNAs of Epstein-Barr virus promote cell cycle progression and prevent apoptosis of primary human B cells. PLoS Pathog. 2010;6:e1001063.
[50] Bahram S, Bresnahan M, Geraghty DE, Spies T. A second lineage of mammalian major histocompatibility complex class I genes. Proc Natl Acad Sci U S A. 1994;91:6259-6263.
[51] Groh V, Bahram S, Bauer S, Herman A, Beauchamp M, Spies T. Cell stress-regulated human major histocompatibility complex class I gene expressed in gastrointestinal epithelium. Proc Natl Acad Sci U S A. 1996;93:12445-12450.
[52] Suarez-Alvarez B, Lopez-Vazquez A, Baltar JM, Ortega F, Lopez-Larrea C. Potential role of NKG2D and its ligands in organ transplantation: new target for immunointervention. Am J Transplant. 2009;9:251-257.
[53] Stern-Ginossar N, Elefant N, Zimmermann A, et al. Host immune system gene targeting by a viral miRNA. Science. 2007;317:376-381.
[54] Nachmani D, Stern-Ginossar N, Sarid R, Mandelboim O. Diverse herpesvirus microRNAs target the stress-induced immune ligand MICB to escape recognition by natural killer cells. Cell Host Microbe. 2009;5:376-385.
[55] Xing L, Kieff E. Epstein-Barr virus BHRF1 micro- and stable RNAs during latency III and after induction of replication. J Virol. 2007;81:9967-9975.
[56] Rani MR, Foster GR, Leung S, Leaman D, Stark GR, Ransohoff RM. Characterization of beta-R1, a gene that is selectively induced by interferon beta (IFN-beta) compared with IFN-alpha. J Biol Chem. 1996;271:22878-22884.
[57] Hutzinger R, Feederle R, Mrazek J, et al. Expression and processing of a small nucleolar RNA from the Epstein-Barr virus genome. PLoS Pathog. 2009;5:e1000547.
[58] Samarsky DA, Fournier MJ, Singer RH, Bertrand E. The snoRNA box C/D motif directs nucleolar targeting and also couples snoRNA synthesis and localization. EMBO J. 1998;17:3747-3757.
[59] Matera AG, Terns RM, Terns MP. Non-coding RNAs: lessons from the small nuclear and small nucleolar RNAs. Nat Rev Mol Cell Biol. 2007;8:209-220.
[60] Huttenhofer A, Brosius J, Bachellerie JP. RNomics: identification and function of small, non-messenger RNAs. Curr Opin Chem Biol. 2002;6:835-843.
[61] Huttenhofer A, Schattner P, Polacek N. Non-coding RNAs: hope or hype? Trends Genet. 2005;21:289-297.
[62] Huttenhofer A, Schattner P. The principles of guiding by RNA: chimeric RNA-protein enzymes. Nat Rev Genet. 2006;7:475-482.
[63] Li JB, Levanon EY, Yoon JK, et al. Genome-wide identification of human RNA editing sites by parallel DNA capturing and sequencing. Science. 2009;324:1210-1213.
[64] Yang W, Chendrimada TP, Wang Q, et al. Modulation of microRNA processing and expression through RNA editing by ADAR deaminases. Nat Struct Mol Biol. 2006;13:13-21.
[65] Kawahara Y, Zinshteyn B, Sethupathy P, Iizasa H, Hatzigeorgiou AG, Nishikura K. Redirection of silencing targets by adenosine-to-inosine editing of miRNAs. Science. 2007;315:1137-1140.
[66] Jia Y, Wang Y, Chao Y, Jing Y, Sun Z, Luo B. Sequence analysis of the Epstein-Barr virus (EBV) BRLF1 gene in nasopharyngeal and gastric carcinomas. Virol J. 2010;7:341.

[67] Suspene R, Aynaud MM, Koch S, et al. Genetic editing of herpes simplex virus 1 and Epstein-Barr herpesvirus genomes by human APOBEC3 cytidine deaminases in culture and in vivo. J Virol. 2011;85:7594-7602.

[68] Edwards RH, Marquitz AR, Raab-Traub N. Epstein-Barr virus BART microRNAs are produced from a large intron prior to splicing. J Virol. 2008;82:9094-9106.

[69] Davis BN, Hata A. microRNA in Cancer---The involvement of aberrant microRNA biogenesis regulatory pathways. Genes Cancer. 2010;1:1100-1114.

[70] Denli AM, Tops BB, Plasterk RH, Ketting RF, Hannon GJ. Processing of primary microRNAs by the Microprocessor complex. Nature. 2004;432:231-235.

[71] Shiohama A, Sasaki T, Noda S, Minoshima S, Shimizu N. Nucleolar localization of DGCR8 and identification of eleven DGCR8-associated proteins. Exp Cell Res. 2007;313:4196-4207.

[72] Suzuki HI, Yamagata K, Sugimoto K, Iwamoto T, Kato S, Miyazono K. Modulation of microRNA processing by p53. Nature. 2009;460:529-533.

[73] Amoroso R, Fitzsimmons L, Thomas WA, Kelly GL, Rowe M, Bell AI. Quantitative studies of Epstein-Barr virus-encoded microRNAs provide novel insights into their regulation. J Virol. 2010;85:996-1010.

[74] Kosaka N, Iguchi H, Ochiya T. Circulating microRNA in body fluid: a new potential biomarker for cancer diagnosis and prognosis. Cancer Sci. 2010;101:2087-2092.

[75] Pegtel DM, Cosmopoulos K, Thorley-Lawson DA, et al. Functional delivery of viral miRNAs via exosomes. Proc Natl Acad Sci U S A. 2010;107:6328-6333.

[76] Gourzones C, Gelin A, Bombik I, et al. Extra-cellular release and blood diffusion of BART viral micro-RNAs produced by EBV-infected nasopharyngeal carcinoma cells. Virol J. 2010;7:271.

[77] Kuppers R. Molecular biology of Hodgkin lymphoma. Hematology Am Soc Hematol Educ Program. 2009:491-496.

17

Animal Models of Lymphoproliferative Disorders Focusing on Waldenström's Macroglobulinemia

Anastasia S. Tsingotjidou
Laboratory of Anatomy and Histology,
Faculty of Veterinary Medicine,
Aristotle University of Thessaloniki
Greece

1. Introduction

Lymphoproliferative disorders (LPDs) represent a heterogeneous group of expanding, monoclonal or oligoclonal, lymphoid cells that occur in the setting of immune dysfunction. They are sometimes equated with "immunoproliferative disorders", but technically LPDs are a subset of immunoproliferative disorders, along with hypergammaglobulinemia and paraproteinemias. Several inherited gene mutations have been identified to cause lymphoproliferative disorders. Acquired and iatrogenic causes are also responsible for the appearance of these diseases.

The most common examples of LPDs are chronic lymphocytic leukemia, acute lymphoblastic leukemia, lymphomas/leukemias (including follicular lymphoma and hairy cell leukemia) and multiple myeloma, although less common LPDs such as post-transplant lymphoproliferative disorder, Waldenström's macroglobulinemia, Wiskott-Aldrich syndrome and Autoimmune LymphoProliferative Syndrome (ALPS) also belong to the same group of disorders.

A few basic current facts for the incidence rates, the prognosis and the treatment of the most common LPDs will be briefly mentioned in the beginning of this chapter. Following that, the recent advances in understanding the pathogenesis of these diseases coming from experimental animal studies will be reviewed in a greater detail. After all, understanding the mechanisms of neoplasia has always been a prerequisite for developing more effective treatments for cancer patients, and the sophisticated animal models available in our days have played a major role in enhancing this knowledge. We have developed an animal model for Waldenström's macroglobulinemia (WM), which is one of the less common LPDs. This will also be presented in detail as an example of the challenges met in developing an animal model that should emulate the human disease, or at least important aspects of it. By introducing core biopsies of WM patients into immunodeficient mice bearing human bone fragments, we established an animal model mimicking important aspects of the disease in humans.

2. Lymphoproliferative disorders

2.1 Chronic lymphocytic leukemia

Chronic lymphocytic leukemia (CLL) is the most common adult leukemia in North America and Europe; it is less frequent in Asia and Africa (Linet et al., 2006). The reported age-adjusted incidence rate of CLL in the United States between 1975 and 2006 was 4.43 per 100,000 persons (Horner et al., 2009). However, because of its long asymptomatic period, the incidence of CLL is under-reported in cancer registries (Dores et al., 2007).

Despite this uncertainty, it is clear that the incidence of CLL rises dramatically with age and that it is more common in men than women (Dores et al., 2007; Redaelli et al., 2004). As the proportion of older people has increased with improved life expectancy in the Western world, the CLL burden has also increased. The American Cancer Society projected 15,490 new cases for 2009, a substantial increase from the 11,168 new cases reported in 2005 (U.S. Cancer Statistics Working group, 2009). The disease burden is also significant in the European Union, with an estimated 46,000 individuals in 2006 living with CLL 5 years post-diagnosis (Watson et al., 2008).

CLL is characterized by a variable clinical course (Rozman & Montserrat, 1995) with some patients having an aggressive malignancy and others a slow, nonprogressive disease and a virtually normal life expectancy. Ideally, a detailed diagnostic workup of a CLL case should include the identification of standardized and reliable prognostic factors. Predicting the outcome of CLL with a statistically significant level of success will provide the basis for individualized therapeutic approaches and patient-adjusted disease management policies. Indeed, several prognostic factors, including serum (Hallek et al., 1999) and cytogenetic alteration markers (Dohner et al., 2000), have been used to assist individual CLL patient prognosis.

2.2 Acute lymphoblastic leukemia

There are two types of acute leukemia: acute myelogenous leukemia (AML) and acute lymphoblastic leukemia (ALL); (Ashfaq et al., 2010). Acute myelogenous leukemia (AML) is a clonal, malignant disease of hematopoietic tissue that is characterized by the proliferation of abnormal (leukemic) blast cells, principally in the marrow, and by impaired production of normal blood cells (Lichtman & Liesveld, 2001). It is the most common acute leukemia affecting adults, and its incidence increases with age. AML accounts for nearly one-third of all new cases of leukemia (Ashfaq et al., 2010).

Acute lymphoblastic leukemia is a neoplastic disease that results from somatic mutation in a single lymphoid progenitor cell at one of several discrete stages of development. The immunophenotype of the leukemic cells at diagnosis reflects the level of differentiation achieved by the dominant clone (Pui, 2001). At diagnosis the leukemic cells not only have replaced normal marrow cells but have disseminated to various extramedullary sites. Studies suggest that the activation of telomerase in leukemic cells contribute to their growth advantage and to disease progression (Ohyashiki et al., 1997; Shay et al., 1996).

ALL represents about 12 percent of all leukemias diagnosed in the US, and 60 percent of all cases occur in persons younger than 20 years (SEER, 1998). ALL is the most common malignancy diagnosed in patients under the age of 15 years, accounting for one-fourth of all cancers and 76 percent of all leukemias in this age group (Gurney et al., 1996). Data from UK showed that there were 691 new cases of ALL and 255 deaths from ALL in 2006 (Cancer Research U.K., 2010). Each year, around 3,250 children are diagnosed with leukemia, of which about 2,400 are ALL cases (Smith et al., 2000). In the USA, survival rate for children with ALL has improved markedly since the early 1970s and is now approximately 80%, but incidence rates have not decreased and have, in fact, increased by 0.8% annually from 1975 to 2007 (SEER, 2010). Worldwide, according to the World Health Organization (WHO), there were 33,142 deaths from leukemia among children under age 15 in 2004, and childhood (<15 years) leukemia caused 1,228,075 disability adjusted life years (WHO, 2010).

Identifying risk factors for childhood leukemia is an important step in the reduction of the overall burden of childhood diseases. Though it has been studied intensively, the etiology of childhood leukemia is not well established. A two-hit model was proposed by Greaves in which prenatal chromosome alterations and postnatal genetic alterations are necessary for childhood leukemia development (Greaves, 2002). Genetic susceptibility and environmental factors play potential roles in this process (Eden, 2010). Ionizing radiation has been significantly linked to childhood leukemia (Bailey et al., 2010). Evidence for an association with benzene exposure or with parental smoking and alcohol consumption is less convincing (Liu et al., 2011) .

Treatment for the majority of ALL subtypes consists of three phases: induction, intensification (consolidation) therapy, and continuation (maintenance) treatment. Although two-thirds of childhood cases are curable with only 12 months of treatment, the vast majority of patients undergo therapy for two years or more (Pui & Evans, 2006). Across medical institutions, chemotherapeutic agents used vary in type and amount, with the most common being methotrexate (MTX), cytosine arabinoside (cytarabine), anthracyclines (such as doxorubicin), asparaginase, mercaptopurine, vincristine, and corticosteroids, presented alone or in combination (Pui & Evans, 2006). Leukemic cells are transported by the circulatory system to nearly every organ system, including the Central Nervous System (CNS). The most common form of CNS prophylaxis was cranial irradiation, or cranial radiation therapy (CRT), which has largely been replaced by intrathecal (IT) and systemic chemotherapy. This change has been made in an effort to eliminate radiation-specific damage to the CNS (Stehbens et al., 1991). Recent regimens have tested whether CRT can be eliminated completely from standard treatment. To date, this has been successful, although alterations in long-term outcome are just beginning to unfold (Pui et al., 2009). Efforts like this are being made to eliminate the possible complications of any form of ALL treatment.

2.3 Lymphomas/leukemias

Despite remarkable advances in diagnosis and treatment, lymphoma continues to rank as a leading cause of cancer-related mortality. Recent cancer statistics for the United States project non-Hodgkin lymphoma (NHL) to be the sixth most commonly diagnosed cancer in 2010 in both men and women, and the eighth and sixth leading cause of cancer-related death in men and women, respectively (Jemal et al., 2010). Based on data from national cancer registries, 65,540 new cases of NHL and 20,210 deaths from NHL are estimated to occur in 2010. In contrast, Hodgkin lymphoma (HL) is less common (8,490 estimated new cases in 2010) and is associated with fewer deaths (1,320 estimated deaths in 2010) (Jemal et al., 2010). In the European Union, reported NHL estimates for the year 2006 were even higher, with 72,800 new cases and 33,000 deaths (Ferlay et al., 2007). In the US, on January 1, 2008, there were approximately 167,000 HL survivors and approximately 454,000 NHL survivors (Howlader et al., 2011). In the Nordic European Countries (NEC: Denmark, Faroe Islands, Finland, Iceland, Norway, Sweden), there were approximately 10,500 HL survivors and approximately 31,500 NHL survivors at the end of 2007 (Engholm et al., 2011). Although there are similarities between these subtypes of lymphoma, the incidence and age of onset are quite different.

Onset of the disease occurs most frequently between the ages of 20 and 35 years. Between 35 and 50 years, it occurs less often especially in females, but from the age of 50 onward there is again a rise in incidence with age (Howlader et al., 2011). The disease occurs predominantly in individuals aged over 45 years and the lifetime prevalence of NHL is one in 50 (Howlader et al., 2011). Due to chemotherapy, radiotherapy and stem cell transplantation, the survival of these patients has improved substantially in the seventies and eighties, but has nowadays leveled off. In effect, most trials focus on maintaining the high level of cure, while reducing the long-term effects of treatment. To date, more than 80% of patients diagnosed with HL are expected to live free of disease for 5 years or more after diagnosis (National Cancer Institute, 2009) The overall 5-year survival rate for all types of NHL (1999–2005) is 50–60%. The statistics vary depending on the cell type, stage of disease at diagnosis, treatment and age of the patient (National Cancer Institute, 2009).

Indolent Non-Hodgkin's lymphoma (NHL) represents a group of incurable slow growing lymphomas that are highly responsive to initial therapy but relapse with less responsive disease (Ardeshna et al., 2003; Horning, 1993; Johnson et al., 1995; Montoto et al., 2002). The landscape for treatment of indolent NHL has dramatically changed with the introduction of rituximab (Rituxan, Genetech, San Francisco, CA). Its greatest impact has been in follicular lymphoma (FL), which constitutes approximately 70% of indolent lymphomas and up to 25% of all cases of NHL (Marcus et al., 2005; The Non-Hodgkin's Lymphoma Classification Project, 1997). Although there are no defined first line therapies for indolent NHL, rituximab has become a standard component in treatment of Follicular Lymphoma (FL) (Friedberg et al., 2009). While indolent lymphoma remains an incurable disease, recent data from the Surveillance Epidemiology and End Results (SEER) database and retrospective analysis of clinical trials in indolent NHL suggest an improved overall survival with the use of rituximab (Fisher et al., 2005; Liu et al., 2006; Pulte et al., 2008). It is hoped that overall survival can be further improved with the use of extended rituximab dosing schedules.

2.4. Multiple Myeloma

Multiple Myeloma (MM) is a B cell malignancy characterized by the presence of bone marrow infiltration by clonal plasma cells that generally secrete a monoclonal component in the serum or urine (Kyle & Rajkumar, 2004). It is the second most frequent hematological malignancy, after non Hodgkin's lymphomas, and accounts approximately for a 10% of all hematological tumors and 1% of all cancers (Petrelli et al., 2009). MM is associated with a constellation of disease manifestations, including osteolytic lesions due to disrupted bone metabolism, anemia and immunosuppression due to loss of normal hematopoietic stem cell function, and end-organ damage due to monoclonal immunoglobulin secretion (Barlogie et al., 2001). The presence of somatic hypermutations of the immunoglobulin variable region genes in myeloma plasma cells suggests that malignant transformation occurs in a B cell that has traversed the germinal centers of lymph nodes. However, the hypoproliferative nature of myeloma has led to the hypothesis that the bulk of the tumor arises from a transformed B cell with the capacity for both self-renewal and production of terminally differentiated progeny (Billadeau et al., 1993; Corradini et al., 1993; Szczepek et al., 1998).

The clinical course of patients requiring therapy for myeloma varies markedly. Even with tandem autotransplants yielding complete remission (CR) rates in excess of 60%. Survival ranges from a few months to greater than 15 years. The extended time (almost 2 years) for those patients to achieve CR, and the even longer time to achieve magnetic resonance imaging (MRI)-CR, strongly suggests enormous tumor cell population heterogeneity in terms of drug responsiveness/resistance (Harousseau et al., 2004).

Differential expression of traditional prognostic factors, such as β2-microglobulin (β2M), albumin, and C-reactive protein (CRP), are thought to be responsible for only a 15%-20% of the outcome heterogeneity of MM. Abnormal metaphase karyotypes, present in one-third of newly diagnosed patients and reflecting stroma independence, have been consistently associated with a rapidly fatal outcome, and fewer than 10% of patients with these abnormalities survive > 5 years (Harousseau et al., 2004).

Advances in molecular cytogenetics have identified primary translocations involving the immunoglobulin heavy chain locus at 14q32 in 40% of patients (Kuehl & Bergsagel; 2002). According to a consensus report of a Paris workshop on myeloma genetics, hyperdiploid and t(11;14)(q13,q32)-positive myeloma are associated with a good prognosis, whereas non-hyperdiploidy, often associated with translocations other than t(11;14) and chromosome 13 deletion, imparts a strikingly dismal prognosis (Fonseca et al., 2004).

2.5 Other lymphoproliferative disorders

Along with Waldenström's macroglobulinemia, there are other LPDs, which are less frequently observed. From this group we will describe in more details the lymphoproliferative disorders detected after bone marrow and organ transplantation. Following this treatment and among patients infected with AIDS, LPDs are believed to result from uncontrolled proliferation of Epstein-Barr virus (EBV)-transformed B-lymphocytes in the setting of immune dysfunction (Cohen, 1991; Deeg & Socié, 1998; Goedert et al., 1998; Hoover, 1992; Kinlen, 1996; Newell et al., 1996; Opelz & Henderson, 1993; Swinnen et al., 1990). Allogeneic bone marrow transplantation, an effective treatment for leukemia and other disorders, produces profound immune deficiency in the early period after transplantation. Post-transplant lymphoproliferative disorders (PTLD) are an uncommon, but frequently fatal, complication of this defective immune function (Bhatia et al., 1996; Deeg & Socié, 1998; Witherspoon et al., 1989). PTLD typically develop in the first 6 months post-transplantantation as clinically aggressive lymphomas of donor origin; most are related to EBV (Deeg & Socié, 1998; Orazi et al., 1997; O'Reilly et al., 1996).

Post-transplant lymphoproliferative disorders are more common if donor and recipient are HLA-mismatched or if T-cell depletion is used for graft-versus-host disease (GVHD) prophylaxis (Curtis et al., 1999). The clinical diagnosis of PTLD may be difficult because it is a spectrum of heterogenous histologic and clinical entities. It may present as an infectious mononucleosis-like illness, with fatigue and lymphadenopathy, or as a febrile illness with leukopenia. Almost all organs may be affected by disease. Because of the progressive nature of PTLD, the key to management may be early or even preemptive treatment with either anti–B-cell monoclonal antibodies (Carpenter et al., 2002; Kuehnle et al., 2000; van Esser et al., 2002) or donor-derived EBV-specific cytotoxic T lymphocytes (CTLs) (Gustafsson et al., 2000; Heslop et al., 1996; Rooney et al., 1998).

3. Animal models of lymphoproliferative disorders

The bulk of LPD-related literature describes the different clinical manifestations encountered and evaluates treatment protocols. Fewer studies focus on dissecting the pathogenesis of LPD by developing animal models. Recent basic research is based on the development of genetically engineered mice or the use of immunodeficient mice as tumor transplant models. A few animal models other than mice have also been reported (miniature swine, zebrafish).

3.1 Chronic lymphocytic leukemia

Chronic lymphocytic leukemia cells require complex microenvironmental and immunologic interactions to survive and proliferate. Such interactions might be best studied in animal models; however, this needs extensive verification. Hofbauer et al. (2011) therefore investigated the composition of the T-cell compartment in the Eμ–*TCL1* transgenic mouse, currently the most widely used murine model for CLL. *TCL1* is a bona fide oncogene, developing a transgenic mouse model where ectopic expression driven by the *lck* promoter in the T cell compartment results in the development of mature T cell leukemias after a long latency period, in a pattern closely resembling human mature T cell leukemia (Virgilio et al., 1998). Immunophenotyping and transplant approaches were used to define T-cell subsets at various stages of CLL. Analogous to human CLL, they observed a skewing of T-cell subsets from naive to antigen-experienced memory T cells that was more pronounced in lymph nodes than in blood. Transplantation of CLL into non-transgenic recipients was feasible without immunosuppression in a pure C57BL/6 background and resulted in the prominent skewing of the T cells of the recipient mice. Both in spontaneously developed CLL and in the transplantation setting, a loss in T-cell receptor diversity was observed, with a relevant number of clonal T-cell populations arising. This suggests that antigen-dependent differentiation toward the T memory pool is initiated by murine CLL cells. In summary, this research team characterized the T-cell phenotypes in the *TCL1* transgenic mouse model and suggested a CLL-dependent antigen-driven skewing of T cells in these mice, making this model valuable for the research of the disease's pathogenesis, since murine CLL cells react similarly with human CLL cells.

The same transgenic mouse (Eμ–*TCL1* transgenic mouse,) was also used by Suljagic et al. (2010). They have investigated whether inhibition of BCR (antigen-dependent B-cell receptor) signaling with the selective Syk inhibitor fostamatinib disodium (R788) had an affect on the growth of the leukemias that develop in the Eμ–*TCL1* transgenic mouse model of CLL. Similarly to human CLL, these leukemias express stereotyped BCRs that react with autoantigens exposed on the surface of senescent or apoptotic cells, suggesting that they are antigen driven. They showed that R788 effectively inhibits BCR signaling *in vivo*, resulting in reduced proliferation and survival of the malignant B cells and significantly prolonged survival of the treated animals. The growth-inhibitory effect of R788 occurs despite the relatively modest cytotoxic effect *in vitro* and is independent of basal Syk activity, suggesting that R788 functions primarily by inhibiting antigen-dependent BCR signals. Importantly, the effect of R788 was found to be selective for the malignant clones, as no disturbance in the production of normal B lymphocytes was observed. Collectively, these data provide further rationale for clinical trials with R788 in CLL and establish the BCR-signaling pathway as an important therapeutic target in this disease.

In another approach, over-expression of human *TCL1*, leads to the development of mature CD19+/CD5+/IgM+ clonal leukemia with a murine disease phenotype similar to the human CLL. Herein, Chen et al. (2009) review their recent study using this *TCL1*-driven mouse model for CLL and corresponding human CLL samples in a cross-species epigenomics approach to address the timing and relevance of epigenetic events occurring during leukemogenesis. They demonstrated that the mouse model recapitulates the epigenetic events that have been reported for human CLL, affirming the power and validity of this mouse model to study early epigenetic events in cancer progression. Epigenetic alterations are detected as early as three months after birth, far before disease manifests at about 11 months of age. These mice undergo NFκ-B repressor complex-mediated inactivation of the transcription factor Foxd3, whose targets become aberrantly methylated and silenced in both mouse and human CLL. Overall, their data suggest the accumulated epigenetic alterations during CLL pathogenesis as a consequence of gene silencing through *TCL1* and NFκ-B repressor complex, suggesting the relevance for NFκ-B as a therapeutic target in CLL.

Another trangenic mouse model for CLL was generated by Santanam et al. (2010). They found that miR-29a is up-regulated in indolent human B-CLL as compared with aggressive B-CLL and normal CD19(+) B cells. To study the role of miR-29 in B-CLL, they generated Eμ-miR-29 transgenic mice overexpressing miR-29 in mouse B cells. Flow cytometric analysis revealed a markedly expanded CD5(+) population in the spleen of these mice starting at 2 months of age, with 85% (34/40) of miR-29 transgenic mice exhibiting expanded CD5(+) B-cell populations, a characteristic of B-CLL. On average, 50% of B cells in these transgenic mice were CD5 positive. At 2 years of age the mice showed significantly enlarged spleens and an increase in the CD5(+) B-cell population to approximately 100%. Of 20 Eμ-miR-29 transgenic mice followed to 24-26 mo of age, 4 (20%) developed frank leukemia and died of the disease. These results suggest that the dysregulation of miR-29 can contribute to the pathogenesis of indolent B-CLL, giving another opportunity to clarify all of its aspects.

The engraftment of cell lines into appropriate mice and/or the injection of fresh cells derived from patients have been used for the development of animal models in different disesases. Here, we describe one animal model where the researchers have developed a novel transplantable xenograft murine model of CLL by engrafting the CLL cell line MEC1 into Rag2(-/-)gamma(c)(-/-)mice. These mice lack B, T, and natural killer (NK) cells, and, in contrast to nude mice that retain NK cells, appear to be optimal recipient for MEC1 cells, which were successfully transplanted through either subcutaneous or intravenous routes. The result is a novel *in vivo* model that has systemic involvement, develops very rapidly, allows the measurement of tumor burden, and has 100% engraftment efficiency. This model closely resembles aggressive human CLL and could be very useful for evaluating both the biologic basis of CLL growth and dissemination as well as the efficacy of new therapeutic agents (Bertilaccio et al., 2010).

Another model has been developed by Aydin et al. (2011), and is exploring the role of CD38 and functionally associated molecular risk factors in a recently described CLL nonobese diabetic/severe combined immunodeficient xenograft model. Intravenous injection of peripheral blood mononuclear cells from 73 patients with CLL into 244 mice resulted in robust engraftment of leukemic cells into the murine spleens detected 4 weeks after transplantation. Leukemic cell engraftment correlated significantly ($P < 0.05$) with markers reflecting disease activity, e.g., Binet stage and lymphocyte doubling time, and the expression of molecular risk factors including CD38, CD49d, ZAP-70, and IgVH mutational status. Increased engraftment levels of CD38+ as compared to CD38- CLL cells could be attributed, in part, to leukemic cell proliferation as evidenced by simultaneous immunostaining of murine spleen sections for Ki-67 and CD20. In short-term (24 h) homing assays, CD38+ CLL cells migrated more efficiently to the bone marrow of the recipient animals than their CD38- counterparts. Finally, the expression of CD38 by the leukemic cells was found to be dynamic in that it was regulated not only by elements of the murine microenvironment but also by co-engrafting non-malignant human T cells. This model could be useful for evaluating the biological basis of CLL growth in the context of the hematopoietic microenvironment as well as for preclinical testing of novel compounds.

Last, but not least we describe the New Zealand Black (NZB) mouse model for CLL. Is a (*de novo)* mouse model of spontaneous CLL (Phillips et al., 1992), in contrast to all other models, which are induced by the expression of exogenous genes (Scaglione et al., 2007). Similar to a subset of human patients who progress from monoclonal B lymphocytosis (MBL) to CLL, NZB mice develop an age-associated progression to CLL. The murine disease is linked to a genetic abnormality in microRNA *mir-15a/16-1* locus, resulting in decreased mature miR-15a/16 (Salerno et al., 2010).

Similar to CLL, the disease in NZB mice is also an age-associated malignant expansion of poly-reactive CD5+ B-1 clones (Caligaris-Cappio & Ghia, 2007; Scaglione et al., 2007). The majority of B-1 clones are IgM+, B220 $(CD45R)^{dim}$ and $CD5^{dim}$, increase with age, and often possess chromosomal abnormalities (Dang et al., 1996). NZB also seem to demonstrate an MBL-like stage at an early age, characterized by multiple clones, as seen in MBL cases reported by Lanasa et al. (2010). High levels of IL-10 are also correlated with the development of these malignant B-1 cells (Ramachandra et al., 1996). This MBL-like state in NZB precedes CLL, and although it exhibits similar manifestations to human MBL, NZB disease always progress to CLL, in contrast to humans who can have an indefinite state of indolent MBL disease (Lanasa et al., 2010). The NZB has also been studied as a model for autoimmunity (Theofilopoulos, 1996). Similar to the autoreactivity associated with CLL autoantibodies (Ghia et al., 2002), the NZB mouse develops a mild autoimmune reaction associated with B cell hyperactivity, resulting in autoimmune hemolytic anemia and antinuclear antibodies (Scaglione et al., 2007).

The diversity of exisitng animal models of CLL leads to multiple options for treatment approaches, which is the end-point of this research.

3.2 Acute lymphoblastic leukemia

The non-obese diabetic/severe combined immunodeficient (NOD/SCID) xenograft mouse model is currently one of the most successful models for studying haematological malignancies such as acute lymphoblastic leukaemia (ALL) (Macor et al., 2008). In this typical tumor transplant model patient bone marrow leukemia cells are directly transplanted into the recipient NOD/SCID mice (Lock et al., 2002). The kinetics of engraftment reflect the human disease, leading to bone marrow (BM) infiltration, followed by migration to the spleen, peripheral blood and other haematopoietic organs (Lock et al., 2002; Kamel-Reid et al., 1989; Nijmeijer et al., 2001). However, for this model to be effective for studying engraftment and therapy responses at the whole genome level, careful molecular characterization is essential.

In the ALL NOD/SCID xenograft model, Samuels et al. (2010) have combined all existing xenograft models and sought to validate species-specific gene expression. Using the human Affymetrix whole transcript platform they analyzed transcriptional profiles from engrafted tissues (e.g. bone marrow, spleen and/or peripheral blood) without prior cell separation of mouse cells and acquired highly reproducible profiles in xenografts from individual mice. The model was further tested with experimental mixtures of human and mouse cells, demonstrating that the presence of mouse cells does not significantly distort expression profiles when xenografts contain 90% or more human cells. In addition, they presented a novel *in silico* and experimental masking approach to identify probes and transcript clusters susceptible to cross-species hybridization. Hence, they demonstrated that species-specific transcriptional profiles can be obtained from xenografts when high levels of engraftment are achieved or with the application of transcript cluster masks. Importantly, this masking approach can be applied and adapted to other xenograft models where human tissue infiltration is lower. This model provides a powerful platform for identifying genes and pathways associated with ALL disease progression and response to therapy *in vivo*.

A genetically defined mouse retroviral transduction/bone marrow transplantation model was used by Medyouf et al. (2010) to investigate the possibility for NOTCH1 to act as a therapeutic target. This is based on the assumption that NOTCH1 is activated by mutation in more than 50% of human T-cell acute lymphoblastic leukemias (T-ALLs) and inhibition of Notch signaling causes cell-cycle/growth arrest. The tumor suppressor phosphatase and tensin homolog (PTEN) is also mutated or lost in up to 20% of cases. It was recently observed among human T-ALL cell lines that PTEN loss correlated with resistance to Notch inhibition, raising concern that patients with PTEN-negative disease may fail Notch inhibitor therapy. They observed primary murine leukemias to remain dependent on NOTCH1 signaling despite Pten loss, with or without additional deletion of p16(Ink4a)/p19(Arf). They also examined 13 primary human T-ALL samples obtained at diagnosis and found no correlation between PTEN status and resistance to Notch inhibition. Furthermore, they noted that Pten loss accelerated disease onset and produced multiclonal tumors, suggesting NOTCH1 activation and Pten loss may collaborate in leukemia induction. Thus, in contrast to previous findings with established cell lines, these results indicate that PTEN loss does not relieve primary T-ALL cells of their "addiction" to Notch signaling. They concluded that refractory/relapsed tumors that have undergone chemotherapy-induced mutation and/or selection may behave differently, but presumably will harbor many other genetic alterations besides PTEN loss. This conclusion, along others of the same research team provide new insight on the therapeutic management of ALL.

Introduction of cells into syngeneic mice is also useful tool for the investigation of ALL and its therapeutic approach. Cultured p185(BCR-ABL)-expressing (p185+) Arf (-/-) pre-B cells injected into healthy syngeneic mice induces aggressive acute lymphoblastic leukemia (ALL) that genetically and phenotypically mimics the human disease (Boulos et al., 2011).

They adapted the Philadelphia chromosome-positive (Ph(+)) ALL animal model for *in vivo* luminescent imaging to investigate disease progression, targeted therapeutic response, and ALL relapse in living mice. Mice bearing high leukemic burdens (simulating human Ph(+) ALL at diagnosis) entered remission on maximally intensive, twice-daily dasatinib therapy, but invariably relapsed with disseminated and/or central nervous system disease. Their research concluded that although non-tumor-cell-autonomous mechanisms can prevent full eradication of dasatinib-refractory ALL in this clinically relevant model, the emergence of resistance to BCR-ABL kinase inhibitors can be effectively circumvented by the addition of "conventional" chemotherapeutic agents with alternate antileukemic mechanisms of action. Thus, preclinical trials using multiple agents underscore the potential value of this murine Ph^{+} ALL model for efficiently and cheaply piloting combination therapies and for elucidating mechanisms of drug resistance, information that is much more difficult to extract from complex human clinical trials.

Other researchers have combined ALL models with exogenous factors, to test their influence in disease. For example, Yun et al. (2010) developed animal models of obesity and leukemia to test whether obesity could directly accelerate acute lymphoblastic leukemia (ALL) using BCR/ABL transgenic and AKR/J mice weaned onto a high-fat diet. Mice were observed until development of progressive ALL. Although obese and control BCR/ABL mice had similar median survival, older obese mice had accelerated ALL onset, implying a time-dependent effect of obesity on ALL. Obese AKR mice developed ALL significantly earlier than controls. The effect of obesity was not explained by WBC count, thymus/spleen weight, or ALL phenotype. However, obese AKR mice had higher leptin, insulin, and interleukin-6 levels than controls, and these obesity-related hormones all have potential roles in leukemia pathogenesis. In conclusion, obesity directly accelerates presentation of ALL, likely by increasing the risk of an early event in leukemogenesis. This is the first study to show that obesity can directly accelerate the progression of ALL. Thus, the observed associations between obesity and leukemia incidence are likely to be directly related to biological effects of obesity.

Smith et al. (2010) used another animal, zebrafish, where malignant cells can be transplanted into sibling animals without the need for immune suppression. Using cell-transplant zebrafish (Langenau et al., 2003) showed that self-renewing cells are abundant in T-ALL and comprise 0.1% to 15.9% of the T-ALL mass. Large-scale single-cell transplantation experiments established that T-ALLs can be initiated from a single cell and that leukemias exhibit wide differences in tumor-initiating potential. T-ALLs can also be introduced into clonal-outcrossed animals, and T-ALLs arising in mixed genetic backgrounds can be transplanted into clonal recipients without the need for major histocompatibility complex matching. Finally, high-throughput imaging methods are described that allow large numbers of fluorescent transgenic animals to be imaged simultaneously, facilitating the rapid screening of engrafted animals. These experiments show that large numbers of zebrafish can be experimentally assessed by cell transplantation and establish new high-throughput methods to functionally interrogate gene pathways involved in cancer self-renewal.

3.3 Lymphomas/leukemias

There are numerous studies utilizing mouse models to study different lymphomas/ leukemias. Here, only a few representative are mentioned, since the thorough report of these models is beyond the scope of this chapter. As with other LPDs, the use of knock-out and/or transgenic mice has been substantial to study lymphomas and leukemias.

The first animal model we describe studies the pathogenesis of multiple hematopoietic malignancies simultaneously. The researchers (Zhang et al., 2011) have generated inducible Pten/Myc double-knockout mice (Pten(-/-)/Myc(-/-)). By comparing the hematopoietic phenotypes of these double-knockout mice with those of Pten(-/-) mice, they found that both sets of animals developed myelo- and lympho-proliferative disorders. Their study suggests that the deregulation of phosphoinositide 3-kinase/Akt signaling in Pten(-/-) hematopoietic cells protects these cells from apoptotic cell death, resulting in chronic proliferative disorders. Since, none of the compound-mutant mice developed acute leukemia or lymphoma, it is concluded that Myc is absolutely required for the development of acute hematopoietic malignancies.

Other researchers (Mukherjee et al., 2011) managed to develop spontaneous T- and B-cell lymphomas, and leukemia in mice: Homozygous deletion of ESPL1 gene that encodes Separase protein (Cohesin protease Separase plays a key role in faithful segregation of sister chromatids by cleaving the cohesin complex at the metaphase to anaphase transition) results in embryonic lethality in mice and Separase overexpression lead to aneuploidy and tumorigenesis. By examining the ESPL1 heterozygosity using a hypomorphic mouse model that has reduced germline Separase activity, they reported that while ESPL1 mutant (ESPL1 (+/hyp)) mice have a normal phenotype, in the absence of p53, mice develop spontaneous T- and B-cell lymphomas, and leukemia with a significantly shortened latency as compared to p53 null mice. Their results indicate that reduced levels of Separase act synergistically with loss of p53 in the initiation and progression of B- and T- cell lymphomas, which is aided by increased chromosomal missegregation and accumulation of genomic instability. ESPL1(+/hyp), p53(-/-) mice provide a new animal model for mechanistic study of aggressive lymphoma and also for preclinical evaluation of new agents for its therapy.

An interesting murine model of diffuse large B-cell lymphoma (DLBCL) described by Yu et al. (2011), uses human DLBCL cell line LY8, to investigate its characteristics of growth pathogenesis and the effect of treatment protocols. LY8 cells were injected subcutaneously into the right flank of nude mice. Harvested tumor tissues were cut into small pieces of 1.5 mm × 1.5 mm × 1.5 mm and implanted subcutaneously into nude mice. Tumor growth was monitored and the histologic characteristics were documented. Expression of LCA, CD20, CD79α, Ki-67, CD3, CD45RO, bcl-6, MUM-1, CD10 and bcl-2 were examined by using immunohistochemistry. IgH clonal rearrangement and status of three microsatellite loci (D14S68, D18S69, D20S199) in the xenografted tumor samples and the parental cell line LY8 were detected using PCR amplification followed by PAGE. The subcutaneous xenograft DLBCL model was successfully established by using cell line LY8, and a stable growth was achieved up to the 9th generation. The tumor in each generation showed similar growth characteristics and the rate of subcutaneous tumor formation was 91.9% (114/124). The tumor growth was observed from the 2nd week after morphological characteristics with those of human DLBCL, and expressed LCA, CD20, CD79α, bcl-6, MUM-1, CD10 and bcl-2. The tumor of xenograft mice and cell line LY8 showed identical IgH rearrangement and microsatellite length. This mouse model recapitulates many features of human DLBCL with high stability and repeatability. Therefore, it provides an ideal animal model for in vivo studies of the biological characteristics and treatment of DLBCL.

Gaurnier-Hausser et al. (2011) set out to determine whether dogs with spontaneous DLBCL (diffuse large B-cell lymphoma) have comparative aberrant constitutive NF-κB activity and to determine the therapeutic relevance of NF-κB inhibition in dogs with relapsed, resistant DLBCL. Constitutive canonical NF-κB activity and increased NF-κB target gene expression were detected in primary DLBCL tissue. NF-κB essential modulator (NEMO)-binding domain (NBD) peptide inhibited this activity and induced apoptosis of primary malignant B cells *in vitro*. Intratumoral injections of NBD peptide to dogs with relapsed DLBCL inhibited NF-κB target gene expression and reduced tumor burden. This work shows that dogs with spontaneous DLBCL share therapeutic relevance of NF-κB inhibition in the treatment of ABC-DLBCL. These results have important translational relevance for ABC-DLBCL treatment in human patients, and dogs with spontaneous DLBCL may represent a clinically relevant, spontaneous, large animal model for human ABC-DLBCL.

Other findings suggest that increasing levels of human-derived IgG in peripheral blood from hu-PBL/SCID mice could be used to monitor EBV-related human B-cell lymphoma development in experimental animals (Tang et al., 2011). Epstein-Barr virus (EBV) has a close association with various types of human lymphomas. Tang et al. (2011) aimed to evaluate the association between human IgG concentration and EBV-associated lymphoma development in huPBL/SCID mice. For that, human peripheral blood lymphocytes (hu-PBL) from EBV-seropositive donors were inoculated intraperitoneally into SCID mouse. Twenty one out of 29 mice developed tumors in their body. Immunohistochemical staining showed that all induced tumors were LCA (leukocyte common antigen) positive, B-cell markers (CD20, CD79a) positive, and T-cell markers (both CD3 and CD45RO) negative. The tumors were diagnosed as human B-cell lymphomas by these morphological and immunohistochemical features. *In situ* hybridization exhibited resultant tumor cells with EBV encoded small RNA-1 (EBER-1). Human-derived IgG could be found in the serum of SCID mice on the 15th day following hu-PBL transplantation, and IgG levels increased as tumor grew in 6 hu-PBL/SCID chimeras. These data suggest that intraperitoneal transfer of hu-PBLs from EBV+ donors to SCID mice leads to high human IgG levels in mouse serum and B cell lymphomas.

3.4 Multiple Myeloma

Plasmacytoma or myeloma can be induced in BALB/c mice by pristane oil or can develop spontaneously in some mouse strains (Potter, 1982; Radl, 1981). In the former, pristane oil induces an oil granuloma cheracterized by a chemically-induced lymphoplasmacytic reaction. This progresses to an autonomously growing plasmacytoma with uncontrolled expression of c-MYC due to its rearrangement. Generally, these plasmacytomas secrete monoclonal immunoglobulin of the IgA isotype. Essential monoclonal gammopathies and a malignancy resembling human plasma cell myeloma may arise spontaneously in inbred mice (Radl et al., 1988; Radl, 1991).

Hence, the Radl model was produced using 5T myeloma cells that arose spontaneously in aged, inbred C57BL/KaLwRijHsd mice and is propagated by the inoculation of these myeloma cells into syngeneic mice. More specifically, in order to develop a better animal model of human myeloma bone disease, Garrett et al. (1997), have established and subcloned a cell line from this murine myeloma and found that it causes osteolytic bone lesions in mice characteristic of human myeloma bone disease. The cell line produces interleukin-6, but grows independent of exogenous interleukin-6. Mice inoculated intravenously with the cultured cells predictably develop an identical disease to the mice injected intravenously with fresh bone-marrow-derived myeloma cells, including monoclonal gammopathy and radiologic bone lesions. They found that some of the mice became hypercalcemic, and the bone lesions are characterized by increased osteoclast activity. They found identical results when they inoculated Nu/Bg/XID mice with cultured murine myeloma cells. Because they can inoculate mice with precise numbers of cells and predict accurately when the mice will develop bone lesions, become hypercalcemic, and die, they considered it as a convenient model for determining the mechanisms by which the myeloma cells cause osteoclast activation in this model of human myeloma bone disease (Garrett et al., 1997; Radl et al., 1979, 1988).

On another approach, researchers made use of two facts:

1. Human myeloma cell lines can survive and disseminate in mice with severe combined immunodeficiency (SCID; Feo-Zuppardi et al., 1992; Huang et al., 1993).
2. Fetal bone implants (SCID-hu) can sustain survival and expansion of primary human myeloma cells from untreated patients with a high success rate (Yaccoby et al., 1998).

Thus, the SCID-hu model is produced, which provides a suitable *in vivo* read out system to study human myeloma biology. Tumor self-renewal capacity can be examined in relation to maturation stage. The contributions of host accessory cells and cytokines to disease manifestation and progression can also be elucidated. It is anticipated that new treatment principles aiming, for example, to inactivate the marrow microenvironment (e.g. bisphosphonates: Aparicio et al., 1998; Shipman et al., 1997) and target neoangiogenesis (e.g. Thalidomide: D' Amato et al., 1994; Singhal et al., 1999) can be evaluated. Another animal model uses adult human bone engraftments into SCID mice. In these mice the engrafted human bone is injected and subsequently populated by fresh tumor cells. In that way a close resemblance to human multiple myeloma has been achieved (Sjak-Shie et al., 1999).

Similar to the extensively tested and validated SCID-hu system, which uses a human fetal bone (Yaccoby et al., 1998, 2002, 2006; Yaccoby & Epstein, 1999), MM cells from the majority of patients grow exclusively in the implanted bone and produce typical myeloma manifestations including stimulation of osteoclastogenesis, suppression of osteoblastogenesis, and induction of severe osteolytic bone disease (Fig. 1). Ethical and scientific concerns regarding the use of human fetal bones in the SCID-hu model of primary human myeloma prompted the researchers to develop a novel system that uses rabbit bones implanted subcutaneously in unconditioned SCID mice. Immunohistochemical analysis of the implanted bone revealed that the majority of bone marrow (BM) microenvironment cells such as blood vessels, osteoclasts and osteoblasts were of rabbit origin. The implanted bones were directly injected with myeloma cells from MM patients. Successful engraftment of unseparated BM cells from 85% of patients and CD138-selected myeloma plasma cells from 81% of patients led to the production of patients' M-protein isotypes and typical myelomamanifestations (osteolytic bone lesions and angiogenesis of rabbit origin; Fig. 1). Myeloma cells grew exclusively in the rabbit bone, but were able to metastasize into another bone at a remote site in the same mouse. Cells from patients with extramedullary disease also grew along the outer surface of the rabbit bones. This demonstrates the ability of SCID-rab model, marked by a nonmyelomatous, nonhuman, and nonfetal microenvironment, to support the growth of CD138-expressing myeloma cells. This system can now be widely used to study the biology of myeloma and its manifestations and to develop novel therapeutic approaches for this disease (Yata & Yaccoby, 2004).

Conclusively, the SCID-hu/rab xenograft model provides a system where primary human myeloma cells can be injected into either a fetal human bone or rabbit bone that is implanted subcutaneously into an immunocompromised mouse (Yaccoby et al., 1998; Yata &Yaccoby, 2004). This model (SCID-rab) has been used since its establishment for different studies, e.g. the effect of anti-DKK1 therapy on bone metabolism and tumor growth in a SCID-rab system, since DKK1 is a key player in MM bone disease and blocking DKK1 activity in myelomatous bones reduces osteolytic bone resorption, increases bone formation, and helps control MM growth (Yaccoby et al., 2007).

The most recent study from Fowler et al. (2009) describes a model of myeloma in which the host microenvironment could be modified genetically. They demonstrated 5T myeloma establishment in recombination activating gene 2 (RAG-2)-deficient mice, which have improper B- and T-cell development. Importantly, these mice can be easily bred with genetically modified mice to generate double knockout mice, allowing manipulation of the host microenvironment at a molecular level. Inoculation of 5TGM1 myeloma cells into RAG-$2^{-/-}$ mice resulted in myeloma development, which was associated with tumor growth within bone and an osteolytic bone disease, as assessed by microcomputed tomography (microCT), histology and histomorphometry. Myeloma-bearing RAG-$2^{-/-}$ mice displayed many features that were similar to both human myeloma and the original Radl 5T model. To demonstrate the use of this model, we have examined the effect of host-derived matrix metalloproteinase 9 (MMP-9) in the development of myeloma in vivo.

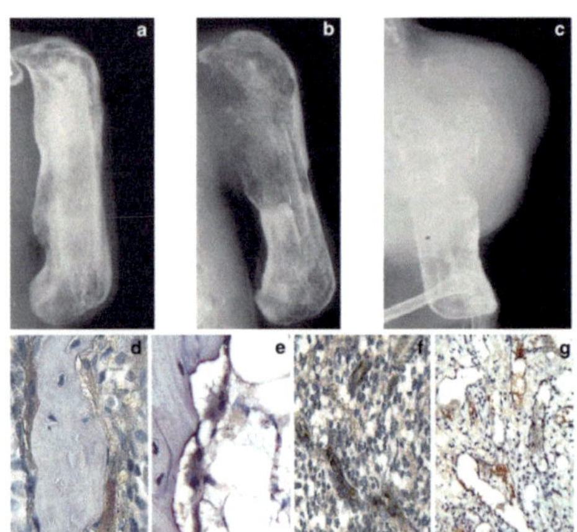

Fig. 1. Growth patterns and typical disease manifestations of myeloma cells in the SCID-rab model. (a, b) Myeloma cells from the majority ofpatients grew exclusively in the rabbit BM (medullary disease). Radiographs (a) before and (b) 12 weeks after myeloma PCs injection show severe resorption of the myelomatous rabbit bone. (c) Myeloma PCs taken from extramedullary disease grew also on the outer surface of the implanted rabbit bone. (d) Increased activity of mulinucleate osteoclasts was detected in myelomatous rabbit bone by staining sections for TRAP. (e) These osteoclasts were of rabbit origin, as revealed by their reactivity with anti-rabbit macrophage antibody. (f, g) Myelomatous rabbit bone sections immunostained with antibody to factor VIII (f) and rabbit CD141 (g) demonstrate increased numbers of tumor-associated microvessels of rabbit origin (From Yata & Yaccoby, 2004, permission pending).

Inoculation of 5TGM1 myeloma cells into mice that are deficient in RAG-2 and MMP-9 resulted in a reduction in both tumor burden and osteolytic bone disease when compared with RAG-2-deficient wild-type myeloma-bearing mice. The establishment of myeloma in RAG-$2^{-/-}$ mice permits molecular examination of the host contribution to myeloma pathogenesis in vivo.

3.5 Other lymphoproliferative disorders

Primates and swine have been used as experimental animals to develop animal models for post-transplant lymphoproliferative disorder (PTLD) one of the less frequently met LPDs.

As previously mentioned, PTLD has been shown to be associated with Epstein-Barr virus (EBV) infection. Although primate animal models of PTLD and the use of molecular markers in its diagnosis had not yet been reported, Schmidtko et al. (2002) designed a study to evaluate the frequency, pathology, and molecular characteristics of PTLD in cynomolgus monkey kidney allograft recipients. Of 160 consecutive primate renal transplants performed, 5.6% developed PTLD 28-103 days after transplantation. In all cases, the lymph nodes were involved and effaced by an atypical polymorphous lymphoid proliferation of EBER+ B cells, diagnostic for PTLD. Focal staining for EBNA-2 was noted in tumor cells. In 67% (six of nine) the PTLD infiltrates were present in extra nodal sites, notably liver (56%), lung (44%), heart (44%), renal allograft (44%), and native kidney (22%). The spleen was infiltrated by PTLD cells in all four animals that had not undergone a pre-transplant splenectomy. The PTLD morphology was similar in all cases and predominantly of the polymorphous type, however, some of these showed areas that appeared minimally polymorphous. No cases of monomorphic PTLD were seen. By *in situ hybridization,* expression of the RNA product, homologous for EBV-encoded RNA (EBER) was identified in the PTLD tumor cells of all cases, indicating latent primate EBV- related infection. This report identifies a novel animal model of EBV associated PTLD in the setting of kidney transplantation, with valuable implications for managing and understanding human PTLD and oncogenesis (Schmidtko et al., 2002).

Barth et al. (2009) developed another non-human primate facial composite tissue allotransplantation model to investigate strategies to achieve prolonged graft survival and immunologic responses unique to these allografts. For this reason, composite facial subunits consisting of skin, muscle, and bone were heterotopically transplanted to mixed lymphocyte reaction-mismatched Cynomolgus macaques. Tacrolimus monotherapy was administered via continuous intravenous infusion for 28 days then tapered to daily intramuscular doses. They concluded that Tacrolimus monotherapy provided prolonged rejection-free survival of composite facial allografts in this non-human primate model but was associated with the development of a high frequency of donor-derived PTLD tumors. The transplantation of a large volume of vascularized bone marrow in composite tissue allografts may be a risk factor for PTLD development.

A high incidence of a PTLD is observed in miniature swine conditioned for allogeneic hematopoietic cell transplantation using a protocol involving T-cell depletion and cyclosporine therapy. Cho et al. (2004), designed a study to assess contributing factors to disease development. Forty-six animals were studied including 12 (26%) that developed PTLD. A number of risk factors for PTLD were examined, including degree of immunosuppression, degree of MHC mismatch and infection by a porcine lymphotrophic herpesvirus (PLHV-1). Flow cytometry was used to measure host and donor T- and B-cell levels in the peripheral blood. Porcine lymphotrophic herpesvirus viral load was determined by quantitative PCR. Animals developing PTLD had significantly lower levels of T cells on the day of transplant. Cyclosporine levels did not differ significantly between animals with and without PTLD. Animals receiving transplants across a two-haplotype mismatch barrier showed an increased incidence of PTLD. All animals with PTLD had significant increases in PLHV-1 viral loads. Porcine lymphotrophic herpesvirus viral copy numbers remained at low levels in the absence of disease. The availability of a preclinical large-animal model with similarities to PTLD of humans may allow studies of the pathogenesis and treatment of that disorder.

Spleen transplantation (SpTx) was also performed in miniature swine across full major histocompatibility complex barriers to study the tolerogenic effect of the spleen (Dor et al., 2004). This study described the development of PTLD after allogeneic SpTx. Recipient pigs underwent whole body irradiation (100 cGy), thymic irradiation (700 cGy), and native splenectomy (day 0), and received a 45-day course of intravenous cyclosporine (trough level 400-800 ng/ml). After SpTx, two of seven pigs developed PTLD (1 donor-type, 1 host-type). These two pigs had greater T cell depletion and higher trough levels of cyclosporine. Early changes that occurred prior to the development of clinical features of PTLD were increased porcine lymphotropic herpesvirus-1 viral loads in blood and tissues, and increased numbers of leukocytes, B cells, and total serum IgM. PTLD can occur after allogeneic SpTx in swine. This model may be useful in studies of the pathogenesis of PTLD.

In another study using miniature swine (Doucette et al., 2007) the Porcine lymphotropic herpesvirus-1 (PLHV-1), a gamma-herpesvirus related to Epstein-Barr virus (EBV) was associated with development of PTLD following allogeneic stem cell or spleen transplantation. Oligonucleotide microarrays were designed based on known open reading frames (ORFs) of PLHV-1. Expression was compared by cohybridization of cDNA from lymph nodes of PLHV-1+ swine after allogeneic spleen transplantation between either: 1) PTLD-affected and PTLD-unaffected swine; or 2) PTLD-affected swine vs. samples from the same animal prior to diagnosis. In PTLD-affected animals, consistent upregulation (nine ORFs) and downregulation (four ORFs) of PLHV-1 mRNA was observed in comparison to those without PTLD. No differences in gene expression were discovered at the time of clinical PTLD diagnosis compared to six to nine days prior to diagnosis in the same animals. This model provides insights into the pathogenesis of PTLD and, by extension, potential diagnostic and therapeutic tools for human EBV-associated PTLD.

4. Waldenström's macroglobulinemia

This disease was first identified by J. Waldenström when he reported two patients with a syndrome of oronasal bleeding, lymphadenopathy, an elevated sedimentation rate, hyperviscosity, normal bone films, cytopenias and a bone marrow with a predominantly lymphoid infiltrate (Waldenström, 1944).

In the Revised European-American Lymphoma (REAL) classification, Waldenström macroglobulinemia (WM) has become viewed as a distinct clinicopathological entity, and is defined largely as a lymphoplasmacytic lymphoma (LPL); (Harris et al, 1994). The Second International Workshop on Waldenström macroglobulinemia attempted to refine further the working definition of the disease within the context of a LPL (Owen et al., 2003). For review, see Ansell et al., 2010.

Despite these efforts, the debate remains within the hematological and hematopathological communities with respect to nosology. These issues of definition have and continue to affect the interpretation of results within and across clinical trials as well as in basic and epidemiological research (Fonseca & Hayman, 2007). The same researchers (Fonseca & Hayman, 2007) used the definition of WM as proposed at the Second International Workshop on WM, with the exception that the original criterion of the presence of any degree of marrow involvement with a lymphoplasmacytoid infiltrate has been modified to allow a distinction to be made between an immunoglobulin (Ig) M monoclonal gammopathy of undetermined significance (MGUS) and WM. This change is based on analyses that have established the prognostic relevance and statistically significant survival differences among IgM MGUS (<10% marrow lymphoplasmacytic infiltrate) and symptomatic/smouldering WM and symptomatic/active WM(≥10% lymphoplasmacytic marrow infiltrate; usually intertrabecular).

Thus, Waldenström macroglobulinemia is a B-cell lymphoproliferative disorder characterized by a lymphoplasmacytic infiltration in the bone marrow or lymphatic tissue and a monoclonal immunoglobulin M protein (IgM) in the serum (Dimopoulos et al., 2005; Owen et al., 2003). Is a rare hematological neoplasm with an overall incidence of approximately 5 cases per 1 million persons per year, accounting for 1–2% of haematological malignancies (Groves et al., 1998; Herrinton & Weiss, 1993).

The median age at diagnosis varies between 63 and 68 years, and most patients (55%-70%) with newly diagnosed disease are men (Dimopoulos et al., 2000). The incidence of Waldenström macroglobulinemia is highest among white people and is rare in other population groups (Benjamin et al., 2003). More specifically, WM is rare in Blacks, who represent only 5% of cases, and it is also rare in those of Mexican-Mestizo descent (Groves et al, 1998; Herrinton & Weiss, 1993; Ruiz-Arguelles et al, 2000). To date, there is no compelling evidence to link WM to specific occupational or environmental exposures, tobacco or alcohol use (Linet et al., 1993).

The aetiology of WM remains unknown. It appears to be primarily a sporadic disease, although there are multiple reports of familial clustering (Blattner et al., 1980; Brown et al., 1967; Elves & Brown, 1968; Getaz & Staples, 1977; McMaster et al., 2005; Ogmundsdottir et al., 1999; Renier et al., 1989; Treon et al., 2006). McMaster et al. (2006) performed a genomewide linkage analysis in 11 high-risk families with WM that were informative for linkage (including a total of 122 individuals with DNA samples). The strongest evidence of linkage was found on chromosomes 1q and 4q (McMaster et al., 2006). Treon et al. (2006) evaluated 257 patients with previously untreated WM and found that 18,7% had at least one first-degree relative with either WM or another B-cell disorder. In addition, those with a familial history had higher percentages of bone marrow involvement, were diagnosed at a younger age, and were more likely to have higher IgM levels upon initial presentation (Treon et al., 2006).

The greatest risk factor for the development of WM is that of having an IgM MGUS. These patients have 46 times greater risk of developing WM than the general population (Kyle et al., 2002). Factors affecting the progression from IgM MGUS to WM are unknown. Infiltration of the bone marrow and extramedullary sites by malignant B cells and elevated IgM levels account for the symptoms associated with this disease. Patients may develop constitutional symptoms, pancytopenia, organomegaly, neuropathy, and symptoms associated with immunoglobulin deposition or hyperviscosity (Dimopoulos et al., 2000; Vijay & Gertz, 2007). However, symptoms vary considerably in individual patients. Although some patients present with the aforementioned symptoms, many are asymptomatic at the time of diagnosis.

Waldenström macroglobulinemia is incurable with current therapy, and half of the patients die of disease progression; median survival is approximately 5 years (Dimopoulos et al., 1999). This disease is diagnosed in many patients at an advanced age, and thus approximately half of the patients die of causes unrelated to Waldenström macroglobulinemia. Because the disease is incurable and the clinical presentations, comorbidities, and causes of death vary substantially, the decision to treat patients and the choice of treatment can be complex. A number of consensus meetings have listed reasonable treatment options (Gertz et al., 2003; Treon et al., 2006; Dimopoulos et al., 2009) but the physician is still faced with a difficult treatment decision in a patient with an uncommon disease.

5. Animal models of Waldenström's macroglobulinemia

In 2003, the Wayne State University Waldenstrom's Macroglobulinemia xenograft model in mice with severe combined immune deficiency (WSU-WM-SCID) was developed (Al-Katib et al., 2003). The WSU-WM-SCID is a model of a more aggressive and resistant WM usually seen toward the late stages of disease. It is, therefore, a particularly useful tool in developing new therapeutic strategies for the more aggressive WM, including targeted therapy, which exploits unique molecular characteristics of tumor cells. The WSU-WM-SCID is the first preclinical animal model available for this disease. It is based on a permanent, EBV-IgMlambda cell line (WSU-WM) established from a patient with a 10-year history of Waldenstrom's macroglobulinemia. These cells are CD5(-)CD10(+)CD19(+)CD20(+)CD22(+) and have t(8;14) (q24;32), t(12;17) (q24;q21), 2p-. WSU-WM cells also express DNA topoisomerase II (alpha and beta), and are bcl(2)(+)bcl(XL)(+)bax(-). Although the tumor has aggressive biological behavior with c-myc-IgH rearrangement, it has retained the salient features of WM. The breakpoint on 8q24 is downstream of c-myc exon 3, which is not usual for Burkitt-type breakpoints. WSU-WM cells also express both secretory (s(u)) and membrane (m(u)) IgM mRNA and secrete IgM in culture supernatant. Histiologically, WSU-WM-SCID xenograft tumors have lymphoplasmacytoid morphology. These features indicate biological, but not histological evolution.

In 2005, Tassone et al., developed a novel *in vivo* model of human WM in severe combined immunodeficient (SCID) mice implanted with human fetal bone chips (SCID-hu mice) into which WM cells from patient bone marrow are engrafted directly into the human bone marrow (huBM) microenvironment. WM cells in SCID-hu mice produced human monoclonal paraprotein (immunoglobulin M [IgM] and/or kappa or lambda chain) detectable in mice sera. Immunohistochemical analysis of human bone retrieved from SCID-hu mice showed infiltration with CD20+, IgM+, and monotypic light chain+ lymphoplasmacytic cells. Mast cells were observed to be associated with the infiltrate in these sections. Treatment of SCID-hu mice bearing WM with rituximab induced tumor regression, associated with a decrease in serum paraprotein. This model, therefore, recapitulates the in vivo biology of WM and allows the study of novel investigational drugs targeting WM cells in the huBM milieu.

Model cell lines are essential tools for investigating the biology and therapeutics of cancer. Approximately 1500 human hematopoietic neoplastic cell lines have been described, covering most major disease entities. Waldenström's macroglobulinemia (WM) is a rare incurable hematological neoplasm from which four cell lines have been derived.

In 2007 a cell line, the BCWM.1 cell line (Ditzel Santos et al., 2007), which was derived from the long-term culture of CD19(+) selected bone marrow lymphoplasmacytic cells isolated from an untreated patient with WM. BCWM.1 cells morphologically resemble lymphoplasmacytic cells (LPC) and propagate in RPMI-1640 medium supplemented with 10% fetal bovine serum. Phenotypic characterization by flow cytometric analysis demonstrated typical WM LPC characteristics: CD5(-), CD10(-), CD19(+), CD20(+), CD23(+), CD27(-), CD38(+), CD138(+), CD40(+), CD52(+), CD70(+), CD117(+), cIgM(+), cIgG(-), cIgA(-), ckappa(-), clambda(+), as well as the survival proteins APRIL and BLYS, and their receptors TACI, BCMA and BAFF-R. Enzyme-linked immunosorbent assay studies demonstrated secretion of IgMlambda and soluble CD27. Karyotypic and multicolor fluorescence in situ hybridization studies did not demonstrate cytogenetic abnormalities. Molecular analysis of BCWM.1 cells confirmed clonality by determination of IgH rearrangements. Inoculation of BCWM.1 cells in human bone marrow chips implanted in severe combined immunodeficient-hu mice led to rapid engraftment of tumor cells and serum detection of human IgM, lambda, and soluble CD27. These studies support the use of BCWM.1 cells as an appropriate model for the study of WM, which in conjunction with the severe combined immunodeficient-hu mouse model may be used as a convenient model for studies focused on both WM pathogenesis and development of targeted therapies for WM.

In 2008, Drexler et al., summarized on the existence of three cell lines, that although are currently used as *in vitro* models, none convincingly pass muster. Mindful that candidate tumor cell lines sometimes arise spuriously by viral immortalization of bystander cells, they reviewed the extent to which WM cell lines portray established disease features in vitro. At closer inspection, it seems that none convincingly displays morphological, immunophenotypic, genotypic or biological features characteristic of WM. Rather it appears that two cell lines (WM1 and BCWM.1) are most probably Epstein-Barr virus-immortalized B-lymphoblastoid cell lines, derived from bystander B-cells. The third cell line (WSU-WM) carries the most common cytogenetic hallmark of Burkitt lymphoma, namely t(8;14)(q24;q32), while none have been shown to carry chromosome 6 deletions recently demonstrated as indicative of disease progression in this entity.

Recently, Hodge et al. (2011) described the establishment of a new WM cell line, MWCL-1. Comprehensive genetic analyses have unequivocally confirmed a clonal relationship between this novel cell line and the founding tumor. MWCL-1 cells exhibit an immunophenotype consistent with a diverse, tumor clone composed of both small B lymphocytes and larger lymphoplasmacytic cells and plasma cells: $CD3^-$, $CD19^+$, $CD20^+$, $CD27^+$, $CD38^+$, $CD49D^+$, $CD138^+$, $cIgM^+$, and κ^+. Cytogenetic studies identified a monoallelic deletion of 17p13 (TP53) in both the cell line and the primary tumor. Direct DNA resequencing of the remaining copy of TP53 revealed a missense mutation at exon 5 (V143A, GTG>GCG). In accordance with primary WM tumors, MWCL-1 cells retain the ability to secrete high amounts of IgM protein in the absence of an external stimulus. The genetic, immunophenotypic, and biologic data presented here confirm the validity of the MWCL-1 cell line as a representative model of WM.

Dr. Janz at Department of Pathology at University of Iowa is currently developing a mouse model of Waldenström's macroglobulinemia. An immunocompetent, transgenic mouse model of human WM that will be useful for preclinical testing of WM drug candidates. Transgenic mouse models of human cancer are experimental model systems that rely on laboratory mice that have been genetically manipulated to render them prone to neoplasms that accurately recapitulate important features of their human cancer counterparts. Model systems of this sort: enable researchers to study the onset and progression of cancer in ways that cannot be pursued in human beings; advance our understanding of the molecular genetic and biological events that contribute to the development and spread of cancer cells; and provide a valuable preclinical platform for evaluating new approaches to treat and prevent cancer in patients. The latter is particularly important in circumstances in which drug testing requires an intact, immunocompetent animal that is able to produce the same kind of tumor microenvironment and recruit the same types of tumor bystander cells commonly found in human patients. To give but one example, therapeutic antibodies target cancer cells by recruiting normal immune cells to the site of attack; thus, the preclinical testing of these antibodies requires strains of laboratory mice that have a normal, fully functioning immune system. To that end, Janz and collaborators are generating a designer model of human WM designated C.IL6/BCL2/AID^{null}. This model combines three crucial pathogenetic factors of human WM - namely the B-lymphocyte growth, differentiation and survival factor IL-6, the cellular oncoprotein BCL-2, and the inability of WM cells to perform immunoglobulin isotype switching (AID^{null}) - on the genetic backgroud of BALB/c (abbreviated as C). Strain C mice are highly susceptible to malignant B-lymphocyte transformation (Diagram 1; http://www.medicine.uiowa.edu Pathology/site/research/ janz/res_projects.html; selected publications of Dr.Janz: de Jong & Janz, 2010; Park et al., 2005).

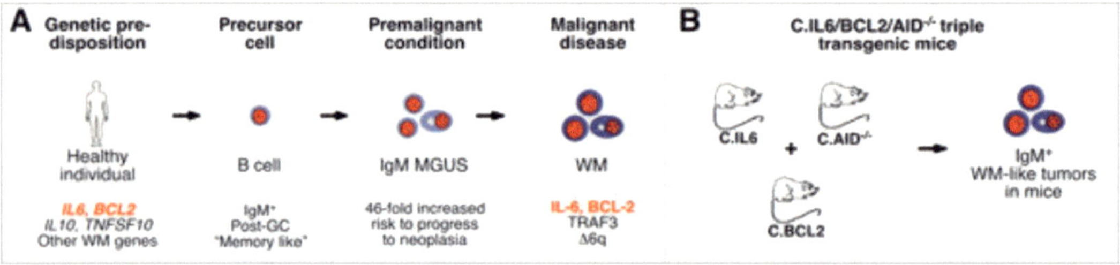

Diagram 1. Schematic overview of the pathogenesis of lymphoplasmacytic lymphoma (LPL)-WM (panel A) and transgenic mouse strains that Janz et al. propose to use for modeling human LPL-WM in mice (panel B).
(A) *IL6* and *BCL2* have been identified as "WM genes" - genes that confer genetic proclivity to the disease (left). Additionally, IL-6 and BCL-2 are major player in the LPL-WM cells (right)
(B) All strains are on the same genetic background of BALB/c (C), an important precondition for intercrossing the various transgenes without jeopardizing crucial practical issues of this project, such as the ability to adoptively transfer fully transformed tumor cells or premalignant B-lineage cells from transgenic mice. We hypothesize that strain C.IL6/BCL2/AID$^{-/-}$ mice will develop IgM$^+$ WM-like tumors.

5.1 Waldenström's macroglobulinemia in NOD/SCID mice

Although important advances have been made in the classification of lymphomas, the remaining discrepancies in WM definition reflect the fact that the pathogenesis of this disease remains largely unknown.

As stated in the previous paragraph, the establishment of reliable animal models will significantly enhance research in dissecting the complicate pathogenesis of WM. In addition, suitable animal models may be used to assess the efficacy of existing treatments and develop novel therapeutic strategies (Al-Katib et al., 1993; 2003). Severe combined immunodeficient (SCID) mice injected with subcutaneous xenografts of neoplastic cells were originally used to study WM. However, the usefulness of these models is limited because they do not recapitulate typical features of WM, such as bone marrow localization. Recently developed SCID mouse WM models overcome this drawback, by utilizing subcutaneous implants of human fetal bone chips. The subsequent injection of bone marrow (BM) aspirates from WM patients directly into the fetal bone implants resulted in successful WM cell engraftment in 69% of animals (Tassone et al., 2005). Although this model offers a potential advantage in that human bone is used, fetal bone, which is at a state of rapid growth, clearly differs from adult bone. It is apparent that there are differences between the bone marrow of a newborn and an adult bone marrow, including apoptotic cells, T cells, B cells and macrophages, developing the microenvironment where the WM cells are being hosted. Not to mention the fact that human bone is made of cells forming temporary anatomical structures, called basic multicellular units that execute bone remodeling, which change with ageing of humans (Seeman, 2008).

Our study was undertaken with the aim to develop a novel non-obese SCID (NOD-SCID) mouse model of WM. For that, pairs of bone particles derived from adult humans were successfully implanted intramuscularly in mice. Each mouse was implanted with a bone fragment taken from a neoplastic disease-free individual in the one hind limb and with a different biopsy taken from a WM patient, in the other. IgM producing neoplastic cells not only retained viability in the bone marrow of the WM bone biopsy but also metastasized to the normal bone marrow of the distant bone implant. The mouse model reported here improves on existing models of WM by recapitulating the adult human bone marrow microenvironment of abnormal WM neoplastic cells.

For this reason, twenty-nine NOD-SCID mice (Charles River Laboratories, France) were used. The animals were housed in static microisolator cages at the bio-containment animal Research Facility of the G. Papanicolaou General Hospital. All experimental procedures and protocols were in accordance with the European Council Directive 86/609 as well as the national and institutional guidelines for animal care.

Cancellous bone core fragments ranging from 16 to 22 mm^3 in size were obtained from the femoral head of neoplastic disease-free adult humans during hip arthroplasty or hemiarthroplasty. Bone fragments were subsequently implanted into the right or left hindlimb muscles of 6 to 8 weeks-old mice (n=23), weighing 25 - 30 grams, as previously described (Tsingotjidou et al., 2001). To test viability of implanted tissue, implants were retrieved from 9 mice that were sacrificed at 4 (n=3), 8 (n=3) and 12 (n=3) weeks post-implantation. Based on previous studies (Boynton et al., 1996) in order to detect hematopoietic cells of human origin mouse anti-human CD45 antibody (1:500; Dako, Carpinteria, CA) was used. Eight to twelve weeks following first bone implantation, the non-implanted hindlimb of the remaining 12 mice was also engrafted with a human bone biopsy taken from WM patients (see flow chart; Diagram 2). For that, bone marrow core needle biopsies (bone biopsies) were obtained from the posterior iliac crest of five patients with active WM during scheduled clinical visits. The biopsy was maintained in RPMI medium until its use. Typically, two implants were produced from each bone biopsy. In one case, however, a single WM bone biopsy was large enough to be the source of 6 implants. All human bone biopsy donors signed Institutional Review Board-approved informed consent forms. Control mice received no implant (n=3) or were implanted only, either with non-WM (n=2) or with WM (n=3) human bone fragments (Diagram 2).

To detect human IgM in the serum of mice, thus providing evidence for presence of human IgM-secreting B-cells or WM cells, mouse blood was collected from the orbital sinus of each mouse monthly during the experiment. Blood serum was serially tested for circulating IgM by ELISA (Diagnostic automation Inc., Calabasas, CA, USA).

Mice were sacrificed at different time points ranging from 1 to 5 months following the implantation of WM bone biopsies (Diagram 2). At necropsy, tissues including femur, tibia, brain, liver, spleen, lungs, kidneys and the WM and non-WM bone grafts were collected and fixed in formalin. Decalcified bones together with other formalin-fixed tissues were processed routinely, embedded in paraffin, sectioned at 5 μm, and stained with haematoxylin and eosin (HE) or immunohistochemistry (IHC). The latter was performed with mouse monoclonal antibodies directed against human CD20 (Biogenex, San Ramon, CA, USA), IgM (Cell Marque, Rocklin, CA, USA), and κ and λlight chains (Novocastra Laboratories, Newcastle-upon-Tyne, UK). Antigens were retrieved with microwave heating in citrate buffer (pH 6) for CD20, or with proteinase K (DAKO, Carpinteria, CA, USA) digestion for 6 minutes at room temperature for IgM and κ or λ chains. Poly-HRP goat anti-mouse IgG (Chemikon, Temecula, CA, USA) was used as secondary antibody. Signal was detected with diaminobenzidine and tissues were counterstained with haematoxylin. Wild type mouse colon along with mesenteric lymph nodes sections were used as negative tissue controls, whereas positive controls were procured from bone biopsy of WM patients not involved in the study. Irrelevant mouse antibodies were used instead of primary antibodies for negative staining controls.

We (Tsingotjidou et al., 2001) and others (Yonou et al., 2001) have previously shown that adult human bone retains viability after engraftment subcutaneously or within the skeletal muscles of immunocompromised mice. In the present study, we first sought to determine whether the above-mentioned model of bone engraftment was successfully reproduced. For that, adult human cancellous bone intramuscular implants were recovered from control SCID mice at 4, 8 or 12 weeks post-implantation for histological evaluation. At four weeks, specimens showed multifocal necrosis and fibrosis. The surface of the human bone was lined by small numbers of osteoblast-like cells and minute amount of newly synthesized osteoid. In contrast, all human bone implants from intramuscularly implanted mice were largely normal at the 8-week time-point. Viable osteocytes and increased numbers of osteoblasts forming adequate amounts of osteoid were evident. However, rare foci of remaining osteonecrotic and fibrotic changes were noticed. At 12 weeks after implantation, the histology of intramuscularly implanted bone was completely restored. The population and spatial distribution of osteoblasts, the amounts of newly formed bone matrix, the restored numbers of viable osteocytes (Fig. 2A) and the presence of active bone marrow cavities (Fig. 2B) were all consistent with normal bone histology. The human origin of haematopoietic cells populating the bone marrow of implants was confirmed by IHC using an antibody against human CD45 that shows no cross-reactivity with mouse CD45 protein (Tsingotjidou et al., 2001; Boynton et al., 1996). No human lymphoid cell was found in murine tissues examined. These results suggest that human bone implant was maintained and thrived in the mouse skeletal muscle environment.

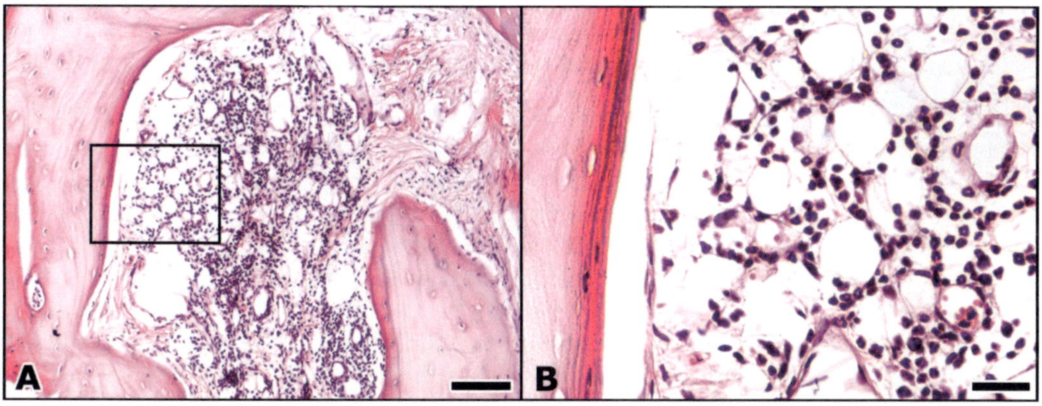

Fig. 2. Non-WM human bone implanted in the hind limb muscles of a NOD-SCID mouse at 12 weeks post-implantation. Higher magnification of the boxed area in A is shown in B. Histology of the human bone is restored. Note new bone formation with viable osteoblasts and bone marrow reconstitution. Haematoxylin & Eosin. Bars, A: 100 μm; B: 25 μm.

Three animals bearing WM bone biopsy alone were sacrificed at 1 (*n*=1), 2 (*n*=1) and 3 (*n*=1) months post implantation (Diagram 2). In all three animals, the bone marrow was diffusely infiltrated by neoplastic cells that had lymphocytic, plasma cell or lymphoplasmacytic phenotype. Tumor cells were often arranged in discrete nodules. Reactive hyperplasia of tumor-associated mast cells was common. Necrotic areas were evident at 1 month post implantation, feature that was diminished afterwards (at 2 and 3 months post implantation).

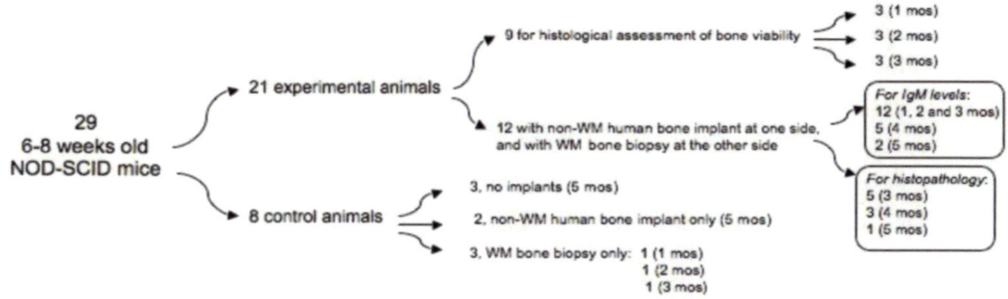

Diagram 2. Flow chart of the experimental design; Time at parentheses indicates the sacrifice point, mos=months

Immunohistochemically, neoplastic cells were CD20 positive. IgM-positive neoplastic cells were also identified in large numbers. Both CD20 and IgM antibodies used for this purpose was against human lymphocytes and IgM. These mice also had elevated IgM in serum at one month following the intramuscular implantation of the biopsy. However, two months post-implantation, blood IgM was moderately-to-markedly reduced. In a single mouse IgM fell to non-detectable levels, while in the remaining moderately elevated IgM was detectable up to three months following the WM bone biopsy implantation, without reaching, however, the high IgM levels encountered at one month post-implantation (Tsingotjidou et al., 2009). Control animals that received no implant (n=3) or were implanted only with non-WM (n=2) showed no elevation in serum IgM throughout the duration of experiment. Upon histological and IHC examination control mice had no detectable lymphocytes or plasma cells in all tissues examined.

Twelve animals (*n*=12) implanted with both WM and non-WM bones were monitored for serum IgM levels throughout the experiment. Necropsies were performed in nine of those (9/12) at 3 (*n*=5), 4 (*n*=3) and 5 (*n*=1) months following implantation of WM bone biopsies (Diagram 2). Histopathological and immunohistochemical analysis of WM implants in these mice (*n*=9) yielded similar results as those described in the control mice bearing WM bone biopsy alone (*n*=3), namely a CD20+, IgM+ neoplastic cell infiltrate. These results indicated that survival of neoplastic cells in this experimental model could be prolonged for at least 5 months post implantation. Interestingly, histopathology and IHC analysis of the controlateral, non-WM implant of 4 out 9 mice revealed that the bone marrow was infiltrated by large numbers of neoplastic cells (Fig. 3). In order to confirm the validity of our findings, clonality by staining against κ- and λ- light chains was documented in two, randomly selected animals (W6 and W10). Cytoplasmic immunolabelling for κ- but not for λ-light chains was evident and restricted specifically and exclusively within the plasmacytic component of the tumor (Fig. 4). Thus, light chain predominance confirmed the clonality of neoplastic cells. Sparsely dispersed IgM positive cells were found in the bone marrow of tibia and femur of one animal (W10). Diffuse infiltration of WM cells was also seen in the liver and kidney of another animal (W44).

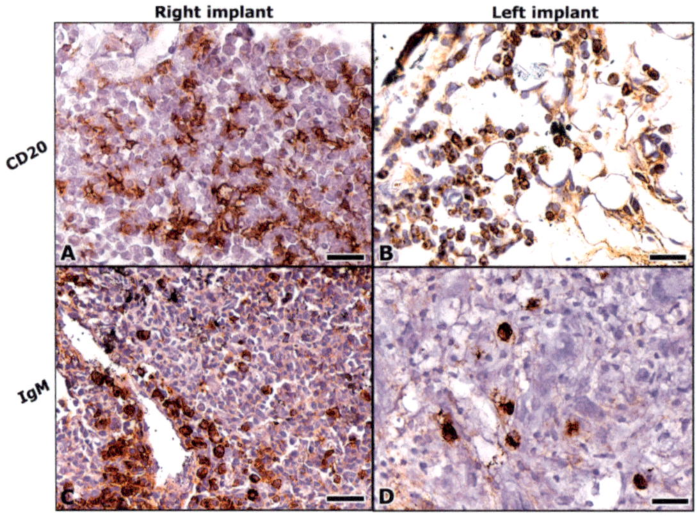

Fig. 3. CD20-specific (A and B) and IgM-specific (C and D) immunohistochemistry of human bone implants. Large numbers of human CD20-positive (A) and IgM-positive (C) WM cells remain viable in the bone marrow of the WM bone biopsy implanted in NOD-SCID mice. CD20-positive (B) and IgM-positive (D) cells could also be detected at the non-WM human bone that was distantly implanted in the same mice. Haematoxylin counterstain, DAB chromogen. Bars: 25 μm.

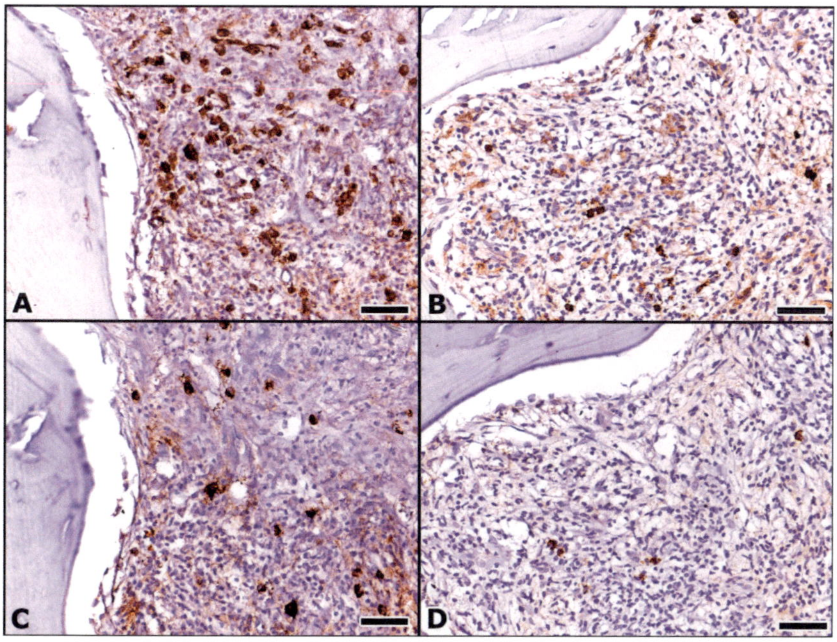

Fig. 4. κ (A and B) and λ (C and D) chain immunophenotyping of neoplastic cells performed in consecutive histological sections taken from both WM (A and C) and non-WM (B and D) bone implants of the same mouse. κ-chain-positive cell predominance in both implants provided evidence for the clonality of neoplastic cells. Haematoxylin counterstain, DAB chromogen. Bars: 50 μm

Serum IgM values in all mice implanted with both WM and non-WM bone biopsies (n=12) correlated with histopathological observations and IHC analysis for neoplastic cell density and metastatic growth. Indeed, mice with increased neoplastic cell burden and controlateral bone implant metastasis (W10, W44, W52 and W6) had increased IgM values in their blood serum (Tsingotjidou et al., 2009). In contrast, mice with sparse neoplastic cells in the WM implant and no evidence of metastasis (W45, W51 and W50) had low or non-detectable levels of serum IgM. It is interesting that 2 out of these 3 mice received implants originating from patients that had the two lowest percentages of bone marrow infiltration by neoplastic cells (20% and 33%) among human bone biopsy donors in this study. In a single mouse (W46), a sudden abolishment of serum IgM levels was observed at the 4th month post implantation of the WM bone (Tsingotjidou et al., 2009). Histological evidence of necrosis found in both implanted bone fragments examined, however, explained this abnormality.

Overall analysis of the monthly records of serum IgM values of mice used in this study reveals that after the second month, there is an overall progressive rise of IgM during months 3 and 4 post implantation of the WM biopsy (Tsingotjidou et al., 2009).

Taken together these results suggest that the WM neoplastic cells in the bone marrow of adult human bone implanted in SCID mice not only survive and grow but also are capable of producing IgM and metastasize (Tsingotjidou et al., 2009). The relatively high value of IgM obtained one month after implantation is considered an artifact attributable to cell damage, as discussed below.

This study described a novel NOD-SCID mouse model of WM. Using the SCID mouse as a vehicle of two human adult bone intramuscular implants we demonstrated that IgM producing WM neoplastic cells retain viability in the bone marrow of the implant originating from WM patients. Interestingly, neoplastic cells not only grew but also metastasized to the normal bone marrow of the second distant bone implant (Fig. 3).

A significant drawback in understanding pathogenesis of WM and developing novel therapeutics is the lack of animal models that recapitulate most features of human WM. Hence, several studies have focused in the development of animal models to study this rare but incurable neoplastic disease. In the past, attempts to grow WM cells *in vitro* or engraft them in immunocompromised mice have failed (Al-Katib et al., 2003). This probably was due to the lack of human bone marrow stromal cells, which are important elements of tumor microenvironment and facilitate both survival and proliferation of WM cells. Recently, however, important advances have been made utilizing SCID mice that were implanted with human fetal bone chips. The bone marrow of fetal bone implants successfully supported the survival and growth of WM cells derived either directly from patients (Tassone et al., 2005) or from a WM cell line that was established for that purpose (Santos et al., 2007). Both those experimental models are important, since they recapitulate a typical feature of the human disease, which is the bone marrow microenvironment-depended growth of WM cells. However, the natural niche of WM cells is the adult and not the fetal bone marrow that both these studies utilized for the engraftment of malignant cells. Adult and fetal bone marrow may differ in the pattern of growth stimuli imparted to WM cells. Although these differences cannot be elucidated, without elaborate research, the murine model of WM proposed in the present study overcomes this skepticism by simply using adult human bone implants.

An interesting observation of this study was that mice implanted with a WM bone fragment, showed elevation of blood IgM one month following the implantation. This peak in IgM levels observed at the first month coincided with the period of maximum damage to the implanted bone particle (Tsingotjidou et al., 2001). This particular elevation, however, may not reflect an active secretion of IgM from WM cells, but rather be due to an initial phase of ischaemic injury leading to WM cell necrosis and subsequent IgM leak. Indeed, histological studies of the human bone implants performed in the present study matched our previous observations (Tsingotjidou et al., 2001), which indicated that 8-12 weeks are needed before implanted bones become adequately vascularized, and restore their pre-transplant normal histology. A similar phenomenon of IgM release is well characterized in human patients following effective anti-neoplastic treatment, due to WM cell damage (Treon et al., 2004). For that reason, only IgM serum values obtained from the second month onwards were taken into consideration and were used as reliable indicators of disease burden of the implanted mice.

The wide range of IgM levels observed in mice of our experiments mimic analogous findings in humans. Accumulated data suggest that the levels of IgM production are highly variable among WM patients. Therefore, such data are valuable for follow-up examinations of individual patients and do not represent a universal indicator of WM burden. Irrespectively of initial IgM levels, however, most mice used in this study showed a similar pattern of IgM fluctuation over time. Following an elevation of IgM at the first month and a subsequent reduction at the second month, which can be considered baseline, there was a progressive rise of IgM during months 3 and 4 post implantation of the WM biopsy.

An interesting feature of the WM murine model presented here is the observed metastasis of the malignant cells. In approximately half of mice implanted with both WM and non-WM bone implants, WM cells metastasized from the affected implant to the healthy one, which was located in the contralateral hindlimb. Human bone, albeit from unrelated individual, was colonized preferentially, since metastasis to murine bone was observed only in a single mouse. Accordingly, existing murine models of WM show either no (Santos et al., 2007) or rare (Tassone et al., 2005) metastases to murine tissues. It is possible, that WM cells engrafted in mice could infrequently acquire novel properties that allow them to traffic, home and survive in murine bone marrow or other tissues. Obviously, accumulated genetic abnormalities driven by a physical selection process, may result in WM cells able to survive in the murine microenvironment. However, these genetic alterations render these cells less appropriate to model metastatic phenomena occurring in human WM, which is predominately an indolent disease. The murine model developed in the present study overcomes inherited disadvantages of existing WM *in vivo* models and better recapitulates metastasis, since it is supporting relocation of primary WM cells derived from patients from one human bone implant to another.

6. Conclusion

The use of bone biopsies taken from different WM patients as implants in SCID mice appears as highly attractive biological system to study aspects of the human disease. The quantitative limitation of harvesting BM particles from patients restricts the possibility to produce large highly homogeneous experimental groups of mice, given the variability of biological behaviour of WM among patients. This fact is exemplified by the results of the present study. Indeed, high levels of serum IgM and infiltration of the contralateral non-WM bone biopsy, by WM cells did not occur consistently in all mice. Hence, we reason that this model may not be suitable for screening specific therapeutic factors of WM. For such studies, the adult bone implant approach might still be considered if the healthy bone was artificially populated with WM cell line. On the other hand, the experimental design used in the present study may be useful for studying the pathogenesis of WM and particularly the interaction with the bone marrow stroma as it exists in the adult bone marrow. It may also be an ideal setting for studying the disease in long term, since the model allows indolent growth in mice, and consequently to assess the pathophysiology of epiphenomena such as neuropathy (work in progress). It is believed that the experimental setting as presented here will contribute to the unraveling of the etiology and pathogenesis of WM to the benefit of the patients.

7. Acknowledgments

This research was supported by the International Waldenström's Macroglobulinemia Foundation (IWMF) grant to A.S.T. We would like to thank Dr. Theofilos Poutahidis for his critical review of the manuscript, and Stergios J. Emmanouilides for his secretarial help.

8. References

Al-Katib, A.R., Mohammad, R., Hamdan, M., Mohamed, A.N., Dan, M. & Smith, M.R. (1993). Propagation of Waldenström's macroglobulinemia cells in vitro and in severe combined immune deficient mice: utility as a preclinical drug screening model. *Blood,* Vol. 81, No. 11, (June, 1993), pp. 3034-3042, ISSN 0006-4971

Al-Katib, A.M., Mensah-Osman, E., Aboukameel, A. & Mohammad, R. (2003). The Wayne State University Waldenstrom's Macroglobulinemia preclinical model for Waldenstrom's macroglobulinemia. *Seminars in Oncology.*, Vol. 30, No. 2, (April, 2003), pp. 313-317, ISSN 0093-7754

Ansell, S.M., Kyle, R.A., Reeder, C.B., Fonseca, R., Mikhael, J.R., Morice, W.G., Bergsagel, P.L., Buadi, F.K., Colgan, J.P., Dingli, D., D,ipenzieri, A., Greipp, P.R., Habermann, T.M., Hayman, S.R., Inwards, D.J., Johnston ,P.B., Kumar, S.K., Lacy, M.Q., Lust, J.A., Markovic, S.N., Micallef, I.N., Nowakowski, G.S., Porrata, L.F., Roy. V., Russell, S.J., Short, K.E., Stewart, A.K,. Thompson, C.A., Witzig, T.E., Zeldenrust, S.R., Dalton, R.J., Rajkumar, S.V. & Gertz, M.A. (2010). Diagnosis and management of Waldenström macroglobulinemia: Mayo stratification of macroglobulinemia and risk-adapted therapy (mSMART) guidelines. *Mayo Clinic Proceedings.*, Vol. 85, No.9, (September, 2010), pp. 824-33, ISSN 0025-6196

Aparicio, A., Gardner, A., Tu, Y., Savage, A., Berenson, J. & Lichtenstein, A. (1998). In vitro cytoreductive effects on multiple myeloma cells induced by bisphosphonates. *Leukemia.*, Vol. 12, No. 2, (February, 1998), pp. 220-229, ISSN 0887-6924

Ardeshna, K.M., Smith, P., Norton, A., Hancock, B.W., Hoskin, P.J., MacLennan, K.A., Marcus, R.E., Jelliffe, A., Vaughan, G., Hudson & Linch, D.C.; British National Lymphoma Investigation. (2003). Long-term effect of a watch and wait policy versus immediate systemic treatment for asymptomatic advanced-stage non-Hodgkin lymphoma: a randomised controlled trial. *Lancet,* Vol. 362, No. 9383, (August, 2003), pp. 516–522, ISSN 0140-6736

Ashfaq, K., Yahaya, I., Hyde, C., Andronis, L., Barton, P., Bayliss, S. & Chen, Y.F. (2010). Clinical effectiveness and cost-effectiveness of stem cell transplantation in the management of acute leukaemia: a systematic review. *Health Technology Assessment,*. Vol. 14, No. 54:iii-iv, ix-xi, pp. 1-141, ISSN 1366-5278

Aydin, S., Grabellus, F., Eisele, L., Möllmann, M., Hanoun, M., Ebeling, P., Moritz, T., Carpinteiro, A., Nückel, H., Sak, A., Göthert, J.R., Dührsen, U. & Dürig, J. (2011). Investigating the role of CD38 and functionally related molecular risk factors in the CLL NOD/SCID xenograft model. *European Journal of Haematology.*, Vol. 87, No. 1, (July, 2011), pp. 10-19:10-9. doi: 10.1111/j.1600-0609.2011.01626.x, ISSN 0902-4441

Bailey, H. D., Armstrong, B. K., De Klerk, N. H., Fritschi, L., Attia, J., Lockwood, L., Milne, E.; Aus-ALL Consortium. (2010). Exposure to diagnostic radiological procedures and the risk of childhood acute lymphoblastic leukemia. *Cancer Epidemiology Biomarkers and Prevention,* Vol. 19, No. 11, (November, 2010), pp. 2897–2909, ISSN 1055-9965

Barlogie, B., Shaughnessy, J., Munshi, N. & Epstein, J. (2001). Plasma cell myeloma. In: *Williams Hematology,* E. Beutler, M. Lichtman, B. Coller, T. Kipps, & U. Seligsohn, (Eds.; ed 6). New York: McGraw-Hill; pp. 1279-1304, ISBN 0-07-116293-3

Barth, R.N., Nam, A.J., Stanwix, M.G., Kukuruga, D., Drachenberg, C.I., Bluebond-Langner, R., Hui-Chou, H., Shipley, S.T., Bartlett, S.T. & Rodriguez, E.D. (2009). Prolonged survival of composite facial allografts in non-human primates associated with posttransplant lymphoproliferative disorder. *Transplantation.,* Vol. 88, No. 11, (December, 2009), pp. 1242-1250, ISSN 0041-1337

Benjamin, M., Reddy, S. & Brawley, O.W. (2003). Myeloma and race: a review of the literature. *Cancer Metastasis Reviews*, Vol. 22, No. 1, (March, 2003), pp. 87-93, ISSN 1573-7233

Bertilaccio, M.T., Scielzo, C., Simonetti, G., Ponzoni, M., Apollonio, B., Fazi, C., Scarfò, L., Rocchi, M., Muzio, M., Caligaris-Cappio, F. & Ghia, P. (2010). A novel Rag2-/-gammac-/--xenograft model of human CLL. *Blood.*, Vol. 115, No. 8, (February, 2010), pp. 1605-1609, ISSN 0006-4971

Bhatia, S., Ramsay, N.K., Steinbuch, M., Dusenbery, K.E., Shapiro, R.S., Weisdorf, D.J., Robison, L.L., Miller, J.S. & Neglia, J.P. (1996). Malignant neoplasms following bone marrow transplantation. *Blood,* Vol. 87, No. 9, (May, 1996), pp. 3633-3639, ISSN 0006-4971

Billadeau, D., Ahmann, G., Greipp, P. & Van Ness, B. (1993). The bone marrow of multiple myeloma patients contains B cell populations at different stages of differentiation that are clonally related to the malignant plasma cell. *Journal of Experimental Medicine,* Vol. 178, No. 3, (September, 1993), pp. 1023-1031, ISSN 0022-1007

Blattner, W.A., Garber, J.E., Mann, D.L., McKeen, E.A., Henson, R., McGuire, D.B., Fisher, W.B., Bauman, A.W., Goldin, L.R. & Fraumeni, Jr, J.F. (1980). Waldenstrom's macroglobulinemia and autoimmune disease in a family. *Annals of Internal Medicine,* Vol. 93, No. 6, (December, 1980), pp. 830–832, ISSN 0003-4819

Boulos, N., Mulder, H.L., Calabrese, C.R., Morrison, J.B., Rehg, J.E., Relling, M.V., Sherr, C.J., & Williams, R.T. (2011). Chemotherapeutic agents circumvent emergence of dasatinib-resistant BCR-ABL kinase mutations in a precise mouse model of Philadelphia chromosome-positive acute lymphoblastic leukemia. *Blood,* Vol. 117, No. 13, (March, 2011), pp. 3585-3595, ISSN 0006-4971

Boynton, E., Aubin, J., Gross, A., Hozumi, N. & Sandhu, J. (1996). Human osteoblasts survive and deposit new bone when human bone is implanted in SCID mouse. *Bone,* Vol. 18, No. 4, (April, 1996), pp. 321-326, ISSN 8756-3282

Brown, A.K., Elves, M.W., Gunson, H.H. & Pell-Ilderton, R. (1967). Waldenstroms macroglobulinaemia. A family study. *Acta Haematologica,* Vol. 38, No. 3, pp. 184–192, ISSN 0001-5792

Caligaris-Cappio, F. & Ghia, P. (2007). The normal counterpart to the chronic lymphocytic leukemia B cell. *Best Practice & Research: Clinical Haematology,* Vol. 20, No. 3 (September, 2007), pp. 385–397, ISSN 1521-6926

Cancer Research, U.K. (2010). Latest UK cancer incidence and mortality summary–numbers. Available from:
http://info. cancerresearchuk.org/cancerstats/incidence/index. htm

Carpenter, P.A., Appelbaum, F.R., Corey, L., Deeg, H.J., Doney, K., Gooley, T., Krueger, J., Martin, P., Pavlovic, S., Sanders, J., Slattery, J., Levitt, D., Storb, R., Woolfrey, A. & Anasetti, C. (2002). A humanized non-FcR–binding anti-CD3 antibody, visilizumab, for treatment of steroid-refractory acute graft-versus-host disease. *Blood,* Vol. 99, No. 8, (April, 2002), pp. 2712-2719, ISSN 0006-4971

Chen, S.S., Sherman, M.H., Hertlein, E., Johnson, A.J, Teitell, M.A., Byrd, J.C. & Plass, C. (2009). Epigenetic alterations in a murine model for chronic lymphocytic leukemia. *Cell Cycle.,* Vol. 8, No. 22, (November, 2009), pp. 3663-3667, ISSN 1538-4101

Cho, P.S., Mueller, N.J., Cameron, A.M., Cina, R.A., Coburn, R.C., Hettiaratchy, S., Melendy, E., Neville, D.M. Jr, Patience, C., Fishman, J.A., Sachs, D.H. & Huang, C.A. (2004).

Risk factors for the development of post-transplant lymphoproliferative disorder in a large animal model. *American Journal of Transplantation*, Vol. 4, No. 8, (August, 2004), pp. 1274-1282, ISSN 1600-6135

Cohen, J.I. (1991). Epstein-Barr virus lymphoproliferative disease associated with acquired immunodeficiency. *Medicine (Baltimore)*, Vol. 70, No. 2, (March, 1991), pp. 137-160, ISSN 0025-7974

Corradini, P., Boccadoro, M., Voena, C. & Pileri, A. (1993). Evidence for a bone marrow B cell transcribing malignant plasma cell VDJ joined to C mu sequence in immunoglobulin (IgG)- and IgA secreting multiple myelomas. *Journal of Experimental Medicine*, Vol. 178, No. 3, (September, 1993), pp. 1091-1096, ISSN 0022-1007

Curtis, R.E., Travis, L.B., Rowlings, P.A., Socié, G., Kingma, D.W., Banks, P.M., Jaffe, E.S., Sale, G.E., Horowitz, M.M., Witherspoon, R.P., Shriner, D.A., Weisdorf, D.J., Kolb, H.J., Sullivan, K.M., Sobocinski, K.A., Gale, R.P., Hoover, R.N., Fraumeni, J.F. Jr, & Deeg, H.J. (1999). Risk of lymphoproliferative disorders after bone marrow transplantation: a multi-institutional study. *Blood*, Vol. 94, No. 7, (October, 1999), pp. 2208-2216, ISSN 0006-4971

D'Amato, R.J., Loughnan, M.S., Flynn, E. & Folkman, J. (1994). Thalidomide is an inhibitor of angiogenesis. *Proceedings of the National Academy of Sciences U S A*, Vol. 91, No. 9, (April, 1994), pp. 4082-4085, ISSN 0027-8424

Dang, A.M., Phillips, J.A., Lin, T. & Raveche, E.S. (1996). Altered CD45 expression in malignant B-1 cells. *Cellular Immunology*, Vol. 169, No. 2, (May, 1996), pp. 196–207, ISSN 0008-8749

Deeg, H.J. & Socié, G. (1998). Malignancies after hematopoietic stem cell transplantation: Many questions, some answers. *Blood*, Vol. 91, No. 6, (March, 1998), pp. 1833-1844, ISSN 0006-4971

Dimopoulos, M.A., Galani, E. & Matsouka, C. (1999). Waldenström's macroglobulinemia. *Hematology/Oncology Clinics of North America*, Vol. 13, No. 6, (December, 1999), pp. 1351-1366, ISSN 0889-8588

Dimopoulos, M.A., Panayiotidis, P., Moulopoulos, L.A., Sfikakis, P. & Dalakas, M. (2000). Waldenström's macroglobulinemia: clinical features, complications, and management. *Journal of Clinical Oncology*, Vol. 18, No. 1, (January, 2000), pp. 214-226, ISSN 0732-183X

Dimopoulos, M.A., Kyle, R.A., Anagnostopoulos, A. & Treon, S.P. (2005). Diagnosis and management of Waldenström's macroglobulinemia. *Journal of Clinical Oncology*, Vol. 23, No. 7, (March, 2005), pp. 1564-1577, ISSN 0732-183X

Dimopoulos, M.A., Gertz, M.A., Kastritis, E., Garcia-Sanz, R., Kimby, E.K., Leblond, V., Fermand, J.P., Merlini. G., Morel, P., Morra, E., Ocio, E.M., Owen, R., Ghobrial, I.M., Seymour, J., Kyle, R.A. & Treon, S.P. (2009). Update on treatment recommendations from the Fourth International Workshop on Waldenström's Macroglobulinemia. *Journal of Clinical Oncology*, Vol. 27, No. 1, (January, 2009), pp. 120-126, ISSN 0732-183X

Ditzel Santos, D., Ho, A.W., Tournilhac, O., Hatjiharissi, E., Leleu, X., Xu, L., Tassone, P., Neri, P., Hunter, Z.R., Chemaly, M.A., Branagan, A.R., Manning, R.J., Patterson, C.J., Moreau, A.S., Ciccarelli, B., Adamia, S., Kriangkum, J., Kutok, J.L., Tai, Y.T., Zhang, J., Pilarski, L.M., Anderson, K.C., Munshi, N., Treon, S.P. (2007).

Establishment of BCWM.1 cell line for Waldenström's macroglobulinemia with productive in vivo engraftment in SCID-hu mice. *Experimental Hematology.*, Vol. 35, No. 9, (September, 2007), pp. 1366-1375, ISSN 0301-472X

Dohner, H., Stilgenbauer, S., Benner, A., Leupolt, E., Kröber, A., Bullinger, L., Döhner, K., Bentz, M. & Lichter, P. (2000). Genomic aberrations and survival in chronic lymphocytic leukemia. *New England Journal of Medicine,* Vol. 343, No. 26, (December, 2000), pp. 1910-1916, ISSN 0028-4793

Dor, F.J., Doucette, K.E., Mueller, N.J., Wilkinson, R.A., Bajwa, J.A., McMorrow, I.M., Tseng, Y.L., Kuwaki, K., Houser, S.L., Fishman, J.A., Cooper, D.K., Huang, C.A. (2004). Posttransplant lymphoproliferative disease after allogeneic transplantation of the spleen in miniature swine. *Transplantation,* Vol. 78, No. 2, (July, 2004), pp: 286-291, ISSN 0041-1337

Dores, G.M., Anderson, W.F., Curtis, R.E., Landgren, O., Ostroumova, E., Bluhm, E.C., Rabkin, C.S., Devesa, S.S. & Linet, M.S. (2007). Chronic lymphocytic leukaemia and small lymphocytic lymphoma: Overview of the descriptive epidemiology. *British Journal of Haematology,* Vol.139, No. 5, (December, 2007), pp. 809–819, ISSN 0007-1048

de Jong, D. & Janz, S. (2010). Anaplastic plasmacytoma of mouse--establishing parallels between subtypes of mouse and human plasma cell neoplasia. *Journal of Pathology,* Vol. 221, No. 3, (July, 2010), pp. 242-247, ISSN 1096-9896

Doucette, K., Dor, F.J., Wilkinson R.A., Martin, S.I., Huang, C.A., Cooper, D.K., Sachs, D.H. & Fishman, J.A. (2007). Gene expression of porcine lymphotrophic herpesvirus-1 in miniature Swine with posttransplant lymphoproliferative disorder. *Transplantation.,* Vol. 83, No. 1, (January, 2007), pp. 87-90, ISSN 0041-1337

Drexler, H.G. & MacLeod, R.A. (2008). Malignant hematopoietic cell lines: in vitro models for the study of Waldenström's macroglobulinemia. *Leukemia Research.,* Vol. 32, No. 11, (November, 2008), pp. 1669-1673, ISSN 0887-6924

Eden, T. (2010). Aetiology of childhood leukaemia, *Cancer Treatment Reviews,* Vol. 36, No. 4, (June, 2010), pp. 286–297, ISSN 0305-7372

Elves, M.W. & Brown, A.K. (1968). Cytogenetic studies in a family with Waldenstrom's macroglobulinaemia. *Journal of Medical Genetics,* Vol. 5, No. 2, (June, 1968), pp. 118–122, ISSN 0022-2593

Engholm, G., Ferlay, J., Christensen, N, Bray, F., Gjerstorff, M.L., Klint, A., Kotlum, J.E., Olafsdottir, E., Pukkala, E. & Storm, H.H. (2010). NORDCAN—Cancer Incidence, Mortality, Prevalence and Prediction in the Nordic Countries, version 3.6. Association of the Nordic Cancer Registries. Danish Cancer Society. Available from: http://www.ancr.nu

Feo-Zuppardi, F.J., Taylor, C.W., Iwato, K., Lopez, M.H., Grogan, T.M., Odeleye, A., Hersh, E.M. & Salmon, S.E. (1992). Long-term engraftment of fresh human myeloma cells in SCID mice. *Blood,* Vol. 80, No. 11, (December, 1992), pp. 2843-2850, ISSN 0006-4971

Ferlay, J., Autier, P., Boniol, M., Heanue, M., Colombet, M. & Boyle, P. (2007). Estimates of the cancer incidence and mortality in Europe in 2006. *Annals in Oncology,* Vol. 18, No. 3, (March, 2007), pp. 581-592, ISSN 0923-7534

Fisher, R.I., LeBlanc, M., Press, O.W., Maloney, D.G., Unger, J.M. & Miller, T.P. (2005). New treatment options have changed the survival of patients with follicular lymphoma.

Journal of Clinical Oncology, Vol. 23, No. 33 (November, 2005), pp. 8447–8452, ISSN 0732-183X

Fonseca, R. & Hayman, S. (2007). Waldenström macroglobulinaemia. *British Journal of Haematology.,* Vol. 138, No. 6 (September, 2007), pp. 700-720, ISSN 0007-1048

Fonseca, R., Barlogie, B., Bataille, R., Bastard, C., Bergsagel, P.L., Chesi, M., Davies, F.E., Drach. J., Greipp, P.R., Kirsch, I.R., Kuehl, W.M., Hernandez, J.M., Minvielle, S., Pilarski, L.M., Shaughnessy, J.D. Jr, Stewart A.K. & Avet-Loiseau, H. (2004). Genetics and cytogenetics of multiple myeloma: a workshop report. *Cancer Research,* Vol. 64, No. 4, (February, 2004), pp.1546-1558, ISSN 0008-5472

Fowler, J.A., Mundy, G.R., Lwin, S.T., Lynch, C.C. & Edwards, C.M. (2009). A murine model of myeloma that allows genetic manipulation of the host microenvironment. *Disease Models & Mechanisms.,* (Vol. 2), No. 11-12, (Nov-Dec, 2009), pp. 604-611, ISSN 1754-8403

Friedberg, J.W., Taylor, M.D., Cerhan, J.R., Flowers, C.R., Dillon, H., Farber, C.M., Rogers, E.S., Hainsworth, J.D., Wong, E.K., Vose, J.M., Zelenetz, A.D. & Link, B.K. (2009). Follicular lymphoma in the United States: first report of the national LymphoCare study. *Journal of Clinical Oncology,* Vol. 27, No. 8, (March, 2009), pp. 1202–1208, ISSN 0732-183X

Garrett, I.R., Dallas, S., Radl, J., & Mundy, G. R. (1997). A murine model of human myeloma bone disease. *Bone.,* Vol. 20, No. 6, (June, 1997), pp. 515-520, ISSN 8756-3282

Gaurnier-Hausser, A., Patel, R., Baldwin, A.S., May, M.J. & Mason, N.J. (2011). NEMO-binding domain peptide inhibits constitutive NF-κB activity and reduces tumor burden in a canine model of relapsed, refractory diffuse large B-cell lymphoma. *Clinical Cancer Research.,* Vol. 17, No. 14, (July, 2011), pp. 4661-4671, ISSN 1078-0432

Gertz, M.A., Anagnostopoulos, A., Anderson, K., Branagan, A.R., Coleman, M., Frankel, S.R., Giralt, S., Levine, T., Munshi, N., Pestronk, A., Rajkumar, V. & Treon, S.P. (2003). Treatment recommendations in Waldenstrom's macroglobulinemia: consensus panel recommendations from the Second International Workshop on Waldenström's Macroglobulinemia. *Seminars in Oncology,* Vol. 30, No. 2, (April, 2003), pp. 121-126, ISSN 0093-7754

Getaz, E.P. & Staples, W.G. (1977). Familial Waldenstrom's macroglobulinaemia: a case report. *South African Medical Journal,* Vol. 51, No. 24, (June, 1977), pp. 891–892, ISSN 0038-2469

Ghia, P., Scielzo, C., Frenquelli, M., Muzio, M., & Caligaris-Cappio, F. (2007). From normal to clonal B cells: Chronic lymphocytic leukemia (CLL) at the crossroad between neoplasia and autoimmunity. *Autoimmunity Reviews,* Vol. 7, No. 2, (December, 2007), pp. 127–131, ISSN 1568-9972

Goedert, J.J., Cote, T.R., Virgo, P., Scoppa, S.M., Kingma, D.W., Gail. M.H., Jaffe, E.S. & Biggar. R.J. (1998). Spectrum of AIDS-associated malignant disorders. *Lancet,* Vol. 351, No. 9119, (June, 1998), pp. 1833-1839, ISSN 0140-6736

Greaves, M. (2002). Science, medicine, and the future: childhood leukaemia. *British Medical Journal,* Vol. 324, No. 7332, pp. 283–287, ISSN 0959-8138

Groves, F.D., Travis, L.B., Devesa, S.S., Ries, L.A. & Fraumeni, J.F. Jr. (1998). Waldenström's macroglobulinemia: incidence patterns in the United States, 1988-1994. *Cancer,* Vol. 82, No. 6, (March, 1998), pp. 1078-1081, ISSN 0008-543X

Gurney, J.G., Davis, S., Severson, R.K., Fang, J.Y., Ross, J.A. & Robison, L.L. (1996). Trends in cancer incidence among children in the U.S. *Cancer*, Vol. 78, No. 3, (August, 1996), pp. 532-541, ISSN 0008-543X

Gustafsson, A., Levitsky, V., Zou, J.Z., Frisan, T., Dalianis, T., Ljungman, P., Ringden, O., Winiarski, J., Ernberg, I., & Masucci, M.G. (2000). Epstein-Barr virus (EBV) load in bone marrow transplant recipients at risk to develop posttransplant lymphoproliferative disease: prophylactic infusion of EBV-specific cytotoxic T cells. *Blood*, Vol. 95, No. 3, (February, 2000), pp. 807-814, ISSN 0006-4971

Hallek, M., Langenmayer, I., Nerl, C., Knauf, W., Dietzfelbinger, H., Adorf, D., Ostwald, M., Busch, R., Kuhn-Hallek, I., Thiel, E. & Emmerich, B. (1999). Elevated serum thymidine kinase levels identify a subgroup at high risk of disease progression in early, nonsmoldering chronic lymphocytic leukemia. *Blood*, Vol. 93, No. 5, (March, 1999), pp.1732-1737, ISSN 0006-4971

Harousseau, J.L., Shaughnessy, J.Jr & Richardson, P. (2004). Multiple myeloma. *Hematology, American Society of Hematology Educational Program*, pp. 237-256, ISSN 1520-4391

Harris, N.L., Jaffe, E.S., Stein, H., Banks, P.M., Chan, J.K., Cleary, M.L., Delsol, G., De Wolf-Peeters, C., Falini, B. & Gatter, K.C. (1994). A revised European-American classification of lymphoid neoplasms: a proposal from the International Lymphoma Study Group [see comments; Review; 296 refs]. *Blood*, Vol. 84, No. 5, (September, 1994), pp. 1361–1392, ISSN 0006-4971

Herrinton, L.J. & Weiss, N.S. (1993). Incidence of Waldenström's macroglobulinemia. *Blood*, Vol. 82, No. 10, (November, 1993), pp. 3148-3150, ISSN 0006-4971

Heslop, H.E., Ng, C.Y.C., Li, C., Smith, C.A., Loftin, S.K., Krance, R.A., Brenner, M.K. & Rooney, C.M. (1996). Long-term restoration of immunity against Epstein-Barr virus infection by adoptive transfer of gene-modified virus- specific T lymphocytes. *Nature Medicine*, Vol. 2, No. 5, (May, 1996), pp. 551-555, ISSN 1078-8956

Hodge, L.S., Novak, A.J., Grote, D.M., Braggio, E., Ketterling, R.P., Manske, M.K., Price Troska, T.L., Ziesmer, S.C., Fonseca, R., Witzig, T.E., Morice, W.G., Gertz, M.A. & Ansell, S.M. (2011). Establishment and characterization of a novel Waldenstrom macroglobulinemia cell line, MWCL-1. *Blood.*, Vol. 117, No. 19, (May, 2011), e190-197, ISSN 0006-4971

Hofbauer, J.P., Heyder, C., Denk, U., Kocher, T., Holler, C., Trapin, D., Asslaber, D., Tinhofer, I., Greil, R. & Egle, A. (2011). Development of CLL in the TCL1 transgenic mouse model is associated with severe skewing of the T-cell compartment homologous to human CLL. *Leukemia*, Vol. 25, No. 9, (September, 2011):1452-1458. doi: 10.1038/leu.2011.111. Epub 2011 May 24, ISSN 0887-6924

Hoover, R.N. (1992). Lymphoma risks in populations with altered immunity—A search for mechanism. *Cancer Research*, Vol. 52, No. suppl. 19, (October, 1992), pp. 5477s-5478s, ISSN 0008-5472

Horner, M.J., Ries, L.A.G., Krapcho, M., Neyman, N., Aminou, R., Howlader, N., Altekruse, S.F., Feuer, E. J., Huang, L., Mariotto, A., Miller, B. A., Lewis, D.R., Eisner, M.P., Stinchcomb, D.G. & Edwards, B.K. (Ed.); (2009). In: *SEER Cancer Statistics Review 1975–2006*. Bethesda, MD: National Cancer Institute; Available from http://seer.cancer.gov/csr/1975_2006/ (based on November 2008 SEER data submission, posted to the SEER web site, 2009)

Horning, S.J. (1993). Natural history of and therapy for the indolent non-Hodgkin's lymphomas. *Seminars in Oncology*, Vol. 20, No. 5, Suppl. 5, (October, 1993), pp. 75–88, ISSN 0093-7754

Howlader, N., Noone, A.M., Krapcho, M., Neyman, N., Aminou, R., Waldron, W., Altekruse, S.F., Kosary, C.L., Ruhl, J., Tatalovich, Z., Cho, H., Mariotto, A., Eisner, M.P., Lewis, D.R., Chen, H.S., Feuer, E.J., Cronin, K.A. & Edwards, B.K. (2010). In: *SEER Cancer Statistics Review, 1975–2008,* National Cancer Institute, Bethesda, MD. Available from: http://seer.cancer.gov/csr/1975_2008/

Huang, Y.W., Richardson, J.A., Tong, A.W., Zhang, B.Q., Stone, M.J. & Vitetta, E.S. (1993). Disseminated growth of a human multiple myeloma cell line in mice with severe combined immunodeficiency disease. *Cancer Research,* Vol. 53, No. 6, (March, 1993), pp. 1392-1396, ISSN 0008-5472

Jemal, A., Siegel, R., Xu, J. & Ward, E. (2010). Cancer statistics, 2010. *CA: A Cancer Journal for Clinicians,* Vol. 60, No. 5, pp. 277-300, ISSN 0007-9235

Johnson, P.W., Rohatiner, A.Z., Whelan, J.S., Price, C.G., Love, S., Lim, J., Matthews, J., Norton, A.J., Amess, J.A. & Lister, T.A. (1995). Patterns of survival in patients with recurrent follicular lymphoma: a 20-year study from a single center. *Journal of Clinical Oncology,* Vol. 13, No. 1, (January, 1995), pp. 140–147. ISSN 0732-183X

Kamel-Reid, S., Letarte, M., Sirard, C., Doedens, M., Grunberger, T., Fulop, G., Freedman, M.H., Phillips, R.A. & Dick, J.E. (1989). A model of human acute lymphoblastic leukemia in immune-deficient SCID mice. *Science,* Vol. 246, No. 4937, (December, 1989), pp. 1597-1600, ISSN 0036-8075

Kinlen, L.J. (1996). Immunologic factors, including AIDS, In: *Cancer Epidemiology and Prevention,* D. Schottenfeld & J.F. Fraumeni Jr, (Eds): (Ed 2), pp. 532-545, ISBN 978-0-19-514961-6, Oxford University Press, New York, NY, USA

Kuehl, W.M. & Bergsagel, P.L. (2002). Multiple myeloma: evolving genetic events and host interactions. *Nature Reviews Cancer,* Vol. 2, No. 3, (March, 2002), pp. 175-187, ISSN 1474-175X

Kuehnle, I., Huls, M.H., Liu, Z., Semmelmann, M., Krance, R.A., Brenner, M.K., Rooney, C.M. & Heslop, H.E. (2000). CD20 monoclonal antibody (rituximab) for therapy of Epstein-Barr virus lymphoma after hemopoietic stem-cell transplantation. *Blood,* Vol. 95, No. 4, (February, 2000), pp. 1502-1505, ISSN 0006-4971

Kyle, R.A., Therneau, T.M., Rajkumar, S.V., Offord, J.R., Larson, D.R., Plevak, M.F. & Melton, III, L.J. (2002). A long-term study of prognosis in monoclonal gammopathy of undetermined significance. *New England Journal of Medicine,* Vol. 346, No. 8, (February, 2002), pp. 564–569, ISSN 0028-4793

Kyle, R.A. & Rajkumar, S.V. (2004). Multiple myeloma. *New England Journal of Medicine,* Vol. 351, No. 18, (October, 2004), pp. 1860–1873, ISSN 0028-4793

Lanasa, M.C., Allgood, S.D., Volkheimer, A.D., Gockerman, J.P., Whitesides, J.F., Goodman, B.K., Moore, J.O., Weinberg, J.B. & Levesque, M.C. (2010). Single-cell analysis reveals oligoclonality among 'low-count' monoclonal B-cell lymphocytosis. *Leukemia,* Vol. 24, No. 1, (January, 2010), pp. 133–140, ISSN 0887-6924

Langenau, D.M., Traver, D., Ferrando, A.A., Kutok, J.L., Aster, J.C., Kanki, J.P., Lin, S., Prochownik, E., Trede, N.S., Zon, L.I. & Look, A.T. (2003). Myc-induced T cell leukemia in transgenic zebrafish. *Science.,* Vol. 299, No. 5608, (February, 2003), pp. 887-890, ISSN 0036-8075

Lichtman, M.A. & Liesveld, J.L. (2001). Acute Myelogenous Leukemia. In: *Williams Hematology,* E. Beutler, M. Lichtman, B. Coller, T. Kipps, & U. Seligsohn, (Eds.; ed 6), pp. 1047-1083, McGraw-Hill, ISBN 0-07-116293-3, New York, NY, USA

Linet, M.S., Humphrey, R.L., Mehl, E.S., Brown, L.M., Pottern, L.M., Bias, W.B. & McCaffrey, L. (1993). A case-control and family study of Waldenstrom's macroglobulinemia. *Leukemia,* Vol. 7, No. 9 (September, 1993), pp. 1363–1369, ISSN 0887-6924

Linet, M.S., Devesa, S.S. & Morgan, G.J. (2006). The leukemias, In: *Cancer Epidemiology and Prevention. 3rd edition,* D. Schottenfeld, & J.F. Fraumeni, (Ed.), 841-871, Oxford University Press, ISBN 978-0-19-514961-6, New York, USA

Liu, Q., Fayad, L., Cabanillas, F., Hagemeister, F.B., Ayers, G.D., Hess, M., Romaguera, J., Rodriguez, M.A., Tsimberidou, A.M., Verstovsek, S., Younes, A., Pro, B., Lee, M,S., Ayala, A., McLaughlin, P. (2006). Improvement of Overall and Failure-Free Survival in Stage IV Follicular Lymphoma: 25 Years of Treatment Experience at The University of Texas M.D. Anderson Cancer Center. *Journal of Clinical Oncology,* Vol. 24, No. 10, (April, 2006), pp. 1582–1589, ISSN 0732-183X

Liu, R., Zhang, L., McHale, C.M. & Hammond, S.K. (2011). Paternal smoking and risk of childhood acute lymphoblastic leukemia: systematic review and meta-analysis. *Journal of Oncology,* 2011:854584. Epub 2011 May, 29, doi:10.1155/2011/854584, ISSN 1687-8450

Lock, R.B., Liem, N., Farnsworth, M.L., Milross, C.G., Xue, C., Tajbakhsh, M., Haber, M., Norris, M.D., Marshall, G.M. & Rice, A.M. (2002). The nonobese diabetic/severe combined immunodeficient (NOD/SCID) mouse model of childhood acute lymphoblastic leukemia reveals intrinsic differences in biologic characteristics at diagnosis and relapse. *Blood,* Vol. 99, No. 11, (June, 2002), pp. 4100-4108, ISSN 0006-4971

Macor, P., Secco, E., Zorzet, S., Tripodo, C., Celeghini, C. & Tedesco, F. (2008). An update on the xenograft and mouse models suitable for investigating new therapeutic compounds for the treatment of B-cell malignancies. *Current Pharmaceutical Design,* Vol. 14, No. 21, pp. 2023-2039, ISSN 1381-6128

Marcus, R., Imrie, K., Belch, A., Cunningham, D., Flores, E., Catalano, J., Solal-Celigny, P., Offner, F., Walewski, J., Raposo, J., Jack, A. & Smith P. (2005). CVP chemotherapy plus rituximab compared with CVP as firstline treatment for advanced follicular lymphoma. *Blood,* Vol. 105, No. 4, (February, 2005), pp. 1417–1423, ISSN 0006-4971

McMaster, M.L., Giambarresi, T., Vasquez, L., Goldstein, A.M. & Tucker, M.A. (2005). Cytogenetics of familial Waldenstrom's macroglobulinemia: in pursuit of an understanding of genetic predisposition. *Clinical Lymphoma,* Vol. 5, No. 4, (March, 2005), pp. 230–234, ISSN 1526-9655

McMaster, M.L., Goldin, L.R., Bai, Y., Ter-Minassian, M., Boehringer, S., Giambarresi, T.R., Vasquez, L.G. & Tucker, M.A. (2006). Genomewide linkage screen for Waldenstrom macroglobulinemia susceptibility loci in high-risk families. *American Journal of Human Genetics,* Vol. 79, No. 4 (October, 2006), pp. 695-701, ISSN 0002-9297

Medyouf, H., Gao, X., Armstrong, F., Gusscott, S., Liu, Q., Gedman, A.L., Matherly, L.H., Schultz, K.R., Pflumio, F., You, M.J. & Weng, A.P. (2010). Acute T-cell leukemias remain dependent on Notch signaling despite PTEN and INK4A/ARF loss. *Blood.,* Vol. 115, No. 6, (February, 2010), pp. 1175-1184, ISSN 0006-4971

Montoto, S., López-Guillermo, A., Ferrer, A., Camós, M., Alvarez-Larrán, A., Bosch, F., Bladé, J., Cervantes, F., Esteve, J., Cobo, F., Colomer, D., Campo, E. & Montserrat, E. (2002). Survival after progression in patients with follicular lymphoma: analysis of prognostic factors. *Annals of Oncology*, Vol. 13, No. 4, pp. 523–530, ISSN 0923-7534

Mukherjee, M., Ge, G., Zhang, N., Huang, E., Nakamura, L.V., Minor, M., Fofanov, V., Rao, P.H., Herron, A. & Pati, D. (2011). Separase loss of function cooperates with the loss of p53 in the initiation and progression of T- and B-cell lymphoma, leukemia and aneuploidy in mice. *PLoS One.*, Vol. 6, No. 7:e22167. Epub 2011 Jul 25, ISSN 1932-6203

National Cancer Institute (2009). General information about adult non-Hodgkin's lymphoma, Available from: http://www.cancer.gov.libproxy.lib.unc.edu/cancertopics/pdq/treatment/adult-non-Hodgkins

Newell, K.A., Alonso, E.M., Whitington, P.F., Bruce, D.S., Millis, J.M., Piper, J.B., Woodle, E.S., Kelly, S.M., Koeppen, H., Hart, J., Rubin, C.M. & Thistlethwaite, J.R. Jr. (1996). Posttransplant lymphoproliferative disease in pediatric liver transplantation. Interplay between primary Epstein-Barr virus infection and immunosuppression. *Transplantation,* Vol. 62, No. 3, (August, 1996), pp. 370-375, ISSN 0041-1337

Nijmeijer, B.A., Mollevanger, P., van Zelderen-Bhola, S.L., Kluin-Nelemans, H.C., Willemze, R. & Falkenburg, J.H. (2001). Monitoring of engraftment and progression of acute lymphoblastic leukemia in individual NOD/SCID mice. *Experimental Hematology,* Vol. 29, No. 3, (March, 2001), pp. 322-329, ISSN 0301-472X

Ohyashiki, J.H., Ohyashiki, K., Iwama, H., Hayashi, S., Toyama, K. & Shay, J.W. (1997). Clinical implications of telomerase activity levels in acute leukemia. *Clinical Cancer Research,* Vol. 3, No. 4, (April, 1997), pp. 619-625, ISSN 0008-5472

Ogmundsdottir, H.M., Sveinsdottir, S., Sigfusson, A., Skaftadottir, I., Jonasson, J.G. & Agnarsson, B.A. (1999). Enhanced B cell survival in familial macroglobulinaemia is associated with increased expression of Bcl-2. *Clinical & Experimental Immunology,* Vol. 117, No. 2, (August, 1999), pp. 252–260, ISSN 0009-9104

Opelz, G. & Henderson, R (1993). Incidence of non-Hodgkin's lymphoma in kidney and heart transplant recipients. *Lancet,* Vol. 342, No. 8886-8887, (December, 1993), pp. 1514-1516, ISSN 0140-6736

Orazi, A., Hromas, R.A., Neiman, R.S., Greiner, T.C., Lee, C.H., Rubin, L., Haskins, S., Heerema, N.A., Gharpure, V., Abonour, R. Srour, E.F., & Cornetta, K. (1997). Posttransplantation lymphoproliferative disorders in bone marrow transplant recipients are aggressive diseases with a high incidence of adverse histologic and immunobiologic features. *American Journal of Clinical Pathology,* Vol. 107, No. 4, (April, 1997), pp. 419-429, ISSN 0002-9173

O'Reilly, R.J., Lacerda, J.F., Lucas, K.G., Rosenfield, N.S., Small, T.N. & Papadopoulos, E.B. (1996). Adoptive cell therapy with donor lymphocytes for EBV-associated lymphomas developing after allogeneic marrow transplants. In: *Important Advances in Oncology,* T.D. De Vita, S. Helman & S.A. Rosenberg (Eds), pp. 149-166, Lippincott-Raven, ISBN 0-7020-1546-6, Philadelphia, PA, USA

Owen, R.G., Treon, S.P., Al-Katib, A., Fonseca, R., Greipp, P.R., McMaster, M.L., Morra, E., Pangalis, G.A., San Miguel, J.F., Branagan, A.R., & Dimopoulos, M.A. (2003). Clinicopathological definition of Waldenstrom's macroglobulinemia: consensus panel recommendations from the Second International Workshop on Waldenström's Macroglobulinemia. *Seminars in Oncology,* Vol. 30, No. 2, (April, 2003), pp. 110-115, ISSN 0093-7754

Park, S.S., Kim, J.S., Tessarollo, L., Owens, J.D., Peng, L., Han, S.S., Tae, Chung, S., Torrey, T.A., Cheung, W.C., Polakiewicz, R.D., McNeil, N., Ried, T., Mushinski, J.F., Morse, H.C. 3rd & Janz, S. (2005). Insertion of c-Myc into Igh induces B-cell and plasma-cell neoplasms in mice. *Cancer Research,* Vol. 65, No. 4 (February, 2005), pp. 1306-1315, ISSN 0008-5472

Petrelli, N.J., Winer, E.P., Brahmer, J., Dubey, S., Smith, S., Thomas, C., Vahdat, L.T., Obel, J., Vogelzang, N., Markman, M., Sweetenham, J.W., Pfister, D., Kris, M.G., Schuchter, L.M., Sawaya, R., Raghavan, D., Ganz, P.A. & Kramer, B. (2009). Clinical Cancer Advances 2009: major research advances in cancer treatment, prevention, and screening–a report from the American Society of Clinical Oncology. *Journal of Clinical Oncology,* Vol. 27, No. 35, (December, 2009), pp. 6052–6069, ISSN 0732-183X

Phillips, J.A., Mehta, K., Fernandez, C. & Raveche, E.S. (1992). The NZB mouse as a model for chronic lymphocytic leukemia. *Cancer Research,* Vol. 52, No. 2, (January, 1992), pp. 437–443, ISSN 0008-5472

Potter, M. (1982). Pathogenesis of plasmacytomas in mice, In: *Cancer: A Comprehensive Treatise,* F. F. Becker, (Ed.), 139, Plenum, New York, NY, USA

Pui, C.-H. (2001). Acute Lymphoblastic Leukemia. In: *Williams Hematology,* E. Beutler, M. Lichtman, B. Coller, T. Kipps, & U. Seligsohn, (Eds.; ed 6), McGraw-Hill; pp. 1141-1161, ISBN 0-07-116293-3, New York, USA

Pui, C. & Evans, W.E. (2006). Treatment of acute lymphoblastic leukemia. *New England Journal of Medicine,* Vol. 354, No. 2, (January, 2006), pp. 166-178, ISSN 0028-4793

Pui, C., Campana, D., Pei, D., Bowman, W.P., Sandlund, J.T., Kaste, S.C., Ribeiro, R.C., Rubnitz, J.E., Raimondi, S.C. Onciu, M., Coustan-Smith, E., Kun, L.E., Jeha, S., Cheng, C., Howard, S.C., Simmons, V., Bayles, A., Metzger, M.L., Boyett, J.M., Leung, W., Handgretinger, R., Downing, J.R., Evans, W.E. & Relling, M.V. (2009). Treating childhood acute lymphoblastic leukemia without cranial irradiation. *New England Journal of Medicine,* Vol. 360, No. 26, (January, 2009), pp. 2730-2741, ISNN 0028-4793

Pulte, D., Gondos, A. & Brenner, H. (2008). Ongoing improvement in outcomes for patients diagnosed as having Non-Hodgkin lymphoma from the 1990s to the early 21st century. *Archives of Internal Medicine,* Vol. 168, No. 5, (March, 2008), pp. 469–476, ISSN 0003-9926

Radl, J., De Glopper, E.D., Schuit, H.R., & Zurcher, C. (1979). Idiopathic paraproteinemia. II. Transplantation of the paraprotein-producing clone from old to young C57BL/KaLwRij mice. *Journal of Immunology,* Vol. 122, No. 2, (February, 1979), pp. 609-613, ISSN 0022-1767

Radl, J. (1981). Animal model of human disease. Benign monoclonal gammopathy (idiopathic paraproteinemia). *American Journal of Pathology,* Vol. 105, No. 1, (October, 1981), pp. 91-93, ISSN 0002-9440

Radl, J., Croese, J.W., Zurcher, C. Van den Enden-Vieveen, M. H. & de Leeuw, A. M. (1988). Animal model of human disease. Multiple myeloma. *American Journal of Pathology,* Vol. 132, No. 3, (September, 1988), pp. 593-597, ISSN 0002-9440

Radl, J. (1991). Four major mechanisms in the development of monoclonal gammopathies. Postulations and facts, *Proceedings of the Third EURAGE Symposium on Monoclonal Gammopathies: Clinical Significance and Basic Mechanisms,* pp. 5, ISBN 907-1021-14-9, Brussels, Belgium, September 18-20, 1991

Ramachandra, S., Metcalf, R.A., Fredrickson, T., Marti, G.E. & Raveche, E. (1996). Requirement for increased IL-10 in the development of B-1 lymphoproliferative disease in a murine model of CLL. *Journal of Clinical Investigation,* Vol. 98, No. 8, (October, 1996), pp. 1788–1793, ISSN 0021-9738

Redaelli, A., Laskin, B.L., Stephens, J.M., Botteman, M.F. & Pashos, C.L. (2004). The clinical and epidemiological burden of chronic lymphocytic leukaemia. *European Journal of Cancer Care (Engl),* Vol.13, No, 3, (July, 2004), pp. 279–287, ISSN 0961-5423

Renier, G., Ifrah, N., Chevailler, A., Saint-Andre, J.P., Boasson, M. & Hurez, D. (1989). Four brothers with Waldenstrom's macroglobulinemia. *Cancer,* Vol. 64, No. 7, (October, 1989), pp. 1554–1559, ISSN 0008-543X

Rooney, C.M., Smith, C.A., Ng, C.Y.C., Loftin, S.K., Sixbey, J.W., Gan, Y., Srivastava, D.K., Bowman, L.C., Krance, R.A., Brenner, M.K. & Heslop, H.E. (1998). Infusion of cytotoxic T cells for the prevention and treatment of Epstein-Barr virus–induced lymphoma in allogeneic transplant recipients. *Blood,* Vol. 92, No. 5, (September, 1998), pp. 1549-1555, ISSN 0006-4971

Rozman, C. & Montserrat, E. (1995). Chronic lymphocytic leukemia. *New England Journal of Medicine,* Vol. 333, No. 16, (October, 1995), pp.1052-1057, ISSN 0028 4793

Ruiz-Arguelles, G.J., Ramirez-Cisneros, F.J., Flores-Martinez, J. & Cernuda-Graham, M.C. (2000). Waldenstrom's macroglobulinemia is infrequent in Mexican Mestizos: experience of a hematological diseases referral center. Revista de Investigación Clínica, Vol. 52, No. 5, (September, 2000), pp. 497–499, ISSN 0034-8376

Salerno, E., Yuan, Y., Scaglione, B.J., Marti, G., Jankovic, A., Mazzella, F., Laurindo, M.F., Despres, D., Baskar, S., Rader, C. & Raveche, E. (2010). The New Zealand black mouse as a model for the development and progression of chronic lymphocytic leukemia. *Cytometry Part B Clinical Cytometry,* Vol. 78, No. Suppl 1, pp. S98-109, ISSN 1552-4949

Samuels, A.L., Peeva, V.K., Papa, R.A., Firth, M.J., Francis, R.W., Beesley, A.H., Lock, R.B. & Kees U.R. (2010). Validation of a mouse xenograft model system for gene expression analysis of human acute lymphoblastic leukaemia. *BMC Genomics.,* Vol. 21, No. 11 (April, 2010), pp. 256, ISSN 1471-2164

Santanam, U., Zanesi, N., Efanov, A., Costinean, S., Palamarchuk, A., Hagan, J.P., Volinia, S., Alder, H., Rassenti, L., Kipps, T., Croce, C.M. & Pekarsky, Y. (2010). Chronic lymphocytic leukemia modeled in mouse by targeted miR-29 expression. *Proceedings of the National Academy of Sciences U S A.,* Vol. 107, No. 27, (July, 2010), pp. 12210-12215, ISSN 0027-8424

Santos, D.D., Ho, A.W., Tournilhac, O., Hatjiharissi, E., Leleu, X., Xu, L., Tassone, P., Neri, P., Hunter, Z.R., Chemaly, M.A., Branagan, A.R., Manning, R.J., Patterson, C.J., Moreau, A.S., Ciccarelli, B., Adamia, S., Kriangkum, J., Kutok, J.L., Tai, Y.T., Zhang, J., Pilarski, L.M., Anderson, K.C., Munshi, N. & Treon, S.P. (2007). Establishment of BCWM.1 cell line for Waldenström's macroglobulinemia with productive in vivo engraftment in SCID-hu mice. *Experimental Hematology,* Vol. 35,. No. 9, (September, 2007), pp.1366-1375, ISSN 0301-472X

Scaglione, B.J., Salerno, E., Balan, M., Coffman, F., Landgraf, P., Abbasi, F., Kotenko, S., Marti, G.E. & Raveche, E.S. (2007). Murine models of chronic lymphocytic leukaemia: role of microRNA-16 in the New Zealand Black mouse model. *British Journal of Haematology*, Vol. 139, No. 5, (December, 2007), pp. 645–657, ISSN 0007-1048

Schmidtko, J., Wang, R., Wu CL, Mauiyyedi, S., Harris, N.L., Della, Pelle, P., Brousaides, N., Zagachin, L., Ferry, J.A., Wang, F., Kawai, T., Sachs, D.H., Cosimi, B.A. & Colvin, R.B. (2002). Posttransplant lymphoproliferative disorder associated with an Epstein-Barr-related virus in cynomolgus monkeys. *Transplantation.*, Vol. 73, No. 9, (May, 2002), pp. 1431-1439, ISSN 0041-1337

Seeman, E. (2008). Bone quality: the material and structural basis of bone strength. *Journal of Bone Mineral Metabolism*, Vol. 26, No. 1, (Epub January, 2008), pp. 1-8, ISSN 0914-8779

SEER Cancer Statisitcs Review, 1973-1995. (1998). National Cancer Institute. Available from: http://seer.cancer.gov/csr/1973_1995/overview.pdf

SEER (Surveillance Epidemiology and End Results); (2010), "SEER Cancer Statistics Review 1975–2007". Available from: http://seer.cancer.gov/csr/1975 2007/results single/sect 28 table.09.pdf.

Shay, J.W., Werbin, H. & Wright, W.E. (1996). Telomeres and telomerase in human leukemias. *Leukemia*, Vol. 10, No. 8, (August, 1996), pp. 1255-1261, ISSN 0887-6924

Shipman, C.M., Rogers, M.J., Apperley, J.F., Russell, R.G. & Croucher, P.I. (1997). Bisphosphonates induce apoptosis in human myeloma cell lines: a novel anti-tumour activity. *Brtish Journal of Haematology*, Vol. 98, No. 3, (September, 1997), pp. 665-672, ISSN 0361-8609

Singhal, S., Mehta, J., Desikan, R., Ayers, D., Roberson, P., Eddlemon, P., Munshi, N., Anaissie, E., Wilson, C., Dhodapkar, M., Zeddis, J. & Barlogie, B. (1999). Antitumor activity of thalidomide in refractory multiple myeloma. *New England Journal of Medicine.*, Vol. 18, No. 341(21), (November, 1999), pp.1565-1571, ISSN 0028-4793

Sjak-Shie, N. N., Tsingotjidou, A. S., Zhang, K., Vescio, R. A., Said, J. W., Lieberman, J. R. & Berenson, J. R. (1999). Development of a SCID-hu animal model that more closely resembles human multiple myeloma. *Blood*, Vol. 94, No. 10, pp. 2447 Part 1 Supp., 1999, ISSN 0006-4971

Smith, A.C., Raimondi, A.R., Salthouse, C.D., Ignatius, M.S., Blackburn, J.S., Mizgirev, I.V., Storer, N.Y. de Jong, J.L., Chen, A.T., Zhou, Y., Revskoy, S., Zon, L.I., & Langenau, D.M. (2010). High-throughput cell transplantation establishes that tumor-initiating cells are abundant in zebrafish T-cell acute lymphoblastic leukemia. *Blood.*, Vol. 115, No. 16, (April, 2010), pp. 3296-3303, ISSN 0006-4971

Smith, M.A., Gloeckler Ries, L.A., Gurney, J.G. & Ross, J.A. (2010). "Leukemia. SEER Pediatric Monograph". Available from: http://seer.cancer.gov/ publications/childhood/leukemia.pdf

Stehbens, J.A., Kaleita, T.A., Noll, R.B., MacLean, W.E. Jr, O'Brien, R.T., Waskerwitz, M.J. & Hammond, G.D. (1991). CNS prophylaxis of childhood leukemia: what are the long-term neurological, neuropsychological, and behavioral effects? *Neuropsychology Review*, Vol. 2, No. 2, (June, 1991), pp. 147-177, ISSN 1040-7308

Suljagic, M., Longo, P.G., Bennardo, S., Perlas, E., Leone, G., Laurenti, L. & Efremov, D.G. (2010). The Syk inhibitor fostamatinib disodium (R788) inhibits tumor growth in the Eμ- TCL1 transgenic mouse model of CLL by blocking antigen-dependent B-cell receptor signaling. *Blood.,* Vol. 116, No. 23, (December, 2010), pp. 4894-4905, ISSN 0006-4971

Swinnen, L.J. Costanzo-Nordin, M.R., Fisher, S.G., O'Sullivan, E.J., Johnson, M.R., Heroux, A.L., Dizikes, G.J., Pifarre, R. & Fisher, R.I. (1990). Increased incidence of lymphoproliferative disorder after immunosuppression with the monoclonal antibody OKT3 in cardiac-transplant recipients. *New England Journal of Medicine,* Vol. 323, No. 25, (December, 1990), pp. 1723-1728, ISSN 0028-4793

Szczepek, A.J., Seeberger, K., Wizniak, J., Mant, M.J., Belch, A.R. & Pilarski, L.M. (1998). A high frequency of circulating B cells share clonotypic Ig heavy-chain VDJ rearrangements with autologous bone marrow plasma cells in multiple myeloma, as measured by single-cell and in situ reverse transcriptasepolymerase chain reaction. *Blood.,* Vol. 92, No. 8, (October, 1998), pp. 2844-2855, ISSN 0006-4971

Tang, Y., He, R., Zhang, Y., Liu, F., Cheng, A., Wu, Y. & Gan, R. (2011). Human-derived IgG level as an indicator for EBV-associated lymphoma model in Hu-PBL/SCID chimeras. *Virology Journal,* Vol. 8, (May, 2011), pp. 213, ISSN 1743-422X

Tassone, P., Neri, P., Kutok, J.L., Tournilhac, O., Santos, D.D., Hatjiharissi, E., Munshi, V., Venuta, S., Anderson, K.C., Treon, S.P. & Munshi, N.C. (2005). A SCID-hu in vivo model of human Waldenström macroglobulinemia. *Blood.,* Vol. 106, No. 4, (August, 2005), pp. 1341-1345, ISSN 0006-4971

The Non-Hodgkin's Lymphoma Classification Project (1997). A clinical evaluation of the International Lymphoma Study Group classification of non-Hodgkin's lymphoma. *Blood,* Vol. 89, No. 11, (June, 1997), pp. 3909–3918, ISSN 0006-4971

Theofilopoulos, A.N. (1996). Genetics of systemic autoimmunity. *Journal of Autoimmunity,* Vol. 9, No. 2, (April, 1996), pp. 207–210, ISSN 0896-8411

Treon, S.P., Branagan, A.R., Hunter, Z., Santos, D., Tournhilac, O. & Anderson, K.C. (2004). Paradoxical increases in serum IgM and viscosity levels following rituximab in Waldenström's macroglobulinemia. *Annals in Oncology,* Vol. 15, No. 10, (October, 2004), pp. 1481-1483, ISSN 0923-7534

Treon, S.P., Gertz, M.A., Dimopoulos, M., Anagnostopoulos, A., Blade, J., Branagan, A.R., Garcia-Sanz, R., Johnson, S., Kimby, E., Leblond, V., Fermand, J.P., Maloney, D.G., Merlini, G., Morel, P., Morra, E., Nichols, G., Ocio, E.M., Owen, R. & Stone, M.J. (2006). Update on treatment recommendations from the Third International Workshop on Waldenström's Macroglobulinemia. *Blood,* Vol. 107, No. 9, (May, 2006), pp. 3442-3446, ISSN 0006-4971.

Tsingotjidou, A.S., Zotalis, G., Jackson, K.R., Sawyers, C., Puzas, J.E., Hicks, D.G., Reiter, R. & Lieberman, J.R. (2001). Development of an animal model for prostate cancer cell metastasis to adult human bone. *Anticancer Research,* Vol. 21, No. 2A, (March-April, 2001), pp. 971-978, ISSN 0250-7005

Tsingotjidou, A.S., Emmanouilides, C.E., Siotou, E., Poutahidis, T., Xagorari, A., Loukopoulos, P., Sotiropoulos, D., Bekiari, C., Doulberis, M., Givissis, P., Fassas, A. & Anagnostopoulos, A. (2009). Establishment of an animal model for Waldenström's macroglobulinemia. *Experimental Hematology,* Vol. 37, No.4, (April, 2009), pp. 469-476, ISSN 0301-472X

U.S. Cancer Statistics Working group. Statistics Working Group (2009). United States Cancer Statistics: 1999–2005 Incidence and Mortality Web-based Report. Atlanta: U.S.

Department of Health and Human Services, Centers for Disease Control and Prevention and National Cancer Institute. Available from: www.cdc.gov/uscs

van Esser, J.W., Niesters, H.G., van der Holt, B., Meijer, E., Osterhaus, A.D., Gratama, J.W., Verdonck, L.F., Löwenberg, B. & Cornelissen, J.J. (2002). Prevention of Epstein-Barr virus-lymphoproliferative disease by molecular monitoring and preemptive rituximab in high-risk patients after allogeneic stem cell transplantation. *Blood,* Vol. 99, No. 12, (June, 2002), pp. 4364-4369, ISSN 0006-4971

Vijay, A. & Gertz, M.A. (2007). Waldenström macroglobulinemia. *Blood,* Vol. 109, No. 12, (June, 2007), pp. 5096-5103, ISSN 0006-4971

Virgilio, L., Lazzeri, C., Bichi, R., Nibu, K., Narducci, M.G., Russo G., Rothstein, J.L. & Croce C. M. (1998). Deregulated expression of TCL1 causes T cell leukemia in mice. *Proceedings of the National Academy of Sciences* USA, Vol. 95, No. 7, (March, 1998), pp. 3885–3889, ISSN 0027-8424

Waldenström, J. (1944). Incipient myelomatosis or 'essential' hyperglobulinemia with fibrinogenopenia: a new syndrome? *Acta Medica Scandinavica,* Vol. 117, pp. 216–222, ISSN 0001-6101

Watson, L., Wyld, P. & Catovsky D. (2008). Disease burden of chronic lymphocytic leukaemia within the European Union. *European Journal of Haematology,* Vol. 81, No. 4, (December 2008), pp. 253–258, ISSN 0902-4441

World Health Organization (2010), "Disease and injury regional estimates for 2004". Available from: http://www.who.int/healthinfo/global_burden_disease/estimates_regional/en/index.html

Witherspoon, R.P., Fisher, L.D., Schoch, G., Martin, P., Sullivan, K.M., Sanders, J., Deeg, H.J., Doney, K., Thomas, D., Storb, R. & Thomas, E.D. (1989). Secondary cancers after bone marrow transplantation for leukemia or aplastic anemia. *New England Journal of Medicine,* Vol. 321, No. 12, (September, 1989), pp. 784-789, ISSN 0028-4793

Yaccoby, S., Barlogie, B. & Epstein, J. (1998). Primary myeloma cells growing in SCID-hu mice: a model for studying the biology and treatment of myeloma and its manifestations. *Blood,* Vol. 92, No. 8, (October, 1998), pp. 2908-2913, ISSN 0006-4971

Yaccoby, S. & Epstein, J. (1999). The proliferative potential of myeloma plasma cells manifest in the SCID-hu host. *Blood.,* Vol. 94, No. 10, (November, 1999), pp. 3576–3582, ISSN 0006-4971

Yaccoby, S, Pearse, R.N., Johnson, C.L., Barlogie, B., Choi, Y. & Epstein, J. (2002). Myeloma interacts with the bone marrow microenvironment to induce osteoclastogenesis and is dependent on osteoclast activity. *British Journal of Haematology,* Vol. 116, No. 2, (February, 2002), pp. 278–290, ISSN 0007-1048

Yaccoby, S., Wezeman, M.J., Zangari, M., Walker, R., Cottler-Fox, M., Gaddy, D., Ling, W., Saha, R., Barlogie, B., Tricot, G., & Epstein, J. (2006). Inhibitory effects of osteoblasts and increased bone formation on myeloma in novel culture systems and a myelomatous mouse model. *Haematologica, Vol.* 91, No. 2, (February, 2006), pp. 192–199, ISSN 0390-6078

Yaccoby, S, Ling, W., Zhan, F., Walker, R., Barlogie, B., Shaughnessy, J.D. Jr. (2007). Antibody-based inhibition of DKK1 suppresses tumor-induced bone resorption and multiple myeloma growth in vivo. *Blood.,* Vol. 109, No. 5, (March 2007), pp: 2106-2111, ISSN 0006-4971

Yata, K., & Yaccoby, S. (2004). The SCID-rab model: a novel in vivo system for primary human myeloma demonstrating growth of CD138-expressing malignant cells. *Leukemia,* Vol.18, No. 11, (November 2004), pp.1891–1897, ISSN 0887-6924.

Yonou, H., Yokose, T., Kamijo, T., Kanomata, N., Hasebe, T., Nagai, K., Hatano, T., Ogawa, Y. & Ochiai, A. (2001). Establishment of a novel species- and tissue-specific metastasis model of human prostate cancer in humanized non-obese diabetic/severe combined immunodeficient mice engrafted with human adult lung and bone. *Cancer Research,* Vol. 61, No. 5, (March, 2001), pp. 2177-2282, ISSN 0008-5472

Yu, B.H., Zhou, X.Y., Zhang, T.C., Zhang, T.M. & Shi, D.R. (2011). Establishment and characterization of a nude mice model of human diffuse large B-cell lymphoma. *Chinese Journal of Pathology* (*Zhonghua Bing Li Xue Za Zhi.),* Vol. 40, No. 4, (April, 2011), pp. 246-250, ISSN 0529-5807

Yun, J.P., Behan, J.W., Heisterkamp, N., Butturini, A., Klemm, L., Ji, L., Groffen, J., Müschen, M. & Mittelman S.D. (2010). Diet-induced obesity accelerates acute lymphoblastic leukemia progression in two murine models. *Cancer Prevention Research (Philadelphia, PA).,* Vol. 3, No. 10, (October, 2010), pp. 1259-1264, ISSN 1940-6215

Zhang, J., Xiao, Y., Guo, Y., Breslin, P., Zhang, S., Wei, W,, Zhang. Z. & Zhang, J. (2011). Differential requirements for c-Myc in chronic hematopoietic hyperplasia and acute hematopoietic malignancies in Pten-null mice. *Leukemia,* Sep. 16. doi: 10.1038/leu.2011.220, ISSN 0887-692

18

Systemic Mastocytosis: An Intriguing Disorder

Antonia Rotolo[1], Ubaldo Familiari[2], Paolo Nicoli[1], Daniela Cilloni[1], Giuseppe Saglio[1] and Angelo Guerrasio[1]
[1]*M.D., Division of Hematology and Internal Medicine,*
[2]*M.D., Pathology Department,*
Department of Clinical and Biological Sciences,
San Luigi Gonzaga Hospital, University of Turin, Turin,
Italy

1. Introduction

Systemic Mastocytosis (SM) is a mast cell (MC) neoplasm of the haematopoietic tissue. It is a rare disorder, but perhaps its prevalence is underestimated, as MC infiltrates may often be undetected. The aim of this chapter is to emphasize the importance of an active and careful work-up through multimodality approaches in order to achieve the diagnosis of SM. This might increase the incidence of SM. Moreover, it must be considered that SM is frequently associated with a second and, in rare cases, a third clonal blood disorder that isn't mast cell derived. Similar cases may be important for the correct initial evaluation and classification, as well as for a better risk stratification and management of patients with haematopoietic malignancies. Therapy could also improve, being personalized and tailored for each single SM patient.

2. Disease overview

Mastocytosis is a disorder characterised by clonal mast cells (MC) proliferation and accumulation. It has been described for the first time in 1869 by Nettleship and Tay as a form of urticaria resulting in a "brownish discoloration". Some years later Ehrlich used "mastzellen" to designate MC (Ehrlich, 1877). The term is derived from the German mästung, that means "to overfeed". In fact, the MCs have metachromatic properties that have been originally attributed to an excessive intake of aniline dye. In 1949 Ellis reported the first observation of MCs infiltrating visceral organs. Hence, several reports allowed standardizing the definition and classification of Mastocytosis.

According to the latest WHO classification Mastocytosis is a myeloproliferative neoplasm (MPN) (Vardiman, 2009). Clonal MCs proliferate, infiltrate and accumulate in skin and/or other organ systems. In Cutaneous Mastocytosis (CM) only skin is involved. In Systemic Mastocytosis (SM) at least one extracutaneous organ is infiltrated. This leads to a heterogeneous clinical presentation.

2.1 Epidemiology

Mastocytosis is a rare disorder. Several studies reported an incidence of 5-10 cases/10^6 people/year. However, there's a risk of underestimation due to the difficulty in getting a diagnosis. Recently Nowak et al. have published results of a monocentric retrospective study, reporting that in most patients mastocytosis was correctly diagnosed over a period of 2 years (up to 11 years in some cases), and often required consultation of three or more clinicians (Nowak, 2011). This was consistent with experiences reported by other authors. There are several possible explanations for such diagnostic delays. First, initial symptoms and signs are usually unspecific and overlap with many other diseases. For instance, at presentation some patients show neurological, psychological and psychiatric symptoms, leading to a misdiagnosis of somatoform disorder instead of mast cell syndrome (Amon, 2010). Second, morphological detection of pathological MCs is not obvious, mainly if they exhibit atypical features, such as hypogranulation or abnormal nuclear morphology (Pardanani, 2011). Moreover, as the second most frequent MC disorder is SM associated with haematological non mast cell disorder (SM-AHNMD), extensive bone marrow involvement by a second haematological neoplasm may obscure or distort MC aggregates (Horny, 2004), delaying or obviating at all the correct diagnosis. Taken together, these observations suggest that clinicians should become more confident with MC syndrome and MC disorders, as clinical suspicion should stimulate further appropriate immunochemical and molecular analysis. According to this, Horny proposed a novel routine approach, using antibodies against neoplastic MC markers in all bone marrow trephines presenting Myelodisplastic Syndrome, Acute Myeloid Leukemia and Chronic Myelomonocytic Leukemia (Horny, 2004).

Mastocytosis is more frequent in children, as CM. Adults represent one third of all cases and they are almost all affected by SM. There are no gender differences in incidence rate and clinical presentation. It can onset at any age, with an incidence peak in the first 2 years of life (Pardanani, 2011). Familiar cases have been occasionally observed. Survival is shorter in SM compared to the general population. However, patients classified according to the WHO 2008 system classification show great differences in demographical and clinical features, prognosis and survival (Lim, 2009). Nevertheless, quality of life is generally poor irrespective to subgroups.

3. Mast cells

Typical MCs are round or oval cells. Their size is small to medium, with a low nucleus/cytoplasm ratio. The nucleus is round or oval, in a central position, with condensed chromatin. The cytoplasm is large with plenty of metachromatic granules. However granules may also be few or lack at all, resulting in hypo-/de-granulated mast cells. Atypical MCs may present an oval nucleus and a hypogranulated cytoplasm. Generally they are spindle-shaped or with prominent projections on membrane surface and their nucleus is eccentric, sometimes with two or more lobes. Cells may appear more immature, with a large size, a high nucleus/cytoplasm ratio and a dispersed chromatin with nucleoli. The grade of immatureness may allow to the diagnosis of mast lineage blasts, characterized by the virtual absence of cytoplasm, with or without metachromatic granules, and fine chromatin with nucleoli.

3.1 Mast cell physiology

Mastocyte is a cell of the immune system. It derives from the haematopoietic stem cell. It is preferentially localized in the skin, respiratory and gastrointestinal mucosa.

MC growth, differentiation, proliferation, survival and activation are mediated by several factors The most important is SCF, that interacts with the tyrosine kinase receptor KIT (CD117 antigen). KIT is a key protein, either in normal or in clonal MCs, and its detection is essential in order to identify MCs and achieve the diagnosis of mastocytosis. Therefore, a multimodality approach should be routinely performed, including flow cytometry, immunochemistry and PCR (see below).

MCs play a main role in type I hypersensitivity reactions. Antigen-IgE complexes bind to the $Fc_{\varepsilon}RI$ on MC membrane and induce MC degranulation. Secretory granules contain histamine, tryptase, proteoglycans, TNF-α and other proteases. Tryptase is the most important mediator: it is virtually present in all MCs, therefore its expression on membrane surface identifies MCs, and serum levels may represent a useful marker of disease (see below).

After MC activation and degranulation, new phospholipid derived mediators are generated (e.g. leukotrienes, prostaglandins and PAF). The clinical manifestations are therefore heterogeneous and depend on the site of reaction. Atopic responses may vary in severeness between transient urticarial eruption and life-threatening anaphylactic shock. Several dermal inflammatory diseases are MC mediated, e.g. atopic dermatitis, bullous pemphigoid and psoriasis. However, MCs have also important physiological fuctions, as they are involved in antimicrobial defense, wound healing, angiogenesis, tumor surveillance and graft tollerance.

4. Pathogenesis

In more than 90% of affected adults a recurrent somatic mutation of *kit* can be detected (Garcia-Montero et al, 2006), suggesting that KIT plays a central role in autonomous proliferation of MC clone as well as in normal mastocytes (Orfao et al., 2007). Usually mutation occurs on exon 17 and results in a substitution of aspartic acid at codon 816 with valine. This mutation affects the tyrosine kinase TK2 domain and activates the receptor independently on ligand binding and dimerisation. According to its high occurrence, WHO diagnostic criteria for SM include *kit*D816V screening. Thus, it should be always investigated in bone marrow or blood or other organs when mastocytosis is suspected. Moreover, *kit*D816V represents an important prognostic factor and should be considered for planning and personalizing the therapeutic strategy.

The same mutation is less frequent in children, with an incidence of 42%. However, also most of the affected children share somatic *kit* point mutations that often involve exon 8 or 9, resulting in changes of the extracellular part of receptor (Bodemer, 2009).

Other mutations have been reported: they usually cluster at exon 11 or 17 affecting the juxtamembrane regulatory domain or TK2 enzymatic domain. Sometimes they've been reported at exons 2, 8, 9, 13 or 14 involving extracellular or TK1 domains. Interestingly, it has been observed a significant correlation between mutation type and disorder class. In fact, these specific genetic alterations have not been detected in different *kit* related neoplasms (e.g. GIST) and seem to be strictly associated with MC disorders (Orfao et al., 2007).

As *kit* is mutated in most patients without subgroup differences, the heterogeneous behaviour of each variant suggests that perhaps several different pathways may be involved in the pathogenesis and progression of the disease. Some authors have demonstrated that NF-κB and cyclin D3 may play a role. (Tanaka A, 2005). In addition, since a second haematological neoplasm is often associated with SM, the pathogenic mechanisms can be more difficult to understand.

Several studies suggests that mastocytosis is a haematopoietic stem cell disease (Horny, 2008). It can be hypothesized that *kit* mutation occurs at the level of leukaemia stem cell, the original clone that is responsible of leukaemia relapse. The occurrence of *kit* mutation confers either proliferative or mast cell lineage differentiative potential. Additional aberrations can then occur in the leukaemia stem cell, leading to the development of the associated myeloid neoplasm. Another possibility is the acquisition of *kit* mutation and transformation of a more mature leukaemia progenitor, resulting in the development of a synchronous mast cell malignancy (Pullarkat, 2003). Even less mature progenitors may be involved as also intra- and peri-lesional B and T cells have been demonstrated to carry the *kit*D816V point mutation. However, in SM patients without any associated clonal lymphoid disease most of the lymphocytes are reactive oligoclonal cells.

5. Clinical findings

Clinical features and course are variable, depending on the site and degree of infiltration and WHO subvariant.

Skin is often involved. Pruritus, erithema and orticarioid lesions usually occurs after mechanic irritation (Darier's sign). Hypercromic and infiltrated lesions affect body trunk, upper and lower limbs in 80% of adults, and head in all children. A frequent symptom is hypotension, often with headache and flushing, sometimes of high grade, resulting in syncope and shock. Diarrhoea is very common, with abdominal pain. Sometimes malabsorption cause a severe worseness of general conditions and must be considered clinically equivalent to organ damage. Bone is always involved: usually patients complain of bone pain, with signs of osteopenia, osteoporosis or atypical atraumatic fracture. Bone marrow infiltration may result in pancytopenia. Organomegaly, in particular enlargement of the lymph nodes, spleen and liver, may be present and causes organ damage (hepatic failure, low levels of albumin, etc.). Neuropsychiatric symptoms could be prevalent at diagnosis and they can be related to disfigurement in appearance: depression, suicide ideation, social and professional inefficiency have been reported (Amon, 2010). Risk of anaphylaxis is increased compared with health population, especially after a trigger exposition (physical exercise, psychic stress, alcohol, NSAID, infections and pregnancy) wich can result in MC activation. Based on this, it is recommended to perform a complete work-up after a first case of a severe anaphylactic reaction, especially in the absence of an evident trigger. Finally, there is a high risk of peptic ulcer. Patients must be closed monitored for all these symptoms in order to prevent complications and improve quality of life with anti-mediator drugs. Moreover, recording symptoms is a key part of staging, as established by WHO, and should drive the correct treatment choice and timing (WHO 2008).

Practically, two groups of clinical findings have been defined, the B and the C group. (Table 1). B stands for "burden of disease" and refers to symptoms that reflect the extension of disease. C stands for "cytoreduction requiring" and refers to signs of organ impairment indicating the need of therapy with cytostatic drugs.

C-findings are due to extensive MC infiltration, with direct organ damage and tissue destruction. The presence of at least one C-finding denotes a high grade disorder, referred as advanced systemic mastocytosis. After excluding any other causes of organ failure, cytoreduction must be considered. Symptoms due to MC infiltrates may be difficult to distinguish from indirect symptoms due to massive mediator release. When relationship between MC infiltration and organ impairment is not clear, patients must be closed monitored with serial dosages of serum tryptase level. An increase trend confirms the progression of the disease and the need of cytoreduction. CD30 expression may also be of help, since a strong positivity in most MCs denotes more likely ASM and MCL, while a weak positivity suggests a diagnosis of ISM. According to this, CD30 may perhaps become a useful tool in grading SM (Valent, 2010).

B-findings related to MC mediators	C-findings due to direct MC infiltration	Organ failure
1. **High MC burden**	**Organopathy**	
Marrow MCs > 30%		
Serum tryptase >200ng/ml		
2. **Dysmyelopoiesis**		
Hypercellular marrow with signs of myelodisplasia or myeloproliferation	Dysmyelopoiesis, with one or more peripheral cytopenias	Severe progressive pancytopenia
3. **Palpable Organomegaly**		
Hepatomegaly	Hepatomegaly with - ascites - abnormal liver function tests - portal hypertension	Progression to liver failure
Splenomegaly	Splenomegaly, with hypersplenism	
Lymph node enlargement	Bone lesions, with - osteolysis - osteoporosis and pathologic fractures	
	Malabsorption, with - hypoalbuminemia - weight loss.	

Table 1. Clinical findings (adapted from Valent *et al.*, 2001).

6. Diagnosis

Mastocytosis must be suspected.

WHO updated diagnostic criteria in 2008. The demonstration of neoplastic MC infiltrates in skin or extracutaneous organ is the *condition sine qua non*. The presence of typical MCs in dermal multifocal aggregates or diffusely infiltrating the skin allows the diagnosis of CM. The involvement of at least one visceral organ denotes SM. However, other criteria must be satisfied, i.e. clinical or biochemical, morphologic, immunophenotypic, molecular (Table 2). This is important to distinguish between any reactive MC proliferation and true clonal MC proliferation, that means Mast Cell Activation Syndrome (MCAS) from Mastocytosis.

Cutaneous mastocytosis (CM) usually presents as maculopapular infiltrates or diffuse erythrodermic rash, with thick skin or multiple nodules. Skin lesions must be biopsied to demonstrate the co-existence of pathological MCs.

The suspicion of mast cell syndrome without any cutaneous signs exclude the diagnosis of CM and requires bone marrow analysis to investigate the possible diagnosis of systemic mastocytosis (SM). Bone marrow biopsy and aspiration should always be performed in such cases as SM involves bone marrow in almost all affected patients. Other specimens may be obtained from other involved organs.

Pathological MCs infiltrates result as aggregates of at least 15 tryptase positive MCs. This is the first major criterion. The following diagnostic steps are BM smear evaluation, flow cytometry characterization and KIT mutational analysis. Finally serum tryptase levels must be dosed.

Cutaneous Mastocytosis	**Typical skin lesions**
• Clinical signs	- Maculopapular cutaneous mastocytosis - Diffuse cutaneous mastocytosis - Mastocytoma
• Microscopic findings	Multifocal or diffuse MC infiltrates
Systemic Mastocytosis	**SM criteria = 1 major + 1 minor or 3 minor criteria**
• Major criterion	Infiltrates of >15 aggregated MCs identified through tryptase immune-histochemistry or other stains in sections obtained from bone marrow or other extracutaneous organs
• Minor criteria	More than 25% spindle shaped MCs in histological sections or more than 25% atypical MCs in BM smear
	Detection of *kit* 816 mutation in BM or blood or any extracutaneous organ
	MC coexpression of CD25 and/or CD2 with CD117
	Serum tryptase levels > 20 ng/ml

Table 2. Proposed criteria to diagnose Mastocytosis (adapted from Valent *et al.*, 2001).

6.1 Histology

The typical histological mast cell lesion consists in focal typical and atypical MC aggregates infiltrating tissues. Giemsa or toluidine blue stains can reveal metachromatic granules, allowing discriminating between spindle mastocytes and fibroblasts.

Skin lesions are characterized by perivascular and periadnexal MC accumulation in upper dermis (Amon, 2010). In bone marrow compact infiltrates are perivascular, sharply demarcated from normal tissue, sometimes intermingled with macrophages and eosinophils. Spindle shaped MCs are often more than 25% of the total MCs. Rarely, infiltration is diffuse, with scattered cells that are difficult to recognize. In particular, in SM-AHNMD it is not unusual for the SM component to be unrecognized due to the extensive infiltration of bone marrow by the AHNMD component. This is commonly seen, for example, in SM-acute leukemia and SM with intense eosinophilic infiltration. Monotonous sheets of blasts may help to detect isolated clonal MCs (Horny, 2004). On the contrary, infiltration due to either reactive benign-looking lymphocytes or low grade lymphomatous cells is usually well defined and spindle mast cells cluster in different nodular lesions (Du, 2010). In some cases reactive well-differentiated lymphocytes have been reported to surround central aggregates of clonal mast cells or to be enclosed within malignant mast cells lesions (Kim, 2010). It must be clearly realized that MCs largely infiltrating malignant cells in haematopoietic disorders are clonal in most synchronous myeloid neoplasia, while they are reactive in all described lymphoid associated disorders so far reported. However, our group observed a case that may perhaps represent the first reported exception to this rule (see below).

Immunochemistry is important to recognize clonal MCs and get the right diagnosis. Spindle-shaped instead of round mast cells are more likely pathological and immunochemical reactions demonstrating co-expression of KIT, tryptase and CD25 enhance the probability of the clonal nature of the MCs (Pardanani et al., 2011).

6.2 Immunophenotyping

Flow cytometry represents the gold standard to identify, enumerate and characterise human MCs. The co-expression of CD2 and/or CD25 with CD117 is a minor WHO criterion to diagnose SM (Valent et al, 2010).

6.3 Molecular studies

Routine diagnostics should include the screening for *kit*D816V. Highly sensitive techniques (e.g. PCR) are recommended as the detection of this specific somatic mutation has been recognized as a valid minor diagnostic criterion by WHO system. *kit*D816V may be found also in myeloid and, less frequently, in lymphoid cells associated within the focal MC lesions, particularly in ASM and MCL. On the contrary, the same finding is rare in SM-AHNMD and depends on the concomitant disorder. In fact, the occurrence of *kit*D816V decreases through CMML, MPN, AML and lymphoproliferative disorders respectively.

Identification of different genetic abnormalities is not requested, since it does not have clinical relevance either for diagnosis or for therapy. However, in case of blood eosinophilia clinicians must consider screening for FIP1L1-PDGFRA fusion protein, since it predicts a great response to imatinib. Other rearrangements involving PDGFRB may be appropriately investigated through conventional cytogenetic analysis, allowing to the diagnosis of the entity defined by WHO as myeloid or lymphoid neoplasms with eosinophilia and abnormalities of PDGFRA, PDGFRB or FGFR1 (WHO 2008).

6.4 Biochemistry

Serum tryptase dosage and levels monitoring are a useful tools for diagnosis (WHO 2008) and follow-up, as they correlate with MC load and activation and disease progression (Pardanani, 2011). Elevated levels of serum tryptase (>20ng/ml) are consistent with the diagnosis, representing the fourth validated minor criterion to be evaluated according WHO system. Very high levels (>200ng/ml) correlate with more aggressive subvariants, severe course and poor prognosis. Anyway, serum tryptase levels are not clinically significant in case of a concomitant myeloid disorder as a proportion of patients affected by AML, CML and MDS usually show high levels of tryptase without any detectable MC disorder.

Serial dosages are recommended after anaphylactic or anaphylactoid episodes to distinguish between a transient elevation and an abnormal persistent increase. In addition, stable levels during follow up are consistent with stable disease (Quintas-Cardama et al., Cancer 2006).

6.5 Further considerations

SM diagnosis requires the presence of the major criterion together with one minor criterion or three isolated minor criteria (Table 2). Subvariants may be classified depending on the percentage of MCs in BM and PB smears and the clinical presentation. More than 20% MCs in BM smear denotes MCL, in the leukemic or aleukemic (more or less than 10% MC in PB smear) subvariants. Less than 20% MCs in BM smear connotes ISM in asymptomatic patients, SSM or ASM in patients suffering from B- or C-findings respectively.

A cytomorphological grading system has been also proposed (Valent et al., 2001). At BM smear analysis MCs may be typical or atypical. Atypical MCs are classified either type I or type II according to the nuclear feature, oval or bi-/polylobed respectively. The proportion of atypical MCs together with metachromatic blasts define the grade of the disorder: high grade > 20%, low grade < 10%, intermediate grade 10-20% MCs (Valent et al., 2001).

There are some peculiar conditions to be considered. First, sometimes a focal MC infiltrate is found without any MC related symptom or sign and coexists with normal skin and bone marrow, denoting a finding of MC tumour. If the growth pattern is destructive and the cytopathologycal grade is high, the diagnosis is of MC sarcoma. Otherwise, a low grade morphology and a respected tissue architecture denotes benign mastocytomas.

Second, MC aggregates may be scattered. This finding is often consistent with reactive MC hyperplasia and occasionally may be observed during the diagnostic approach for non MC hematologic diseases. A WHO entity is SM-AHNMD, where a myelo-/lymphoproliferative disorder coexists with a clonal MC growth. Myeloid neoplasms usually share the peculiar pattern of diffuse cells proliferation admixed with malignant mast cells, on the contrary lymphoid clones are clearly distinct, with a well-cut separation between the two clonal components, and generally the demonstration of SM in the bone marrow is an occasional histological finding in patients with a previous diagnosis of LNH in a lymph node (Schipper et al, 2011). Thus, a diffuse MC infiltration in the fields of LNH always suggests a reactive MC hyperplasia (Valent, 2001).

Also AHNMD is recommended to be investigated for biomolecular markers, in order to get a complete characterization and evaluate the event of therapeutic targets.

With regard to MCL, histology must refer to bone marrow areas away from spicules and the proportion of blasts must be cytomorphologically evaluated on the bone marrow smear. Thus histological detection of even more than 20% of blasts is not enough to make a diagnosis of MCL (Valent, 2010).

7. Classification and prognosis

MC disorders are classified in two groups: cutaneous and systemic. The former seems to have a good prognosis (Koga et al., 2011), the latter shows a poor prognosis. More precisely, in case of systemic involvement the observed survival is shorter than general population. The median overall survival is about 5 years (Pardanani et al., 2009), with excess deaths occurring between the third and the fifth year after diagnosis (Pardanani et al., 2011). However, prognosis is heterogeneous among SM subgroups and correlates with the WHO system. In fact, stratifying by the WHO classes, the Kaplan-Meier analysis allows distinguishing between an indolent and a rapidly progressive course. In the first case there is not a significant difference between affected patients and matched controls. By contrast, in the so-called aggressive forms median survival ranges between 2 and 41 months, depending on the variant (Pardanani et al. 2009).

7.1 CM

Cutaneous mastocytosis (CM) is a disorder characterized by accumulation of clonal mast cells isolated in the skin. Dermatologists are used to differentiate some clinical variants based on macroscopic presentation. Maculopapular Cutaneous Mastocytosis denotes the most frequent form, often described as urticaria pigmentosa (UP). It is the typical manifestation of CM, with disseminated small plaques. Sometimes lesions limits appear undefined and skin may be extensively involved, leading to the clinical condition referred as Diffuse Cutaneous Mastocytosis. Children rather than adults may carry a single blistering lesion known as solitary Mastocytoma, that generally goes to spontaneous regression with time. Other rare variants occur almost exclusively during childhood, with aspects of infiltration (bullae, plaques or nodules) or hyperpigmentation (Telangiectasia Macularis Eruptiva Perstans or TMEP) with or without erythema (Amon et al., 2010).

7.2 SM

Systemic mastocytosis (SM) is a disorder classified among Myeloproliferative Neoplasms by WHO in 2008. Unlike CM, clinical SM variants have been universally accepted and included in the international classification system since 2001. In addition, in 2010 Pardanani et al. published results of an observational study on 342 patients, leading to a formal validation of the WHO classification. Thus, SM subgroups are clinical evidence-based entities, with clear definition, characteristic features, definite prognosis and tailored management indications, beyond the clinical usage.

7.2.1 ISM

Indolent systemic mastocytosis (ISM) is the most frequent variant in adults (46%). Patients are young (median age 49) and usually show urticarioid skin lesions, gastrointestinal symptoms and MC mediator related syndrome. Almost all affected patients show bone marrow involvement, but no B- nor C- findings. Prognosis is very good, life expectancy is similar to general population, but quality of life is definitely poor. No progression risk has been observed, thus no cytoreduction has to be considered and only management of symptoms is needed (Valent et al., 2010).

7.2.2 SSM

Smoldering systemic mastocytosis is a recent subvariant of ISM. B-findings are always present, C-findings never. It is defined by high burden of MC (tryptase levels more than 200 ng/mL), enlarged spleen and/or lymph nodes, multilineage myelodysplasia or myeloid proliferation in the absence of diagnostic criteria for MDS, MPD, LMMC or AML. c-kit D816V should be detected in at least one non MC lineage. 14% of the patients with ISM are SSM affected individuals. They are older than typical ISM variant. Constitutional symptoms are almost constant. 23% patients are affected by a subvariant defined by isolated bone marrow involvement (BMM, Bone Marrow Mastocytosis), often associated with severe MC mediators related syndrome, including anaphylaxis. Prognosis is good, expected survival is even more than ten years, so symptomatic treatment may be enough. However, it must be stated that median survival is significantly inferior in SSM than in ISM (120 *versus* 301 months respectively). Moreover, there is an up to 18% risk of progression to aggressive subvariants as ASM, MCL and SM-AHNMD. Thus, patients must be strictly monitored, in order to switch to a cytoreductive therapeutic program if required. Cytoreduction is indicated even in absence of aggressive SM variants, if tryptase reach levels greater than 1000 ng/mL or symptoms show a worsening trend. Also, recurrent anaphylaxis unresponsive to immunotherapy or without specific IgE suggests that splenectomy or cytoreduction are needed for a better control of MC burden. This is in order to prevent a severe adverse event, as well as in myeloproliferative disorders hydroxyurea is administered to prevent deep venous thrombosis/pulmonary embolism (Valent et al., 2010).

7.2.3 ASM

Aggressive systemic mastocytosis is less frequent (12%) and occurs generally in adults. It is defined by the presence of at least one C-finding, associated with constitutional symptoms and visceromegaly, particularly of liver, spleen and lymph nodes. Prognosis is poor, with an overall median survival of 41 months. Leukemic transformation occurs in 5% of the patients. Affected patients must be always treated. Treatment depends on clinical course. According to time to progression, patients should be stratified in slowly and rapidly progressing. In the first case the natural history is similar to SSM. In the second case the disease is difficult to control and its behavior is similar to MCL: early blasts may increase, satisfying diagnostic criteria for leukemia. In addition, in some *kit*D816V patients the same mutation may become undetectable with progression. This is somewhat similar to disease progression in acute myeloid leukemia. In slowly progressing ASM milder therapeutic options may be considered, while rapidly progressing ASM always requires heavy chemotherapeutic approaches, according to the rapid multiorgan failure occurring in such patients. Tryptase levels usually increase every day, reflecting the poor clinical course (Valent et al., 2010).

7.2.4 MCL

Mast cell leukemia is the most rare variant, virtually limited to adulthood. In Pardanani's analysis it occurred in 1% of the patients. Median survival is 2 months. Usually MC blasts infiltrate extensively BM, with a range of 60-90%. High intensity chemiotherapy has to be administered, but patients generally result refractory (Valent et al., 2010).

7.2.5 SM-AHNMD

Systemic mastocytosis with an associated non-mast cell lineage disease (SM-AHNMD) is an heterogeneous and intriguing group of haematological malignancies, in which clonal proliferation of mast cells is associated with a second and, in rare cases, a third (Kim, 2010) clonal blood disorder that is not mast cell derived (Horny, 2008; Pardanani, 2010).

SM-AHNMD accounts for 40% of all cases of SM. About 89% of the patients show concomitant myeloid neoplasms: MPN (45%), CMML (29%) and MDS (23%). Among MPN, there is a high prevalence FIP1L1-PDGFRA related HES. In the remaining cases (21%) SM is associated with lymphoma, myeloma, CLL or amyloidosis. Prognosis is poor, with a median overall survival of 31 months in patients with MPN compared to 15, 13 and 11 months in patients with CMML, MDS and AML respectively. Transformation in MC leukemia occurs more frequently in SM-MDS (29%) (Pardanani, 2010).

WHO diagnostic criteria for SM remain valid, except for elevated serum tryptase levels, as they could be very high also in patients affected by AML, MDS and MPS without MC disorders.

The pathogenesis is not clear: in SM associated with myeloid malignancies mast cells and myeloid cells seem to originate from the same clone (Pardanani, 2009; Garcia-Montero 2006); according to this, in SM-LMMC *kit*D816V has been shown in both components. However, in SM-AML the leukemic counterpart generally lacks of *kit* mutation, suggesting a different origin for the two clones. At the opposite, in SM associated with lymphoid proliferative disease a distinct clonal origin has been demonstrated at least in some cases (Kim, 2007). Moreover, it has been hypothesized that malignant mast cells may support and promote the growth of the associated lymphoid disorder (Merluzzi, 2010).

Lymphoid proliferation as AHNMD component has been rarely observed. More precisely, B cell lymphomas associated with SM usually are low grade. To the best of our knowledge, the occurrence of SM and synchronous high grade lymphoma has been reported so far only by Schipper *et al.*, which described a case of SM associated with diffuse large B cell lymphoma (SM-DLBCL) (Schipper, 2011). Interestingly, we observed another patient, which is unlike to represent an accidental case. In our patient the diagnosis of mast cell disease was made concurrently with that of lymphoma, but we cannot state whether both the malignancies were synchronous or occurred at different time. In addition, the morphological evaluation of the bone marrow revealed a peculiar pattern of diffuse large B-cells proliferation admixed with malignant mast cells (fig. 1). Compared to what we observed, in Schipper *et al.* reported a sharp separation between the two clonal components, with the histological demonstration of SM in the bone marrow and DLBCL in a lymph node at different time. According to typical morphological findings, mastocytes appeared either solitary or clustered in a separate contest from malignant B cell. By contrast, our case of SM with concurrent large cell lymphoma seems to be unusual because of the great overlap between the two clonal populations of large B lymphocytes and mastocytes. Indeed, in our case, the lymphoid component resulted histologically atypical and new, as diffusely infiltrating within the malignant proliferating mast cells.

As expected, our case was positive for the D816V mutation in exon 17 like the vast majority of SM. Unfortunately, we do not know whether this mutation occurred also in clonal B cells, since they were not sorted from bone marrow specimen for DNA extraction. Therefore it is not possible to rule out any hypothesis about the pathogenesis of such an association.

On the therapeutical side, in SM-AHNMD it is recommended to treat SM as pure SM and AHNMD as pure AHNMD (Valent, 2003; Valent 2010). Accordingly, it is important a complete molecular characterization of both the disorders (Valent et al., 2010).

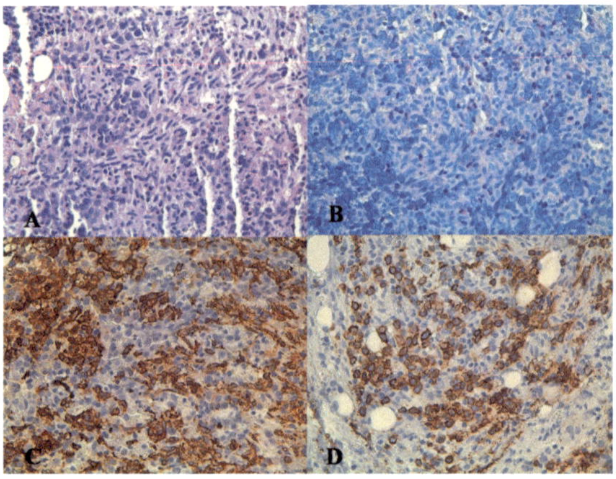

Fig. 1. **A-B** Bone marrow sections stained with haematoxylin and eosin (A) and Giemsa (B), 40x. **C-D** Immunohistochemistry on bone marrow sections with antibodies against tryptase to detect mast cells (C) and antibodies against CD79a to detect B lymphocytes (D), 40x. A great overlap between lymphocytes and mast cells lesions is observed, resulting in a diffuse proliferation of B-cells admixed with mast cells.

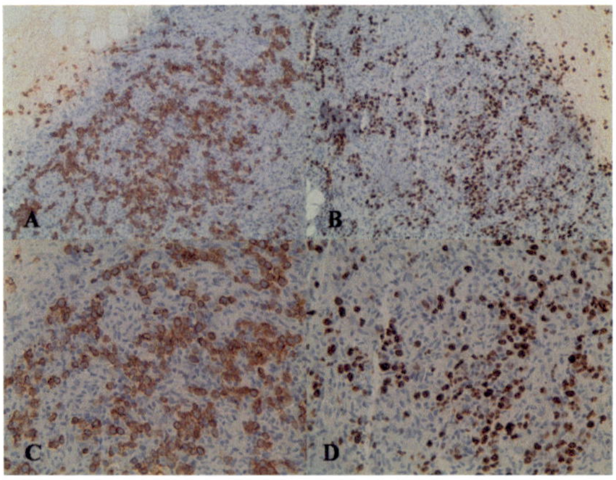

Fig. 2. Immunoperoxidase staining detecting large B lymphocytes, positive for CD79a (A, 20x; C, 40x) and exhibiting nuclear Ki-67 reactivity (B, 20x; D, 40x).

8. Treatment

To date Mastocytosis is incurable, thus clinicians should personalize treatment for each patients in order to reduce symptoms and complications (Molderings et al., 2011).

Exposition to triggers (animal venoms, extreme temperatures, mechanical irritation, alcohol, medications, etc.) should be avoided, but often no clear trigger may be identified, therefore active therapy must be considered (Valent et al., 2010).

Treatment in Mastocytosis may be symptomatic or cytoreductive. Symptoms could be managed with both non specific and tailored drugs. Cytoreduction should be considered if symptoms are refractory to basic therapy, rapidly worsening or life-threatening, or in the presence of complications (C-finding).

In summary, in CM and ISM therapeutic approach may be just symptomatic. In advanced forms of SM schedules must be personalized, depending on progression risk. In SSM and slowly progressing ASM IFNα and 2CdA may be appropriated. In rapidly progressing ASM, MCL and SM-AHNMD high intensity chemotherapy and allogeneic bone marrow transplantation represent the current therapeutic approach.

8.1 Symptomatic treatment

The so-called basic therapy consists in antihistaminic medications and MC membrane stabilizers. Usually relief occurs many days or weeks after the introduction of a new drug, therefore the persistence of symptoms does not justify an earlier shift to others therapeutic schedules. As each new drug can trigger a hypersensitive reaction, one drug at a time should be introduced (Quintas-Cardama et al., 2006).

When first line fails, immunomodulating agents may be considered, such as prednisone, cyclosporine, methotrexate, and azathioprine (Quintas-Cardama et al., 2006). IFNα might be combined with prednisone, but it generally represents the first line agent for cytoreduction in ASM.

Omalizumab, a humanized murine antibody targeted to IgE, is now available as an experimental option (Quintas-Cardama et al., 2006). It seems to control MC activation syndrome also in patients resistant to conventional fist line therapy. Recently, Molderings *et al.*, reporting their experience in four patients, showed its good risk-benefit profile. Two patients benefit a rapid remission, the third had a progressive improvement, only the fourth suffered from a worsening in MC-mediators syndrome (Molderings et al., 2011). Such isolated experience suggests that omalizumab could represent a new promising option.

Epinephrine on demand remains the gold standard during life-threatening anaphylactic or anaphylactoid episodes.

8.2 Cytoreductive treatment

Cytoreduction consists in single (IFNα and 2CdA) or multidrug (Fludarabine, Cytarabine, Mitoxantrone) approaches.

Usually IFNα represents the first line of treatment in slowly progressing variants. Cladribine is the second line, sometimes associated with novel agents (e.g. Imatinib).

In rapidly progressing variants Mito FLAG must be considered, with or without a previous treatment with 2CdA, in order to perform HSCT as soon as possible. In these cases BMT represents the only effective strategy to cure mastocytosis. If patient is ineligible, experimental trials remain the next option. Palliation is the last choice.

8.3 Novel agents

8.3.1 Tyrosine kinase inhibitors

Tyrosine kinase inhibitors have been under investigation since several years, particularly imatinib, dasatinib and midostaurin. Some clinical trials have been performed and many reports have been described. Target therapy has been observed to reduce both MC proliferation and infiltration, and sometimes to normalize BM histology. However, mediators related syndrome improved or got complete remission just in isolated reports.

8.3.1.1 Imatinib

Among the TK inhibitors, Imatinib is the most studied molecule. Low doses of Imatinib can inhibit wild type KIT. However, since D816V alters the kinase domain conformation, inhibiting steric interaction between the drug and the TK domain, efficacy of imatinib on *kit*D816V SM is still controversial. A phase II study conducted by Vega-Ruiz *et al.*, showed that imatinib has no significant clinical activity in patients carrying the D816V mutation. By contrast, in a different phase II trial Droogendij *et al.* observed an apparent remission in 11 *kit*D816V positive SMs (Droogendij et al., 2006). Some authors underline that concomitant use of prednisone may perhaps justify their results (Vega-Ruiz et al., 2009). Nevertheless, in some of these patients the observed reduction of symptoms was only transient. The case of SM with wild type kit or other sporadic mutations is different, since the conformational structure of the TK domain does not seem to be impaired. Moreover, these patients usually show an objective response, consisting in reduction of seric tryptase levels and bone marrow MC percentage (Vega-Ruiz, 2009). In summary, on one hand available data seem to suggest that imatinib is active against sporadic *kit* mutations, on the other hand the activity on *kit*D816V is not well established yet. Accordingly, in 2006 FDA approved the use of imatinib in adults with ASM without the D816V mutation.

Imatinib is also a potent competitive inhibitor of PDGFR and has been demonstrated to be either active or effective in FIP1L1/PDGFRA related HES. Consequently, SM patients with blood eosinophilia are recommended to be screened for this fusion protein. However, cardiogenic shock has been reported in patients with HES after the start of therapy with imatinib. Such an adverse event could be easily avoided by concomitant administration of corticosteroids during the first one or two weeks of treatment, mostly in case of echocardiographic abnormalities or high serum troponin levels at baseline.

Nilotinib is another TK inhibitor that has shown an in vitro activity against *kit* similar to imatinib, but no clinical experiences have been reported yet (Quintas-Cardama et al., Cancer 2006).

8.3.1.2 Dasatinib

Dasatinib is a dual SRC/ABL kinase inhibitor that is more potent than imatinib also against KIT. Preliminary data from either preclinical or clinical studies seemed to suggest a key role in SM, independently on mutational state of *kit* (Shah et al., 2006). However, data are too limited to draw any conclusion and the efficacy of dasatinib still remains controversial. Some authors described long lasting histological responses (Verstovsek et al, 2007) and both groups of patients with wild type and *kit*D816V improved in symptoms and quality of life. Wild type kit and *kit*D816V improved in symptoms and quality of life. It has been proposed a weekly dose escalation from 20 mg QD up to 100 mg QD during the first month of therapy (Rondoni et al., 2007). The proportion of responses may increase administering a dose of 120 mg QD in case of suboptimal or no response after three months of therapy. Based on this, the GIMEMA group is conducting an Italian multicenter phase II study in which subjects with SM are treating with a continuous regimen of dasatinib at a starting dose of 20 mg once daily. The primary endpoint is the evaluation of clinical response in terms of proportion of subjects experiencing a regression in B/C findings and mediator-related symptoms. The secondary endpoints include duration of response, progression free survival and time to response (GIMEMA, 2008).

8.3.1.3 Midostaurin

Midostaurin is a multi-kinase inhibitor with a demonstrated *in vitro* activity against KIT, but there are only sporadic observations of effectiveness *in vivo*. Gotlib *et al.* reported a case of MCL associated with MDS/MPD who received a transient benefit from administration of midostaurin (Gotlib et al., 2005). More interestingly, midostaurin seems to exhibit a synergic activity with nilotinib (Quintas-Cardama et al., 2006), suggesting a more attracting role of these small molecules, as useful tools to combine in multidrug strategies in order to avoid the resistance to single agent approaches.

8.3.1.4 Other TK inhibitors

Several more small molecules have been identified as potential agents against MC diseases: e.g. ATP analogs (OSI-930, MLN518, PD180970, PD180970, PD173955, AP23464 and AP23848), indolinone-based products (SU11652, SU11654 and SU11655) or quinoxaline derivatives (AGL2043). To date there are no data on clinical tolerability and efficacy yet (Quintas-Cardama et al., 2006).

8.3.2 Monoclonal antibodies

Monoclonal antibodies might play a crucial role in the future. The antiCD25 antibody conjugated with the pseudomonas exotoxin-A generates a potent immunotoxin with proapoptotic activity, associated with a significant reduction in the number of MCs (Valent et al., 2004). The effect is similar to that reported by other authors after in vitro exposure to Ontak, also known as denileukin diftitox, consisting in recombination of CD25 ligand and diphtheria toxin. Based on data on Ontak preclinical activity as well as clinical effectiveness in cutaneous T-cell lymphoma, there are ongoing phase II trials to test Ontak also in SM patients.

Other monoclonal antibodies are under investigation in Mastocytosis: the antiCD25 Daclizumab and Basiliximab, the antiCD33 Gemtuzumab with the toxic compound calicheamicin and the antiCD87 and antiCD45 antibodies, conjugated to $_{131}$I radioisotope or diphtheria toxin (Quintas-Cardama et al., Cancer 2006).

8.3.3 mTor inhibitors

mTor inhibitors have been tested since it has been demonstrated, both *in vitro* and *in vivo,* that the mTor pathway is active in SM and contributes to MC survival, growing and proliferation (Kim et al, 2008). Preclinical observations suggest that mTor inhibitors act against clonal MCs. Particularly, rapamycin inhibits selectively the mTor pathway, either in fresh MCs collected from KITD816V patients or in KITD816 cell lines. Hence, everolimus was tested in a clinical trial, but it did not show any apparent significant effectiveness. Perhaps some more experiences must be collected to determine whether mTor inhibitors may play any role in SM (Quintas-Cardama et al., 2006).

8.3.4 Future perspectives in SM therapy

Apoptosis still remains an attractive way to be investigated. Several drugs have shown some activity on Bcl-2 family members, as bortezomib, obatoclax and geldanamycin. The first one acts promoting Bim expression, the second one is known as BH3-mimetic (Aichberger et al., 2009), the last one inhibits the hsp90-bcl2 complex (Quintas-Cardama et al., 2006).

9. Conclusion

SM is a rare disorder, but its prevalence might be underestimated. Afar from drafting a complete and exhaustive review on mastocytosis, the aim of this chapter was to remark the relevance of SM. Clinical suspicion is really important and multimodality approaches must be considered to get the right diagnosis. Then, treatment must be personalized for each patient, accordingly with a careful and complete characterization of the disease.

Prospectively, two major challenges still have to be faced in SM research: first, the molecular and cellular pathogenesis; second, the definition of new strategies of treatment. About the former goal, we do believe that reporting new cases may be of great usefulness and is needed to better understand the nature of the disorder. In order to this, the case we described may perhaps represent a paradigmatic example. Referring to treatment, several novel agents are under investigation. However, preliminary clinical data seem to suggest that the use of a single drug may be insufficient. That means that a multidrug strategy is needed within a multitarget approach.

10. References

Aichberger, KJ.; Gleixner, KV.; Mirkina, I.; Cerny-Reiterer, S.; Peter, B.; Ferenc, V.; Kneidinger, M.; Baumgartner, C.; Mayerhofer, M.; Gruze, A.; Pickl, W F.; Sillaber, C. & Valent, P. (2009) Identification of proapoptotic Bim as a tumor suppressor in neoplastic mast cells: role of KIT D816V and effects of various targeted drugs, *Blood*, vol.114, no.26, pp.5342-5351, doi: 10.1182/blood-2008-08-175190

Amon, U.; Hartmann, K.; Horny, HP. & Nowak, A. (2010) Mastocytosis - an update *JDDG*; Vol.8, pp.695–712, DOI: 10.1111/j.1610-0387.2010.07482.x

Bodemer, C.; Hermine, O.; Palmérini, F.; Yang, Y.; Grandpeix-Guyodo, C.; Leventhal, PS.; Hadj-Rabia, S.; Nasca, L.; Georgin-Lavialle, S.; Cohen-Akenine, A.; Launay, JM.; Barete, S.; Feger, F.; Arock, M.; Catteau, B.; Sans, B.; Stalder, JF.; Skowron, F.; Thomas, L.; Lorette, G.; Plantin, P.; Bordigoni, P.; Lortholary, O.; de Prost, Y.;

Moussy, A.; Sobol, H.& Dubreuil, P. (2010) Pediatric mastocytosis is a clonal disease associated with D816V and other activating c-KIT mutations. *J Invest Dermatol*, Vol.130, pp.804–15.

González de Olano D, Alvarez-Twose I, Esteban-López MI, Sánchez-Muñoz L, de Durana MD, Vega A, García-Montero A, González-Mancebo E, Belver T, Herrero-Gil MD, Fernández-Rivas M, Orfao A, de la Hoz B & Castells MC, Escribano L. (2008) Safety and effectiveness of immunotherapy in patients with indolent systemic mastocytosis presenting with Hymenoptera venom anaphylaxis. *J Allergy Clin Immunol.* Vol.121(2), pp.519-526

Droogendijk. HJ.; Kluin-Nelemans, HJC.; van Doormaal, JJ.; Oranje, AR.; van de Loosdrecht, AA. & van Daele PLA (2006) Imatinib mesylate in the treatment of systemic mastocytosis - A phase II trial. *Cancer*, Vol.107, pp.345-351.

Du, S.; Rashidi, HH.; Le, DT.; Kipps, TJ.; Broome, HE. & Wang, HY. (2010) Systemic Mastocytosis in association with chronic lymphocytic leukaemia and plasma cell myeloma. *Int J Clin Exp Pathol*, Vol.3, No.4, pp.448-457.

Ehrlich P. (1877) Berträge zur Kenntnis der anilifarbungen und ihrer Verwendung in der microscopischem Technik. *Arch. Mikros. Anat.* Vol.13, pp.163-77.

Ellis, JM. (1949) Urticaria pigmentosa: a report of a case with autopsy. *AMA Arch Pathol,* Vol.48(5) , pp. 426–435.

Garcia-Montero, AC.; Jara-Acevedo, M.; Teodosio, C.; Sanchez, ML.; Nunez, MR.; Prados, A., Aldanondo, I.; Sanchez, L.; Dominguez, M.; Botana, LM.; Sanchez-Jimenez, F.; Sotlar, K.; Almeida, J.; Escribano, L. & Orfao, A. (2006) KIT mutation in mast cells and other bone marrow hematopoietic cell lineages in systemic mast cell disorders: a prospective study of the Spanish Network on Mastocytosis (REMA) in a series of 113 patients, *Blood,* Vol.108, pp.2366-2372, DOI 10.1182/blood-2006-04-015545

Gotlib, J.; Berube, C.; Growney, JD.; Chen, CC.; George, TI.; Williams, C.; Kajiguchi, T.; Ruan, J.; Lilleberg, SL.; Durocher, JA.; Lichy, JH.; Wang, Y.; Cohen, PS.; Arber, DA.; Heinrich, MC.; Neckers, L.; Galli, SJ.; Gilliland, DG. & Coutre SE. (2005) Activity of the tyrosine kinase inhibitor PKC412 in a patient with mast cell leukemia with the D816V KIT mutation. *Blood*. Vol.106, pp.2865–2870.

Gotlib J, George TI, Corless C, Linder A, Ruddell A, Akin C, DeAngelo DJ, Kepten I, Lanza C, Heinemann H, Yin O, Gallagher N, Graubert T (2008) The Kit tyrosine kinase inhibitor midostaurine (PKC412) exhibits a high response rate in aggressive systemic mastocytosis (ASM): interim results of a phase II trial. *Blood*, Vol.110, No. 11, pp.3536, ISSN 0006-4971.

Hissard, R.; Moncourier, L. & Jacquet, J. (1951) Study of a case of mastocytosis, *Ann Med Interne (Paris)*, Vol.52, No.6, pp. 583-607.

Horny, HP.; Sotlar, K.; Sperr, WR. & Valent, P. (2004) Systemic mastocytosis with associated clonal haematological non-mast cell lineage, diseases: a histopathological challenge. *J Clin Pathol,* Vol.57, pp.604–608.

Horny, HP.; Sotlar, K. & Valent P. (2007) Mastocytosis: state of the art. *Pathobiology*, Vol.74, pp.121–32.

Horny, HP.; Sotlar, K.; Valent, P. & Hartmann, K. (2008) Mastocytosis. A disease of the Hematopoietic Stem Cell. *Dtsch Arztebl Int.*, Vol.105, No.40, pp.686–692. doi:10.3238/arztebl2008.0686

Kim Y, Weiss L, Chen Y & Pullarkat V (2007) Distinct clonal origins of systemic mastocytosis and associated B-cell lymphoma *Leukemia* Research Vol.31, No.12, pp.1749-1754.

Kim, MK.; Kuehn, HS.; Metcalfe, DD. & Gilfillan, AM. (2008) Activation and Function of the mTORC1 Pathway in Mast Cells *J Immunol*, Vol.180, pp.4586-4595.

Koga, H.; Kokubo, T.; Akaishi, M.; Iida, K. and Korematsu, S. (2011) Neonatal Onset Diffuse Cutaneous Mastocytosis: A Case Report and Review of the Literature *Pediatric Dermatology* Vol.28,No.5, pp.542–54

Metcalfe, DD. (2008) Mast cells and mastocytosis. *Blood,* Vol.112, pp.946–56

Merluzzi, S.; Frossi, B.; Gri, G.; Parusso, S.; Tripodo, C.; & Pucillo, C. (2010), Mast cells enhance proliferation of B lymphocytes and drive their differentiation toward IgA-secreting plasma cells *Blood;* Vol.115, No.14, pp.2810-2817.

Middelkamp Hup, MA.; Heide, R.; Tank, B.; Mulder, PGH. & Oranje, AP. (2002) Comparison of mastocytosis with onset in children and adults *Journal of the European Academy of Dermatology and Venereology,* Vol.16, No.2, pp.115–120. doi:10.1046/j.1468-3083.2002.00370.x

Molderings, GJ.; Brettner, S.; Homann, J.; Afrin, LB. (2011) Mast cell activation disease: a concise practical guide for diagnostic workup and therapeutic options. *Journal of Hematology & Oncology,*4:10, available from http://www.jhoonline.org/content/4/1/10

Molderings, GJ.; Raithel, M.; Kratz, F.; Azemar, M.; Haenisch, B.; Harzer. S. & Homann, J. (2011) Omalizumab treatment of systemic mast cell activation disease: experiences from four cases. *Intern Med.* Vol.50, No.6, pp.611-5

Nettleship, E. &Tay, W.(1869) Rare forms of urticaria. *Br Med J,* Vol.2, pp.323-330.

Nowak, A.; Gibbs, BF. & Ulrich Amon, U. (2011) Pre-inpatient evaluation on quality and impact of care in systemic mastocytosis and the influence of hospital stay periods from the perspective of patients: a pilot study JDDG. *Journal der Deutschen Dermatologischen Gesellschaft* Vol.9, No.7, pp.525–532. doi*:* 10.1111/j.1610-0387.2011.07638.x

Orfao, A., Garcia-Montero, AC.; Sanchez, L. & Escribano, L for the Spanish Network on Mastocytosis (REMA) (2007) Recent advances in the understanding of mastocytosis: the role of KIT mutations, *British Journal of Haematology,* Vol.138, pp.12–30, doi:10.1111/j.1365-2141.2007.06619.x

Pardanani, A.; Kim, KH.; Lasho, TL.; Finke, C.; McClure, RF.; Li, CY. & Teffery, A. (2009) Prognostically relevant breakdown of 123 patients with systemic mastocytosis associated with other myeloid malignancies. *Blood,* Vol.114, pp.3769-3772.

Pardanani A, Tefferi A. Proposal for a revised classification of systemic mastocytosis (2010) *Blood* Vol.115, No.13, pp.2720-1.

Pardanani, A (2011) Systemic mastocytosis in adults: 2011. update on Diagnosis, Risk-stratification and Management, *American Journal of Hematology,* Vol.86, No.4, pp.362–371

Parikh, SA.; Kantarjian, HM.; Richie, MA.; Cortes, JE.& Verstovsek, S (2010) Experience with everolimus (RAD001), an oral mammalian target of rapamycin inhibitor, in patients with systemic mastocytosis. *Leuk Lymph,* Vol.51,pp.269-274.

Quintas-Cardama, A.; Aribi, A.; Cortes, J.; Giles, F.J.; Kantarjian, H. & Verstovsek, S. (2006) Novel Approaches in the Treatment of Systemic Mastocytosis, *Cancer,* Vol.107, No.7, pp. 1429-39 doi: 10.1002/cncr.22187

Rondoni, M.; Paolini, S.; Colarossi, S.; Piccaluga, PP.; Papayannidis, C.; Palandri, F.; Laterza, C.; De Rosa F.; Pregno, P.; Gatto, S.; Ottaviani, E.; Saglio, G.; Cilloni, D.; Pane, F.; Triggiani, M.; Soverini, S., Zaccaria, A.; Baccarani, M & Martinelli G. (2007) Response to Dasatinib in Patients with Aggressive Systemic Mastocytosis with D816V Kit Mutation. *ASH Annual Meeting Abstracts* 2007 110: 3562.

Schipper, EM.; Posthuma, W.; Snieders, I.; & Brouwer, R.E. (2011). Mastocytosis and diffuse large B-cell lymphoma, an unlikely combination, *Neth J Med.* Vol.69, No.3, pp.132-4.

Shah, NP.; Lee, FY.; Luo, R.; Yibin, J.; Donker, M. & Akin, C. (2006) Dasatinib (BMS-354825) inhibits KITD816V, an imatinib-resistant activating mutation that triggers neoplastic growth in most patients with systemic mastocytosis. *Blood,* Vol.108, pp.286-291.

Sotlar, K.; Fridrich, C.; Mall, A.; Jaussi, R.; Bültmann, B.; Valent, P.& Horny, HP. (2002) Detection of c-kit point mutation Asp-816→Val in microdissected pooled single mast cells and leukemic cells in a patient with systemic mastocytosis and concomitant chronic myelomonocytic leukemia. *Leuk Res,* Vol.26, pp.979–984.

Tanaka, A.; Konno, M.; Muto, S.; Kambe, N.; Morii, E.; Nakahata, T.; Itai, A. & Matsuda, H. (2005) A novel NF-kB inhibitor, IMD-0354, suppresses neoplastic proliferation of human mast cells with constitutively activated c-kit receptors. *Blood.* Vol.2005, No.105, pp.2324–23

Taylor, ML.; Sehgal, D.; Raffeld, M.; Obiakor, H.; Akin, C.; Mage; RG. & Metcalfe, DD. (2004) Demonstration that mast cells, T cells, and B cells bearing the activating kit mutation D816V occur in clusters within the marrow of patients with mastocytosis. *Journal of Molecular Diagnostics,* Vol.6, No.4, pp.335-42. PMID:15507672, doi:10.1186/1756-8722-4-10

Travis, WD.; Li, CY.; Yam, LT.; Bergstralh, EJ.& Swee, RG (1988) Significance of systemic mast cell disease with associated hematologic disorders. *Cancer,* Vol.62, pp.965–972.

Triggiani, M.; Multicenter, Open-Label, Single Arm Phase II Clinical Trial of Dasatinib in the Treatment of Systemic Mastocytosis Writing Committee: Martinelli, G.; Merante, S.; Rondoni, M.; Zanotti, R.; Pagano, L.; Musto, P.; Cilloni, D.; Pulsoni, A.; Colarossi, S.; Venditti, A.; Amadori, S.; Beghini, A.; Cairoli, S.; Morra, E.; Pane, F.; Saglio, G. & Baccarani, M. Available from *ClinicalTrials.gov*

Valent, P.; Horny, HP.; Escribano, L.; Longley; BJ.; Li, CY.; Schwartz, LB.; Marone, G.; Nun˜ez, R.; Akin, C.; Sotlar, K.; Sperr, WR.; Wolff, K.; Brunning, RD.; Parwaresch RM.; Austen, KF.; Lennert, K.; Metcalfe, DD.; Vardiman, JW.; Bennett, JM.; (2001), Diagnostic criteria and classification of mastocytosis: a consensus proposal, *Leukemia Research,* Vol.25, pp.603–625

Valent, P.; Akin, C.; Sperr, WR.; Horny, HP.; Arock, M.; Lechner, K.; Vardiman, JW. & Metcalfe, DD.; Diagnosis and treatment of systemic mastocytosis: state of the art. (2003) *Br J Haematol* Vol.122,No.5, pp.695–717.

Valent, P.; Ghannadan, M.; Akin, C.; Krauth, MT.; Selzer, E.; Mayerhofer, M.; Sperr, WR.; Arock, M.; Samorapoompichit. P.; Horny, HP. & Metcalfe, DD. (2004) On the way to targeted therapy of mast cell neoplasms: identification of molecular targets in neoplastic mast cells and evaluation of arising treatment concepts. *Eur J Clin Invest.* Vol.34, No.2, pp.41–52.

Valent, P.; Sperr, WR. & Akin, C. (2010) How I treat patients with advanced systemic mastocytosis, *Blood,* Vol.116, pp.5812-5817

Valent, P.; Cerny-Reiterer, S.; Herrmann, H.; Mirkina, I.; George, TI.; Sotlar, K.; Sperr, WR. & Horny, HP. (2010) Phenotypic heterogeneity, novel diagnostic markers, and target expression profiles in normal and neoplastic human mast cells *Best Practice & Research Clinical Haematology* Vol.23, pp.369–378, doi: 10.1016 / j.beha.2010.07.003

Vardiman, JW.; Thiele, J.; Arber, DA.; Brunning, RD.; Borowitz, MJ.; Porwit, A.; Harris, NL.; Le Beau, MM.; Hellström-Lindberg, E.; Tefferi, A. & Bloomfield, CD. (2009) The 2008 Revision of the WHO Classification of Myeloid Neoplasms and Acute Leukemia: Rationale and Important Changes, *Blood,* available from bloodjournal.hematologylibrary.org, doi:10.1182/blood-2009-03-209262 ISSN 1528-0020

Vega-Ruiz A, Cortes JE, Sever M, Manshouri T, Quintás-Cardama A, Luthra R, Kantarjian HM, Verstovsek S (2009) Phase II study of imatinib mesylate as therapy for patients with systemic mastocytosis. *Leuk Res,* Vol.33, pp.1481-1484.

Verstovsek, S.; Tefferi, A.; Cortes, J.; Susan O'Brien, S.; Garcia-Manero, G.; Pardanani, A.; Akin, C.; Faderl, S.; Ma n s h o u r i , T.; Thomas, D. & Kantarjian, H. (2007) Phase II Study of Dasatinib in Philadelphia Chromosome-Negative Acute and Chronic Myeloid Diseases, Including Systemic Mastocytosis. *Clin Cancer Res* Vol.2008; No.14, pp.3906-3915, doi:10.1158/1078-0432.CCR-08-036

Part 3

Hematology in the Clinic

19

Targeting the Minimal Residual Disease in Acute Myeloid Leukemia: The Role of Adoptive Immunotherapy with Natural Killer Cells and Antigen-Specific Vaccination

Sarah Parisi and Antonio Curti
Department of Hematology and Oncological Sciences "L. and A. Seràgnoli", University of Bologna, Bologna Italy

1. Introduction

Acute myeloid leukemia (AML) is a neoplastic disorder characterized by the clonal expansion of non-lymphoid hematopoietic progenitor cells with failure of normal hematopoiesis. Several biological and clinical parameters have been identified at diagnosis to classify different AML subtypes with different prognosis. In this view, genetic abnormalities confer the most important prognostic information. Therapeutic interventions based on conventional or high-dose chemotherapy have significantly improved the complete remission (CR) rates of acute leukemia. However, a significant portion of responding patients still harbors a minimal residual disease (MRD), which is often resistant to further pharmacological treatments and ultimately leads to disease relapse and progression. Although allogeneic stem cell transplantation may significantly improve the clinical results of AML patients who achieved complete remission, such approach has several and important limitations and is not applicable to all the patients. For these reasons, novel therapeutic approaches to improve the clinical outcome of AML patients are under investigation, and treatments with high compliance such as adoptive and active immunotherapy are desirable. Aim of the present work will be to focus the most relevant insights in the field. In particular, we will report about the use of natural killer (NK) cells as a means of adoptive immunotherapy against neoplastic cells, including AML. Moreover, we will discuss the role of vaccines against leukemia with particular emphasis on the immunogenicity of novel and promising leukemia-associated antigens.

2. Acute Myeloid Leukemia

Acute myeloid leukemia (AML) is a hematopoietic malignant disease rising from neoplastic transformation of myeloid stem cells. This causes the alteration of the normal cell differentiation and proliferation systems, resulting in the accumulation in bone marrow and peripheral blood of non-functional myeloid cells termed myeloblasts. AML may arise *de novo* or secondary to pre-existing myelodysplasia or previous chemotherapies.

Myeloblasts lack the normal proliferation systems and their over-proliferation and accumulation in bone marrow and peripheral blood cause lack of production of hematopoietic normal cells, this resulting in peripheral deficiency of platelets, neutrophils and hemoglobin.

Prognosis of AML depends on multiple factors: age at diagnosis (age>60 years is a poor prognostic factor), hyperleukocytosis, cytogenetic status and molecular specific characteristics are the most important ones.

AML can occur at every age, but its incidence increases with age (median age at presentation: 65 years). It has an annual incidence of 3.6 per 100,000. This incidence increases with age, rising to 16.3 per 100,000 per year in the over 65 age group. Older adults typically have a highly inferior prognosis and an increased risk of therapy-related toxicity and mortality.

Conventional treatment of AML is based on chemotherapy regimens and consists of several well-defined phases: the first one is the CR-induction cycle, based on the administration of 3 days-anthacycline associated with 7 days-cytarabine. Its aim is to 'empty' bone marrow and allow the normal hematopoietic cells repopulation.

Response rates with conventional chemotherapy range from 60% to 85% in young adults (age < 60 years), but more than 50% of these patients are going to relapse, with a five-year overall survival of 40%. Older patients with a diagnosis of AML have a poorer prognosis, with less than 10% of long survivers; this is due to biological unfavorable risk factors, such as unfavorable cytogenetics, which are more frequent in the elderly (Leith et al. 1997).

One of the main cause of relapse in patients who achieved complete remission after chemotherapy is the persistance of a small amount of leukemic cells termed MRD. Minimal residual disease detection became one of the main tasks for hematologists; immunophenotypical and molecular markers able to discriminate normal cells from blastic cells allow the detection of residual leukemic cells not detected by morphologic examinations.

After the induction therapy two or more consolidation cycles are needed in order to eradicate leukemic cells completely. Allogeneic stem cell transplantation is one of the most effective consolidation therapy, even if it is feasible only for fit patients and only if a suitable HLA-matched donor is available.

Moreover, allogeneic stem cell transplantation is highly effective if performed after obtaining first CR, while its efficacy is poor in case of relapsed/refractory patients.

Only young and fit patients can undergo stem cell transplantation because of its significantly high toxicity, mortality and morbidity rates.

Attempts to effectively prime and sustain anti-tumor immunity against leukemic cells have recently provided promising preclinical and clinical results. Results from allogeneic stem cell transplantation (SCT) represent the main evidence that leukemic cells are targets of the immune system. In fact, since the first clinical observation that allogeneic SCT offered a clinical advantage over autologous transplantation due to a graft-versus-leukemia (GVL) effect, much more attention has been given to the role of adoptive immunotherapy over conditioning regimen as a means to eradicate tumor cells. In particular, donor lymphocyte infusions (DLIs) are capable to restore a durable complete remission. Such results are the proof of principle of the crucial activity of anti-tumor immunity in controlling the growth of leukemic cells.

3. Adoptive immunotherapy with natural killer cells

Human NK cells are a subset of PB lymphocytes defined by the expression of CD56 or CD16 and the absence of the T-cell receptor (CD3) (Robertson et al, 1990). They recognize and kill transformed cell lines in an MHC-unrestricted fashion and play a critical role in the innate immune response. Several studies demonstrated that NK function, which is distinct from the MHC-restricted cytolytic activity of T cells, may be relevant for the immune control of tumor development and growth. Although NK cell killing is MHC-unrestricted, NK cells display a number of activating and inhibitory receptors that ligate MHC molecules to modulate the immune response (Lanier et al, 1998). NK cell receptors that recognize antigens at the HLA-A, -B, or -C loci are members of the immunoglobulin super family and are termed killer immunoglobulin receptors or KIRs (Farad et al, 2002). Engagement of these NK cell receptors results in stimulation or inhibition of NK cell effector function, which ultimately depends on the net effect of activating and inhibitory receptors (Figure 1).

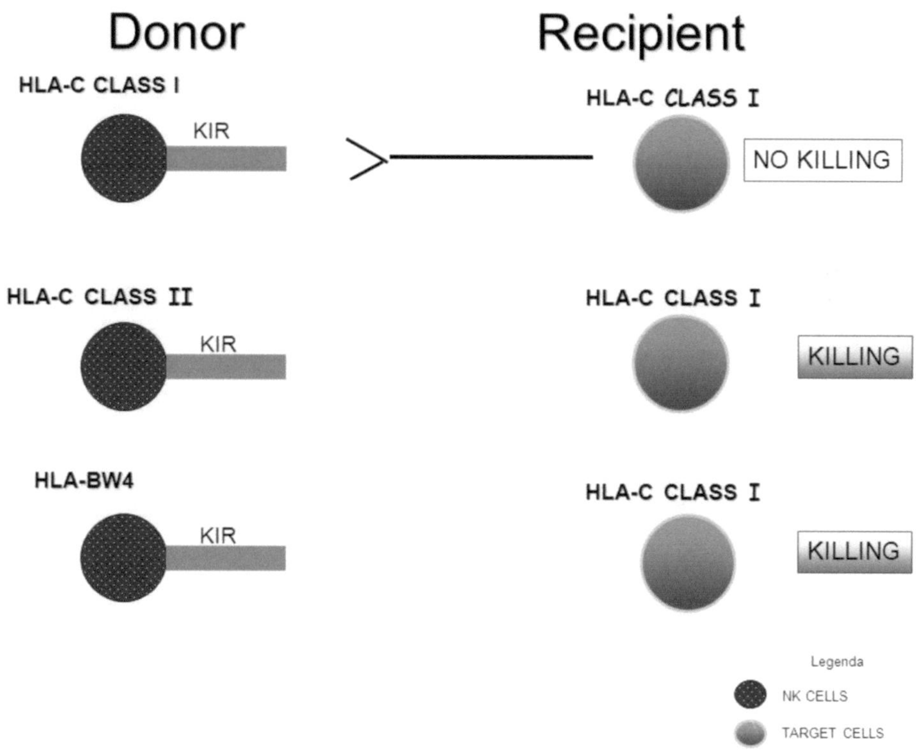

Clinical trials attempting to utilize the anti-tumor effect of NK cells have met only modest success due to the lack of understanding of receptors and ligands which determine whether NK cells will be activated or suppressed. On the contrary, data from haploidentical T-cell depleted transplantation suggest that KIR mismatch with tumor MHC may significantly impact on tumor cell killing, particularly in AML (Ruggeri et al, 2002). In fact, these studies show that AML patients with KIR ligand mismatch are significantly protected against leukemia relapse. In addition, preclinical and clinical investigations demonstrated that haploidentical KIR-mismatched NK cells play the main role as anti-leukemia effector cells and they exert their cytotoxic activity within 4-5 days (Ruggeri et al 2002, Ruggeri et al, 1999). In particular, high risk AML patients with a KIR-ligand mismatch in the graft-versus-host (GVDH) direction had a relapse rate of 0% compared to KIR-ligand matched patients who had a relapse rate of 75%. Given these results, haploidentical KIR-mismatch NK cells administered to AML patients as cell-based immunotherapy may induce NK cell-mediated killing of leukemia cells resulting in the elimination of residual disease in high risk AML patients. Furthermore, alloreactive mismatched NK cells facilitate hematopoietic engraftment after infusion of haploidentical stem cells, and inhibit the onset of GVHD by targeting host antigen-presenting cells (Ruggeri et al, 2002). Of note, the differential expression of activating ligands on hematopoietic and not hematopoietic tissues may provide an additional explanation for the observed GVL effect in the absence of GVHD.

Partially purified haploidentical NK cells have been already used clinically and labeled with ^{111}In to track, in vivo, their kinetics and organ distribution in patients with renal cancer (Brand et al, 2004). A seminal study demonstrated that up to 1.5 x 10^7/haploidentical NK cells/Kg can be safely infused in AML and cancer patients following Fludarabine/ Cyclophosphamide (Flu/Cy) immunosuppressive chemotherapy and, in some cases, clinical responses without GVHD had been observed (Miller et al, 2005). Interestingly, circulating haploidentical NK cells were found, in selected patients, up to 28 days after infusion especially when exogenous IL-2 was given for 9 doses. In vivo expansion of NK cells was correlated with a high IL-15 serum concentration. In particular, in this study, 19 poor risk AML patients were reported who had received a cell population containing a median of $8.5 \pm 0.5 \times 10^6$ and $1.75 \pm 0.3 \times 10^5$ NK and T cells, respectively. Five out of 19 patients achieved CR. NK cells adoptive immunotherapy was well tolerated and hematological and non hematological toxicity were mainly related to the immunosuppressive regimen and IL-2 administration. The maximum tolerated dose of NK cells was not achieved and GVHD was not observed despite the relatively high number of haploidentical T cells infused. However, it should be noted that NK cells were only partially purified after a single round of depletion of $CD3^+$ cells which resulted in less than 2 logs reduction of T cells.

More recently, a study of haploidentical KIR-HLA mismatched NK cell transplantation in childhood AML reported that NK cell therapy prolonged disease-free and overall survival (Rubnitz et al, 2010). In this pediatric cohort of AML patients, who underwent NK therapy after an immunosuppressive regimen, the 2-year event-free survival was 100%. Notably, all the children were considered at low-risk of relapse, with a significant fraction harboring good-prognosis cytogenetics. Furthermore, as children weigh less than adults, the median number of infused NK cells was significantly higher than in adult trial and the separation procedure consisted in highly purified NK cells. These differences may partially explain the discrepancy in clinical results and suggest that in adult patients the clinical effect of NK therapy may be implemented by increasing the number of infused NK cells.

We recently published the results of a clinical trial of adoptive immunotherapy with haploidentical KIR-mismatched NK cells in elderly patients with AML (Curti et al, 2011).

Thirteen AML patients, 5 with active disease, 2 in molecular relapse and 6 in morphological complete remission (CR);(median age 62 years, range 53-73) received highly purified $CD56^{+}CD3^{-}$ NK cells from haploidentical KIR-ligand mismatched donors after fludarabine/ cyclophosphamide immunosuppressive chemotherapy, followed by IL-2. The median number of infused NK cells was 2.74 x 10^{6}/Kg. T cells were under 10^{5}/Kg. No NK cell-related toxicity, including GVHD, was observed. One of the 5 patients with active disease achieved transient CR, whereas 4/5 patients had no clinical benefit. Both patients in molecular relapse achieved CR which lasted for 9 and 4 months, respectively. Three/6 patients in CR are disease-free after 34, 32 and 18 months. After infusion, donor NK cells were found in the peripheral blood of all evaluable patients (peak value on day 10). They were also detected in bone marrow in some cases. Donor-versus-recipient alloreactive NK cells were demonstrated *in vivo* by the detection of donor-derived NK clones that killed recipient's targets. Adoptively transferred NK cells were alloreactive against recipient's cells, including leukemia. Taken together, these data demonstrate that infusion of purified NK cells is feasible in elderly patients with high risk AML.

4. Vaccination against acute myeloid leukemia: WT1 as a novel promising antigen

During the last years a number of studies have demonstrated that tumor-associated antigens (TAA) may be recognized by the immune system leading to the activation of tumor-specific cytotoxic T lymphocytes (CTLs) with the potential to eradicate tumor cells. Moreover, during the last decade the role of dendritic cells (DCs) as natural adjuvants of immune response has been deeply elucidated. The identification of a wide number of TAA, together with new insights into the mechanisms underlying the activation of anti-tumor immune response, has led to the development of novel anti-tumor vaccination strategies which are currently under investigation in the clinical setting. In AML, some TAA, such as PRAME, Wilms' tumor gene (WT1), proteinase 3 have been recently identified. In particular, WT1, which is a zinc-finger transcription factor expressed during normal ontogenesis, is significantly over-expressed in acute and chronic myeloid leukemia and myelodysplastic syndromes and it appears as an attractive target for immunotherapy.

WT1-specific antibodies against the N-terminus portion of the WT1 protein have been found in the sera of AML patients, but not in healthy donors, suggesting that anti-WT1-specific immune response is present in these patients. Preclinical studies have clearly demonstrated that peptides from WT1 may be used to generate in vitro a WT1-specific cytotoxic response (Li et al, 2005; Pinilla-Ibarz et al, 2006; Oka et al, 2000). While a number of WT1-derived CD8 T-cell epitopes have been reported, two peptides, namely HLA-A0201-restricted peptide 126–134 and HLA-A24-restricted peptide 235–243, have been studied extensively. Since murine and human WT1 are similar, WT1 126 and WT1 235 have also been tested in animal models. B6 mice were injected with WT1 peptides and analyzed for the induction of a T-cell and B-cell mediated immune responses against WT1. This analysis revealed that WT1 vaccination induced WT1-specific immunity, which was also capable to delay in vivo the growth of tumor cell lines, naturally overexpressing WT1. Recently, a National Cancer Institute Pilot Project assigned to WT1 the position of best and most suitable target antigen for cancer immunotherapy, due to a number of characteristics, such as its therapeutic function, immunogenicity and expression level (Cheever et al, 2009)

These data have prompted several groups to investigate the role of WT1 as a tumor-antigen in the clinical setting of cancer immunotherapy. Particularly, Oka et al conducted phase I clinical trials using peptide WT1-235 (CMTWNQMNL) and its analogue (CYTWNQMNL) for patients with overt leukemia from MDS, MDS with myelofibrosis and AML (Oka et al, 2004). Vaccination was performed by injecting 0.3–3 mg of native or analogue peptide 235 emulsified with the adjuvant Montanide ISA51. The vaccination resulted in an increase in WT1-specific CTLs followed by a rapid reduction in leukemic blast cells. No serious toxicity was observed, but leukemic blasts relapsed after the vaccination was stopped. Recently, these investigators reported that biweekly injection of AML patients with either native or analogue peptide 235 along with Montanide and GM-CSF resulted in three patients remaining in CR for 4 years (Tsuboi et al, 2007). The WT1-235 peptide has also been shown to induce HLA-A0201-restricted CTL (Pinilla-Ibarz, 2006). Keilholz et al first reported that vaccination of a patient with recurrent AML, using HLA-A0201-restricted WT1 peptide 126 along with KLH as an adjuvant, induced CR (Mailander et al, 2004). No haematological or renal toxicities were observed. Rezvani et al reported a phase I clinical trial in patients with AML, CML and MDS, using combined HLA-A0201-binding peptide vaccines from PR1 169–177 and WT1 126–134. Their results show that the emergence of $PR1^+$ or $WT1^+CD8^+$ T cells in patients who received WT1 vaccine was associated with a decrease in WT1 mRNA expression, suggesting a vaccine-driven anti-leukemia effect (Rezvani et al, 2008). An analogue to WT1 peptide 126–134 was generated by substituting R for Y at the position 2 anchor motif (named WT1-A1) (Pinilla-Ibarz et al, 2006). This analogue peptide generated a more potent CD8 T-cell response which recognized and lysed $WT1^+$ leukemia cells in vitro. In addition to the HLA-A0201 and -A24 vaccines derived from WT1 protein, Asemissen et al identified a highly immunogenic HLA-A1-binding WT1 peptide (317–327) that is processed and able to induce a CD8 T-cell response in healthy donors and patients with haematological malignancies (Asemissen et al, 2006).

The German group reported about their phase 2 trial of WT1 peptide vaccination in patients with AML and MDS (Keilholz et al, 2009). Vaccination consisted of GM-CSF subcutaneously days 1 to 4, and WT1126-134 peptide and 1 mg keyhole limpet hemocyanin on day 3. Seventeen AML patients and 2 refractory anemia with excess blasts patients received a median of 11 vaccinations. Treatment was well tolerated. Objective responses in AML patients were 10 stable diseases (SDs) including 4 SDs with more than 50% blast reduction and 2 with hematologic improvement. An additional 4 patients had clinical benefit after initial progression, including 1 CR and 3 SDs. WT1 mRNA levels decreased at least 3-fold from baseline in 35% of patients. In 8 of 18 patients, WT1-tetramer$^+$ T cells increased in blood and in 8 over 17 patients in bone marrow, with a median frequency in bone marrow of 0.18% at baseline and 0.41% at week 18. This WT1 vaccination study provides immunologic, molecular, and preliminary evidence of potential clinical efficacy in AML patients, warranting further investigations.

Other approaches include the use of autologous DCs, generated from leukemia patients in CR and loaded with tumor antigens and/or the differentiation of leukaemia blasts into leukemic DCs. In particular, Van Tendeloo et al reported the results of a phase I/II clinical trial of WT1 vaccination based on antigen-loaded DCs with the induction of complete and molecular responses in some cases (Van Tendeloo et al, 2010). These results are promising. However, the clinical experience with DC-based vaccines targeting WT1 is far too limited and future studies are highly warranted to assess the role and the efficacy of these strategies of active immunotherapy in the clinical management of MRD in AML.

5. Conclusion

In conclusion, the clinical results of AML patients, especially if elderly, are particularly dismal, although the achievement of CR with MRD after combined chemotherapy appears as possible in the majority of patients. Unfortunately, the persistence of MRD leads to progression and patients ultimately die. For these reasons, alternative approaches for the prevention of relapse in CR patients are necessary and are currently under active investigation. In particular, the role of immunological therapies in the post-remission management of adult AML patients, such as NK therapy and active immunization against relevant tumor rejection antigens, including WT1, have been recently exploited with promising results in terms of immunological and clinical responses. Further studies (phase II-III) are highly warranted to really evaluate the role of such approaches and their impact on overall survival of AML patients.

6. References

[1] Asemissen A, U. Keilholz and S. Tenzer et al., Identification of a highly immunogenic HLA-A*01-binding T cell epitope of WT1, Clinical Cancer Research 12 (2006), pp. 7476–7482.

[2] Brand JM, Meller B, Von Hof K, et al. Kinetics and organ distribution of allogeneic natural killer lymphocytes transfused into patients suffering from renal cell carcinoma. Stem Cells and Development 2004; 13: 307-314.

[3] Cheever MA, Allison JP, Ferris AS, Finn OJ, Hastings BM, Hecht TT, Mellman I, Prindiville SA, Viner JL, Weiner LM, Matrisian LM.The prioritization of cancer antigens: a national cancer institute pilot project for the acceleration of translational research. Clin Cancer Res. 2009 Sep 1;15(17):5323-37.

[4] Curti A, Ruggeri L, D'Addio A, et al. Successful transfer of alloreactive haploidentical KIR ligand-mismatched natural killer cells after infusion in elderly high-risk acute myeloid leukemia patients. Blood. 2011 Jul 25. [Epub ahead of print]

[5] Farad SS, Fehniger T, Ruggeri L, et al. Natural killer cell receptors:new biology and insights into graft versus leukemia effect. Blood. 2002; 100: 1935-1947.

[6] Keilholz U, Letsch A, Busse A, Asemissen AM, Bauer S, Blau IW, Hofmann WK, Uharek L, Thiel E, Scheibenbogen C.A clinical and immunologic phase 2 trial of Wilms tumor gene product 1 (WT1) peptide vaccination in patients with AML and MDS. Blood. 2009 Jun 25;113(26):6541-8.

[7] Lanier LL. NK cell receptors. Annu Rev Immunol. 1998; 16: 359-393.

[8] Leith CP, Kopecky KJ, Godwin J, et al. Acute myeloid leukemia in the elderly: assessment of multidrug resistance (MDR1) and cytogenetics distinguishes biologic subgroups with remarkably distinct responses to standard chemotherapy. A Southwest Oncology Group study. Blood. 1997 May 1;89(9):3323-9.

[9] Li Z, Oka Y, Tsuboi A, Masuda T, Tatsumi N, Kawakami M, Fujioka T, Sakaguchi N, Nakajima H, Fujiki F, Udaka K, Oji Y, Kawase I, Sugiyama H. WT1(235), a ninemer peptide derived from Wilms' tumor gene product, is a candidate peptide for the vaccination of HLA-A*0201-positive patients with hematopoietic malignancies. Int J Hematol. 2005 Dec;82(5):458-459.

[10] Mailänder V, Scheibenbogen C, Thiel E, Letsch A, Blau IW, Keilholz U. Complete remission in a patient with recurrent acute myeloid leukemia induced by

vaccination with WT1 peptide in the absence of hematological or renal toxicity. Leukemia. 2004 Jan;18(1):165-166.
[11] Miller JS, Soignier Y, Panoskaltsis-Mortari A, et al. Successful adoptive transfer and in vivo expansion of human haploidentical NK cells in patients with cancer. Blood. 2005;105(8):3051-3057.
[12] Oka Y, Tsuboi A, Taguchi T, Osaki T, Kyo T, Nakajima H, Elisseeva OA, Oji Y, Kawakami M, Ikegame K, Hosen N, Yoshihara S, Wu F, Fujiki F, Murakami M, Masuda T, Nishida S, Shirakata T, Nakatsuka S, Sasaki A, Udaka K, Dohy H, Aozasa K, Noguchi S, Kawase I, Sugiyama H. Induction of WT1 (Wilms' tumor gene)-specific cytotoxic T lymphocytes by WT1 peptide vaccine and the resultant cancer regression. Proc Natl Acad Sci U S A. 2004 Sep 21;101(38):13885-13890.
[13] Oka Y, Udaka K, Tsuboi A, Elisseeva OA, Ogawa H, Aozasa K, Kishimoto T, Sugiyama H.Cancer immunotherapy targeting Wilms' tumor gene WT1 product. J Immunol. 2000 Feb 15;164(4):1873-1880.
[14] Pinilla-Ibarz J, May RJ, Korontsvit T, Gomez M, Kappel B, Zakhaleva V, Zhang RH, Scheinberg DA. Improved human T-cell responses against synthetic HLA-0201 analog peptides derived from the WT1 oncoprotein. Leukemia. 2006 Nov;20(11):2025-2033.
[15] Rezvani K, A.S.M. Young and S. Mielke et al., Leukemia-associated antigen specific T-cell responses following combined PR1 and WT1 peptide vaccination in patients with myeloid malignancies, Blood 111 (2008), pp. 236–242.
[16] Robertson MJ, Ritz J. Biology and clinical relevance of human natural killer cells. Blood. 1990; 76: 2421-2438.
[17] Rubnitz JE, Inaba H, Ribeiro RC, et al. NKAML: a pilot study to determine the safety and feasibility of haploidentical natural killer cell transplantation in childhood acute myeloid leukemia. J Clin Oncol. 2010;28(6):955-959.
[18] Ruggeri L, Capanni M, Casucci M, et al. Role of natural killer cell alloreactivity in HLA-mismatched hematopoietic stem cell transplantation. Blood. 1999; 94: 333-339.
[19] Ruggeri L, Capanni M, Urbani E, et al. Effectiveness of donor natural killer cell alloreactivity in mismatched hematopoietic transplants. Science. 2002; 295: 2097-2100.
[20] Tsuboi A, Oka Y, Nakajima H, et al. Long-term follow-up of three patients with acute myeloid leukemia with minimal residual disease who were treated with WT1 vaccination. In: Third international conference on WT1 in human malignancies, Berlin Sept 20-21, 2007.
[21] Van Tendeloo VF, Van de Velde A, Van Driessche A, et al. Induction of complete and molecular remissions in acute myeloid leukemia by Wilms' tumor 1 antigen-targeted dendritic cell vaccination Proc Natl Acad Sci U S A. 2010 Aug 3;107(31):13824-9.

20

The Ubiquitin-Proteasomal System and Blood Cancer Therapy

Xinliang Mao and Biyin Cao
Cyrus Tang Hematology Center, Soochow University
P.R.China

1. Introduction

The ubiquitin-proteasomal system (UPS) is critical for the regulation of protein homeostasis and is composed of the protein ubiquitination system and proteasomal degradation system. Protein ubiquitination is referred to the process that the small protein ubiquitin is covalently tagged to a specific substrate protein. Once a protein is ubiquitinated, its structural conformation, cellular location, and biological function will change accordingly, or it will be delivered into the 26S proteasome complex for degradation by specific proteases. The UPS is extensively involved in nearly all the important cell biological activities, such as cell metabolism, cell proliferation, glycogen synthesis, immunological process, organogenesis, etc. (Ciechanover, 1998; Haglund and Dikic, 2005; Kirkin and Dikic, 2010).

The UPS system is also widely associated with various diseases, such as inflammation, arthritis, heart disease and cancers (Ciechanover et al., 2000). For example, the proteasome has emerged as a milestone target for cancer therapy, which was further demonstrated by the discovery of the proteasome inhibitor bortezomib for the therapy of multiple myeloma (Kisselev and Goldberg, 2001; Richardson et al., 2003). Recently, in addition to the proteasome, the protein ubiquitination pathway is also being developed as a novel target for anti-cancer drugs (Bedford et al., 2011 ; Colland, 2010). In this chapter, we will discuss the UPS system, its biological implications, and associated targeted drug discovery for hematological malignancies.

2. The ubiquitin-proteasomal system (UPS)

The UPS is composed by at least 6 components, including ubiquitin (Ub), ubiquitin-activating enzymes (UBA, E1), ubiquitin-conjugating enzymes (UBC, E2), ubiquitin ligases (E3), proteasomes, and deubiquitinases (Dub) (Figure 1). The substrate proteins are first tagged with a ubiquitin chain under the guidance of E1, E2 and E3, and the produced polyubiquitinated proteins are then transferred to 26S proteasomes where it is degraded by the 20S core particles.

2.1 Ubiquitination

Ubiquitin is a ubiquitinously expressed small protein composed of 76 amino acids and it plays a central role in the UPS system. It can be linked to a substrate protein with the

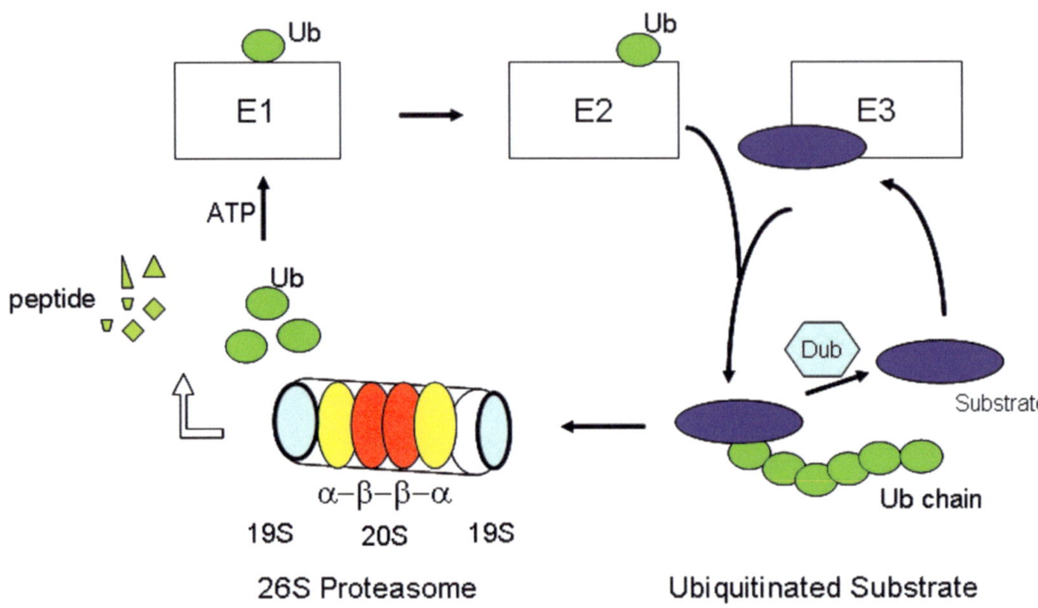

Fig. 1. The ubiquitination-proteasomal system (UPS). The UPS is composed of 6 components, including ubiquitin (Ub), ubiquitin-activating enzyme (E1), ubiquitin-conjugating enzyme (E2), ubiquitin ligase (E3), deubiquitinases (Dub) and proteasomes.

assistance of E1, E2, and E3, and can be removed from the target protein by Dubs. Ubiquitin is highly conserved and is expressed in most species but it is only found in eukaryotic organisms. This strong sequence conservation suggests that ubiquitin plays a very fundamental role in maintaining cell function and in species evolution. Actually, ubiquitin is involved in all aspects of cell biology and activities by regulating its extensive substrate proteins. Proteins will undergo turnover, translocation or conformational changes after they are covalently attached a ubiquitin, which is called ubiquitination, one of the most important post-translational modifications of proteins, where the carboxylic acid of the terminal glycine from the di-glycine motif in the activated ubiquitin forms an amide bond to the epsilon amine of the lysine in the substrate proteins (Ciechanover et al., 2000). In the 76 amino acids, there are 6 lysine residues (K) including K6, K11, K27, K29, K33, K48, and K63 as shown in Figure 2. These lysine residues are responsible for ubiquitin attachment to the target proteins. Theoretically, any lysine residues in a protein could be linked a ubiquitin, including ubiquitin itself, however, the biological function may differ and it depends on the ubiquitination status (Haglund and Dikic, 2005).

Ubiquitination can be categorized into three classes based on the tagged ubiquitin (Haglund and Dikic, 2005; Ye and Rape, 2009): i) monoubiquitination: proteins are bound to a single ubiquitin, ii) multiubiquitination or poly-monoubiquitination: proteins are tagged with several single ubiquitin molecules; iii) polyubiquitination: proteins are attached with poly-ubiquitin chains. These differences of ubiquitination on target proteins will regulate a variety of cellular processes, including protein degradation, signal transduction, membrane trafficking, DNA repair, chromatin remodelling, peroxisome biogenesis and viral budding (Ye and Rape, 2009). For example, polyubiquitin chain occurring at the 11th (K11) and 48th

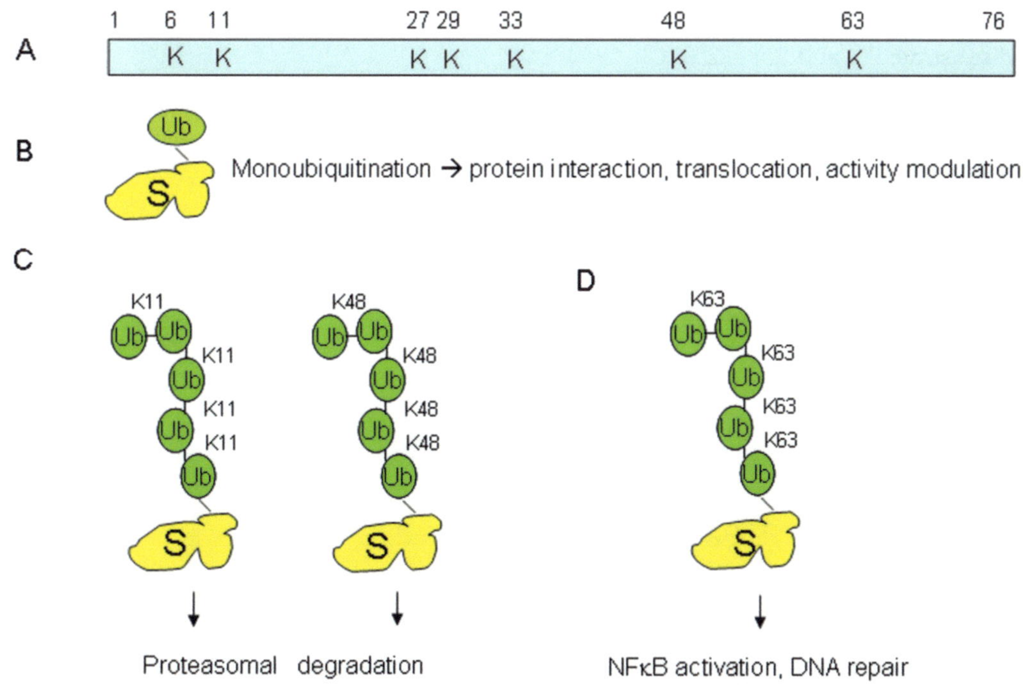

Fig. 2. Protein ubiquitination and functional modulation. There are 7 lysine (K) residues in 76 amino acids of ubiquitin and each could be further conjugated to a specific protein (A). Monoubiquitination (B) regulates protein conformation, cellular localization and protein interaction. Proteins tagged with polyubiquitin-chains occurring at K11 or K48 (C) are subject to degradation in the 26S proteasome. Polyubiquitination at K63 (D) activates NFκB function and is involved in DNA repair.

lysine (K48) of ubiquitin is mainly involved in protein degradation, but the K63 polyubiquitination is mainly responsible for modification of protein function and involved in signal transduction, including regulation of NFκB signal pathway, DNA repair and targeting to the lysosome (Ye and Rape, 2009). For other proteins polyubiquintinated at K6, 27, 29 or 33, whether they are involved in protein degradation or DNA repair is largely unknown (Ye and Rape, 2009)(Figure 2).

2.2 Ubiquitining enzymes

The ubiquitination process is an ATP-dependent enzymatic reaction and requires at least 3 types of enzymes, including E1, E2 and E3 as described earlier, thus the ubiquitination process is alternatively known as the E1-E2-E3 cascade. In the process of ubiquitination, ubiquitin is first activated by E1 using ATP as an energy source to form a ubiquitin-adenylate intermediate. Subsequently, the ubiquitin is transferred to the cysteine residue, the E1 active site, resulting in a thioester linkage between the C-terminal carboxyl group of ubiquitin and the E1 cysteine sulfhydryl group. Secondly, the activated ubiquitin is transferred from E1 to the cysteine of an E2 via a trans(thio)esterification reaction. Finally, the ubiquitination cascade creates an isopeptide bond between a lysine of the target protein and the C-terminal glycine of ubiquitin with the coordination of an E3 which identifies specific recognition modules in the target protein and is capable of interaction with both E2 and substrate (Ye and Rape, 2009).

In human genome, there are only two genes encoding E1, whilst E2 is encoded by 60-100 genes, and there are ~ 1000 different E3 genes (Deshaies and Joazeiro, 2009; Schulman and Harper, 2009). E1 activates ubiquitin at the top level, and transfers activated ubiquitin to different E2. E3s identify individual substrates and specifically ligate E2-Ub complex to a certain target protein. These enzymes form a hierarchical structure (Figure 3) and control the whole ubiquitination process. In this ubiquitination cascade, E1 binds to dozens of E2s, which bind to hundreds of E3s, and E3s specifically target thousands of substrate proteins.

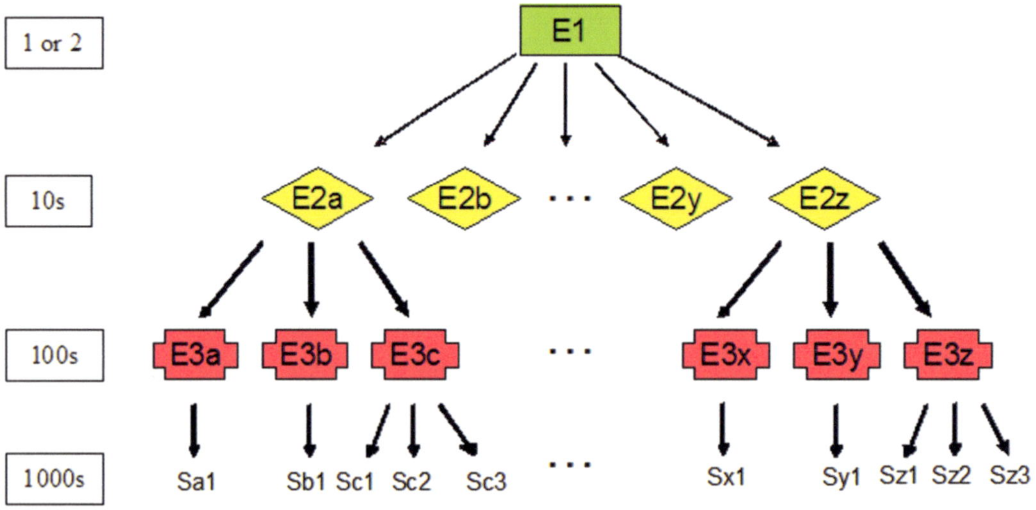

Fig. 3. E1, E2 and E3 form an enzymatic cascade for protein ubiquitination. One single E1 initiates the whole ubiquitination process, by activating Ub and transferring it to E2. There are around 100 E2s in human. Each E2 will deliver activated Ub to one or several E3s which are a large family of around 1000 members. E3s specifically identify target proteins (substrates) and attach Ub to individual proteins.

There are around 100 Dubs in human cells which cleave the ubiquitin-protein bonds thus regulating ubiquitin-dependent metabolic pathways (Colland, 2010). Polyubiquitinated proteins are deubiquitinated by Dubs immediately before degradation in the proteasome. In addition to ubiquitin recycling, Dubs are also involved in processing of ubiquitin precursors, in proofreading of protein ubiquitination and in disassembly of inhibitory ubiquitin chains.

2.3 The proteasome system

The 26S proteasome is a large protein complex with molecular weight more than 2000 kilodalton and it is composed of one 20S core particle and two 19S regulatory particles, where the core particle is made up of two α units (at the two ends) and two β units (in the middle). Each of these units is composed of 7 ring-like subunits thus the total 28 subunits stack up to form a hollow cylinder (Figure 1). The α subunits N-termini form a gate and serve as docking domains for the regulatory particles that block unregulated access of substrates to the interior cavity (Smith et al., 2007). Proteins are lysed in the core particle but proteases are only found in the interior surface of the β units, especially β1, β2 and β5. Although these proteases share a common mechanism, each subunit dominants its distinctive catalytic activity due to interatomic contacts with local residues near the active sites of each subunit. β1, β2, and β5 mainly present caspase-like, trypsin-like, and chymotrypsin-like activity, respectively. Each catalytic β subunit also possesses a conserved lysine residue required for proteolysis. The proteasomes catalyze thousands of polyubiquitinated proteins, therefore, they are critical in regulatory protein function and cell activity.

3. The UPS is extensively involved in hematological malignancies

3.1 Protein ubiquitination in blood cancers

Heavy ubiquitination levels of proteins, associated with overactivation of E1, have been observed both in leukemia cell lines and primary acute leukemia cells compared with the normal blood cells (Bedford et al., 2011; Xu et al., 2010). Additionally, blood cancer-specific proteins are also regulated by the UPS. For example, multiple myeloma (MM) tumor cells are recurrently associated with several chromosomal translocations that result in overexpression of transcription factors involved in the UPS pathway such as c-Maf, MafB, and fibroblast growth factor receptor 3 (FGFR3), which converge dysregulation of D-cyclins (Bergsagel and Kuehl, 2005). All these proteins could be poly-ubiquitinated and degraded in proteasomes. D-type cyclins are ubiquitinated under the coordination of SCF E3 ligase complex. The fibroblast growth factor receptor FGFR3 could also be ubiquitinated. In chronic leukemia, FGFR3 undergoes ubiquitination by c-Cbl, a RING finger domain-containing E3 ligase. In chronic leukemia cells, the specific BAR-ABL fusion protein is ubiquitinated by c-CBL. Targeting at c-CBL, arsenic induces degradation of BCR-ABL (Mao et al., 2010).

3.2 Ubiquitination enzymes and blood cancers

E1 is responsible for the first step of the ubiquitination process by activating ubiquitin and is overexpressed in all leukemia and MM cell lines and primary samples. When E1 is knocked down, these leukemia and MM cells will go to apoptosis (Xu et al., 2010). Several E2s have been reported to be involved in MM development. For example, CDC34, the cell cycle regulator, is highly expressed in MM patient cells and cell lines in contrast to normal cells (Block et al., 2001). CDC34 has been implicated in the ubiquitination of p27 (Kip1), IκBα, Wee1, and MyoD, thus facilitating the degradation of these proteins by 26S proteasomes and modulating cell cycle progression. Inhibition of CDC34 enzymatic activity abrogates interleukin-6-induced protection against dexamethasone-induced MM cell apoptosis.

Ubiquitin ligase E3s are the largest family in the UPS system. Various E3s are involved in leukemia, myeloma and lymphomas (Bernassola et al., 2008). For example, XIAP, the representative of the RING finger family of E3s, and Mdm2, the primary E3 ligase for p53 ubiquitination (Jones et al., 2008), are overexpressed in various leukemic and myeloma cells and contribute to cell proliferation and anti-apoptotic activity. XIAP is also the most important enzyme that inhibits caspase-3, -6, and -7 activities and confers to drug resistance. Skp2 is another important E3 ligase. In CML cells, BCR-ABL fusion oncogene frequently upregulate Skp2 expression via transcriptional activation, while treatment of Bcr-Abl kinase inhibitor imatinib led to G1 growth arrest accompanied with reduced Skp2 expression (Chen et al., 2011). SKP2 contributes to increased p27(Kip1) turnover, cell proliferation, and a poor prognosis in many tumor types (Zhan et al., 2007).

3.3 Deubiquitinases and blood cancers

Attached ubiquitin can be removed by a ubiquitin protease from targeted protein. USP9X is one of the most studied deubiquitinases and is probably involved in deubiquitination from oncoprotein MCL-1. Increased USP9X expression correlates with increased MCL1 protein in human follicular lymphomas and diffuse large B-cell lymphomas (Schwickart et al., 2010). Moreover, patients with multiple myeloma overexpressing USP9X have a poor prognosis. Knockdown of USP9X increases MCL1 polyubiquitination, which enhances MCL1 turnover and cell killing by the BH3 mimetic ABT-737, an inhibitor of MCL1 (Schwickart et al., 2010). Thus, USP9X has been identified as an effective prognostic and therapeutic target. Another important Dub is CYLD, which is a negative regulator of NFκB. CYLD is located in the 16q12 and its lower expression in MM cells is highly associated with deletion of 16q. In T cell leukemia, the Notch/Hes1 pathway sustains NFκB activation through CYLD repression. In MM cells highly expressing NFκB, both the DNA copy number and protein expression of CYLD are markedly decreased. On the other hand, when treated with proteasome inhibitors such as MG132, CYLD will be accumulated in MM cells. CYLD presents as a tumor suppressor deubiquitinase and restoration of CYLD will sensitize cancer cell apoptosis (Jin et al., 2008).

3.4 Proteasomes and blood cancers

Several lines of evidence have shown that proteasome subunits in both leukemia and MM cells are abnormally higher than those normal or untransformed counterparts (Kumatori et al., 1990). Immunohistochemical staining shows considerably increased concentrations of proteasomes in leukemic cells from the bone marrow of patients with various types of leukemia and the predominant localization of these proteasomes in the nuclei. Moreover, enzyme immunoassay and Northern blot analysis indicate that the concentrations of proteasomes and their mRNA levels are consistently much higher in a variety of malignant human hematopoietic cell lines than in resting peripheral lymphocytes and monocytes from healthy adults. Proteasome expression is also increased in normal blood mononuclear cells during blastogenic transformation induced by phytohemagglutinin; their expression increased in parallel with induction of DNA synthesis and returned to the basal level with progress of the cell cycle. These findings strongly suggest that proteasomes are associated with cell cycle progression. Later studies demonstrated that proteasomes regulate a serial of cell cycle proteins, including p27, pRb, cyclin D, p53, p27, pro-apoptotic Bcl-2 family members, as well as the most important transcription factor in cell proliferation, NFκB (Kisselev and Goldberg, 2001). Importantly, leukemia and myeloma cells are more sensitive to proteasome inhibitors. An early study found that the IC_{50} to inhibit cell proliferation in lymphoma is 5 times lower than normal T cells when treating cells with lactacystin, a classic and typical inhibitor of proteasomes (Delic et al., 1998). Another study indicated that B-CLL cells are about 10 times more sensitive to lactacystin than normal peripheral B lymphocytes. These results strongly suggest that proteasomes could be used as a drug target for myeloma and lymphoma therapy.

4. Discovery of bortezomib and its application in MM therapy

4.1 Discovery of bortezomib as a treatment for myeloma

Proteasomes are critical for cancer cells, therefore they could be used as a drug target for cancer therapy. Efforts are first made to develop such kinds of inhibitors for MM therapy. The seminal contribution came from Myogenic which developed a series of proteasome inhibitors, including MG132, one of the most common proteasome inhibitors currently used in research, and MG-341, which was renamed PS-341 and was further developed as a promising drug candidate for cancer therapy. PS-341 alone achieved an overall remission rate of 35% in refractory and/or relapse myeloma patients, when it was used in combination with other drugs such as cyclophosphamide and dexamethasone, the ORR could reach around 90% or greater. Following several large and multi-center clinical trials, PS-341 was approved by Food and Drug Administration of USA for MM in 2003, and for mantle cell lymphoma in 2006. PS-341 is now known as its general name bortezomib based on its chemical structure and is marketed as Velcade®. Recent studies also demonstrated that bortezomib might be particularly active against the active B cell-like diffuse large B cell lymphoma (ABC-DLBCL). ABC-DLBCL has a worse survival after upfront chemotherapy and is characterized by constitutive activation of the NFκB pathway, which can inhibit chemotherapy. Although bortezomib alone has no activities on ABC-DLBCL, when administrated with chemotherapeutics, such as R-CHOP or DA-EPOCH-B, it achieved a superior overall response and survival according to a clinical study of 49 patients. Although ABC-DLBCL and GCB-DLBCL have similar poor outcome by regular chemotherapeutics, ABC-DLBCLs are more sensitive to bortezomib. Bortezomib presented a high responsive rate (83% *vs* 13%) and median overall survival (10.8 *vs* 3.4 months) in ABC compared with GCB-DLBCL, respectively (Dunleavy et al., 2009). It is predictable that bortezomib as an inhibitor of NFκB pathway will be developed for other cancer therapy.

4.2 Molecular mechanisms of bortezomib in the treatment of myeloma

Bortezomib is a dipeptide containing phenylalanine and leucine in which the carboxylic group is replaced by a boronic acid group (-RB(OH)2) (Figure 4).

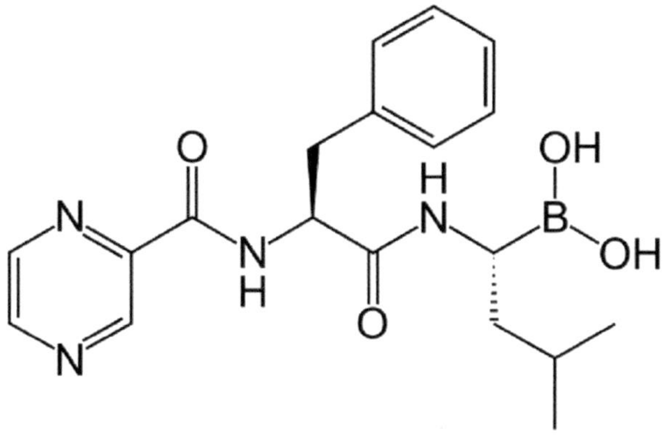

Fig. 4. The chemical structure of bortezomib. Bortezomib is a dipeptide made up of phenylalanine and leucine in which boronic acid group replaces the carboxyl group.

Bortezomib is a potent inhibitor of proteasomes. Mechanistically, its active boron acid group competitively and reversibly binds to the catalytic site of the 26S proteasome with high affinity and specificity. Specifically, the boric acid group of bortezomib binds to and blocks the catalytic threonine residue in the β subunits of the 20S core particle. Inhibition of proteasome results in accumulation of several important tumor suppressor proteins, including p21, p27, p53, PTEN, and IκBα. IκBα is an inhibitor of NFκB, the most important transcription factor in regulating cell proliferation. Normally, IκBα is bound to NFκB and inhibits its activity. The IκBα stability is regulated via the UPS pathway. Once IκBα is degraded, NFκB will be librated and translocated into the neucleus where it binds to the promoters of various genes and initiates their transcription and expression. IκBα/NFκB signaling plays a critical role in bortezomib-induced cell apoptosis. Bortezomib also interrupts the interaction of Mdm2 and its substrate p53, thus restoring p53 function and leading to cell apoptosis. Moreover, bortezomib directly acts on MM cells and alters cellular interactions and cytokine secretion in the bone marrow (BM) millieu to inhibit tumor cell growth, induce apoptosis, and overcome drug resistance. Specifically, bortezomib inhibits the paracrine growth of human MM cells by decreasing their adherence to bone marrow stromal cells (BMSCs) and related NFκB-dependent induction of interleukin-6 secretion in BMSCs, as well as inhibiting proliferation and growth signaling of residual adherent MM cells (Hideshima et al., 2001).

4.3 Pitfalls of bortezomib in MM treatment

Although bortezomib has made a great success in the treatment of MM and MCL, it is not a perfect drug, and some critical features prevent its application (Kumar and Rajkumar, 2008; Oerlemans et al., 2008). Firstly, it is unstable and it retains its activity for 4-8 hrs after re-constituted, thus having to be used within 8 hours. Secondly, the drug is administrated via *i.v.* injection which should be performed by a nurse at a clinic or in a hospital, which largely increases the cost of the health care system.

Thirdly, the therapeutic window of bortezomib is very narrow. The therapeutic dosage is 1.3 mg/m^2 body surface, it will produce dose-dependent toxicity when the dose reaches 1.5 mg/m^2. These adverse effects and toxicity include myelosuppression which leads to anemia, neutropenia and thrombocytopenia, and bortezomib-induced peripheral neuropathy, which occurs in more than 30% patients and this kind of neuropathy is sometimes even worse to affect patients' daily activity (Richardson et al., 2006). Although these kinds of adverse effects are recoverable when the drug is discontinued, some patients couldn't endure the severe effects. Recent studies suggest that some important genes (such as *RHOBTB2* and *SOX8*) involved in the development of the nervous system (especially the peripheral nervous system) are upregulated by bortezomib after one cycle therapy (Cavo et al., 2010).

Lastly, drug resistance is becoming an emerging issue. Although 35% of refractory and relapsed myeloma patients are generally responsive after bortezomib treatment, there are only 4% patients with a complete remission outcome and 65% had no response. There are several underlying issues for bortezomib resistance. Firstly, the resistance to bortezomib is associated with overexpression of β5 subunits of 20S core particles, which leads to impaired binding of bortezomib and decreased proteasome inhibition. For example, K562 cells with a high level of β5 are more resistant to bortezomib than other cell lines such as OCI-AML2 expressing low levels of β5 (Li et al., 2010). Secondly, bortezomib resistance is also associated with mutations in β5 gene. A DNA sequencing analysis in bortezomib-resistant cells revealed that the G322A mutation in PSMB5 gene leads to an Alanine→ Threonine change, which largely confers resistance because threonine is the target of bortezomib (Oerlemans et al., 2008). In a Jurkat cell model, mutations such as C323T and G326A are also reported (Lu et al., 2008). Thirdly, overexpression of other anti-apoptotic genes such as PSMD4 (Shaughnessy et al., 2010), a non-ATPase subunit of the proteosomal 19S regulator, and heat shock protein 27 (HSP27) (Chauhan et al., 2003), an important gene protecting cell against apoptosis, are also found to be associated with resistance to bortezomib. Recently, an siRNA screen identified several important molecular modulators that sensitize bortezomib-induced cell apoptosis, including proteasome subunits PSMA5, PSMB2, PSMB3, and PSMB7 (Zhu et a., 2011), this is quite reasonable because these genes directly modulate the proteasome function. To be noted, the Cyclin-dependent kinase 5 (CDK5) and other 11 genes were also identified from this screen, but their detailed roles in bortezomib-induced cell death are yet to be studied. A most recent study demonstrated that impaired bortezomib binding to mutant β5 subunit of the proteasome is the underlying basis for bortezomib resistance in leukemia cells, while proteasome subunit overexpression is an essential compensatory mechanism for the impaired catalytic activity of these mutant proteasomes (Franke et al., 2011).

5. Development of novel proteasomal inhibitors

Currently, several classes of novel proteasome inhibitors have been developed and some have been moved to advanced clinical trials for the treatment of various blood cancers, such as leukemia, lymphoma, and myeloma. Although they share some common features, these novel inhibitors of proteasomes could be classified as: highly selective and irreversible, orally active, non-competitive, and natural products. The details are shown in Table 1.

5.1 Highly selective and irreversible novel inhibitors of proteasomes

Several promising novel proteasomal inhibitors have been extensively investigated *in vivo*, *in vitro*, and in clinical settings. Compared with bortezomib, these agents are highly selective and irreversible, such as carfilzomib, NPI-0052, and PI-083.

5.1.1 Carfilzomib

Carflizomib, or PR-171, is a tetrapeptide epoxyketone and a selective and irreversible proteasome inhibitor that primarily targets the chymotrypsin-like (CT-L) subunits in both the constitutive proteasome (c20S, β5) and the immunoproteasome (i20S, LMP7) (Parlati et al., 2009). Inhibition of proteasome-mediated proteolysis results in an accumulation of polyubiquitinated proteins, which may lead to cell cycle arrest, induction of apoptosis, and inhibition of tumor growth. Compared with bortezomib, carfilzomib displays minimal cross reactivity on off-target enzymes, good tolerability and little side effects in multiple open-label clinical trials (O'Connor et al., 2009). In patients with relapsed or refractory multiple myeloma, twice-weekly consecutive-day single-agent carfilzomib 20 mg/m^2 , escalating to 27 mg/m^2 the second cycle was associated with a 54% overall response rate in bortezomib-naive patients and a 26% overall response rate in bortezomib and immunomodulatory drug refractory patients. The overall response rate is 20% higher than that with single bortezomib treatment. The U.S. Food and Drug Administration has granted fast track designation for carfilzomib to develop as a potential treatment of patients with relapsed and refractory multiple myeloma.

Drugs	Features	R&D Stage	Institutes
Highly selective and irreversible			
Carfilzomib (PR-171)	Epoxomicin analog Minimal activity against off-target enzymes Lymphoid neoplasms and multiple myeloma	Phase III for MM Phase I for solid tumors	Proteolix Onyx
Marizomib (NPI-0052 Salinospormide A)	Marine product, β-lactone-γ-lactam family More potent than Bortezomib MM, lymphomas, leukemias and solid tumors	Phase II for myeloma	Nereus Pharmaceuticals, Inc.
PI-083	From Streptomyces matensis Thr21,Gly47, Ala 49 of β5, Asp114 of β6 Cancer-selective proteasome inhibitor Myeloma, lung cancer, breast cancer	Preclinical	Moffitt Cancer Center
Orally active			
CEP-18770	Boronic-acid based More sustained Pharmacodynamics Competes with bortezomib Few side effects during treatment	Phase II for myeloma	Cephalon
PR-047	c20S, i20S >80% inhibition in most tissues High oral bioavailability		Proteolix
Non-comparative inhibitors on 20S proteasomes			
Clioquinol 5-Amino-8-hydroxyl-quine (5AHQ)	Binding to a subunits of 20S Non-competitive inhibition Overcome resistance to Bortezomib	Phase I	University Health Network
Natural Products			
Pristimerin	Isolated from Celastrus and Maytenus spp. Tripernoid family C6 of Pristimerin interacts with hydroxyl group of N-terminal Thr of c20S Inhibits IKK, suppresses NFκB, cyclin D	Preclicical	Mayo Clinic
EGCG (-)-epigallocatechin-3-gallate	From green tea Ester bond of EGCG attacked by N-terminal Thr of 20S Competitively inhibits Proteasome with Bortezomib	Preclinical	Not available

Table 1. Novel Proteasome inhibitors against blood cancers

5.1.2 Marizomib

Marizomib (NPI-0052 or salinosporamide A) is a structurally and pharmacologically unique β-lactone-γ-lactam proteasome inhibitor produced by a marine actinomycete *Salinispora tropica* (Macherla et al., 2005). Unlike bortezomib, marizomib irreversibly binds to proteasomes and inhibits all three protease activities, including chymotrypsin-like (CT-L, β5), trypsin-like (T-L, β2), and caspase-like (C-L,β1). This nature is responsible for its slower efflux, longer duration of action, and greater cytotoxicity (Obaidat et al.). Preclinical studies suggest that marizomib is a more potent inducer of apoptosis in myeloma cells than bortezomib, and demonstrates activity in bortezomib resistant cell lines as well. In addition to MM, marizomib has been evaluated in models for MCL, Waldenstrom's macroglobulinemia (WM), chronic and acute lymphocytic leukemia, glioma, colorectal and pancreatic cancers, and has exhibited synergistic activities in tumor models in combination with bortezomib, and various histone deacetylase inhibitors (B et al., 2011; Singh et al., 2010). Marizomib has been moved to Phase II clinical trials and achieved very good responses. In a Phase I study of 17 patients with relapsed and relapsed/refractory multiple myeloma, Drug- related adverse events have consisted principally of mild-to-moderate fatigue, nausea and diarrhea. More importantly, NPI-0052 does not appear to induce peripheral neuropathy or myelosuppression associated with bortezomib treatment (Hofmeister et al., 2009).

5.2 Orally active inhibitors of proteasomes: CEP-18770, PR-047 and ONX-0912

The *i.v.* administration of bortezomib largely increases the workload of the physicians and other medical staff and largely increases the healthcare budget. Therefore, orally active inhibitors of proteasomes are of great interest. Currently, several such orally active drugs have been developed, including CEP-18770, PR-047 and ONX-0912.

5.2.1 CEP-18770

CEP-18770 is a novel orally-active inhibitor of the chymotrypsin-like activity of the proteasome that down-modulates the NFκB activity (Piva et al., 2008). CEP-18770 induces apoptotic cell death in MM cell lines and in primary purified CD138-positive explant cultures from untreated and bortezomib-treated MM patients. Importantly, CEP-18770 exhibits a favorable cytotoxicity profile toward normal human epithelial cells, bone marrow progenitors, and bone marrow-derived stromal cells. Both intravenous and oral administration of CEP-18770 resulted in a sustained pharmacodynamic inhibition of proteasome activity in tumors relative to normal tissues, complete tumor regression of MM xenografts and improved overall median survival in a systemic model of human MM. In addition, CEP-18770 has a strong antiangiogenic activity *in vitro*, and potently represses RANKL-induced osteoclastogenesis. A recent study suggests that CEP-18770 enhances the anti-myeloma activity of bortezomib and melphalan which suggests a combinatorial regimen for MM therapy (Piva et al., 2008; Sanchez et al., 2010). This agent has moved to clinical trials for relapsed or refractory multiple myeloma (http://clinicaltrials.gov/ct2/show/NCT01348919) or for solid tumors and non-Hodgin's lymphomas (http://clinicaltrials.gov/ct2/show/NCT00572637).

5.2.2 PR-047

PR-047 is also an orally active inhibitor that selectively inhibits CT-L activity of both the constitutive proteasome (β5) and immunoproteasome (LMP7) and demonstrated an absolute bioavailability of up to 39% in rodents and dogs. It was well tolerated with repeated oral administration at doses resulting in >80% proteasome inhibition in most tissues and elicited an antitumor response equivalent to intravenously administered carfilzomib in multiple human tumor xenograft and mouse syngeneic models (Zhou et al., 2009). The favorable pharmacologic profile supports its further development for the treatment of malignant diseases.

5.2.3 ONX-0912

Like carfilzomib, ONX-0912 is also an epoxyketone compound with novel selective, irreversible inhibition activity to the immunopreteasome and constituent 20S particles. ONX-0912 displays great oral activity (Chauhan et al., 2010). Primary WM cells expressing higher level of 20S are more responsive to ONX-0912 (Roccaro et al., 2010). ONX-0912 induces WM cell apoptosis through c-JNK activation, NFκB inhibition, caspase cleavage, and initiation of the unfolded protein response. Moreover, ONX-0912 also reduce the secretion of BM-derived interleukin-6 (IL-6) and insulin-like growth factor 1 (IGF-1), thus inhibiting BM-induced Akt phosphorylation and phosphorylated extracellular signal-related kinase activation in WM cells. In addition to blood cancers, ONX-0912 also displays potent anticancer activity in solid tumors and a Phase I study of ONX 0912 administered orally in patients with advanced refractory or recurrent solid tumors is under evaluation (http://clinicaltrials.gov/ ct2/show/NCT01129349).

5.3 Non-classic inhibitors: Clioquinol and 5-amino-8-hydroxyl-quinoline

Most of the proteasomal inhibitors competitively bind to the β subunits of 20S proteasome, for example, MG-132, bortezomib, and carfilzomib. Recently, we found that a group of quinoline-based agents including clioquinol, chloroquine, 5-amino-8-hydroxyl quinoline (5AHQ), and metfloquinoline display potent inhibition on proteasomal catalytic activity by a non-competitive manner (Li et al., 2010; Mao et al., 2009). Further studies indicated that these agents bind to the α subunits other than β subunits of the 20S core particle as bortezomib or MG-132 does. In analysis of its binding to purified 20S archaeal proteasomes from *Thermoplasma acidophilium* by using nuclear magnetic resonance (NMR) technology, chloroquine binds to the α subunits with 260 Å distance from β active sites. Notably, chloroquine and MG132 can bind the proteasome simultaneously, further establishing that they exploit two completely separate binding pockets (Sprangers et al., 2008).

The interaction of 5AHQ with α_7– α_7 produced clear spectral changes localized to residues Ile159, Val113, Val87, Val82, Leu112, Val89, Val134, Val24 and Leu136, which are inside the antechamber. In contrast, MG132 which binds the proteolytic chamber produces shifts in the beta rings of the full proteasome. Binding to the α subunit, 5AHQ leads to a conformational change of the core particle and displays a non-competitive inhibition on proteasome. 5AHQ preferentially induced cell death in primary myeloma and leukemia cells compared with normal hematopoietic cells. More importantly, 5AHQ overcomes the resistance to bortezomib and is equally cytotoxic to human myelomonocytic leukemia THP1/BTZ500 cells which are 237-fold more resistant to bortezomib than wild-type THP1 cells because of the overexpression and mutation of the bortezomib-binding β5 subunits (Li et al., 2010). Therefore, a group of quinoline-based small molecules can inhibit proteasomal activity in a non-cannoical manner. Because of their low toxicity and novel inhibition mechanism, these compounds could be developed for MM and leukemia therapy. Currently, clioquinol has been moved to clinical trials for refractory acute myeloid leukemia.

5.4 Natural proteasomal inhibitors: Pristimerin and EGCG

Except for small chemical compounds or peptide reagents, several natural products have been identified and evaluated for MM treatment in both *in vivo* and *in vitro* assays. The most promising candidate could be NPI-0052 or marizomib isolated from a marine actinomycete *Salinispora tropica* as described above. Here we discuss two more agents in this category pristimerin and (-)-epigallocatechin-3-gallate (EGCG).

5.4.1 Prisitmerin

Pristimerin belongs to the tripernoid family and is isolated from a traditional Chinese medicine called *Celastrus* and *Maytenus spp.* Nucleophilic susceptibility and *in silico* docking studies show that C6 of pristimerin is highly susceptible towards a nucleophilic attack by the hydroxyl group of N-terminal threonine of the proteasomal chymotrypsin subunit. This interaction leads to an inhibition of the chymotrypsin-like activity of a purified rabbit 20S proteasome (Yang et al., 2008). Pristimerin displayed similar inhibition activity in purified rabbit 20S proteasomes and in human prostate cancer cell lysates (Tiedemann et al., 2009). The IC_{50}s are 2.2 and 3.0 μM *in vitro* and *in vivo*, respectively. The treatment of pristimerin in prostate cancer cells resulted in the accumulation of ubiquitinated proteins and three proteasome target proteins, Bax, p27 and IκBα. However, myeloma cells are more sensitive to pristimerin. Pristimerin potently inhibits both IKK and the proteasome in MM cells with an IC_{50} of 100 nM. Pristimerin causes overt suppression of constitutive NFκB activity in myeloma cells that may mediate its suppression of cyclin D, thus inducing myeloma cell apoptosis.

5.4.2 (-)-epigallocatechin-3-gallate (EGCG)

EGCG is one of the polyphenols found in green tea extract and inhibits proteasomal activity (Golden et al., 2009). The ester bond of EGCG is attacked by the N-terminal threonine residue of the proteasome, forming a covalent EGCG-proteasome complex which has been confirmed by high performance liquid chromatography (HPLC) analysis. Recent studies found that EGCG competitively inhibits proteasomal activity in a same manner as bortezomib does, thus neutralizing the inhibiting activity of bortezomib and other boronic acid-based proteasome inhibitors. Therefore, green tea polyphenols block the anticancer effects of bortezomib and green tea is not encouraged for myeloma patients who are using bortezomib (Golden et al., 2009). However, a recent study didn't find antagonism of bortezomib in preclinical *in vivo* experiments, where EGCG or ascorbic acid plasma concentrations are commensurate with dietary or supplemental intake and suggest that patients receiving bortezomib treatment do not need to avoid normal dietary consumption of green tea, vitamin C-containing foods, or EGCG or vitamin C dietary supplements (Bannerman et al., 2011).

6. Targeting at ubiquitination and deubiquitination systems for blood cancer treatment

Proteasomes are critical components of both cancer cells and normal tissues because they determine the fate of most of the proteins and therefore inhibition of proteasome will also lead to normal cell stress and apoptosis. Thus inhibition of proteasomes indiscriminately raises levels of hundreds of proteins regardless to their anticancer effect. Thus, proteasomal inhibitors are a double-edged sword because they kill cancer cells, simultaneously, kill normal cells. Because proteasome-coupled protein ubiquitination is more specific, inhibition of certain enzymes involved in protein ubiquitination will be a more pertinent target for cancer drug development. There are four kinds of enzymes, E1, E2, E3 and Dubs which contain thousands of members in total. Currently, with the exception of E2, inhibitors of these other enzymes have been identified and are being evaluated for the treatment of hematological malignancies.

6.1 Targeting at E1 for hematological malignancies

E1 or Ubiquitin-activating enzyme (UBA) controls the protein ubiquitination by activating ubiquitin using ATP as an energy supplier. Knockdown of E1 by small interfering RNA (siRNA) strategy decreases the abundance of ubiquitinated proteins in leukemia and myeloma cells and induced cell death (Xu et al., 2010). Blood cancer cells including leukemia and myeloma are more sensitive to E1 inhibitors. A small molecule PYZD-4409, an inhibitor of E1, can abolish protein ubiquitination, thus inducing endoplasmic reticulum (ER) stress, and leading to cancer cell apoptosis. PYZD-4409 also displayed ideal anti-leukemia activity *in vivo* without untoward toxicity by decreasing tumor volume and weight (Xu et al., 2010). However, the same concern may arise as that already seen in bortezomib because there is only a single E1 protein in humans.

6.2 Targeting at E3 for blood cancer therapies

The E3 ligases are the largest family in the UPS system. E3s are the primary determinant of substrate specificity and represent the largest and most diverse class of Ub/Ub-like regulatory enzymes. There are 600-1000 potential E3s responsible for E2 binding, substrate recognition, and regulatory functions. Targeting the ubiquitin ligases promises more specificity because most E3s tag only a few proteins for destruction. Such drugs can, in theory, block degradation of its specific substrate proteins. Currently, interfering with E3-substrate interaction is one of the leading strategies for anti-cancer drugs targeting at UPS.

One of the most promising E3s is Skp2, the F-box protein that controls degradation of p27, an important tumor suppressor gene (Zhan et al., 2007). Skp2 levels are abnormally high in leukemia and myeloma cells, therefore, blocking Skp2 activity might reasonably be expected to stop cancer cell proliferation. CpdA is such an inhibitor of Skp2 by preventing incorporation of Skp2 into the SCF Skp2 ligase, CpdA induces G1/S cell-cycle arrest as well as SCF Skp2- and p27-dependent cell killing (Chen et al., 2008). In models of MM, CpdA overcomes resistance to dexamethasone, doxorubicin, and melphalan, as well as to bortezomib, and also acted synergistically with this proteasome inhibitor. Importantly, CpdA is active against patient-derived plasma cells and both myeloid and lymphoblastoid leukemia blasts, and showed preferential activity against neoplastic cells while relatively sparing other marrow components (Chen et al., 2008).

Another interesting E3 is MdM2 which regulates p53 ubiquitination. Several inhibitors of MdM2 have been identified, such as Nutlins (Stuhmer et al., 2005) and MI-63 (Ding et al., 2006; Samudio et al., 2010). By disrupting the interaction of MdM2 and p53, both Nutlins and MI-63 can restore p53 which further tends to promote arrest of cell cycle and apoptosis. These drugs are effective in inducing apoptosis of MM cells which express wild-type p53, unfortunately, it won't work in cancer cells with mutated or deleted p53.

6.3 Targeting at deubiquitinases

Just like E3s, deubiquitinases play a tumor-suppressing or -promoting role dependent on its targeting protein. For example, USP9X is an oncoprotein enzyme that removes ubiquitin from the anti-apoptotic protein MCL-1 (Sun et al., 2011). MCL1 is overexpressed in most blood cancer cells, and is highly associated with cancer cell proliferation and protects cancer cells from apoptosis (Sun et al., 2011). MCL1 is degraded by proteasomes after poly-ubiquitination. High expression of USP9X is seen in leukemia and MM cells. A small molecule called WP1130 (Kapuria et al., 2010) has been identified as a partly selective Dub inhibitor by directly inhibiting activity of USP9x, USP5, USP14, and UCH37, which are known to regulate survival protein stability and 26S proteasome function. WP1130-mediated inhibition of tumor-activated Dubs results in downregulation of antiapoptotic and upregulation of proapoptotic proteins, such as Mcl-1 and p53, thus leading to cancer cell death (Kapuria et al., 2010).

Although large-scale inhibitors of ubiquitination enzymes are yet to fully develop, successful E3 and Dub inhibitors have established the proof-of-principle that inhibition of ubquitinating/deubiquitinating enzymes is novel and potentially powerful strategy to develop anti-blood cancer drugs and is surely an area that will expand greatly in the future.

7. Summary

The ubiquitin-proteasome system has been widely investigated in the association of hematological malignancies, it is extensively involved in the development and therapy of blood cancers, including leukemia, lymphoma and multiple myeloma. Targeting at the UPS specific genes/proteins, several novel drugs have been developed including the first-approved proteasome inhibitor-bortezomib in the treatment of myeloma and mantle cell lymphoma. The upcoming years will witness the introduction of more potent and more patient-friendly next generations of UPS inhibitors such as carfilozomib and inhibitors of ubiquitinating/deubiquitinating enzymes for the treatment of blood cancer patients.

8. Acknowledgment

This project was partly supported by the Priority Academic Program Development of Jiangsu Higher Education Institutions (PAPD).

9. References

B CP, M XA, K CA, Baritaki S, BerkFers C, Bonavida B, Chandra J, Chauhan D, C. Cusack J J, Fenical W, I MG, Groll M, P RJ, K SL, G KL, McBride W, D JM, C PM, S TCN, Oki Y, Ovaa H, Pajonk F, P GR, A MR, C MS, M AS, Valashi E, Younes A, & Palladino

MA (2011). Marizomib, a proteasome inhibitor for all seasons: preclinical profile and a framework for clinical trials. Current Cancer Drug Targets 11(3):254-284.

Bannerman B, Xu L, Jones M, Tsu C, Yu J, Hales P, Monbaliu J, Fleming P, Dick L, Manfredi M, Claiborne C, Bolen J, Kupperman E, & Berger A (2011) Preclinical evaluation of the antitumor activity of bortezomib in combination with vitamin C or with epigallocatechin gallate, a component of green tea. Cancer Chemotherapy and Pharmacology.

Bedford L, Lowe J, Dick LR, Mayer RJ, & Brownell JE (2011) Ubiquitin-like protein conjugation and the ubiquitin-proteasome system as drug targets. Nature reviews 10(1):29-46.

Bergsagel PL and Kuehl WM (2005) Molecular pathogenesis and a consequent classification of multiple myeloma. Journal of Clinical Oncology 23(26):6333-6338.

Bernassola F, Karin M, Ciechanover A, & Melino G (2008) The HECT family of E3 ubiquitin ligases: multiple players in cancer development. Cancer Cell 14(1):10-21.

Block K, Boyer TG, & Yew PR (2001) Phosphorylation of the human ubiquitin-conjugating enzyme, CDC34, by casein kinase 2. The Journal of Biological Chemistry 276(44):41049-41058.

Cavo M, Tacchetti P, Patriarca F, Petrucci MT, Pantani L, Galli M, Di Raimondo F, Crippa C, Zamagni E, Palumbo A, Offidani M, Corradini P, Narni F, Spadano A, Pescosta N, Deliliers GL, Ledda A, Cellini C, Caravita T, Tosi P , & Baccarani M (2010) Bortezomib with thalidomide plus dexamethasone compared with thalidomide plus dexamethasone as induction therapy before, and consolidation therapy after, double autologous stem-cell transplantation in newly diagnosed multiple myeloma: a randomised phase 3 study. Lancet 376(9758):2075-2085.

Chauhan D, Li G, Shringarpure R, Podar K, Ohtake Y, Hideshima T, & Anderson KC (2003) Blockade of Hsp27 overcomes Bortezomib/proteasome inhibitor PS-341 resistance in lymphoma cells. Cancer Research 63(19):6174-6177.

Chauhan D, Singh AV, Aujay M, Kirk CJ, Bandi M, Ciccarelli B, Raje N, Richardson P, & Anderson KC (2010) A novel orally active proteasome inhibitor ONX 0912 triggers in vitro and in vivo cytotoxicity in multiple myeloma. Blood 116(23):4906-4915.

Chen JY, Wang MC, & Hung WC (2011) Bcr-Abl-induced tyrosine phosphorylation of Emi1 to stabilize Skp2 protein via inhibition of ubiquitination in chronic myeloid leukemia cells. Journal of Cellular Physiology 226(2):407-413.

Chen Q, Xie W, Kuhn DJ, Voorhees PM, Lopez-Girona A, Mendy D, Corral LG, Krenitsky VP, Xu W, Moutouh-de Parseval L, Webb DR, Mercurio F, Nakayama KI, Nakayama K, & Orlowski RZ (2008) Targeting the p27 E3 ligase SCF(Skp2) results in p27- and Skp2-mediated cell-cycle arrest and activation of autophagy. Blood 111(9):4690-4699.

Ciechanover A (1998) The ubiquitin-proteasome pathway: on protein death and cell life. The EMBO Journal 17(24):7151-7160.

Ciechanover A, Orian A, & Schwartz AL (2000) The ubiquitin-mediated proteolytic pathway: mode of action and clinical implications. Journal of Cellular Biochemistry 34:40-51.

Colland F (2010) The therapeutic potential of deubiquitinating enzyme inhibitors. Biochemical Society Transactions 38(Pt 1):137-143.

Delic J, Masdehors P, Omura S, Cosset JM, Dumont J, Binet JL, & Magdelenat H (1998) The proteasome inhibitor lactacystin induces apoptosis and sensitizes chemo- and radioresistant human chronic lymphocytic leukaemia lymphocytes to TNF-alpha-initiated apoptosis. British Journal of Cancer 77(7):1103-1107.

Deshaies RJ and Joazeiro CA (2009) RING domain E3 ubiquitin ligases. Annual Review of Biochemistry 78:399-434. Ding K, Lu Y, Nikolovska-Coleska Z, Wang G, Qiu S, Shangary S, Gao W, Qin D, Stuckey J, Krajewski K, Roller PP, & Wang S (2006) Structure-based design of spiro-oxindoles as potent, specific small-molecule inhibitors of the 12MDM2-p53 interaction. Journal of Medicinal Chemistry 49(12):3432-3435.

Dunleavy K, Pittaluga S, Czuczman MS, Dave SS, Wright G, Grant N, Shovlin M, Jaffe ES, Janik JE, Staudt LM, & Wilson WH (2009) Differential efficacy of bortezomib plus chemotherapy within molecular subtypes of diffuse large B-cell lymphoma. Blood 113(24):6069-76.

Franke NE, Niewerth D, Assaraf YG, van Meerloo J, Vojtekova K, van Zantwijk CH, Zweegman S, Chan ET, Kirk CJ, Geerke DP, Schimmer AD, Kaspers GJ, Jansen G, & Cloos J (2011) Impaired bortezomib binding to mutant β5 subunit of the proteasome is the underlying basis for bortezomib resistance in leukemia cells. Leukemia Sept 23 [Epub ahead of print].

Impaired bortezomib binding to mutant β5 subunit of the proteasome is the underlying basis for bortezomib resistance in leukemia cells.

Golden EB, Lam PY, Kardosh A, Gaffney KJ, Cadenas E, Louie SG, Petasis NA, Chen TC, & Schonthal AH (2009) Green tea polyphenols block the anticancer effects of bortezomib and other boronic acid-based proteasome inhibitors. Blood 113(23):5927-5937.

Haglund K and Dikic I (2005) Ubiquitylation and cell signaling. The EMBO journal 24(19):3353-3359.

Hideshima T, Richardson P, Chauhan D, Palombella VJ, Elliott PJ, Adams J, & Anderson KC (2001) The proteasome inhibitor PS-341 inhibits growth, induces apoptosis, and overcomes drug resistance in human multiple myeloma cells. Cancer Research 61(7):3071-3076.

Jin W, Chang M, Paul EM, Babu G, Lee AJ, Reiley W, Wright A, Zhang M, You J, & Sun SC (2008) Deubiquitinating enzyme CYLD negatively regulates RANK signaling and osteoclastogenesis in mice. The Journal of Clinical Investigation 118(5):1858-1866.

Jones RJ, Chen Q, Voorhees PM, Young KH, Bruey-Sedano N, Yang D, & Orlowski RZ (2008) Inhibition of the p53 E3 ligase HDM-2 induces apoptosis and DNA damage--independent p53 phosphorylation in mantle cell lymphoma. Clinical Cancer Research 14(17):5416-5425.

Kapuria V, Peterson LF, Fang D, Bornmann WG, Talpaz M, & Donato NJ (2010) Deubiquitinase inhibition by small-molecule WP1130 triggers aggresome formation and tumor cell apoptosis. Cancer research 70(22):9265-9276.

Kirkin V and Dikic I (2010) Ubiquitin networks in cancer. Current Opinion in Genetics & Development 21(1):21-28.

Kisselev AF and Goldberg AL (2001) Proteasome inhibitors: from research tools to drug candidates. Chemistry & Biology 8(8):739-758.

Kumar S and Rajkumar SV (2008) Many facets of bortezomib resistance/susceptibility. Blood 112(6):2177-2178.

Kumatori A, Tanaka K, Inamura N, Sone S, Ogura T, Matsumoto T, Tachikawa T, Shin S, & Ichihara A (1990) Abnormally high expression of proteasomes in human leukemic cells. Proceedings of the National Academy of Sciences of the United States of America 87(18):7071-7075.

Li X, Wood TE, Sprangers R, Jansen G, Franke NE, Mao X, Wang X, Zhang Y, Verbrugge SE, Adomat H, Li ZH, Trudel S, Chen C, Religa TL, Jamal N, Messner H, Cloos J, Rose DR, Navon A, Guns E, Batey RA, Kay LE, & Schimmer AD (2010) Effect of noncompetitive proteasome inhibition on bortezomib resistance. Journal of the National Cancer Institute 102(14):1069-1082.

Lu S, Yang J, Song X, Gong S, Zhou H, Guo L, Song N, Bao X, Chen P, & Wang J (2008) Point mutation of the proteasome beta5 subunit gene is an important mechanism of bortezomib resistance in bortezomib-selected variants of Jurkat T cell lymphoblastic lymphoma/leukemia line. The Journal of Pharmacology and Experimental Therapeutics 326(2):423-431.

Macherla VR, Mitchell SS, Manam RR, Reed KA, Chao TH, Nicholson B, Deyanat-Yazdi G, Mai B, Jensen PR, Fenical WF, Neuteboom ST, Lam KS, Palladino MA, & Potts BC (2005) Structure-activity relationship studies of salinosporamide A (NPI-0052), a novel marine derived proteasome inhibitor. Journal of Medicinal Chemistry 48(11):3684-3687.

Mao JH, Sun XY, Liu JX, Zhang QY, Liu P, Huang QH, Li KK, Chen Q, Chen Z, & Chen SJ (2010) As4S4 targets RING-type E3 ligase c-CBL to induce degradation of BCR-ABL in chronic myelogenous leukemia. Proceedings of the National Academy of Sciences of the United States of America 107(50):21683-21688.

Mao X, Li X, Sprangers R, Wang X, Venugopal A, Wood T, Zhang Y, Kuntz DA, Coe E, Trudel S, Rose D, Batey RA, Kay LE, & Schimmer AD (2009) Clioquinol inhibits the proteasome and displays preclinical activity in leukemia and myeloma. Leukemia 23(3):585-590.

O'Connor OA, Stewart AK, Vallone M, Molineaux CJ, Kunkel LA, Gerecitano JF, & Orlowski RZ (2009) A phase 1 dose escalation study of the safety and pharmacokinetics of the novel proteasome inhibitor carfilzomib (PR-171) in patients with hematologic malignancies. Clinical Cancer Research 15(22):7085-7091.

Obaidat A, Weiss J, Wahlgren B, Manam RR, Macherla VR, McArthur K, Chao TH, Palladino MA, Lloyd GK, Potts BC, Enna SJ, Neuteboom ST, & Hagenbuch B (2011) Proteasome Regulator Marizomib (NPI-0052) Exhibits Prolonged Inhibition, Attenuated Efflux, and Greater Cytotoxicity than Its Reversible Analogs. The Journal of Pharmacology and Experimental Therapeutics 337(2):479-486.

Oerlemans R, Franke NE, Assaraf YG, Cloos J, van Zantwijk I, Berkers CR, Scheffer GL, Debipersad K, Vojtekova K, Lemos C, van der Heijden JW, Ylstra B, Peters GJ, Kaspers GL, Dijkmans BA, Scheper RJ, & Jansen G (2008) Molecular basis of bortezomib resistance: proteasome subunit beta5 (PSMB5) gene mutation and overexpression of PSMB5 protein. Blood 112(6):2489-2499.

Parlati F, Lee SJ, Aujay M, Suzuki E, Levitsky K, Lorens JB, Micklem DR, Ruurs P, Sylvain C, Lu Y, Shenk KD, & Bennett MK (2009) Carfilzomib can induce tumor cell death through selective inhibition of the chymotrypsin-like activity of the proteasome. Blood 114(16):3439-3447.

Piva R, Ruggeri B, Williams M, Costa G, Tamagno I, Ferrero D, Giai V, Coscia M, Peola S, Massaia M, Pezzoni G, Allievi C, Pescalli N, Cassin M, di Giovine S, Nicoli P, de Feudis P, Strepponi I, Roato I, Ferracini R, Bussolati B, Camussi G, Jones-Bolin S, Hunter K, Zhao H, Neri A, Palumbo A, Berkers C, Ovaa H, Bernareggi A, & Inghirami G (2008) CEP-18770: A novel, orally active proteasome inhibitor with a tumor-selective pharmacologic profile competitive with bortezomib. Blood 111(5):2765-2775.

Richardson PG, Barlogie B, Berenson J, Singhal S, Jagannath S, Irwin D, Rajkumar SV, Srkalovic G, Alsina M, Alexanian R, Siegel D, Orlowski RZ, Kuter D, Limentani SA, Lee S, Hideshima T, Esseltine DL, Kauffman M, Adams J, Schenkein DP, & Anderson KC (2003) A phase 2 study of bortezomib in relapsed, refractory myeloma. The New England Journal of Medicine 348(26):2609-2617.

Richardson PG, Briemberg H, Jagannath S, Wen PY, Barlogie B, Berenson J, Singhal S, Siegel DS, Irwin D, Schuster M, Srkalovic G, Alexanian R, Rajkumar SV, Limentani S, Alsina M, Orlowski RZ, Najarian K, Esseltine D, Anderson KC, & Amato AA (2006) Frequency, characteristics, and reversibility of peripheral neuropathy during treatment of advanced multiple myeloma with bortezomib. Journal of Clinical Oncology 24(19):3113-3120.

Roccaro AM, Sacco A, Aujay M, Ngo HT, Azab AK, Azab F, Quang P, Maiso P, Runnels J, Anderson KC, Demo S, & Ghobrial IM (2010) Selective inhibition of chymotrypsin-like activity of the immunoproteasome and constitutive proteasome in Waldenstrom macroglobulinemia. Blood 115(20):4051-4060.

Samudio IJ, Duvvuri S, Clise-Dwyer K, Watt JC, Mak D, Kantarjian H, Yang D, Ruvolo V, & Borthakur G (2010) Activation of p53 signaling by MI-63 induces apoptosis in acute myeloid leukemia cells. Leukemia & Lymphoma 51(5):911-919.

Sanchez E, Li M, Steinberg JA, Wang C, Shen J, Bonavida B, Li ZW, Chen H, & Berenson JR (2010) The proteasome inhibitor CEP-18770 enhances the anti-myeloma activity of bortezomib and melphalan. British Journal of Haematology 148(4):569-581.

Schulman BA, & Harper JW (2009) Ubiquitin-like protein activation by E1 enzymes: the apex for downstream signalling pathways. Nature Review Molecular Cell Biology 10(5):319-331.

Schwickart M, Huang X, Lill JR, Liu J, Ferrando R, French DM, Maecker H, O'Rourke K, Bazan F, Eastham-Anderson J, Yue P, Dornan D, Huang DC, & Dixit VM (2010) Deubiquitinase USP9X stabilizes MCL1 and promotes tumour cell survival. Nature 463(7277):103-107.

Shaughnessy JD, Jr., Qu P, Usmani S, Heuck CJ, Zhang Q, Zhou Y, Tian E, Hanamura I, van Rhee F, Anaissie E, Epstein J, Nair B, Stephens O, Williams R, Waheed S, Alsayed Y, Crowley J, & Barlogie B (2011) Pharmacogenomics of bortezomib test-dosing identifies hyperexpression of proteasome genes, especially PSMD4, as novel high-risk feature in myeloma treated with total therapy 3. Blood. May 31. [Epub ahead of print].

Singh AV, Palladino MA, Lloyd GK, Potts BC, Chauhan D, & Anderson KC (2010) Pharmacodynamic and efficacy studies of the novel proteasome inhibitor NPI-0052 (marizomib) in a human plasmacytoma xenograft murine model. British Journal of Haematology 149(4):550-559.

Smith DM, Chang SC, Park S, Finley D, Cheng Y, & Goldberg AL (2007) Docking of the proteasomal ATPases' carboxyl termini in the 20S proteasome's alpha ring opens the gate for substrate entry. Molecular cell 27(5):731-744.

Sprangers R, Li X, Mao X, Rubinstein JL, Schimmer AD, & Kay LE (2008) TROSY-based NMR evidence for a novel class of 20S proteasome inhibitors. Biochemistry 47(26):6727-6734.

Stuhmer T, Chatterjee M, Hildebrandt M, Herrmann P, Gollasch H, Gerecke C, Theurich S, Cigliano L, Manz RA, Daniel PT, Bommert K, Vassilev LT, & Bargou RC (2005) Nongenotoxic activation of the p53 pathway as a therapeutic strategy for multiple myeloma. Blood 106(10):3609-3617.

Sun H, Kapuria V, Peterson LF, Fang D, Bornmann WG, Bartholomeusz G, Talpaz M, & Donato NJ (2011) Bcr-Abl ubiquitination and Usp9x inhibition block kinase signaling and promote CML cell apoptosis. Blood 117(11):3151-3162.

Tiedemann RE, Schmidt J, Keats JJ, Shi CX, Zhu YX, Palmer SE, Mao X, Schimmer AD, & Stewart AK (2009) Identification of a potent natural triterpenoid inhibitor of proteosome chymotrypsin-like activity and NF-kappaB with antimyeloma activity in vitro and in vivo. Blood 113(17):4027-4037.

Xu GW, Ali M, Wood TE, Wong D, Maclean N, Wang X, Gronda M, Skrtic M, Li X, Hurren R, Mao X, Venkatesan M, Beheshti Zavareh R, Ketela T, Reed JC, Rose D, Moffat J, Batey RA, Dhe-Paganon S, & Schimmer AD (2010) The ubiquitin-activating enzyme E1 as a therapeutic target for the treatment of leukemia and multiple myeloma. Blood 115(11):2251-2259.

Yang H, Landis-Piwowar KR, Lu D, Yuan P, Li L, Reddy GP, Yuan X , & Dou QP (2008) Pristimerin induces apoptosis by targeting the proteasome in prostate cancer cells. Journal of Cell Biochemistry 103(1):234-244.

Ye Y and Rape M (2009) Building ubiquitin chains: E2 enzymes at work. Nature Review Molecular Cell Biology 10(11):755-764.

Zhan F, Colla S, Wu X, Chen B, Stewart JP, Kuehl WM, Barlogie B, & Shaughnessy JD, Jr. (2007) CKS1B, overexpressed in aggressive disease, regulates multiple myeloma growth and survival through SKP2- and p27Kip1-dependent and -independent mechanisms. Blood 109(11):4995-5001.

Zhou HJ, Aujay MA, Bennett MK, Dajee M, Demo SD, Fang Y, Ho MN, Jiang J, Kirk CJ, Laidig GJ, Lewis ER, Lu Y, Muchamuel T, Parlati F, Ring E, Shenk KD, Shields J, Shwonek PJ, Stanton T, Sun CM, Sylvain C, Woo TM, & Yang J (2009) Design and synthesis of an orally bioavailable and selective peptide epoxyketone proteasome inhibitor (PR-047). Journal of Medicinal Chemistry 52(9):3028-3038.

Zhu YX, Tiedemann R, Shi CX, Yin H, Schmidt JE, Bruins LA, Keats JJ, Braggio E, Sereduk C, Mousses S, & Stewart AK (2011) RNAi screen of the druggable genome identifies modulators of proteasome inhibitor sensitivity in myeloma including CDK5. Blood 117(14):3847-57.

21

Heparin-Induced Thrombocytopenia

Kazuo Nakamura
Nihon Pharmaceutical University
Japan

1. Intoduction

Heparin is an effective anti-coagulant for the prevention of venous thromboembolism and for the treatment of venous thrombosis and pulmonary embolism (Girolami et al., 2003; Hirsh et al., 2004; Shantsila et al., 2009). It is often used for patients with unstable angina and acute myocardial infarction, and for patients who have undergone vascular surgery (Battistelli et al., 2010). The administration of heparin frequently induces a reduction in platelet counts. This phenomenon is called heparin-induced thrombocytopenia (HIT) and be classified as either type I or II. To avoid confusion between the syndromes, "HIT type I" has been changed to "non-immune heparin associated thrombocytopenia", and ''HIT type II'' is simply called ''HIT''.

The origin of non-immune heparin associated thrombocytopenia is not yet completely understood, though it is thought to be caused by heparin-induced platelet clumping (Fabris et al., 1983; Chong & Ismail, 1989). Thrombocytopenia of this type is mild (platelet count, >100 x 10^9 cells/L), not progressive, nor associated with bleeding or thrombosis (Salzman et al., 1980), and is independent of any immune reaction (Chong et al., 1993a; Burgess & Chong, 1997; Shantsila et al., 2009). It is characterized by a transitory, slight and asymptomatic reduction in platelet count, occurring during the first 1-2 days of heparin administration. This phenomenon gradually resolves without interruption of heparin administration, and platelet counts gradually rises to pre-treatment levels within a few days without special treatment. Non-immune heparin associated thrombocytopenia may be related to the direct binding of heparin to platelet membranes (Salzman et al., 1980; Fabris et al., 1983; Chong & Ismail, 1989).

In this view, the term HIT refers only to HIT type II. HIT is associated with a heparin-related immune reaction. It is a prothrombotic disease initiated by administration of heparin, and is related to antibody-mediated platelet activation causing thrombin generation and thrombotic complications. Thrombocytopenia is common in hospitalized patients, occurring in up to 58% of critically ill individuals, and can be caused by a variety of factors (Strauss et al., 2002). HIT, which is associated with significant morbidity and mortality if unrecognized, can be regarded as a very severe side effect of a drug, (Chong, 1992; Aster, 1995; Chong, 2003). Unfortunately, HIT often remains unrecognized, undiagnosed, and untreated, a problem that can be rectified with increased awareness and a high degree of suspicion for HIT. Current treatment recommendations are based on recent advances in research on the pathophysiology and the natural history of HIT (Jang & Hursting, 2005). HIT should be considered a clinicopathologic syndrome (Warkentin et al., 1998; Warkentin, 2002, 2003) since its diagnosis is based on both clinical criteria, such as thrombocytopenia and thrombosis, and laboratory data, such as platelet count dynamics and the detection of HIT antibodies (Shantsila et al., 2009).

However, HIT is often difficult to diagnose because of the following phenomena: 1) nonimmune heparin-associated thrombocytopenia occurs in 10-30% of patients receiving heparin (Blank et al., 2002); 2) HIT antibody seroconversion is observed in the absence of thrombocytopenia or other clinical sequelae; and 3) enzyme-linked immunosorbent assay (ELISA) detects both clinically irrelevant (non-pathogenic) and clinically relevant (pathogenic) antibodies (Shantsila et al., 2009). Seroconversion of anti-HIT antibody without thrombocytopenia or other clinical sequela is not considered HIT, whereas a diagnosis of HIT can be made when anti-HIT antibody formation is accompanied by an otherwise unexplained platelet count fall, or by skin lesions at heparin injection sites or acute systemic reactions after intravenous injection of heparin (Bartholomew et al., 2005). Furthermore, HIT formation may also be related to the occurrence of venous limb gangrene occurring in HIT patients treated with oral anticoagulants (Warkentin, 1996a). A mnemonic device, the "4 **T**s" of HIT, has been developed to remember the salient clinical features of HIT, thus facilitating patient assessment and HIT diagnosis (Warkentin & Heddle, 2003): the degree of ***T***hrombocytopenia, the ***T***iming of the platelet fall, the presence of ***T***hrombosis or other sequelae, and o***T***her potential causes of thrombocytopenia (Lillo-Le Louët et al., 2004; Denys et al., 2008; Gruel et al., 2008).

Despite the utility of this memory device, severe morbidity and mortality in HIT patients persists because of lack of awareness accompanied by a delayed diagnosis. Thus, we have developed the following chapter to provide an overview of HIT, focusing particularly on the epidemiology, pathophysiology, diagnosis, laboratory evaluation, and treatment.

2. Overview of HIT

HIT type II, namely, HIT, is immune-mediated and associated with a risk of thrombosis. It develops in approximately 5-10% of patients treated with heparin and is characterized by a significant reduction in platelets (levels fall by 30% or more), generally after the fifth day of therapy (Warkentin et al., 1998; Warkentin, 2002). Although, this phenomenon is usually resolved by therapy within 5-15 days, some cases may require months of treatment (Chong, 1992; Warkentin et al., 1998; Warkentin, 2002).

Platelet count monitoring is recommended for heparin-treated patients in whom the risk of HIT is high (e.g., postoperative patients) or intermediate (e.g., medical or obstetric patients receiving a prophylactic dose of heparin or postoperative patients receiving antithrombotic prophylaxis) (Chong et al., 1993a; Jang & Hursting, 2005). Shantsila et al. (2009) have recommended measurement of platelet counts before, and 24 h after, initiation of heparin therapy in patients who have received heparin within the past 100 days. Platelet counts should also be performed every 2-3 days in intermediate-risk patients, every other day in high-risk patients, and immediately in patients with systemic, cardiorespiratory, or neurologic symptoms that occur within 30 min after an intravenous injection of heparin.

HIT should be suspected when thrombocytopenia ($<$15-20 $\times$ 10^9 cells/L, or a $>$50% decrease in platelet count) occurs during heparin administration, typically 5-14 days after initiation of heparin administration (Warkentin & Kelton, 2001a); however, very severe thrombocytopenia (platelet count <15-20 × 10^9 cells/L) is generally not due to HIT. Routine platelet count monitoring for HIT may be appropriate in a least some clinical situations, and it may be reasonable to stratify the intensity of need for platelet count monitoring in relation to the risk of HIT.

Although it is difficult to predict which heparin-exposed patients will develop HIT, one consistent factor is a property of heparin preparation. HIT antibodies occur at higher levels in patients given bovine unfractionated heparin (UFH) than in those treated with porcine UFH or low molecular weigh heparin (LMWH) (Green et al., 1984; Bailey et al., 1986; Monreal et al., 1989; Rao et al., 1989; Warkentin et al., 1995; Warkentin et al., 2003a; Lee & Warkentin, 2004; Denys et al., 2008; Gruel et al., 2008).

HIT antibody formation is also influenced by the medical circumstances in which heparin is administered. For example, approximately 20% of heparin-exposed patients develop HIT antibodies after orthopedic surgery, while as many as 70% develop antibodies after receiving a cardiopulmonary bypass (CPB) (Amiral et al., 1996a). However, it can be difficult to compare results across studies because of differences in duration and route of anticoagulant administration, as well as patient group composition (Lee et al., 2004).

3. Epidemiology

There is a need for studies on HIT incidence. The work that has been done is sufficient, and they have so many differences that it is difficult to compare results across studies in order to uncover broader trends. Most HIT studies are retrospective, and differ with respect to patient characteristics, type of heparin preparation, duration of therapy, definition of thrombocytopenia, and laboratory tests used for confirm thrombocytopenia diagnosis (Schmitt & Adelman, 1993; Magnani, 1993; Chong, 2003). Despite these problems, it is possible to draw some general conclusions about HIT epidemiology.

There are 3 characteristic profiles in the timing of the onset of thrombocytopenia. Approximately 70% of HIT patients are classified as "typical-onset HIT". In these patients, platelet counts begin to decrease (serocnversion and initial platelet count fall) within 5-10 days after beginning heparin treatment (Warkentin & Kelton, 2001a). Approximately 25-30% of HIT patients are classified as having "Rapid-onset HIT", which occurs when platelet counts fall abruptly within 24 h of starting heparin therapy (Warkentin & Kelton, 2001a; Lubenow et al., 2002). "Rapid-onset HIT" is strongly associated with recent heparin exposure, usually within the preceding 100 days (Warkentin & Kelton, 2001a; Lubenow et al., 2002). Because of the previous exposure, patients already have circulating HIT antibodies, which cause platelet counts to fall quickly once heparin is re-administered. The last category of HIT, affecting approximately 3-5% of HIT patients, is "delayed-onset HIT" in which the onset of thrombocytopenia begins several days after completion of heparin treatment (Warkentin & Kelton, 2001b; Rice et al., 2002; Warkentin & Bernstein, 2003; Warkentin, 2004a). This type of syndrome is often clinically severe, as it is associated with high-titer, platelet-activating HIT antibodies that do not require ongoing heparin administration to exert their pathogenic effect (Rice et al., 2002). Furthermore, this type may occur in patients exposed to minimal amounts of heparin, although it has also been observed in patients exposed to large amounts of heparin during coronary artery bypass grafting (Rice et al., 2002; Jackson et al., 2006). Rarely, patients who received intravenous heparin develop acute inflammatory or cardiorespiratory symptoms and signs within 30 min (Warkentin, 2007).

HIT severity is mainly determined by the extent of thrombotic complications (Girolami et al, 2003). Many HIT patients develop thrombosis after receiving as an antithrombotic prophylaxis (Warkentin, 1996a; Wallis et al., 1999). The thrombotic event is frequently a worsening of pre-existing thrombosis in heparin-treated HIT patients, and this worsening of thrombosis may cause a new thromboembolic complication (Magnani, 1993; Warkentin & Kelton, 1990, 1996; Nands et al., 1997); this has been observed in approximately 20% of cases (Wakentin, 2004a). Development of a new thrombus or extension of an existing thrombus during treatment with prophylactic or therapeutic UFH or LMWH should always raise a suspicion of HIT (Shantsila et al., 2009). The first event to be associated with HIT was arterial thrombosis, which seems to be more frequent in patients with cardiovascular disease (Nands et al., 1997); venous complications may be common in patients undergoing post-surgical prophylaxis (Rhodes et al., 1973; Magnani, 1993; Warkentin & Kelton, 1996;). In most cases, arterial complications manifest as thromboses of the large vessels, leading to gangrene and limb amputation, stroke, myocardial infarction, and cardiac thrombosis (Warkentin & Kelton, 1990; Boshkov et al., 1993; Fondu, 1995; Chong, 1995).

Approximately 10-20% of patients who develop HIT while receiving subcutaneous injections of heparin experience skin lesions, ranging from painful erythematous plaques to skin necrosis, at the injection sites (Warkentin, 2004a; Chong, 1995). Skin lesions have been observed in patients without thrombocytopenia but with circulating HIT antibodies (Warkentin, 1996b). Occasionally, HIT associated with intravenous heparin injection also manifests as an acute systemic reaction developing within 5-30 min after heprin administration (Ansell et al., 1986; Popov et al., 1997; Warkentin, 2004a).

Estimates of HIT prevalence among heparin-treated patients differ depending on heparin type. Fabris et al. (2000) found that laboratory-confirmed HIT occurs in approximately 2% of patients receiving UFH. Among patients given therapeutic doses of bovine UFH, HIT has been observed in approximately 5% of patients. This is a much higher rate than that observed in patients given procine UFH (1%). Prophylactic doses of porcine heparin have been reported to cause HIT in <1% of patients (Warkentin & Kelton, 1990). However, risk of HIT is relatively low in medical and obstetric patients receiving LMWH (Fabris et al., 2000). For instance, Warkentin (2004a) reorted that HIT was observed in 2.7% of patients treated with subcutaneous UFH injection, but in no patients receiving LMWH; further, thrombotic complications were more frequent in the former group (88.9%) than in the latter (17.8%). Both the bovine/procine UFH and the LMWH data were collected from medical patients receiving LMWH or UFH as "flushes", *e.g.*, oncology patients with indwelling catheters (Mayo et al., 1990; Kadidal et al., 1999). A randomized controlled trial that compared use of porcine UFH with LMWH after hip replacement surgery found that HIT was significantly less common among patients who received the latter treatment (Lee & Warkentin, 2004; Warkentin, 2004a).

4. Pathophysiology

Francis and colleagues have reported that HIT antibody formation in cardiac surgery patients who received procine UFH was significantly lower than those with bovine UFH (Francis et al., 2003). The IgG fraction of HIT patients serum has been found to cause *in vitro* platelet aggregation in the presence of therapeutic amounts of heparin (Rhodes et al., 1973), indicating that HIT has an immunologic etiology (Amiral et al., 1998; Warkentin et al., 2000).

Green *et al.* (1978) reported that immunoglobulin-heparin complexes form only in the presence of platelets (Green et al., 1978), and several platelet proteins have been proposed as the receptors of heparin-dependent antibodies (Lynch & Howe, 1985). Multiple studies have found that the pro-aggregating effect of heparin depends on the degree of sulfation and the molecular weight of the heparin (Geinacher et al., 1992; Geinacher et al., 1993; Kelton et al., 1994) and is mediated by the release of platelet alpha-granules (Gruel et al., 1993), which contain platelet factor 4 (PF4), a small, positively charged molecule produced by megakaryocytes. Although its biological function is unknown, it has been identified as the main co-factor of heparin (Amiral et al., 1992, Gentilini et al., 1999); it also binds to endothelial-surface glycosaminoglycans, *e.g.*, heparin sulfate (Visentin et al., 1994; Cines et al., 2007). Normal blood levels of PF4 are very low, as it is only released into circulation following weak platelet activation. However, PF4 levels may be high in specific clinical circumstances, such as prosthetic hip or cardiac surgery, which are associated with platelet activation (Greinacher et al., 1994a). When heparin binds with PF4, it undergoes a conformational change and becomes immunogenic, leading to the generation of anti-heparin/PF4 antibodies, namely, HIT antibodies (Suh et al., 1998; Ziporen et al., 1998). The PF4/heparin ratio is important for the constitution of the multimolecular antigenic complex, and the optimal PF4/heparin ratio has been reported to range from 4-6:1 (Kelton et al., 1994; Visentin et al., 1994; Amiral et al., 1995; Cines et al., 2007). The immunogenicity of heparin-PF4 conjugates may form the biological basis for differences in immunogenicity between bovine and porcine sources of heparin: Bovine lung heparin has longer polysaccharide chains and a higher degree of sulfation, which could increase reactivity with PF4 (Boshkov et al., 1993).

HIT antibodies activate platelets and stimulate an immunomedited endothelial lesion, followed by the appearance of thrombocytopenia and/or thrombosis (Fondu, 1995; Greinacher, 1995; Warkentin et al., 1998; Cines et al., 2007). Platelet activation is primarily caused by binding between the immunocomplex and FcγRIIa (CD32) receptors (Adelman et al., 1989; Anderson et al., 1995; Baglin, 2001), leading to degranulation and the release of pro-coagulant substances (*e.g.*, serotonin, histamine, and adenosine diphosphate), thromboxane biosynthesis, an influx of Ca^{2+}, and the generation of highly pro-thrombotic phospholipid microparticles (Chong et al., 1981; Chong et al., 1989a; Warkentin & Kelton, 2001a). The immunocomplex can bind to Fc receptors on the surfaces of monocytes, neutrophils, and endothelial cells, and the binding of the immunocomplex to so many types of cells can contribute to the profound thrombin generation seen in patients with HIT. Thrombin generation can be enhanced by HIT activation of monocytes and endothelial cell tissue factor on the surface of monocytes and endothelial cells (Visentin et al., 1994; Warkentin, 1999; Newman & Chong, 2000; Pouplard et al., 2001; Arepally & Mayer, 2001). These thrombotic processes may lead to a hypercoagulable state, thus increasing the risk of severe and extensive thromboembolic complications in many patients. Additional activation of platelets by thrombin and other released agonists results in a further increase in the numbers of FcγRIIa receptors on the platelet surface, facilitating even more platelet activation (Chong et al., 1993b; Anderson et al., 1995). However, some reports have indicated that platelet activation can be blocked by the FcγRIIa receptor-specific monoclonal antibody (IV.3) (Kelton et al., 1988; Visentin et al, 1994).

While IgG-class HIT antibody can be detected in most HIT patients, IgA and IgM HIT antibodies can be found in only a small portion of patients (Suh et al., 1997; Amiral et al.,

1996b). Given that IgA and IgM antibodies do not activate platelets in the presence of heparin *in vitro*, and that they are unable to bind FcγRIIa, their presence in HIT patients could simply be coincidental, though IgM and IgA are not able to bind to FcγRIIa (Amiral et al., 1996a; Amiral et al., 1996b; Amiral et al., 1996c; Blank et al., 1997). These data suggest that platelet activation occurs independently of the IgG FcγRIIa receptor. After heparin administration is interrupted, the HIT antibody gradually disappears; laboratory tests for HIT antibodies are usually "negative" or "weakly positive" at 100 days (Shantsila et al., 2009). For HIT to develop at this point, the HIT antibody would need to form again (Lubenow et al., 2002; Rice et al., 2002). Harris et al. (2008) have reported an association between the PLA2 polymorphism of glycoprotein IIIa and the risk of thrombosis in patients with HIT antibodies.

5. Diagnosis of HIT

The diagnosis of HIT should be based both on clinical criteria, such as the presence of thrombocytopenia and thrombosis, and laboratory data, such as platelet count dynamics and detection of HIT antibodies. However, it may be difficult to establish a general diagnostic protocol, given the lack of a readily accessible standard laboratory test and the frequent detection of elevated anti-HIT antibody levels in heparin-treated patients that display no clinical features of the disease (Arepally & Ortel, 2006).

In the majority of patients with HIT, thrombocytopenia is defined as an otherwise unexplained >50% drop in the platelet count (Warkentin et al., 2008a); thrombocytopenia is generally of moderate severity, and median platelet count is approximately 50-60 x 10^9 platelets/L (Jackson et al., 2006). In HIT patients, platelet counts are generally < 20 x 10^9 platelets/L. Clinical presentation of HIT in patients with profound thrombocytopenia can be rapidly progressive and include the development of disseminated intravascular coagulation and microvascular thrombotic complications (Ortel, 2009). Patients are likely to suffer from HIT when their platelet counts drop to less than 50% of normal levels and when they present with thrombosis or skin lesions at heparin injection sites (Jackson et al., 2006). Generally, platelet count decreases and/or thrombotic events begin 5–10 days after the initiation of heparin therapy in heparin-hypersensitive individuals, and platelet count in thrombocytopenic patients may not return to initiation levels until several days later (Warkentin & Kelton, 2001a). In patients who have undergone operation, the expected pattern would show a return of normal platelet count immediately after surgery, followed by an unexpected drop (Warkentin, 2003). Persistent thrombocytopenia following cardiac bypass surgery is usually not a result of HIT, but instead may stem from other causes, such as postoperative complications. However, postoperative thrombocytopenia lasting for >5 days without an apparent alternative cause may be the result of HIT (Lillo-Le et al., 2004).

Several diagnostic algorithms have been developed to provide a more systematic approach to the diagnosis of HIT. Patients can be assigned an HIT score using the "**4 Ts,**" an assessment protocol and memory device focused on the salient clinical features of HIT: degree of **T**hrombocytopenia (maximum points for a platelet count fall of >50% or a nadir of 20–100 × 10^9/L), the **T**iming of the fall in platelet count (maximum points for an onset of 5–10 days after initiation of heparin treatment or within 1 day if there has been recent heparin exposure), the presence of **T**hrombosis or other sequelae (maximum points for new thrombosis, skin lesions, or acute systemic reactions), and o**T**her causes of thrombocytopenia excluded (maximum points for no other cause event) (Warkentin, 2003, Warkentin et al., 2003b, Bryant et al., 2008). The "4 Ts" is useful for following the recommendation of Warkentin and Heddle, who suggest the employment of a clinical decision–making model to establish a pretest probability for HIT in patients who receive UFH or LMWH (Warkentin & Heddle, 2003). A diagnostic score for HIT after cardiopulmonary bypass surgery has also been proposed (Lillo-Le et al., 2004). Other studies have demonstrated the usefulness of combining the 4Ts score with laboratory testing when diagnosing HIT (Lillo-Le et al., 2004; Denys et al., 2008; Gruel et al., 2008); laboratory tests can also be used independently for confirming a clinical diagnosis.

5.1 Laboratory testing

Laboratory testing is necessary to confirm the diagnosis of HIT, and is most helpful in these patients clinically assessed to be at intermediate high clinical risk of HIT (Arepally & Ortel, 2006). Patients who have undergone cardiopulmonary bypass surgery frequently have elevated antiheparin/PF4 antibody levels; among these individuals, testing should not be used to "screen" patients for HIT or evaluate patients assessed to have a low pre-test probability for HIT (Warkentin et al., 2008a). Although a lot of laboratory tests are available for detection of heparin-PF4 antibody, these tests have several advantages and disadvantages. Blood sampling for the detection of HIT antibodies was performed in patients with clinically suspected HIT on days 5 to 14 following the initiation of heparin therapy (Warkentin et al., 2008a). Although HIT antibodies are detectable in the blood for several weeks after heparin administration, discontinuation of heparin administration, samples should be collected as soon as possible because antibody levels can decrease quite rapidly.

The first test developed for diagnosing HIT was the platelet aggregation test, which uses citrated platelet-rich plasma (PRP) and standard platelet aggregometry (Warkentin, 2004b). The platelet aggregation test is able to provide results quickly (Kelton et al, 1988), although results of this test is more influenced by heparin concentrations and donor platelet variability compared to those of ^{14}C-serotonin release assay (SRA) (Warkenin & Kelton, 1990; Chong, 1992, 1995). Accordingly, to increase sensitivity and specificity, test conditions need to be optimized– instance, by washed platelets (Chong et al., 1993a; Greinacher et al., 1994a; Pouplard et al., 1999a). Washed platelet activation assays, such as the platelet SRA, (Sheridan et al., 1986; Warkentin et al., 1992; Warkentin, 2001; Price E et al., 2007), and the heparin-induced platelet activation test (Greinacher et al., 1991; Greinacher et al,. 1994a) are used by a few reference laboratories. In these assays, it is necessary to use of apyrase in a wash step for maintenance of platelet reactivity to HIT antibodies, and to resuspend in a calcium- and magnesium-containing buffer (Polgár et al., 1998; Warkentin, 2001). The major limitation of this method is its technically demanding nature (Warkentin, 2000), which limits its use to a few reference laboratories. In most clinical laboratories, immunological tests such as ELISA are used because they are easy to perform, have a rapid turnaround time, and are highly sensitive (Price et al., 2007). There are 2 PF4-dependent antigen assays that are commercially available for detecting HIT antibodies (Amiral et al., 1992; Collins et al., 1997; Warkentin, 2000; Warkentin et al., 2001): the Asserachrom (Stago, Asnières, France), which detects antibodies that react with PF4-heparin complexes, and the GTI-PF4 (GTI, Brookfield, WI, USA), which detects antibodies that react with PF4 bound to polyvinyl sulfonate.

Prospective studies have shown that, among HIT antibody classes, only HIT-IgG antibodies have very high sensitivity for diagnosing clinical HIT (Warkentin et al., 2000; Lindhoff-Last et al., 2001). Detection of PF4-heparin antibodies is performed as followed. Unbound material is removed, and a chromogen is added to label the bound conjugate, producing a yellow color, read at 405 nm. The amount of yellow produced at the end point, as indicated by the optical density (OD), is proportional to the amount of antibody present. A positive result is reported if OD reading is 0.400 or more. Higher ELISA OD results have been shown to significant correlation of the serotonin release assay results and an increased risk for thrombosis in patients with HIT (Warkentin et al., 2008b). Furthermore, the ELISA results are most useful when combined with a clinical scoring system (Janatpour et al., 2007). Zwicker et al (2004) have reported that higher ELISA OD measurements correlated significantly with thrombosis, and patients with isolated HIT (HIT in the absence of thrombosis) and an OD level of 1.0 or more had a 6-fold increased risk of thrombosis compared with patients who had OD levels between 0.4 and 0.99 (Zwicker et al, 2004). The sensitivity of the ELISA for PF4-heparin antibodies is greater than functional assays (Greinacher et al., 1994b; Amiral et al., 1995; Pouplard et al., 1999b), though a "positive" result may not denote the same magnitude of thrombotic risk.

5.2 Laboratory data from 2 potential HIT patients

We examined 2 patients who experienced thrombocytopenia after being given UFH during percutaneous transluminal coronary angioplasty (PTCA) and cardiac surgery. For both individuals, we tested for HIT by measuring platelet aggregability and quantifying levels of both anti-heparin-PF4 complex antibody (anti-HIT antibody) and thrombin-antithrombin III complex (TAT). Platelet aggregation in response to 0.2 μg/mL collagen was measured using Born's turbidimetric methods (Born GVR, 1962), and quantified by light transmission, as previously reported (Toyohira et al., 1995; Kariyazono et al., 1997; Nakamura et al., 1999); platelet aggregation activity was evaluated as percent maximum aggregation (MA). First samples were prepared by incubating the PRP of suspected HIT patients with UFH (0.2 IU/mL), and second samples were prepared by separately adding plasma from the 2 patients to the PRP of healthy volunteers at a ratio of 1:1, then adding UFH (0.2 IU/mL). We then used a commercial ELISA kit (GTI Diagnostics, Waukesha, WI, NJ, USA) to measure anti-heparin antibodies in these samples.

As shown in Figure 1, platelet aggregation was much higher in the first set of sample than in the first control sample (without UFH); in other words, heparin had a strong positive effect on aggregation. As a result, MA of second sample was 68% (Figure 2), and showed strong aggregation. The ELISA results indicated significantly higher OD values for the 2 potential HIT patients than in the healthy volunteers. Furthermore, remarkably high levels of circulating TAT and TNF-alpha were found in the plasma of the suspected HIT patients. Our laboratory data indicate the likelihood that anti-HIT antibodies were present in the plasma of both patients. Furthermore, these data demonstrate the marked acceleration of blood coagulation in these patients, suggesting an increased risk of thrombosis.

These findings support previous reports that many HIT patients are hypercoagulable and have greatly elevated levels of TAT (Warkentin et al., 1997; Greinacher et al., 2000); furthermore, this helps explain the strong relationship between HIT and venous or arterial thrombosis (Warkentin & Kelton, 2001a).

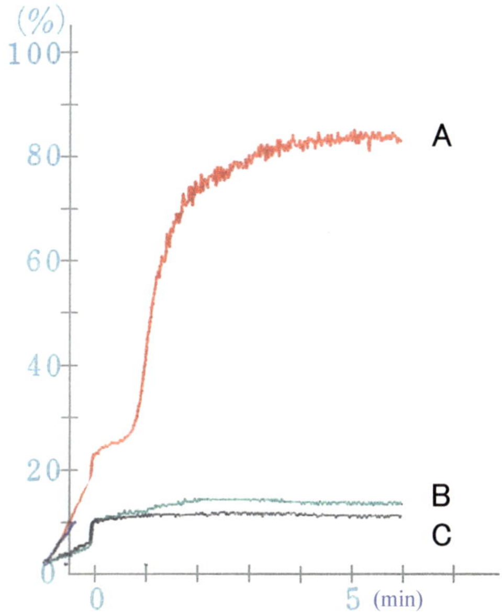

Fig. 1. Platelet aggregation was stimulated by 0.2 µg/mL collagen. In case A's PRP incubated without UFH (first control sample) (C). In healthy volunteer's PRP incubated with UFH (second control sample) (B). In case A's PRP incubated with UFH (A).

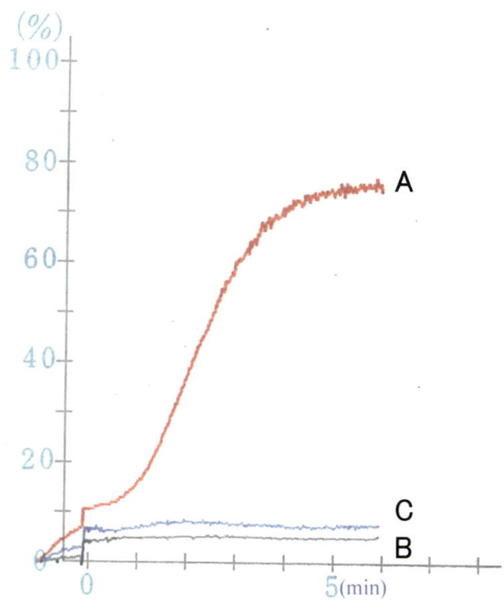

Fig. 2. Anti-heparin antibody was detected by turbidimetric method. Collagen (0.2 µg/mL) was used as agonist. In case A's PRP incubated without UFH (first control sample) (C). In healthy volunteer's PRP was mixed with case A's plasma following incubation without UFH (third control sample) (B). In healthy volunteer's PRP was mixed with case A's plasma following incubation with UFH (A).

Given these findings, we propose a model for the pathophysiological mechanism of HIT (Figures 3 and 4). This model helps explain observations that the hypercoagulable state, coupled with endothelial cell dysfunction due to injury from heparin antibody, activated platelets, leukocytes, platelet microparticles, atherosclerosis or medical intervention, can lead to arterial thrombosis (Walenga et al., 2000). Furthermore, the model is supported by the report that anti-HIT antibodies bind to and directly activate microvascular endothelial cells, whereas binding to and activating macrovascular endothelial cells requires pre-activation by platelets or TNF-alpha (Walenga et al., 2004).

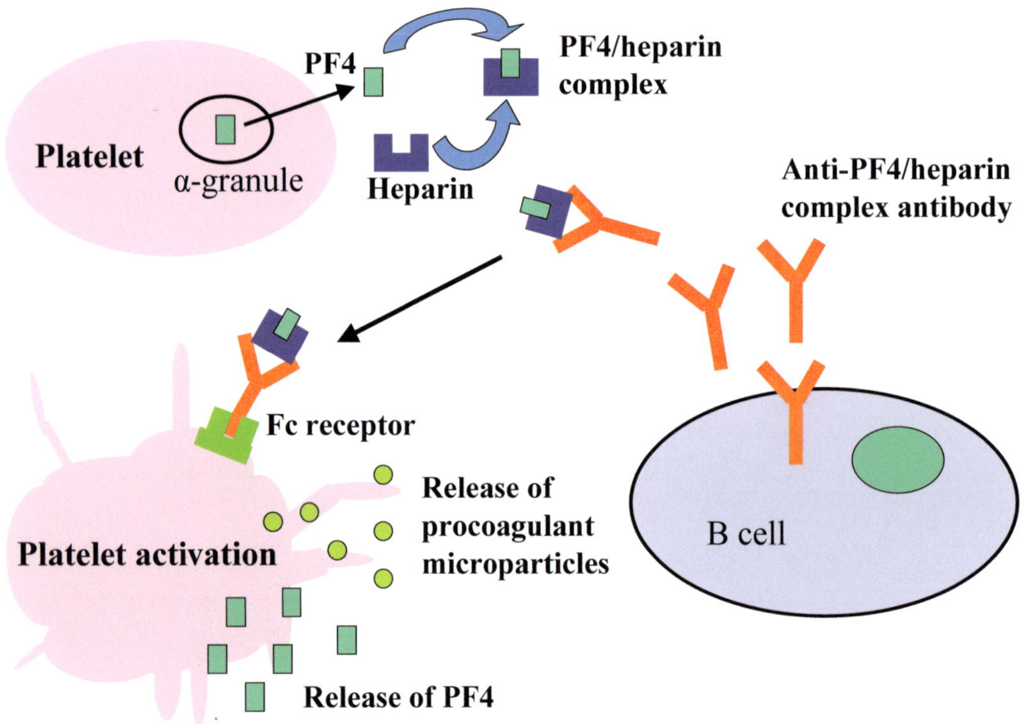

Fig. 3. Pathophysiological mechanism of HIT (1). Stage 1; binding of heparin to PF4 induces the formation of a neoepitope. Stage 2; an immune response against the PF4/heparin complex induces antibody formation. Stage 3; the complex of PF4/heparin and specific antibody associates with platelets via binding of the antibody Fc part to the platelet immunoglobulin receptor FcγRIIa (CD32), representing the major stage in platelet activation in HIT. Stage 4; activated platelets shed procoagulant microparticles which enhance thrombin generation.

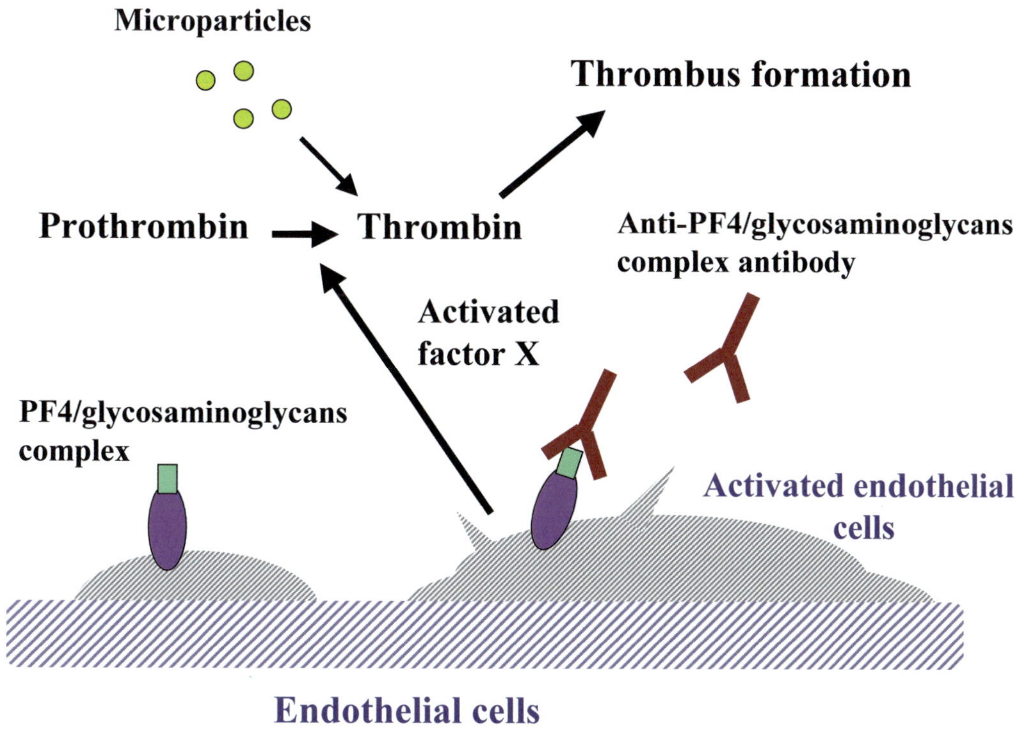

Fig. 4. Pathophysiological mechanism of HIT (2). Stage 5; binding of released PF4 to heparan sulfate of endothelial cell induces the formation of PF4/glycosaminoglycans complex on the surface of endothelial cell. Stage 6; PF4/glycosaminoglycans complex antibody binds to PF4/glycosaminoglycans complex on the surface of endothelial cell, and activates endothelial cell. Stage 7; activation of endothelial cells lead to the release of activated factor X. Stage 8; thrombin generation induces thrombus formation.

6. Management of HIT

All heparins must be avoided when treating patients suspected to have HIT; even exposure to very low amounts of heparin through heparin-coated catheters and heparin flushes used to maintain intravenous lines may trigger HIT (Laster et al., 1989). Likewise, preparations of LMWH can induce severe HIT, though they do so less frequently than UFH (Warkentin et al., 2003a; Warkentin & Greinacher, 2003; Walenga et al., 2004). Further, the cross-reactivity rate between heparin and LMWH is so high that LMWH is not recommended for the treatment of HIT patients (Chong, 2003; Warkentin et al., 2008a). Alternative anticoagulant therapy must be initiated immediately, both for HIT patients diagnosed with thrombocytopenia alone or with thromboembolism (Warkentin & Greinacher, 2004). In patients in whom treatment was delayed until an HIT diagnosis could be confirmed by laboratory tests, the incidence of new thrombosis was approximately 10-fold higher than in individuals treated promptly with a direct thrombin inhibitor (Greinacher et al., 2000).

Marked decreases of platelet counts in HIT patients require anticoagulation with an effective antithrombotic drug that does not cross-react *in vivo* with the circulating anti-heparin/PF4 antibodies. There are currently 3 thrombin inhibitors available for patients with HIT: lepirudin, argatroban, and bivalirudin, all of which directly bind and inactivate thrombin. Prospective cohort studies have been performed to investigate the efficacy and major bleeding endpoints for lepirudin (Greinacher et al., 1999a; Greinacher et al., 1999b; Lubenow et al., 2004; Lubenow et al., 2005) and argatroban (Lewis et al., 2001; Lewis et al., 2003) in patients with HIT complicated by thrombosis. When respective historical control data were taken into consideration, composite end point risk rates and new thrombosis risk rates were 0.48 and 0.28 for lepirudin, respectively, and 0.75 and 0.45 for argatroban, respectively. The corresponding absolute event rates were 19.2% (lepirudin) and 42.3% (argatroban) for the composite end point, and 7.0% (lepirudin) and 15.5% (argatroban) for new thrombosis. Patients who received lepirudin were less likely to require amputation than those who were given argatroban. Fatal bleeding after treatment with lepirudin has been found to range from 1.2% of patients (in a prospective study) to 3.9% of patients (in a retrospective observational study) (Lubenow et al., 2005; Tardy et al., 2006). Danaparoid and fondaparinux may also be used to manage HIT (Warkentin et al., 2008a). When abrupt decreases in platelet count (to $<10 \times 10^9$ clls/L) are observed in patients who underwent angioplasty and were treated with a combination of heparin and glycoprotein IIb/IIIa antagonist, the recommended antagonist is always glycoprotein IIb/IIIa (Shantsila et al., 2009)

6.1 Lepirudin

Lepirudin, a recombinant form of hirudin, is a direct, specific, and irreversible inhibitor of thrombin that is administered via intravenous injection (Greinacher & Lubenow, 2001). The Biggest drawback of Lepirudin is that it must be accompanied by the strict laboratory monitoring: activated partial thromboplastin time (aPTT) monitoring should be performed at 4-h intervals until it is clear that patients have reached a steady state within the normal range of values (Warkentin et al., 2008b). Moreover, patients should be informed that they have received lepirudin, since fatal anaphylactic reactions have been reported in patients re-exposed to lepirudin during a second round of intravenous treatment (Greinacher et al., 2003). Although similar bleeding rates have been observed in lepirudin-treated patients and historical control subjects, this drug has been found to significantly reduce the combined end point of death, limb amputation, and new thromboembolic complications in patients with HIT associated thrombosis (Greinacher et al., 1999a; Greinacher et al., 1999b).

6.2 Argatroban

Argatroban is a synthetic L-arginine-derived direct thrombin inhibitor that reversibly binds to the thrombin active site. Argatroban is administered by intravenous injection, with dose adjustment to maintain aPTT at 1.5-3.0 times the baseline value (Gosselin et al., 2004). It has been reported that, in HIT patients without thrombosis, treatment with argatroban produces a significant reduction in the composite end point, such as all-cause death, all-cause limb amputation, and new thrombosis at 37 days (Lewis et al., 2001; Lewis et al., 2003). In HIT patients who underwent lower extremity revascularization, the composite end point of deaths, urgent revascularization, and limb amputations developed in 25% of patients treated with argatroban, and 6% of patients had major bleeding episodes (Baron et al., 2008). Restoration of platelet counts is universally observed within 6–7 days of the initiation of argatroban therapy (Bartholomew et al., 2007). Some precautions are required when argatroban infusion is overlapped by warfarin anticoagulant therapy, although argatroban causes a further substantial increase in the international normalized ratio (INR). In addition, careful thought should be given to the participation of direct thrombin inhibitor to the patient's INR.

6.3 Danaparoid

Danaparoid is approved as an alternative anticoagulant for HIT in many countries. Danaparoid, a heparinoid with predominantly anti-Xa activity and some anti-IIa activity, is a mixture of three glycosaminoglycans such as heparin sulfate, dermatan sulfate, and chondroitin sulfate. Danaparoid presents its anticoagulant effect by catalyzing the inactivation of factor Xa in the presence of antithrombin, and has a unique property of specific suppression of HIT antibody-induced platelet activation that is not observed with other drugs used for HIT treatment (Chong et al., 1989b). Tardy-Poncet et al. reported that major bleeding episodes in those patients treated with danaparoid were significantly fewer compared with those treated with lepirudin (Tardy-Poncet et al., 1999). Among the drugs used for the treatment of HIT, danaparoid is the only drug whose efficacy and safety have been confirmed by a prospective randomized controlled study (Chong et al., 2001).

6.4 Bivalirudin

Bivalirudin, which is not approved as an HIT treatment, is a 20-amino acid polypeptide with sequence homology to hirudin. Campbell et al. (2000) reported 94% procedural success in a series of 17 percutaneous coronary intervention patients who were given bivalirudin as a treatment for HIT (Campbell et al., 2000). In the Anticoagulant Therapy with Bivalirudin to Assist in the Performance of Percutaneous Coronary Intervention in Patients with HIT (or ATBAT) multicenter open-label trial (Mahaffey et al., 2003), clinical percutaneous coronary intervention success, defined as the absence of death, emergency bypass surgery, or Q-wave infarction, was achieved in 96% of patients treated with bivalirudin; further, patients displayed a low rate of bleeding. Cumulatively, these results indicate that bivalirudin therapy is safe and effective during percutaneous coronary intervention.

6.5 Fondaparinux

Fondaparinux, a synthetic pentasaccharide with potent indirect anti-Xa inhibitor properties, is used only a limited number of patients with HIT. The generation of HIT-related antigen depends on the polysaccharide chain length (Amiral et al., 1995). Because patients have a very low risk of developing HIT while receiving fondaparinux (Warkentin et al., 2005), platelet count monitoring is not needed during administration of this drug. Despite these advantages, fondaparinux cannot be recommended for in the treatment of HIT until there are more data demonstrating its efficacy and safety (Rota et al., 2008; Lobo et al., 2008).

7. Conclusion

Heparin is one of the most widely used and valuable anticoagulants for the treatment and prophylaxis of thrombotic complications. However, HIT is not only a common but also a serious complication of heparin therapy with a high rate of morbidity and mortality. Its prompt clinical and laboratory recognition is necessary to stop heparin administration immediately and start an alternative anticoagulant. HIT antibody test results must be interpreted in the appropriate context of the available clinical information. Furthermore, additional diagnostic information is available as a result of considering the magnitude of a given positive test result. The diagnosis of HIT should be clearly recorded in the patient's notes and marked as a serious allergy.

8. References

Adelman B, Sobel M, Fujimura Y, Ruggeri ZM, & Zimmerman TS. (1989). Heparin-associated thrombocytopenia: observations on the mechanism of platelet aggregation. *J Lab Clin Med*, 113, 2, (Feb 1989), pp.204-210.

Amiral J, Bridey F, Dreyfus M, Vissoc AM, Fressinaud E, et al. (1992). Platelet factor 4 complexed to heparin is the target for antibodies generated in heparin-induced thrombocytopenia. *Thromb Haemost*, 68, 1, (Jun 1992), pp.95-96.

Amiral J, Bridey F, Wolf M, Boyer-Neumann C, Fressinaud E, et al. (1995). Antibodies to macromolecular platelet factor 4-heparin complexes in heparin-induced thrombocytopenia: a study of 44 cases. *Thromb Haemost*, 73,11, (Jan 1995), pp.21-28.

Amiral J, Marfaing-Koka A, Poncz M, & Meyer D. (1998). The biological basis of immune heparin-induced thrombocytopenia. *Platelets*, 9, 2, (1998), pp.77-91.

Amiral J, Marfaing-Koka A, Wolf M, Alessi MC, et al. (1996c). Presence of autoantibodies to interleukin-8 or neutrophil-activating peptide-2 in patients with heparin-associated thrombocytopenia. *Blood*, 88, 2, (Jul 1996), pp.410–416.

Amiral J, Peynaud-Debayle E, Wolf M, Bridey F, Vissac AM, et al. (1996a). Generation of antibodies to heparin-PF4 complexes without thrombocytopenia in patients treated with unfractionated or low-molecular-weight heparin. *Am J Hematol*, 52, 2, (Jun 1996), pp.90-95.

Amiral J, Wolf M, Fischer A, Boyer-Neumann C, Vissac A, et al. (1996b). Pathogenicity of IgA and/or IgM antibodies to heparin-PF4 complexes in patients with heparin-induced thrombocytopenia. *Br J Haematol*, 92,4, (Mar 1996), pp.954–959.

Anderson CL, Chacko GW, Osborne JM, & Brandt JT. (1995). The Fc receptor for immunoglobulin G (Fc gamma RII) on human platelets. *Semin Thromb Hemost*, 21, 1, (1995), pp.1-9.

Ansell JE, Clark WP Jr, Compton CC. (1986). Fatal reactions associated with intravenous heparin. *Drug Intell Clin Pharm*, 20, 1, (Jun 1986), pp.74-75.

Arepally GM, & Mayer IM. (2001). Antibodies from patients with heparin-induced thrombocytopenia stimulate monocytic cells to express tissue factor and secrete interleukin-8. *Blood*. 98, 4, (Aug 2001), pp.1252-1254.

Arepally GM, & Ortel TL. (2006). Clinical practice. Heparin-induced thrombocytopenia. *N Engl J Med*, 355, 8, (Aug 2006), pp.809-817.

Aster RH. (1995). Heparin-induced thrombocytopenia and thrombosis. *N Engl J Med*, 332, 20, (May 1995), pp. 1374–1376.

Baglin TP. (2001). Heparin induced thrombocytopenia thrombosis (HIT/T) syndrome: diagnosis and treatment. *J Clin Pathol*, 54, 4, (Apr 2001), pp.272-274.

Bailey RT Jr, Ursick JA, Heim KL, Hilleman DE, & Reich JW. (1986). Heparin-associated thrombocytopenia: a prospective comparison of bovine lung heparin, manufactured by a new process, and porcine intestinal heparin. *Drug Intell Clin Pharm*, 20, 5, (May 1986), pp.374-378.

Baron SJ, Yeh RW, Cruz-Gonzalez I, Healy JL, Pomerantsev E, et al. (2008). Efficacy and safety of argatroban in patients with heparin induced thrombocytopenia undergoing endovascular intervention for peripheral arterial disease. *Catheter Cardiovasc Interv*, 72, 1, (Jul 2008), pp.116–120.

Bartholomew JR, Begelman SM, & Almahameed A. (2005). Heparin-induced thrombocytopenia: principles for early recognition and management. *Cleve Clin J Med*, 72, (Suppl 1), (Apr 2005), pp.S31-S36.

Bartholomew JR, Pietrangeli CE, & Hursting MJ. (2007). Argatroban anticoagulation for heparin-induced thrombocytopenia in elderly patients. *Drugs Aging*, 24, 6, (Jun 2007), pp.489–499.

Battistelli S, Genovese A, & Gori T. (2010). Heparin-induced thrombocytopenia in surgical patients. *Am J Surg*, 199, 1, (Jan 2010), pp.43-51.

Blank M, Cines DB, Arepally G, Eldor A, Afek A, et al. (1997). Pathogenicity of human anti-platelet factor 4 (PF4)/heparin in vivo: generation of mouse anti- PF4/heparin and induction of thrombocytopenia by heparin. *Clin Exp Immunol*, 108, 2, (May 1997), pp.333-339.

Blank M, Shoenfeld Y, Tavor S, Praprotnik S, Boffa MC, et al. (2002). Anti-platelet factor 4/heparin antibodies from patients with heparin-induced thrombocytopenia provoke direct activation of microvascular endothelial cells. *Int Immunol*, 14, 2, (Feb 2002), pp.121-129.

Born GVR. (1962). Aggregation of blood platelets by adenosine diphosphate and its reversal. *Nature*, 194, (Jun 1962), pp.927-929.

Boshkov LK, Warkentin TE, Hayward CP, Andrew M, & Kelton JG. (1993). Heparin-induced thrombocytopenia and thrombosis: clinical and laboratory studies. *Br J Haematol*. 84, 2, (Jun 1993), pp.322-328.

Bryant A, Low J, Austin S, & Joseph J. (2008). Timely diagnosis and management of heparin-induced thrombocytopenia in a frequent request, low incidence single centre using clinical 4T's score and particle gel immunoassay. *Br J Haematol*, 143, 5, (Dec 2008), pp.721-726.

Burgess JK, & Chong BH. (1997). The platelet proaggregating and potentiating effects of unfractionated heparin, low molecular weight heparin and heparinoid in intensive care patients and healthy controls. *Eur J Haematol*, 58, 4, (Apr 1997), pp.279-285.

Campbell KR, Mahaffey KW, Lewis BE, Weitz JI, Berkowitz SD, et al. (2000). Bivalirudin in patients with heparin-induced thrombocytopenia undergoing percutaneous coronary intervention [abstract]. *J Invasive Cardiol*, 12, (Suppl F), (Dec 2000), pp.14F–19F.

Chong BH, & Ismail F. (1989). The mechanism of heparin-induced platelet aggregation. *Eur J Haematol*, 43, 3, (Sep 1989), pp.245-251.

Chong BH, Burgess J, & Ismail F. (1993a). The clinical usefulness of the platelet aggregation test for the diagnosis of heparin-induced thrombocytopenia. *Thromb Haemost*, 69, 4, (Apr 1993), pp.344-350.

Chong BH, Grace CS, & Rozenberg MC. (1981). Heparin-induced thrombocytopenia: effect of heparin platelet antibody on platelets. *Br J Haematol*, 49, 4, (Dec 1981), pp.531-540.

Chong BH, Ismail F, Cade J, Gallus AS, Gordon S, Chesterman CN. (1989a). Heparin-induced thrombocytopenia: studies with a new low molecular weight heparinoid, Org 10172. Blood, 73, 6, (May 1989), pp.1592-1596.

Chong BH, Ismail F, Cade J, Gallus AS, Gordon S, et al. (1989b). Heparin-induced thrombocytopenia: studies with a new low molecular weight heparinoid, Org 10–172. *Blood*, 73, 6, (May 1989), pp.1592–1596.

Chong BH, Pilgrim RL, Cooley MA, & Chesterman CN. (1993b). Increased expression of platelet IgG Fc receptors in heparin induced thrombocytopenia. *Blood*, 81, 4, (Feb 1993), pp.988–993.

Chong BH. (1995). Heparin-induced thrombocytopenia. *Br J Haematol*, 89, 3, (1995), pp.431-439.

Chong BH. (2003). Heparin-induced thrombocytopenia. *J Thromb Haemost*, 1, 7, (Jul 2003), pp.1471–1478.

Chong BH. Heparin-induced thrombocytopenia. (1992). *Aust N Z J Med*, 22, 2, (Apr 1992), pp.145-152.

Cines DB, Rauova L, Arepally G, Reilly MP, McKenzie SE, et al. (2007). Heparin-induced thrombocytopenia: an autoimmune disorder regulated through daynamic outoantigen assembly/disassembly. *J Clin Apheresis*, 22, 1, (Feb 2007), pp.31-36.

Collins JL, Aster RH, Moghaddam M, Piotrowski MA, Strauss TR, et al. (1997). Diagnostic testing for heparin-induced thrombocytopenia (HIT): an enhanced platelet factor 4 complex enzyme linked immunosorbent assay (PF4ELISA). *Blood*, 90, (suppl), p.461a.

Denys B, Stove V, Philippé J, & Devreese K. (2008). A clinical-laboratory approach contributing to a rapid and reliable diagnosis of heparin-induced thrombocytopenia. *Thromb Res*, 123, 1, (Jan 2008), pp.137-145.

Fabris F, Fussi F, Casonato A, Visentin L, Randi M, et al. (1983). Smith MR, Girolami A. Normal and low molecular weight heparins: interaction with human platelets. *Eur J Clin Invest*, 13, 2, (Apr 1983), pp.135-139.

Fabris F, Luzzatto G, Stefani PM, Girolami B, Cella G, et al. (2000). Heparin-induced thrombocytopenia. *Haematologica*, 85, 1, (Jun 2000), pp.72-81.

Fondu P. (1995). Heparin-associated thrombocytopenia: an update. *Acta Clin Belg*, 50, 6, (1995), pp.343-357.

Francis JL, Palmer GJ 3rd, Moroose R, & Drexler A. (2003). Comparison of bovine and porcine heparin in heparin antibody formation after cardiac surgery. Ann Thorac Surg, 75, 1, (Jun 2003), pp.17-22.

Gentilini G, Kirschbaum NE, Augustine JA, Aster RH, & Visentin GP. (1999). Inhibition of human umbilical vein endothelial cell proliferation by the CXC chemokine, platelet factor 4 (PF4), is associated with impaired downregulation of p21(Cip1/WAF1). *Blood*, 93, 1, (Jun 1999), pp.25-33.

Girolami B, Prandoni P, Stefani PM, Tanduo C, Sabbion P, et al. (2003). The incidence of heparin-induced thrombocytopenia in hospitalized medical patients treated with subcutaneous unfractionated heparin: a prospective cohort study. *Blood*, 101, 8, (April 2003), pp.2955-2959.

Gosselin RC, Dager WE, King JH, Janatpour K, Mahackian K, et al. (2004). Effect of direct thrombin inhibitors, bivalirudin, lepirudin, and argatroban, on prothrombin time and INR values. *Am J Clin Pathol*, 121, 4, (Apr 2004), pp.593–599.

Green D, Harris K, Reynolds N, Roberts M, & Patterson R. (1978). Heparin immune thrombocytopenia: evidence for a heparin-platelet complex as the antigenic determinant. *J Lab Clin Med*, 91, 1, (Jun 1978), pp.167-175.

Green D, Martin GJ, Shoichet SH, DeBacker N, Bomalaski JS, et al. (1984). Thrombocytopenia in a prospective, randomized, double-blind trial of bovine and porcine heparin. *Am J Med Sci*, 288, 2, (Sep 1984), pp.60-64.

Greinacher A, & Lubenow N. (2001). Recombinant hirudin in clinical practice: focus on lepirudin. *Circulation*, 103, 10, (Mar 2001), pp.1479–1484.

Greinacher A, Amiral J, Dummel V, Vissac A, Kiefel V, et al. (1994b). Laboratory diagnosis of heparin-associated thrombocytopenia and comparison of platelet aggregation test, heparin-induced platelet activation test, and platelet factor 4/heparin enzyme-linked immunosorbent assay. *Transfusion*, 34, 5, (May 1994), pp.381-385.

Greinacher A, Eichler P, Lubenow N, Kwasny H, & Luz M. (2000). Heparin-induced thrombocytopenia with thromboembolic complications: meta-analysis of 2 prospective trials to assess the value of parenteral treatment with lepirudin and its therapeutic aPTT range. *Blood*, 96, 3, (Aug 2000), pp.846-851.

Greinacher A, Janssens U, Berg G, Böck M, Kwasny H, et al. (1999a). Lepirudin (recombinant hirudin) for parenteral anticoagulation in patients with heparin-induced thrombocytopenia: Heparin-Associated Thrombocytopenia Study (HAT) investigators. *Circulation*, 100, 6, (Aug 1999), pp.587–593.

Greinacher A, Lubenow N, & Eichler P. (2003). Anaphylactic and anaphylactoid reactions associated with lepirudin in patients with heparin-induced thrombocytopenia. *Circulation*, 108, 17, (Oct 2003), pp.2062–2065.

Greinacher A, Michels I, & Mueller-Eckhardt C. (1992). Heparin-associated thrombocytopenia: the antibody is not heparin specific. *Thromb Haemost*, 67, 5, (May 1992), pp.545-549.

Greinacher A, Michels I, Kiefel V, Mueller-Eckhardt C. (1991). A rapid and sensitive test for diagnosing heparin-associated thrombocytopenia. *Thromb Haemost*, 66, 6, (Dec 1991), pp.734-736.

Greinacher A, Michels I, Liebenhoff U, Presek P, & Mueller-Eckhardt C. (1993). Heparin-associated thrombocytopenia: immune complexes are attached to the platelet membrane by the negative charge of highly sulphated oligosaccharides. *Br J Haematol*, 84, 4, (Aug 1993), pp.711-716.

Greinacher A, Pötzsch B, Amiral J, Dummel V, Eichner A, et al. (1994a). Heparin-associated thrombocytopenia: isolation of the antibody and characterization of a multimolecular PF4-heparin complex as the major antigen. *Thromb Haemost*, 71, 2, (Feb 1994), pp.247-251.

Greinacher A, Völpel H, Janssens U, Hach-Wunderle V, Kemkes-Matthes B, Eichler P, et al. (1999b). Lepirudin provides safe and effective anticoagulation in patients with heparin-induced thrombocytopenia: a prospective study. *Circulation*, 99, 1, (Jan 1999), pp.73–80.

Greinacher A. (1995). Antigen generation in heparin-associated thrombocytopenia: the nonimmunologic type and the immunologic type are closely linked in their pathogenesis. *Semin Thromb Hemost*, 21, 1, (1995), pp.106-116.

Gruel Y, Boizard-Boval B, & Wautier JL. (1993). Further evidence that alpha-granule components such as platelet factor 4 are involved in platelet-IgG-heparin interactions during heparin-associated thrombocytopenia. *Thromb Haemost*, 70, 2, (Aug 1993), pp.374-375.

Gruel Y, Régina S, & Pouplard C. (2008). Usefulness of pretest clinical score (4Ts) combined with immunoassay for the diagnosis of heparin-induced thrombocytopenia. Curr Opin Pulm Med, 14,5, (Sep 2008), pp.397-402.

Harris K, Nguyen P, & Van Cott EM. (2008). Platelet PLA2 polymorphism and the risk for thrombosis in heparin-induced thrombocytopenia. *Am J Clin Pathol*, 129, 2, (Feb 2008), pp.282-286.

Hirsh J, Heddle N, & Kelton JG. (2004). Treatment of heparin-induced thrombocytopenia: a critical review. *Arch Intern Med*, 164, 4, (Feb 2004), pp.361-369.

Jackson MR, Neilson WJ, Lary M, Baay P, Web K, & ET AL. (2006). Delayed-onset heparin-induced thrombocytopenia and thrombosis after intraoperative heparin anticoagulation: four case reports. *Vasc Endovasc Surgery*, 40, 11, (Jun-Feb 2006), pp.67-70.

Janatpour KA, Gosselin RC, Dager WE, Lee A, Owings JT, et al. (2007). Usefulness of optical density values from heparin-platelet factor 4 antibody testing and probability scoring models to diagnose heparin-induced thrombocytopenia. *Am J Clin Pathol*, 127, 3, (Mar 2007), pp.429-433.

Jang IK, & Hursting MJ. (2005). When heparins promote thrombosis: review of heparin-induced thrombocytopenia. *Circulation*, 111, 20, (May 2005), pp.2671-2683.

Kadidal VV, Mayo DJ, & Horne MK. (1999). Heparin-induced thrombocytopenia (HIT) due to heparin flushes: a report of three cases. *J Intern Med*. 246, 3, (Sep 1999), pp.325-329.

Kariyazono H, Nakamura K, Shinkawa T, Moriyama Y, Toyohira H, et al. (1997). Inhibitory effects of antibiotics on platelet aggregation in vitro. *Hum Exp Toxicol*, 16, 11, (Nov 1997), pp.662-666.

Kelton JG, Sheridan D, Santos A, Smith J, Steeves K, et al. (1988). Heparin-induced thrombocytopenia: laboratory studies. *Blood*, 72, 3, (Sep 1988), pp.925-930.

Kelton JG, Smith JW, Warkentin TE, Hayward CP, Denomme GA, & Horsewood P. (1994). Immunoglobulin G from patients with heparin-induced thrombocytopenia binds to a complex of heparin and platelet factor 4. Blood, 83, 11, (Jun 1994), pp.3232-3239.

Laster JL, Nichols WK, & Silver D. (1989). Thrombocytopenia associated with heparin-coated catheters inpatients with heparin-associated antiplatelet antibodies. *Arch Intern Med*, 149, 10, (Oct 1989), pp.2285–2287.

Lee DH, & Warkentin TE. (2004). Frequency of heparin-induced thrombocytopenia. In: Warkentin TE. Greinacher A. eds. Heparin-induced thrombocytopenia. 3rd ed. New York, NY: Marcel Dekker, pp.107-148

Lewis BE, Wallis DE, Berkowitz SD, Matthai WH, Fareed J, et al. (2001). Argatroban anticoagulant therapy in patients with heparin-induced thrombocytopenia. *Circulation*, 103, 14, (Apr 2001), pp.1833–1843.

Lewis BE, Wallis DE, Leya F, Hursting MJ, & Kelton JG; Argatroban-915 Investigators. (2003). Argatroban anticoagulation in patients with heparin-induced thrombocytopenia. *Arch Intern Med*, 163, 15, (Aug 1003), pp.1849–1856.

Lillo-Le Louët A, Boutouyrie P, Alhenc-Gelas M, Le Beller C, Gautier I, et al. (2004). Diagnostic score for heparin-induced thrombocytopenia after cardiopulmonary bypass. *J Thromb Haemost*, 2, 11, (Nov 2004), pp.1882-1888.

Lindhoff-Last E, Gerdsen F, Ackermann H, & Bauersachs R. (2001). Determination of heparin–platelet 4–IgG antibodies improves diagnosis of heparin-induced thrombocytopenia. *Br J Haematol*, 113, 4, (Jun 2001), pp.886–890.

Lobo B, Finch C, Howard A, & Minhas S. (2008). Fondaparinux for the treatment of patients with acute heparin-induced thrombocytopenia. *Thromb Haemost*, 99, 1, (Jan 2008), pp.208–214.

Lubenow N, Eichler P, Lietz T, & Greinacher A; Hit Investigators Group. (2005). Lepirudin in patients with heparin-induced thrombocytopenia: results of the third prospective study (HAT-3) and a combined analysis of HIT-1, HAT-2, and HAT-3. *J Thromb Haemost*, 3, 11, (Nov 2005), pp.2428–2436.

Lubenow N, Eichler P, Lietz T, Farner B, Greinacher A. (2004). Lepirudin for prophylaxis of thrombosis in patients with acute isolated heparin-induced thrombocytopenia: an analysis of 3 prospective studies. *Blood*, 104, 10, (Nov 2004), pp.3072-7.

Lubenow N, Kempf R, Eichner A, Eichler P, Carlsson LE, et al. (2002). Heparin-induced thrombocytopenia: temporal pattern of thrombocytopenia in relation to initial use or reexposure to heparin. *Chest*, 122, 1, (Jul 2002), pp.37-42.

Lynch DM, & Howe SE. (1985). Heparin-associated thrombocytopenia: antibody binding specificity to platelet antigen. *Blood*, 66, 5, (Nov 1985), pp.1176-1181.

Magnani HN. (1993). Heparin-induced thrombocytopenia (HIT): an overview of 230 patients treated with orgaran (Org 10172). *Thromb Haemost*, 70, 4, (Oct 1993), pp.554-561.

Mahaffey KW, Lewis BE, Wildermann NM, Berkowitz SD, Oliverio RM, et al. (2003). The anticoagulant therapy with bivalirudin to assist in the performance of percutaneous coronary intervention in patients with heparin-induced thrombocytopenia (ATBAT) study. *J Invasive Cardiol*, 15, 11, (Nov 2003), pp.611-616.

Mayo DJ, Cullinane AM, Merryman PK, & Horne MK 3rd. (1990). Serologic evidence of heparin sensitization in cancer patients receiving heparin flushes of venous access devices. *Support Care Cancer*, 7, 6, (Nov 1990), pp.425-427.

Monreal M, Lafoz E, Salvador R, Roncales J, & Navarro A. (1989). Adverse effects of three different forms of heparin therapy: thrombocytopenia, increased transaminases, and hyperkalaemia. *Eur J Clin Pharmacol,* 37, 4, (1989), pp.415-418.

Nakamura K, Kariyazono H, Moriyama Y, Toyohira H, Kubo H, et al. (1999). Effects of sarpogrelate hydrochloride on platelet aggregation, and its relation to the release of serotonin and P-selectin. *Blood Coagul Fibrinolysis*, 10, 8, (Dec 1999), pp.513-519.

Nand S, Wong W, Yuen B, Yetter A, Schmulbach E, et al. (1997). Heparin-induced thrombocytopenia with thrombosis: incidence, analysis of risk factors, and clinical outcomes in 108 consecutive patients treated at a single institution. *Am J Hematol*, 56, 1, (Sep 1997), pp.12-16.

Newman PM, & Chong BH. (2000). Heparin-induced thrombocytopenia: new evidence for the dynamic binding of purified anti-PF4-heparin antibodies to platelets and the resultant platelet activation. *Blood*, 96, 1, (Jul 2000), pp.182-187.

Ortel TL. (2009). Heparin-induced thrombocytopenia: when a low platelet count is a mandate for anticoagulation. *Hematology (Am Soc Heamatol Educ Prog)*, pp.225-232.

Polgár J, Eichler P, Greinacher A, Clemetson KJ. (1998). Adenosine diphosphate (ADP) and ADP receptor play a major role in platelet activation/aggregation induced by sera from heparin-induced thrombocytopenia patients. *Blood*, 91, 2, (Jun 1998), pp.549-554.

Popov D, Zarrabi MH, Foda H, & Graber M. (1997). Pseudopulmonary embolism: acute respiratory distress in the syndrome of heparin-induced thrombocytopenia. *Am J Kidney Dis*, 29, 3, (Mar 1997), pp.449-452.

Pouplard C, Amiral J, Borg JY, Laporte-Simitsidis S, Delahousse B, et al. (1999b). Decision analysis for use of platelet aggregation test, carbon 14-serotonin release assay, and heparin-platelet factor 4 enzyme-linked immunosorbent assay for diagnosis of heparin-induced thrombocytopenia. *Am J Clin Pathol*, 111, 5, (May 1999), pp.700-706.

Pouplard C, Iochmann S, Renard B, Herault O, Colombat P, et al. (2001). Induction of monocyte tissue factor expression by antibodies to heparin-platelet factor 4 complexes developed in heparin-induced thrombocytopenia. *Blood*, 97, 10, (May 2001), pp.3300-3302.

Pouplard C, May MA, Iochmann S, Amiral J, Vissac AM, et al. (1999a). Antibodies to platelet factor 4-heparin after cardiopulmonary bypass in patients anticoagulated with unfractionated heparin or a low-molecular-weight heparin : clinical implications for heparin-induced thrombocytopenia. *Circulation*, 99, 19, (May 1999), pp.2530-2536.

Price E, Hayward C, Moffat K, Moore J, Warkentin T, et al. (2007). Laboratory testing for heparin-induced thrombocytopenia is inconsistent in North America: a survey of North American specialized coagulation laboratories. *Thromb Haemost*, 98, 6, (Dec 2007), pp.1357-1361.

Rao AK, White GC, Sherman L, Colman R, Lan G, et al. (1989). Low incidence of thrombocytopenia with porcine mucosal heparin. A prospective multicenter study. *Arch Intern Med*, 6, (Jun 1989), 149, pp.1285-1288.

Rhodes GR, Dixon RH, & Silver D. (1973). Heparin induced thrombocytopenia with thrombotic and hemorrhagic manifestations. *Surg Gynecol Obstet*, 136, 3, (Mar 1973), pp.409-416.

Rice L, Attisha WK, Drexler A,& Francis JL. (2002). Delayed-onset heparin-induced thrombocytopenia. *Ann Intern Med*, 136, 3, (Feb 2002), pp.210-215.

Rota E, Bazzan M, & Fantino G. (2008). Fondaparinux-related thrombocytopenia in a previous low-molecular-weight heparin (LMWH)-induced heparin-induced thrombocytopenia (HIT). *Thromb Haemost*, 99.4, (Apr 2008), pp.779-781.

Salzman EW, Rosenberg RD, Smith MH, Lindon JN, & Favreau L. (1980). Effect of heparin and heparin fractions on platelet aggregation. *J Clin Invest*, 65, 1, (Jan 1980), pp.64-73.

Schmitt BP, & Adelman B. (1993). Heparin-associated thrombocytopenia: a critical review and pooled analysis. *Am J Med Sci*, 305, 4, (Apr 1993), pp.208-215.

Shantsila E, Lip GY, & Chong BH. (2009). Heparin-induced thrombocytopenia. A contemporary clinical approach to diagnosis and management. *Chest*, 135, 6, (June 2009), pp.1651-1664.

Sheridan D, Carter C, Kelton JG. (1986). A diagnostic test for heparin-induced thrombocytopenia. *Blood*, 67, 2, (Jan 1986), pp.27-30.

Strauss R, Wehler M, Mehler K, Kreutzer D, Koebnick C, et al. (2002). Thrombocytopenia in patients in the medical intensive care unit: bleeding prevalence, transfusion requirements, and outcome. *Crit Care Med*, 30, 2, (Aug 2002), pp.1765–1771.

Suh JS, Aster RH, & Visentin GP. (1998). Antibodies from patients with heparin-induced thrombocytopenia/thrombosis recognize different epitopes on heparin: platelet factor 4. *Blood*, 91, 1, (Feb 1998), pp.916-922.

Suh JS, Malik MI, Aster RH, & Visentin GP. (1997). Characterization of the humoral immune response in heparin- induced thrombocytopenia. *Am J Hematol*, 54, 3, (Mar 1997), pp.196-201.

Tardy B, Lecompte T, Boelhen F, Tardy-Poncet B, Elalamy I, et al. (2006). Predictive factors for thrombosis and major bleeding in an observational study in 181 patients with heparin-induced thrombocytopenia treated with lepirudin. *Blood*, 108, 5, (Sep 2006), pp.1492–1496.

Tardy-Poncet B, Tardy B, Reynaud J, Mahul P, Mismetti P, et al. (1999). Efficacy and safety of danaparoid sodium (ORG 10172) in critically ill patients with heparin-associated thrombocytopenia. *Chest*, 115, 6, (Jun 1999), pp.1616–1620.

Toyohira H, Nakamura K, Kariyazono H, Yamada K, Moriyama Y, et al. (1995). Significance of combined use of anticoagulants and antiplatelet agents in the early stage after prosthetic valve replacement. *Kyobu Geka*, 48, 9, (Aug 1995), pp.749-755.

Visentin GP, Ford SE, Scott JP, & Aster RHJ. (1994). Antibodies from patients with heparin-induced thrombocytopenia/thrombosis are specific for platelet factor 4 complexed with heparin or bound to endothelial cells. *Clin Invest*, 93, 1, (Jun 1994), pp.81-88.

Walenga JM, Jeske WP, & Messmore HL. (2000). Mechanisms of venous and arterial thrombosis in heparin-induced thrombocytopenia. *J Thromb Thrombolysis*, 10, (Suppl), pp.S13-S20.

Walenga JM, Jeske WP, Prechel MM, & Bakhos M. (2004). Newer insights on the mechanism of heparin-induced thrombocytopenia. *Semin Thromb Hemost*, 30, (Suppl1), (Feb 2004), pp.S57-S67.

Wallis DE, Workman DL, Lewis BE, Steen L, Pifarre R, et al. (1999). Failure of early heparin cessation as treatment for heparin-induced thrombocytopenia. *Am J Med*, 106, 6, (Jun 1999), pp.629-635.

Warkentin TE, & Bernstein RA. (2003). Delayed-onset heparin-induced thrombocytopenia and cerebral thrombosis after a single administration of unfractionated heparin [letter]. *N Engl J Med*, 348, 11, (Mar 2003), pp.1067-1069.

Warkentin TE, & Greinacher A. (2004). Heparin-induced thrombocytopenia: recognition, treatment, and prevention. *Chest*, 126, (suppl 3), (Sep 2004), pp.311S-337S.

Warkentin TE, & Heddle NM. (2003). Laboratory diagnosis of immune heparin-induced thrombocytopenia. *Curr Hematol Rep*, 2, 2, (Mar 2003), pp.148-157.

Warkentin TE, & Kelton JG. (1990). Heparin and platelets. *Hematol Oncol Clin North Am*, 4, 1, (Feb 1990), pp.243-264.

Warkentin TE, & Kelton JG. (1996). A 14-year study of heparin-induced thrombocytopenia. *Am J Med*, 101, pp.502-507.

Warkentin TE, & Kelton JG. (2001a). Temporal aspects of heparin-induced thrombocytopenia. *N Engl J Med*, 344, 17, (Apr 2001), pp.1286-1292.

Warkentin TE, & Kelton JG. (2001b). Delayed-onset heparin-induced thrombocytopenia and thrombosis. *Ann Intern Med*, 135, 7, (Oct 2001), pp.502-506.

Warkentin TE, Aird WC, & Rand JH. (2003b). Platelet-endothelial interactions: sepsis, HIT, and antiphospholipid syndrome. *Hematology (Am Soc Heamtol Educ Prog)*, pp.497-519.

Warkentin TE, Chong BH, & Greinacher A. (1998).Heparin-induced thrombocytopenia: towards consensus. *Thromb Haemost*, 79, 1, (Jun 1998), pp.1-7.

Warkentin TE, Cook RJ, Marder VJ, Sheppard JA, Moore JC, et al. (2005). Anti-platelet factor 4/heparin antibodies in orthopedic surgery patients receiving antithrombotic prophylaxis with fondaparinux or enoxaparin. *Blood*, 106, 12, (Dec 2005), pp.3791–3796.

Warkentin TE, Elavathil LJ, Hayward CP, Johnston MA, Russett JI, et al. (1997). The pathogenesis of venous limb gangrene associated with heparin-induced thrombocytopenia. *Ann Intern Med*, 127, 9, (Nov 1997), pp.804-812.

Warkentin TE, Greinacher A, Koster A, & Lincoff AM; American College of Chest Physicians. (2008a). Treatment and prevention of heparin-induced hrombocyotopenia. American College of Physicians evidence-based clinical practice guidelines (8th edition). *Chest*, 133, (suppl 6), (Jun 2008), pp.340S-380S.

Warkentin TE, Hayward CP, Smith CA, Kelly PM, Kelton JG. (1992). Determinants of donor platelet variability when testing for heparin-induced thrombocytopenia. *J Lab Clin Med*, 120, 3, (Sep 1992), pp.371-379.

Warkentin TE, Levine MN, Hirsh J, Horsewood P, Roberts RS, et al. (1995a). Heparin-induced thrombocytopenia in patients treated with low-molecular-weight heparin or unfractionated heparin. *N Engl J Med*, 332, 20, (May 1995), pp.1330-1335.

Warkentin TE, Roberts RS, Hirsh J, & Kelton JG. (2003a). An improved definition of immune heparin-induced thrombocytopenia in postoperative orthopedic patients. *Arch Intern Med*, 163, 20, (Nov 2003), pp.2518-2524.

Warkentin TE, Sheppard J, Moore J, Sigouin CS, & Kelton J. (2008b). Quantitative interpretation of optical density measurements using PF4-dependent enzyme-immunoassays. *J Thromb Haemost*, 6, 8, (Aug 2008). pp.1304-1312.

Warkentin TE, Sheppard JA, Horsewood P, Simpson PJ, Moore JC, et al. (2000). Impact of the patient population on the risk for heparin-induced thrombocytopenia. *Blood*, 96, 5, (Sep 2000), pp.1703-1708.

Warkentin TE. (1996a). Heparin-induced thrombocytopenia: IgG-mediated platelet activation, platelet microparticle generation, and altered procoagulant/ anticoagulant balance in the pathogenesis of thrombosis and venous limb gangrene complicating heparin-induced thrombocytopenia. *Transfus Med Rev*, 10, 4, (Oct 1996), pp.249-258.

Warkentin TE. (1996b). Heparin-induced skin lesions. *Br J Haematol*, 92, 2, (Feb 1996), pp.494-497.

Warkentin TE. (1999). Generation of platelet-derived microparticles and procoagulation activity by heparin-induced thrombocytopenia IgG/serum and other IgG platelet agonists: a comparison with standard platelet agonists. *Platelets*. 10, 5, (1999), pp.319-326.

Warkentin TE. (2000). Laboratory testing for heparin-induced thrombocytopenia. *J Thromb Thromblysi*, 10, (suppl 1), (Nov 2000), pp.S35-S45.

Warkentin TE. (2001). Laboratory testing for heparin-induced thrombocytopenia. In: Warkentin TE. Greinacher A. eds. Heparin-induced thrombocytopenia. 2nd ed. New York, NY: Marcel Dekker Inc; pp.231-269.

Warkentin TE. (2002). Platelet count monitoring and laboratory testing for heparin-induced thrombocytopenia. *Arch Pathol Lab Med*, 126, 11, (Nov 2002), pp.1415-1423.

Warkentin TE. (2003). Heparin-induced thrombocytopenia: pathogenesis and management. *Br J Haematol*, 121, 4, (May 2003), pp.535-555.

Warkentin TE. (2004a). Clinical picture of heparin-induced thrombocytopenia. In: Warkentin TE. Greinacher A. eds. Heparin-induced thrombocytopenia. 3rd ed. New York, NY: Marcel Dekker, pp.53-106.

Warkentin TE. (2004b) Laboratory testing for heparin-induced thrombocytopenia. In: Warkentin TE. Greinacher A. eds. Heparin-induced thrombocytopenia. 3rd ed. New York, NY: Marcel Dekker, pp.271-311.

Warkentin TE. (2007). Clinical picture of heparin-induced thrombocytopenia. In: Warkentin TE. Greinacher A. eds. Heparin-induced thrombocytopenia. 4rd ed. New York, NY: InformaHealthcare USA, pp.21-66.

Ziporen L, Li ZQ, Park KS, Sabnekar P, Liu WY, Arepally G, et al. (1998). Defining an antigenic epitope on platelet factor 4 associated with heparin-induced thrombocytopenia. *Blood*, 92, 9, (Nov 1998), pp.3250–3259.

Zwicker JI, Uhl L, Huang WY, Shaz BH, Bauer KA. (2004). Thrombosis and ELISA optical density values in hospitalized patients with heparin-induced thrombocytopenia. *J Thromb Haemost*. 12, 2, (Dec 2004), pp.2133-2137.

22

Converting Hematology Based Data into an Inferential Interpretation

Larry H. Bernstein[1,*], Gil David[2], James Rucinski[3] and Ronald R. Coifman[2]
[1]*Triplex,*
[2]*Yale University Department of Mathematics,*
Program in Applied Mathematics, New Haven, CT,
[3]*New York Methodist Hospital-Weill-Cornell, Brooklyn, NY*
USA

1. Introduction

The most commonly ordered test used for managing patients worldwide is the hemogram, with or without the review of a peripheral smear. The measured features in a standard hemogram has undergone modification of the over the last 30 years with an expansion to the panel of tests. The initial hemogram was the hemoglobin, hematocrit, and total white cell count, to which platelet count, lymphocytes and neutrophils were added as the necessary vital dye stains and the resolution were substantially improved. The revolutionary Coulter principle used impedance of the cells passing through a narrow window. Newer instruments may used both impedance and/or flow cytometric principles. Yet the accurate identification of reticulocytes, measurement of cellular hemoglobin, measurement of immature granulocytes, lymphoid or myeloblasts, identification of clumped platelets interfering with identification of large platelets were all challenges to overcome. The hemogram provides a vital window to visualize the cellular changes associated with the production, release or suppression of the formed elements from the blood forming organ to the circulation. In this chapter, we shall not be concerned with the specific use of the hemogram in assessing disorders to the coagulation pathways or its use in detection of hematological and non-hematological tumors. Rather in the hemogram we can view data reflective of a broad spectrum medical conditions affecting most patients presenting to a physician who are then referred to a specialist for example in hematology-oncology or infectious diseases.

The theme of what we are about to present is that once we go beyond qualitative changes to the morphology of the cellular components of blood, we have also to consider their quantitative characteristics expressed as measurements of size, density, and concentration, which results in more than a dozen composite variables, including the mean corpuscular volume (MCV), mean corpuscular hemoglobin concentration (MCHC), mean corpuscular hemoglobin (MCH), total white cell count (WBC), total lymphocyte count, neutrophil count (mature granulocyte count and bands), monocytes, eosinophils, basophils, platelet count, and mean platelet volume (MPV), and flags to denote blasts, reticulocytes, platelet clumps, and so on. If you were to add the comprehensive metabolic panel, which includes monovalent and divalent cations and anions, total CO2, total protein and albumin, to name a few, there is a potential for information overload to the physician. These data in turn have to be comprehended in context with vital signs, key symptoms, and an accurate medical history. Consequently, the limits of memory and cognition are tested in medical practice on a daily basis. In this chapter we will discuss problems in the interpretation of data generated by automated laboratory diagnostic machinery, as experienced by the physician, and how through better design of the software (middleware) that presents this data the situation could be improved.

2. The current status of the physician-laboratory interface

The clinical laboratory has several divisions. Microbiology and anatomic pathology are the oldest, and they are the least automated, but they have rigorous definitions for their interpretation, as is true for immunohematology. Hematology and chemistry are the most automated, but their interpretations are more difficult than the other disciplines. To start with we will consider automated chemistry, hematology, and immunology with large high-throughput sample platforms. These analyzers have enhanced performance by interface with middleware, which have embedded rules to accept or reject a test result based on a result lying outside an assigned confidence limit, or based on a difference from a previous measurement within an assigned time interval in hours or days. A middleware is a minicomputer installed either between an instrument and a laboratory information system or between an instrument and a hospital information system. The middleware handles an enormous transaction rate of test workflow that would otherwise compete with physician interactions in trying to access the data output. The middleware also carries out on-line quality control checks, monitors the completion of panel accessions, and does "delta" checks for excessive differences between measurements taken in sequence. Further, depending on whether a test is measured from unclotted and unspun blood, or from plasma or serum fraction, hematology, chemistry and immunology testing are tested with different turnaround times (time from receipt to time to report). In all of these cases, tests from different core "instruments" or laboratory "facilities" of laboratory testing have to be interpreted without conflict in the production "silo" (the term refers to a separate mode of production that is separate from and not interoperable with other information sources).

3. Data overload and unstructured

The computer architecture that the physician uses to view the results is not open-architecture, and the middleware solutions used to overcome the problem are insufficient in that the data is not recombined from the rigid lists into a structured format that readily enables the physician to interpret the report. Consequently the results are more often than not presented as the designer would prefer, and not as the end-user would like. In order to optimize the interface for physician, the system would have a "front-to-back" design, with the call up for any patient ideally consisting of a dashboard design that presents the crucial information that the physician would likely act on in an easily accessible manner. The problem of the user having to adjust to what the system confronts them with is described by Didner (1) in an internal Bell Labs memo approved for external release. The key point being that each item used has to be closely related to a corresponding criterion needed for a decision. Currently, improved design is heading in that direction. In removing this limitation the output requirements have to be defined before the database is designed to produce the required output. The ability to see any other information, or to see a sequential visualization of the patient's course would be steps to home in on other views. In addition, the amount of relevant information, even when presented well, is a cognitive challenge unless it is presented in a disease- or organ-system structure. So the interaction between the user and the electronic medical record has a significant effect on practitioner time, ability to minimize errors of interpretation, facilitate treatment, and manage costs. This is a correction for a view from the mere transmission of a body of automated tests that are generated at sites not near to the patient, often with a high priority reporting required from the operating room, the emergency room, or the intensive care units in order to make triage decisions or to adjust fluids or make treatment decisions.

The reality is that clinicians are challenged by the need to view a large amount of data, with only a few resources available to know which of these values are relevant, or the need for action on a result, or its urgency. An approach (2,3), called the foresighted-practice guideline, aligned with concepts developed by Lawrence Weed (4). Weed emphasizes that the information infrastructure was lacking at the time of his writing (1997), and that tools are needed to extend the mind's capability to process large numbers of relevant variables. The challenge then becomes how fundamental measurement theory can lead to the creation at the point of care of more meaningful actionable presentations of results (5). WP Fisher (6) refers to the creation of a context in which computational resources for meeting the challenges will be incorporated into the electronic medical record. The one which he chooses is a probabilistic conjoint (Rasch) measurement model (7), which uses scale-free standard measures and meets data quality standards. He illustrates this by fitting a set of data provided by Bernstein (19)(27 items for the diagnosis of acute myocardial infarction (AMI) to a Rasch multiple rating scale model testing the hypothesis that items work together to delineate a unidimensional measurement continuum. The results indicated that highly improbable observations could be discarded, data volume could be reduced based on its internal consistency, and that consistency could be used to increase the ability of the care provider to interpret the data. The use of a computer-derived algorithm has been shown to aid the physician (8,9). A huge amount of progress has occurred regarding model construction and validation in the last 11 years. An ordinal regression (adjacent category logit model)(10) used on the AMI problem (11) is superceded by a Latent Class Model of Jay Magidson and Jeroen Vermunt (LatentGOLD, Statistical Innovations, Medford, MA)(12). The LatentGOLD has LC Cluster models, DFactor models, and LC Regression models and has the advantage of allowing performance of LC analyses on data containing more than just a few variables. It uses the fundamental methods of model fit (13,14) established as Alaike (AIC)(14,15,16) and Bayes (BIC)(14) information criteria. These have not been applied to classifying a large and complex medical data set.

4. Classified data a separate issue from automation

On the other hand, automation itself may not be as important as the critical value of the information provided. The disciplines required in blood banking and in microbiology have only been recently automated, but their importance is readily understood with the exception of an error in blood sample, or its contamination. To an extent, blood screening has become a large scale production to service the user population.

The classification of blood types emerged at the turn of the last century firstly as a result of the work of Paul Ehrlich (17) establishing a groundwork for immunology, and then later Karl Landsteiner's seminal work in laying the foundation for the blood groups (17). These works resulted in a well-defined classification of a set of identified blood group antigens and the absence of antibody in the individual's serum against the blood type, with the exception of auto-antibody reactions.

4.1 Microbiology classification

Microbiology classification has its origin in the taxonomic principles set down by Bergey's Manual of Determinative Bacteriology, which originated in 1857, and is maintained by Bergey's Trust. It is guided by observable features that are key for separating groups and subgroups. The kind of features that we readily identify are gram stain positivity, colonies on agar, cocciform or bacillary shape, outer capsule, motility, the clusters formed, the metabolic features in growth media, and even the expected antibiotic reactivity. Thus, we have an example: in Table 1.

GROUP 4
Description: Gram Negative, Aerobic/Microaerophilic rods and cocci
Key differences are: pigments/fluorescent, motility, growth requirements, denitrification,
morphology, and oxidase, read Genera descriptions
Examples: Acinetobacter, Pseudomonas, Beijerinckia
GROUP 5
Description: Facultatively Anaerobic Gram negative rods
Key differences are: growth factors, morph., gram rxn., oxidase rxn., read Genera descriptions
Examples: Family Enterobacteriaceae and Vibrionaceae
GROUP 17
Description: Gram-Positive Cocci
Key differences are: oxygen requirements, morph., growth requirements (45°C and supplements), read Genera descriptions
Examples: Micrococcus, Staphylococcus, Streptococcus, Enterococcus, Lactococcus

Table 1. Typical classes of bacteria

Table 1 does not further divide into subclasses, which requires metabolic differentiation in growth media.

4.2 Feature extraction

This further breakdown in the modern era is determined by genetically characteristic gene sequences that are transcribed into what we measure. Eugene Rypka contributed greatly to clarifying the extraction of features in a series of articles, which set the groundwork for the methods used today in clinical microbiology (18,19). The method he describes is termed S-clustering, and will have a significant bearing on how we can view hematology data. He describes S-clustering as extracting features from endogenous data that amplify or maximize structural information to create distinctive classes. The method classifies by taking the number of features with sufficient variety to map into a theoretic standard. The mapping is done by a truth table, and each variable is scaled to assign values for each: message choice. The number of messages and the number of choices forms an N-by N table. He points out that the message choice in an antibody titer would be converted from 0 + ++ +++ to 0 1 2 3. In looking at laboratory values the practitioner separates any test by low normal moderately-high high. Even though there may be a large number of measured values, the variety is reduced by this compression, even though there is risk of loss of information. Yet the real issue is how a combination of variables falls into a table with meaningful information. He describes how syndromic classification is uniquely valuable for clinical laboratory information by amplifying information in the course of making a pattern-identifiable syndromic classification. Rudolph, Bernstein and Babb (20) used it for the diagnosis of acute myocardial infarction.

5. Optimal weighting and value assigned to predictor variables

We are interested in classifying data as essential for determining optimal decision limits for tests, and for analyzing variable combinations that are essential and optimal for separating the groups that are separated with fewest errors. This is only possible by reducing data uncertainty. We are concerned with accurate assignment into uniquely variable groups by information in test relationships. One determines the effectiveness of each variable by its contribution to information gain in the system. The reference or null set is the class having no information. Uncertainty in assigning to a classification is only relieved by providing sufficient information. One determines the effectiveness of each variable by its contribution to information gain in the system. The possibility for realizing a good model for approximating the effects of factors supported by data used for inference owes much to the discovery of Kullback-Liebler distance or "information" (21), and Akaike (22) found a simple relationship between K-L information and Fisher's maximized log-likelihood function (23).

5.1 Advances in applied mathematics

Perhaps the current exponential growth of knowledge since the mapping of the human genome a decade ago has been enabled by parallel advances in applied mathematics, which has not been a part of the entrance competencies for premedical education, and is now taught to some extent in medical and postmedical education for a better understanding of modern clinical trials. The knowledge and use of the science of complexity in much of what we encounter is brought to account by Ray Kurzweill (24). In a univariate universe, we have significant control in visualizing data because we can be confident in separating unlike data by methods that rely on distributional assumptions, although errors in assignment can be substantial. The median (by rank order assignment is the best method of assignment under the circumstances). In reality, there is likely to be a different assignment of predictor values given an association with a different disease entity. In order to better define the target output another variable is necessary. As we attend to more associated outputs, the number of predictors is expanded. Now we begin to have multiple classes delineated by the confidence limits of the conjoint predictors. As the number of separate categories increases, the size of the database has to increase to limit the error in the so called model representation.

5.2 Complexity

As the complexity of models have increased to using several predictors for at least two outputs, and the dependencies are not clear, the models used for analysis of the data are derived by tables and use of the goodness of fit. The development of the Akaike Information Criterion (15,16,21,22,23) brought together two major disciplines that had separate developments, information theory and statistics. The powerful tools now available are not dependent on distributional assumptions, and allow classification and prediction. In fact modeling today has a primary goal of finding an underlying structure in studied data sets. A sequence of exploratory programs have been developed by Statistical Innovations, a Boston based company founded by Jay Magidson focused on classification problems with complex data sets, encompassing a mixture of nominal and continuous predictors, and where there is a high complexity with the data sample size may approach the number of predictors (COREXpress® , Latent GOLD® 4.5, LG-Syntax Module, Latent GOLD® Choice , SI-CHAID® , GOLDMineR). Many articles can be cited concerning these advances (25-32). Further, IBM has introduced a software program for Predictive Analytics available in 2011.

6. Prior experience in similarly developed taxonomies can be applied to hematology

We consider a novel approach to medical inference to have considerable parallel with work in bacterial taxonomy, or the rapidly growing work in genomics, proteomics, and translational medicine. In the diagnosis of anemia, we divide these into microcytic, normocytic and macrocytic. We also consider whether there is proliferation of marrow precursors, whether there is domination of a cell line, and whether there is a suppression of hematopoiesis. This gives us a two dimensional model. Then we consider another, the release into the blood of immature cells, for intermediate to the blast stage. Keep in mind that the thalassemias (and hemoglobin H disease) are characterized by moderate to severe microcytosis, and there is no anisocytosis (variation in size), and being a genetic disorder in production of globin chains, there is a high RBC count, whereas, iron deficiency anemia (IDA) differs by lack of iron incorporation into hemoglobin so that there is a low MCV, anisocytosis, and a low RBC count so that the ratio (Mentzer's index) of the MCV/RBC is very low with thalassemia, but not in IDA. We shall elaborate more on the creation of an evidence-based inference-engine that can substantially interpret the data at hand and convert it in real time to a "knowledge-based opinion", which is improvable from what exists today by incorporating clinical features and duration of onset into the model.

The evaluation of platelet abnormalities is somewhat more limited, but addresses the disorders of platelet numbers and of platelet size, and clumping. This does not discern abnormalities of platelet function (like von Willebrands, or drug induced). When platelets decrease abruptly with disseminated intravascular coagulation (DIC), as in sepsis or with massive trauma, the evidence is pretty good.

6.1 Hematopoiesis

Figure 1 is a pictorial diagram of hematopoietic cell lineages that are readily found in texts and cells are delineated further by identification of cell differentiation (CD) antigens. This lineage is expressly important for both the innate response and the humoral response to injury. Our knowledge of the innate response has become more and more intimately associated with long term metabolic effects, constitution, and chronic inflammation.

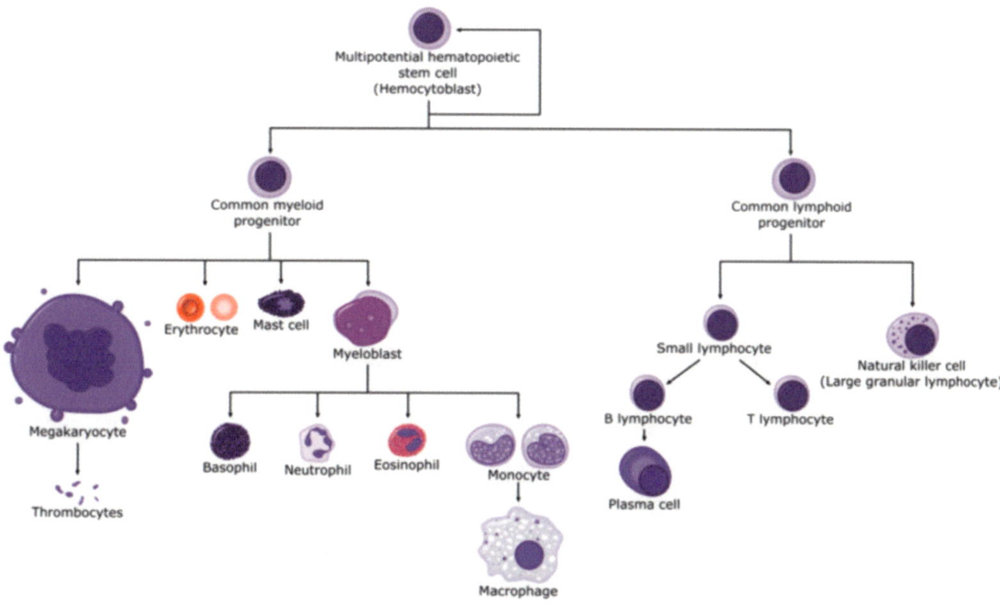

Fig. 1. A common depiction of the evolution of the myeloid and lymphoid cell lines from a multipotential hematopoietic stem cell. The platelets, red blood cells, mast cells and myeloid series are depicted as derived from a common myeloid progenitor cell. A branching from the myeloblast gives the granulocytic cells and the monocyte. Promyelocyte, metamyelocyte and myelocyte are intermediates not shown (band neutrophil is viewed as a neutrophil). The lymphocyte series is being more defined (as the myelocytic) that the naïve depiction by cell differentiation (CD) markers, and interactions are being investigated by cytokine, chemokine and cell signaling pathways.

Figure 1 shows a primary separation into a lymphocytic and a myeloid series. Note that the erythrocyte series and platelets are shown to be in lineage from a myeloid progenitor cell. It is conceivable that this picture is an oversimplification, but in clinical application, it is readily understood. This makes sense with respect to the uncommon evolution of myeloid metaplasia into erythroleukemia, but the diagram doesn't have an obvious connection for myelofibrosis, except for in the monocyte-macrophage linkage.

6.2 Peripheral smear

The peripheral smear is only viewed on the basis of flagged features seen on the hemogram. Blasts, indicative of release of very immature lymphocytes or myeloblasts are flagged and have to be reviewed by a pathologist before release, or done by the hematology supervisor and retained for pathologist review. In the case of children, there are numerous lymphocytes, and there may also be normoblasts and reticulocytes released from an active marrow. The presence of small mononuclear cells can be correctly identified by an experienced morphologist, but not necessarily by an automated cell counter. Consequently, proportionately more peripheral smears are evaluated for children than for adults. The greatest problem in the childhood age group is infection or sepsis. The lymphocyte and reticulocyte counts are very high in the infant, and the peak age for acute lymphocytic leukemia is at two years old. This makes it far more difficult to identify myelocytes and metamyelocytes (not shown in Figure 1), indicators of myeloid proliferation, in children than adults (33). The band neutrophil has been used to signify a left shift in myelopoiesis associated with sepsis, but it is quite variable and has been largely disregarded. This has accounted for the use of an automated cell counter that is also a flow cytometer for improved recognition of immature neutrophils below the band count. In the case of the red cell series (not shown) we classify first based on the RBC count, and then on the cell size. By these measures we have a decrease in mature red cell count based on WHO standards, adjusting for menstruation and pregnancy in women. We at the same time consider whether the RBC is normocytic, microcytic, or macrocytic and/or megaloblastic. What about increased or decreased production? Thalassemia is characterized by small cells that are neither hypochromic, or decreased in the peripheral circulation. Platelets may be large, they may be excessive in number, or they may be significantly decreased.

7. Extension of conditions and presentation to the electronic medical record (EMR)

We have published on the application of an automated inference engine (34) to the Systemic Inflammatory Response (SIRS), a serious infection, or emerging sepsis. We can report on this without going over previous ground. Of considerable interest is the morbidity and mortality of sepsis, and the hospital costs from a late diagnosis. If missed early, it could be problematic, and it could be seen as a hospital complication when it is not. Improving on previous work, we have the opportunity to look at the contribution of a fluorescence labeled flow cytometric measurement of the immature granulocytes (IG)(35), which is now widely used, but has not been adequatedly evaluated from the perspective of diagnostic usage. We have done considerable work on protein-energy malnutrition (PEM)(36-38), to which the automated interpretation is currently in review (39). Of course, the cholesterol, lymphocyte count, serum albumin provide the weight of evidence with the primary diagnosis (emphysema, chronic renal disease, eating disorder), and transthyretin would be low and remain low for a week in critical care. This could be a modifier with age in providing discriminating power.

7.1 Design of EMR

The current design of the Electronic Medical Record (EMR) is a linear presentation of portions of the record by services, by diagnostic method, and by date, to cite examples. This allows perusal through a graphical user interface (GUI) that partitions the information or necessary reports in a workstation entered by keying to icons. This requires that the medical practitioner finds the history, medications, laboratory reports, cardiac imaging and EKGs, and radiology in different workspaces. The introduction of a DASHBOARD, a visual panel of essential information on the computer screen that is widely used in business organizations, has allowed a presentation of drug reactions, allergies, primary and secondary diagnoses, and critical information about any patient the care giver needing access to the record. The advantage of this innovation is obvious. The startup problem is what information is presented and how it is displayed, which is a source of variability and a key to its success.

7.2 Dashboard

We are proposing an innovation that supercedes the main design elements of a DASHBOARD and utilizes the conjoined syndromic features of the disparate data elements. So the important determinant of the success of this endeavor is that it facilitates both the workflow and the decision-making process with a reduction of medical error. This has become extremely important and urgent in the 10 years since the publication "To Err is Human" (40), and the newly published finding that reduction of error is as elusive as reduction in cost. Whether they are counterproductive when approached in the wrong way may be subject to debate.

7.3 Syndromic classification

In order to clarify the concept of syndromic classification we make a distinction between lists of diseases that are assigned to abnormal test results and can be appended to test results. The oldest application has been in the identification of bacteria after culture isolation using growth in defined media that identify genetically determined metabolic pathways characteristic for each organism. A solid foundation in this work was elaborated by Rypka (18, 19). This was made less complicated by the genetic complement that defines its function. We introduce an AUTOMATED inference engine processing the data and making an interpretation available to the ordering physician and can anticipate an enormous impact on diagnosis and treatment. It addresses the complexity of inputs and enables rather than disables the practitioner. The method identifies outliers and combines data according to commonality of features. In some cases there may be conditions that are aggregated by similarity and dissimilarity into variants of the same condition with different treatment responses. How can we have confidence that we can successfully approach this problem in a new way? In the first place we are able to construct an interpretation of the composite data that is consistent with how a practitioner views multisystem pathophysiology in service of clinical decision-making.

8. A new inference methodology identifies and classifies anomalies

The main mathematical breakthroughs are provided by accurate patient profiling and inference methodologies in which anomalous subprofiles are extracted and compared to potentially relevant cases. Our methodologies organize numerical medical data profiles into demographics and characteristics relevant for inference and case tracking. As the model grows and its knowledge database is extended, the diagnostic and the prognostic become more accurate and precise.

As an example, inputs from test data such as hematology results are processed for anomaly characterization and compared with similar anomalies in a data base of 30,000 patients, provide diagnostic statistics, warning flags, and risk assessment. These are based on past prior experience, including: diagnostics and treatment outcomes (collective experience). The system was trained on this database of patients, built the learning knowledge base and used to analysis and diagnosis 5,000 new patients. Our system identified successfully the main risks with very high accuracy (more than 96%) and very low false rate (less than 0.5%)(34).

9. Representation and conclusion

The main benefit is a real time assessment as well as diagnostic options based on comparable cases, flags for risk and potential problems as illustrated in Figure 2. Figure 2 depicts the following case acquired on 04/21/10. The patient was diagnosed by our system with severe SIRS.

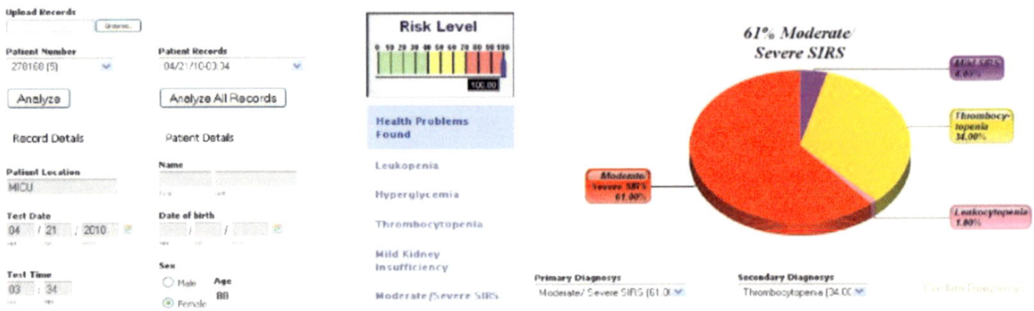

Fig. 2. The depiction of a patient diagnosed with severe systemic inflammatory response syndrome (SIRS), which may evolve into multiple organ failure (MODS), and death by circulatory collapse (systemic shock) if not arrested, depending on systemic functional reserve and successive stress. The far right is a pie chart of measured effects, and primary and secondary diagnoses. The middle lists the diagnoses found above which there is a scale with the risk. The left is patient demographics.

We anticipate that the effect of implementing this diagnostic amplifier would result in higher physician productivity at a time of great human resource limitations, safer prescribing practices, rapid identification of unusual patients, better assignment of patients to observation, inpatient beds, intensive care, or referral to clinic, shortened length of patients ICU and bed days.

10. References

[1] Didner RS. Back-to-Front systems design: A guns and butter approach. Unpublished research, 1979. Bell Laboratories, Piscataway, NJ 08854.

[2] Naegele TA, Wetzler HP. The foresighted practice guideline model: A win-win solution. http://www.swcp.com

[3] Naegele TA. Practice guidelines and clinical decision making. J Osteopath Med. March 1993:53-8.

[4] Weed L. New Connections between medical knowledge and patient care. Brit Med J 1997; 315:231-5.

[5] Haux R. Health information systems - past, present, future. Int J Med Inform. 2006; 75(3-4):268-81. Epub 2005 Sep 19.

[6] Fisher, W. P., Jr., Bernstein, L. H., Qamar, A., Babb, J., Rypka, E. W., & Yasick, D. (2002, February). At the bedside: Measuring patient outcomes. Advance for Administrators of the Laboratory, 11(2), 8, 10 [http://laboratory-manager.advanceweb.com/Article/At-the-Bedside-7.aspx].

[7] Fisher, W. P., Jr., & Burton, E. (2010). Embedding measurement within existing computerized data systems: Scaling clinical laboratory and medical records heart failure data to predict ICU admission. Journal of Applied Measurement, 11(2), 271-287.

[8] Linacre JM. Many-Facet Rasch Measurement. 1994. Mesa Press. Chicago,IL.

[9] Qamar A, McPherson C, Babb J, Bernstein LH, et al. The Goldman algorithm revisited: prospective evaluation of a computer-derived algorithm versus unaided physician judgement in suspected acute myocardial infarction. Amer Heart J 1999; 138:705-9.

[10] Goldman L, Weinberg M, Weisberg M, Olshen R, Cook EF, Sargent RK, Lamas GA, Dennis C, Wilson C, Deckelbaum L, Fineberg H, Stiratelli R. A computer-derived protocol to aid in the diagnosis of emergency room patients with acute chest pain. N Engl J Med 1982;307:588-596.

[11] Bernstein LH, Qamar A, McPherson R, Zarich S. Evaluation of a new graphical ordinal regression model (GOLDminer) in the diagnosis of myocardial infarction utilizing clinical features and laboratory data. http://www.statisticalinnovations.com/products/goldminer_tutorial2.html

[12] Magidson, J. and Vermunt, J.K. Latent class models for clustering: A comparison with K-means. Canadian Journal of Marketing Research, 2002; 20, 36-43.

[13] Browne MW, Cudeck R. Alternative ways of assessing model fit. In Testing Structural Equation Models (Bollen KA, Long JS, eds). 1993. Chapter 6. pages 1-34. SAGE Publishers, Inc. Newbury Park, CA. ISBN 0-8039-9507-8 (pbk).

[14] Raftery AE. Baysian model selection in structural equation models. In Testing Structural Equation Models (Bollen KA, Long JS, eds). 1993. Chapter 7. pages 163-179. SAGE Publishers, Inc. Newbury Park, CA. ISBN 0-8039-9507-8 (pbk).

[15] Akaike H. Factor analysis and AIC. Psychometrika 1987; 52:317-332.

[16] Bozdogen H. Model selection and Akaike's information criteria (AIC): the general theory and irs analytical extensions. Psychometrika 1987; 52:345-370.

[17] JW Goding. Emergence of the concept of complementarity and binding between antigen and antibodies: Contributions of Ehrlich and Landsteiner. In (JW Goding) Monoclonal Antibodies. Principles and Practice. Antibody Response. Elsevier Ltd 1996. Chapter 2. pages 7-25. (ISBN 978- 0 -12-287023-1).

[18] Rypka EW. Methods to evaluate and develop the decision process in the selection of tests. In Nakamura R. ed. Clinics in Laboratory Medicine.Phila.: WB Saunders Co.1992; 12(2):351-86.

[19] Rypka EW, Madar DA. A system for detecting emerging events: the systems-cybernetics approach. Presentation: Research Association of Medical and Biological Organizations (RAMBO). Biology department, University of New Mexico, Albuquerque, NM. July 17, 1996.

[20] Rudolph RA, Bernstein LH, Babb J. Information induction for predicting acute myocardial infarction. Clin Chem 1988; 34:2031-8.

[21] Kullback S, Liebler RA. On information and sufficiency. Annals of Math Statistics 1951; 22:79-86.

[22] Akaike H. Information theory as an extension of the maximum likelihood principle. In BN Petrov and F Csaki, Eds. Second International Symposium on Information Theory. Akdemiai Kiado, Budapest. 1973; 267-281.

[23] Fisher RA. On the Mathematical Foundations of Theoretical Statistics. Philosophical Transactions of the Royal Society of London. A. 1922; 222:309-368.
[24] Kurzweill R. The Singularity is Near: When Humans Transcend Biology. 2005. Viking Press. ISBN 0670033847.
[25] Jaynes ET. Bayesian Methods: General Background, ' In Maximum Entropy and Bayesian Methods in Applied Statistics.(Justice JH, ed). 1986, pp 1-26. Cambridge University Press.
[26] Skilling J. Classic maximum entropy. In Maximum Entropy and Bayesian Methods in Applied Statistics.Skilling J, ed. 1989. Pp 45-52. Kluwer Publishers, Norwell, MA.
[27] Burnham, K. P., and D. R. Anderson. 1998. Model selection and inference: a practical information-theoretic approach. Springer-Verlag, New York, New York, USA. 353 pp.
[28] Malakoff D. Bayes offers a 'new' way to make sense of numbers. Science 1999; 286:1460–64.
[29] Magidson J, Vermunt JK. Comparing Latent Class Factor Analysis with the traditional approach in Data Mining. In Bozdogan, ed. Statistical Datamining and Knowledge Discovery. 2004. Chapter 22, pg 373. CRC Press.
[30] Vermunt JK, Magidson. In Latent Class Models for Classification. Computational Statistics and Data Analysis. 2003:531-533.
[31] Magidson J. Latent Class (Finite Mixture) Segments. How to find themand what to do with them. Sensometrics, Rotterdam. 2010. Presentation.
[32] http://statisticalinnovations.com/products/latentgold_v4.html.
[33] Roehrl MH, Lantz D, Sylvester C, Wang JY. Age-dependent reference ranges for automated assessment of immature granulocytes and clinical significance in an outpatient setting. Arch Pathol Lab Med 2011; 135(4):471-77.
[34] David G, Bernstein L, Coifman RR. Generating evidence based interpretation of hematology screens via anomaly characterization. The Open Clinical Chemistry Journal 2011; 4:101-6.
[35] Bernstein LH, Rucinski J.Measurement of Granulocyte Maturation May Improve the Early Diagnosis of the Septic State. Clin Chem Lab Med 2011; 49 (in press) Doi 10.1515/CCLM.2011688
[36] Brugler L, DiPrinzio MJ, Bernstein L. The five year evolution of a malnutrition treatment program in a community hospital. J Comm J Qual Improv 1999; 25(4):191-206.
[37] Brugler L, Stankovic A, Bernstein L, Scott F, OSullivan-Maillet J. The role of visceral protein markers in protein calorie malnutrition. Clinical Chemistry and Laboratory Medicine 2002; 12:1360–1369.
[38] Brugler L, Stankovic AK, Schlefer M, Bernstein L. A simplified nutrition screen for hospitalized patients using readily available laboratory and patient information. Nutrition 2005; 21:650–658.
[39] David G, Bernstein L, Coifman RR. The Automated Malnutrition Assessment. Nutrition Nut-11-00351 (Elsevier) in review
[40] Executive Summary. To Err Is Human. (Kohn LT, Corrigna JM, Donaldson MS, eds.) Committee on Quality of Healthcare in America. IOM. National Academy Press 2000. Washington, DC. http// www.nap.edu/books/0309068371/html. ISBN 978-0-309-06837-6.

23

The Effects of Splenectomy and Autologous Spleen Transplantation on Complete Blood Count and Cell Morphology in a Porcine Model

Nina Poljičak-Milas[1], Anja Vujnović[2], Josipa Migić[3], Dražen Vnuk[4] and Matko Kardum[1]
[1]*Faculty of Veterinary Medicine, Department of Pathophysiology, University of Zagreb*
[2]*Croatian Veterinary Institute*
[3]*Pliva d.o.o.*
[4]*Faculty of Veterinary Medicine, Surgery, Orthopedics and Ophthalmology Clinic, University of Zagreb*
Croatia

1. Introduction

Spleen, as a part of hematopoietic and immune system, plays an important role in the life cycle of blood cells. There are three major functions of the spleen and these are handled by three different tissues within the spleen. Reticuloendothelial tissue is responsible for removing old or damaged erythrocytes and cell debris from the blood stream. This same tissue may participate in hematopoiesis when there is an increased need for red blood cells and is a place where young erythrocytes produced in bone marrow undergo the process of maturation before releasing into the blood stream. Venous sinusoids along with the ability of the spleen to contract, provides a means for expelling the contained blood to meet increased circulatory demands in certain animals. White pulp provides lymphocytes and a source of plasma cells and hence antibodies for the cellular and humoral specific immune defenses (Dyce et al., 2002; Teske, 2000).

Splenectomy is a surgical removal of the spleen that may be carried out in patients whose spleen has been ruptured by trauma or damaged by other pathological processes such as cancer, infections or some autoimmune diseases (Tillson, 2003). However, total removal of the spleen may lead to side effects such as postsplenectomy infections and sepsis, due to the decreased production of antibodies and phagocytes or thrombosis, due to elevated platelet count in blood (Bessler et al., 2004; Khan et al., 2009; Miko et al., 2003; Timens & Leemans, 1992). Also, many studies report increased count of morphologically abnormal erythrocytes, immature red blood cells and pathologic erythrocyte inclusions in the peripheral blood of various species following splenectomy as a result of the loss of splenic filtrating function (Haklar et al., 1997; Resende et al., 2002; Traub et al., 1987). In addition, it has been reported that removal of the spleen causes significantly higher increase of reticulocyte count than other surgeries. This suggests that spleen may somehow hormonally regulate the release of red blood cells into circulation, thus after removal of spleen bone marrow releases more red blood cells as well as more immature erythrocytes into the blood stream (Knežević et al., 2002; Lorber, 1958). Splenectomy also causes changes in number of white blood cells with subsequent leukocytosis (Bessler et al., 2004; Karagülle et al., 2007). Initial transient neutrophilia is followed by the persistent lymphocytosis and monocytosis. Increased leukocytosis accompanied by the significant left shift is found in patients, and often there are myelocytes or other precursor in the granulocytic series in their peripheral blood (Labar & Hauptmann, 1998; Tang et al., 2003; Zhang et al., 2002).

Severe postoperative infections after removal of the spleen prompted a development of alternative methods to conserve functions of the spleen. Autologous spleen transplantation is a method of choice after total splenectomy in order to preserve splenic immune and hematopoietic functions (Marques et al., 2003; Patel et al., 1981). The effectiveness of splenic autotransplant depends on many factors and is still controversial (Theodorou et al., 2007). Studies done on rats, mice, rabbits and men report that autotransplantat's capability of recovering its primary function highly depends on the volume of transplanted spleen tissue (Karagülle et al., 2007; Miko et al., 2003; Resende & Petroianu, 2003; Tang et al., 2003).

In the recent years there is a close cooperation between Faculty of Veterinary Medicine and Medical faculty in University of Zagreb. Because of close interests that both faculties have, combined projects and seminars have been established. One of the best examples was education of Medical faculty surgeons for laparoscopic cholecystectomy, liver lobectomy, laminectomy, and for experimental wounds surgery on our faculty, in the Clinic for Surgery, Orthopedics and Ophthalmology. These operative procedures were carried out on pigs because of its similarity in organs size. In recent years, a xenotransplantation of pig organs to nonhuman primates is being investigated. In order to prolong survival of primates that have received porcine xenografts, the same animals underwent a splenectomy to prevent humorally mediated immunological damage (Cozzi et al., 2000). In order to save human lives, it is important not only to master the precise surgical technique, but also to recognize all the factors that may affect the rejection or return of physiological functions of organs after transplantation.

The aim of this study was to evaluate the effects of total splenectomy and autologous spleen transplantation in a porcine model on complete blood count and cell morphology. Also, we aimed to determine the functional effectiveness of autotransplanted splenic tissue by its capacity to remove erythrocyte having Howell-Yolly bodies from the blood stream.

2. Materials and methods

2.1 Animals, anaesthesia and surgery

The experimental protocol was approved by the Department of Veterinary Science, Ministry of Agriculture, Republic of Croatia and was conducted in accordance with the guidelines for the treatment of laboratory animals. Nineteen pigs of either sex, aged three months, weighing 19-26 kg were used in the experiment. Food was withheld from all the pigs 12 h and water 2 h before the experiment. All animals were premedicated with 2 mg/kg i.m. of xylazine (Xylapan, Vetoquinol, Bern, Switzerland), and left auricular vein was catheterized percutaneously for continuous infusion of lactated Ringer's solution at a rate of 10 ml/kg/h (Infusion pump BIOF 3000, Biotron CO, Kangwondo, South Corea) during surgical procedures and for the administration of drugs. Anaesthesia was induced with 5 mg/kg i.v.

of ketamine (Ketaminol 10, Intervet, Boxmeer, The Netherlands) and 10 μg/kg i.v. fentanyl (Fentanyl-Jannsen, Jannsen Pharmaceutica, Beerse, Belgium), and animals were intubated, connected to a circle system and maintained on spontaneous ventilation. Anaesthesia was maintained with 1.5% isoflurane (Forane, Abbott, Queenborough, UK) and oxygen and continuous intravenous infusion of fentanyl in a dose of 0.8 μg/kg/min. Supplemental doses of ketamine were applied during surgery to maintain sufficient anaesthesia depth. Preoperative antibiotic prophylaxis was administered using 20 mg/kg ampicillin and sublactam *i.v.* (Penactam, Krka, Novo Mesto, Slovenia).

After anaesthesia induction, animals were randomly divided into three groups: sham-operated pigs with spleens intact (control group, n=6), splenectomized pigs (n=6), and splenectomized pigs with small fragments of 20% mass of the spleen autotransplanted into the greater omentum (n=7).

2.2 Blood sampling and experimental protocol

Two blood samples of each pig were taken from the *v. auricularis lateralis* just before surgery and on the first, fifth, twelfth and twenty sixth day postoperatively. Exceptionally, blood samples for reticulocyte, and differential white blood cell counting were also taken on the fortieth postoperative day. First sample was collected into the Vacutainer® tubes containing K_3EDTA anticoagulant (BD-Vacutainer, Plymouth PL6 7BP UK) and the other was taken without anticoagulant and was used to make blood smears. Hematological parameters: red blood cell count (RBC), white blood cell count (WBC), hemoglobin concentration (Hgb), hematocrit (Htc), mean corpuscular volume (MCV), mean corpuscular hemoglobin (MCH), mean corpuscular hemoglobin concentration (MCHC), red blood cell distribution width (RDW), platelet count (PLT) and mean platelet volume (MPV) were determined using automated blood analyzer (SERONO-9120 Baker System). Reticulocyte counting was done on brilliant cresyl blue stained blood smears, and differential leukocyte count and morphological changes of blood cells were determined by identifying 200 consecutive leukocytes on May Grünwald stained blood smears using immersion objective with 1000x enlargement of the light microscope (Olympus BX 41). The frequency of blood cells immature precursor, degenerative neutrophils or increased reactive lymphocytes is reported as a few (5% to 10%) or moderate (11% to 30%). Similarly, semi quantitative evaluation of red blood cell morphology based on average number of abnormal cells per 1000x microscopic monolayer field was used to assess morphological changes in erythrocyte (Weiss, 1984).

The results were statistically analyzed by calculating mean values, standard deviation, and coefficient of variability, and were presented in tables as the mean values ± standard deviation. The significance of the differences between the results was verified using the Student *t*-test and Statistica 7.1 computer programme.

3. Results

3.1 Red blood cell count (RBC), hemoglobin (Hgb) and hematocrit (Htc)

Total red blood cell count in sham-operated pigs was significantly decreased only on the fifth day postoperatively compared to the value before surgery. In splenectomized pigs red blood cell count was significantly lower on the first, fifth, twelfth and twenty sixth day postoperatively compared to the value before surgery. In pigs with autologous splenic transplants, red blood cell count was significantly decreased on the fifth and twelfth day after surgery compared to the value before surgery. Hemoglobin and hematocrit values in sham-operated pigs were significantly decreased on the fifth day postoperatively compared to the values before surgery. Splenectomized pigs showed significantly lower values of these parameters on the fifth, twelfth and twenty sixth day postoperatively compared to the values before surgery. In pigs with splenic autotransplants, hemoglobin and hematocrit values were significantly decreased on the first, fifth and twelfth day after surgery compared to the values before surgery (Table 1.).

3.2 Mean corpuscular volume (MCV), mean corpuscular hemoglobin (MCH), mean corpuscular hemoglobin concentration (MCHC) and red blood cell distribution width (RDW)

There were no statistical differences of mean corpuscular volume value in sham-operated pigs before and after surgery. Compared to the value before surgery mean corpuscular volume value showed significant raise in splenectomized pigs on the twelfth and twenty sixth day postoperatively, and in contrast autotransplanted pigs showed significantly decreased value of mean corpuscular volume on the first, fifth and twelfth day postoperatively. There were no statistical differences of mean corpuscular hemoglobin value in sham-operated pigs before and after surgery while mean corpuscular hemoglobin concentration value was significantly higher on the twelfth day after surgery compared to preoperative value. In splenectomized pigs significant raise in values of both parameters was noted on the fifth day postoperatively when compared to the values of these parameters before surgery. In pigs with splenic autotransplants mean corpuscular hemoglobin value was significantly decreased on the first and twelfth day after surgery, but the mean corpuscular hemoglobin concentration value was significantly raised on the fifth day after surgery when compared to preoperative values. There were no noted significant changes of red blood cell distribution width values except in sham-operated pigs on the twenty sixth day postoperatively when compared to the same value before surgery (Table 1.).

3.3 Total and differential white blood cell count

In group with autotransplanted splenic tissue on the fifth postoperative day total white blood cell count dropped significantly in comparison with the preoperative value as well as in comparison with the value measured in the control group on the same day of experiment. After this, on the twelfth and twenty sixth day of the experiment, significant increase of white blood cell count in comparison with the preoperative value was noted in all experimental groups of pigs (Table 1.). Changes in absolute differential count of segmented neutrophils followed the same pattern as those in the total white blood cell count during whole experimental period in each of the groups of pigs.

Compared to the value right before surgery, rise in absolute count of unsegmented neutrophils was noted, with significant increase on the first and twelfth day in the control group, first and fifth day in splenectomized group and first, twelfth and twenty sixth day in group with autotransplanted splenic tissue (Table 2.).

Although absolute number of lymphocytes was decreasing postoperatively in all experimental groups of pigs, it was significantly decreased only on the fifth day in splenectomized group and in this group it remained at low values until the end of experimental period. In contrast, on the twelfth postoperative day absolute number of lymphocytes in control and autotransplanted group started to rise, even exceeding preoperative levels.

Relative differential number of monocytes ranged from one to eight percent in all blood smears. Still, statistical analysis showed significant decrease of absolute number of monocytes on the fifth day after the surgery in control group compared to the value before operation and twelfth day after splenectomy compared to the control group of the same day. Relative differential number of eosinophils on blood smears ranged from zero to twelve percent in all groups. Only statistically significant shift in the absolute number of eosinophils occurred on the first day after the surgery in control group compared to values before the surgery. Relative number of basophils in all groups ranged from one and three percent and statistically significant increase in number was found on the fifth day in the group with autotransplanted tissue compared to the values before surgery and control group of the same day (Table 2.).

3.4 Ratio of absolute differential number of neutrophils and lymphocytes (N/L)

Compared with the preoperative values, significantly elevated neutrophil/lymphocyte ratio was recorded in the control group on the first, fifth and twelfth postoperative day. In splenectomized pigs significant elevation of neutrophil/lymphocyte ratio in respect to preoperative value, as well as in respect to the value of control group on the same day of the experiment, appeared on the fifth day postoperatively and it remained on the significantly higher values till the end of experimental period. On the twelfth day of the experiment significant decrease of neutrophil/lymphocyte ratio in comparison with the sham-operated pigs on the same day was reported in group with autotransplanted splenic tissue (Table 3.).

		Before surgery	Days after surgery			
			1st	5th	12th	26th
WBC 10^9/L	Sham-operation		27.33±9.26	24.94±11.60	**38.95±5.88	**28.14±0.42
	Splenectomy	22.26±3.82	20.26±3.32	26.37±9.01	*39.23±12.09	*27.13±7.57
	Autotransplantation		23.87±0.21	*18.13±4.53+	***34.9±6.75	**28.91±3.18
RBC E*10^{12}/L	Sham-operation		7.22±0,52	***5.85±0.55	6.84±0.16	5.09±1.79
	Splenectomy	6.89±0.11	*6.33±0.42$^+$	***5.19±0.44$^+$	**3.01±1.49$^+$	*4.73±0.97
	Autotransplantation		6.35±0.29$^+$	**5.20±1.12	*5.92±0.94$^+$	4.55±1.18
Hgb g/L	Sham-operation		134.5±14.14	**109.4±9.19	125.75±4.27	99.5±29.44
	Splenectomy	126.71±5.66	120.6±10.61$^+$	***101.83±7.22	**69.75± 18.53^{++}	*106.33±8.96
	Autotransplantation		*112.57±4.95^{++}	**93.57±19.61$^+$	**106.57± 16.29^{++}	85.5±13.28

		Before surgery	Days after surgery			
			1st	5th	12th	26th
Htc L/L	Sham-operation	0.39±0.01	0.42±0.05	***0.33±0.03	0.38±0.01	0.30±0.09
	Splenectomy		0.37±0.03^{+}	***0.30±0.03^{+}	*0.21±0.07^{+}	*0.32±0.04
	Autotransplantation		*0.35±0.02^{+}	**0.28±0.07	**0.33±0.05^{+}	0.26±0.04
MCV fL	Sham-operation	56.92±0.78	57.87±2.33	56.56±1.13	55.7±1.3	59.8±2.66
	Splenectomy		59.04±1.48	58.57±2.54	*69.7±8.58^{+}	*68.67±6.22
	Autotransplantation		*54.6±1.34^{++}	**53.84±1.93^{+}	*54.57±1.58	57.25±3.14
MCH pg	Sham-operation	18.41±0.57	18.63±0.49	18.74±0.28	18.4±0.65	19.85±1.21
	Splenectomy		19.1±0.42	***19.65±0.57^{+}	22.13±2.81	23±3.01
	Autotransplantation		*17.74±0.26^{+}	17.99±0.62	*17.81±0.59	19.2±2.08
MCHC g/L	Sham-operation	323.57±4.95	322.67±2.83	330.8±1.41	*330.25±4.11	331.5±5.19
	Splenectomy		323.6±1.41	**335.5±8.19	344.48±13.08	333.33±6.59
	Autotransplantation		324.86±8.49	*334.71±12.45	326.29±5.5	335.5±6.35
RDW %	Sham-operation	23.01±0.07	23.2±3.39	22.54±2.83	22.7±2.14	*21.85±0.17
	Splenectomy		23.08±3.54	23.62±3.5	24.48±4.43	23.4±1.17
	Autotransplantation		23.87±2.69	23.43±1.32	22.93±1.11	22.15±0.87
PLT E*10⁹/L	Sham-operation	551.92±359.72	509.33±16.26	554±46.67	389.33±19.43	272±125.73
	Splenectomy		400±147.35	534.25±381.81	***96±25.94^{+++}	286.33±219.21
	Autotransplantation		587.67±326.51	690±431.74	445.53±405.88	223±114.28
MPV fL	Sham-operation	10.49±1.2	10.8±2.12	10.5±0.21	11.4±1.08	12.6±1.42
	Splenectomy		11.33±0.79	***11.65±0.87^{+}	*12.63±1.08	10.97±1.37
	Autotransplantation		***12.43±0.42^{+}	***12.5±0.57^{++}	12.45±0.92	12.7±1.63

All values are presented as mean values ± standard deviation.
Statistical difference with respect to the value before surgery:*P<0.05; **P<0.01; ***P<0.001.
Statistical difference with respect to the value in sham operated pigs on the same day of experiment: $^{+}$P<0.05; $^{++}$P<0.01; $^{+++}$P<0.001.

Table 1. White blood cell count (WBC), red blood cell count (RBC), blood hemoglobin concentration (Hgb), hematocrit (Htc), mean corpuscular volume (MCV), mean corpuscular hemoglobin (MCH), mean corpuscular hemoglobin concentration (MCHC), platelet count (PLT), mean platelet volume (MPV) and red blood cell distribution width (RDW) in the peripheral blood of observed pigs during the experiment

		Before surgery	Days after surgery			
			1st	5th	12th	26th
Segmented neutrophils	Sham-operation	7.52±3.93 31.3% (6-50%)	13.12±6.85 44.7% (7-64%)	12.15±9.85 47.2% (39-63%)	**19.10±3.80 48.5% (41-54%)	**10.99±3.21 39.17% (31-49)
	Splenectomy		5.67±7.08 27.4% (14-61%)	11.32±10.00 41.3% (22-54%)	**24.38±13.99 61.75% (55-68%)	*14,00±3.28 48.5% (40-60%)
	Auto-transplantation		8.34±4.27 34.3% (18-56%)	*4.20±0.74++ 22.1% (8-36%)	*14.07±5.08 38.9% (11-55%)	*11.77±4.51 39.9% (18-57%)
Band neutrophils	Sham-operation	0.58±0.40 2.6% (1-5%)	*1.57±0.19 5.5% (4-8%)	0.63±0.13 2.8% (0-8%)	**1.53±0.05 4.0% (3-6%)	0.32±0.22 1.2% (0-3%)
	Splenectomy		**1.85±0.80 9.8% (5-15%)	**3.67±2.83++ 14.5% (5-28%)	1.58±2.18 4.5% (0-10%)	0.67±0.40 2.25% (0-4%)
	Auto-transplantation		**1.84±0.21 7.9% (4-18%)	1.00±0.39 5.7% (1-14%)	*1.41±0.06 3.9% (2-8%)	*1.64±0.08+ 5.43% (0-12%)
Lymphocytes	Sham-operation	13.06±2.88 61.2% (43-86%)	11.94±2.04 47.2% (28-85%)	11.61±2.29 47.6% (37-54%)	*16.81±2.67 43.7% (36-51%)	*15.54±3.82 55.2% (45-63%)
	Splenectomy		11.62±3.44 57.0% (29-70%)	**9.39±4.88 36.3% (29-49%)	12.52±6.33 31.5% (28-36%)	12.50±0.63+ 45.0% (36-56%)
	Auto-transplantation		12.93±3.51 54.3% (36-69%)	11.96±1.77 66.7% (51-86%)	**17.86±6.51 52.6% (36-79%)	14.22±1.50 50.1% (29-70%)
Monocytes	Sham-operation	0.33±0.27 1.4% (0-3%)	0.36±0.03 1.3% (1-2%)	**0.09±0.13 0.4% (0-1%)	0.48±0.06 1.2% (1-2%)	0.56±0.43 1.8% (0-7%)
	Splenectomy		0.36±0.03 2.2% (0-8%)	0.57±0.75 2.0% (1-3%)	0.18±0.22+ 0.5% (0-1%)	0.49±0.20 1.7% (0-5%)
	Auto-transplantation		0.28±0.38 1.3% (0-3%)	0.36±0.12 2.0% (0-5%)	0.53±0.51 1.6% (0-4%)	0.28±0.32 1.0% (0-3%)
Eozynophils	Sham-operation	0.75±0.60 3.3% (0-9%)	**0.21±0.18 1.0% (0-3%)	0.41±0.27 1.8% (0-4%)	0.95±0.45 2.2% (0-6%)	0.63±1.05 2.3% (0-5%)
	Splenectomy		0.71±0.31 3.4% (1-5%)	1.29±0.22 5.3% (1-12%)	0.48±0.66 1.5% (0-3%)	0.58±0.48 2.3% (0-4%)
	Auto-transplantation		0.48±0.38 2.3% (0-5%)	0.44±0.24 2.3% (0-3%)	0.83±0.06 2.6% (1-5%)	0.85±0.72 3.0% (1-6%)
Basophyls	Sham-operation	0.03±0.07 (0-1%)	0.10±0.02 (0-1%)	0.04±0.02 (0-1%)	0.08±0.23 (0-1%)	0.10±0.21 (0-1%)
	Splenectomy		0.04±0.14 (0-1%)	0.13±0.03 (0-2%)	0.08±0.21 (0-1%)	0.07±0.02 (0-1%)
	Auto-transplantation		0.00±0 (0%)	*0.18±0.14+ (0-3%)	0.20±0.22 (0-2%)	0.15±0.14 (0-2%)

Absolute differential values (10^9/L) are presented as mean values ± standard deviation
Relative differential values (%) are presented as mean value, and minimum and maximum values in the brackets
Statistical difference with respect to the value before surgery:*P<0.05; **P<0.01; ***P<0.001.
Statistical difference with respect to the value in sham operated pigs on the same day of experiment: $^{+}$P<0.05; $^{++}$P<0.01; $^{+++}$P<0.001.

Table 2. Absolute and relative white blood cell differential count in the peripheral blood of observed pigs during the experiment

	N/L ratio				
	Day 0	Day 1	Day 5	Day 12	Day 26
Sham-operation	0.61	*1.39	*1.09	*1.25	0.76
Splenectomy	0.61	0.83	**1.62^{+}	***2.13^{++}	*1.18
Autotransplantation	0.61	0.89	0.45^{++}	0.93	1.09

Statistical difference with respect to the value before surgery: *P<0.05; **P<0.01; ***P<0.001.
Statistical difference with respect to the value in sham operated pigs on the same day of experiment: $^{+}$P<0.05; $^{++}$P<0.01; $^{+++}$P<0.001.

Table 3. Ratio of absolute differential number of neutrophils and lymphocytes (N/L) in the peripheral blood of observed pigs during the experiment

3.5 Platelet number (PLT) and mean platelet volume (MPV)

There were no statistical differences in platelet count in sham-operated and autotransplanted pigs, while on the twelfth postoperative day platelet count in splenectomized pigs was significantly lower in comparison with the platelet count before surgery, and to the value in the control group at the same experimental day. There were no statistical differences of mean platelet volume value in sham-operated pigs before surgery and the value of mean platelet volume on days after surgery. In splenectomized pigs significantly higher mean platelet volume value was noted on the fifth and twelfth day postoperatively. In autotransplanted pigs statistical differences were noted on the first and fifth day after the surgery in comparison with the value before surgery (Table 1.).

3.6 Reticulocyte count (RTC)

Prior to surgeries, reticulocyte count in all experimental pigs ranged within 0.5 to 1.5 %. On the first postoperative day reticulocyte count was significantly increased (2 to 4 %) when compared to the value before surgeries and it continued to grow simultaneously in all experimental groups on the fifth (4 to 8 %), twelfth (6 to 8 %) and twenty sixth (6 to 9 %) postoperative day. On the fortieth day after the surgery, reticulocyte count continued to increase in splenectomized (7 to 16 %) and autotransplanted pigs (7 to 18 %), while at the same time it began to decrease in sham-operated pigs (2 to 3 %), although was still significantly higher when compared to the preoperative value. Corrected reticulocyte count (reticulocyte production index - RPI) is shown in Table 4., and was extremely high on twenty sixth experimental day in splenectomized and autotransplanted pigs (Table 4.).

	RPI				
	Day 0	Day 1	Day 5	Day 12	Day 26
Sham-operation	0.5	1.2	2.3	3.3	1.1
Splenectomy	0.5	1.0	2.0	1.8	4.5
Autotransplantation	0.5	1.0	2.0	1.9	4.0

Table 4. Reticulocyte production index (RPI) in experimental pigs

3.7 Morphological changes of red blood cells

Polychromasia (the heterogeneous staining of red blood cells), as well as increased number of Howell-Jolly bodies (nuclear remnants found in red cells) were present on the blood films of all experimental groups, regardless of the surgical procedures, although both of these morphological changes were more manifested and frequent in pigs with total splenectomy. Five to seven erythrocytes containing Howell-Jolly bodies were found per 1000x microscopic monolayer field on the blood smears of splenectomized pigs. Erythroblasts (immature, nucleated red cells) sporadically appeared on the blood films of splenectomized pigs and pigs with transplanted autologous splenic tissue on all postoperative days. Abnormally shaped erythrocytes, such as leptocytes and codocytes, were found only on the blood smears of splenectomized pigs from the twelfth to the fortieth postoperative day.

3.8 Morphological changes of white blood cells

Neither morphological changes nor precursor cells were found on the blood films of experimental pigs prior to surgeries. On the first postoperative day a few (one to three %) reactive lymphocytes and a few (two to five %) metamyelocytes were found on each smear of control pigs. Similar results were found in the splenectomized group, but number of metamyelocytes was higher than in the control group (three to five %). Results found in group with autotransplanted tissue were almost identical to those in splenectomized group of pigs.

On the fifth day after the surgery reactive lymphocytes were found at only one blood smear from the control group, but blood smears of other two groups contained averagely three to four reactive lymphocytes. Splenectomized group had the largest number of metamyelocytes (four to six %), and also contained dividing cells, while in the group with autotransplanted tissue number of metamyelocytes was smaller (two to five %).

On the twelfth day after the surgery reactive lymphocytes became rarer, and were found only on one smear of splenectomized group, but still on almost all smears (one to two %) in the group with autotransplanted tissue. Metamyelocytes appeared sporadically on the blood smears of each experimental group. Twenty-six days after surgeries reactive lymphocytes were no longer noted on blood smears, and number of found metamyelocytes was decreasing until the fortieth postoperative day when they completely disappeared.

4. Discussion

4.1 Hematocrit, hemoglobin and erythrocyte count

Sham operated pigs exhibited the fastest recovery of hematologic values after surgery. Although red blood cell values of autotransplanted group were significantly lower when compared to sham operated pigs, postoperative blood regeneration took less time than in splenectomized pigs. In contrast to other two surgical procedures, total splenectomy resulted in a greater decrease of red blood cell values, even below physiological values (according to Jain (1993)), which persisted for a longer period (Diagram 1.). Hemoglobin and hematocrit values changed codependently with the changes of red blood cell count in all experimental groups on all postoperative days (Diagram 2., 3.). Postoperative oligocythemia, followed by decrease of hemoglobin and hematocrit, as the result of blood loss is a very well known founding. Durance of postoperative blood regeneration depends on many factors (e.g. degree of tissue lesion and trauma, blood loss and availability of hematopoiesis activating substances). The significant decrease of erythrocyte values and long postoperative recovery after total splenectomy and autotransplantation of splenic tissue have been documented in mice (Sipka et al., 2006), dogs (Lorber, 1958) and humans (Knežević et al., 2002). Results of this study suggest that observed decrease of erythrocyte values and postoperative recovery in each experimental group were in accordance with severity of surgical traumas (sham-operation, splenectomy and transplantation of autologous splenic tissue).

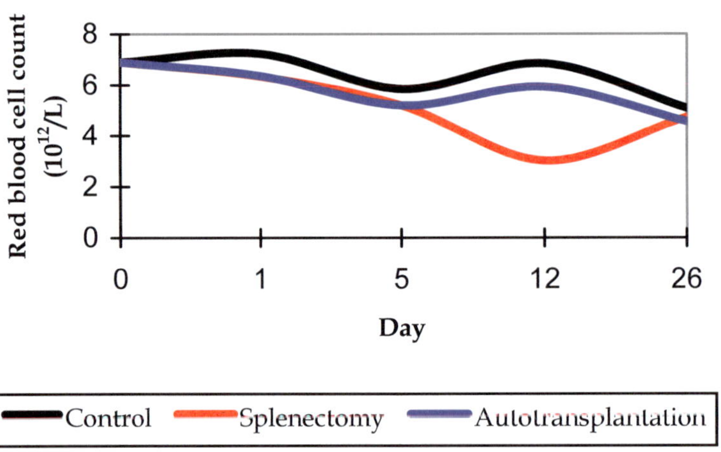

Diagram 1. Changes in red blood cell count in the blood of experimental pigs during the experiment

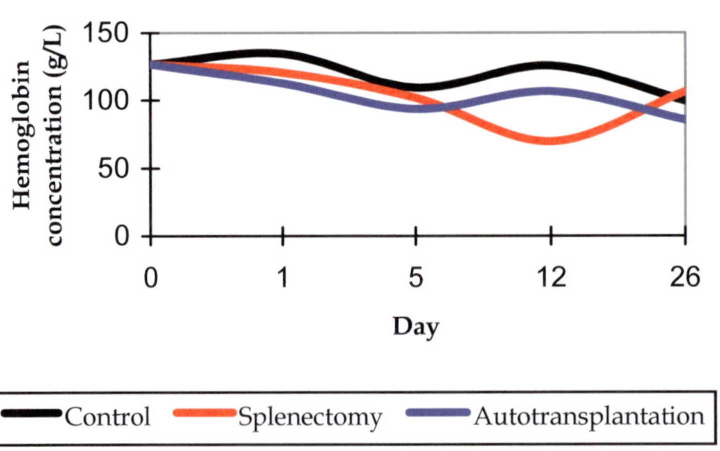

Diagram 2. Changes in blood hemoglobin concentration of experimental pigs during the experiment

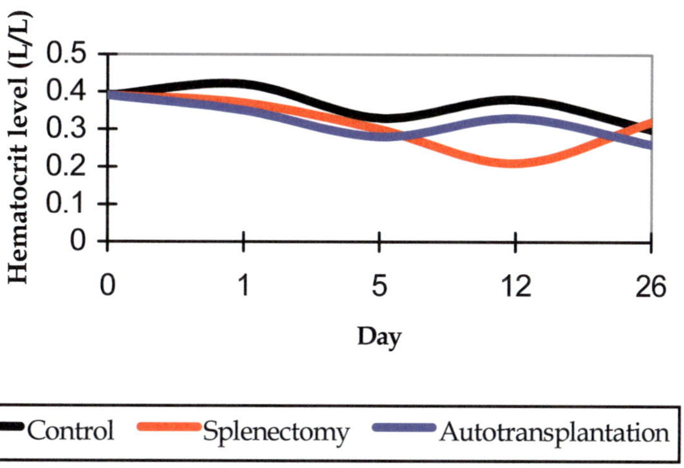

Diagram 3. Changes in hematocrit level in the blood of experimental pigs during the experiment

4.2 Mean corpuscular volume, mean corpuscular hemoglobin and mean corpuscular hemoglobin concentration

As previous experiments report, splenectomized patients of different species have higher mean corpuscular volume values than autotransplanted and sham-operated patients (Knežević at al., 2002, Lorber, 1958). The aging erythrocytes undergo changes in their plasma membrane which make them retain the fluid inside the cell, thus aged erythrocytes have higher mean corpuscular volume values. Total splenectomy leads to increased number of circulating old red blood cells. This, combined with significant reticulocytosis, led to high mean corpuscular volume values of splenectomized pigs in this study (Diagram 4.). Lower postoperative value of mean corpuscular volume in autotransplanted pigs was expected as the result of significantly lower concentration of hemoglobin. Surgical trauma and blood loss led to inadequate iron supply for the developing erythroblasts and consequently to limited hemoglobin synthesis. The red blood cell membrane shrinks to fit its hemoglobin content, thus volume of the cell decreases.

4.3 Total and differential white blood cell count

Leukocytosis, characterized by neutrophilia, initial lymphocytopenia and later recovery of lymphocyte count, was recorded postoperatively in all experimental groups (Diagram 5., 6., 7.). Increase in total leukocyte count after splenectomy and autotransplantation of splenic tissue as well as persistent leukocytosis are main characteristics of white blood cell count in mice (Bessler et al., 2004), rabbits (Karagülle et al., 2007) and humans (Zhang et al., 2002). However, in present study the differences in the degree of leukocytosis among the groups were not detected, except on the fifth postoperative day when a significant decline in the total number of leukocytes in pigs with a transplanted tissue was established compared to the control group at the same day of the experiment. Therefore, present leukocytosis has not been regarded as a change specific for splenectomy or autotransplantation rather than a post-injury inflammatory response due to tissue lesions during operation.

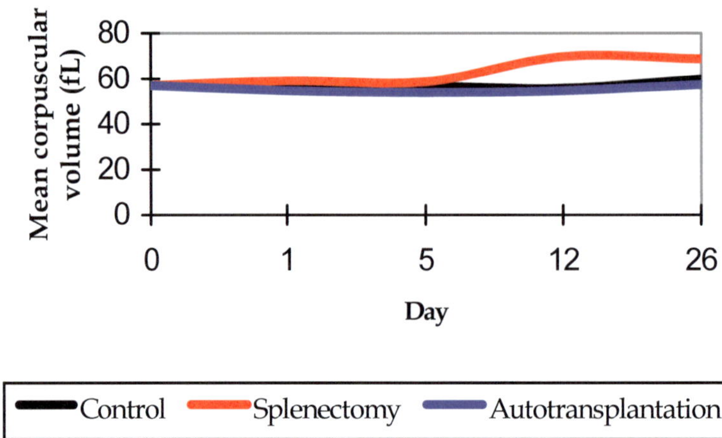

Diagram 4. Changes in erythrocyte mean corpuscular level of experimental pigs during the experiment

Due to differential leukocyte count in various species following splenectomy diverse reports were published. Some authors find an increase neutrophil and lymphocyte count Tarnuzi & Smiley (1967), other significantly higher lymphocyte count while neutrophil count remained unchanged (Bessler at al., 2004). Opposite to that, Sipka at al. (2006) found a significant increase in neutrophil count while lymphocyte count remained unchanged. However, some researches found none significant changes in differential neutrophil and lymphocyte count in blood after splenectomy or autotransplantation of splenic tissue (Resende & Petroianu, 2003; Shokouh-Amiri at al., 1990). In present study there does not seem to be a unique form of changes in differential blood count after splenectomy and autotransplantation of the spleen so we can conclude that the pattern of recorded changes in each experimental group corresponded with the degree of immune response of circulating white blood cells and stress caused by the surgical procedure.

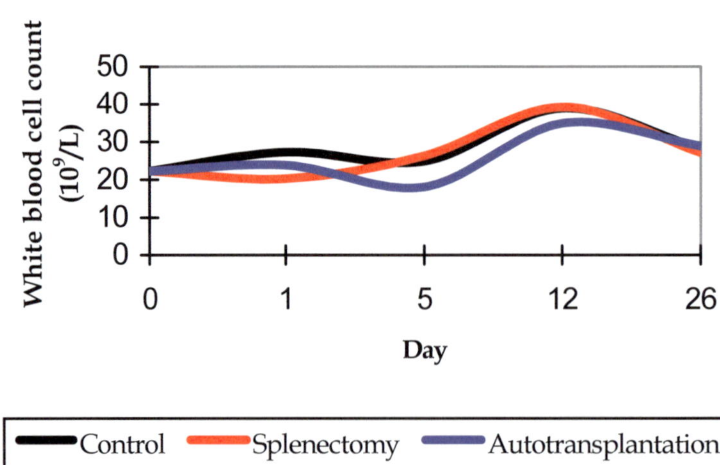

Diagram 5. Changes in total leukocyte count in the blood of experimental pigs during the experiment

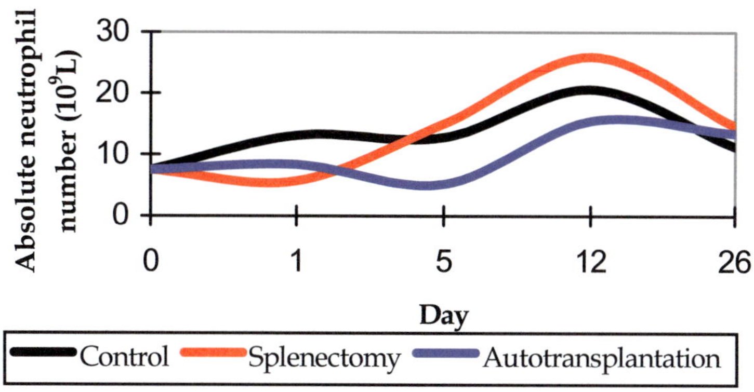

Diagram 6. Changes in absolute neutrophil number in the blood of experimental pigs during the experiment

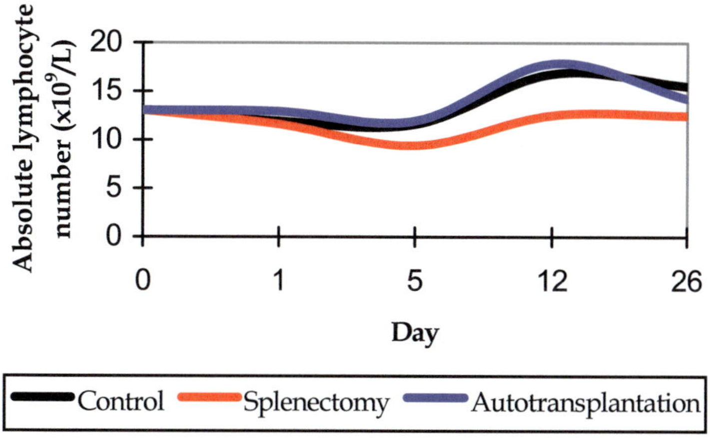

Diagram 7. Changes in absolute lymphocyte number in the blood of experimental pigs during the experiment

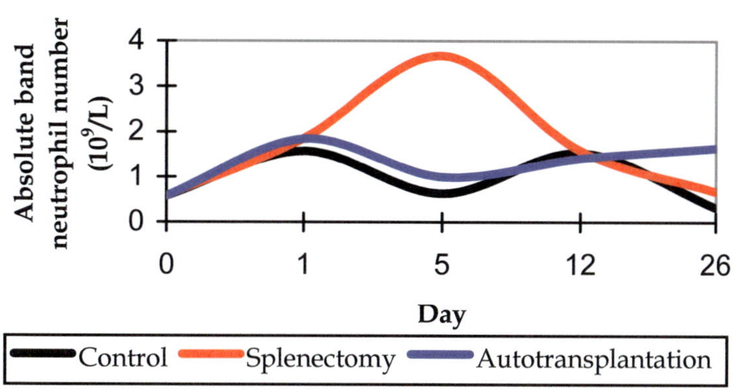

Diagram 8. Changes in absolute band neutrophil number in the blood of experimental pigs during the experiment

Apart from changes found in absolute neutrophil count, there were also changes in number of band neutrophils. Before the surgeries, relative band neutrophil count found on blood smears was 2.6 % in average. Compared to that value, it was evident that amount of band neutrophil increased during postoperative period in all groups. The largest increase was found in group of splenectomized pigs, where up to 28 % band neutrophils per smear were found (Diagram 8.). Increased number of band neutrophils, subsequent with findings of granulocyte precursors and dividing cells, suggest an increased bone marrow activity and release of immature cells, as well as their mobilization from the marginal pool.

4.4 Ratio of absolute differential number of neutrophils and lymphocytes

As it is well known, significant neutrophilia and lymphocytopenia occur as an immediate immune response following multiple traumas, surgical procedures, endotoxemia and sepsis. Since duration, pattern and degree of this immune response highly depend on the extensiveness and severity of surgical procedure, ratio of neutrophils and lymphocytes (N/L) can be considered as a reliable indicator of the immune response progress (Zahorec, 2001). Although both, sham-operated and splenectomized group of pigs in our study had significant postoperative increases in neutrophil/lymphocyte ratio (Diagram 9.), the change was more pronounced in splenectomized group indicating that splenectomy imposed greater stress on the organism than sham operation. The lowest value of neutrophil/lymphocyte ratio during the research was recorded on the fifth postoperative day in the group of autotransplanted piglets. Described decrease came as a result of concurrent lymphocytopenia and neutropenia on the fifth day of the experiment in the blood of piglets with splenic autotransplants.

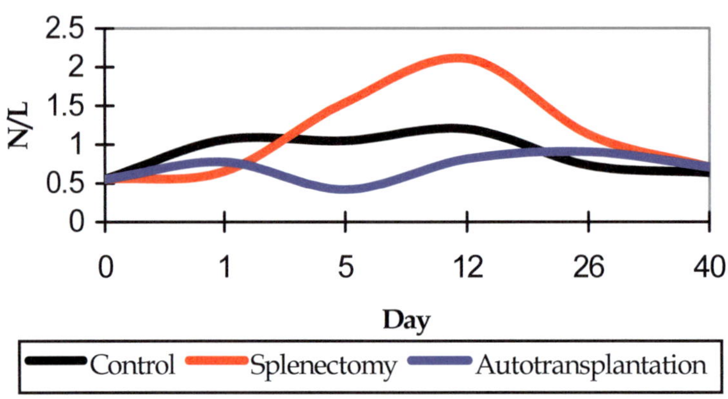

Diagram 9. Changes in ratio of absolute number of segmented neutrophils and lymphocytes (N/L) in the blood of experimental pigs during the experiment

4.5 Platelets

Diverse reports on the platelet level in various species following splenectomy have been published. The response has been reported to be either unchanged (Resende & Petroianu,

2003; Resende et al., 2002) or increased (Karagülle et al., 2007; Knežević et al., 2002; Miko et al., 2003). As one third of total platelets is physiologically sequestered in the spleen, and spleen is also the site of platelet destruction, it is expected, that after their removal, thrombocytosis will develop. In contrast, this study demonstrates significant decrease of platelet number in splenectomized animals (Diagram 10.). As documented, total splenectomy leads to decreased number of T-lymphocytes (Smith et al., 1999; Westermann & Pabst, 1986) which are essential factors in the production of platelets (Mazur, 1987), so we can conclude that this could be the reason of thrombocytopenia that has shortly occurred in splenectomized group of this study.

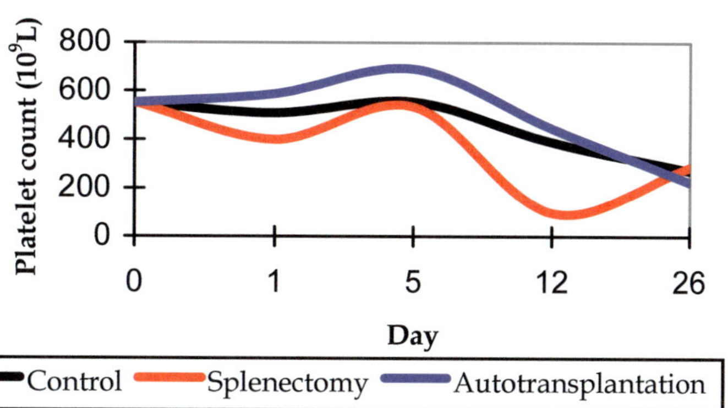

Diagram 10. Changes in platelet count in the blood of experimental pigs during the experiment

4.6 Reticulocytes

Usually, the degree of reticulocytosis is related to the magnitude of hemorrhage during the surgery. Also, many studies report that reticulocytosis following splenectomy is more significant than following other surgical procedures (Knežević et al., 2002; Miko et al., 2003). All experimental groups in this study had the same rate of reticulocytosis growth until twenty sixth day after surgeries when accelerated recovery from acute postoperative anemia was observed in the control group of pigs, suggesting that the least blood loss and surgical trauma occurred during the sham operation (Diagram 11.). In contrast, number of reticulocytes in the pheripheral blood of splenectomized and autotransplanted pigs continued to grow on the twenty sixth and fortieth postoperative day as the result of inadequate blood filtration and prolonged life span of reticulocytes, as well as the loss of splenic humoral control mechanism responsible for releasing young red blood cells into the blood stream. Because of the different intensity of anemia determined in the experimental pig groups, the reticulocyte production index was calculated to avoid erroneously elevated reticulocyte count (Table 4.). On the first postoperative day reticulocyte production index 1 in all three groups of pigs showed insufficient response of bone marrow to compensate postoperative anemia. From fifth to twelfth postoperative day reticulocyte production index in splenectomized and autotransplanted pigs was increased, but still insufficient for compensation of anemia. At the same time, higher reticulocyte production index (over 3) in control group was matched with recovery of red blood cell count. On the twenty sixth postoperative day, data indicates extremely high values of reticulocyte production index in splenectomized and autotransplanted pigs, but that was probably due to increased reticulocyte production in bone marrow, and inadequate blood filtration and prolonged life span of reticulocytes, as well as the loss of splenic humoral control, as mentioned before.

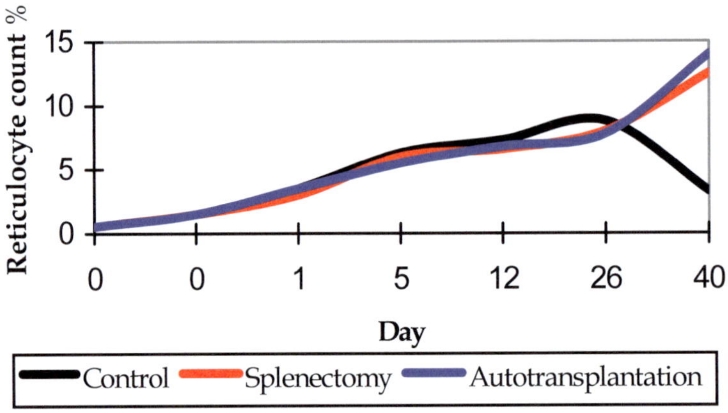

Diagram 11. Average percentage of reticulocytes in the peripheral blood of observed pigs during the experiment

4.7 Erythrocyte morphology

The main developments found in this study were the creation of leptocytes and codocytes and increased number of Howell-Jolly bodies in the peripheral blood of splenectomized pigs (Picture 1.). This founding is in accordance with the results of previous studies on various species, so we can conclude these changes were specific for splenectomized patients. Some authors use the number of erythrocytes containing Howell-Jolly bodies to assess preservation of spleen's blood filtering function (Patel et al., 1981; Resende & Petroianu, 2003; Resende et al., 2002), but number of oxidatively modified erythrocytes containing Heinz bodies can also be used for that purpose (Haklar et al., 1997). Polychromasia and increased number of circulating erythroblasts (Picture 2.) came as a side effect of significant reticulocytosis in all experimental groups. More frequent occurance of morphologically abnormal red blood cells on the blood films of autotransplanted pigs when compared with sham-operated pigs suggests that the autologous splenic tissue was not able to filtrate the blood effectively.

There is still controversy about the effectiveness of regenerated splenic tissue, but the one conclusion of all researches done is common, that functionality and histological restitution of the transplanted splenic tissue depends on the amount of successfully transplanted mass of spleen (Haklar et al., 1997; Sipka, et al., 2006; Tang et al., 2003). In the present research the implant in overall amount of 20 % has not been enough for keeping filtration function of healthy spleen, which correlates with researches from Tang et al. (2003), who find that architecture of red and white pulp, as well as restitution of cardiovascular system is not sufficient for another seven months after transplantation.

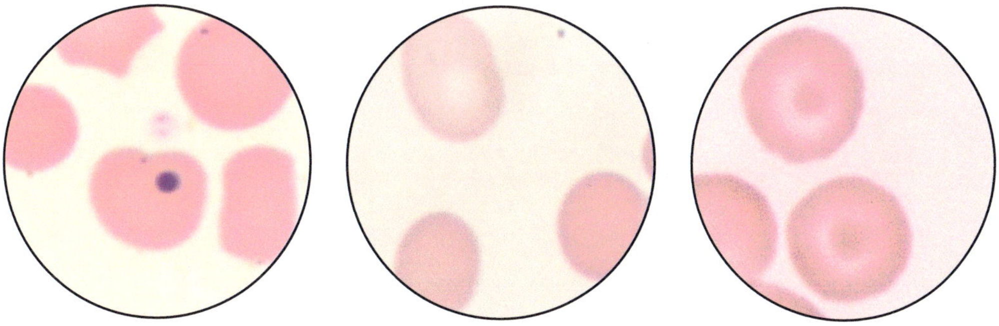

Picture 1. Erythrocyte containing Howell-Jolly bodies, leptocyte and codocytes

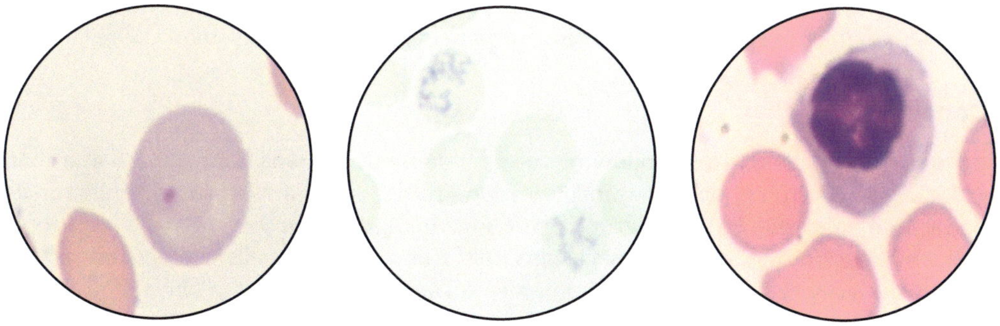

Picture 2. Polychromatophyl, reticulocyte and acydofile erythroblast

4.8 Morphological changes of white blood cells

On the first and fifth day of the experiment morphological evaluation of white blood cells revealed the presence of reactive, granulated and cytotoxic lymphocytes on the blood films of all experimental groups (Picture 3.). After this, morphologically altered lymphocytes appeared only on the twelfth postoperative day on the blood smears of pigs with autotransplanted splenic tissue. Most likely, in this case, inflammatory cascade and production of cytokines were triggered as a response to extensive tissue lesions following autotransplantation, thus leading to the greater number of morphologically altered lymphocytes in the peripheral blood. Metamyelocytes, and dividing cells appeared

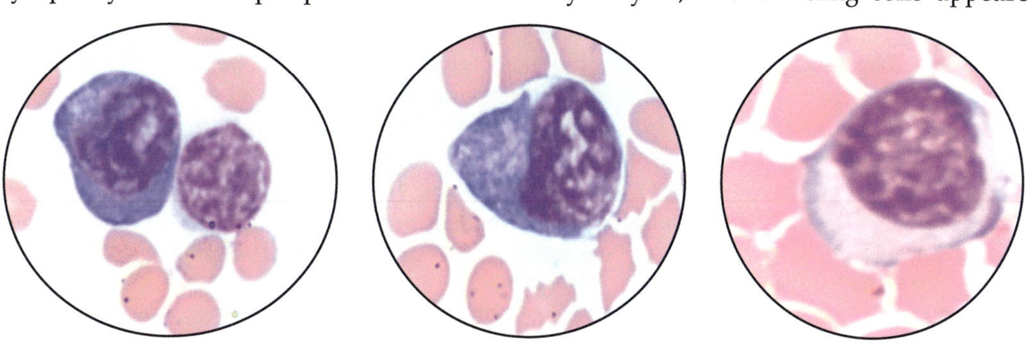

Picture 3. Reactive lymphocytes

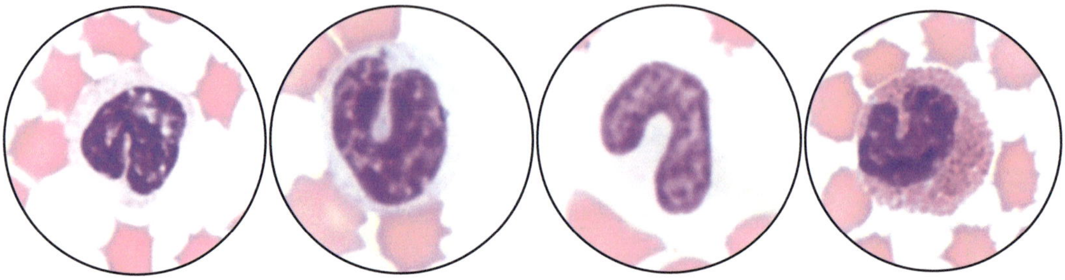

Picture 4. Metamyelocyte, band neutrophils and band eozynophil

sporadically in the peripheral blood of all experimental animals until the twelfth day, but they were most commonly found on the blood smears of splenectomized piglets, with the highest frequency on the fifth day of the experiment (Picture 4.). These results correspond with those reported in splenectomized human patients (Labar & Hauptman, 1998).

5. Conclusion

All groups showed leukocytosis following the operation but this was not regarded as a change specific for splenectomy or autotransplantation, rather than a post-injury inflammatory response due to tissue lesions during operation. Increased number of band neutrophils, subsequent with findings of granulocyte precursors and dividing cells, suggest an increased bone marrow activity and release of immature cells, as well as their mobilization from the marginal pool. Anemia and reticulocytosis found in blood samples of all three groups of pigs may have been physiological results showing the classical postoperative organism reaction to blood loss and surgical trauma. On the other side, frequenter appearance of variations in red blood cell morphology such as appearance of leptocytes, codocytes and Howell-Jolly bodies on the blood smears of splenectomized pigs when compared with other two experimental groups suggests that this was a change specific for splenectomy. More frequent occurance of morphologically abnormal red blood cells on the blood films of autotransplanted pigs compared with sham-operated pigs suggests that the autologous spleen tissue was not able to filtrate the blood effectively. The mass of implant in overall amount of 20% has not been sufficient for keeping filtration function of healthy spleen, therefore should the amount of transplanted mass of spleen be increased.

6. References

Bessler, H., Bergman, M., Salman, H., Beilin, B. & Djaldetti, M. (2004). The relationship between partial splenectomy and peripheral leukocyte count. *Journal of Surgical Research,* 122, No. 1, (November 2004), pp. (49–53). ISSN 0022-4804

Cozzi, E., Bhatti, F., Schmoeckel, M., Chavez, G., Smith, K. G. C., Zaidi, A., Bradley, J., Thiru, S., Goddard, M., Vial, C., Ostilie, D., Wallwork, J., White, D.J.G. & Friend, P. (2000). Long-term survival of nonhuman primates receiving life-supporting transgenic porcine kidney xenografts. *Transplantation,* 70, No.1, (July 2000), pp. (15-21). ISSN 0041-1337

Dyce, K.M., Sack, W.O. & Wensing C.J.G. (2002). *Textbook of veterinary anatomy.* (3rd ed.) Saunders Ltd, ISBN 721689663, Philadelphia, London, New York, St. Louis, Sydney, Toronto.

Haklar, G., Demirel, M., Peker, O., Eskitürk, A., Işgör, A., Söyletir, G. & Yalçin, A.S. (1997). The functional assessment of autotransplanted splenic tissue by its capacity to remove oxidatively modified erythrocytes. *Clinica Chimica Acta*, 258, No. 2, (February 1997), pp. (201–208). ISSN 0009-8981

Jain, N.C. (1993). *Essentials of Veterinary Hematology*. Williams and Wilkins, ISBN 0-8121-1437, USA.

Karagülle, E., Hoşcoşkun, Z., Kutlu, A.K., Kaya, M. & Baydar, S. (2007). The effectiveness of splenic autotransplantation: an external study. *Turkish Journal of Trauma & Emergency Surgery*, 13, No. 1, (October 2007), pp. (13-19). ISSN 1306-696

Khan, P.N., Nair, R.J., Olivares, J., Tingle, L.E. & Li, Z. (2009). Postsplenectomy reactive thombocytosis. *Baylor University Medical Center Proceedings*, 22, No.1, (January 2009), pp. (9-12). Available from: http://www.ncbi.nlm.nih.gov/pmc/articles/PMC2626351/?tool=pubmed

Knežević, S., Stefanović, D., Petrović, M., Djordjević, Z., Matić, S., Artiko, V., Milovanović, A. & Popović, M. (2002). Autotransplantation of the spleen. *Acta Chirurgica Jugoslavica*, 49, No. 3, pp. (101-106). ISSN 0354-950X

Labar, B. & Hauptmann, E. (1998). *Hematologija*. Školska knjiga, ISBN 953-0-30598-2, Zagreb.

Lorber, M. (1958). The Effects of Splenectomy on the Red Blood Cells of the Dog with Particular Emphasis on the Reticulocyte Response. *Blood*, 13, No 10, (October 1958), pp. (972-985). ISSN 0006-4971

Marques, R.G., Petroianu, A. & Coelho, J.M.C.O. (2003). Bacterial phagocytosis by macrophage of autogenous splenic implant. *Brazilian Journal of Biology*, 63, No. 3, (August 2003), pp. (491-495). ISSN 1519-6984 Available from: http://www.scielo.br/scielo.php?pid=S1519-69842003000300015&script=sci_arttext&tlng=es

Mazur, E.M. (1987). Megakaryocytopoiesis and platelet production. *Experimental Hematology*, 15, No. 4, (May 1987), pp. (340-350). ISSN 0301-472X

Miko, I., Brath, E., Nemeth, N., Toth, F.F., Sipka, S., Kovacs, J., Sipka S., Fachet, J., Furka, A., Furka, I. & Zhong, R. (2003). Hematological, hemorheological, immunological, and morphological studies of spleen autotransplantation in mice: preliminary results. *Microsurgery*, 23, No. 5, (October 2003), pp. (483–488). ISSN 0974-3227

Patel, J., Williams, J.S., Shmigel, B. & Hinshaw, J.R. (1981). Preservation of splenic function by autotransplantation of traumatized spleen in man. *Surgery*, 90, No. 4, (October 1981), pp. (683–688). ISSN 0039-6060

Resende, V., Petroianu, A. & Junior, W. C. T. (2002). Autotransplantation for treatment of severe splenic lesions. *Emergency Radiology*, 9, No. 4, (August 2002) pp. (208–212). ISSN 1438-1435

Resende, V. & Petroianu, A. (2003). Functions of the splenic remnant after subtotal splenectomy for treatment of severe splenic injuries. *The American Journal of Surgery*, 185, No. 4, (April 2003), pp. (311–315). ISSN 0002-9610

Sipka, S. Jr., Bráth, E., Tòth, F. F., Fabian, A., Krizsan, C., Barath, S., Sipka, S., Nemeth, N., Balint, A., Furka, I. & Mikò, I. (2006). Distribution of peripheral blood cells in mice after splenectomy or autotransplantation. *Microsurgery*, 26, No. 1, (January 2006), pp. (43-49). ISSN 0033-8419.

Smith, E., DeYoung, N.J. & Drew, P.A. (1999). Immune cell subpopulations in regenerated splenic tissue in rats. *ANZ. Journal of Surgery*, 69, No. 7, (July 1999), pp. (522-525). ISSN 1445-2197.

Shokouh-Amiri, M. H., Kharazmi, A., Rahimi-Saber, S., Hansen, C. P. & Jensen, S. L. (1990). Phagocyte function after splenic autotransplantation. *Archives of Surgery,* 125, No. 5, (May 1990), pp. (595–597). ISSN 0004-0010

Tarnuzi,A. & Smiley, R.K.(1967). Hematologic effects of splenic implants. Blood. 29. No. 3, (August 1966), pp. (373-384). ISSN 0006-4971

Tang, W.H, Wu, F.L., Huang, M.K. & Friess, H. (2003). Splenic tissue autotransplantation in rabbits: no restoration of host defense. *Langenbecks Archives of Surgery*, 387, No. 9-10, (January 2003), pp. (379-385). ISSN 1435-2443

Teske, E. (2000). Leukocytes - Lymphocytes, In: *Schalm's Veterinary Hematology*, Feldman, B. F., Zinkel, J. G., Jain, N. C. Eds., pp. (223–228). Lippincott Williams & Wilkins, ISBN 0-683-30692-8, Philadelphia, Baltimore, New York, London, Buenos Aires, Hong Kong, Sidney, Tokyo.

Theodorou, G. L., A. Mouzaki, Tsiftsis, D., Apostolopoulou, A., Mougiou, A., Theodori, E., Vagianos, C. & Karakantza M. (2007). Effect of non-operative management (NOM) of splenic rupture versus splenectomy on the distribution of peripheral blood lymphocyte populations and cytokine production by T cells. *Clinical and Experimental Immunology*, 150, No. 3, (October 2007), pp. (429-436). Available from: http://www.ncbi.nlm.nih.gov/pmc/articles/PMC2219385/

Timens, W. & Leemans, R. (1992). Splenic autotransplantation and the immune system. *Annals of Surgery*, 215, No. 3, (March 1992), pp. (256-260). ISSN 0003-4932

Tillson, D.M. (2003). Spleen. In: *Textbook of Small Animal Surgery*, Slatter, D.H, Ed., pp. (1046-1062), Saunders Co. LTd, ISBN 9780721686073, Philadelphia.

Traub, A., Giebnik, G.S., Smith, C., Kuni, C.C., Brekke, M.L., Edlund, D. & Perry, J.F. (1987). Splenic reticuloendothelial function after splenectomy, spleen repair, and spleen autotransplantation. *The New England Journal of Medicine,* 317, No. 25, (December 1987), pp. (1559-1564). ISSN 1533-4406

Weiss, D.J. (1984). Uniform evaluation and semiquantitative reporting of hematologic data in veterinary laboratories. Cited in: *Atlas of veterinary hematology. Blood and Bone Marrow of Domestic animals,* Harvey J.W., pp. (18-19). W.B. Saunders Co., ISBN 0-7216-6334-6, USA

Westermann, J. & Pabst, R. (1986). Autotransplantation of splenic fragments: lymphocyte subsets in blood, lymph nodes and splenic tissue. *Clinical & Experimental Immunol*ogy, 64, No. 1, (April 1986), pp. (188-194). ISSN 1365-2249.

Zahorec, R. (2001). Ratio of neutrophil to lymphocyte counts — rapid and simple parameter of systemic inflammation and stress in critically ill. *Bratislava Medical Journal*, 102, No.1, (January 2001), pp. (5–14). ISSN 0006-9248. Available from: http://www.bmj.sk/2001/10201-01.PDF

Zhang, H., Chen, J., Kaiser, G.M., Mapudengo, O., Zhang, J., Exton, M. S. & Song, E. (2002). The Value of Partial Splenic Autotransplantation in Patients with Portal Hypertension. *Archives of Surgery*, 137, No.1, (January 2002), pp. (89–93). ISSN 0004-0010

24

Physiological Factors in the Interpretation of Equine Hematological Profile

K. Satué[1], A. Hernández[1] and A. Muñoz[2]
[1]*Department of Animal Medicine and Surgery, School of Veterinary Medicine, Cardenal Herrera-CEU University, Valencia*
[2]*Department of Animal Medicine and Surgery, Equine Sport Medicine Centre, School of Veterinary Medicine, University of Córdoba*
Spain

1. Introduction

Cellular components of the blood reflect specific changes in an organ or body system or more often, a general response of the individual to some physiological or pathological conditions. In this chapter, we will review the main physiological factors that should be considered when interpreting equine hematological profiles. The interpretation of the hematological profile in conjunction with history and physical findings directs the clinician in the selection of other diagnostic, imaging and sampling techniques. Additionally, a hematological profile provides invaluable information concerning the severity of the disease and the response to a treatment, and it helps in establishing a prognosis. Further, horses can have different hematological disorders, making hematology important in equine medicine. A special consideration should be made for equine athletes, since the assessment of a hematological profile is pivotal in the diagnosis of a reduced performance.

2. Erythron

2.1 Introduction and specific characteristics of the equine erythrocytes

The term erythron refers to red cell precursors, the tissues in which production takes place and mature erythrocytes themselves and its functional unit, the red blood cell (RBC). The erythron is assessed from peripheral blood samples, by calculating the number of circulating RBC, hemoglobin concentration (HB), packed cell volume (PCV), volumetric indices, such as mean corpuscular volume (MCV), mean corpuscular hemoglobin (MCH) and mean corpuscular hemoglobin concentration (MCHC), a morphological examination at microscopic level (Messer, 1995; Kramer, 2000) and sometimes, examination of the bone marrow (Lording, 2008). When interpreting an equine hematological profile, some specific characteristics of this species should be kept in mind.

PCV unstable. The horse is somewhat unique compared to most other mammalians in that the spleen is a very capacious organ, storing between 6 and 12 L of red-cell-rich blood at rest (Persson, 1967; McKeever et al., 1993). Large numbers of RBCs temporally sequestered in the spleen can be rapidly transferred into the circulation in response to excitement (handling, venipuncture, loss blood, twitching, and pain) and intense exercise (Persson, 1967; 1983). This response is induced by the release of catecholamines and therefore, the resting PCV in horses should be carefully assessed under different excitation levels (Persson, 1967; Schalm and Carlson, 1982). By contrast, tranquilizers and anesthetics decreased circulating RBCs, because of splenic sequestration (Jain, 1986). Comparable changes are not found in splenectomized horses following excitement and strenuous exercise or tranquilization (Kunugiyama et al., 1997).

The intensity of changes in circulating RBC in relation to spleen activity depends on individual variations, age, breed and fitness level and in the case of exercise, duration and intensity. The time required for RBCs to return to resting values is dependent on the degree of the excitement, and it can vary from 40 to 60 minutes to up to several hours (Jain, 1986).

Rouleaux formation and erythrocyte sedimentation rate. Rouleaux formation is the result of the aggregation of RBCs in linear stacks and depends on the number of RBCs and their tendency to aggregate. Rouleaux formation is a characteristic finding in healthy horses, as a result of weak surface changes on RBC membranes (Brockus et al., 2003). There is a positive correlation between the rate of rouleaux formation and the rate of setting of RBCs in anticoagulated blood (erythrocyte sedimentation rate). Rouleaux formation is accentuated in some diseases associated with hyperproteinemia, because high concentrations of plasma proteins, particularly fibrinogen and immunoglobulins, have an insulating effect that reduces the RBC surface membrane charge, promoting RBC aggregation (Schalm and Carlson, 1982; Brockus et al., 2003).

Autoagglutination can be seen in some horses without hemolysis as a result of cold antibodies, with a maximal activity at 4-20°C or as a result of unfractioned heparin treatment (Monreal et al., 1995). Macroscopically, agglutination has a granular appearance and microscopically, appears as grape-like clusters of RBCs. It should be differentiate from rouleaux by using the saline dilution test. Typically a 1:2 dilution will disperse rouleaux but not the autoagluttinated RBCs. Infrequently, a higher dilution (up to 1:10) may be needed to disperse rouleaux. Agglutination causes erroneous MCV values and RBC numbers determined by impedance, because the aggregates may interfere with the electronic or optical evaluation of the erythrocytes. Pre-treating cell suspensions from agglutinated heparin-treated horses with trypsin might reverse the agglutination, improving the accuracy of cell counts (Grondin and Dewitt, 2010).

Absence of peripheral signs of regeneration. Life span of equine RBC in the circulation is approximately 140 to 150 days (Schalm and Carlson, 1982). RBCs are released from bone marrow as mature cells and the horse is unique in failing to release reticulocytes into peripheral blood when there is a regenerative response to hemorrhage or hemolysis. Therefore, morphological features indicative of regeneration, such as reticulocytes and polychromasia are rare in equine blood films. Reticulocyte counts may be performed on marrow aspirates in anemic horses. Values greater than 5% are consistent with accelerated erythropoiesis. Further, in those cases where anemia derives from decreased erythropoiesis, bone marrow examination may identify the cause and enable to carry out a definitive diagnosis (Schalm and Carlson, 1982).

The only indication of maximally stimulated erythropoiesis in routine hematology data is anisocytosis and increased MCV (by up to 10 to 15 fl above baseline levels for an individual horse) (Jain, 1986). Other way to evaluate regeneration is to interpret RBC distribution width or RDW. It is a coefficient of the degree of anisocytosis of circulating RBCs. This parameter will be increased in anemias with significant macrocytosis and/or microcytosis. The RDW is wider in healthy horses than in other species, and normal values range between 14 and 25% (Kramer, 2000). Similarly, assays of RBC creatine concentrations enable a more accurate evaluation of the erythropoietic response in horses. Mean RBC creatine concentration is significantly higher in young RBC populations (Wu et al., 1983), it shows a positive correlation with the reticulocyte count in bone marrow aspirates and a negative correlation with myeloid-erythroid ratio (Lording, 2008). However, it is not a common clinical procedure.

The response to hemolysis is greater than following hemorrhage, although the regenerative capability of horses is relatively poor compared with other species (Brockus et al. 2003). Complete recovery from very severe hemolytic or hemorrhagic anemia may take approximately 1 to 2 months and 2 to 3 months respectively (Lumsden et al., 1975a,b).

Howell-Jolly bodies. They are nuclear remnants of DNA that occasionally are seen in healthy equine peripheral blood films. They are small, round, purple inclusions. Increased number can be seen with enhanced erythropoiesis and with decreased or compromised splenic function (Schalm and Carlson, 1982; Kramer, 2000; Grondin and Dewitt, 2010).

RBC morphology. Equine RBC is relatively small compared to other animal species, with a mean diameter of 5-6 µm and a MCV of approximately 40 to 52 fl (Lassen and Swardson, 1995; Kramer, 2000; Grondin and Dewitt, 2010). They exhibit a mild degree of anisocytosis and RBC size may differ between horse breeds. Breeds dedicated to sport, such as Thoroughbred racehorses or Standardbred horses have an MCV lower than other breeds. Because HB is spread over a larger number of cells, the total surface of the red cell mass is increased. This adaptation of sport equine breeds appears to be a mean to achieve an easier gas exchange during exercise (Allen and Powell, 1983; Kramer, 2000).

2.2 Physiological factors influencing erythron in horses

2.2.1 Sampling handling

In relation to the anticoagulant used, blood parameters in horses are not altered after anticoagulation in heparin-lithium or EDTA. On the contrary, when using sodium citrate, most hematological parameters significantly decrease, compared with the other anticoagulants (Sharif et al., 2010).

Once the blood sample has been taken, another parameter to consider is the time to conduct the blood test. This should be done as soon as possible, preferably within the first 6 hours after collection, in order to avoid the damage caused by storage. The most common change associated with storage is an increase in the RBC size, a fact that artefactually leads to increased MCV and PCV (Allen et al., 1988). However, within limitations in some hematological parameters, equine blood samples stored in EDTA at 4ºC for a maximum of 72 hrs may be adequate for blood tests (Sharif et al., 2010).

Exposure of the sample to high temperatures or direct sunlight can cause hemolysis, resulting in altered RBC values (Rose and Hodgson, 1994).

2.2.2 Accuracy of measurements

The accuracy of the determinations results from the characteristics of the equipment of analysis. Therefore, it is very important to know the sources of errors according to the type of equipment. It has been recommended to conduct repeated measurements, allowing a more reliable interpretation of the results (Persson, 1975; Jain, 1993; Rose and Hodgson, 1994). In fact, Persson (1975) described a variation of up to 30% in baseline HB in three Standardbred horses in which blood samples were obtained in 7 consecutive days.

2.2.3 Attitude and degree of excitement of the horse

Another aspect that might influence the interpretation of RBC parameters is the attitude and the degree of excitement the horse has before and during blood withdrawal (Rose and Hodgson, 1994). Excitement leads to a rise in circulating RBC, HB and PCV. This is the result of the splenic contraction produced by the release of adrenaline and noradrenaline (Kurosawa et al., 1998). The main limiting factor is the time to collect the blood sample. Venipuncture for longer than 30 sec significantly alters the hemograma, as it involves splenic mobilization, resulting from the actions of the sympathetic-adrenal and hypothalamic-pituitary axis (Persson, 1967; Kurosawa et al., 1998).

There are many physiological factors that cause stress in the horse, such as exercise (whether in training or competition), adverse environmental conditions, particularly high heat and humidity, but also dust and very cold or windy weather, long-distance transport, insufficient rest between athletic events, lack of sleep at shows (e.g. late night events or activity in the boarding barn, stall too small for the horse to lie down and rest comfortably), new experiences during training or competition, confinement, removal from familiar environment and social group, changes in daily routine when traveling and at shows, strange environments (e.g. boarding at shows), presence and activity of strange horses and people at shows and increased stress levels in the handlers and rider and weaning, among others (Friend, 2001).

2.2.4 Method of venipuncture

An early study showed that the use of vacuum tubes for blood collection can cause cell damage (Archer, 1977). The use of higher gauge needles leads to satisfactory results according to most of the authors (Jeffcott, 1977; Messer, 1995). In our experience, additional care should be having in blood samples taken in maximally exercised horses in order to avoid hemolysis. Recently, it has been demonstrated that there are not significant differences when comparing hematological parameters obtained using two different methods: venipuncture and intravenous catheter (May et al., 2010).

2.2.5 Feeding

Another factor to take into account when interpreting equine erythrogram is the food and the time of blood sampling in relation to time of feeding. Significant increases in PCV and total plasma proteins (TPP) are found in animals after be fed. This fact has been associated with loss of fluids through the saliva and other gastrointestinal fluids, as well as fluid shifts from the circulation to the gastrointestinal system (Kerr and Snow, 1982). Similarly, there are variations in RBC parameters in horses subjected to different nutritional regimes (Greppi et al., 1996), as well as in animals which common salt is added to the food, supplied 8 hrs before blood collection. In main lines, it is recommended to avoid collecting blood samples within 3 hrs of feeding a large concentrate meal or hay ration or at least ensure that samples are collected at the same time each day.

2.2.6 Circadian biological rhythms

RBC parameters exhibit diurnal infradian, circadian and ultradian rhythms, both in athletic and sedentary horses (Gill and Rastawicka, 1986). Gill and Rastawicka (1986) described elevations in PCV and HB overnight in comparison to light time. Hauss (1994) relates this variation to the influence exerted by alternation between periods of light and darkness on erythropoiesis. After that, Greppi et al. (1996) corroborated these results, and they also found a significant effect of biological rhythms in TPP.

2.2.7 Gender

Hematological differences linked to gender seem to have limited importance in horses. Indeed, minor differences between adult females and males have been reported. However, the results of research in this field are subjected to controversy. Males have slightly higher RBC, HB and PCV, while females have higher MCH and MCHC (Jain, 1986; Hernández et al., 2008; Satué et al., 2009). By contrast, Gill and Rastawicka (1986) observed in Thoroughbred racehorses and Quarter Horses that RBC, PCV and HB were higher in mares than in males. Persson and Ullberg (1974) had reported that baseline hematologic values were higher in stallions than in mares and geldings, probably because of the effect of androgens on erythropoiesis. However, this feature was not seen during exercise in this paper. The authors explained these results indicating that mares and geldings established a hypokinetic circulation with increased oxygen uptake by active muscle during exercise (Persson and Ullberg, 1974).

2.2.8 Season

Season is an exogenous factor that modulates the dynamic of blood components in horses, both in cycling and pregnant mares (Gill and Wanska, 1978; Gill and Kownacka, 1979; Satué, 2004; Satué et al., 2011). Indeed, the patterns of seasonal changes on RBC, HB and PCV in Thoroughbreds and Arabian horses have showed decreased values in winter (Gill and Wanska, 1978; Gill et al., 1979). In Carthusian mares, Satué et al. (2011) confirmed these results. RBC, PCV and MCV in summer were significantly higher than in spring, autumn and winter. However, HB in spring was significantly higher and MCV and MCH in spring and summer were significantly lower than in other seasons, without modifications in MCHC (Satué et al., 2011). These variations could be related to the effect of some factors, such as the breeding season (Satué et al., 2011). Furthermore, these patterns could be subjected to a different degree of tolerance to the cold, and dissimilar changes in ambient temperatures in different locations (Ruiz et al., 2004). It has been suggested that intense cold decreases RBC due to the reduction in the half-life (Ruiz et al., 2004).

2.2.9 Altitude

Horses subjected to high altitude have significantly higher RBC, HB and PCV values, compared to animals that live at less altitude. It is considered a compensatory mechanism for the lower content of oxygen in the atmospheric air, which is proportionally reduced to the altitude (Wickler and Anderson, 2000).

2.2.10 Age

The influence of age on hematological parameters have been evaluated in different horse breeds (Ralston et al., 1988; McFarlane et al., 1998; Cebulj-Kadunc et al., 2002; 2003; Satué, 2004; Hernández et al., 2008; Satué et al., 2009). Most of the studies on age with hematology have focused on foals from birth to 4 years of age (Harvey et al., 1984; Jain, 1993), even though geriatric horses have received much attention recently, probably because of the increase of the age population (McFarlane et al., 1998).

Newborn foals have RBCs of fetal origin, large size and high RBC, HB and PCV. These parameters are reduced sharply within 12-24 hrs of life, then decline more gradually over the subsequent 2 weeks, and after that, they remain in the lower limit of the adult reference internal during the first year of life (Jain, 1986; Harvey, 1990; Grondin and Dewitt, 2010). The initial hematological changes in foals at birth are thought to be due to the increase in fetal RBC destruction, inadequate iron supplementation, needed for HB synthesis, catecholamine release and expansion of plasma volume as adjustments of fluid balance as a result of the osmotic effect of colostral immunoglobulins. Declines in these values are attributed to decreased RBC survival time, decreased iron delivery to the bone marrow, decreased stimulus for erythropoietin production as a result of higher HB saturation, increased blood oxygen content, and enhanced delivery of oxygen to the tissues due to lower 2,-3 diphosphoglycerate concentrations (Harvey, 1990). Normal adult hematological values are attained at 1-2 years of age. MCV are high at birth and then decrease, reaching its lowest values at 3-5 months of age (Jain, 1986; Harvey, 1990). They do not increase to adult values until approximately 1 year of age (Harvey, 1990). Microcytosis in foals has been attributed to a decrease in serum iron as a result of increased demand for growth. These RBCs may be too small to be recognized as erythrocytes by some impedance counts, hence generating erroneous MCV, RBC and PCV values. Mild anisocytosis is also a typical finding in young foals (Harvey, 1990). MCHC remains constant after birth and is similar to adult values (Harvey, 1990).

Stewart et al. (1970) found that PCV and HB were lower in foals younger than 2 years. Between 3 and 4 years of age, there was a gradual increase in MCV and MCH and since HB and PCV remained unchanged during this period, the increase in MCV was accompanied by a slight reduction in RBC. In Carthusian pregnant mares and in Spanish Purebred horses, Hernández et al. (2008) and Satué et al. (2009) found a reduction of RBC with a compensatory increase in MCV and MCH associated with aging. These results agree with those presented for other equine breeds, such as Standardbreds (Jain, 1986; Ralston et al., 1988), Lipizziano (Cebulj-Kadunc et al., 2002) and wild horses (Plotka et al., 1988). However, McFarlane et al. (1998) found a decreasing trend in geriatric horses, without achieving statistical significance. This fact was linked to a reduced regenerative capacity of the bone marrow (McFarlane et al., 1998).

As indicated before, increased MCV appears to be a common finding associated with aging in the horse (Ralston et al., 1988; McFarlane et al., 1998; Satué, 2004) and it has been explained as the result of changes in the dynamics of maturation of the RBCs (McFarlane et al., 1998).

2.2.11 Breed

Breed in horses exerts a significant effect on the erythron. Light horse breeds or 'hot-blooded breeds' have higher RBC, HB and PCV and blood volume compared to draft horses or 'cold-blooded breeds' (Jain, 1993; Kramer, 2000; Grondin and Dewitt, 2010). Thus, PCV as low as 24% can be found in healthy draft horses and pony breeds. Further, Thoroughbreds have smaller MCV than draft horses. Breeds ancestrally closer have minor differences in HB, MCH and MCHC (Jain, 1986). American miniature horses have lower RBC, HB and PCV but higher MCV, MCH and MCHC than other breeds (Harvey et al., 1984). Donkeys have similar RBC, HB and PCV than ponies, but much higher MCV (Jeffcott, 1977).

2.2.12 Exercise

Exercise has variable effects on the erythrogram, depending on exercise duration and intensity (short-term high intensity or maximal exercise and long-term low intensity or submaximal prolonged exercise), fitness and training levels and environmental conditions. In main lines, exercise results in increased RBC, HB and PCV. At the onset of the exercise, this rise derives from the mobilization of splenic RBC under the influence of the catecholamines. The direct effect of this increased RBC is a greater oxygen transport capacity and therefore, aerobic performance. Both the intensity and the duration of the exercise determine the magnitude of the catecholamine response (Kurosawa et al., 1998). The extent of the increase in PCV is a function of the exercise intensity in maximal exercises and in increasing-intensity exercises and a linear relationship between PCV and speed has been described (Persson, 1983; Muñoz et al., 1998; 1999). This relationship is maintained until the maximum PCV is achieved (60-65%) (Persson, 1983).

Even though the majority of the increase in PCV in high-intensity exercises is due to the splenic contraction, exercise-induced fluid shifts also have a role. A decrease of 5-10% in plasma volume is expected in short-term and in incremental-intensity exercises (McKeever et al., 1993; Muñoz et al., 1998). This reduction is attributed to the loss of sweat in order to dissipate heat produced by muscle contraction and to the exchange of fluids between the different body compartments, because of changes in blood pressure (McKeever et al., 1993; Muñoz et al., 1998; 1999).

The rise in PCV during exercise is linked to higher HB and RBC. If we consider the importance of increased HB in the oxygen transport capacity, it is plausible to think that increased PCV, HB and RBC leads to higher aerobic capacity and therefore, exercise performance (Muñoz et al., 1997). Indeed, several studies carried out in splenectomized horses have demonstrated a marked reduction in exercise performance (McKeever et al., 1993; Kunugiyama et al., 1997). On the other hand, there is a close relationship between increased PCV and blood viscosity. As a consequence, there should be a limit in the elevation of PCV that offsets improved oxygen-carrying capacity (Muñoz et al., 1997). This fact has been implied in the loss of performance of horses with red cell hypervolemia (Funkquist et al., 2000).

Other changes associated with brief maximal exercises are small increases in MCV and decreases in MCH and MCHC. Additionally, RBC in blood samples obtained after this type of exercise seems to be more resistant to osmotic stress (Smith et al., 1989), although a later study found a reduced RBC deformability (Geor et al., 1992).

On the other hand, prolonged submaximal exercise or endurance exercise leads to moderate increase in PCV, associated with loss of fluids because of the quantitative importance of sweating. In this case, the increased PCV, HB and RBC are good indices of dehydration. We have found that endurance horses with PCV higher than 50% are disqualified from competition and some of them require intensive intravenous fluid therapy (Muñoz et al., 2010; Trigo et al., 2010). The increase in PCV should be equal to the increase in TPP. In these cases where PCV increases and TPP remains unchanged, other reasons different from dehydration should be considered in order to explain these results. In fact, we found that the most rapid endurance horses in competitions can have higher PCV than the slower horses. Other reason that can lead to increased PCV in endurance horses is pain. We studied 13 endurance horses that had increased PCV (PCV> 52%) with non-increased TPP (TPP<7.2 g/dl) during a competition. One of them had laminitis, 2 had heart arrhythmias, 2 had colic, 3 were retired from competition by the owners and the remaining 5 were able to finish the competition (Trigo et al., 2010).

2.2.13 Training

Although training has limited effects on RBC parameters at rest, some differences are found between horses undergoing high-intensity and endurance training. Speed-trained horses have higher RBC, HB and PCV, which is considered an adaptation for a greater demand for oxygen uptake, stimulating RBC production. However, it is very difficult to obtain a 'true' basal blood sample in these horses, because of their demeanor and nervous temperament. The increased excitability of a horse as it gets fitter could result in elevations of RBC, HB and PCV values (McKeever et al., 1993). On the other hand, regular monitoring of the hemogram during training has little value for assessing the fitness of the horse, but it is very helpful in order to detect subclinical problems that can significantly reduce exercise performance. Decreases in PCV have been reported as a consistent finding in horses with viral respiratory tract disease and in gastric ulcers (McGowan, 2008; Nieto et al., 2009).

In Standardbred trotters, prolonged and/or intensive training can result in an excessive increase in red cell mass, phenomenon known as red cell hypervolemia, which results in a significant reduction of racing performance. Some authors have related the hypervolemia with overtraining (Golland et al., 2003). It has been hypothesized that increased blood viscosity leads to reduced capillary perfusion and inadequate utilization of oxygen by contracting muscles.

By contrast, endurance-trained horses have lower resting RBC, PCV and HB than sprint-trained horses (Muñoz et al., 2010; Robert et al., 2010; Trigo et al., 2010). In fact, in our experience, is very common to find PCV as low as 30-32% in endurance healthy horses with good performance (Muñoz et al., 2010). There are two main reasons to explain these results. Firstly, it has been indicated that feeding fibrous diets might increase water consumption and then plasma volume (Robert et al., 2010). The second reason is the effect of a greater release of aldosterone, which promotes water and electrolyte-conserving mechanisms in the kidneys and gastrointestinal tract (McKeever et al., 2002). These changes appear at the beginning of the training program, with retention of water and electrolytes after only 3 days of endurance training (McKeever et al., 2002). The advantage of plasma expansion in endurance horses is to provide extra total body water for the maintenance of cardiovascular and thermoregulatory stability during prolonged exercise in order to compensate the significant losses associated with sweating (McKeever et al., 2002; Robert et al., 2010). Despite these results, it is clear that hematological measurements are of little value in assessing the fitness or progress of endurance horses in training.

2.2.14 Reproductive status

The researchers that have evaluated the hematological changes resulting from pregnancy in the mare have provided controversial results. Studies in Thoroughbred, Arabian, Carthusian, Brazilian and Breton pregnant mares have described a significant increase in RBC parameters during pregnancy (Berlink et al., 2000; Satué, 2004; Satué et al., 2008). There is not a reasonable explanation to justify these results, although it has been hypothesized that the increased fetal metabolic requirements might condition this response (Satué, 2004). In an early study, a mild anemia appeared at the end of pregnancy (Trum, 1952). This result agrees with studies carried out in pregnant women (Bailit et al., 2007) and other animal species (Steinhardt et al., 1994; Zvorc et al., 2006). The decrease of RBC parameters in pregnancy has been associated with an absolute gain of plasma, RBC and HB. As the increase in RBC and HB is slower than the rise in plasma, a relative oligocythemia is found, despite the increased erythropoietin concentration probably derived from placental prolactin. The hypervolemia of pregnancy has been associated with water and sodium retention after an activation of the renin-angiotensin-aldosterone axis, stimulated by estrogens (Satué and Domingo, 2008). The hypervolemia of pregnancy is necessary in order to meet the demands of the gravid uterus, to protect the mother and the fetus from the harmful effects of decreased venous return and to prevent the mother from suffering the adverse effects of blood loss during delivery (McMullin et al., 2003).

It has been suggested that iron deficiency anemia is common in the pregnant mare. Detlef (1985) studied the effect of iron supplementation in pregnant mares compared with untreated control mares. In the treated mares, RBC and HB were not changed during pregnancy, whereas a decline in RBC parameters was found in the control group. Additionally, the foals born from supplemented mothers had higher HB and RBC than the foals born from the untreated mares (Detlef, 1985).

Near the parturition, RBC parameters do not change (Taylor-Macallister et al., 1997). After delivery, RBC parameters increase slightly, until the total blood volume is restored by releasing the attachments and fetal fluids. On the other hand, lactation induces a reduction in RBC, HB and PCV (Harvey et al., 1994; 2005).

2.2.15 Administration of sedatives-tranquilizers

The administration of tranquilizing compounds, such as phenothiazine derivatives (acepromazina, chlorpromazine...) and adrenergic α-2 agonists (xylazine, romifidine, detomidine...) significantly affect the RBC parameters. These drugs lead to a relaxation of the smooth muscle in the splenic capsule, promoting the storage of RBC (Jeffcott, 1977). Further, these drugs, after an initial short phase of hypertension, have a prolonged hypotensive effect. Hypotension leads to increased plasma volume, with the subsequent hemodilution and reduced RBC parameters at rest (Jain, 1986).

3. Leukon

The term leukon refers to the set of data derived from total and differential count of white blood cells (WBC) and the analysis of WBC morphology (Grondin and Dewitt, 2010). Circulating WBC represents the outcome of the dynamic production of the bone marrow, the release of the cells to the peripheral blood and, the storage in different organs or pools.

Cells can coexist in different stages of maturation, being fully mature cells (neutrophils, NEU, eosinophils, EOS, monocytes, MON, lymphocytes, LYM and basophils, BAS) and immature (band neutrophils, metamyelocytes, myelocytes and progranulocytes) (Messer, 1995; Welles, 2000; Grondin and Dewitt, 2010).

3.1 Neutrophils

The release of NEU from the bone marrow into the circulated depends on the tissue demands and the production of different humoral substances. After passing into the blood, NEU can be in the circulating pool or stored in the marginal pool (in the endothelium of several organs, such as lungs or intestine). Three main locations of the NEU can be described: 1) Bone marrow. There is a proliferating population of NEU, including promyelocytes, myelocytes, metamyelocytes, and mature ENU, prepared for release into peripheral blood; 2) Blood. In the blood compartment, mature NEU appear as round cells, 10-15 μm of diameter, with clear cytoplasm, neutral or granules stain pink and with the nucleus polymorphic and segmented and the chromatin arranged in the form of knots; 3) Tissues. In inflammatory processes, there is a release of chemotactic substances that promotes NEU migration from the vascular bed into the tissues. Marginal pool of NEU adheres to the vascular endothelium, mainly in the small vessels. This fact facilitates the migration to the tissues, while serving as a reserve, so there is a continuous exchange between circulating and marginal pools (Lassen and Swardson, 1995; Grondin and Dewitt, 2010; Smith, 2000; Welles, 2000).

Barr bodies (sex chromatin lobe/ drumstick) can be recognized in females and resemble a small purple body attached to the nucleus by a thin chromatin strand. Further, in peripheral blood, both mature and immature or band NEU can be found. Equine band NEUs are less frequently seen because horses do not exhibit marked left shifts during inflammatory insults compared to dogs and cats. In cases of bacterial infection, the band NEUs might represent between 1 and 10% of the total WBC differential count (Welles, 2000). Band NEUs have a polymorphic nucleus, without constrains, with a less condensed chromatic pattern than the segmented NEUs. The cytoplasm is similar to this of the mature NEU (Jain, 1993; Welles, 2000). Hypersegmented NEUs are rarely seen in healthy and they have five or more lobes separated by filaments. Prolonged storage of blood may lead to the artefactual development of hypersegmented NEUs. Idiopathic hypersegmentation of NEUs have been described in Quarter Horses that lacked evidences of clinical disease. Hyposegmented NEUs have also been reported in apparently healthy Arabian horses, which were diagnosed as Pelger-Huët anomaly (Grondin et al., 2007).

Circulating NEUs have a half-life of 10.5 hours, renewing approximately 1.5 times per day (Lassen and Swardson, 1995; Welles, 2000). Then, they leave the bloodstream and migrate into the tissues. It is a unidirectional movement, because they do not return to the peripheral circulation. In the tissues, NEUs are functional for 1 to 2 days, and then, they are fagocyted by the monocyte-macrophage system or by the mucosal surfaces (Welles, 2000).

3.2 Lymphocytes

LYM are the second largest population of circulating WBCs, after NEUs and the main components of the immune system. They are smaller than NEUs and the other granulocytes, with a dark-staining nuclei, coarse chromatin pattern and scant amount of blue cytoplasm. The mature cell has a diameter of 7-12 µm, an eccentric, round nucleus with a notch on some occasions (Latimer and Rackich, 1992). LYMs are made up to 38-66% T cells, 17-38% B cells with the remaining being null cells (Tizard, 2009). Occasionally, larger LYMs are present, and they have smooth chromatin patterns and large amounts of pale blue cytoplasm (Jain, 1986). Reactive LYMs or immunocytes are rarely seen in health. They are slightly larger than small LYMs, with scalloped nuclear margins, moderately aggregated chromatin, scant to moderate amounts of intensely basophilic cytoplasm and sometimes, they have a pale-staining Golgi zone (Latimer, 1999; Grondin and Dewitt, 2010).

The half-life of LYMs varies between 20 and 200 days (Schalm and Carlson, 1982), with a mean duration of transit through the blood of 30 hrs. Blood LYMs have the ability to recirculate in the blood, lymphatic channels, lymphoid and peripheral tissues and they are able to have mitosis, allowing amplification of the immune response (Jain, 1986; Latimer, 1999; Welles, 2000). Most of the LYMs are originated in the peripheral lymphoid tissues, and only a small percentage comes from central lymphoid tissues, i.e. bone marrow and thymus. The circulation time depends on the LYM subtype and the tissue of origin. T cells circulate more rapidly than B cells and migration through the splenic parenchyma is faster than through the lymph nodes (Hopkins and McConnell, 1984).

3.3 Eosinophils

EOS are cells slightly larger than neutrophils that contain large, reddish-orange granules in the cytoplasm, often obscuring the nuclei and giving a raspberry-like appearance, with a pale blue cytoplasm (Kramer, 2000; Smith, 2000). The lobulated nucleus seldom shows fine filamentation. Degranulated EOSs are vacuolated and are rarely seen in health (Latimer, 1999; Grondin and Dewitt, 2010). The amount of EOS in peripheral blood is low, because most of these cells migrate into tissues, such as the bronchial mucosa, gastrointestinal tract…The half-life of circulating EOS is about 2 to 12 hrs (Latimer, 1999; Young, 2000).

3.4 Monocytes

MON are the largest WBC in circulation, with a large, broad, variable in shape nuclei (oval, bilobed, horseshoe) with lacy chromatin and gray-blue cytoplasm with small azurophilic granules. The cytoplasm can also have a few clear vacuoles of variable size, located in the cell periphery and with a foamy appearance (Jain, 1993; Bienzle, 2000). After their production in the bone marrow, MON are released into the bloodstream. In circulation, they distributed between the circulating and marginal pools, with a ratio of 1/3.5 between them. This ratio remains constant in different physiological states and in response to disease. The mean circulating MON life is about 8.4 hrs, and there is not exchange at the tissue level and blood. In the tissues, the MONs mature into macrophages, a transformation that is accompanied by changes in ultrastructure, in the appearance of cellular receptors or by metabolic changes. The half-life of macrophages ranges from several days to months (Bienzle, 2000; Welles, 2000).

3.5 Basophils

BAS are cells slightly larger than the NEUs, with a lobulated nucleus, although to a lesser extent than NEUs, a cytoplasm from blue to gray, with large amounts of granules distributed irregularly, and with an intense purple stain that vary in size and shape and can mask the nucleus (Jain, 1993; Kramer, 2000).

3.6 Physiological factors influencing leukogram in horses

There are two main WBC responses, physiological leukocytosis and stress leukocytosis. Physiological leukocytosis refers to changes in circulating WBC associated with the intervention of the sympathetic-adrenal axis resulting from splenic contraction in cases of fear, excitement, or high intensity exercise. There is a mobilization of the marginal pool of NEUs and/or LYM, because of a reduction in NEU adherence capacity, increased blood flow through the microvasculature and splenic contraction (Latimer, 1999). These events result in leukocytosis with mature neutrophilia and/or lymphocytosis. In some cases, eosinophilia and monocytosis are also found (Snow et al., 1983; Welles, 2000). These changes are transient and the marginal pool of NEUs is restored again in 20-30 min after the onset of the response and the LYM counts returned to baseline after 1 hr (Rossdale et al., 1982).

Stress leukocytosis is associated with cortisol release under certain stressful situations. This hormone induces neutrophilia without left shift, lymphopenia and eosinopenia. Neutrophilia derives from the mobilization from the marginal pool, the reduced ability to migrate from the blood to the peripheral tissues and the increased mobilization of the population of bone marrow reserve. Lymphopenia is the result of LYM sequestration from lymphoid tissues and the eosinophenia derives from the marginalization of EOS in the blood vessels and the decreased release from the bone marrow (Caracostas et al., 1981; Welles, 2000). This response appears between 2 and 4 hours after the elevation of the endogenous cortisol concentrations or after exogenous administration of corticoids (Rossdale et al., 1982; Burguez et al., 1983). Normal values are recovered in 24 hrs. This response has been also found after an endurance exercise and in response to a great variety of pathological processes (Welles, 2000).

3.6.1 Breed

Minor differences have been found among equine breeds in relation to WBC, with the hot-blooded horses having higher WBC compared to cold-blooded horses (Jain, 1986; Harvey et al., 1984). Thoroughbreds and Arabian have a mean NEU/LYM ratio of 1.0, whereas cold-blooded horses and miniature horses have ratios of 1.7 and 0.67, respectively (Jain, 1986).

3.6.2 Time of the day

In Thoroughbred racing horses, Allen and Powell (1983) described that LYM count has higher in the evenings and lower in the mornings. These findings have been attributed to the circadian variations in the release of endogenous corticoids. It is well known that maximum cortisol concentrations appear in the morning (McKeever, 2011).

3.6.3 Gender

WBC and granulocytes are higher in females than in stallions, as recently found in Spanish Purebred horses (Hernández et al., 2008; Satué et al., 2009). On the contrary, previous researchers performed in warm-blooded horse breeds reported higher values in males and in females (Lassen and Swardson, 1995; Cebulj-Kadunc et al., 2002). Other study failed to find significant differences between sexes (Lacerda et al., 2006).

3.6.4 Age

NEU number is low in the fetus (<1,500/µl, before 300 days of gestation), increases after birth in response to cortisol (8,000/µl) and then decrease to mean adult values (4000/µl) at about 4-6 months of age. Band NEU do not exceed 150/µl in healthy foals (Harvey, 1990; Allen et al., 1998). Foals born at term have higher NEU count than foals born prematurely. LYM numbers in foals are low at birth (average 1,400/µl), increase to 5,000/µl at 3 months of age, and reach adult values at 1 year of age (Jain, 1986; Harvey, 1990). LYMs further decline during adulthood while NEU count remains the same, resulting in a higher NEU/LYM ratio in aged horses compared to foals (Jain, 1986). The ratio NEU/LYM reaches values of 2/1 in geriatric horses (Jain, 1993; Lassen and Swardson, 1995; Hernández et al., 2008). The progressive trend towards lymphopenia in geriatric horses is characterized by a reducing in B cells CD4+ and CD8+, in relation to immune senescence (Smith et al., 2002; Hernández et al., 2008; Satué et al., 2010).

EOSs are not routinely detected in the fetus and in foals at birth, achieving a mean of 400/µl by 4 months of age (Harvey, 1990). EOSs count increases with aging due to prolonged exposure to allergens through life (Jain, 1993; Satué et al., 2009). However, McFarlane et al. (1998), Cebulj-Kadunc et al. (2003) and Hernández et al. (2008) did not found differences in EOS count between young and adult horses. Band NEU, MON and BAS do not seem to change with aging in horses (Harvey, 1990; Jain, 1993; Lassen and Swardson, 1995; Cebulj-Kadunc et al., 2003; Satué, 2004; Hernández et al., 2008).

3.6.5 Exercise

WBC show different responses according to the type of exercise. Sprint exercise is associated with leukocytosis because of neutrophilia but mainly because of lymphocytosis, with a decrease in NEU/LYM ratio. These changes are likely secondary to catecholamine release and splenic contraction. At 3 hr after exercise, there is an increase in NEU/LYM ration, because the increase of NEU and decrease in LYM associated with cortisol concentrations. The NEU/LYM ratio returns to baseline values by 6 hrs after exercise (Snow et al., 1983).

Endurance exercise is associated with leukocytosis, resulting from a neutrophilia and lymphopenia (Snow et al., 1982). Probably this is combined effect of increased circulating corticosteroids and splenic contraction. Horses that completed an endurance event at a faster speed have higher NEU/LYM ration than slower horses (Trigo et al., 2010). Additionally, it has been demonstrated that exhausted endurance horses had left shift in the NEUs and significantly lymphopenia (Trigo et al., 2010).

3.6.6 Training

Total WBC is unchanged during training for racing and for endurance events. In addition, there are no alterations in the proportions of the different WBC populations. Some overtrained horses develop eosinophenia together with clinical signs of disease, and this result has led to the hypothesis that EOSs may be a more sensitive indicator of training stress than other types of WBCs (Tyler-McGowan et al., 1999). It is important to take into account that decreased NEU count and later, increased LYM count is consistent with systemic or respiratory disease, that are common causes of loss of performance in trained horses (McGowan, 2008).

3.6.7 Reproductive status

Although in main lines, estrous cycle and pregnancy do not change substantially the leukogram (Berlink et al., 2000; Da Costa et al., 2003), some studies have found a reduction in WBC, NEU and EOS counts during pregnancy (Satué, 2004; Satué et al., 2010). The reduction in WBC in Thoroughbred mares appears during the first 4 months of pregnancy, with a trend toward increase from half of pregnancy and it is maintained until the time of delivery (Gill et al., 1994). During delivery, leukocytosis with neutrophilia, lymphopenia and eosinopenia appear, in association with the hypothalamic-pituitary-adrenal stimulation and glucocorticoid release (Silver et al., 1984; Harvey et al., 1994). However, this idea has not been confirmed by all the authors (Taylor-Macallister et l., 1997). Finally, lactation induces leucopenia with an intensity proportional to the degree of stress during the period of maximum milk production (Harvey et al., 1994).

4. Platelets

Platelets or thrombocytes are cytoplasmic fragments of megakariocytes. Equine platelets stain very lightly with Wright-Giemsa stain and sometimes can be difficult to discern on blood films. They are round, oval or elongate, measuring 2.5-3.5 µm in diameter, with light blue cytoplasm with fine azurophilic granules (Kramer, 2000). The survival time of equine platelets in circulating blood is 4-7 days (Jain, 1993). Equine platelet concentrations are some of the lowest reported for mammals. Finding 6-10 platelets/field of high resolution in a peripheral blood film indicates an adequate platelet concentration. Mean platelet volume (MCV) and mean platelet mass have been reported in horses: 4.3-5.6 fl and 0.47-0.96 10^6/fl respectively (Boudreaux and Ebbe, 1998).

Morphologically, giant platelets, greater than the diameter of a RBC, are associated with accelerated thrombocytopoiesis. Platelet clumping indicates platelet activation and aggregation during blood collection, and might lead to erroneously low platelet concentrations. EDTA-dependent pseudo thrombocytopenia has been reported in a Thoroughbred gelding (Hinchcliff et al., 1993).

4.1 Physiological factors influencing platelets in horses

4.1.1 Anticoagulant

The use of EDTA as anticoagulant, although it can produce aggregation in normal situations, it is more common in patients with severe gastrointestinal disease due to platelet activation by circulating endotoxins and formation of aggregates of platelets and leukocytes (Hinchliff et al., 1993; Saigo et al., 2005).

4.1.2 Blood sample collection and analytical time

Repeated venipuncture, alterations in blood flow or delay in carrying out the analysis alter platelet count. It is advisable to perform the analysis within the first 2 hrs after collection, as MPV can be altered if the EDTA-sample is kept refrigerated. On the other hand, it is interesting to use sodium citrate as an anticoagulant in order to measure platelet size (Sellon, 1998; Seghatchian, 2006).

4.1.3 Breed

In Quarter Horses, Jeffcott (1977) found that the number of platelets in this breed was higher than in other equine breeds. A clear explanation for this result is lacking, although factors others than the breed should be taken into consideration.

4.1.4 Age

Platelet numbers in foals do not change during the first year of life. In adult horses, age determines a progressive decrease in platelet count (Ralston et al., 1988; Jain, 1993; Satué, 2004; Satué et al., 2009), as well as in other species (Zinkl et al., 1990). By contrast, other studies in horses did not agree with these results (McFarlane et al., 1998).

4.1.5 Exercise and training

The effect of exercise on platelet parameters seems to be intensity dependent. Short brief or maximal exercise results in significant increases in platelet numbers, whereas moderate exercise does not appear to alter platelet numbers (Bayly et al., 1983). Further, some studies reported reduced platelet aggregability in response to high-intensity exercise (Bayly et al., 1983), but other authors described increased aggregability and activation of platelets (Kingston et al., 2002). One possible explanation for the diverse results is the modifications in blood pH and hemoconcentration, with changes in ionized calcium concentrations and platelet activity. In addition, and given many of the methodological and technical problems when working with equine platelets, it is unknown if training alters platelet function.

4.1.6 Reproductive status

In human beings, laboratory animals and female elephants, a marked activation of the megakaryopoiesis has been found at the end of pregnancy. This fact continues during the initial weeks after delivery, possibly in association with high concentrations of estrogen, progesterone and other steroid hormones (Jackson et al., 1992). In the mare, most of the studies concluded that pregnancy does not exert significant effects on circulating platelets (Harvey et al., 1994; Berlink et al., 2000). However, Satué (2004) and Satué et al. (2010) described a progressive decline in platelet numbers during pregnancy in Carthusian broodmares. Hormonal dynamic during pregnancy, coupled with increased levels of thromboxane B2 produced by the placenta, chorion and amnion.

While in other species delivery leads to thrombocytosis (Suárez et al., 1988; Jackson et al., 1992), mares during delivery do not develop significant changes in platelet numbers (Harvey et al., 1994). This response is attributed to the combined effect of stress and increased release of estrogen, progesterone and other steroid hormones. Finally, lactation does not exert evident influence of circulation platelet numbers in mares (Harvey et al., 1994; Satué, 2004).

5. Conclusion

Hematological profile is frequently used in horses as an aid for the diagnosis and/or consequences of systemic, infectious and some parasitic diseases. It can also provide significant information about the response to treatment, the severity of the process and the metabolic state of an animal. Despite the wide use of hematology, interpretation is challenging because many exogenous and endogenous factors significantly modify blood parameters. The present chapter reviews the current knowledge of the influence of physiological factors on erythrocytes, leukocytes and platelets in horses.

6. References

Allen, A.L., Myers, S.L., Searcy, G.P. & Fretz, P.B. (1998). Hematology of equine fetuses with comparison to their dams. *Veterinary Clinical Pathology.*, Vol. 27, (September 1998), pp. 93-100, ISSN: 0275-6382.

Allen, B.V. & Powell, D.G. (1983). Effects of training and time of day of blood sampling on the variation of some common haematological parameters in the normal throroughbred racehorses. In: *Equine Exercise Physiology*. Snow, D.H., Persson, S.G.B. & Rose, R.J. (eds.), pp. 328-335, Granta Editions, ISBN: 0-7020-2857-6, Cambridge, England.

Allen, B.V. (1988). Relationships between the erythrocyte sedimentation rate, plasma proteins and viscosity, and leucocyte counts in thoroughbred racehorses. *Veterinary Record.*, Vol. 1, Nº 22, (April 1988), pp. 329-332, ISSN: 2042-7670.

Archer, R.K. (1977). Technical methods. In: *Comparative Clinical Haematology*. Archer, R.K. & Jeffcott, L.B. (eds.), pp. 537-586, Blackwell Scientific Publications, ISBN: 1078-8956, Oxford.

Bailit, J.L., Doty, E. & Todia, W. (2007). Repeated hematocrit measurements in low risk pregnant women. *Journal of Reproduction Medicine,* Vol. 52, Nº 7, (July 2007), pp. 619-622, ISSN: 0024-7758.

Bayly, W.M., Meyers, K.M., Keck, M.T., Huston, L.J. & Grant, B.D. (1983). Exercise-induced alterations in haemostasis in thoroughbreds horses. In: *Equine Exercise Physiology*. Snow, D.H., Persson, S.G.B., Rose, R.J. (eds.), pp. 336-343, Granta Editions, ISBN: 0-7020-2857-6, Cambridge, England.

Berlink, B., Correa, J., Evangelista, A., Peixoto, R. & Penteado, C. (2000). Constituintes hematimétricos do sangue de éguas gestantes de raça árabe. *Veterinaria Noticias*, Vol. 6, Nº 1, (Marzo 2000), pp. 51-55, ISSN: 0104-3463.

Bienzle, D. (2000). Monocytes and macrophages. In: *Schalm´s Veterinary Hematology*. Feldman, B.F., Zinkl, J.G., Jain, N.C. (eds.), pp. 318-320, Lippincott Williams & Wilkins, ISBN: 978-0-8138-1798-9, Iowa, U.K.

Boudreaux, M.K. & Ebbe, S. (1998). Comparison of platelet number, mean platelet volume and platelet mass in five mammalian species. *Comparative Haematolology International*, Vol. 8, nº 1, (March 1998), pp. 16-20, ISSN: 0938-7714.

Brockus, C.W. & Anderasen, C.B. Erythrocytes. In: *Duncan and Prasse´s Veterinary Laboratory Medicine: Clinical Pathology*. Latimer, K.S., Mahaffey, E.A. & Prasse, K.W. (eds.), pp. 3-45, Iowa State Press, ISBN 0813820146, Iowa, U.K.

Burguez, P.N., Ousey, J., Cash, R.S. & Rossdale, P.D. (1983). Changes in blood neutrophil and lymphocyte counts following administration of cortisol to horses and foals. *Equine Veterinary Journal*, Vol. 15, Nº 1, (January 1983), pp. 58-60, ISSN: 2042-3306.

Caracostas, M.C., Moore, W.E. & Smith, J.E. (1981). Intravascular neutrophilic granulocyte kinetics in horses. *American Journal of Veterinary Research,* Vol. 42, Nº 4, (April 1981), pp. 623-625, ISSN: 0002-9645.

Cebulj-Kadunc, N., Bozic, M., Kosec, M. & Cestnik, V. (2002). The influence of age and gender on haematological parameters in Lipizzan horses. *Journal of Veterinary Medicine Serie A, Physiology, Pathology and Clinic Medicine,* Vol. 49, N° 4, (May 2002), pp. 217-221, ISSN: 0931-184X.

Cebulj-Kadunc, N., Kosec, M. & Cestnik, V. (2003). The variations of white blood cell count in Lipizzan horses. *Journal of Veterinary Medicine Serie A, Physiology, Pathology and Clinic Medicine,*Vol. 50, N° 5, (June 2003), pp. 251-253, ISSN: 0931-184X.

Da Costa, R.P., Carvalho, H., Agrícola, R., Alpoim-Moreira, J., Martins, C. & Ferreira-Dias, G. (2003). Peripheral blood neutrophil function and lymphocyte subpopulations in cycling mares. *Reproduction in Domestic Animals,* Vol. 38, N° 6, (December 2003), pp. 464-469, ISSN: 1439-0531.

Detlef, C. (1985). Untersuchungen uber das rote blutbild und der eisenversorgunganzei genden parameter bei stuten und deren fohlen im peripartalen abschnitt unter besonderer berucksichtigung einer eisensubstitution. *Inaugural Dissertation zur Erlangung des Doktorgrades bei dem Fachbereich* Veterinarmedizin und Tierzucht der Justus-Liebig-Universitat zu Gieben.

Friend, T.H. (2001). Dehydration, stress and water consumption of horses during long-distance commercial transport. *Journal of Animal Science,* Vol. 78, N° 10, (October 2000), pp. 2568-2580, ISSN 0021-8812.

Funkquist, P., Nyman, G. & Persson, S.G. (2000). Haemodynamic response to exercise in Standardbred trotters with red cell hypervolaemia. *Equine Veterinary Journal,* Vol.32, No.5 (September 2000), pp. 426-431, ISSN 2042-3306.

Geor, R.J., Weiss, D.J., Burris, S.M. & Smith, C.M. (1992). Effects of furosemide and pentoxifylline on blood flow properties in horses. *American Journal of Veterinary Research,* Vol.53, No.11 (November 1992), pp. 2043-2049, ISSN 0002-9645.

Gill, J. & Kownacka, M. (1979). Seasonal changes in erythrocyte, hemoglobin and leukocyte indexes in pregnant mares of thoroughbred horses. *Bulletin of the Academy Polish Science and Biology,* Vol. 27, N° 2, (June 1979), pp. 143-148, ISSN 0001-4141.

Gill, J. & Rastawicka, M. (1986). Diurnal changes in the hematological indices in the blood of racing Arabian horses. *Polskie Archiwum Weterynaryjne.,* Vol. 26, N° 1 (November 1986), pp. 169-179, ISSN 0079-3647.

Gill, J. & Wanska, E. (1978). Seasonal changes in erythrocyte, hemoglobin and leukocyte indexes in barren mares of thoroughbred horses. *Bulletin of the Academy Polish Science and Biology,* Vol. 26, N° 5, pp. 347-53, ISSN 0001-4141.

Gill, J., Flisinska-Bojanowska, A. & Grzelkowska, K. (1994). Diurnal and seasonal changes in the WBC number, neutrophil percentage and lysozyme activity in the blood of barren, pregnant and lactating mares. *Advances in Agricultural Sciences.,* Vol. 3, N° 1, pp. 15-23, ISSN 0021-8596.

Gill, J., Szwarocka-Priebe, T., Krupska, U. & Peplowska, Z. (1979). Seasonal changes in haematological indices, protein and glycoprotein levels and in activity of some enzymes in Arabian horses. *Bulletin of the Academy Polish Science and Biology,* Vol. 26, N° 10, (Feb 1979), pp. 719-723, ISSN 0001-4141.

Golland, L.C., Evans, D.L., McGowan, C.M., Hodgson, D.R. & Rose, R.J. (2003). The effects of overtraining on blood volumes in Standardbred racehorse. *Equine Vet. J.,* Vol. 165, N° 3, (May 2003), pp. 228-232, ISSN 2042-3306.

Greppi, G.F., Casini, L., Gatta, D., Orlandi, M. & Pasquini, M. (1996). Daily fluctuations of haematology and blood biochemistry in horses fed varying levels of protein. *Equine Veterinary Journal,* Vol. 28, N° 5, (September 1996), pp. 350-353, ISSN 2042-3306.

Grondin, T.M. & Dewitt, S.F. (2010). Normal hematology of the horse and donkey. In: *Schalm´s Veterinary Hematology.* Weiss, D.J. & Wardrop, K.J. (eds.), pp. 821-828, Wiley Blackwell Inc., ISBN 978-0-8138-1798-9, Ames, I.A.

Grondin, T.M., Dewitt, S.E. & Keeton, K.S. (2007). Pelger-Hüet anomaly in an Arabian horse. *Veterinary Clinical Pathology.,* Vol. 36, N° 3, (September 2007), pp. 306-310, ISSN 0275-6382.

Harvey, J.W. (1990). Normal hematologic values. In: *Equine Clinical Neonatology.* Koterba, A.M., Drummond, W.H. & Kosch, P.C. (eds.), pp. 561-570, Lea & Febiger, ISBN 0812111842, Philadelphia.

Harvey, J.W., Asquith, R.L., Pate, M.G., Kipivelto, J., Chen, C.L. & Ott, E.A. (1994). Haematological findings in pregnant, postparturient and nursing mares. *Comparative Hematology International,* Vol. 4, N° 1, (April, 1994), pp. 25-29, ISSN 0938-7714.

Harvey, J.W., Pate, M., Kivipelto, J. & Asquith, R. (2005). Clinical biochemistry of pregnant and nursing mares. *Veterinary Clinical Pathology,* Vol. 34, N° 3, (September 2005), pp. 248-254, ISSN 0275-6382.

Harvey, R.B., Hambright, M.B. & Rowe, L.D. (1984). Clinical biochemical and hematologic values of the American Miniature Horse: reference values. *American Journal of Veterinary Research,,* Vol. 45, N° 5, (May 1984), pp. 987-990, ISSN 0002-9645.

Hauss, E. (1994). Chronobiology of circulating blood cells and platelets. In: *Biological Rhythms in Clinical and Laboratory Medicine.* Touitou, Y. & Hauss, E. (eds.), pp. 504-526, Springer-Verlag, ISBN 9783540544616, N.Y.

Hernández, A.M., Satué K.; Lorente, C.; Garcés, C. & O`connor J.E. (2008). The influence of age and gender on haematological parameters in Spanish Horses. *Proceeding of Veterinary European Equine Meeting - XIV SIVE Congress,* Venice (Italy).

Hinchcliff, K.W., Kociba, G.J. & Mitten, L.A. (1993). Diagnosis of EDTA-dependent pseudothrombocytopenia in a horse. *Journal of American Veterinary Medical Association,* Vol. 203, N° 12, (December 1993), pp. 1715-1716, ISSN 0003-1488.ç

Hopkins, J. & McConnell, I. (1984). Immunological aspects of lymphocyte recirculation. *Veterinary Immunology and Immunopathology,* Vol. 6, N° 1, (May 1984), pp. 3-33, ISSN 0165-2427.

Jackson, C.W., Steward, S.A., Ashmun, R.A. & McDonald, T.P. (1992). Megakaryocytopoiesis and platelet production are stimulated during late pregnancy and early postpartum in the rat. *Blood,* Vol. 79, N° 7, (April 1992), pp. 1672-1678, ISSN 0006-4971.

Jain, N.C. (1986). The horse. Normal haematologic with comments on response to disease. In: *Schalm's Veterinary Hematology.* Jain N.C. (ed.), pp. 140-177, Lea & Febiger, ISBN 0812109422 9780812109429, Philadelaphia, USA.

Jain, N.C. (1993). Comparative hematology of common domestic animals. In: *Essentials of Veterinary Hematology,* Jain N.C. (ed.), pp. 19-53, Lea & Febiger, ISBN 0-6121-1437-X, Philadelphia.

Jeffcott, L.B. (1977). Clinical haematology of the horse. In: *Comparative Clinical Haematology.* Archer, R.K. & Jeffcott, L.B. (eds.), pp. 161-213, Blackwell Scientific Publications, ISBN 1618-5641, Oxford, U.K.

Kerr, M.G. & Snow, D.H. (1982). Alterations in haematocrit, plasma proteins and electrolytes in horses following the feeding of hay. *Veterinary Record*, Vol. 110, pp. 538-540, ISSN 0042-4900.

Kingston, J.K., Bayly, W.M., Sellon, D.C., Meyers, K.M. & Wardrop, K.J. (2002). Effects of formaldehyde fixation on equine platelets using flow cytometric methods to evaluate markers of platelet activation. *American Journal of Veterinary Research*, Vol. 63, N° 6, (June 2002), pp. 840-844, ISSN 0002-9645.

Kramer, J.W. (2000). Normal hematology of the horse. In: *Shalm's Veterinary Hematology*. Feldman, B.F., Zinkl, J.G. & Jain, N.C. (eds.), pp. 1069-1074, Williams & Wilkins, ISBN: 978-0-8138-1798-9, Philadelphia, UK.

Kunugiyama, I., Ito, N., Narizuka, M., Kataoka, S., Furukawa, Y., Hiraga, A., Kai, M. & Kubo, K. (1997). Measurement of erythrocyte volumes in splenectomized horses and sham-operated horses at rest and during maximal exercise. *Journal of Veterinary Medical Science*, Vol. 59, N° 9, (September 1997), pp. 733-737, ISSN 0916-7250.

Kurosawa, M., Nagata, S., Takeda, F., Mima, K., Hiraga, A., Kai, M. & Taya, K. (1998). Plasma catecholamine, adrenocorticotropin and cortisol responses to exhaustive incremental treadmill exercise of the thoroughbred horse. *Journal of Veterinary Medical Science*, Vol. 9, N° 1, (December 1998), pp. 9-18, ISSN 0737-0806.

Lacerda, L., Campos, R., Sperb, M., Soares, E.; Barbosa, E., Rerreira, R., Santos, V. & González, F.H. (2006). Hematological and biochemical parameters in three high performance horse breeds from southern Brazil. *Archives of Veterinary Science.*, Vol. 11, N° 2, (October 2006), pp. 40-44, ISSN 1517-784X.

Lassen, E.D. & Swardson, C.J. (1995). Hematology and hemostasis in the horse: normal functions and common abnormalities. *Veterinary Clinics of North America: Equine Practice*, Vol. 11, N° 3, (Dec 1995), pp. 351-389, ISSN 0749-0739.

Latimer, K.S. & Rakich, P.M. (1992). Peripheral blood smears. In: *Cytology and Hematology of the Horse.* Cowell, R.L. & Tyler, R.D. (eds.), pp. 191-235, American Veterinary Publications, ISBN 0-323-01317-1, California, USA.

Latimer, K.S. (1999). Leukocytic hematopoiesis. In: *Equine Medicine and Surgery*. King, C. (ed.), pp. 1992-2001, Mosby, ISSN 9780815117438, St. Louis, USA.

Lording, P.T. (2008). Erythrocytes. *Veterinary Clinics of North America: Equine Practice*, Vol. 24, N° 2, (August 2008), pp. 225-237, ISSN 0749-0739.

Lumsden, H.J., Valli, V.E., McSherry, B.J., Robinson, G.A. & Claxton, M.J. (1975, a). The kinetics of hematopoiesis in the light horse III. The hematological response to hemolytic anemia. *Canadian Journal of Comparative Medicine*, Vol. 39, N° 3, (July 1975), pp. 332-339, ISSN 0008-4050.

Lumsden, H.J., Valli, V.E., McSherry, B.J., Robinson, G.A. & Claxton, M.J. (1975, b). The kinetics of hematopoiesis in the light horse II. The hematological response to hemorrhagic anemia. *Canadian Journal of Comparative Medicine,*, Vol. 39, N° 3, (July 1975), pp. 324-331, ISSN 0008-4050

May, M.L., Nolen-Walston, R.D., Utter, M.E. & Boston, R.C. (2010). Comparison of hematologic and biochemical results on blood obtained by jugular venipuncture as compared with intravenous catheter in adult horses. *Journal of Veterinary Internal Medicine*, Vol.24, No.6, (November-December 2010), pp. 1462-1466, ISSN 1939-1676.

McFarlane, D., Sellon, D.C. & Gaffney, D. (1998). Hematologic and serum biochemical variables and plasma corticotropin concentration in healthy aged horses. *American*

Journal of Veterinary Research, Vol. 59, N° 9, (October 1988), pp. 1247-1251, ISSN 0002-9645.

McGowan, C. (2008). Clinical pathology in the racing horse: the role of clinical pathology in assessing fitness and performance in the racehorse. *Veterinary Clinics of North America: Equine Practice*, Vol.24, No.2, (August, 2008), pp. 405-421, ISSN 0749-0739.

Mckeever, K.H. (2011). Endocrine alterations in the equine athlete: an update. *Veterinary Clinics of North America: Equine Practice*, Vol. 27, N° 1, (April 2011), pp. 197-218, ISSN 0749-0739.

McKeever, K.H., Hinchcliff, K.W., Reed, S.M. & Robertin, J.T. (1993). Role of decreased plasma volume in haematocrit alterations during incremental treadmill exercise in horses. *American Journal of Physiology* Vol. 265, N° 2, (August 1993), pp. 404-408, ISSN 0363-6135.

McKeever, K.H., Scali, R., Geiser, S. & Kearns, C.F. (2002). Plasma aldosterone concentration and renal sodium excretion are altered during the first days of training. *Equine Veterinary Journal*, Vol.32, N°34, (September 2002), pp. 524-532, ISSN 2042-9645

McMullin, M.F., White, R., Lappin, T., Reeves, J. & Mackenzie, G. (2003). Haemoglobin during pregnancy: relationship to erythropoietin and haematinic stats. *European Journal of Haematology*, Vol. 71, N° 1, (July 2003), pp. 44-50, ISSN 1600-0609.

Messer, NT. (1995). The use of laboratory tests in equine practice. *Veterinary Clinics of North America: Equine Practice*, Vol. 11, N° 3, (December 1995), pp. 345-350, ISSN 0749-0739.

Monreal, L., Villatoro, A.J., Monreal, M., Espada, Y., Anglés, A.M. & Ruiz-Gopegui, R. (1995). Comparison of the effects of low - molecular - weight and unfractioned heparin in horses. *American Journal of Veterinary Research.*, Vol. 56, N° 10, (October 1995), pp. 1281-1285, ISBN 0002-9645.

Muñoz, A., Riber, C., Trigo, P., Castejón-Riber, C., Castejón, F.M. (2010). Dehydration, electrolyte imbalances and renin-angiotensin-aldosterone-vasopressin axis in successful and unsuccessful endurance horses. *Equine Veterinary Journal*, Vol.42, No.38, (November 2010), pp, 83-90, ISSN 2042-3306.

Muñoz, A., Santisteban, R., Rubio, M.D., Agüera, E.I., Escribano, B.M. & Castejón, F.M. (1998). Locomotor, cardiocirculatory and metabolic adaptations to training in Andalusian and Anglo-Arabian horses. *Research in Veterinary Science*, Vol.66, No.1, (February 1998), pp. 25-31, ISSN 0034-5288.

Muñoz, A., Santisteban, R., Rubio, M.D., Riber, C., Agüera, E.I. & Castejón, F.M. (1999). Locomotor response to exercise in relation to plasma lactate accumulation and heart rate in Andalusian and Anglo-Arabian horses. *Veterinary Research Communications*, Vol.23, No6, (October, 1999), pp. 369-384, ISSN 0165-7380.

Muñoz, A., Santisteban, R., Rubio, M.D., Vivo, R., Agüera, E.I., Escribano, B.M. &, Castejón, F.M. (1997). The use of functional indexes to evaluate fitness in Andalusian horses. *Journal of Veterinary Medical Science*, Vol.59, No.9, (September 1997), pp. 747-752, ISSN 0916-7250.

Nieto, J.E., Snyder, J.R., Vatistas, N.J. & Jones, J.H. (2009). Effect of gastric ulceration on physiologic responses to exercise in horses. American *Journal of Veterinary Research*, Vol.70, No.6, (June 2009), pp. 787-795, ISSN 0002-9645.

Persson, S.G.B. & Ullberg, L. (1974). Blood volume in relation to exercise tolerance in trotters. *Journal of South African Veterinary Association*, Vol. 45, N° 4, pp. 293-299, ISSN 0038-2809.

Persson, S.G.B. (1967). On blood volume and working capacity in horses. *Acta Physiologica Scandinava, Suppl.*, Vol. 19, pp. 1-189, ISSN 0302-2994.

Persson, S.G.B. (1975). The circulatory significance of the splenic red cell pool. *Proceeding of the 1st International Symposium on Equine Hematology*, Michigan State University, East Lansing.

Persson, S.G.B. (1983). Evaluation of exercise tolerance and fitness in the performance horse. In: *Equine Exercise Physiology*. Snow, D.H., Persson, S.G.B. & Rose, R.J. (eds.), pp. 441-447, ISBN 1478-0615, Granta Editions, Cambridge, U.K.

Plotka, E.D., Eagle, T.C., Gaulke, S.J., Tester, J.R. & Siniff, D.B. (1988). Hematologic and blood chemical characteristics of feral horses from three management areas. *Journal of Wild Diseases*, Vol. 24, N° 2, (April 1988), pp. 231-239, ISSN 0090-3558.

Ralston, S.L., Nockels, C.F. & Squires, E.L. (1988). Differences in diagnostic test results and haematologic data between aged and young horses. *American Journal of Veterinary Research*, Vol. 49, N° 8, (August 1988), pp. 1387-1392, ISSN 0002-9645.

Robert, C., Goachet, A.G., Fraipont, A., Votion, D.M., Van Erck, E. & Leclerc, J.C. (2010). Hydration and electrolyte balance in horses during an endurance season. *Equine Veterinary Journal*, Vol.42, No.38, (November 2010), pp, 98-104, ISSN 2042-3306.

Rose, R.J. & Hodgson, D.R. (1994). Hematology and biochemistry. In: *The Athletic Horse: Principles and Practice of Equine Sports Medicine.* Hodgson, D.R. & Rose, R.J. (eds.), pp. 63-76, ISBN 0721637590, W.B. Saunders Company, Philadelphia.

Rossdale, P.D., Burguez, P.N. & Cash, R.S. (1982). Changes in blood neutrophil-lymphocyte ratio related to adrenocortical function in the horse. *Equine Veterinary Journal*, Vol. 14, N° 4, (October 1982), pp. 293-298, ISSN 2042-3306.

Ruiz, G., Rosenmann, M. & Cortes, A. (2004). Thermal acclimation and seasonal variations of erythrocyte size in the Andean mouse Phyllotis xanthopygus rupestres. *Comparative Biochemistry and Physiology A*, Vol. 139, N° 4, (December 2004), pp. 405- 409, ISSN 1095-6433.

Saigo, K., Sakota, Y. & Masuda, Y. (2005). EDTA-dependent pseudothrombocytopenia: clinical aspects and laboratory tests. *Rinsho Byor.*, Vol. 53, N° 7, (July 2005), pp. 646-653, ISSN 0047-1860.

Satué, K. & Domingo, R. (2008). Microhematocrit values, total proteins and electrolytes concentrations in Spanish Purebred mares during pregnancy. *Proceedings of 10th Annual Congress of the European Society of Veterinary Clinical Pathology (ESVCP) and the 8th Biennial Congress of the International Society for Animal Clinical Pathology (ISACP), European Society of Veterinary Clinical Pathology*, 30 september-3 october, CAB Abstracts, Barcelona (Spain).

Satué, K. & Domingo, R. (2011). Longitudinal study of the renin-angiotensin-aldosterone system in purebred Spanish broodmares during pregnancy. *Theriogenology*, Vol.75, No.7, (April 2011), pp. 1185-1194, ISSN 0093-691X.

Satué, K. (2004). Hematología en la yegua Pura Raza Española de Estirpe Cartujana. *Doctoral Thesis.* Departament of Animal Medicine and Surgery. CEU-Cardenal Herrera University.

Satué, K., Blanco, O. & Muñoz, A. (2009). *Age-related differences in the hematological profile of Andalusian broodmares of Carthusian strain.* Veterinarny Medicine, *Vol. 54, N° 4, (April 2009), pp. 175–182, 2009, ISSN 8750-7943.*

Satué, K., Hernández A. & Lorente, C. (2008). Erythrocyte parameters in Spanish horse: influence of age and gender. *Proceedings of 10th Annual Congress of the European Society of Veterinary Clinical Pathology (ESVCP) and the 8th Biennial Congress of the International Society for Animal Clinical Pathology (ISACP), European Society of Veterinary Clinical Pathology,* 30 september-3 october, CAB Abstracts, Barcelona (Spain).

Satué, K., Hernández, A., Lorente, C. & O´Coonor, J.E. (2010). *Immunophenotypical characterization in Andalusian horse: variations with age and gender.* Veterinary Immunology and Immunopathology, *Vol. 133, N° 2, (February 2010), pp. 219-227, ISSN 0165-2427.*

Satué, K., Muñoz, A. & Montesinos, P. (2011). Seasonal variations in the erythrogram in pregnant Carthusian mares. *Proceeding of 13th conference of the ESVCP/ECVCP, 9TH conference of AECCP, 12TH ACCP and ASVCP,* 31 Aug-3 Sept, Dublin (Ireland).

Schalm, O.W. & Carlson, G.P. (1982). The blood and the blood forming organs. In: *Equine Medicine and Surgery*. pp. 377-414, American Veterinary Publications.

Seghatchian, J. (2006). A new platelet storage lesion index based on paired samples, without and with EDTA and cell counting: comparison of three types of leukoreduced preparations. *Transfusion Apher. Science,* Vol. 35, N° 3, (December 2006), pp. 283-292, ISSN 1473-0502.

Sellon, D.C. (1998). Thrombocytopenia in horses. *Equine Veterinary Education,* Vol. 10, N° 3, (June 1998), pp. 133-139, ISSN 0957-7734.

Sharif, M., Ameri, M., Moshfeghi, S., Sharifi, H., Mohammad, S. & Mohsen, S. (2010). Artifactual changes in haematological variables in equine blood samples stored at different temperatures and various anticoagulants. *Comparative Clinical Pathology,* pp. 1-4, (October 2010), ISSN 1618-565X.

Silver, M., Ousey, J.C. & Dudan, F.E. (1984). Studies on equine prematurity 2: post natal adrenocortical activity in relation to plasma adrenocorticotrophic hormone and catecholamine levels in terms and premature foals. *Equine Veterinary Journal,* Vol. 16, N° 4, (July 1984), pp. 278-286, ISSN 2042-3306.

Smith, G.S. (2000). Neutrophils. In: *Schalm´s Veterinary Hematology. Feldman*, B., Zinkl, J. & Jain, N. (eds.), pp. 281-298, Williams & Wilkins, ISBN: 978-0-8138-1798-9, Philadelphia, UK.

Smith, J., Erickson, H. & Debowes, R. (1989). Changes in circulating equine erythrocytes induced by brief, high speed exercise. *Equine Veterinary Journal,* Vol. 21, N° 6, (November 1989), pp. 444-446, ISSN 2042-3306.

Smith, J.E., Erickson, H.H., Debowes, R.M. & Clark, M. (1989). Changes in circulating equine erythrocytes induced by brief, high-speed exercise. *Equine Veterinary Journal,* Vol.21, No6, (November 1989), pp. 444-446, ISSN 2042-3306.

Smith, R. III, Chaffin, K., Cohen, N. & Martens, R.J. (2002). Age-related changes in lymphocyte subset in Quarter Horse foals. *American Journal of Veterinary Research,* Vol. 63, N° 4, (April 2002), pp. 531-536, ISSN 0002-9645.

Snow, D.H., Kerr, M.G., Nimmo, M.A. & Abbott, E.M. (1982). Alterations in blood, sweat, urine and muscle composition during prolonged exercise in the horse. *Veterinary Record,* Vol. 110, Nº 16, (April 1982), pp. 377-384, ISSN 0042-4900.

Snow, D.H., Ricketts, S.W. & Douglas, T.A. (1983). Post-race biochemistry in thoroughbreds. In: *Equine Exercise Physiology.* Snow, D.H., Persson, S.G.B., Rose, R.J. (eds.), pp. 389-399, Granta Editions, ISBN: 0-7020-2857-6, Cambridge, England.

Steinhardt, M., Thielscher, H.H. von Horn, T., von Horn, R., Ermgassen, K., Ladewig, J. & Smidt, D. (1994). The hemoglobin concentration in the blood of dairy cattle of different breeds and their offspring during the peripartum period. *Tierärztliche Practice,* Vol. 22, Nº 2, (April 1994), pp. 129-135, 1994, ISSN 0303-6286.

Stewart, G.A., Clarkson, G.T. & Steel, J.D. (1970). Hematology of the race horse and factors affecting interpretation of the blood count. *Proceeding of the Annual Convention of the American Association of Equine Practitioners,* pp 70, . pp: 17. COMPLETAR ANA ¡¡¡¡.

Suárez, C.R., Gonzalez, J., Menéndez, C., Fareed, J., Fresco, R. & Walenga, J. (1988). Neonatal and maternal platelets: activation at time of birth. *American Journal of Hematology,* Vol. 29, Nº 1, (September 1988): 18-21, ISSN 0361-8609.

Taylor-Macallister, C., Macallister, C.G., Walker, D. & Aalseth, D. (1997). Haematology and serum biochemistry evaluation in normal postpartum mares. *Equine Veterinary Journal,* Vol. 29, Nº 3, (May 1997), pp. 234-235, ISSN 2042-3306.

Tizard, J.R. (2009). *Veterinary Immunology: an introduction* (8th ed.), Saunders Elsevier, ISBN 0721601367, St. Louis, Missouri.

Trigo, P., Castejón, F.M., Riber, C. & Muñoz, A. (2010). Use of biochemical parameters to predict metabolic elimination in endurance rides. *Equine Veterinary Journal,* Vol.42, No.38, (November 2010), pp, 142-146, ISSN 2042-3306.

Trum, B.F. (1952). Normal variances in horse blood due to breed, age, lactation, pregnancy and altitude. *American Journal of Veterinary Research,* Vol. 13, Nº 49, (October 1952), pp. 514-519, ISSN 0002-9645.

Tyler-McGowan, C.M., Golland, L.C., Evans, D.L., Hodgson, D.R. & Rose, R.J. (1999). Haematological and biochemical responses to training and overtraining. *Equine Veterinary Journal. Suppl.,* Vol. 30, Nº, (October 1999), pp. 621-625, ISSN 2042-3306.

Welles, E. (2000). Clinical interpretation of equine leucograms. In: *Schalm´s Veterinary Hematology.* Feldman, D.F., Zinkl, J.G., Jain, N.C. (eds.), pp. 405-410, Williams & Wilkins, ISBN: 978-0-8138-1798-9, Philadelphia, UK.

Wickler, S.J. & Anderson, T.P. (2000). Hematological changes and athletic performance in horses in response to high altitude (3.000 m). *American Journal of Physiology Regulatory Integrative Comparative Physiology,* Vol. 279, Nº 4, (November 2000), pp. 1176-1181, ISSN 1522-1490.

Wu, M.J., Feldman, B.F. & Zinkl, J.G. (1983). Using red blood cell creatinine concentration to evaluate the equine erythropoietic response. *American Journal of Veterinary Research,* Vol. 44, Nº 8, (August 1983), pp. 1427-1432, ISSN 0002-9645.

Young, K.M. (2000). Eosinophils. In: *Schalm´s Veterinary Hematology.* Feldman, D.F., Zinkl, J.G., Jain, N.C. (eds.), pp. 297-307, Williams & Wilkins, ISBN: 978-0-8138-1798-9, Philadelphia, UK.

Zinkl, J., Mae, D., Guzmán, P., Farver, T. & Humble, J. (1990). Reference ranges and the influence of age and sex on hematological and serum biochemical values in donkeys (*Equus asinus*). *American Journal of Veterinary Research,* Vol. 51, N° 3, (March 1990), pp. 408-413, ISSN 0002-9645.

Zvorc, Z., Mrljak, V., Susic, V. & Gotal, J.P. (2006). Haematological and biochemical parameters during pregnancy and lactation in sows. *Veterinarski Arhives,* Vol. 76, N° 3, (June 2006), pp. 245-253, ISSN 0372-5480.